H·O·L·T

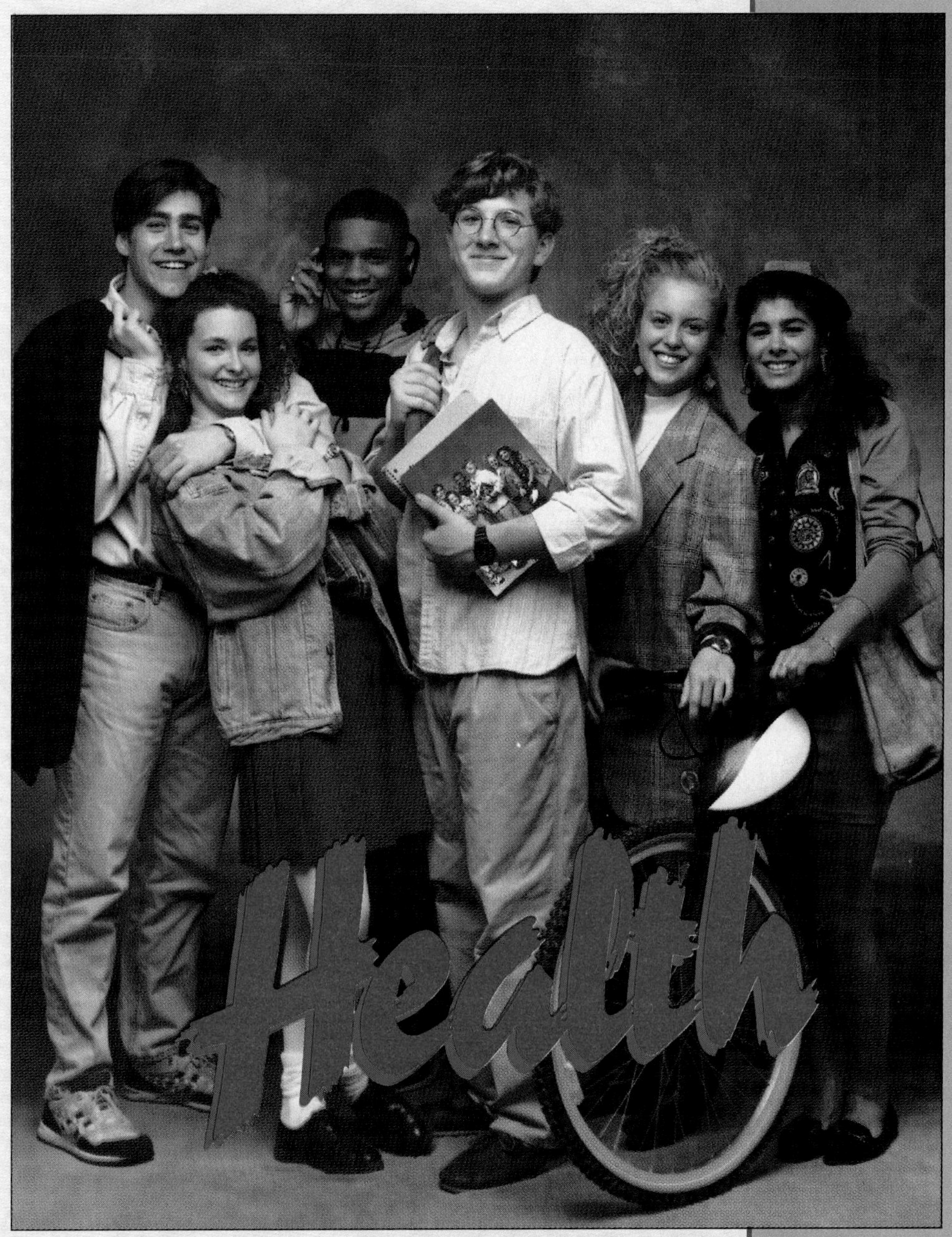

Annotated Teacher's Edition

JERROLD GREENBERG ED.D.
UNIVERSITY OF MARYLAND
COLLEGE PARK, MD

ROBERT GOLD, PH.D.
UNIVERSITY OF MARYLAND
COLLEGE PARK, MD

ACKNOWLEDGMENTS

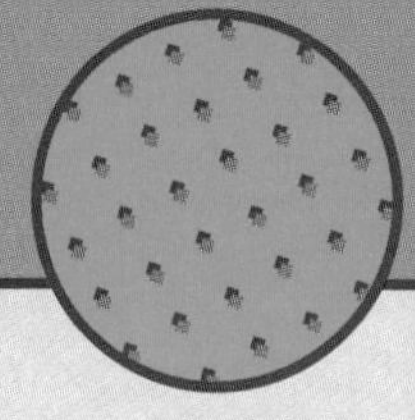

Contributing Authors

Clint Bruess, Ed.D.
University of Alabama at Birmingham
Birmingham, AL

George Dintiman, Ph.D.
Virginia Commonwealth University
Richmond, VA

Susan Laing
Southeast Regional Medical Education Center
Birmingham, AL

Contributing Writers

Letitia Blalock
Writer
Austin, TX

Beverly Bradley, Ph.D., R.N., C.H.E.S.
Supervisor of Health Programs
San Francisco Unified School District
San Francisco, CA

Deborah Fortune, Ph.D.
University of North Carolina
Department of Health and Physical Education
Charlotte, NC

Molly Gardner
Writer
Austin, TX

Susan Hammack
Managing Director
Disease Prevention News
Texas Department of Health
Austin, TX

Jacquelyn Jarzem, Ph.D.
Instructor
Austin Community College
Austin, TX

Carolyn Parks, Ph.D.
Cleveland State University
Department of HPERD
Cleveland, OH

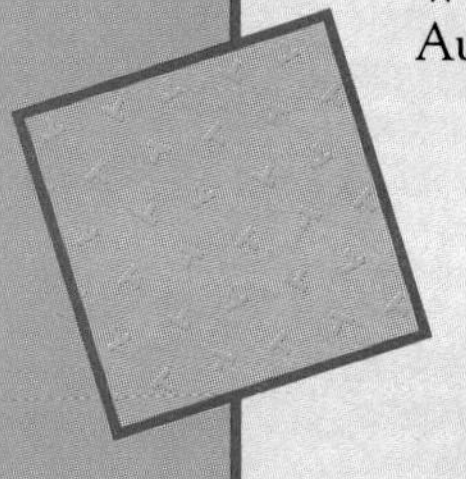

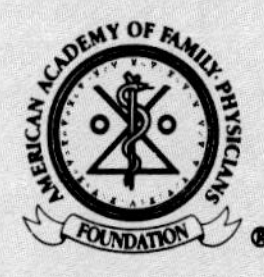

THIS HEALTH EDUCATION MATERIAL HAS BEEN REVIEWED FAVORABLY BY THE AMERICAN ACADEMY OF FAMILY PHYSICIANS FOUNDATION

Printed in the United States of America

ISBN 0-03-075326-0

1 2 3 4 5 6 041 96 95 94 93

Reviewers

Robert Ball, Ph.D.
Self-Esteem Consultant
Sacramento, CA

Diane Brinkman, M.D.
Obstetrician
Seton Hospital
Austin, TX

Cathy Brown
Executive Director
Rainbow Days, Inc.
Dallas, TX

Hugh Buchanan, Jr.
Health Teacher
Lilburn, GA

Michael Byrd
Health Teacher
Austin, TX

Alan Combs, Ph.D.
Professor of Pharmacology
and Toxicology
University of Texas
Austin, TX

Laurie Corwin
Health Teacher
Dallas, TX

Ileana Corbel-de la Garza
Public Education Director
Austin Rape Crisis Center
Austin, TX

Kathryn Danos
Health Teacher
Wales, MA

Jesse Flores
Youth Advocacy
Austin, TX

Linda Fox-Simmons
Registered Dietitian
Nutrition and Health Training
Alternatives
Austin, TX

Dian Gilham
American Cancer Society
Austin, TX

Rueben Gonzales
Division of Pharmacology
& Toxicology
University of Texas
Austin, TX

Frances Hamm
Executive Director
Faulkner Center
Austin, TX

Cynthia Hanes
Registered Dietitian
Austin Regional Clinic
Austin, TX

Hans Haydon
Austin-Travis County Health
Department
Austin, TX

Susan Hoff
Director of Direct Services
Rainbow Days, Inc.
Dallas, TX

Michael Jaworski, M.D.
Psychiatrist
Austin, TX

Alvanetta Jones
Health Teacher
Dallas, TX

John Mathis
Health Teacher
Klamath, OR

Jane Maxwell
Director for Planning and Evaluation
Texas Commission on Alcohol
and Drug Abuse
Austin, TX

Wendy McGinty
Physician's Assistant
Austin, TX

Paula Mohler
Physical Therapist
Texas Orthopedics
Austin, TX

Forrest Pettigrew, MSW-CSW
Austin, TX

Betty Phillips, M.D.
Psychologist
Fort Bragg Army Base
Fayetteville, NC

Frances Poteet
Health Teacher
El Paso, TX

Paula Rogge, M.D.
Family Practitioner
Austin, TX

Elizabeth Rutledge, M.D.
Urologist
Austin, TX

Lynn Silton
Self Esteem Strategies
Palo Alto, CA

Sandra Sinclair, D.D.S.
Dentist
Austin, TX

Ellen Smith, M.D.
Austin Gynecological
Oncology Association
Austin, TX

Paul Stubbs, D.D.S.
President, Dental Association of Texas
Austin, TX

Pamela Swan, Ph.D.
Department of Kinesiology
University of Colorado–Boulder
Boulder, CO

David Techner
Grief Counselor
West Bloomfield, MI

Lynn Thompson-Haas
Austin Rape Crisis Center
Austin, TX

Mary Tonelli, M.D.
Grayson Co. Health Dept.
Sherman, TX

Lily Townsend
Health Teacher
Pensacola, FL

Virginia Uribe, Ph.D.
Project 10
Fairfax High School
Los Angeles, CA

Tracy Watkins
Health Teacher
Coral Gables, FL

Sara Williman
Health Teacher
Van Wert, OH

Steve Wilson, M.D.
Orthopedic Associates
Round Rock, TX

Lloyd Wong
Health Teacher
Riverside, CA

Mark White, CSW-ACP
Austin, TX

Gary Zelazny, M.D.
Dermatologist
Austin, TX

Table of Contents

PRESENTS THE DECISION-MAKING MODEL USED THROUGHOUT THE TEXT.

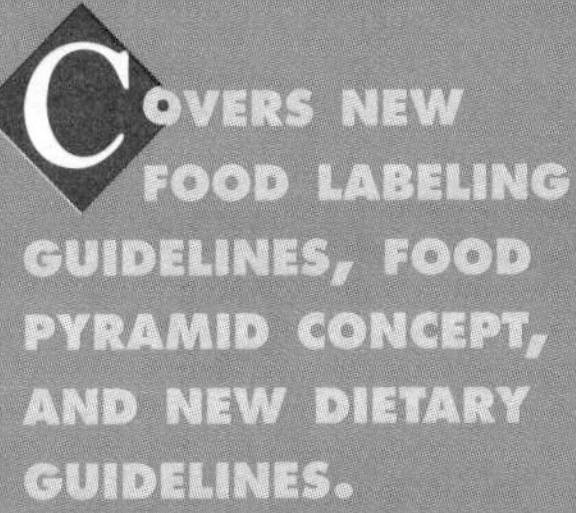

COVERS NEW FOOD LABELING GUIDELINES, FOOD PYRAMID CONCEPT, AND NEW DIETARY GUIDELINES.

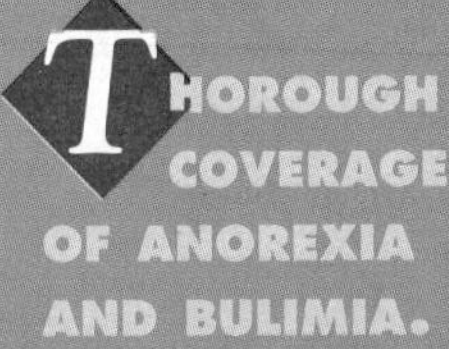

THOROUGH COVERAGE OF ANOREXIA AND BULIMIA.

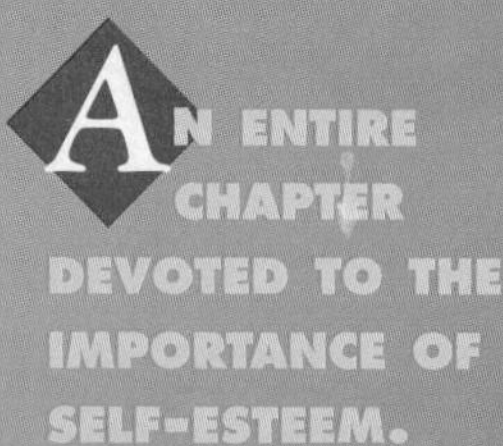

An entire chapter devoted to the importance of self-esteem.

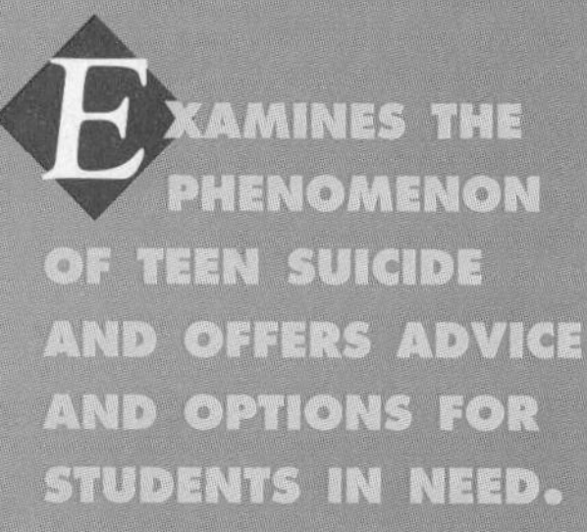

Managing stress and the factors that cause it through relaxation techniques.

Examines the phenomenon of teen suicide and offers advice and options for students in need.

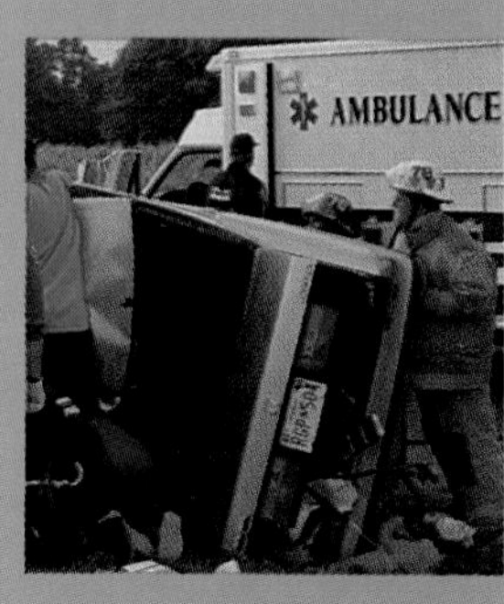

INCLUDES HARD FACTS ON DRUNKEN DRIVING, AND A COMPASSIONATE LOOK AT CODEPENDENCY.

OFFERS ADVICE ON HOW TO QUIT USING TOBACCO, AS WELL AS THE REASONS NEVER TO START.

IN-DEPTH DISCUSSION ON THE NATURE OF ADDICTION AND THE DANGER OF ILLICIT DRUGS TO INDIVIDUALS AND SOCIETY.

UNIT FIVE

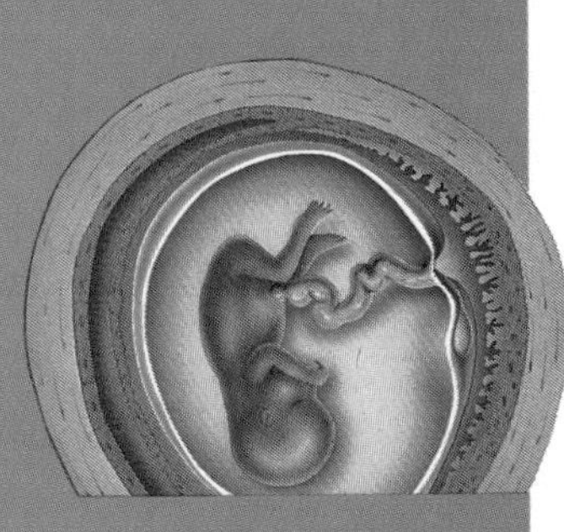

Emphasizes the importance of peer relationships, and presents specific steps on ways to resolve conflicts through communication and respect.

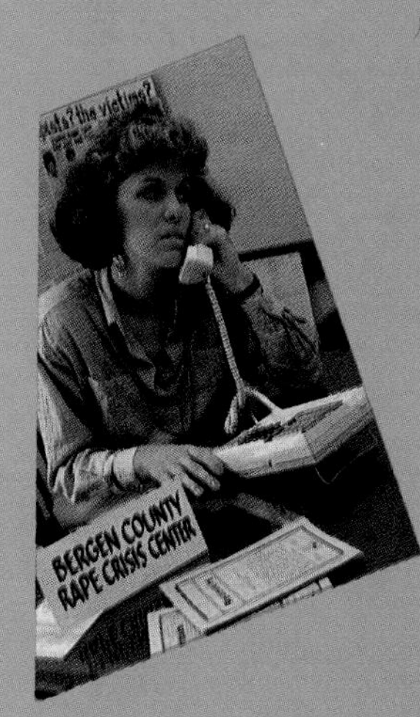

Includes blunt discussions of date rape and gang violence.

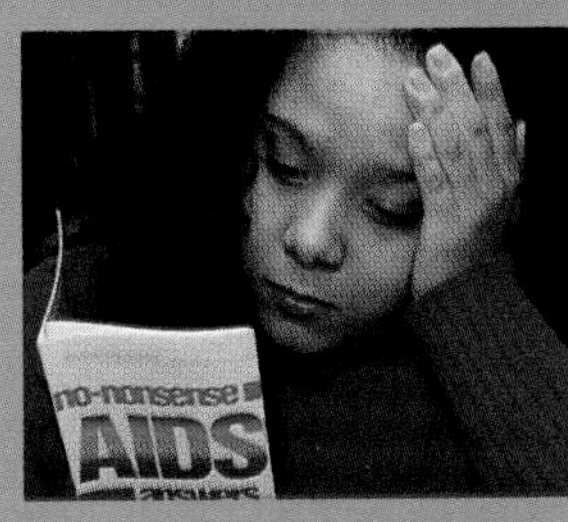

UP-TO-DATE INFORMATION ON THE NATURE OF THE DISEASE, HOW IT IS TRANSMITTED, AND WHAT BEHAVIORS ARE SAFE AND UNSAFE.

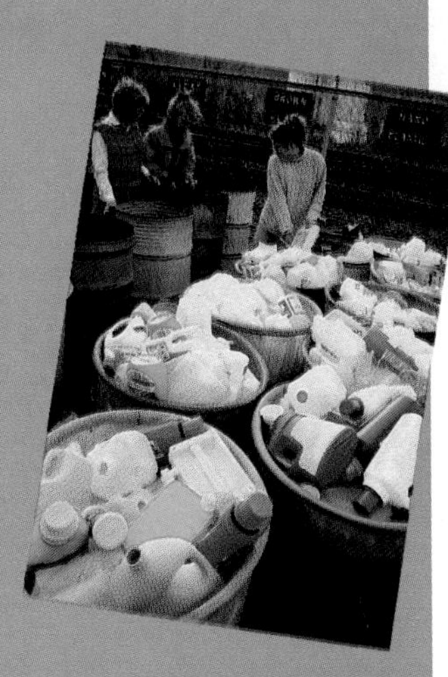

Body Systems Handbook

Health Careers Handbook

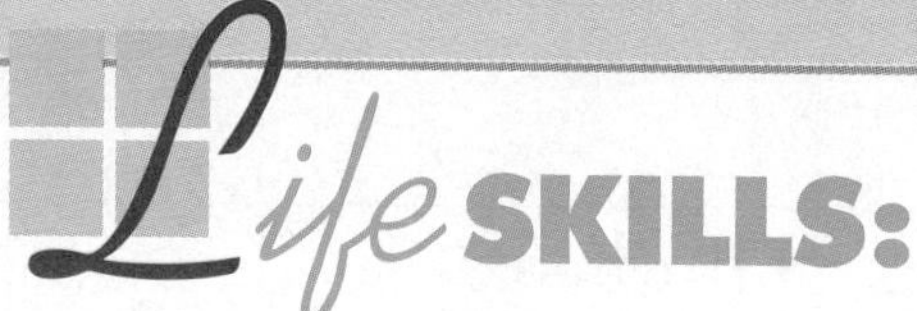

Life SKILLS:

What Would You Do? Making Responsible Decisions

Cultural DIVERSITY

Check Up

H · O · L · T

Health

Philosophy and Objectives

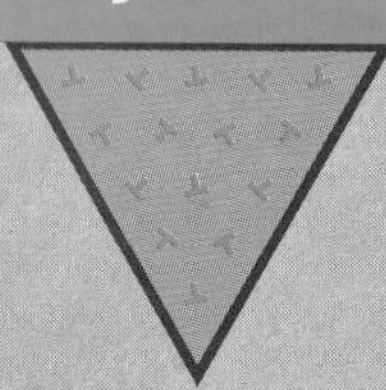

THE HEALTH CURRICULUM AND TODAY'S TEENS

The changing focus of the high school health curriculum over the last 10 years has been dramatic. The role of the health teacher has become critically important in helping students adjust and adapt to the challenges of adolescence because no single age group is more subject to avoidable health risks. No single age group is in more need of a quality health course than adolescents. Our goal is to provide the instructional support you need to present a health course that meets the needs of today's teens by focusing on health issues from an adolescent perspective.

From page one of *Holt Health*, you'll see it's different. Your students will want to read the text because its relevant to them. They'll want to discuss what they've read because its relevant to how they live today. As a result, The *Holt Health* classroom is highly interactive. Life Skills and decision-making skills form the core of the program. Students apply these skills in making choices on health and lifestyle issues.

Establishing Links to the Community
The *Holt Health* program recognizes that health education is not restricted to the school environment. Throughout *Holt Health*, students are expected to look at resources in the community related to particular health issues.

"I'm trying to make my own decisions now and not do things just because my friends are doing them."
Beatriz

Section **7.4** *Seeking Help*

Objectives

- *Describe the signs of mental and emotional health problems.*
- *List community resources that help with mental and emotional problems.*
  LIFE SKILLS: Using Community Resources
- *Differentiate among types of treatment for mental and emotional problems.*

Blood Alcohol Level's Effect on Death Risk

BAL	Chance of Dying
.02—.04	1.5 times as likely
.05—.09	11 times as likely
.10—.14	48 times as likely
.15+	380 times as likely

(FIGURE 13-11) **Drinking alcohol in any amount can put a person's life in danger.**

Breaking the Law
People under 21 break a law every time they have any alcohol (except under special circumstances, such as religious purposes). Like all crimes, getting caught drinking alcohol under the age of 21 can lead to arrest, a fine, and even a criminal record. Many teenagers have decided that they'd rather not risk their futures by drinking alcohol now. In addition, driving while under the influence of alcohol is illegal for people of all ages. A person does not have to be in an accident in order to be caught driving drunk—the driver of any car exceeding the speed limit or noticeably weaving through traffic is subject to inspection and a possible blood alcohol level test.

Losing Control
One of the best reasons not to drink is that alcohol can make a person lose control. Drinking to the point of intoxication can remove inhibitions completely. As a result, drunk people may find themselves doing things they regret.

For example, Krystal and Claudio are the school's most popular couple. Wherever they go is *the* place to be. Whatever they do, everyone wants to do too. It's a secret, but one thing they *haven't* done is have sexual intercourse.

Claudio lives with his grandmother, who happens to be out of town for the weekend. He takes advantage of this opportunity, and throws the year's wildest party. By the end of the night, everyone is very drunk, including Claudio and Krystal. The house is severely damaged: the stereo is broken beyond repair, and part of the carpet has been badly burned.

Claudio doesn't know any of this yet, because Krystal has suddenly decided she's ready to have sex with him. The two of them have stumbled to his bedroom.

Hours later, Claudio wakes up, horrified and ashamed. He hadn't wanted it to be like that. How could he have been so stupid? He knows they both made a mistake and that it's too late to go back now. What if Krystal gets pregnant? What about sexually transmitted diseases? Claudio knows that if they hadn't been drunk, they wouldn't have lost control.

Teenagers who drink are much more likely to get pregnant and also to suffer sexually transmitted diseases, such as AIDS, than those who don't. In fact, teenagers who use alcohol make up one of the fastest growing groups of people with AIDS in the United States.

Standards Set by Parents or Guardians
Many teenagers decide not to drink because they want to abide by the standards set by their parents or guardians. Chances are that a lot of students in your class have decided not to drink for this reason.

An Alcohol-Free Life
People who choose not to drink do so because they like being sober. They find that being drunk interferes with a lot of activities they enjoy—like taking part in sports, or going to the movies, or socializing with friends, or reading. Being sober allows them to get the most out of the things that make them happy.

What Would You Do?

Making Responsible Decisions

He Doesn't *Seem* Drunk
You're at a party, and it's getting late. Your friend Cliff, who drove you to the party, tells you he's sober enough to take you home. He doesn't seem drunk at all, but you know he's had at least four or five drinks. What would you do?

Remember to use the decision-making steps:

1. State the Problem.
2. List the Options.
3. Imagine the Benefits and Consequences.
4. Consider Your Values.
5. Weigh the Options and Decide.
6. Act.
7. Evaluate the Results.

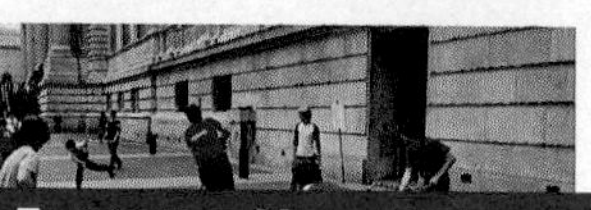

270 CHAPTER 13 ALCOHOL: A DANGEROUS DRUG

ALCOHOL 271

ENGAGING NARRATIVE

The harsh realities confronting today's teens are presented through compelling and compassionate scenarios.

HOLT HEALTH: THE SELF-HELP BOOK FOR TEENS

Building Self-Esteem

People who feel good about themselves by their very nature can readily identify and avoid unhealthy risk-taking behaviors. Recognizing this fact, you will find a full chapter on self-esteem in the *Holt Health* program. This chapter helps students recognize their own self worth and the importance of acting responsibly toward others. Teens today are so heavily influenced by the media. They are consistently bombarded with images and models of how to look and act. *Holt Health* breaks through the stereotypes in helping students learn to appreciate themselves as individuals and appreciate the diversity among people.

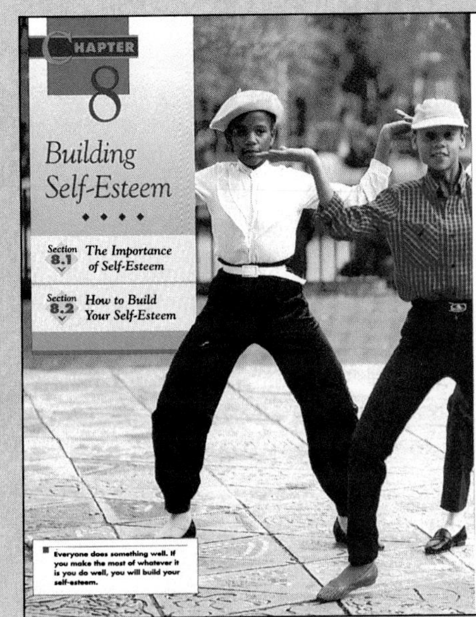

Lindsey feels ugly and unlikable. She compares herself with the models in the fashion magazines and wishes she could be as thin. When she looks in the mirror, she sees a chubby girl. Yet Lindsey is 5'3" tall and weighs only 105 lbs. She isn't really chubby at all. She constantly fantasizes about being popular, but feels that she doesn't have a chance. She is very shy and doesn't often talk to other students because she is afraid they won't like her.

Lindsey realizes that many people her age feel the way she does. However, she has made a silent promise to herself to find ways to feel better about herself and her life.

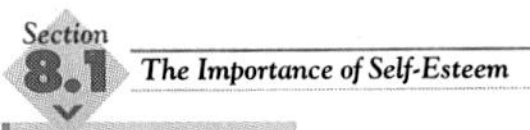

Section 8.1 The Importance of Self-Esteem

Objectives

- *Define self-esteem.*
- *Describe how self-esteem develops.*
- *Explain how media messages can affect one's self-esteem.*
- *Assess your own self-esteem.* **LIFE SKILLS: Assessing Your Health**

Self-esteem is your pride in and acceptance of yourself. It is your sense of personal worth. When you feel worthwhile, you are able to make good decisions, experience acceptance from others, and give and receive love.

Lindsey has decided to improve her self-esteem. To do so, she must learn to respect herself, consider herself worthy, and avoid comparing herself with others.

Your self-esteem influences your relationships with your family, friends, teachers, and bosses. It affects how you do in school and at work. Low self-esteem can be very damaging, and has been linked to serious problems such as alcohol and drug abuse, eating disorders, suicide, and other self-destructive behaviors.

How Self-Esteem Develops

The development of self-esteem begins at birth. Early on, our feelings about ourselves tend to be a reflection of how we are treated by the people most important in our lives—usually our parents or guardians. We learn to see ourselves as we think they see us.

Most parents love their children and wouldn't knowingly do anything to damage their child's self-esteem. But parents are only human. Sometimes they don't say exactly what they mean. For example, a

self-esteem: *pride in and acceptance of yourself; your sense of personal worth.*

8.1 THE IMPORTANCE OF SELF-ESTEEM 177

Cultural DIVERSITY

Social Support and African-American Churches

You read at the beginning of this chapter that having good relationships with others—having social support—is an important part of being mentally healthy. Different people find this support in different ways. For many African-Americans, churches serve as an important base of social support.

In fact, African-American churches have a long history of providing support and a sense of community to their members. Almost from the beginning, the churches served as community centers where African-Americans could gather to socialize. In the segregated past, their churches were often the *only* public buildings where they could have large gatherings.

People still come together at churches for services, weddings, baptisms, concerts, suppers, socials, plays, parties, meetings, discussion groups, educational programs, and sports like basketball and softball. Most African-American churches are open at least four nights a week to accommodate all these events.

At times, the support African-American churches give is more than social; families in financial trouble often go to their churches for housing, clothing, and money. Recently, some churches have even begun addressing their members' health-care needs.

In addition, churches have played a crucial role in the ongoing battle against racial discrimination. In the 1800s, African-American churches were active in the movement to abolish slavery. They were also part of the "underground railroad" that helped escaped slaves find their way to freedom.

Later, black religious institutions furnished much of the leadership for the civil rights movement. Two of the most important leaders of that time, Martin Luther King, Jr., and Malcolm X, began their civil rights work as religious leaders. King was a Baptist minister and Malcolm X was a speaker for the Nation of Islam. Today, African-American churches continue to work for social justice.

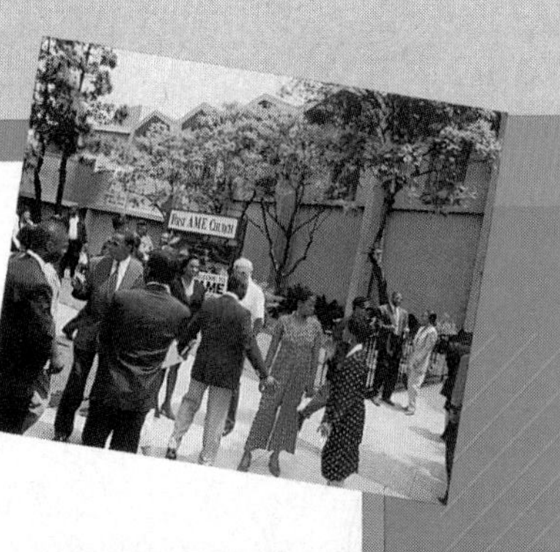

CULTURAL DIVERSITY

Holt Health reflects the diversity among people, not only in appearance, but in attitudes and beliefs. Throughout the text, students encounter the message to treat all others with dignity and respect. In special Cultural Diversity features, students examine the cultural norms related to health issues.

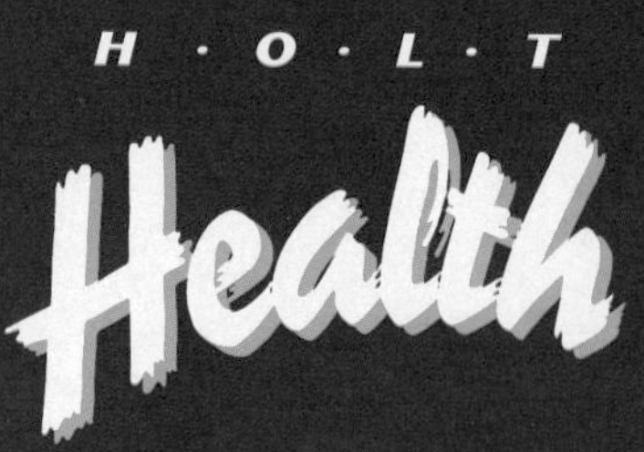

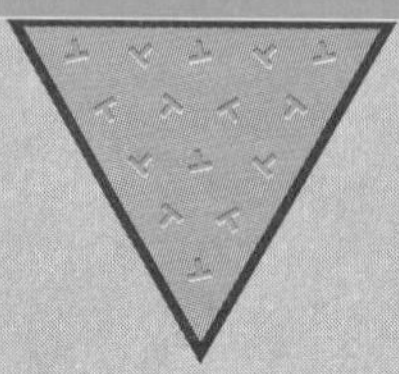

Life Skills Development

The purpose of any health course is to develop subject area content in a way that applies to daily life for life. Unlike other courses in the school curriculum, one's quality of life is intimately tied to avoiding health risks. Those risks can only be identified through health instruction. The development of Life Skills in *Holt Health* is an integral part of the total course. To emphasize the development of these skills, you will find them clearly labeled in the Life Skills feature pages throughout the text. The feature strand can be divided into the following categories that correspond to most curriculum objectives.

Life Skills Categories:

Solving Problems
Coping
Setting Goals
Resisting Pressure
Assessing Your Health
Intervention Strategies
Using Community Resources
Communicating Effectively
Being A Wise Consumer
Making Responsible Decisions
Practicing Self-Care

Section 13.2 Teenagers and Alcohol

Objectives

- *Name two reasons why some people drink.*
- *Name four reasons not to drink.*
- *Discuss myths and facts about alcohol.*
- *Name at least three ways you could refuse alcohol if a friend offers it to you.*
  LIFE SKILLS: Resisting Pressure
- *Use the decision-making steps to decide whether to take a ride with someone who has been drinking.*
  LIFE SKILLS: Making Responsible Decisions

Life Skills Objectives

Life Skills development is part of the instructional objectives for a lesson.

What Would You Do?

Making Responsible Decisions

You Made a Promise

Julia is your best friend. She has been acting depressed lately because her boyfriend broke up with her. Julia came to you and told you that she is thinking about killing herself. But she made yo[...] one.

After you talk with h[...] should tell anyone about[...] promise not to and she *is*[...] you do?

Remember to use th[...] decision-making ste[...]

1. State the Problem.
2. List the Options.
3. Imagine the Benefits and Consequences.
4. Consider Your Values.
5. Weigh the Options and Decide.
6. Act.
7. Evaluate the Results.

Developing Decision-Making Skills

The decision-making strand in the program is introduced in Chapter 2. This model is consistently applied throughout the program in the What Would You Do? features. What Would You Do? is a subset of Making Responsible Decisions from the Life Skills strand.

Life Skills Features

These pages in the pupil's text include activities to develop the eleven lifeskills in the program.

LifeSKILLS: Assessing Your Health

Self-Esteem Scale

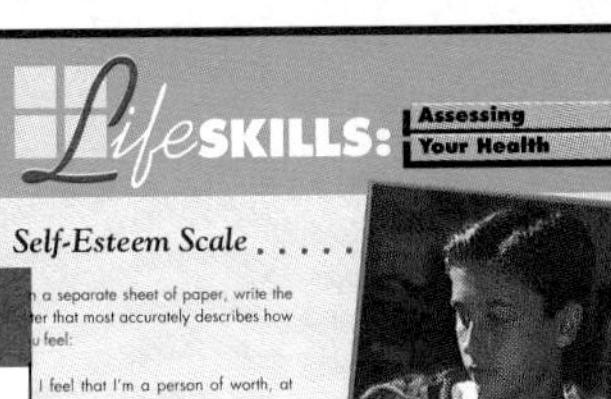

...n a separate sheet of paper, write the ...ter that most accurately describes how ...u feel:

1. I feel that I'm a person of worth, at least equal to others.
   a. Strongly agree
   b. Agree
   c. Disagree
   d. Strongly disagree
2. I feel that I have a number of good qualities.
   a. Strongly agree
   b. Agree
   c. Disagree
   d. Strongly disagree
3. All in all, I am inclined to ... that I am a fail...
   ...
   c. Disagree
   d. Strongly disagree
5. I feel I do not have much to be proud of.
   a. Strongly agree
   b. Agree
   c. Disagree
   d. Strongly disagree
6. I take a positive attitude toward myself.
   a. Strongly agree
   b. Agree
   c. Disagree
   d. Strongly disagree
7. On the whole, I am satisfied with myself.
   a. Strongly agree
   b. Agree
   c. Disagree
   d. Strongly disagree
8. I wish I could have more respect for myself.
   a. Strongly agree
   b. Agree
   c. Disagree
   d. Strongly disagree
9. I certainly feel useless at times.
   a. Strongly agree
   b. Agree
   c. Disagree
   d. Strongly disagree
10. At times I think I am no good at all.
    a. Strongly agree
    b. Agree
    c. Disagree
    d. Strongly disagree

Scoring. To score the scale and derive a measure of your self-esteem, follow these instructions.

1. The positive responses for questions 1–3 are:
   question 1: (a) or (b)
   question 2: (a) or (b)
   question 3: (c) or (d)
   If you answered two or three of these questions positively, give yourself 1 point.
2. The positive responses for questions 4 and 5 are:
   question 4: (a) or (b)
   question 5: (c) or (d)
   If you answered either one or both of these questions positively, give yourself 1 point.
3. If your answer to question 6 was (a) or (b), give yourself 1 point.
4. If your answer to question 7 was (a) or (b), give yourself 1 point.
5. If your answer to question 8 was (c) or (d), give yourself 1 point.
6. If your answer to question 9 or 10 or both was (c) or (d), give yourself 1 point.

Add up all the points you gave yourself.

The range of scores on this self-esteem scale is 0–6. The higher the score, the more positive your self-esteem.

semen may remain in the woman's vagina for quite a while after intercourse. Therefore, more women than men become infected with HIV from vaginal intercourse.

Oral Intercourse With an Infected Person Oral intercourse, also called oral sex, is contact between one person's mouth and another person's genitals. The viruses can be passed to either partner through tiny cuts or through the mucous membranes of the mouth and genitals.

Anal Intercourse With an Infected Person Anal intercourse is when a man puts his penis into the anus of another person. It is possible for either partner to transmit the virus to the other. HIV can get through the mucous membranes of the anus, the rectum, or the opening in the penis.

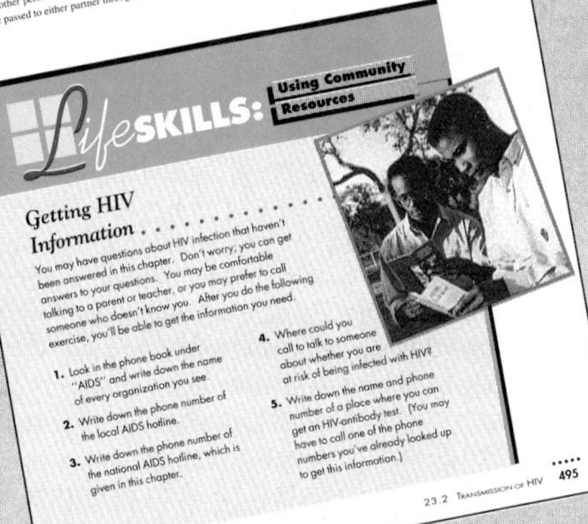

LifeSKILLS: Using Community Resources

Getting HIV Information

You may have questions about HIV infection that haven't been answered in this chapter. Don't worry; you can get answers to your questions. You may be comfortable talking to a parent or teacher, or you may prefer to call someone who doesn't know you. After you do the following exercise, you'll be able to get the information you need.

1. Look in the phone book under "AIDS" and write down the name of every organization you see.
2. Write down the phone number of the local AIDS hotline.
3. Write down the phone number of the national AIDS hotline, which is given in this chapter.
4. Where could you call to talk to someone about whether you are at risk of being infected with HIV?
5. Write down the name and phone number of a place where you can get an HIV-antibody test. (You may have to call one of the phone numbers you've already looked up to get this information.)

23.2 Transmission of HIV 495

Life Skills Worksheets

These creative activities extend and reinforce the skill development in the pupil's text. They are part of the Teaching Resources for the program.

Chapter 14

Tobacco: Hazardous and Addictive

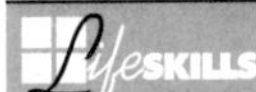

ACTIVITY A: Communicating Effectively

Different Ways to Communicate With Smokers

To protect themselves from cigarette smoke, nonsmokers need to learn how to communicate effectively with smokers about maintaining a smoke-free environment. How would you respond to each of the following situations?

1. Lara was walking down the hall at school when she caught a whiff of cigarette smoke. She followed the smell and saw a younger student snuffing out a cigarette inside her locker. What would you do if you were Lara and why?
2. Juan drove up to a self-service gas station and noticed that the woman at the pump next to his was smoking as she pumped gas into her car. What would you do if you were Juan? Why?
3. Cheryl's aunt is in the hospital recovering from kidney surgery. While Cheryl is visiting, her aunt's hospital roommate lights up a cigarette. Cheryl doesn't know if smoking is permitted or not in her aunt's hospital room, but she knows smoke makes her aunt uncomfortable. What would you do if you were Cheryl?
4. As you are waiting for your bus at the corner bus stop, you notice your neighbor, who is in her sixth month of pregnancy, light a cigarette. What would you do? Why?

Life Skills 14A 5

Life Skills Check

1. **Using Community Resources**
   You need to find out if something you are doing is risky behavior for HIV. You feel that you cannot talk to your parents or any of your teachers or counselors. In fact, you feel that you cannot talk about this to anyone you know. How could you get the information you need?
2. **Resisting Pressure**
   You are being pressured by your boyfriend or girlfriend to have sexual intercourse. In talking about this situation with a friend, she tells you that you have nothing to worry about if you use a condom. How would you respond to this statement?

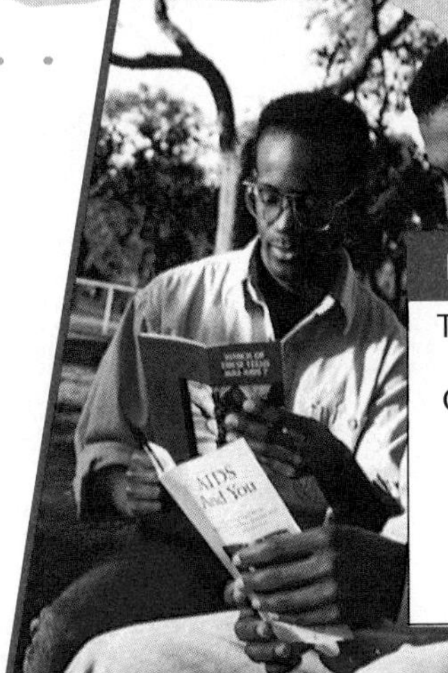

Life Skills Assessment

To ensure that the skills are being mastered, every Chapter Review contains a series of questions in the Life Skills Check section. These questions measure students abilities to apply what they've learned.

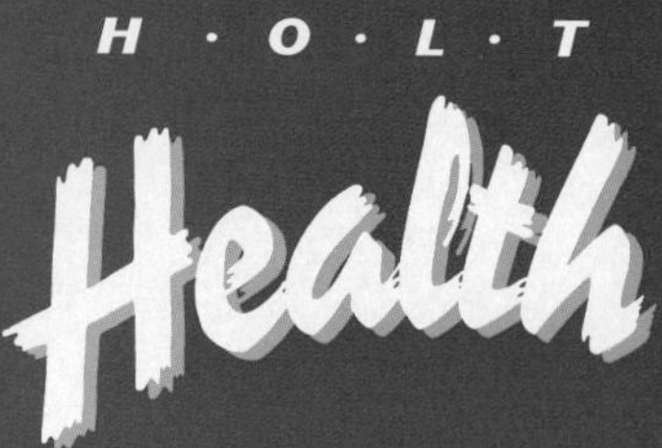

Your Partner in Quality Health Instruction

Instructional Aids

The *Holt Health* program provides a number of unique features designed to meet the instructional challenges you face in teaching high school health.

right for them.

Question Box

Have students write out any questions they have about how to make good decisions. The Que... Box provides them an opportunity to ... questions anonym... To ensure that stu... with questions are... embarrassed to be... writing, have thos... do not have ques... write something ... such as somethin... already know abo... decision making... the paper instead...

20 MA...

The Question Box

The true goal of the health course should be to encourage dialogue and deal with the burning questions students have about themselves and their health. To address this goal The *Holt Health* Question Box is a feature that opens every chapter. Students submit anonymously any questions they may have about the topics they will be covering in the chapter. You can then build your lesson plans to deal with students' questions and start a dialogue concerning any issues they need to discuss.

Section 8.2 Lesson Plan

MOTIVATE

Journal 8C
Expectations of Yourself

This may be done as a warm-up activity. Most teenagers feel dissatisfied with the... some degree, often be...

completing this statement: "I would feel really good about myself if I ___." Then ask that they explain to themselves whether they think this expectation is reasonable, and why.

TEACH

Reinforcement
Fighting Low Self-Esteem

Taking responsibility for how th...

The Journal

A wellness approach to health requires that the course be highly introspective in nature. The Journal provides a vehicle for students to privately reflect and express their feelings and opinions on many health issues. Often the Journal is used to record answers to warm-up activities that begin lessons. Students then use these answers to contribute to the class discussion once the class begins. The Journal is referred to throughout the Annotated Teacher's Edition, and is part of the *Holt Health* Teacher's Resource Binder.

Plan for Action

List the greatest stressors in your life at this time and devise a plan to lower your stress level using the suggestions in this chapter.

Plan for Action

Plan a balanced weekly exercise program to fit you own personal needs.

Plan for Action

Friends and family can support a dying person and each other. List three things you can do in the future to help a dying friend.

Chapter Review 225

Plan for Action

A health program is effective if the education the student receives causes a positive change in lifestyle or behavior. Unless that change occurs, the instruction has fallen on deaf ears. Plan for Action helps you assess behavioral change. Each Plan for Action in the Chapter Review requires students to build a daily life plan that reflects their understanding of the ideas and concepts in the chapter.

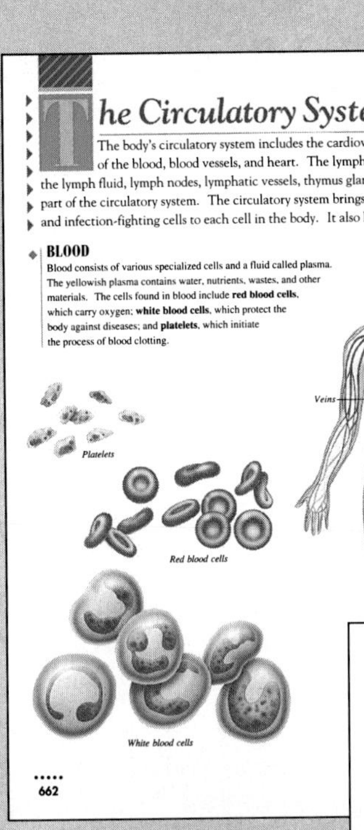
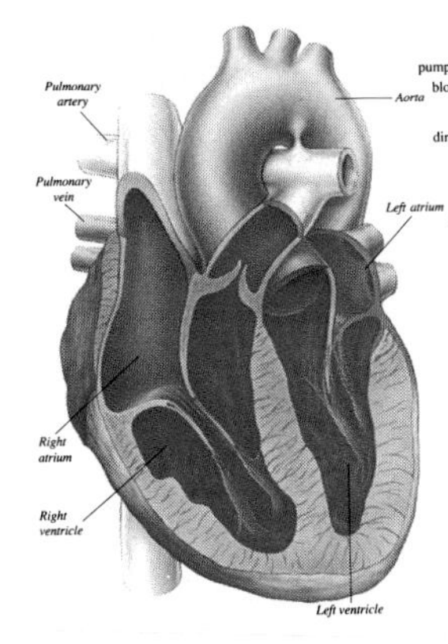
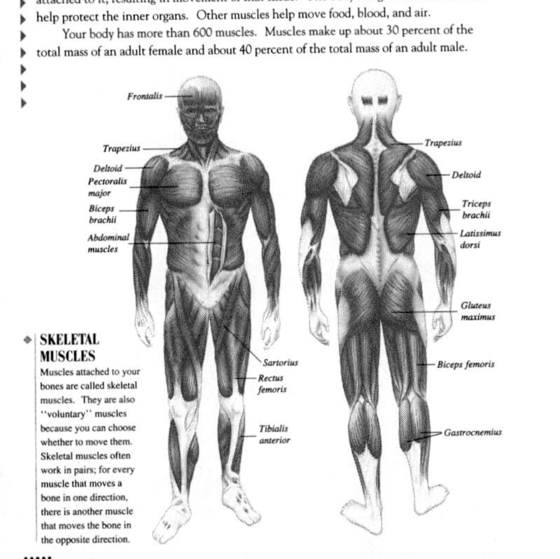
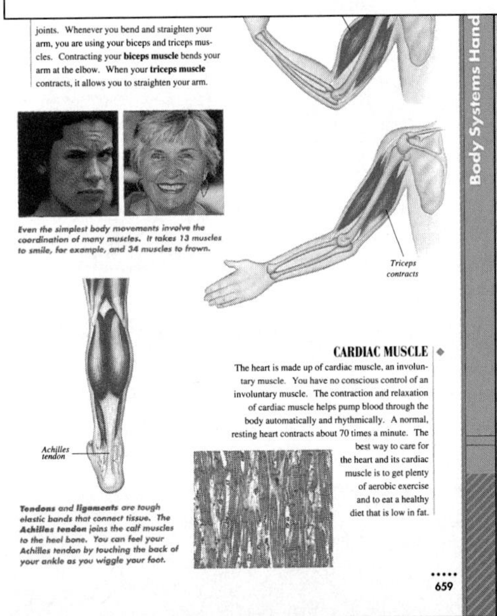

Teaching Human Body Systems

Holt Health is a wellness approach focused on everyday living. In keeping with that philosophy, you will find all the technical background on human body systems in a convenient handbook. This structure gives you the flexibility to integrate the coverage of a particular body system as needed with a core chapter. For example, when studying Chapter 4, Nutrition Principles, you could have students use the Handbook to review the parts and functions of the digestive system.

Personal Issues ALERT

Today's students come from very diverse backgrounds and as such they have had very diverse experiences. The likelihood of having a student that has had direct experience with abuse, violence, addiction, and even AIDS is very high. To assist you in covering potentially sensitive areas, a text chapter opens with a Personal Issues ALERT with notes on covering potentially sensitive subjects in the chapter.

H · O · L · T

Health

Your Partner in Quality Health Instruction

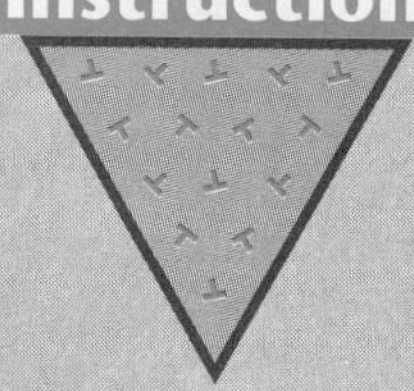

HOLT HEALTH ANNOTATED TEACHER'S EDITION

TEACHER'S INTERLEAF PAGES

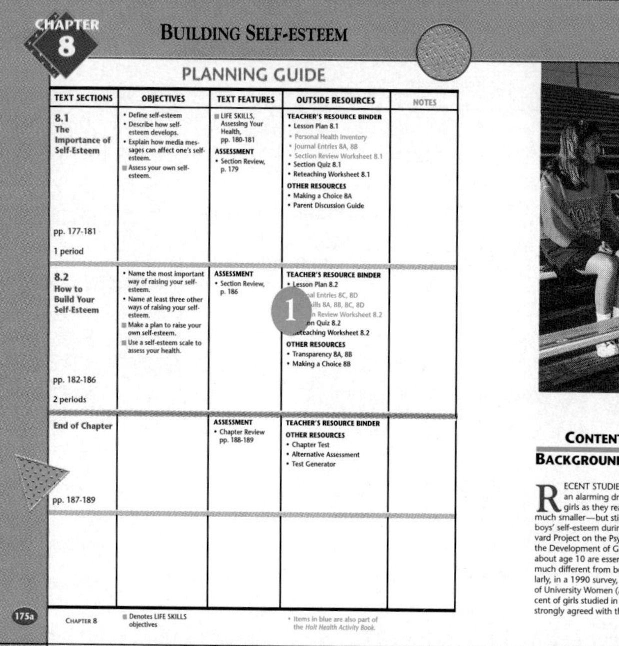

CHAPTER 8 BUILDING SELF-ESTEEM

PLANNING GUIDE

TEXT SECTIONS	OBJECTIVES	TEXT FEATURES	OUTSIDE RESOURCES	NOTES
8.1 The Importance of Self-Esteem pp. 177-181 1 period	• Define self-esteem • Describe how self-esteem develops. • Explain how media messages can affect one's self-esteem. • Assess your own self-esteem.	LIFE SKILLS, Assessing Your Health, pp. 180-181 ASSESSMENT • Section Review, p. 179	TEACHER'S RESOURCE BINDER • Lesson Plan 8.1 • Personal Health Inventory • Journal Entries 8A, 8B • Section Review Worksheet 8.1 • Section Quiz 8.1 • Reteaching Worksheet 8.1 OTHER RESOURCES • Making a Choice 8A • Parent Discussion Guide	
8.2 How to Build Your Self-Esteem pp. 182-186 2 periods	• Name the most important way of raising your self-esteem. • Name at least three other ways of raising your self-esteem. • Make a plan to raise your own self-esteem. • Use a self-esteem scale to assess your health.	ASSESSMENT • Section Review, p. 186	TEACHER'S RESOURCE BINDER • Lesson Plan 8.2 • Journal Entries 8C, 8D • Skills 8A, 8B, 8C, 8D • Section Review Worksheet 8.2 • Section Quiz 8.2 • Reteaching Worksheet 8.2 OTHER RESOURCES • Transparency 8A, 8B • Making a Choice 8B	
End of Chapter pp. 187-189		ASSESSMENT • Chapter Review pp. 188-189	TEACHER'S RESOURCE BINDER OTHER RESOURCES • Chapter Test • Alternative Assessment • Test Generator	

PLANNING GUIDES

Organize All Your Materials

1 The Planning Guides help you in selecting all the appropriate materials for a text section. You also see at-a-glance all the supplements you can select from when covering a particular chapter.

CONTENT BACKGROUND

Keeps You Up-To-Date

2 You'll find a content background article for each chapter in the Teacher's Interleaf.

PLANNING FOR INSTRUCTION

3 **Key Facts** gives you a quick overview of the important ideas of the chapter.

4 **Myths and Misconceptions** helps you dispell faulty thinking students may have on a subject.

5 **Vocabulary** highlights those terms you want students to master in working through the chapter.

6 **Special Needs Strategies** provide alternative instructional methods for students with low abilities or limited English skills.

7 **Enrichment Strategies** help you in providing challenging projects for taking the class or groups of students into more depth on a subject.

Teacher's Wrap

***Holt Health* Instructional Model**

The instructional model for *Holt Health* consists of three phases.

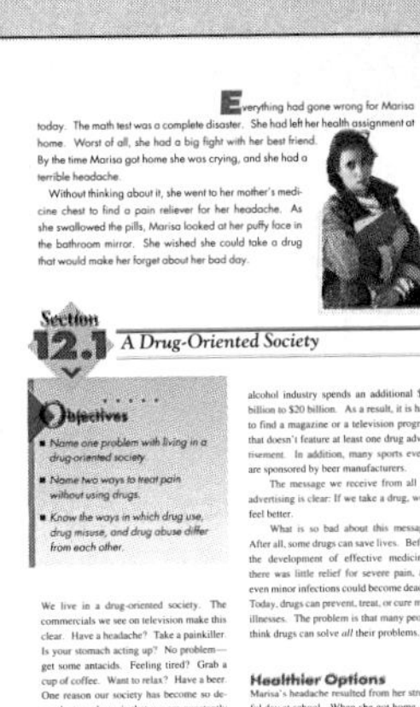

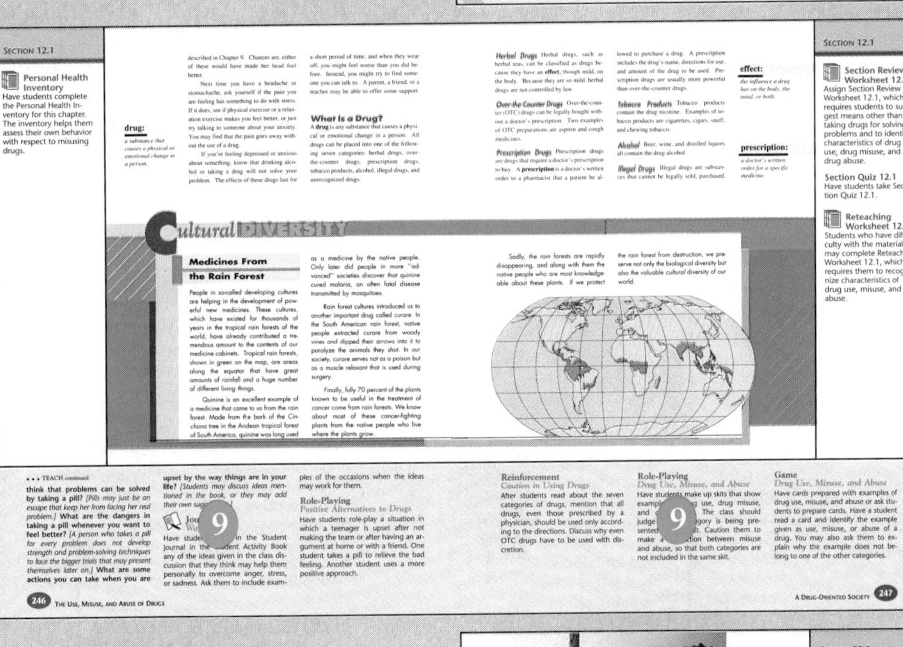

8 Phase 1: Motivate

Self-Reflection and Assessment of Prior Knowledge

You'll find specific features in the Annotated Teacher's Edition for beginning the chapter and each lesson with the Question Box or Journal.

9 Phase 2: Teach

Processing Information

This stage of instruction focuses on the strategies you use to cover the key concepts of the chapter. The Annotated Teacher's Edition gives you a wide range of highly interactive strategies including class discussion, cooperative learning activities, role playing, games, reinforcement strategies, and journal writing activities.

10 Phase 3: Assess

Evaluate Understanding

This stage of instruction focuses on evaluating student's understanding of the subject matter. *Holt Health* provides a number of strategies including Section Reviews, Chapter Reviews, Closure Activities, and Alternative Assessment Strategies. To learn more about the complete assessment plan for *Holt Health* turn to page 24T.

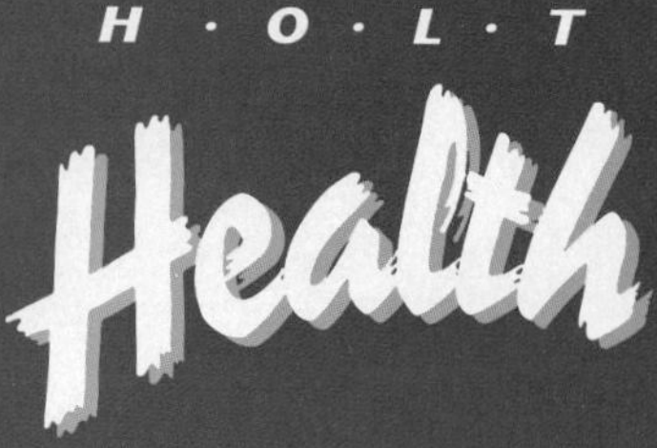

TEACHING RESOURCE SUPPLEMENTS (IN COPYMASTER FORM)

The *Holt Health* program provides the following supplements to support class discussion, group interaction, and individualized instruction for today's dynamic health classroom.

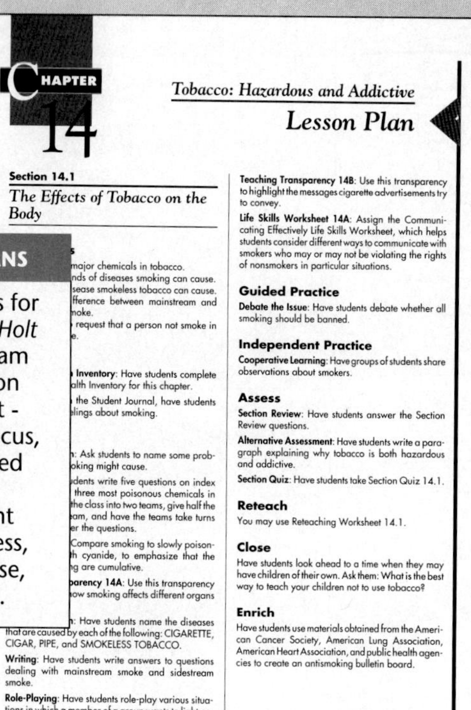

CHAPTER 14

Tobacco: Hazardous and Addictive

Lesson Plan

Section 14.1

The Effects of Tobacco on the Body

...major chemicals in tobacco.
...nds of diseases smoking can cause.
...sease smokeless tobacco can cause.
...fference between mainstream and ...moke.
... request that a person not smoke in ...e.

...**Inventory**: Have students complete ...alth Inventory for this chapter.
... the Student Journal, have students ...elings about smoking.

...: Ask students to name some prob...oking might cause.
...dents write five questions on index ... three most poisonous chemicals in ...the class into two teams, give half the ...am, and have the teams take turns ...er the questions.
...Compare smoking to slowly poison...h cyanide, to emphasize that the ...g are cumulative.
...**parency 14A**: Use this transparency ...ow smoking affects different organs

...: Have students name the diseases that are caused by each of the following: CIGARETTE, CIGAR, PIPE, and SMOKELESS TOBACCO.

Writing: Have students write answers to questions dealing with mainstream smoke and sidestream smoke.

Role-Playing: Have students role-play various situations in which a member of a group wants to light up.

Teaching Transparency 14B: Use this transparency to highlight the messages cigarette advertisements try to convey.

Life Skills Worksheet 14A: Assign the Communicating Effectively Life Skills Worksheet, which helps students consider different ways to communicate with smokers who may or may not be violating the rights of nonsmokers in particular situations.

Guided Practice

Debate the Issue: Have students debate whether all smoking should be banned.

Independent Practice

Cooperative Learning: Have groups of students share observations about smokers.

Assess

Section Review: Have students answer the Section Review questions.

Alternative Assessment: Have students write a paragraph explaining why tobacco is both hazardous and addictive.

Section Quiz: Have students take Section Quiz 14.1.

Reteach

You may use Reteaching Worksheet 14.1.

Close

Have students look ahead to a time when they may have children of their own. Ask them: What is the best way to teach your children not to use tobacco?

Enrich

Have students use materials obtained from the American Cancer Society, American Lung Association, American Heart Association, and public health agencies to create an antismoking bulletin board.

Lesson Plan 14.1 1

LESSON PLANS

Detailed plans for teaching the *Holt Health* program using a lesson cycle format - Objectives, Focus, Teach, Guided Practice, Independent Practice, Assess, Reteach, Close, and Enrich.

CHAPTER 8

Building Self-Esteem

Journal Entries

ACTIVITIES C and D

Section 8.2 *How to Build Your Self-Esteem*

C. Complete this statement about yourself: I would feel really good about myself if I ...

Explain to yourself whether your expectation is reasonable. Give reasons.

D. Write about one or more things you do well. Explain how you acquired the skill and how it makes you feel about yourself.

8 Journal Entries 8C and 8D

JOURNAL ENTRIES

Writing prompts and activities for student self-reflection to assess feelings and attitudes on a health topic.

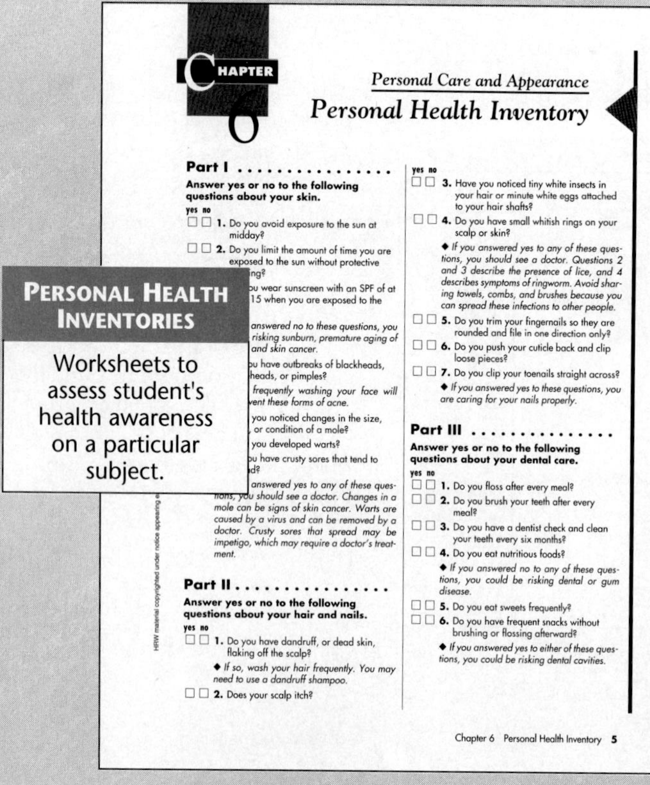

CHAPTER 6

Personal Care and Appearance

Personal Health Inventory

Part I . . . .

Answer yes or no to the following questions about your skin.

yes no

☐ ☐ **1.** Do you avoid exposure to the sun at midday?

☐ ☐ **2.** Do you limit the amount of time you are exposed to the sun without protective ...ing?

...ou wear sunscreen with an SPF of at ...15 when you are exposed to the ...

... answered no to these questions, you ... risking sunburn, premature aging of ... and skin cancer.

...ou have outbreaks of blackheads, ...heads, or pimples?

... frequently washing your face will ...ent these forms of acne.

... you noticed changes in the size, ... or condition of a mole?

... you developed warts?

...u have crusty sores that tend to ...d?

... answered yes to any of these questions, you should see a doctor. Changes in a mole can be signs of skin cancer. Warts are caused by a virus and can be removed by a doctor. Crusty sores that spread may be impetigo, which may require a doctor's treatment.

Part II . . . .

Answer yes or no to the following questions about your hair and nails.

yes no

☐ ☐ **1.** Do you have dandruff, or dead skin, flaking off the scalp?

◆ *If so, wash your hair frequently. You may need to use a dandruff shampoo.*

☐ ☐ **2.** Does your scalp itch?

yes no

☐ ☐ **3.** Have you noticed tiny white insects in your hair or minute white eggs attached to your hair shafts?

☐ ☐ **4.** Do you have small whitish rings on your scalp or skin?

◆ *If you answered yes to any of these questions, you should see a doctor. Questions 2 and 3 describe the presence of lice, and 4 describes symptoms of ringworm. Avoid sharing towels, combs, and brushes because you can spread these infections to other people.*

☐ ☐ **5.** Do you trim your fingernails so they are rounded and file in one direction only?

☐ ☐ **6.** Do you push your cuticle back and clip loose pieces?

☐ ☐ **7.** Do you clip your toenails straight across?

◆ *If you answered yes to these questions, you are caring for your nails properly.*

Part III . . . .

Answer yes or no to the following questions about your dental care.

yes no

☐ ☐ **1.** Do you floss after every meal?

☐ ☐ **2.** Do you brush your teeth after every meal?

☐ ☐ **3.** Do you have a dentist check and clean your teeth every six months?

☐ ☐ **4.** Do you eat nutritious foods?

◆ *If you answered no to any of these questions, you could be risking dental or gum disease.*

☐ ☐ **5.** Do you eat sweets frequently?

☐ ☐ **6.** Do you have frequent snacks without brushing or flossing afterward?

◆ *If you answered yes to either of these questions, you could be risking dental cavities.*

Chapter 6 Personal Health Inventory 5

PERSONAL HEALTH INVENTORIES

Worksheets to assess student's health awareness on a particular subject.

CHAPTER 15

Alcohol: A Dangerous Drug

Personal Pledge

In this chapter I have learned that:

- while alcohol is widely advertised and legally used, it addicts and kills people, damages their bodies, and is associated with crime and family violence;
- anyone under the legal drinking age who drinks alcohol is breaking the law and can be arrested;
- alcohol quickly affects the brain when it is consumed;
- beer and wine have the same effect as hard liquor;
- it is dangerous to drive after only one drink;
- alcohol reduces inhibitions and coordination, decreases judgment and control, and slows reflexes in the short term;
- alcohol can cause liver diseases, heart disease, brain damage and memory loss, and contribute to cancers in the long term;
- alcoholics often deny they have a problem with alcohol, but they can be helped throug[h] such programs as Alcoholics Anonymous.

Therefore, I have decided to abstain from alcohol as long as I am under the legal drinking age; to use alcohol very carefully, if at all, after that; to monitor myself for signs of alcohol dependency or addiction; and to get help if I need it. Furthermore, I will try to persuade others not to drink and drive, not to ride with a driver who has been drinking, and to get appropriate help if needed.

X ____________________
Signature

34 Personal Pledge

PERSONAL PLEDGE

Opportunities for students to demonstrate their commitment to healthy decisions and avoiding high-risk behaviors.

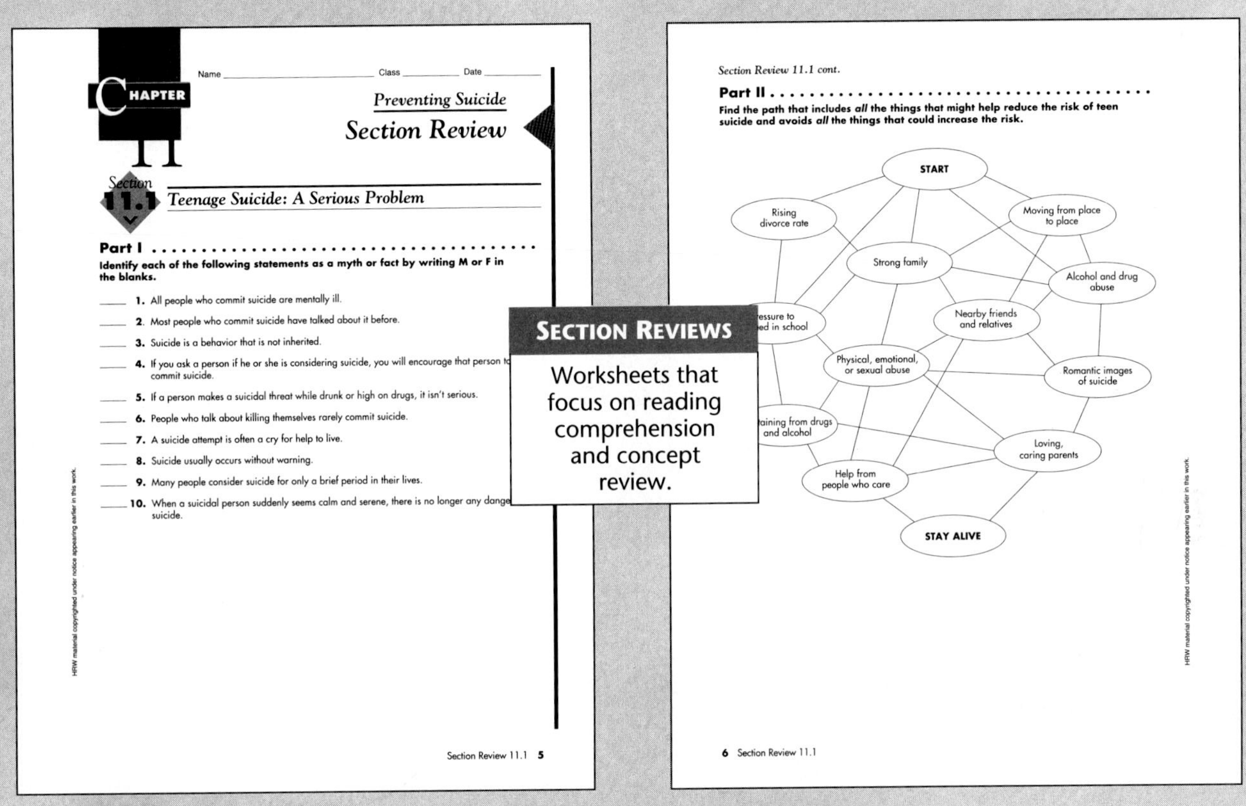

Name ______________ Class ________ Date ________

CHAPTER 11

Preventing Suicide

Section Review

Section 11.1 Teenage Suicide: A Serious Problem

Part I

Identify each of the following statements as a myth or fact by writing M or F in the blanks.

_____ 1. All people who commit suicide are mentally ill.

_____ 2. Most people who commit suicide have talked about it before.

_____ 3. Suicide is a behavior that is not inherited.

_____ 4. If you ask a person if he or she is considering suicide, you will encourage that person to commit suicide.

_____ 5. If a person makes a suicidal threat while drunk or high on drugs, it isn't serious.

_____ 6. People who talk about killing themselves rarely commit suicide.

_____ 7. A suicide attempt is often a cry for help to live.

_____ 8. Suicide usually occurs without warning.

_____ 9. Many people consider suicide for only a brief period in their lives.

_____ 10. When a suicidal person suddenly seems calm and serene, there is no longer any danger of suicide.

HRW material copyrighted under notice appearing earlier in this work.

Section Review 11.1 5

Section Review 11.1 cont.

Part II

Find the path that includes *all* the things that might help reduce the risk of teen suicide and avoids *all* the things that could increase the risk.

HRW material copyrighted under notice appearing earlier in this work.

6 Section Review 11.1

SECTION REVIEWS

Worksheets that focus on reading comprehension and concept review.

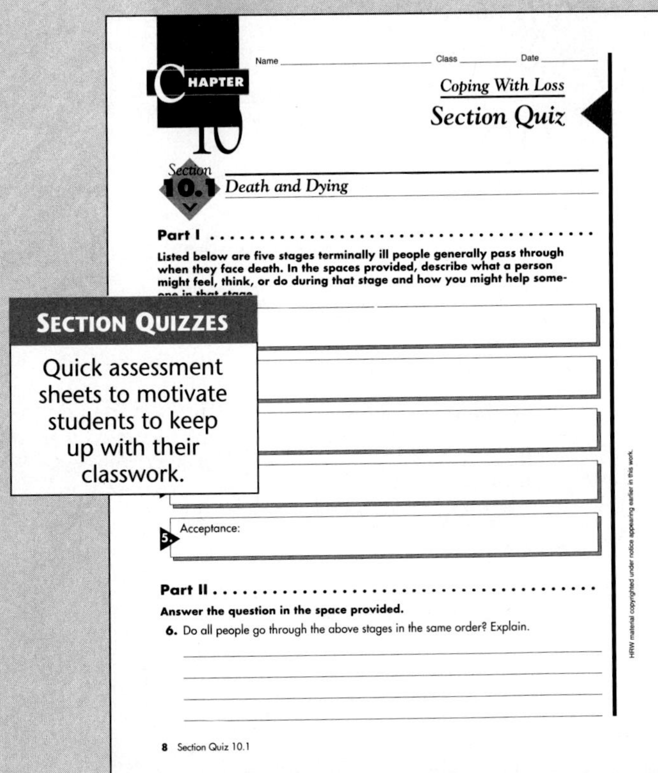

Name ______________ Class ________ Date ________

CHAPTER 10

Coping With Loss

Section Quiz

Section 10.1 Death and Dying

Part I

Listed below are five stages terminally ill people generally pass through when they face death. In the spaces provided, describe what a person might feel, think, or do during that stage and how you might help some-one in that stage.

5. Acceptance:

Part II

Answer the question in the space provided.

6. Do all people go through the above stages in the same order? Explain.

HRW material copyrighted under notice appearing earlier in this work.

8 Section Quiz 10.1

SECTION QUIZZES

Quick assessment sheets to motivate students to keep up with their classwork.

CHAPTER 14

Tobacco: Hazardous and Addictive

LIFE SKILLS

ACTIVITY A: Communicating Effectively

Different Ways to Communicate With Smokers

To protect themselves from cigarette smoke, nonsmokers need to communicate effectively with smokers about maintaining a smok[e-free environ]ment. How would you respond to each of the following situation[s]

1. Lara was walking down the hall at school when she caught a whiff of cigare[tte smoke. She followed] the smell and saw a younger student snuffing out a cigarette inside her locke[r. What would you do if] you were Lara and why?

2. Juan drove up to a self-service gas station and noticed that the woman at th[e next pump was] smoking as she pumped gas into her car. What would you do if you were Ju[an?]

3. Cheryl's aunt is in the hospital recovering from kidney surgery. While Chery[l was visiting, her aunt's] hospital roommate lights up a cigarette. Cheryl doesn't know if smoking is p[ermitted in her] aunt's hospital room, but she knows smoke makes her aunt uncomfortable. What would you do if you were Cheryl?

4. As you are waiting for your bus at the corner bus stop, you notice your neighbor, who is in her sixth month of pregnancy, light a cigarette. What would you do? Why?

HRW material copyrighted under notice appearing earlier in this work.

Life Skills 14A 5

LIFE SKILLS

To extend the Life Skills core of the text, these worksheets provide practice and reinforcement activities for the eleven life skills in the program.

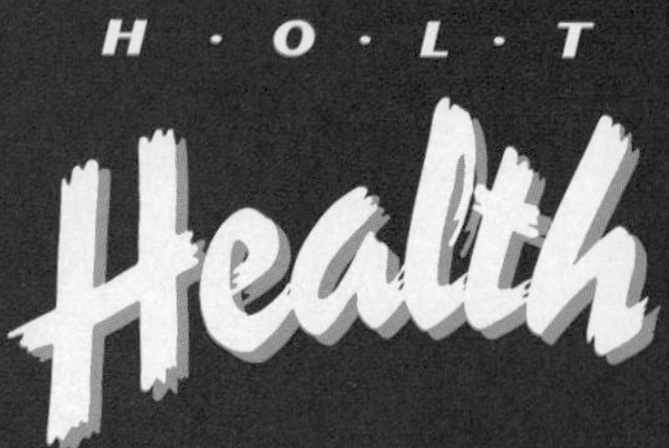

TEACHING RESOURCE SUPPLEMENTS (IN COPYMASTER FORM)

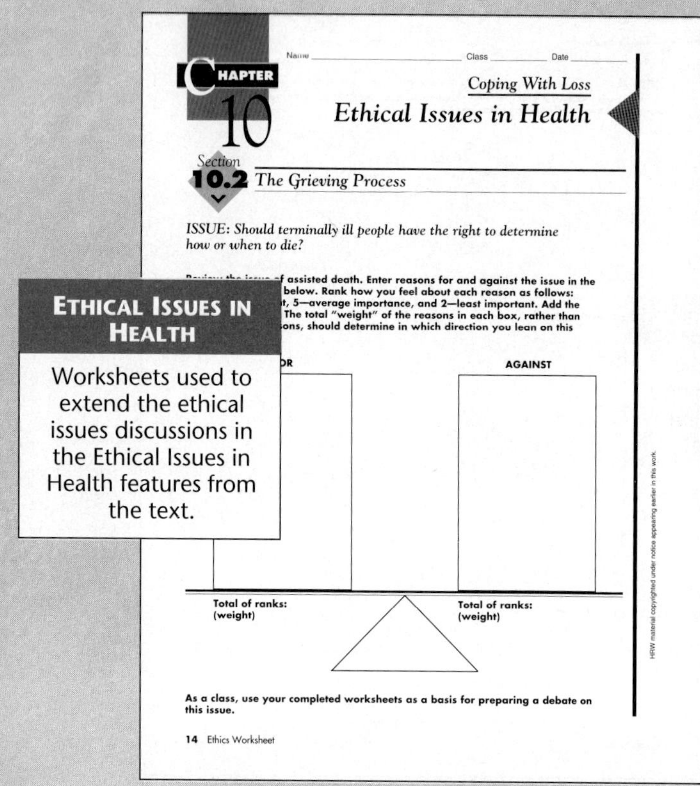
Name ______ Class ______ Date ______

CHAPTER 10

Coping With Loss

Ethical Issues in Health

Section 10.2 The Grieving Process

ISSUE: Should terminally ill people have the right to determine how or when to die?

Review the issue of assisted death. Enter reasons for and against the issue in the ... below. Rank how you feel about each reason as follows: ...t, 5—average importance, and 2—least important. Add the ... The total "weight" of the reasons in each box, rather than ...ons, should determine in which direction you lean on this ...

FOR	AGAINST
Total of ranks: (weight)	Total of ranks: (weight)

As a class, use your completed worksheets as a basis for preparing a debate on this issue.

14 Ethics Worksheet

HRW material copyrighted under notice appearing earlier in this work.

ETHICAL ISSUES IN HEALTH

Worksheets used to extend the ethical issues discussions in the Ethical Issues in Health features from the text.

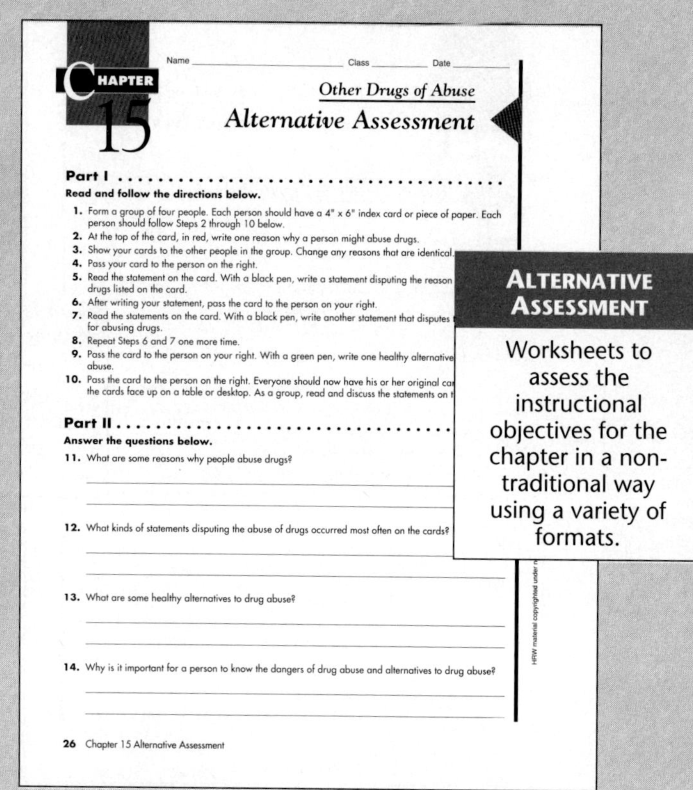
Name ______ Class ______ Date ______

CHAPTER 15

Other Drugs of Abuse

Alternative Assessment

Part I

Read and follow the directions below.

1. Form a group of four people. Each person should have a 4" x 6" index card or piece of paper. Each person should follow Steps 2 through 10 below.
2. At the top of the card, in red, write one reason why a person might abuse drugs.
3. Show your cards to the other people in the group. Change any reasons that are identical.
4. Pass your card to the person on the right.
5. Read the statement on the card. With a black pen, write a statement disputing the reason ... drugs listed on the card.
6. After writing your statement, pass the card to the person on your right.
7. Read the statements on the card. With a black pen, write another statement that disputes ... for abusing drugs.
8. Repeat Steps 6 and 7 one more time.
9. Pass the card to the person on your right. With a green pen, write one healthy alternative ... abuse.
10. Pass the card to the person on the right. Everyone should now have his or her original car... the cards face up on a table or desktop. As a group, read and discuss the statements on t...

Part II

Answer the questions below.

11. What are some reasons why people abuse drugs?
12. What kinds of statements disputing the abuse of drugs occurred most often on the cards?
13. What are some healthy alternatives to drug abuse?
14. Why is it important for a person to know the dangers of drug abuse and alternatives to drug abuse?

26 Chapter 15 Alternative Assessment

HRW material copyrighted under ...

ALTERNATIVE ASSESSMENT

Worksheets to assess the instructional objectives for the chapter in a non-traditional way using a variety of formats.

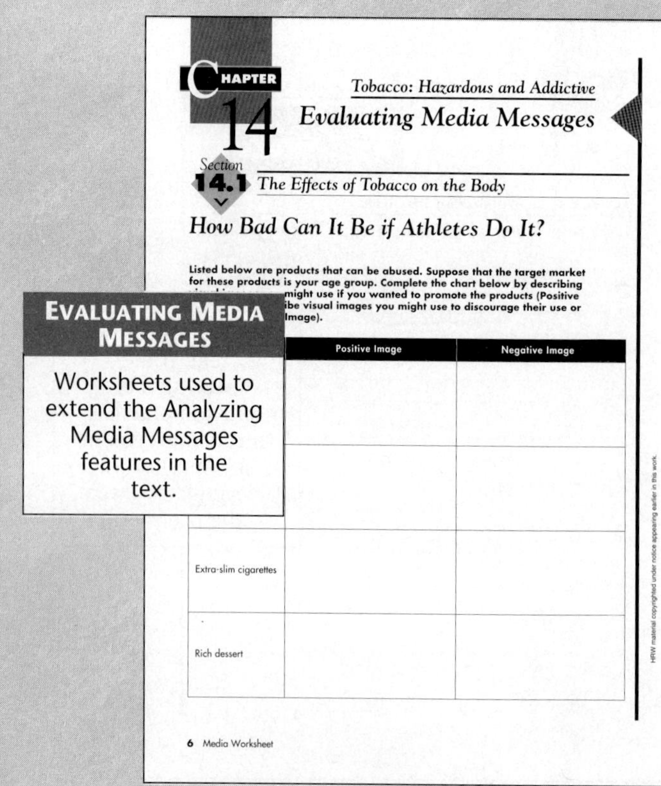
CHAPTER 14

Tobacco: Hazardous and Addictive

Evaluating Media Messages

Section 14.1 The Effects of Tobacco on the Body

How Bad Can It Be if Athletes Do It?

Listed below are products that can be abused. Suppose that the target market for these products is your age group. Complete the chart below by describing ... might use if you wanted to promote the products (Positive ...be visual images you might use to discourage their use or ...Image).

	Positive Image	Negative Image
Extra-slim cigarettes		
Rich dessert		

6 Media Worksheet

HRW material copyrighted under notice appearing earlier in this work.

EVALUATING MEDIA MESSAGES

Worksheets used to extend the Analyzing Media Messages features in the text.

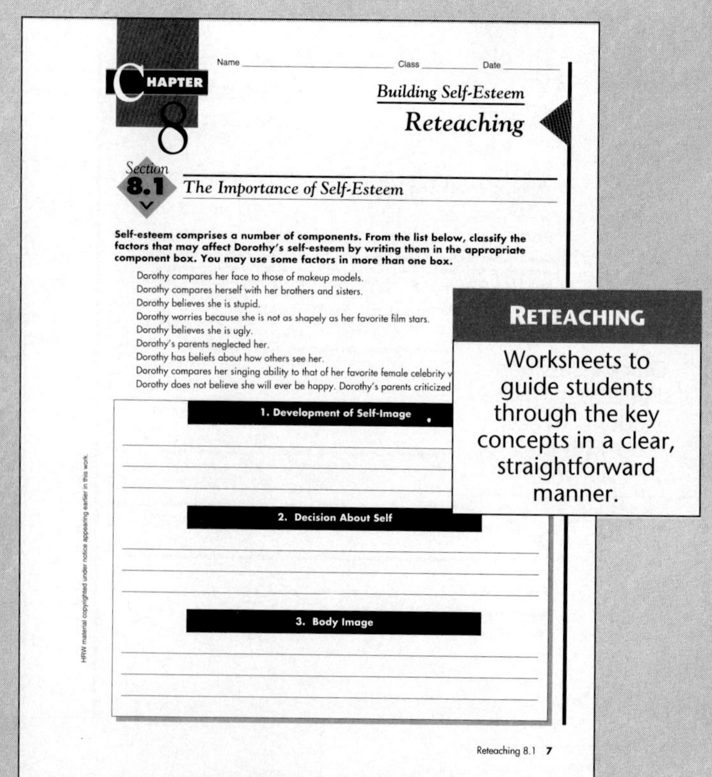
Name ______ Class ______ Date ______

CHAPTER 8

Building Self-Esteem

Reteaching

Section 8.1 The Importance of Self-Esteem

Self-esteem comprises a number of components. From the list below, classify the factors that may affect Dorothy's self-esteem by writing them in the appropriate component box. You may use some factors in more than one box.

Dorothy compares her face to those of makeup models.
Dorothy compares herself with her brothers and sisters.
Dorothy believes she is stupid.
Dorothy worries because she is not as shapely as her favorite film stars.
Dorothy believes she is ugly.
Dorothy's parents neglected her.
Dorothy has beliefs about how others see her.
Dorothy compares her singing ability to that of her favorite female celebrity ...
Dorothy does not believe she will ever be happy. Dorothy's parents criticized ...

1. Development of Self-Image

2. Decision About Self

3. Body Image

Reteaching 8.1 7

HRW material copyrighted under notice appearing earlier in this work.

RETEACHING

Worksheets to guide students through the key concepts in a clear, straightforward manner.

Name ____________ Class ________ Date ________

CHAPTER 14

Tobacco: Hazardous and Addictive

Chapter Test

Part I

Match the terms on the left with the definitions on the right.

____ **1.** cancer
____ **2.** carbon monoxide
____ **3.** cardiovascular disease
____ **4.** chronic bronchitis
____ **5.** cilia
____ **6.** emphysema
____ **7.** mainstream smoke
____ **8.** sidestream smoke

a. tiny hairs that line the bronchial tubes
b. smoke that is inhaled directly into the mouth and lungs through a cigar, pipe, or cigarette
c. a gas that is found in tobacco smoke and interferes with the blood's ability to carry oxygen
d. a disease caused by the formation ... deadly cells that attack and replac...
e. an inflammation of the bronchial t... the production of excessive mucus
f. smoke that enters the environment ... tobacco
g. disease of the heart and blood ves...
h. a disease in which the air sacs of t... tured or torn

Part II

Write the letter of the correct answer in the blank.

____ **9.** The chemical in tobacco that is a psychoactive substance and is addictive i...
a. tar c. carbon monoxide
b. nicotine d. nitrogen dioxide

____ **10.** The chemical in tobacco smoke that is made up of solid particles that contribute to the destruction of cilia and respiratory disease is
a. carbon monoxide c. tar
b. ammonia d. nicotine

____ **11.** Which of the following is *not* true of lung cancer?
a. It causes over 120,000 deaths per year.
b. It is the most common cause of cancer deaths among American women.
c. The risk of developing it can be greatly reduced by not smoking or breathing smoke.
d. Its connection to cigarette smoking is unclear.

____ **12.** Smoking is directly related to and can increase one's risk for
a. heart attack c. stroke
b. kidney cancer d. all of the above

Chapter Test

Each 3-page test thoroughly covers the instructional objectives for the chapter using multiple choice, matching, and essay items.

Chapter 14 Test cont.

____ **13.** Jason's father has been smoking for many years. His lungs have trouble absorbing oxygen from the air and pushing out carbon dioxide. As a result, Jason's father is always short of breath. Jason's father most likely has
a. bronchitis c. lung cancer
b. emphysema d. respiratory failure

____ **14.** The most dangerous use of tobacco is
a. pipe smoking c. cigarette smoking
b. tobacco chewing d. breathing others' smoke

____ **15.** Using smokeless tobacco—chewing tobacco and snuff—can put one at greater risk for
a. emphysema c. mouth cancer
b. lung cancer d. all of the above

____ **16.** The tobacco smoke that rises from a lit pipe is called
... smoke c. mainstream smoke
...am smoke d. filtered smoke

...es *not* smoke. However, she works in an office where several co-workers smoke ...all day long. Which of the following is *not* true of Angela?
...ld be no worse off if she herself smoked.
... passive smoker.
... risk for lung cancer.
...bject to sidestream smoke.

...just found out she is pregnant. She and her husband, Jeff, smoke. They would be ...p smoking because
... can cause a miscarriage
...loping fetus could be born too early if Katya continued to smoke
...ugh Katya may stop smoking, the smoke from Jeff's cigarettes could affect the ...
...e above

____ **14.** Rodger and his friends started smoking cigarettes in sixth grade. The strongest influence on them was most likely from
a. their peers c. advertisements
b. their parents d. a professional athlete

____ **20.** Which of the following is least likely to encourage a young person to quit smoking?
a. Friends who don't smoke
b. A desire to participate in sports
c. Knowledge about the health consequences of smoking
d. Parents who smoke but tell their children not to smoke

Chapter 14 Test cont.

____ **21.** At first, Ellen thought it was glamorous to smoke. But now she's tired of being short of breath and coughing every morning. If she quits she will
a. stop coughing and feel better
b. enable the cilia in her bronchial tubes to repair themselves
c. immediately reduce her risk for lung and other cancers
d. all of the above

____ **22.** Paula works in a high-stress job. She and most of her co-workers smoke. It will be particularly hard for her to quit because
a. Cigarette smoking leads to the use of other drugs.
b. Her stress cannot be handled in other ways.
c. She may have little support from the people she is with all day.
d. She will have to breathe sidestream smoke.

____ **23.** Which of the following would probably *not* help Paula stop successfully?
a. Spontaneously throw away her cigarettes one day at work
b. Gradually cut down the number of cigarettes she smokes
c. Talk with her doctor about a nicotine patch
d. Wait until she is on vacation to stop smoking

Part III

Answer the question in the space provided.

24. Most doctors' offices and hospitals have adopted a nonsmoking policy. How might they justify this policy?

Activity Book

This consumable workbook contains the following items from the Teacher's Resource Binder.

Journal Entries
Personal Inventories
Life Skills
Section Reviews
Evaluating Media Messages
Ethical Issues in Health

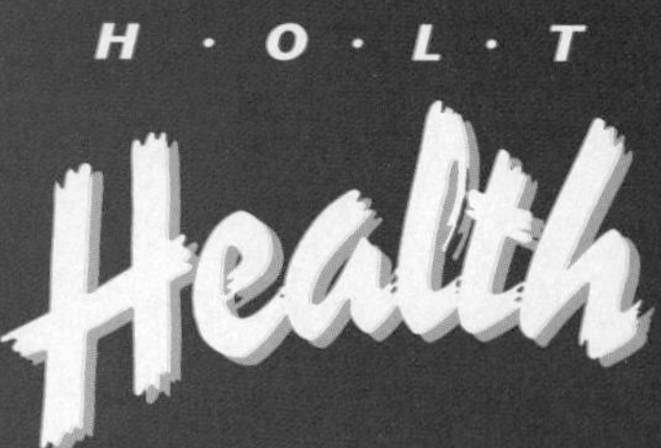

Teaching Resource Supplements

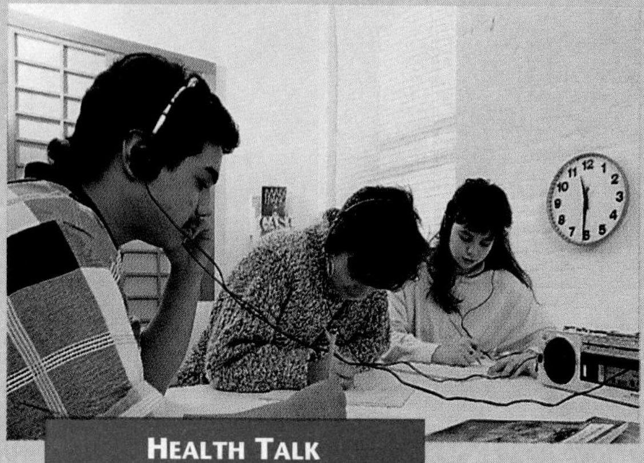

Health Talk English/Spanish Audiocassettes

This audio program addresses the needs of auditory learners or students with English language difficulties. Each audio program reviews key concepts in English or Spanish and includes audio questions to assess comprehension.

Test Generators

This teacher utility software can be used to construct customized chapter tests from a bank of over 1200 items. Available for Macintosh® and IBM® and compatible PC's.

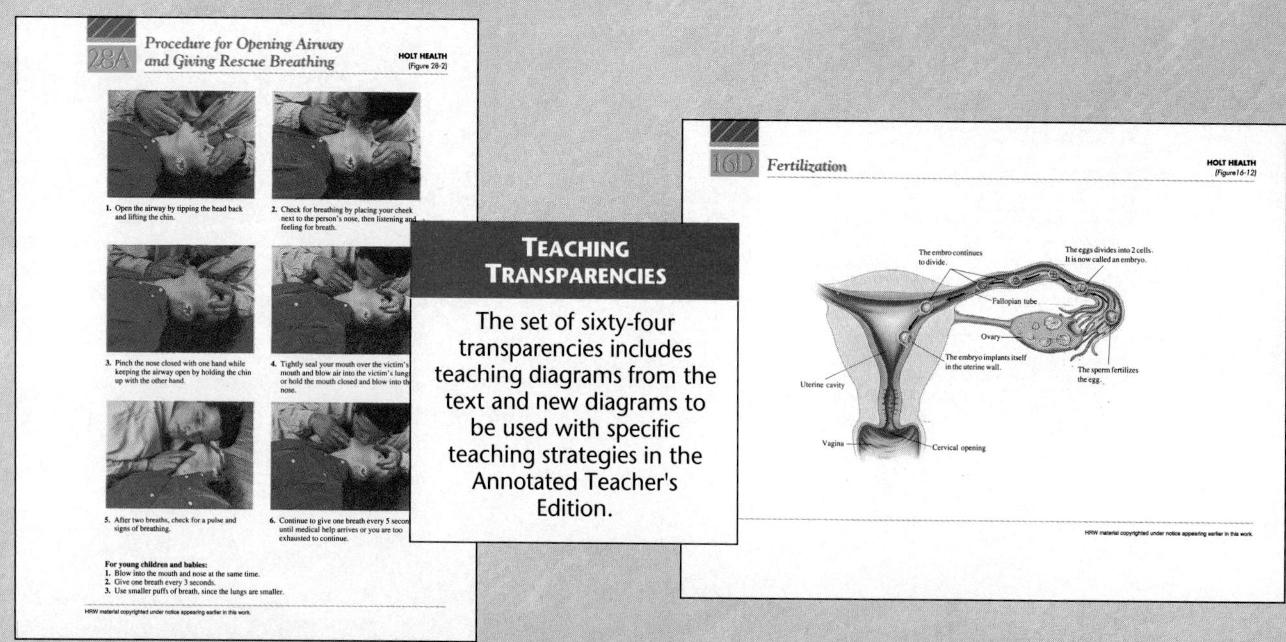

Teaching Transparencies

The set of sixty-four transparencies includes teaching diagrams from the text and new diagrams to be used with specific teaching strategies in the Annotated Teacher's Edition.

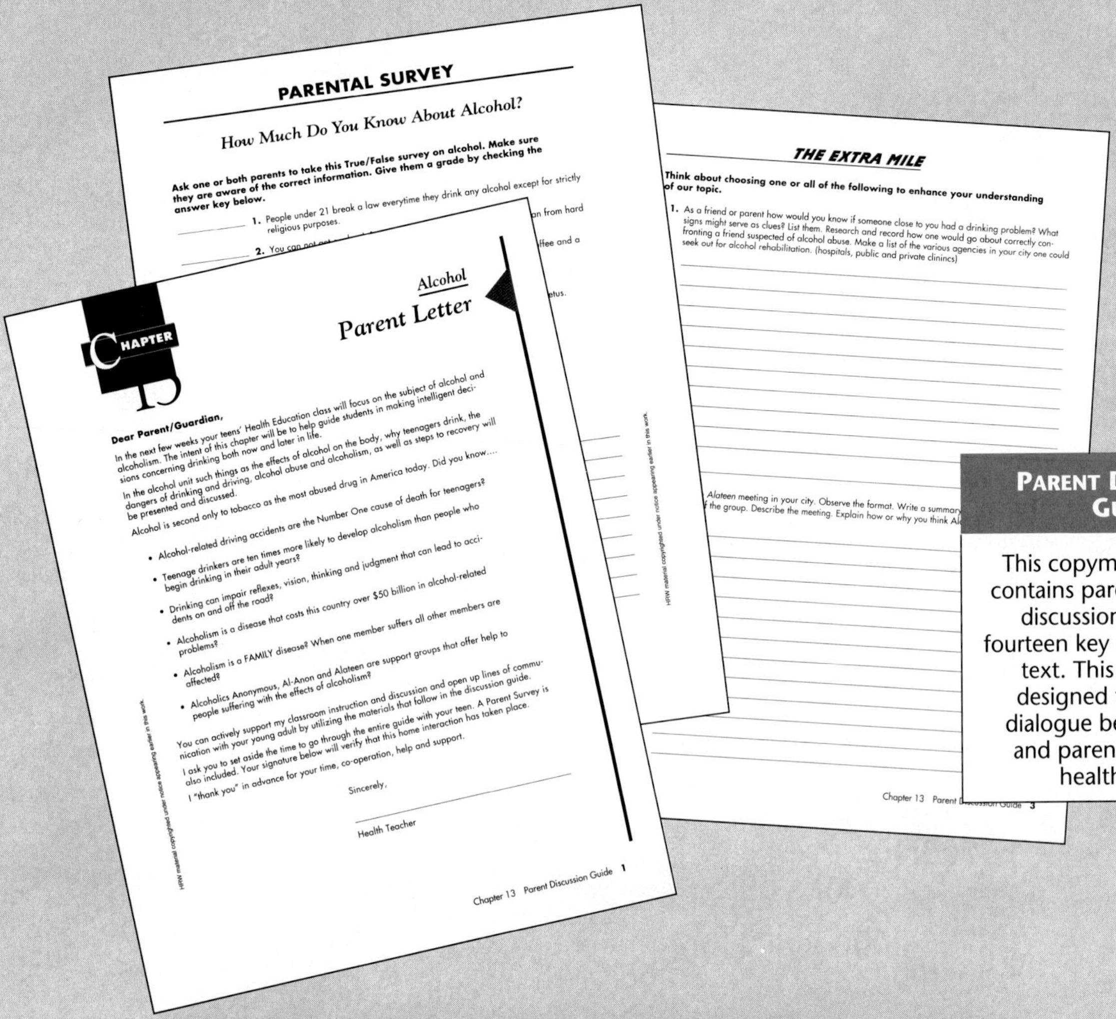

PARENTAL SURVEY

How Much Do You Know About Alcohol?

Ask one or both parents to take this True/False survey on alcohol. Make sure they are aware of the correct information. Give them a grade by checking the answer key below.

_____ 1. People under 21 break a law everytime they drink any alcohol except for strictly religious purposes.

_____ 2. You can not ...

THE EXTRA MILE

Think about choosing one or all of the following to enhance your understanding of our topic.

1. As a friend or parent how would you know if someone close to you had a drinking problem? What signs might serve as clues? List them. Research and record how one would go about correctly confronting a friend suspected of alcohol abuse. Make a list of the various agencies in your city one could seek out for alcohol rehabilitation. (hospitals, public and private clinincs)

... Alateen meeting in your city. Observe the format. Write a summary ... the group. Describe the meeting. Explain how or why you think Al...

Chapter 13 Parent Discussion Guide 3

CHAPTER 13

Alcohol

Parent Letter

Dear Parent/Guardian,

In the next few weeks your teens' Health Education class will focus on the subject of alcohol and alcoholism. The intent of this chapter will be to help guide students in making intelligent decisions concerning drinking both now and later in life.

In the alcohol unit such things as the effects of alcohol on the body, why teenagers drink, the dangers of drinking and driving, alcohol abuse and alcoholism, as well as steps to recovery will be presented and discussed.

Alcohol is second only to tobacco as the most abused drug in America today. Did you know....

- Alcohol-related driving accidents are the Number One cause of death for teenagers?
- Teenage drinkers are ten times more likely to develop alcoholism than people who begin drinking in their adult years?
- Drinking can impair reflexes, vision, thinking and judgment that can lead to accidents on and off the road?
- Alcoholism is a disease that costs this country over $50 billion in alcohol-related problems?
- Alcoholism is a FAMILY disease? When one member suffers all other members are affected?
- Alcoholics Anonymous, Al-Anon and Alateen are support groups that offer help to people suffering with the effects of alcoholism?

You can actively support my classroom instruction and discussion and open up lines of communication with your young adult by utilizing the materials that follow in the discussion guide.

I ask you to set aside the time to go through the entire guide with your teen. A Parent Survey is also included. Your signature below will verify that this home interaction has taken place.

I "thank you" in advance for your time, co-operation, help and support.

Sincerely,

Health Teacher

Chapter 13 Parent Discussion Guide 1

PARENT DISCUSSION GUIDE

This copymaster booklet contains parent letters and discussion guides for fourteen key chapters in the text. This program is designed to stimulate dialogue between teens and parents on critical health issues.

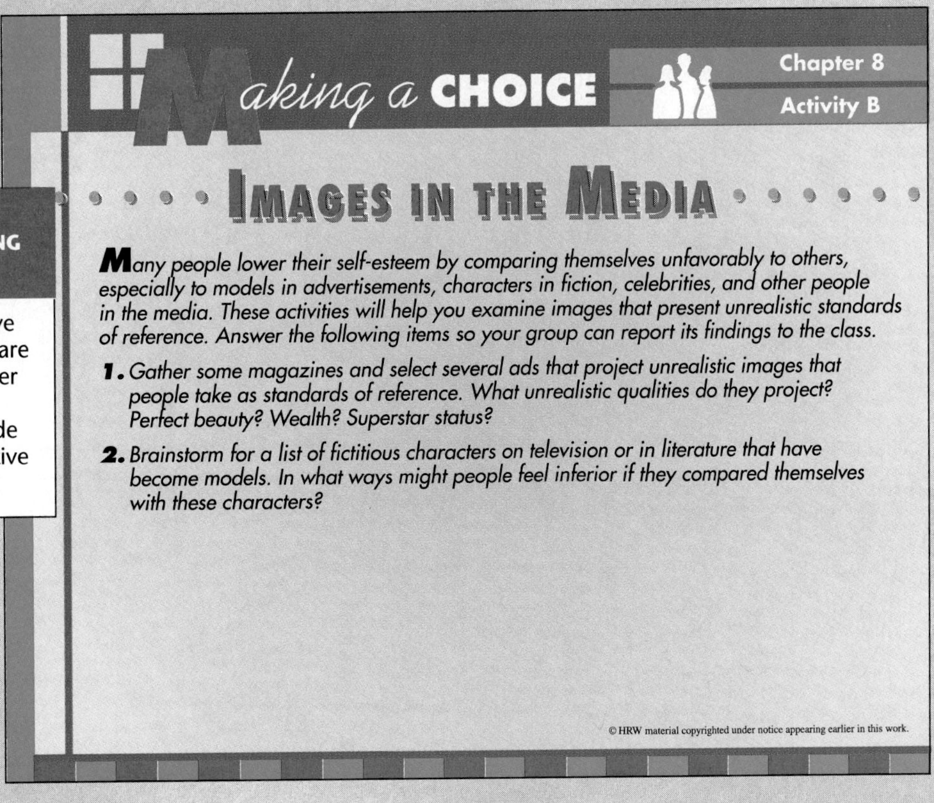

Making a CHOICE

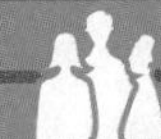

Chapter 8

Activity B

IMAGES IN THE MEDIA

Many people lower their self-esteem by comparing themselves unfavorably to others, especially to models in advertisements, characters in fiction, celebrities, and other people in the media. These activities will help you examine images that present unrealistic standards of reference. Answer the following items so your group can report its findings to the class.

1. *Gather some magazines and select several ads that project unrealistic images that people take as standards of reference. What unrealistic qualities do they project? Perfect beauty? Wealth? Superstar status?*
2. *Brainstorm for a list of fictitious characters on television or in literature that have become models. In what ways might people feel inferior if they compared themselves with these characters?*

MAKING A CHOICE COOPERATIVE LEARNING STRATEGIES

Boxed set of cooperative learning activites. There are two activities per chapter and 6 copies of each activity so you can divide the class into 6 cooperative groups.

UNIT 1

INTRODUCTION TO HEALTH AND WELLNESS

CHAPTER OVERVIEWS

CHAPTER 1

HEALTH AND WELLNESS: A QUALITY OF LIFE

This chapter introduces the concept of wellness and describes the five components of health—physical, social, mental, emotional, and spiritual. It provides a health-illness continuum on which students can plot their total health status. The chapter explains the relationships of health, self-esteem, social support, and physical fitness to wellness. In the second section, students are introduced to the idea of making healthy decisions by looking at teen health risks and completing a survey.

CHAPTER 2

MAKING RESPONSIBLE DECISIONS

Students learn how responsible decision making is related to health and wellness. The leading causes of death in young people and older people are discussed and related to the short-term and long-term consequences of health-related decisions. A decision-making model is presented. Students follow a fictional character through the process of decision making using the model. Then they are asked to apply the model to a real or invented situation of their own.

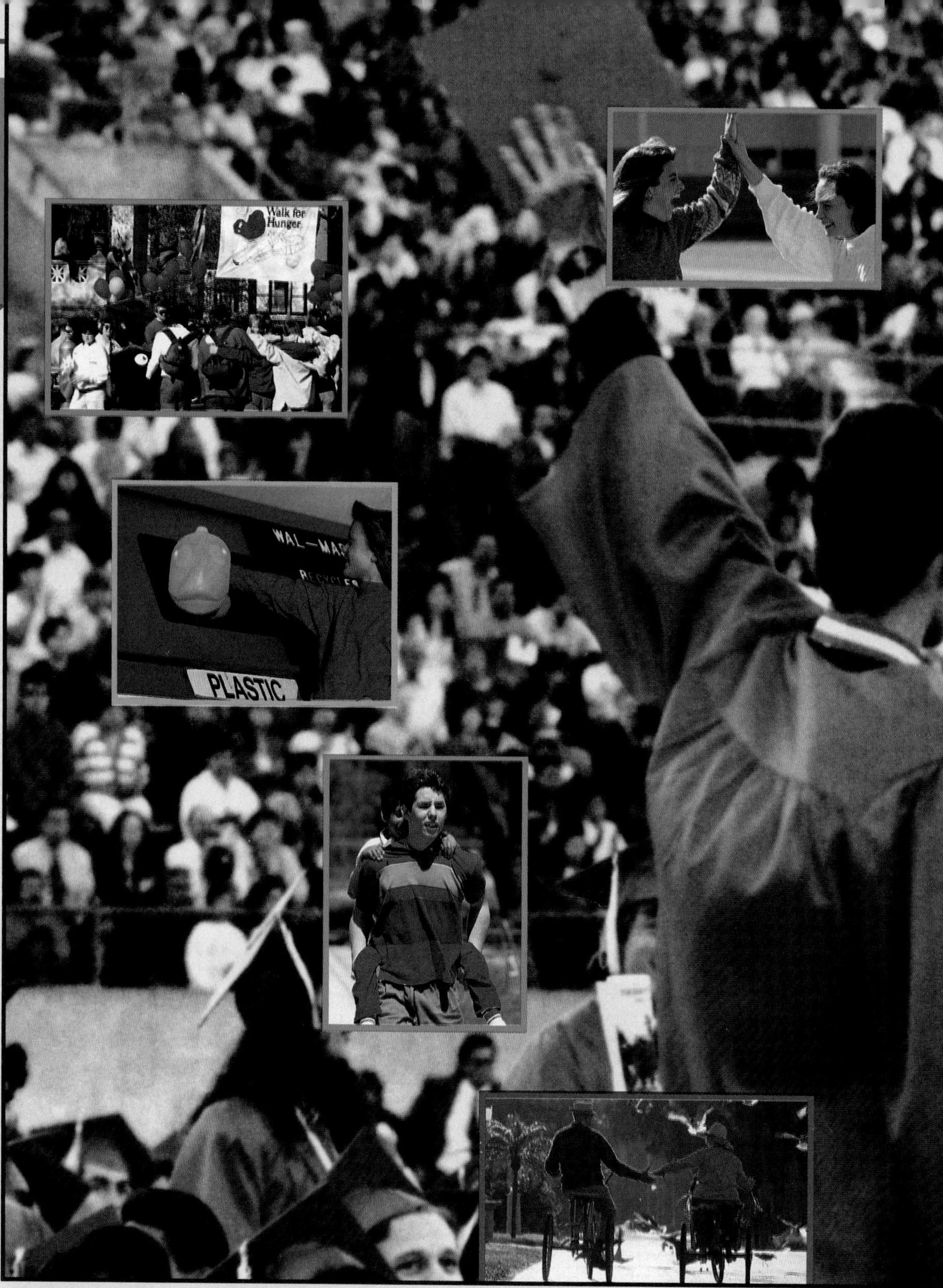

UNIT ONE

INTRODUCTION TO HEALTH AND WELLNESS

CHAPTER 1

HEALTH AND WELLNESS: A QUALITY OF LIFE

CHAPTER 2

MAKING RESPONSIBLE DECISIONS

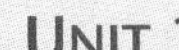

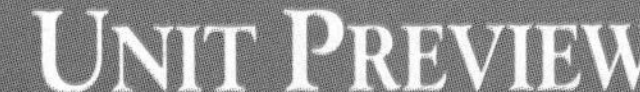

UNIT PREVIEW

This unit helps students understand what constitutes health and how it is related to total wellness. Through gaining this understanding, assessing their own health, and identifying their health risk factors, students begin thinking about managing their own health. The most important component of health management is responsible decision making. A decision-making model is provided to help students in this process. The five major health themes are emphasized throughout the unit, as indicated on the chart below.

THEMES TRACE

	WELLNESS	BUILDING SELF-ESTEEM	DECISION MAKING	DEVELOPING LIFE-MANAGEMENT SKILLS	ACCEPTANCE OF DIVERSITY AMONG PEOPLE
Chapter 1	pp. 4–16	p. 9	pp. 5–6	pp. 8–9, 14–16	pp. 6–7
Chapter 2		p. 28	pp. 20–33	pp. 29–30	p. 26

Health and Wellness: A Quality of Life

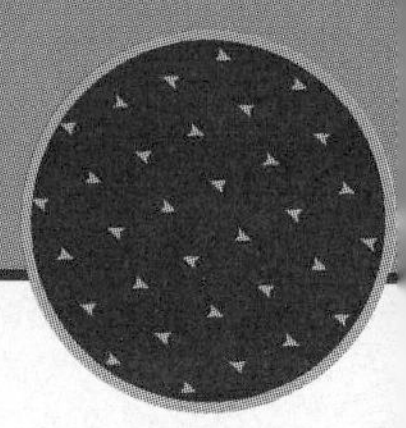

PLANNING GUIDE

TEXT SECTIONS	OBJECTIVES	TEXT FEATURES	OUTSIDE RESOURCES	NOTES
1.1 Health and You pp. 5-10 2 periods	• Explain how the five components of health provide a picture of overall health. • Describe the difference between wellness and health. ■ Plot your current state of health on the health-illness continuum. • Describe the ways in which self-esteem, social support, health, and wellness are related. • Describe the health benefits of physical fitness.	**ASSESSMENT** • Section Review, p. 10	**TEACHER'S RESOURCE BINDER** • Lesson Plan 1.1 • Personal Health Inventory • Journal Entry 1A • Life Skills 1A • Section Review 1.1 • Section Quiz 1.1 • Reteaching 1.1 **OTHER RESOURCES** • Making a Choice 1A	
1.2 Health Concerns in the United States pp. 11-16 2 periods	• Compare the leading causes of death for teens with the leading causes for adults. • Compare the leading causes of death today with those of 100 years ago. ■ Identify your health risk factors.	■ Life SKILLS: Assessing Your Health, pp. 14-16 **ASSESSMENT** • Section Review, p. 13	**TEACHER'S RESOURCE BINDER** • Lesson Plan 1.2 • Journal Entry 1B • Section Review 1.2 • Section Quiz 1.2 • Reteaching 1.2 **OTHER RESOURCES** • Making a Choice 1B • Transparency 1A	
End of Chapter pp. 17-19		**ASSESSMENT** • Chapter Review, pp. 18-19	**TEACHER'S RESOURCE BINDER** • Chapter Test • Alternative Assessment **OTHER RESOURCES** • Test Generator	

■ Denotes LIFE SKILLS objectives

• Items in blue are also part of the *Holt Health Activity Book.*

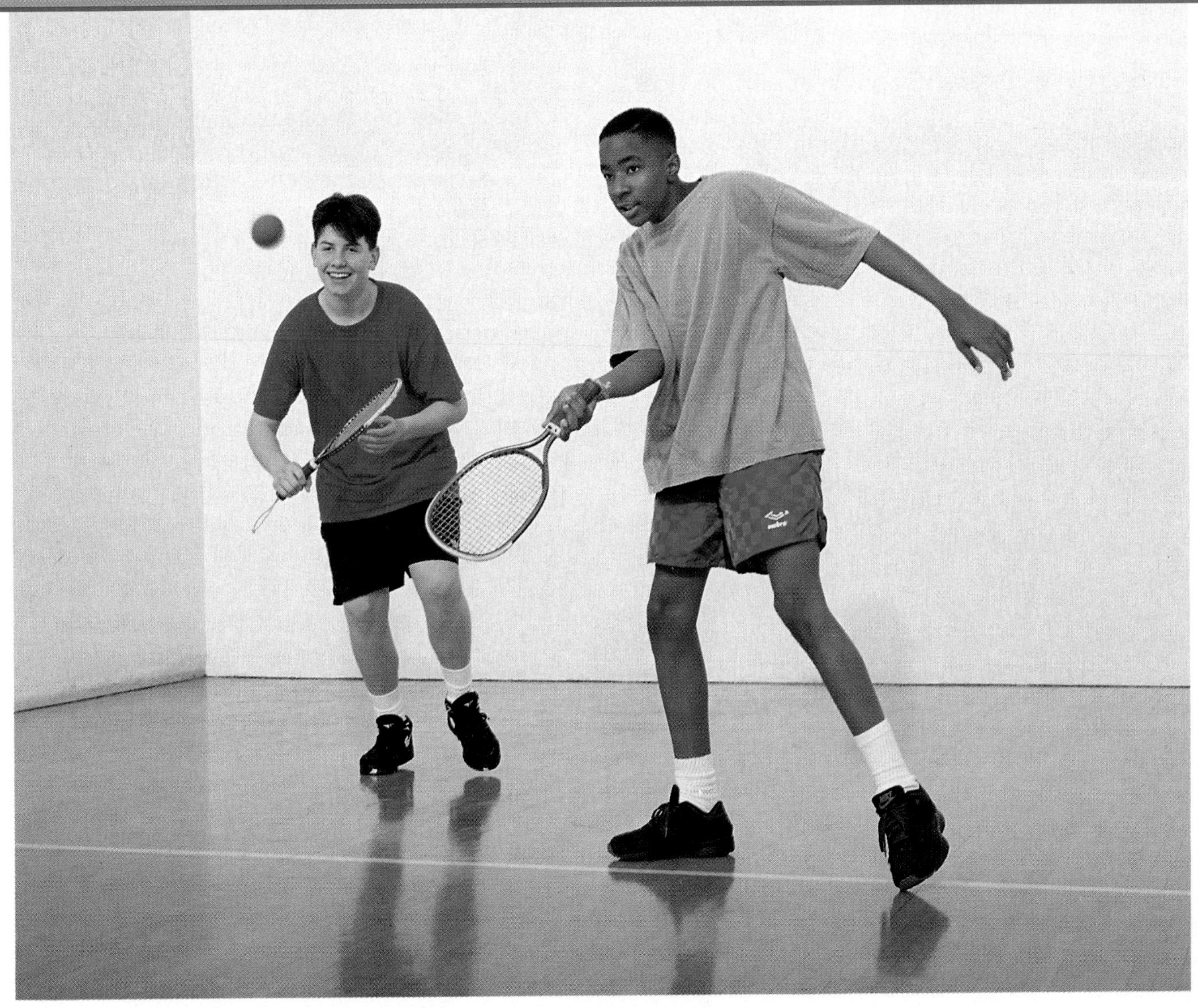

Content Background The Wellness Business

As the cost of medical care has risen in the United States, the preventive medicine and fitness industry has grown. The public is starting to realize that the physician's ability to heal is limited by the patient's lifestyle choices and the availability of funds to pay for services. They know it is less costly to maintain good health than to repair it. Taken together, the resources devoted to the maintenance of optimal health can be called the wellness industry. In its broad outlines, it takes in skiing and meditation, saunas and swimming pools—with the aim of promoting good health, fitness, and the enjoyment of physical, mental, and social activities.

One segment of the industry is live-in treatment programs for weight management, smoking cessation, chemical dependency, stress reduction, and lifestyle change. People who attend live-in programs may have given up on remedial, symptomatic medical treatment by physicians, or may be following doctors' orders to improve their behavior. Residential treatment programs help them learn about health and develop new habits under the close supervision of a trained staff. These programs are costly because of the staff, facilities, and licensing required to operate them; many people who need such programs cannot afford them. Medical insurance will pay for specific services within these programs, such as the medical tests and physicians' services, but will not pay for the health education and lodging provided by these programs because they cannot measure the quality of the results. This could be shortsighted. The costs for cardiac bypass surgery, for example, exceed the costs of residential treatment programs by more than five to one. Economically it makes better sense for an insurance carrier to pay the lower cost of a preventive program, but the system does not currently permit it.

Another part of the wellness business is the health club industry. Only one out of two people who start an exercise program stay with it for more than six months. A health club can provide the social and physical atmosphere and financial pressure to help you stick with a program. Health clubs have started to replace bars as places for people to meet and socialize. Costs to belong to these establishments vary. Many clubs have a one-time initiation fee plus monthly payments. (The initiation fees can vary from \$50 to \$1,000. The yearly dues range from \$100 to \$1,500.) The fees depend on the location of the club and the ratio of staff and square footage to membership. Club staff can be certified by various agencies, and clubs may belong to national associations—both of which serve to raise quality standards. In competition with health clubs, some country clubs, business schools, and corporations are now starting to add fitness facilities. Along with exercise facilities, the health clubs are adding other services—food, tournaments, league play, camps, massage, newsletters, clothing and equipment shops, hair and tanning salons, and child care.

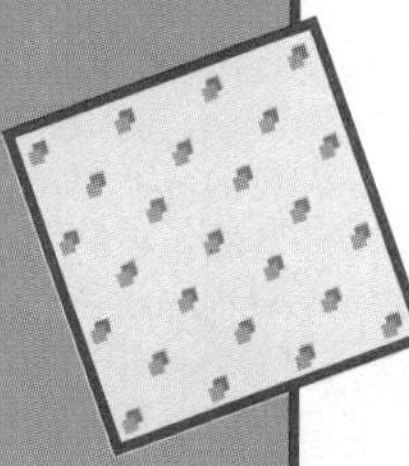

Resorts are another entire industry that has grown up around the need to get away, to enjoy recreation, and to relax. These places now provide a variety of courses such as photography, furniture making, pottery, and children's arts. Residential spas offer complete diet, exercise, and relaxation programs. And many soothing treatments are available—massage, mud baths, scrubs, and facials—which relax a person both mentally and physically. Home spas and saunas can have a similar effect.

With lifestyle changes, diet, relaxation, and recreation, people keep themselves healthy and fit—and away from doctors' offices. The healthy choices and changes people make in their daily lives add up to preventive medicine.

PLANNING FOR INSTRUCTION

KEY FACTS

- **The five major components of health—physical, social, mental, emotional, and spiritual—must be in balance for you to be truly healthy.**
- **Health is the state of well-being that comes from realizing your potential in each of the five components of health. Optimal health is known as wellness.**
- **Achieving wellness involves making the right choices and behaving in a way that maximizes your health.**
- **Self-esteem, or feeling good about yourself, is important to health and wellness.**
- **Social support helps you to manage stressors without becoming ill.**
- **Teens are exposed to very serious health issues; however, some of them involve decisions that a teen can control.**
- **The leading causes of death at the beginning of this century were communicable diseases, such as pneumonia, tuberculosis, and influenza. Now, the leading causes of death are heart disease and cancer, both of which can be the result of people's lifestyle choices.**

MYTHS AND MISCONCEPTIONS

MYTH: If you are physically fit, you are perfectly healthy.

Some people are physically fit but are not socially, mentally, emotionally, and spiritually healthy.

MYTH: Some people can't help getting heart disease or cancer.

Heart disease and cancer can be the result of people's lifestyle choices. If people would exercise regularly, eat properly, have periodic medical exams, avoid the use of tobacco, and manage stress effectively, the number of deaths from heart disease and cancer could be greatly reduced.

MYTH: Teens today are a lot healthier than teens were 80 or 90 years ago because of the advances of medicine.

In some respects this is true. However, health problems of teens today differ from those of the past, and some new ones are life-threatening.

VOCABULARY

Essential: The following vocabulary terms appear in boldface type.

physical health	wellness
social health	self-esteem
mental health	social support
emotional health	physical fitness
spiritual health	communicable disease
health	

Secondary: Be aware that the following terms may come up during class discussion.

transition	coordination
components	premature death
stressful situations	sexually transmitted disease
depression	lifestyle
unifying force	quarantine
spiritual potential	food and water sanitation
well-being	
health-illness continuum	
cardiorespiratory endurance	

FOR STUDENTS WITH SPECIAL NEEDS

LEP Students: Appoint a team of students who have a grasp on what total health means. Have them draw up a questionnaire that can be used to assess a student's health profile. (Questions might include: Do you enjoy doing things with other people? Are you comfortable with the way your body looks and feels? When you want to, can you tell people how you feel? Do you have enough energy for your daily activities? for sports?) When the questionnaire is ready, the team can use it on a one-on-one basis, posing the questions to LEP students and making sure they understand what total health comprises. Then have the LEP students switch roles and ask the questions of those who prepared the questionnaire.

Less-Advanced Students: Ask students to analyze the Life Skills Health Risks Survey and list each section of the survey under one of the five components of health. Discuss with students any disagreements about which component is emphasized in a section.

ENRICHMENT

- Have students choose a book or movie they have enjoyed that recalls a person's struggle toward one aspect of health. This will give students the opportunity to review what is meant by total health, while at the same time preparing them to become more aware of an aspect of health that is portrayed in an interesting novel or film. Ask them to outline the steps in the struggle of the character, noting how he or she responded. Tell students to write a paragraph about what they learned from the character's story.
- Arrange for a speaker who can address teen health problems. The speaker may be a counselor, a health care worker, a spiritual guide, an athletic coach or player, or a teen club advisor. Have students prepare questions they would like the speaker to address. The questions can be submitted anonymously and should be given to the speaker beforehand.
- Ask students to write a story about a teen with a health problem who struggled and overcame it or learned to live a productive life with the problem. Topics might include learning to get along with parents or peers, life after parents divorce, coping with alcohol abuse in the family, overcoming low self-esteem, getting help for depression, controlling anger, forming worthwhile relationships, and living with a physical health problem.

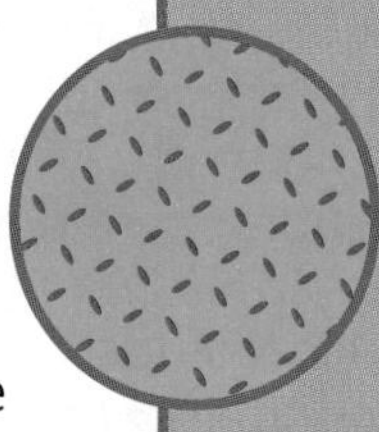

CHAPTER 1 CHAPTER OPENER

GETTING STARTED

Using the Chapter Photograph
Ask students how the person in the picture presents an image of wellness. Have them discuss what they think it means to be healthy. Is health purely a matter of physical well-being? What other things contribute to it?

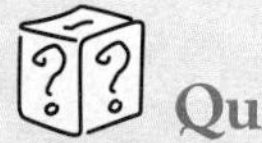

Question Box
Have students anonymously write out any questions they have about health and wellness, as it pertains to teens and their families, and put them in the Question Box. To ensure that students with questions are not embarrassed to be seen writing, have students who do not have questions write a fact they already know about health and wellness on the paper instead.

Preview the questions and then answer them at appropriate points in the chapter. You may wish to allow students to write additional questions as they go through the chapter.

Personal Issues *ALERT*
The discussion of health or wellness may make students uncomfortable. They may have a health problem or someone close to them who is ill. They may feel that everyone will think they are different or unacceptable because of these problems. Prepare the class to be respectful of privacy and sensitive to the feelings of others. Help them see that there are many aspects to good health and that someone with a physical health problem may more than compensate in the other aspects of health.

CHAPTER 1

Health and Wellness: A Quality of Life

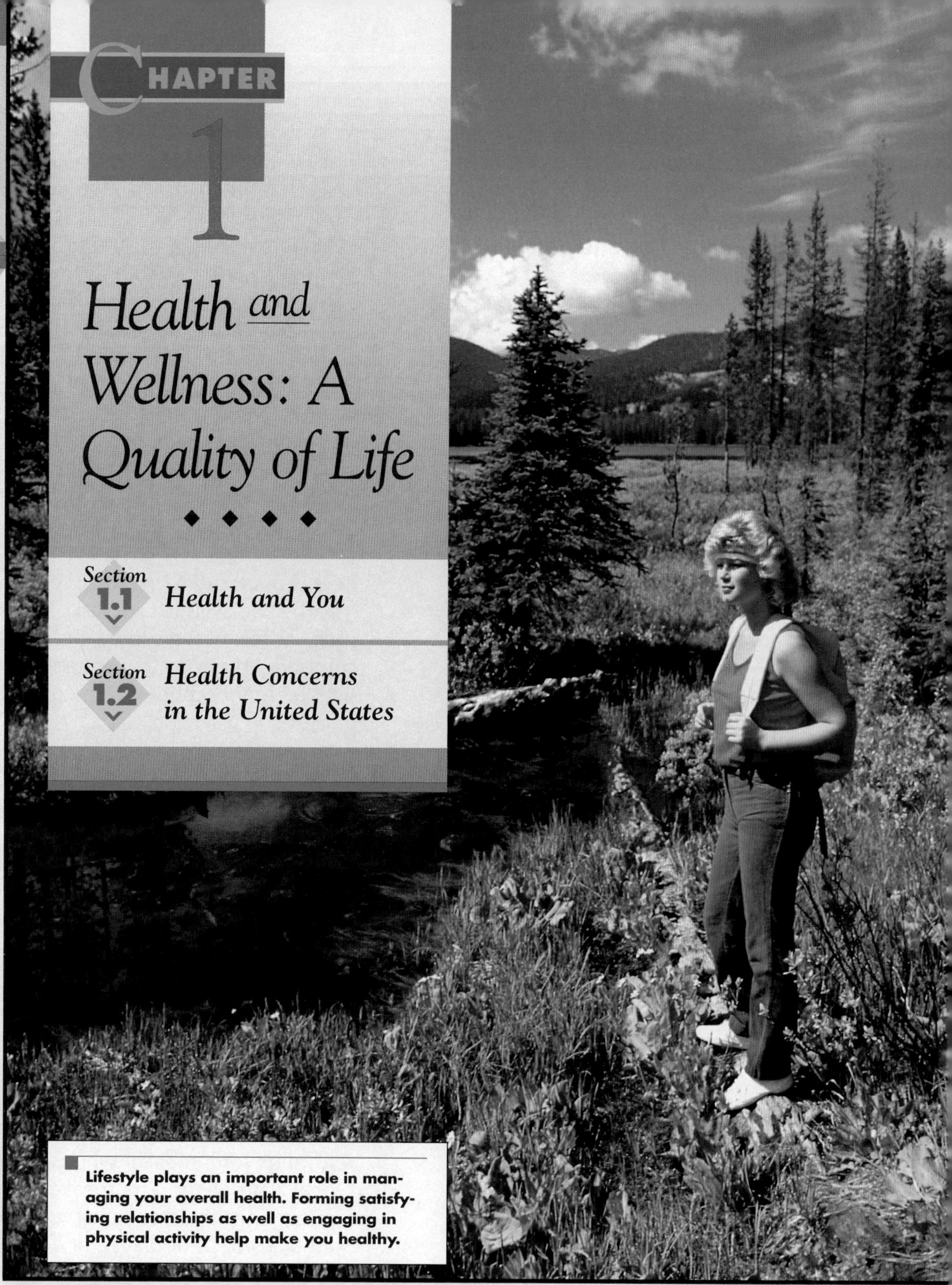

Lifestyle plays an important role in managing your overall health. Forming satisfying relationships as well as engaging in physical activity help make you healthy.

Tara looked at her schedule. Fourth-period health was coming up next. Now that was the last class she felt like taking. Health class in grade school had been boring. Memorizing parts of the body and reading about diseases was not something she looked forward to doing again.

Right now all she could think about were the problems at home. Her mother's drinking was getting worse. Everything seemed to fall apart during the divorce. Her parents continued to argue all the time and Tara really felt caught in the middle. Her younger sister was talking about running away. Tara felt helpless in dealing with it all. Who could she turn to?

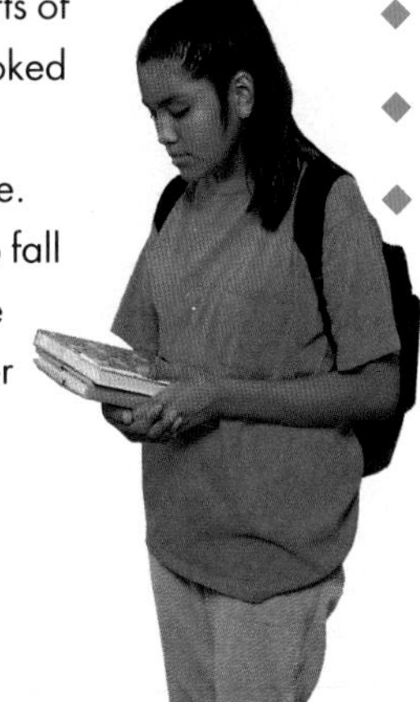

Section 1.1 Health and You

Objectives

- *Explain how the five components of health provide a picture of overall health.*
- *Describe the difference between wellness and health.*
- *Plot your current state of health on the health-illness continuum.*
  LIFE SKILLS: Assessing Your Health
- *Describe the ways in which self-esteem, social support, health, and wellness are related.*
- *Describe the health benefits of physical fitness.*

You are at one of the most exciting yet challenging times of your life. You are no longer a child who requires constant care and the closeness of family. Your adult identity is in the early stages of formation. Your body is changing as you make this transition from child to adult. Your relationships with your friends and family are changing too. You want to spend more time with your friends and less with your family. Your family may be adjusting well to your need for independence or you may feel that you are still being treated like a child. The teen years are a time of adjustment to many new freedoms and responsibilities. It can also be a time of tremendous conflict in your relationships with your family and friends. During this time, you will establish habits and views that you will carry with you throughout your life.

You are faced with many choices that can have a major effect on your future. Should you smoke? Or, maybe you are already smoking. Should you drink alcohol? Or, maybe you have already tried alcohol. What about drugs? It is rare for a teen in the United States to get through high school

Background
Choosing a Healthy Lifestyle

Most subjects taught in school increase a student's knowledge and experience. The study of health can impart more than knowledge and experience. It can set the course for a change of lifestyle that should lead to a fuller, more rounded life. When students make the proper decisions that lead to a healthy lifestyle, they improve the quality of their own life, cause a positive impact on the lives of those near them, and prolong the time they have to lead productive lives.

Section 1.1 Lesson Plan

MOTIVATE

Journal 1A
Concerns About Health

This may be done as a warm-up activity. Encourage students to record their concerns about their own health, or that of someone close to them, in the Student Journal in the Student Activity Book. They may wish to write down their feelings about the story of Tara.

Cooperative Learning
Tara's Problems

Have students form groups to discuss the problems Tara is facing and how this might affect her health. Ask them to tell how they might react to the same problems. Have them offer suggestions of what Tara can do to get help.

TEACH

Class Discussion
Components of Health

Write on the chalkboard: Health is not just the absence of disease. **What does this mean?** *[People can be without physical problems and still not be healthy if, for example, they are mentally or emotionally ill.]* **When might you be without physical disease and still not have physical health?** *[If you do not*

Background
Health as Adaptation
Health is the successful adaptation to each challenge—physical, mental, emotional, or spiritual—in the everyday environment. These adaptations may be in response to genetic makeup, microbes, carcinogens, pollutants, pressures, and problems. A diabetic can adapt to a genetic health hazard by using insulin and adhering to a special diet. Many health-conscious people avoid contact with known carcinogens and pollutants when possible. A teenager can make healthful choices and interact with others to create a healthful environment.

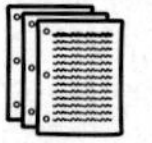

Personal Health Inventory
Have students complete the Personal Health Inventory for this chapter. The inventory helps them assess their knowledge about health before taking this course.

without having to make decisions on these health-related issues.

You may now be experiencing problems in your life that have a profound effect on your health both now and in the future. The story about Tara in the introduction to this chapter is an example. Tara's family is not functioning properly. Everyone is under a lot of stress. Tara's mother has an alcohol abuse problem. Tara and her family need help. One goal of this course is to give you the knowledge you need to work through problems like these, should you be going through them now or sometime in the future. Throughout the text, you will be encouraged to seek help when you can't resolve a problem on your own. You will find out where in your community you can get help for yourself or others close to you. This course will put you in an active role in managing your health.

Describing Health

How do you generally respond when someone asks ''How are you?'' If you respond that you are ''fine,'' take a moment to write down what you think it means to feel fine. If you respond in some other way, write down what your response really means. If you are not fine, are you sick? Now look at your description. How you feel is really part of describing your health.

Cultural DIVERSITY

Being Healthy—What Does It Mean?

Health—like beauty—means different things to different cultures. In the United States, slender people are generally viewed as healthy. In eastern Europe and parts of Asia, however, a thin person would be considered unhealthy and would be urged to eat more. Mental health can also be defined culturally. Before the fall of the Soviet Union, those who opposed the ruling government were considered insane, and many political dissidents were sent to mental hospitals. Before the women's movement, women in America who were not content with home and children were labeled neurotic and were routinely given tranquilizers to pacify them. A bank clerk in Milwaukee who hears voices makes an appointment with a mental health therapist, but an Inuit shaman expects to hear voices and relies on sage advice from the invisible world.

Remedies for treating illness can also be culturally based. In some Jewish households, chicken soup is more than just a comfort food. It is considered a ''medicine'' for various illnesses. Garlic, familiar as a tasty addition to salad dressing and pizza sauce, has in many cultures been relied upon as a medicine. It has been called ''Russian penicillin,'' but its use as a medical remedy spans many cultures—from ancient Mesopotamia to the most up-to-date of New Age pharmacies. An accountant in Arizona might buy a bottle of vitamin tablets or make an appointment with her doctor for a checkup if she is feeling run-down,

• • • TEACH continued

have a disease but you lack physical fitness; you might not have energy to do homework, engage in outside activities, and socialize with friends. If so, you are not physically healthy.] **How would you describe people who are socially healthy?** *[People who are socially healthy have friends with whom they spend time and discuss problems. They interact well with people and have satisfying relationships.]* **How can you tell if someone is mentally healthy?** *[If someone has a sense of self-worth, is open to new ideas, and can cope with stressful situations, he or she has good mental health.]* **What is meant by spiritual health?** *[People have spiritual health if they are working to find peace with themselves and those around them, either with the help of religion or by relying on their own individual life purpose .]*

Role-Playing
Being Emotionally Healthy
Have students role-play a particular problem or a difficult situation in which one member of the group exemplifies good emotional health by accepting that problem as a challenge. Have them also role-play the same situation in which one member of the group shows poor emotional health by becoming overly angry or depressed by the problem.

Health was once thought to be the absence of disease. Health is now described in much broader terms, because we know so much more about what it takes to be healthy. There are five major components of health—physical health, social health, mental health, emotional health, and spiritual health. All five components must be in balance for you to be truly healthy.

Physical Health **Physical health** covers those aspects of health related directly to the body. Your weight, strength, and the way your body functions are physical characteristics that are part of your physical health. The absence of disease is part of physical health. Being physically healthy means you can get through your day at school and still have the energy to do your homework, engage in outside activities, and socialize with friends. Developing your physical fitness improves your physical health.

Audra is on the track and volleyball teams. She gets a lot of exercise and picks foods that keep her performance level high. Her boyfriend, Josh, has been smoking for two years. Because he smokes, Josh often skips meals and snacks throughout the day instead. He had five colds last winter alone. Audra is obviously doing a better job than Josh in attending to her physical health.

physical health:
your physical characteristics and the way your body functions.

while her Chinese counterpart might rely solely on ginseng root as a tonic. A housewife in West Virginia has her choice of these, but might choose the ginseng because her mother and grandmother both dug the roots themselves and prepared them for use by relying on an old family recipe.

Some remedies that the western world once condemned as superstition are now enjoying a new respectability. The ancient Chinese healing art of acupuncture is now being used in the West to relieve pain. Many western physicians and scientists refused to accept acupuncture as anything more than mind over matter until first-hand observation of the results changed their opinions. Now several kinds of treatment apply the meridians and pressure points of acupuncture for pain relief.

Good health is a matter of mind, body, and spirit working together in balance and harmony. *Hozro*, or harmony, is the aim of the Navajo *hataali*. The Blessing Way ceremony to bring patients back into balance using chants and meditation. Harmony is also the aim of holistic healing methods, in which all levels of an individual are brought into balance. Thus, health becomes a connecting flow of vitality throughout all parts of an individual's life and thought.

Cultural diversity can add a rich, new dimension to your view of health and wellness. But you must remain open to new ideas.

Section 1.1

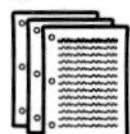

Life Skills Worksheet 1A

Determining Your Health History

Assign Life Skills Worksheet 1A, which has students complete a health history for themselves.

Making a Choice 1A

Assessing Attitudes

Assign the Assessing Attitudes card. The card asks students to consider which statements reflect attitudes that are emotionally healthy.

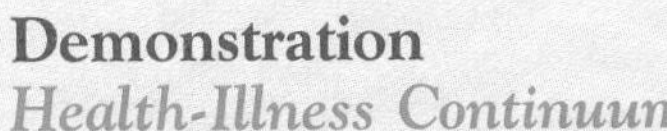

Demonstration
Health-Illness Continuum

Make a health-illness continuum for the bulletin board. Pass out index cards. Ask students to write on the cards an activity that will help them move in the right direction along the continuum. Their activities may be expressed in the affirmative (eating right) or stated negatively (not using alcohol). Have them tape their cards to appropriate places on the continuum. After students have attached their cards, discuss how engaging in any harmful activities would hinder their progress on the continuum to health.

Role-Playing
Benefits of Social Support

Have students work in groups of three or four to act out a situation in which a friend is doing poorly in school because of problems at home. Have one student present the problem; have the others provide support or suggest where the troubled friend can obtain support. After students act out their parts, have the class discuss the feelings of each of the players. Have students suggest alternative ways to help the friend.

Cooperative Learning
Sharing Health Experiences

Have students form groups to develop a radio campaign focusing public attention on wellness. They should write 10-, 30-, and 60-second spots promoting their ideas of the concept of wellness. Have students perform their

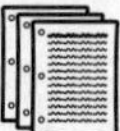

Section Review Worksheet 1.1

Assign Section Review Worksheet 1.1, which requires students to identify components of health.

Section Quiz 1.1

Have students take Section Quiz 1.1.

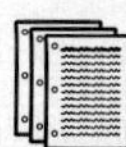

Reteaching Worksheet 1.1

Students who have difficulty with the material may complete Reteaching Worksheet 1.1, which allows them to play a game that reinforces the components of health.

social health: *interactions with people to build satisfying relationships.*

spiritual health: *maintaining harmonious relationships with other living things and having spiritual direction and purpose.*

health: *state of well-being that comes from a good balance of the five aspects of health.*

wellness: *optimal health in each of the five aspects of health.*

mental health: *the ability to recognize reality.*

emotional health: *expressing feelings in an appropriate way.*

Social Health Being socially healthy means you have friends and others with whom you discuss your problems and with whom you spend time. Your **social health** involves interacting well with people and the environment and having satisfying relationships. Your social health development started when you were a toddler and began interacting with peers. However, it is during the teen years that your social skills really develop. Taking an active role in your community and helping others is also part of the social aspect of your health.

Colby is just a great guy to be around. He's friendly, funny, and always makes you feel comfortable. He seems to get along with most everyone. Tyler is really shy. He's very quiet in class and hopes people don't notice him. He spends most of his time by himself, though he does eat lunch sometimes with Jim. Tyler would really like to get to know Kaleigh, a girl in his history class, but he feels too uncomfortable to just walk up to Kaleigh and begin talking. He's even thought of asking Jim what he might do or say, but he just hasn't gotten around to it. Colby seems to have a good grasp of his social health. Tyler won't feel completely healthy until he is more comfortable interacting with people.

Mental Health Your ability to recognize reality is described as **mental health.** Being mentally healthy means you are open to learning new things and accepting new ideas. You have a sense of self-worth and tolerate things that are different. You can cope with stressful situations because you know that stress is a part of life that you can manage. You work to develop your individual strengths and minimize your weaknesses.

Emotional Health Your ability to control feelings so that they are expressed in an appropriate way defines your **emotional health.** While everyone experiences bad feelings at one time or another, emotionally healthy people can overcome the difficulties. An emotionally healthy person enjoys life and views hardships or difficulties as challenges. An emotionally healthy person can express anger without violence and sadness without serious depression.

Spiritual Health **Spiritual health** involves your relationship to other living things and the role of spiritual direction in your life. This description means various things to people. For some people, spiritual health is defined by a religion. For others, it involves understanding your individual purpose in life. Being spiritually healthy means you are working to achieve your spiritual potential, to find harmony in living. You are at peace with yourself and those around you.

Health and Wellness

These five aspects of health contribute to your total health picture. It should be obvious that if you are physically fit, but you cannot get along with your teachers and parents, then you are not completely healthy. If you are very active in your church, synagogue, and community, but feel depressed and anxious most of the time, you are not healthy. **Health** can now be formally defined as the state of well-being that comes from realizing your potential in each of the five aspects of health. Optimal health is described by the term **wellness**. A state of wellness is achieved by looking at your total health picture from a positive perspective.

Health-Illness Continuum Your total health can be described by a plot on the health-illness continuum shown in Figure 1-1. Plotting your health position on the continuum should involve looking at your health status in each of the five aspects of health. The right side of the continuum represents optimum health or wellness.

• • • TEACH continued

announcements for the class or record them to make a class tape.

Extension

Promoting Health in the Community

Ask students to find community groups that sponsor activities intended to promote physical, mental, emotional, social, and spiritual health. Have them collect posters and brochures that describe and illustrate the activity and the sponsoring group. Display the materials on the bulletin board.

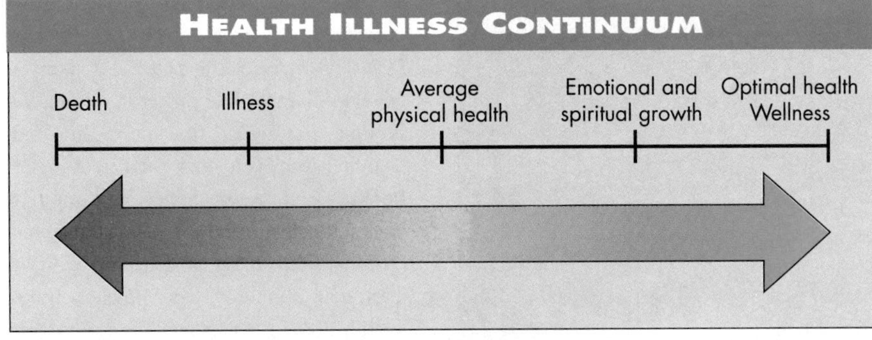

(FIGURE 1-1) **Your health status on the continuum depends on how well you attend to each of the five areas that make up your total health picture.**

Achieving wellness involves making choices and behaving in ways that benefit your health. Making life-threatening choices like abusing alcohol or extreme dieting puts you on the left side of the continuum, which is the path to illness or an early death.

Self-Esteem and Wellness In order to achieve wellness, you have to feel good about yourself. Feeling good about yourself is called having positive **self-esteem**. You can be free of disease, you can get good grades in school, you can have nice friends, and be physically fit, but if you don't feel good about yourself you have not reached a state of wellness. In fact, when you get to Chapter 9, Managing Stress, you will discover that low self-esteem can actually make you physically ill. The stress you feel from not feeling good about yourself reduces your ability to fight off disease. So how you feel about yourself is related not only to your mental and emotional health, but is also related to your physical health.

Self-esteem is such an important component of health and wellness that it is a theme of this book. Chapter 8 focuses on self-esteem and what you can do to improve your self-esteem if you need to. Throughout this book you will see surveys that help you recognize your strengths and weaknesses. You will be given ideas on how to highlight your strengths and improve your weaknesses. But you should also become more accepting of yourself and of characteristics that you might see as negative. You need to recognize that everyone has some flaws.

Wellness Involves Social Support It is quite clear to people in the health profession that people need people. In fact, there is a name given to the benefits one gets from

self-esteem:

feeling good about yourself and your abilities.

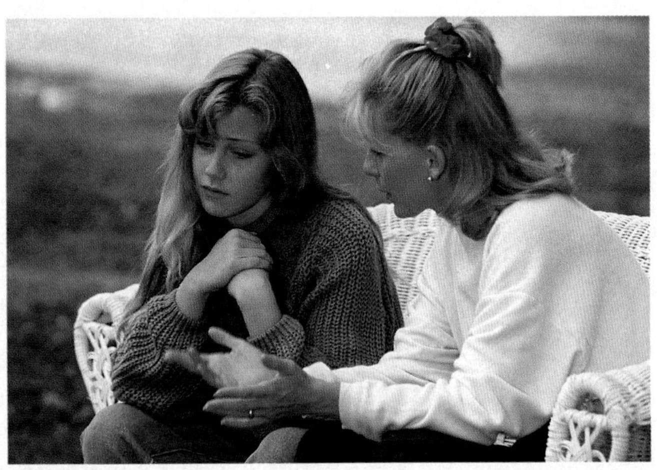

(FIGURE 1-2) **Building relationships and receiving support from others is essential to your overall health and wellness.**

Review Answers

1. Answers may include: if a person is not physically healthy, he or she may not be able to see or spend time with friends. This could affect social health and cause stress. If the person cannot control this stress, it may affect mental and emotional health. If the person has a serious illness, he or she may lose or question faith.

2. To be healthy, one must have a balance of good physical, social, mental, emotional, and spiritual health. To reach a state of wellness, one must feel good about oneself.

Answers to Questions 1 and 2 are on p. 9.

3. Being physically fit helps a person stay physically healthy and control weight and stress. Controlling stress helps improve a person's mental and emotional health. If the person gets exercise in activities that require group participation, such as team sports, he or she also improves social health. All of these factors help a person feel good about himself or herself and in this way improve self-esteem.

4. Answers may include people students trust, such as friends, family members, teachers, school counselors, and religious leaders.

5. Answers should reflect ways of improving physical, social, mental, emotional, and/or spiritual health.

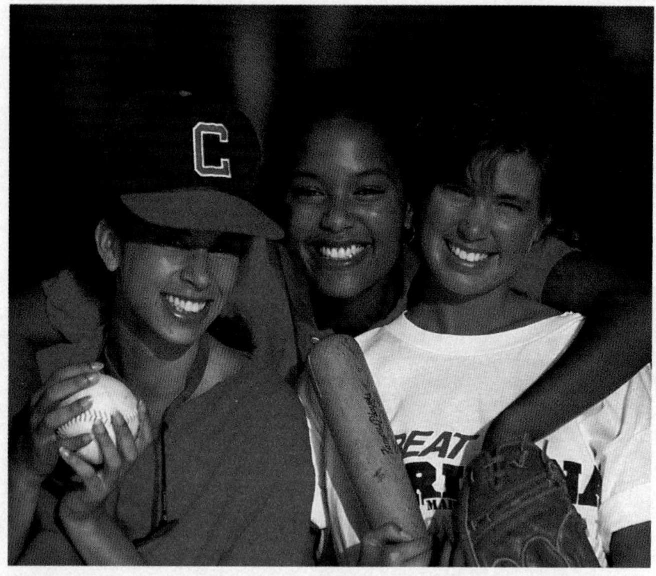

(FIGURE 1-3) **Physical activity can improve your physical health as well as provide for your social health.**

social support: *deriving positive feelings from sharing life situations with others.*

talking to others about joys, sorrows, problems, and stressors. It's called **social support**. It is now well known that a lot of stress in your life can make you physically sick. However, if you have social support, it is more likely you'll be able to manage stressors without becoming ill. Hasn't there been a time when you felt better about a bad situation after discussing it with a friend or relative? Throughout this course you will be encouraged to seek the help or advice of someone you can trust when you are having a problem. The purpose of this course is to give you a set of skills that will enable you to live a healthy lifestyle. Employing these skills when needed throughout your life keeps you on the path to wellness.

physical fitness: *a state in which your body can meet daily life demands.*

Wellness and Physical Fitness **Physical fitness** is a state in which your body can meet the daily demands of living. It means you have a healthy heart, blood vessels, and lungs (cardiorespiratory endurance), and that you have sufficient muscular strength, endurance, flexibility, agility, balance, and coordination. People who are fit have fewer heart attacks and are less likely to develop diseases like diabetes. When you become physically fit, you're not only healthier but you look and feel better. Looking and feeling better also improves your self-esteem, and you have already read how important that is. In Chapter 3 you will learn how to improve your physical fitness by developing a personal fitness program and then working to stick to it.

There is much you can do if you make up your mind to do it. Your potential is unlimited. Bob Weiland realized this when he decided to compete in the Marine Corps Marathon. It took him 79 hours and 57 minutes to complete the 26.2 miles. Despite having lost his legs in Vietnam and having to propel himself with his hands and no wheelchair, Bob finished the course. Now that is wellness!

Review

1. *How might a physical health problem, such as a disease, affect the other components of your health?*
2. *Why is self-esteem so important to overall health?*
3. *How can being physically fit improve your self-esteem?*
4. *List the people you use for social support.*
5. ***Critical Thinking*** *List two things you could do to improve your position on the health-illness continuum.*

ASSESS

Section Review

Have students answer the Section Review questions.

Alternative Assessment

Realizing Your Health Potential

Have students explain what is meant by realizing their potential in each of the five aspects of health. They might come up with a range of examples showing least healthy to most healthy behavior in an area. For instance, is it emotionally healthier to express anger by throwing something or by talking the problem out?

Closure

Self-Esteem/Health Relationship

Have students write a letter to a friend who shows signs of low self-esteem, explaining to him or her how this might be the cause of health problems.

Section 1.2 Health Concerns in the United States

Objectives

- *Compare the leading causes of death for teens with the leading causes for adults.*
- *Compare the leading causes of death today with those of 100 years ago.*
- *Identify your health risk factors.*
  - **LIFE SKILLS: Assessing Your Health**

At the beginning of this century, the major health issue confronting teens was premature death due to disease. Today you face many more serious health issues than those of your great-grandparents. Interestingly enough, most of the health issues affecting teens are related to lifestyle. The choices you make about how you live have a direct impact on your overall health.

Teen Health Issues

One in five teens in the United States has at least one serious health problem. The suicide rate for teens is now three times what it was 20 years ago. One in three high school seniors has gotten drunk, which may explain why the leading cause of death among teens is car accidents. Figure 1-5 gives some additional teen health statistics like the fact that each year 2.5 million teens are infected with a sexually transmitted disease. This statistic is especially alarming when you realize that one of those diseases is AIDS. There is currently no cure for AIDS, no vaccine against AIDS, and it is always fatal. Given some of these facts, it seems that at this time of your life, you are exposed to a great many more health risks than those of your great-grandparents.

Another goal of this course is to help you successfully manage those risks. You will look at all the possible consequences of abusing alcohol. You will learn ways to manage the various stressful situations you encounter, so that you don't feel you have to turn to alcohol to solve your problems or to feel good. You will see how diet and exercise can give you a more positive attitude, so that you are better able to deal with the challenges of living. You will study an effective model that you can use when making various decisions in your life. You will learn the importance of seeking help for problems you cannot solve. And, you will

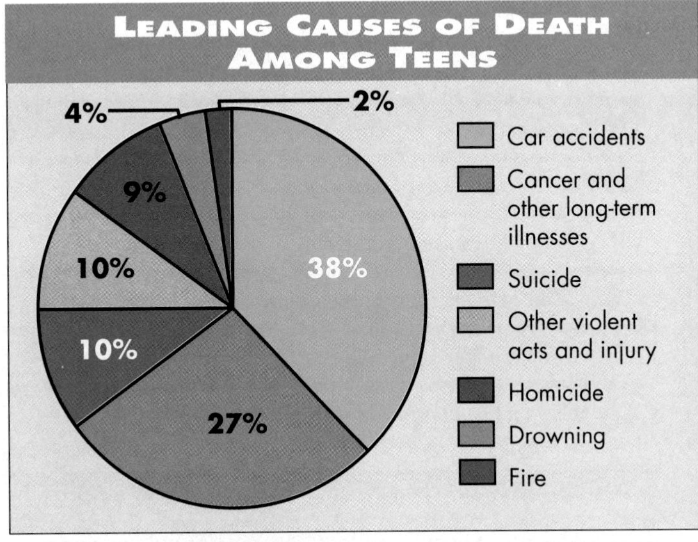

(FIGURE 1-4) **Most teen deaths could be prevented with improved health education.**

SECTION 1.2

Background

Preventive Health Care

Most Americans have been oriented toward crisis health care. When they are sick, they concentrate on getting well. More recently, interest has turned to preventive health care. This approach has a much broader goal than overcoming a particular illness. Preventive health care focuses on removing the obstacles to good health before a person becomes ill, and on promoting wellness in all its aspects. Preventive care helps a person postpone, or even avoid, many illnesses altogether.

Section 1.2 Lesson Plan

MOTIVATE

Journal 1B

Teen Health Problems

This may be done as a warm-up activity. Encourage students to record in the Student Journal in the Student Activity Book their opinions about some of the most pressing health issues facing teens today.

TEACH

Writing

Health Issues for Teens

Have students write brief essays about one of the teen health issues for which statistics are given in the text. They should choose one about which they have knowledge or strong feelings. They could begin by outlining the issue as they see it, and follow up with ideas for working on the problem.

Class Discussion

Causes of Death: Today and 100 Years Ago

Have students look at the graph of the causes of death in the United States today and in 1900. Ask them to speculate why diseases such as pneumonia and influenza are no longer major causes of death. Then ask, **Why do you think heart disease and cancer have increased so noticeably as causes of death today?** *[People's work*

Making a Choice 1B

Looking at Causes of Death

Assign the Looking at Causes of Death card. The card asks students to discuss strategies that could be used to reduce the number of teen deaths due to certain causes.

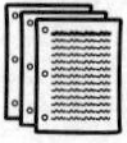

Section Review Worksheet 1.2

Assign Section Review Worksheet 1.2, which requires students to complete sentences about health concerns in the United States.

Section Quiz 1.2

Have students take Section Quiz 1.2.

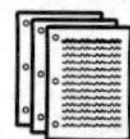

Reteaching Worksheet 1.2

Students who have difficulty with the material may complete Reteaching Worksheet 1.2, which requires students to identify leading causes of death.

find out where in your community you can go for help.

National Health Risks

communicable disease: *a disease that is passed on by another person or organism.*

Pneumonia, tuberculosis, and influenza (flu) were the leading causes of death in the United States in the early part of this century. These three diseases fall into the category of **communicable diseases,** which means a person can get the disease from someone else. The government responded to this health problem by enacting laws on quarantine (isolation of disease victims), sewage disposal, and food and water sanitation. These actions caused a significant reduction in the number of people that got communicable diseases.

Figure 1-6 shows a comparison of causes of death early in the century with those of today. Heart disease and cancer have replaced pneumonia and tuberculosis as the leading causes of death. Heart disease and cancer can be the result of people's lifestyle choices. Experts agree that if people would exercise regularly, eat properly, have periodic medical exams, avoid the use of tobacco, and manage stress effectively, the number of deaths from heart disease and cancer would be greatly reduced.

Teen Health Statistics

Teen Health Statistics
12% of teens have mental disorders severe enough to require treatment
61% of teens report feelings of deep depression and hopelessness
45% of teens report they have trouble coping due to stressful situations at home or school
36% of teens feel they have no future to look forward to
34% of teens have considered suicide
14% of teens have attempted suicide
30% of teens smoke regularly
35% of teens have tried marijuana
8% of teens have tried cocaine
Over 50% of teens report having had sexual intercourse
Over 1 million teens become pregnant each year
2.5 million teens contract a sexually transmitted disease each year

FIGURE 1-5 **Teen health problems are widespread and varied. All these statistics involve health-related decisions that you can control in managing your own health.**

Developing Life Skills

Health professionals and medical professionals now stress prevention as their guiding principle to achieving wellness. Community health specialists have taken a more active role in educating the public concerning healthy living practices and disease prevention. Many hospitals and clinics now sponsor health education programs for the public that focus on diet, exercise, stress reduction, and emotional well being. It is believed that these programs will help reduce health care costs by getting people to accept more responsibility for their health.

In keeping with the prevention philosophy, Life Skills pages throughout this text to help you apply what you learn in this class. The first Life Skills, on page 14, helps you identify your potential health risks.

Stopping to assess your behavior or feelings about a subject or issue may be a difficult task, but it is something that you will be frequently asked to do in this course. A journal will be a handy place to record this information. You may not want to admit that you are having trouble coping

• • • TEACH continued

and lifestyles have changed drastically. Lack of exercise, improper diet, smoking, and failure to manage stress are the main causes of heart disease and cancer.] **Which lifestyle changes could help teens avoid some of the causes of death on the graph for today?** *[Eating more healthful foods and exercising regularly would help them avoid heart disease; staying clear of alcohol and drugs would help them avoid accidents and liver disease; not smoking would prevent lung disease; and getting help when depressed would discourage suicide.]*

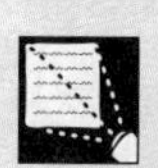

Teaching Transparency 1A
Heart Disease—Leading Killer

Use this transparency to discuss how deadly heart disease is for Americans. Discuss the following facts:

- Almost one in two Americans dies of cardiovascular disease.
- In 1988, heart disease killed almost as many Americans as cancer, accidents, pneumonia, influenza, and all other causes of death combined.
- More than one in four Americans suffer from some form of cardiovascular disease.
- About 175,000 Americans under the age of 65 die each year from cardiovascular disease.
- Someone in the United States dies from cardiovascular disease every 32 seconds.

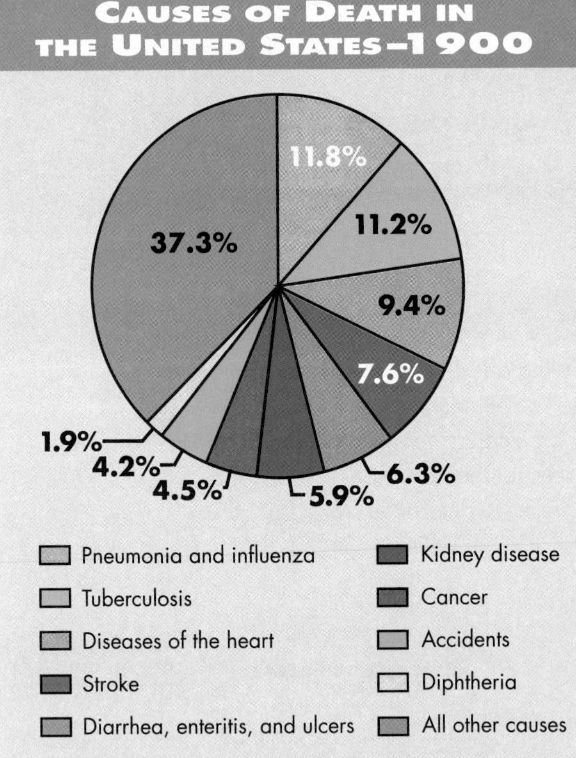

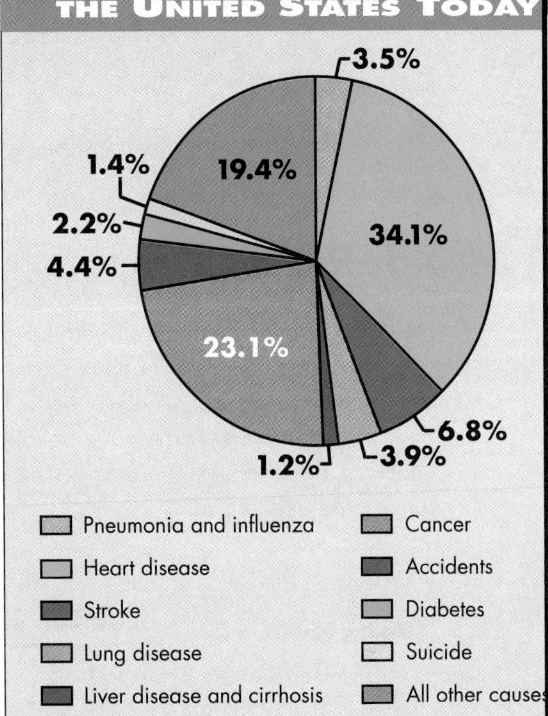

(FIGURE 1-6) **Today most leading causes of death could be prevented by changes in lifestyle.**

with a situation at home or that you are under too much pressure from friends or family. You may be much more comfortable expressing these feelings in the journal.

Keep a copy of your answers to this first Life Skills survey in your journal. Complete the survey again at the end of the course to find out if you have reduced your health risks. Other Life Skills pages will cover the following areas.

- Solving Problems
- Coping
- Setting Goals
- Resisting Pressure
- Assessing Your Health
- Using Community Resources Effectively
- Communicating Effectively
- Being A Wise Consumer
- Making Responsible Decisions
- Practicing Self-Care

Review

1. *List three health-related decisions that you might make in the next year.*
2. *In what ways do the leading causes of death for teens differ from those of adults?*
3. ***Critical Thinking*** *Why are health problems today so different from those that affected people 100 years ago?*

Review Answers

1. Answers will vary. Some answers might be: do not drink, do not drive with someone who has been drinking, do not put myself at risk from a sexually transmitted disease or a pregnancy, talk to a trusted friend or family member about my concerns, do not smoke, do not use drugs. Accept any answer that moves students toward optimal health.

2. Leading causes of death for teens involve accidents that are related to alcohol and drug use and increased risk taking. Leading causes of death among adults are related to lifestyle issues such as exercise, diet, use of tobacco, and stress.

3. Health problems 100 years ago were caused mostly by communicable diseases, which have been brought under control and almost eliminated by better sanitation and immunizations. Different types of health problems have emerged, most directly related to lifestyle.

Point out to students that lifestyle choices they make now can greatly reduce their risk of developing cardiovascular disease in the future.

Debate the Issue

Changing Lifestyle: Is It Worth It?

Divide the class into two teams to debate the question: If having good health means changing your lifestyle, is it worth the effort? Students on both sides of the argument should support their positions with information about how a change of lifestyle can affect the health of teens. Encourage students to express their own opinions on the topic after the debate is over.

Writing

Open Letter to Teens

Encourage students to write an open letter to teens, based on the health statistics in this section. Have them include what impressed them most about the statistics and the consequences if these trends continue. Let them share their letters in small groups or with the class.

Extension

Healthy Choices

Have students notice which foods sold in the school cafeteria or restaurants are healthful and which are less healthful. Have them prepare humorous posters that encourage students to choose healthful foods.

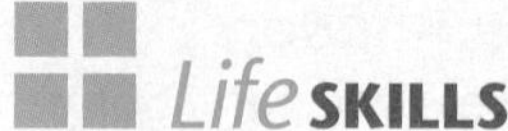

Health Risks Survey

Have students identify their behavior in each of the six sections in the Health Risks Survey by writing on a separate piece of paper the number that corresponds to their usual practice. Have students do this exercise independently, in order to benefit from the experience.

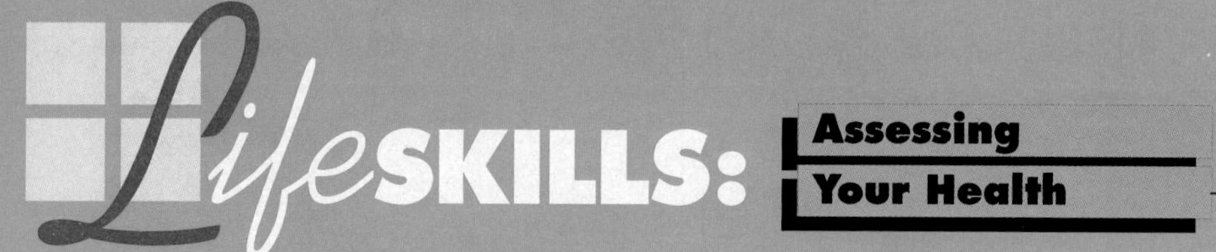

Health Risks Survey

The United States government developed the following questionnaire to help people assess their health behavior and their health risks. The questionnaire has six sections. Answer each item on a separate piece of paper by listing the number corresponding to the answer that describes your behavior. Then add the numbers you have circled to determine your score for that section.

Eating Habits	Almost Always	Sometimes	Almost Never
1. I eat a variety of foods each day, such as fruits and vegetables; whole grain breads and cereals; lean meats, dairy products, dry peas and beans; and nuts and seeds.	4	2	0
2. I limit the amount of fat, saturated fat, and cholesterol I eat (including fats in meats, eggs, butter, cream, shortenings, and organ meats such as liver).	2	1	0
3. I limit the amount of salt I eat by not adding salt at the table, avoiding salty snacks, and having my meals cooked with only small amounts of salt.	2	1	0
4. I avoid eating too much sugar (especially frequent snacks of sticky candy or soft drinks).	2	1	0
Your Eating Habits Score:			

Exercise and Fitness	Almost Always	Sometimes	Almost Never
1. I maintain a comfortable weight, avoiding overweight or underweight.	3	2	0
2. I exercise vigorously for 15 to 30 minutes at least three times a week (examples include running, swimming, brisk walking).	3	2	0
3. I do exercises that enhance my muscle tone for 15 to 30 minutes at least three times a week (examples include yoga and calisthenics).	2	1	0
4. I use part of my leisure time to participate in individual, family, or team activities that increase my level of fitness (such as gardening, bowling, golf, or baseball.	2	1	0
Your Exercise and Fitness Score:			

ASSESS

Section Review

Have students answer the Section Review questions.

Alternative Assessment

Time of Regrets

Have students make up a skit featuring an elderly person dying of heart disease who sees himself in various scenes as a teen—taking his first smoke, getting no exercise, eating fatty foods. Have students discuss which lifestyle changes might have helped this person to avoid heart disease.

Closure

Changing Lifestyle

Have students explain in their own words how changes in lifestyle could mean better health.

Stress Control

	Almost Always	Some-times	Almost Never
1. I enjoy school or other work I do.	2	1	0
2. I find it easy to relax and express my feelings freely.	2	1	0
3. I recognize early, and prepare for, events or situations likely to be stressful for me.	2	1	0
4. I have close friends, relatives, or others whom I can talk to about personal matters and call on for help when needed.	2	1	0
5. I participate in group activities (such as church/ synagogue or community organizations) or hobbies that I enjoy.	2	1	0

Your Stress Control Score: ______

Safety

	Almost Always	Some-times	Almost Never
1. I wear a seat belt while riding in a car.	2	1	0
2. I avoid driving, or getting in a car with someone else who is driving, while under the influence of alcohol and other drugs.	2	1	0
3. I obey the traffic rules and observe the speed limit when driving or ask others to do so when driving in a car with them.	2	1	0
4. I am careful when using potentially harmful products or substances (such as household cleaners, poisons, and electrical devices).	2	1	0
5. I avoid smoking in bed.	2	1	0

Your Safety Score: ______

Alcohol and Drug Use

	Almost Always	Some-times	Almost Never
1. I avoid drinking alcoholic beverages.	4	2	0
2. I avoid using alcohol or other drugs (especially illegal drugs) as a way of handling stressful situations or the problems of my life.	3	1	0
3. I read and follow the label directions when using prescription and over the counter drugs.	3	1	0

Your Alcohol and Drug Score: ______

Tobacco Use

	Almost Always	Some-times	Almost Never
1. I avoid smoking cigarettes.	4	1	0
2. I do not use chewing tobacco, smoke a pipe, or smoke cigars.	3	1	0
3. I avoid areas where others are smoking.	3	1	0

Your Cigarette Smoking Score: ______

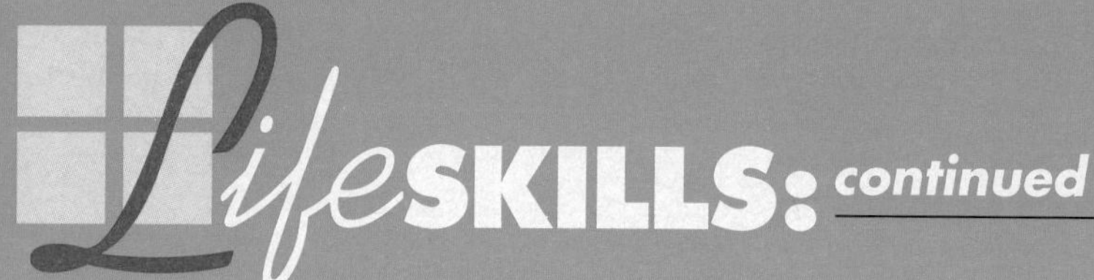

Your Health Score

Make sure you have figured your score for each of the six sections. Use the scale that follows for assessing each section.

Tabacco Use	Alcohol and Drug Use	Eating Habits	Exercise and Fitness	Stress Control	Safety
10	10	10	10	10	10
9	9	9	9	9	9
8	8	8	8	8	8
7	7	7	7	7	7
6	6	6	6	6	6
5	5	5	5	5	5
4	4	4	4	4	4
3	3	3	3	3	3
2	2	2	2	2	2
1	1	1	1	1	1

Interpreting Your Scores

Scores of **9 or 10** are excellent! You are putting your knowledge to work for you by practicing good health habits.

Scores of **6 - 8** indicate your health practices in this area are good, but there is room for improvement. Look again at the items you answered with a "Sometimes" or an "Almost Never." What changes can you make to improve your score?

Scores of **3 - 5** mean you have behaviors that put your health at risk.

Scores of **0 - 2** mean you may be taking serious, unnecessary risks with your health. This course will make you aware of the risks and what to do about them.

Fill out this survey again at the end of your health course. Our goal is to give you the information you need to improve your scores.

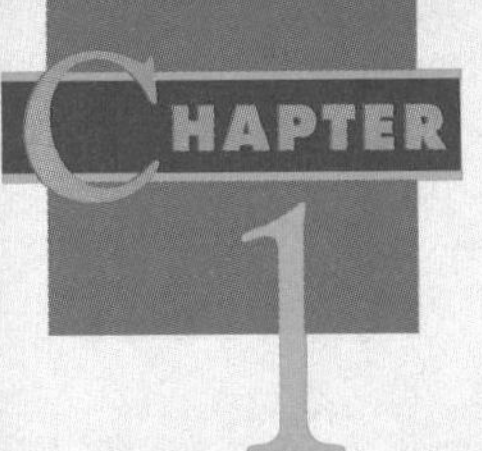

Highlights

Summary

- Health is more than the absense of disease; it is the state of mental, physical, and social well-being.
- The concept of health requires a balance of five components: physical health, social health, mental health, emotional health, and spiritual health.
- A state of wellness is achieved by looking at your total health picture from a positive perspective.
- Making choices and behaving in a way that maximizes your health are the strongest influences on your level of wellness.
- To achieve wellness, you have to feel good about yourself.
- If you have social support, it is more likely you'll be able to manage stressors without becoming ill.
- Most of the health issues affecting teens are related to lifestyle.
- The major health dangers for teenagers today include accidents, suicide, homicide, unwanted pregnancy, and sexually transmitted diseases.

Vocabulary

physical health your physical characteristics and the way your body functions.

social health interactions with people to build satisfying relationships.

mental health the ability to recognize reality.

emotional health expressing feelings in an appropriate way.

spiritual health belief in some force or order in nature.

health state of well-being that comes from a good balance of the five aspects of health.

wellness optimal health in each of the five aspects of health.

self-esteem feeling good about yourself and what you can do.

social support deriving positive feelings from sharing life situations with others.

physical fitness a state whereby your body can meet daily life demands.

communicable disease getting a disease from another person or organism.

Chapter 1 Highlights Strategies

Summary

Have students read the summary to reinforce the concepts they learned in Chapter 1.

Vocabulary

Have students write a letter to a friend describing what is included in the study of health. Ask students to use the vocabulary words from Chapter 1 in their letters.

Extension

Have students make health and wellness posters to be displayed throughout the community, in youth centers, libraries, banks, and storefronts. The posters should show some aspect of health related to teens, and should convey some of the problems young people have today, and ways to help teens with these problems.

CHAPTER 1 ASSESSMENT

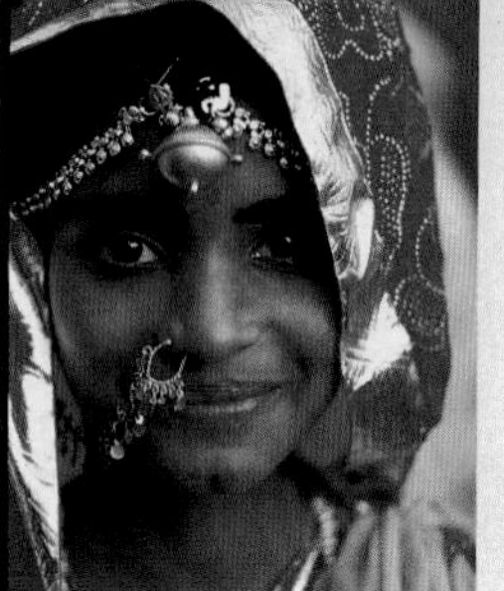

CHAPTER 1

Chapter Review

CHAPTER REVIEW

Concept Review

1. health
2. physical health
3. social health
4. spiritual health
5. health-illness continuum
6. self-esteem
7. social support
8. physical fitness
9. heart disease, cancer
10. choices

Expressing Your Views

Sample responses:

1. Somewhere near "Average Health"
2. More people are working out at health clubs or developing their own fitness program, which might include exercises such as walking, jogging, swimming, and cycling.
3. Abusing alcohol and other drugs, unprotected sexual intercourse
4. Being involved in an accident with another car or with a pedestrian. This accident could lead to injury or death. The risks of being involved in an accident and being injured can be reduced by wearing a seat belt, not driving while under the influence of alcohol or drugs or riding in a car with someone else driving under the influence of alcohol and other drugs, obeying traffic rules, and observing the speed limit when driving, as well as asking others to do these things when you are riding in a car with them.

Life Skills Check

Sample student responses:

1. Eat a healthy diet that is low in fat, salt, and sugar; maintain a comfortable weight and exercise regularly; learn to control stress; avoid smoking cigarettes; avoid drinking alcoholic beverages; avoid using drugs, especially illegal drugs; and practice safety behaviors, such as wearing a seat belt when riding in a car.
2. Someone from my support group, such as parents, a teacher, a counselor, a coach, or a religious leader
3. Lists and evaluations will vary for each student.

Concept Review

1. The well-being of your body, your mind, and your relationships with other people is called ________.
2. ________ refers to the care of your body and the way your body functions.
3. The way people get along with one another and make and keep friends is called ________.
4. ________ involves the belief in some unifying force over nature.
5. A special scale that shows your total health has many levels is called a ________.
6. Feeling good about yourself is called having a positive ________.
7. The benefit one gets from talking about joys, sorrows, problems, and stressors is called ________.
8. ________ means you have a healthy heart, blood vessels, and lungs.
9. Pneumonia and tuberculosis have been replaced by ________ and ________ as the leading causes of death in the U.S. today.
10. The ________ you make about how you live have a direct impact on your overall health.

Expressing Your Views

1. Benton is 15 years old. He has started to exercise regularly, has lowered his fat intake, and has stopped drinking alcohol. Where would you place him on the Wellness Continuum?
2. What are some of the indications that Americans are becoming more fitness oriented?
3. Most of the health issues facing teens today are determined by lifestyle. In your opinion, what are the two risk behaviors that will most influence a teen's health?
4. Demetra just received her driver's license. What are some of the risks involved in driving a car? What do you think Demetra could do to reduce the risks?

Chapter 1 Assessment

Life Skills Check

1. Assessing Your Health
You are content with your current state of wellness, but you would like to make sure you are healthy in the years to come. What are some things you could do now to ensure your future well-being?

2. Assessing Your Health
Lately you have not been getting along with your friends or family. The stress in your life is sometimes almost overwhelming. Often you just want to be alone. Who could you talk to? Explain your choice.

3. Assessing Your Health
Keep a list of all your choices and activities for one day. Then think of ways to add more activity to your normal day. Choose two or three of these and try them for four days. Evaluate your performance.

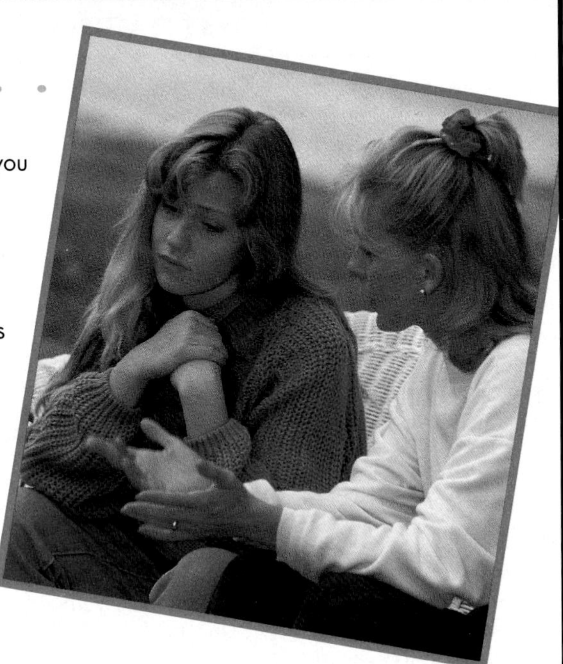

Projects

1. Interview a person over age 50 and a person over age 70 to find out what health problems were most common during their teenage years. Prepare a brief report to the class comparing what you learned in the two interviews with what you learned in this chapter about health problems facing teens today.
2. Collect newspaper or magazine pictures that depict healthful or wellness behaviors and harmful behaviors. Glue these pictures on a poster board. Show your poster to the class and discuss how advertisements can influence your health choices both positively and negatively.

Plan for Action

Your level of health and wellness affects every aspect of your day-to-day life. Develop a month-long plan to improve your personal level of wellness using the Health Risks Survey in the Life SKILLS feature.

Projects
Have students plan and carry out the projects for health and wellness within the school and community.

Plan for Action
Have students role-play a situation in which they have just heard of a friend's suicide. They also happen to know someone else who is very depressed and decide to work together to help this teen by providing support and help in finding adult assistance.

Assessment Options

Chapter Test
Have students take the Chapter 1 Test.

Alternative Assessment
Have students do the Alternative Assessment activity for Chapter 1.

Test Generator
The Test Generator (Macintosh® or IBM® format) contains an additional 50 assessment items for this chapter.

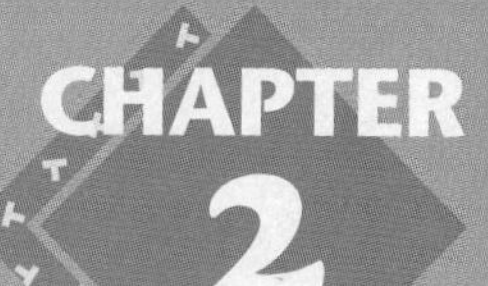

MAKING RESPONSIBLE DECISIONS

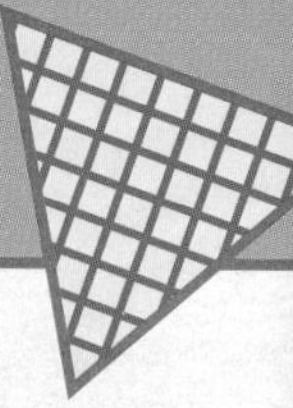

PLANNING GUIDE

TEXT SECTIONS	OBJECTIVES	TEXT FEATURES	OUTSIDE RESOURCES	NOTES
2.1 **Why Does Health Involve So Many Decisions?** pp. 21-23 1 period	• Name the top three causes of death of people ages 15–24. • Explain how decisions made today can affect how long you live. • Name the top three causes of death of people ages 55–64. • Explain how decisions made today can affect your quality of life when you are older.	**ASSESSMENT** • Section Review, p. 23	**TEACHER'S RESOURCE BINDER** • Lesson Plan 2.1 • Personal Health Inventory • Journal Entries 2A • Life Skills Worksheet • Section Review Worksheet 2.1 • Section Quiz 2.1 • Reteaching Worksheet 2.1 **OTHER RESOURCES** • Transparencies 2A, 2B, 2C • Parent Discussion Guide	
2.2 **How to Make a Responsible Decision** pp. 24-30 2 periods	• Name the steps of the decision-making model presented in this chapter. • Discuss the importance of values to responsible decision making. ■ Demonstrate the ability to use a decision-making model to make a responsible decision.	• What Would You Do?, p. 29 **ASSESSMENT** • Section Review, p. 30	**TEACHER'S RESOURCE BINDER** • Lesson Plan 2.2 • Journal Entries 2B, 2C, 2D • Media Worksheet • Section Review Worksheet 2.2 • Section Quiz 2.2 • Reteaching Worksheet 2.2 **OTHER RESOURCES** • Transparency 2D • Making a Choice 2A, 2B	
End of Chapter pp. 31-33		**ASSESSMENT** • Chapter Review, pp. 32-33	**TEACHER'S RESOURCE BINDER** **OTHER RESOURCES** • Chapter Test • Alternative Assessment • Test Generator • English/Spanish Audiocassette 1	

■ Denotes LIFE SKILLS objectives

• Items in blue are also part of the *Holt Health Activity Book.*

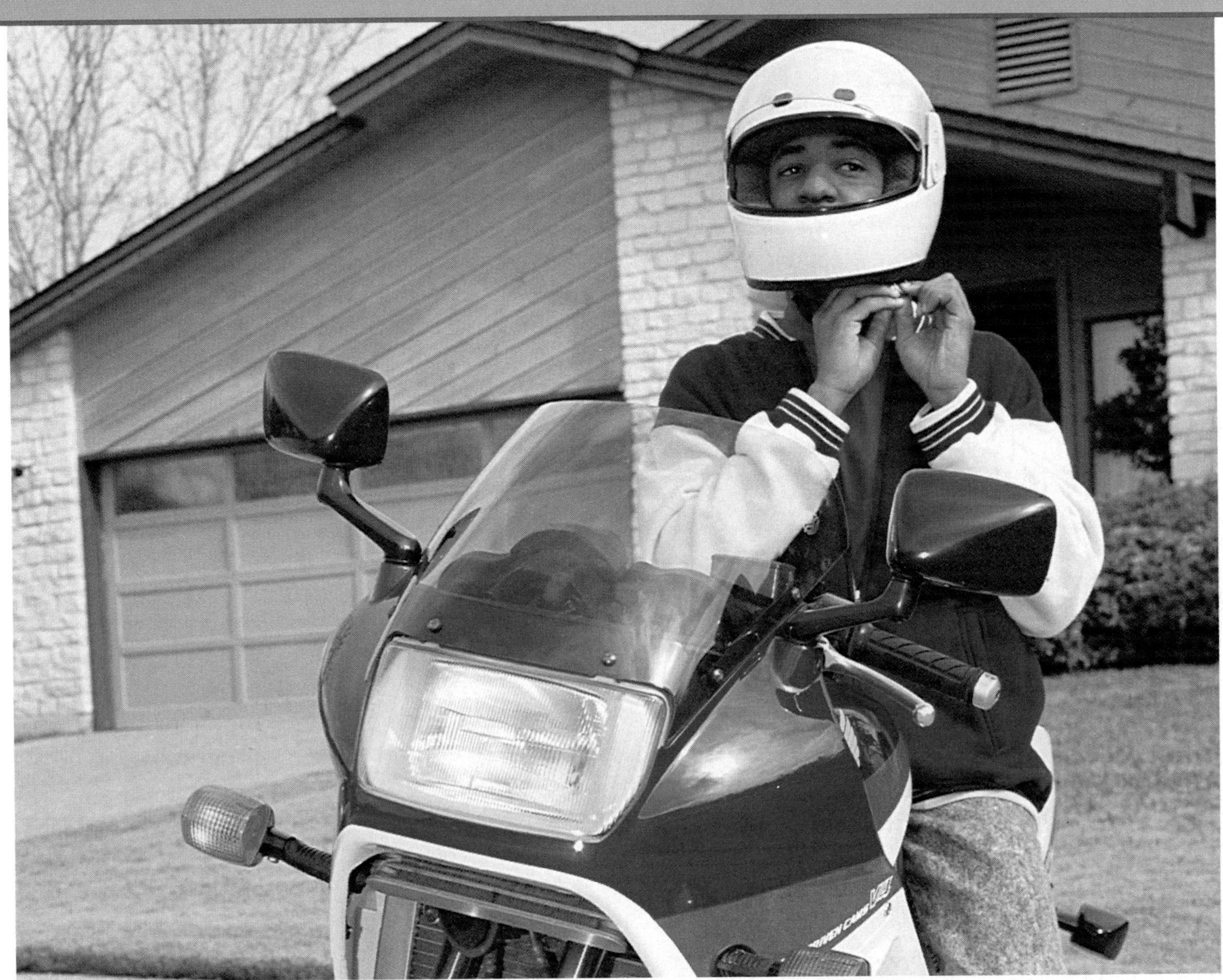

CONTENT BACKGROUND

Making Responsible Decisions

EVEN THOUGH STUDIES SHOW THAT contemporary teenagers share their parents' values and opinions more often than they disagree with them, adults are in general less available than they once were to guide their sons and daughters in the decision-making process. To a large extent, this is due to the fact that 40 to 50 percent of today's teenagers live in single-parent homes, usually headed by working mothers.

According to studies published by the National Adolescent Health Survey (NASHS), a large percentage of teenagers do make responsible decisions even with less guidance. But, the survey also indicates that most adolescents engage in behaviors that place them at risk at some times.

One category included in the NASHS study was "Injury Prevention." The survey indicates that although many students know what they should do in given situations to avoid disabling or fatal injuries, many do not take precautions. For example, 92 percent of teenagers who ride bicycles never wear helmets. Sixty-two percent of teenagers surveyed said that their friends would think that wearing a helmet is a silly thing to do. According to the same study, only 41 percent of the students surveyed wore seat belts the last time they rode in a passenger vehicle such as a car, van, or truck. Nearly the same percentage (39 percent) said that they had ridden in a vehicle driven by a person who had just used drugs or alcohol.

More than eight out of ten respondents, or 83 percent, said that they had taken an alcoholic drink at least one time themselves. Forty-two percent of teenagers surveyed said they had drunk alcohol in the past month, and 32 percent said that they had had five or more alcoholic drinks on a single occasion during the preceding 2 weeks. Yet 43 percent said they believe their friends would disapprove of their drinking alcohol occasionally and the same percentage said that a person who has five or more alcoholic drinks once or twice each weekend is at great risk.

The results of the NASHS and other studies indicate that over half of all adolescents in the United States are participating in high-risk behavior. We can expect these behaviors to change only if we allow young people to practice using decision-making models—such as the one presented in the chapter—in a classroom, where incorrect choices will not threaten them.

PLANNING FOR INSTRUCTION

KEY FACTS

- **Responsible decision making provides a measure of control over personal health.**
- **Lifestyle choices contribute directly to quality of life and length of life. Some consequences of these choices are immediate; others are long-term.**
- **The leading causes of death among young people 15 to 24 years old are accident, homicide, and suicide. Choosing to use alcohol or drugs increases the odds of being hurt or killed in one of these ways.**
- **A person born in the United States today has a life expectancy of 76 years.**
- **The leading causes of death among people 55 to 64 years old are cancer, heart disease, and stroke.**
- **Responsible decisions may be made by using a decision-making model: (1) stating the problem, (2) listing the options, (3) thinking through the benefits and consequences of each option, (4) considering your values, (5) weighing the options and making a decision based on those options, (6) acting to implement the decision, and (7) evaluating the results.**
- **A good decision is one made responsibly, not just one that has an immediate happy result.**
- **Some decisions must be made under pressure, with no time for thinking through consequences. To be prepared for such situations, practice decision-making skills in advance and consider values first.**

MYTHS AND MISCONCEPTIONS

MYTH: No one can help you make decisions; you must make them for yourself.
In fact, talking over choices with a friend or an adult whose judgment you trust may be helpful. The friend may see the situation more objectively, provide further insight, or be able to suggest options you haven't thought about.

MYTH: The best decision is the one with the best immediate outcome.
An action that has a pleasant immediate outcome may have disastrous results in the long term. On the other hand, some decisions result in unpleasant consequences for the short term but good results in the future.

MYTH: If the outcome isn't what I expected, I made the wrong decision.
Events beyond a person's control may cause unexpected or undesired results. It doesn't mean a poor choice was made, just that the actions of others or outside circumstances prevented the desired outcome.

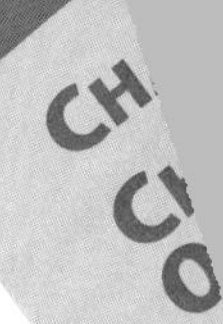

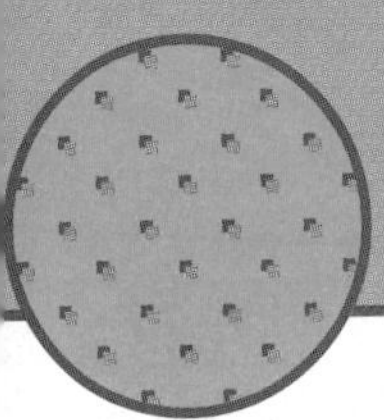

VOCABULARY

Essential: The following vocabulary terms appear in boldface type:

life expectancy
quality of life
decision-making model
values

Secondary: Be aware that the following terms may come up during class discussion:

lifestyles
short-term consequences
long-term consequences
emphysema
options

FOR STUDENTS WITH SPECIAL NEEDS

Visual Learners: Students may benefit from a display of images that focus on lifestyle decisions. Such images might be paired and could include pictures of alcoholic beverages versus healthful drinks; young people watching television versus exercising or participating in sports; foods high in fat and sugar versus those high in fiber, complex carbohydrates, and vitamins; teens in gangs versus teens in positive-action organizations (e.g., SADD). The display might be organized around a key phrase such as "Decisions for Life."

Auditory Learners: Have students form small groups. Provide each group with a cassette tape on which a young person's lifestyle decision is described. (Examples might include opting not to go to college, deciding to work 30 hours a week during high school, buying a motorcycle, taking up smoking, cutting out fatty foods.) Have each group discuss the likely short-term and long-term effects of the decision they heard on the tape. After ranking the most important effects, students can record their responses and a statement telling whether they think the decision was responsible. The class can listen to each group's tape and discuss their reactions.

ENRICHMENT

- Invite a counselor or health professional from a local health department, clinic, or hospital to speak to the class about the health outcomes of poor lifestyle decisions. Such a resource can provide first-hand observations about (anonymous) case histories and an objective perspective about health choices that have dramatic short-term and long-term results.
- Have students write open-ended scripts about situations calling for quick decisions. They can use these scripts to prepare skits to perform for other classes. The audience could be asked to choose the decision they want made, with actors trying to show probable outcomes for various decisions. They might build in "freeze frames" at key moments in order to point out steps in the decision-making process and to allow for audience reaction.

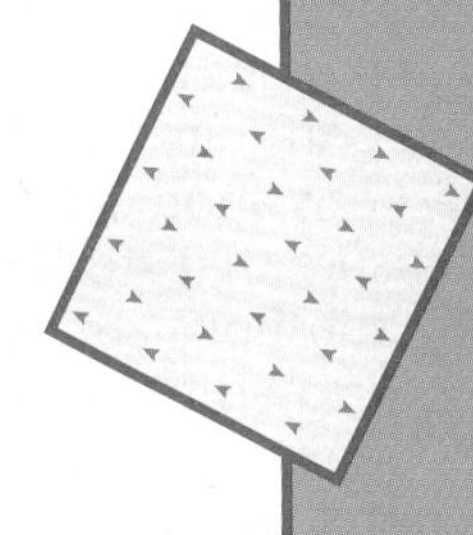

APTER 2
APTER
PENER

GETTING STARTED

Using the Chapter Photograph
Ask students to list some decisions the people in the photograph might have made before coming to the party or may have to make before it ends. List them on the chalkboard. Then ask students to pick out those decisions that might have serious consequences and to explain why. Have them name and discuss several other key decisions young people must make. Tell the class that this chapter will discuss the importance of responsible decision making and provide a model for making decisions that are right for them.

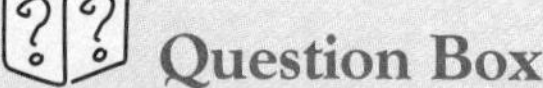

Question Box
Have students write out any questions they have about how to make good decisions. The Question Box provides them with an opportunity to ask questions anonymously. To ensure that students with questions are not embarrassed to be seen writing, have those who do not have questions write something else—such as something they already know about decision making—on the paper instead.

CHAPTER 2

Making Responsible Decisions

◆ ◆ ◆ ◆

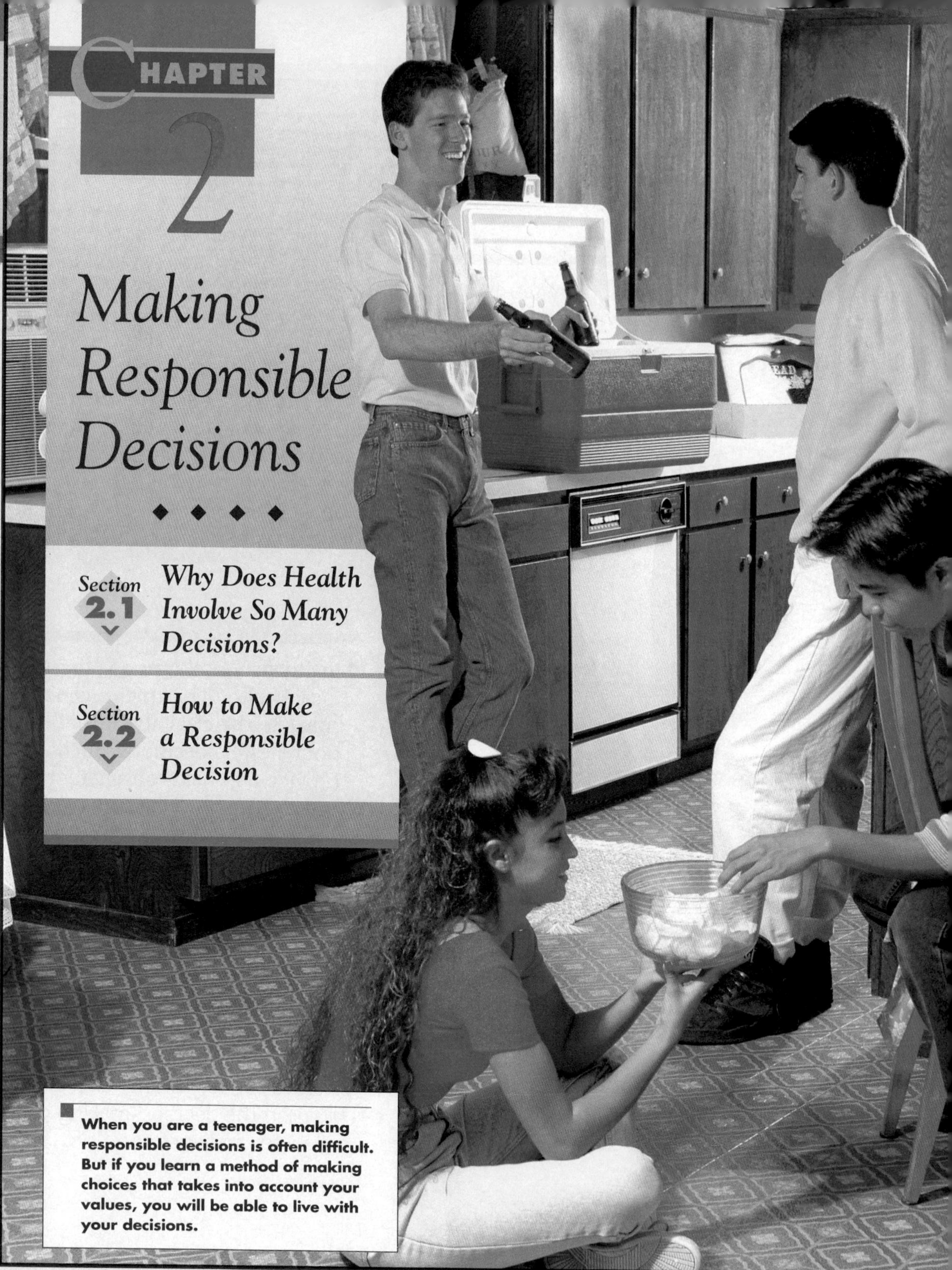

When you are a teenager, making responsible decisions is often difficult. But if you learn a method of making choices that takes into account your values, you will be able to live with your decisions.

Preview the questions and then answer them at appropriate points in the chapter. You may wish to allow students to write additional anonymous questions as they go through the chapter.

Personal Issues *ALERT*
Discussion of important lifestyle decisions (such as alcohol consumption and drug use) may make some students uncomfortable. Those who are coping with alcoholism or addiction, or who have family members who are coping with either, may withdraw or respond angrily. Keep in mind that these students may have no control over the situation. They may also feel that revealing any personal information would show disloyalty to family. Prepare the class to respect privacy and to show sensitivity toward those who reveal information about their personal lives.

Richard can't decide what to do. His friend Nicole asked him if he wanted to go to a party with Nicole and her friend Selena this Saturday night. Nicole said the beer would be flowing freely. Richard wants to go because he has been attracted to Selena for a long time. He always wanted to ask her out but was afraid she would turn him down. Going to this party would be the perfect way to get to know her without putting his pride on the line. But Richard has a big problem. He made up his mind last year that he didn't want to drink. His brother was arrested twice for drunken driving and finally went into an alcoholism treatment program. Even though his brother seems to be doing much better now, Richard doesn't want to go through what his brother did. So far he's been able to stick to his decision. But if he goes to this party he knows he'll be tempted to drink, especially if Nicole and Selena are drinking. What should he do? What would you do?

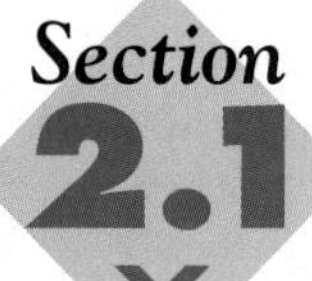

Why Does Health Involve so Many Decisions?

Objectives

- *Name the top three causes of death of people ages 15–24.*
- *Explain how decisions made today can affect how long you live.*
- *Name the top three causes of death of people ages 55–64.*
- *Explain how decisions made today can affect your quality of life when you are older.*

This is not the first time that Richard has had to make a difficult choice. Each day *everyone* faces decisions. Some choices are pretty easy to make—like deciding which shoes to wear, or which shoe to put on first. But other decisions have important consequences for your health, and these are often the difficult ones to make. In this chapter you'll learn a method for making responsible decisions that you can use for the rest of your life.

Responsible decision making is an important part of health; the choices you make give you a great deal of control over your own health.

The decisions you make could be more important to your health than any other factor. Your lifestyle—your way of living—could affect your health more than the traits you inherited from your parents, more than your environment, and more than the kind of health care you get.

Sometimes the choices you make affect your health immediately. Other times, the consequences are not seen until many

Section 2.1

Background
Statistics

Students may be interested in these facts: Three-fourths of young people's deaths from accidental injury are due to automobile accidents; alcohol is a causative factor for half of these. Half of all fatal car crashes involving youths occur at night (but 80 percent of young drivers' travel is done during daylight). When a young person enters high school, his or her odds of dying in an auto accident increase 400 percent. Teens have the worst record of any age group when it comes to using seat belts. Teens who drink and drive stand a greater chance of being in a crash than adults who drink and drive.

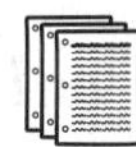

Personal Health Inventory

Have students complete the Personal Health Inventory for this chapter. The inventory helps them assess whether they make responsible decisions.

Section 2.1 Lesson Plan

MOTIVATE

Journal 2A
Richard's Dilemma

This may be done as a warm-up activity. Have students write down their reactions in the Student Journal in the Student Activity Book to Richard's dilemma. Ask them to tell what they would decide and to explain why.

TEACH

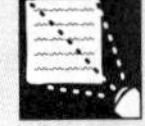

Teaching Transparency 2A
Leading Causes of Death

Show the transparency which is a graph of leading causes of death for people 55 to 64 years old (Figure 2-1). Have students visualize a specific city or geographic area in your state whose population approximates the total number of deaths represented by the graph. **Why do so many people die prematurely?** *[Students may suggest drug and alcohol use, sedentary and stressful lifestyles, poor diet, job hazards, dangerous and overpopulated neighborhoods.]*

Reinforcement
Prevention of Accidents

Some students may be shocked by the statistics in Figure 2-1. Tell students that the total number of teen deaths each year is low compared to the number of deaths in other age groups. Many

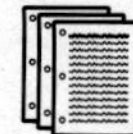

Life Skills Worksheet 2A

Suicide Prevention

Assign the Suicide Prevention Life Skills Worksheet, which requires students to determine what suicide prevention services are available in their community.

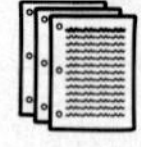

Section Review Worksheet 2.1

Assign Content Review Worksheet 2.1, which requires students to identify short-term and long-term consequences of various health decisions and to list how the decisions would affect their life expectancy and quality of life.

Section Quiz 2.1

Have students take Section Quiz 2.1.

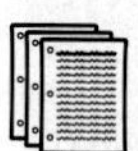

Reteaching Worksheet 2.1

Students who have difficulty with the material may complete Reteaching Worksheet 2.1, which requires them to identify the major causes of death in two age groups and to identify factors that adversely affect life expectancy and quality of life.

years later. The choice that Richard has to make about the party is one that can have both short-term and long-term consequences for his health.

Short-Term Consequences of Health Decisions

The short-term consequences of health decisions can be dramatic. You may be surprised to learn that the top three causes of death among young people are not illnesses at all. Almost half of the deaths in this age group are caused by accidents! As Figure 2-1 shows, the top three causes of death among people 15 to 24 years old are:

life expectancy: *the number of years a person can reasonably be expected to live.*

1. accidental injury
2. homicide
3. suicide

These causes of death are often directly related to the choices a person makes. If someone chooses to ride a bicycle without a helmet, for example, he or she is more likely to be seriously injured in an accident than a person who decides to wear a helmet. And if Richard decides to go to the party and then ends up drunk, he is at a greater risk of becoming involved in an accident than if he had avoided the temptation to drink.

It has been shown that the use of alcohol and drugs greatly increases the chances that a person will experience serious injury, be involved in violence, or commit suicide. So one of the best decisions a young person can make is to abstain from (not use) drugs and alcohol.

A person born in the United States today has a **life expectancy** of 76 years. In other words, the number of years a person could reasonably be expected to live is 76 years. What if a young woman with a life expectancy of 76 years decided to ride her bicycle without a helmet, was hit by a car, and died at the age of 18? That decision would cost her 58 years of life.

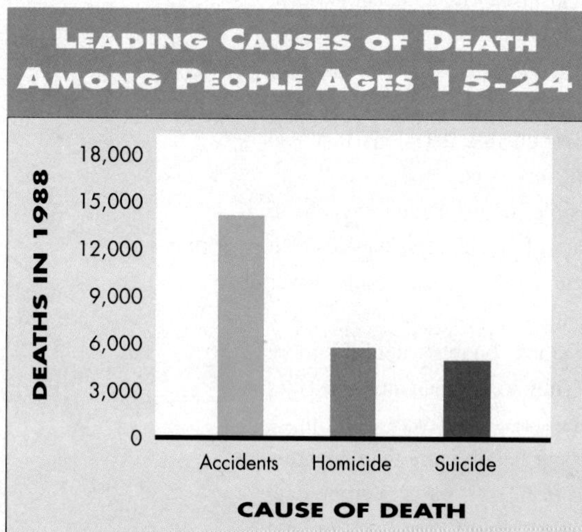

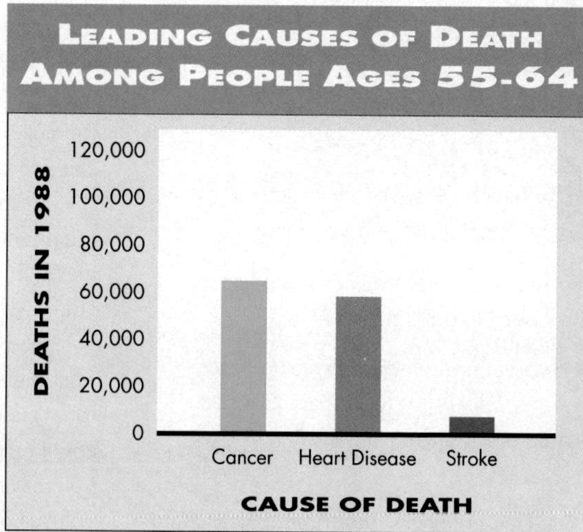

(FIGURE 2-1) **These charts show the leading causes of death for young people (left) and for older people (right). The decisions you make now can affect your health immediately *and* later in your life. (Source: United States Department of Health and Human Services.)**

• • • TEACH continued

accidental deaths among teens are tragic because they are preventable. Ask them to speculate about ways that accidents can be prevented.

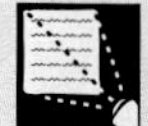

Teaching Transparency 2B
Leading Causes of Death

Show the transparency which is a graph of leading causes of death for people 15 to 24 years old (Figure 2-1). Have students discuss specific choices by young people that might lead to death by accident, homicide, or suicide. **Why do you think most deaths at this age are due to accident?** *[Students may suggest inexperience in driving, experimentation with alcohol or drugs, greater willingness to participate in risky activities, carelessness.]*

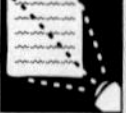

Teaching Transparency 2C
Causes of Cancer

Use this transparency to discuss the causes of cancer. Ask students to identify what percentage of cancers are a result of bad health decisions, and are therefore preventable.

Extension
Checking the Statistics

Have students visit a local hospital or county coroner's office to find out

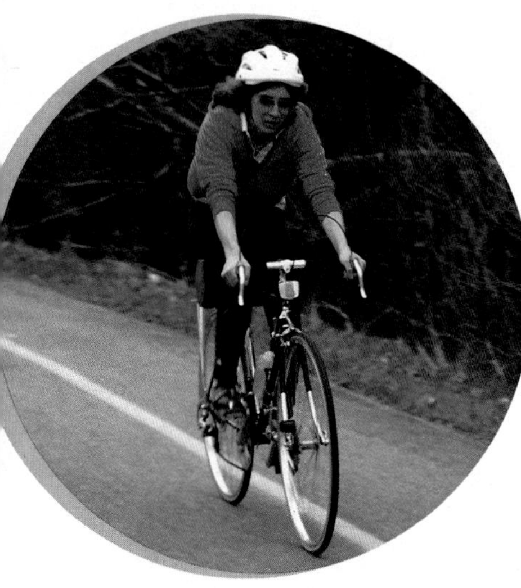

(FIGURE 2-2) **Health decisions can have immediate consequences. A decision to wear a helmet while bicycling can save your life.**

Long-Term Consequences of Health Decisions

Some decisions might not have immediate consequences for your health, but they can determine what your life will be like when you are older. Look again at Figure 2-1. The top three causes of death among people between the ages of 55 and 64 are:

1. cancer
2. heart disease
3. stroke

Each of these causes of death is often the result of choices made early in life. If you choose to smoke, for instance, you are much more likely to get lung cancer than a nonsmoker. Smoking begun in the teenage years and continued over long periods of time is the cause of most deaths due to lung cancer.

Suppose a man succeeded in living all the years of his life expectancy. But during the last 20 of those years he was always sick and in pain. He had emphysema, a lung disease, as a result of smoking cigarettes since the age of 16. Even though he lived a *long* life, his **quality of life** was poor. Quality of life is the degree to which a person lives life to its fullest capacity with enjoyment and reward.

quality of life: *the degree to which a person lives life to its fullest capacity with enjoyment and reward.*

If Richard's brother hadn't taken steps to recover from his alcoholism, he could have developed any number of ailments that would have severely damaged his quality of life. You are not likely to have a good quality of life if you smoke for 40 years and get emphysema. Similarly, you probably won't have a good quality of life if you develop heart disease as a result of poor diet and inadequate exercise.

You may not be able to do all the things you would like to do in your later years unless you make healthy choices now. The decisions you make today will influence not only how long you live, but also how you *feel* years from now.

Review

1. *Name the top three causes of death of people ages 15–24.*
2. *Explain how decisions made today can affect how long you live.*
3. *Name the top three causes of death of people ages 55–64.*
4. *Explain how decisions made today can affect your quality of life when you are older.*
5. ***Critical Thinking*** *If Richard's brother hadn't decided to quit drinking, how do you think his quality of life would be affected if he lived into his fifties?*

SECTION 2.1

Review Answers

1. Accidental injury, homicide, suicide
2. Decisions concerning safety, such as wearing a helmet when riding a bicycle or wearing a seat belt when riding in a car, can protect a person from serious injury and even death. Also, decisions to not drink and not use drugs can greatly reduce a person's risk of being involved in an accident or developing health problems. Accept any reasonable answer.
3. Cancer, heart disease, stroke
4. Decisions that affect one's health—such as smoking, drinking alcohol, using drugs, getting little or no exercise, and eating a poor diet—can decrease the quality of life as a person gets older.
5. Richard's brother might have developed ailments that would be damaging to his overall health and quality of life. For example, his ailments might prevent him from keeping a steady job. His life expectancy might also be reduced. Accept any reasonable answer.

about death rates and causes of death for young people in their community. They might ask whether statistics have been compiled for the county and compare their data with that in the text.

ASSESS

Section Review

Have students answer the Section Review questions.

Alternative Assessment

Have students write a paragraph analyzing a decision that could lead to poor quality of life decades from now. They should describe the decision, list specific health outcomes, and explain the short-term or long-term effects of the decision.

Closure

Wellness Contract

Have students draw up a wellness contract aimed at a specific goal for fostering good health. It may be aimed at good nutrition, exercise, avoidance of tobacco and other drugs, or any other behavior that they wish to commit to. Suggest that they include the goal (with a specific time span), the action they will take to reach the goal, a calendar for keeping track of results, a space for evaluating results, and a date and signature line.

Background
Cognitive Dissonance
Psychologists use a concept called cognitive dissonance in describing people's tendency to reconcile contradictory information about themselves. This concept is helpful in thinking about what happens when a person analyzes the consequences of a decision. If the outcome of a decision is positive (the person has success, remains healthy, feels good, and so on) the person may credit the decision, whether or not the decision was in fact wise. If the outcome is negative (the person has an accident, becomes ill, loses a job), he or she may assess the outcome irrationally, either blaming outside forces incorrectly or generalizing the failure inappropriately. If a person does not assess a decision realistically, he or she may come to false and even damaging (destructive) conclusions.

Section 2.2 How to Make a Responsible Decision

Objectives
- *Name the steps of the decision-making model presented in this chapter.*
- *Discuss the importance of values to responsible decision making.*
- *Demonstrate the ability to use a decision-making model to make a responsible decision.*
  LIFE SKILLS: Making Responsible Decisions

decision-making model: *a series of steps that helps a person make a responsible decision.*

Why is it necessary to teach people how to make decisions? Don't people just naturally learn how? No, it doesn't always work that way. Many people—perhaps most of us—have great difficulty making decisions, and then worry about it long after the choice has been made. ''Did I do the right thing?'' they wonder. ''What if I had made the other decision?'' A lot of people need specific instructions before they know how to make responsible decisions.

A Decision-Making Model
In this section you'll see how Richard uses a **decision-making model** to make his choice. A decision-making model is a series of steps that helps a person make a responsible decision.

The decision-making model used in this textbook is shown in Figure 2-4. Follow along as you see Richard go through the steps to make his decision.

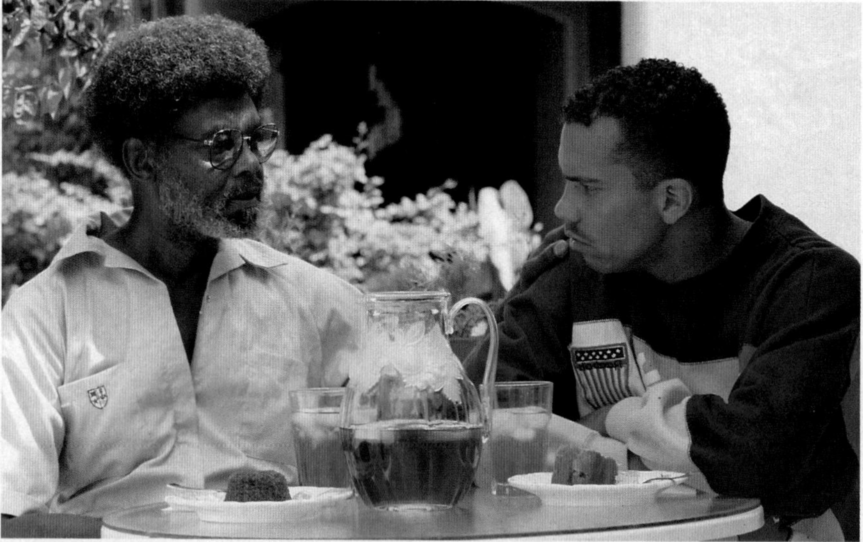

(FIGURE 2-3) **When making a difficult decision, it often helps to talk with someone you trust, such as a parent, teacher, counselor, or friend.**

Section 2.2 Lesson Plan

MOTIVATE

Journal 2B
Difficult Decisions

Direct students to the Student Journal to write about a decision they had difficulty making and then worried about afterward.

Role-Playing
Making the Right Decision

Have students select one or more of the following scenarios to role-play:
- A friend offers a ride to two teens. The car already has six passengers. Without a ride, the two teens will have a 2-mile walk to the beach.
- Your best friend went to a game instead of doing homework and asks to borrow your homework before class.
- Richard goes to the party, where everyone wants him to drink beer.

Encourage participants to resolve each scenario. Discuss what might happen next as a result of their decisions.

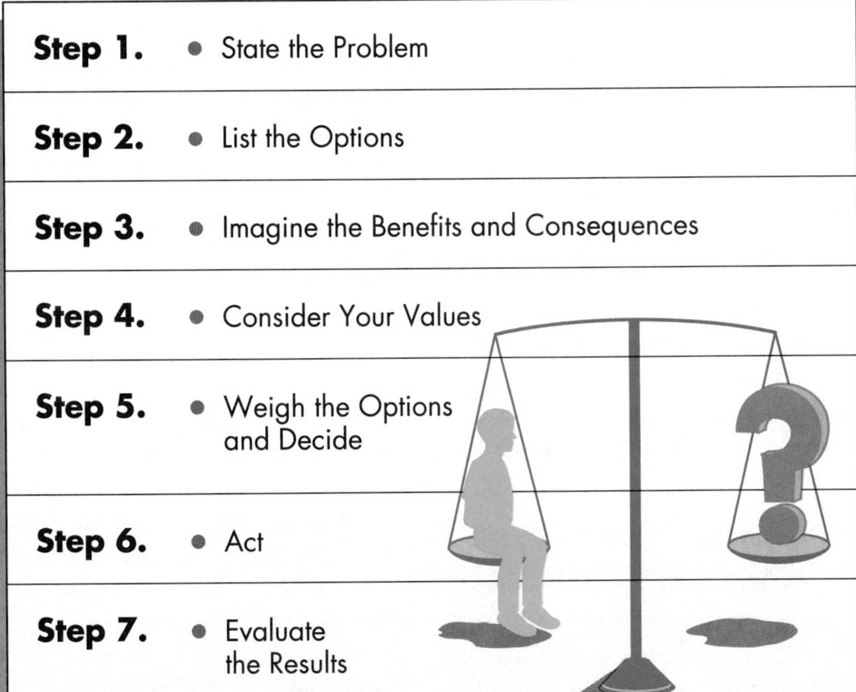

(FIGURE 2-4) **A decision-making model is a series of steps that helps a person make a responsible decision. Richard used the steps shown above to make his decision about the party.**

Step 1. State the Problem The first step in making a decision is to state the problem clearly. This is how Richard states his problem: "Should I go to the party even though I don't want to drink?"

Step 2. List the Options Before deciding what to do, Richard needs to list all the options. As he sees it, these are his options:

1. Go to the party and hope that he isn't tempted to drink.
2. Stay home and watch reruns of "Who's the Boss?"

Not very appealing options. Surely there are other alternatives. Well, Richard thinks, he could tell Nicole and Selena ahead of time that he isn't going to drink. That way they might not try to pressure him into drinking. So now he has a third option:

3. Go to the party, but tell Nicole and Selena ahead of time that he is not going to drink.

Richard can't think of any more options. It seems that he will have to choose among these three. But that's not necessarily true. A person in the middle of trying to solve a problem may not be able to *recognize* all the options.

If Richard discusses his problem with other people, however, they may be able to think of other options or at least provide additional information. In this case, Richard talks to his good friend Carlos about his dilemma. Carlos tells him he has heard that

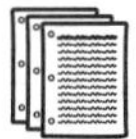

Making a Choice 2A

When Others Are Drinking

Assign the When Others Are Drinking card. The card asks students to role-play a situation in which a couple decide what to do at a party where drinking is occurring.

Evaluating the Media Worksheet

What is a Media Message?

Have students complete the Evaluating the Media worksheet for Unit 1.

TEACH

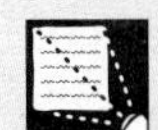

Teaching Transparency 2D
Decision-Making Model

Show the transparency of the steps in the decision-making model (Figure 2-4). **Which steps do you think are most important? Which do you think could be left out? Why? When do you think using this model would be most helpful?**

Class Discussion
Consulting Others

Ask students how they would decide whom to talk to when trying to make an important decision. You might place the following factors on the board and encourage them to think of others.

- knows me well
- is an expert on the subject
- has common sense and good judgment
- knows the situation or has made a similar decision

Have students discuss the relevance of each factor to decision-making .

Journal 2C
People You Trust

Have students write in the Student Journal the names of responsible people whom they trust and could talk to about important decisions. Then ask them to write down their reasons for choosing these people.

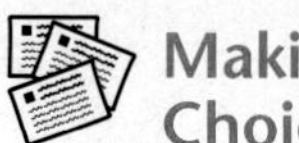

Making a Choice 2B

Values

Assign the Values card. The card requires students to consider how individual values may differ among students and to discuss the effects of making decisions that are inconsistent with one's values.

values: *a person's strong beliefs and ideals.*

Selena doesn't drink either. Richard hadn't even considered that possibility. ''What about going to a movie?'' Carlos suggests. ''That way you can see Selena but not have to worry about drinking.'' So now he has a fourth option:

4. Persuade Nicole and Selena to go to a movie instead of the party.

If Selena doesn't drink, Richard thinks, he might have a pretty good chance of getting the girls to change their plans.

Having someone to talk to whose opinions you trust is a valuable asset. It's important to remember, though, that you don't want to be persuaded to do something that isn't good for you.

Step 3. Imagine the Benefits and Consequences of Each Option Many people have the hardest time with this step because they don't want to think about all the painful things that could happen as a result of choosing some of their options. But that's why this step is so important. In the long run, it's less painful to just imagine the consequences of a bad decision than to actually *experience* the consequences.

Take some time and carefully think through the benefits and negative consequences of each of your options. Make separate lists of the short-term consequences and the long-term consequences. A solution that solves the immediate problem might have terrible consequences later. And a solution that has uncomfortable consequences at first can be the best one in the long run.

Figure 2-5 shows the possible benefits and negative consequences that Richard imagined during his decision-making process. Remember that this is how *Richard* saw his situation. If you had Richard's problem, your lists of benefits and consequences might be entirely different.

Step 4. Consider Your Values The next step in making a responsible decision is to think about how each option fits with your **values.** There are many definitions of the word ''values,'' but when you see the word in this book it means a person's strong beliefs and ideals.

Your values allow you to choose between good and bad, and between right and wrong. Your values show the kind of person you are and what you care most about.

A person's values develop over time and are influenced by the teachings of family, culture, and religious and spiritual leaders. It's important to realize that not everyone will share your values. Each person develops his or her own value system, based on individual life experiences. However, there are some values that seem to be important to people from many backgrounds and cultures. These values, which are sometimes called ''universal values,'' are:

- honesty
- trustworthiness
- responsibility to oneself and others
- self-control
- social justice

Richard feels that the value most relevant to his problem is responsibility to himself and others. It is very important to Richard to protect himself from harm. It is also important to him to avoid needlessly hurting his family. If he developed a drinking problem like his brother's, it would cause his family a lot of pain.

He also recognizes that his problem involves self-control. He had vowed to himself that he would not drink, and he doesn't want to break his promise to himself by losing control.

When Richard looks over his list of options, he sees that Option 2 and Option 4 fit his values. If he chooses either of these options, he will be certain not to drink.

• • • TEACH continued

Class Discussion
Ranking Values

Have students study the bulleted list of "universal values" and rank them from most important to least important. If a value that is important to them is not listed, ask them to add it. Tally the class opinions on the chalkboard. Stress that people's values differ, just as students' opinions about the relative importance of specific values differ.

Demonstration
Values and Behavior

Ask students to draw a visual map by using arrows to represent the relationship between personal values and behavior. You might copy the clearest visual map on the chalkboard or on an overhead transparency. Then trace the path on the visual as students name a value and suggest a behavior that proceeds from it.

Reinforcement
Deciding on a Plan

For the following situation, ask students to suggest a plan Maria could follow to help her carry out her decision:

> Maria decides that she is going to exercise regularly to lose weight and get in shape. She feels good about her decision. A month later, however, she still has not begun to exercise.

Richard's Options

FIGURE 2-5

Options	Possible Benefits	Possible Short-Term Negative Consequences	Possible Long-Term Negative Consequences
1. *Go to the party and hope that I am not tempted to drink.*	*I will be sure to spend the evening with the girls.*	*I may drink and feel guilty about it.* *I may drink and lose the chance to go out with Selena, since she doesn't drink.* *I may drink and end up in a dangerous situation, such as driving while drunk.*	*If I drink after I've decided not to drink, I could become a problem drinker like my brother. The negative consequences of being a problem drinker would take all day to list. Some of them are increased risk of injuries, physical illness, emotional depression, and damaged relationships with people I care about.*
2. *Stay at home and watch reruns of "Who's the Boss".*	*I will not have to deal with the pressures to drink alcohol.* *I will keep my promise to myself about not drinking.*	*I will not get to spend the evening with the girls.*	*The girls might think I'm no fun.*
3. *Go to the party but tell Nicole and Selena ahead of time that I am not going to drink.*	*I will have a better chance of keeping my promise to myself about not drinking than if I choose Option 1.*	*I might drink anyway and have the same possible short-term consequences of Option 1.*	*If I drink, I have the same possible long-term consequences of Option 1.* *In addition, I might lose the respect of Nicole and Selena if I drink after I said I would not.*
4. *Persuade Nicole and Selena to go to a movie instead of the party.*	*I will get to spend the evening with the girls.* *I will know that Nicole and Selena would rather spend time with me than go to the party.* *I will keep my promise to myself about not drinking.* *I may improve my chances with Selena, since she doesn't drink.*	*Nicole and Selena might insist on going to the party, with or without me.* *If I do convince them to go to the movie instead, they may still feel a little upset about not going to the party.*	*If they don't want to go to the movie, the girls might think I'm no fun.*

Section Review Worksheet 2.2

Assign Section Review Worksheet 2.2, which requires students to order the steps in the decision-making model and to explain various steps in a decision-making scenario.

Section Quiz 2.2

Have students take Section Quiz 2.2

(Students may suggest some of the following: Decide on specific exercises she enjoys and can realistically do. Plan an exercise schedule that fits into her daily schedule. Ask a friend to exercise with her regularly. Make a chart to show improvements. Allow herself a small reward for each goal reached.)

Debate the Issue

Decisions Under Pressure

Have the class divide into two teams to argue each side of the following question: When you have to make a decision quickly, under pressure, should you always go with your first, instinctive response? Students on both sides should support their arguments with information they have learned about decision making and values. Have students suggest guidelines they think are important in making quick decisions under pressure.

Extension

Observing Decision Making

Students who need practice in making decisions can benefit from observing the process. Suggest that students sit in on student council or town council meetings. They may also interview several adults about the processes they use to make major decisions.

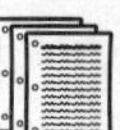

Reteaching Worksheet 2.2

Students who have difficulty with the material may complete Reteaching Worksheet 2.2, which requires them to identify various steps in a decision-making scenario.

Step 5. Weigh the Options and Decide The next step is to weigh your options and make the decision. Carefully examine the possible benefits and negative consequences of each option. Which option has the most benefits and the fewest negative consequences? Pay special attention to the long-term consequences of the options.

Most important, remember what you learned in Step 4—how the options fit your values. If you have trouble deciding between two options that seem equally desirable, choose the one that better reflects your strong beliefs and ideals. There is a very practical reason to act in accordance with one's values: When people go against their values, they are likely to feel bad about themselves. Always ask yourself, ''How will I feel about myself later if I choose this option?''

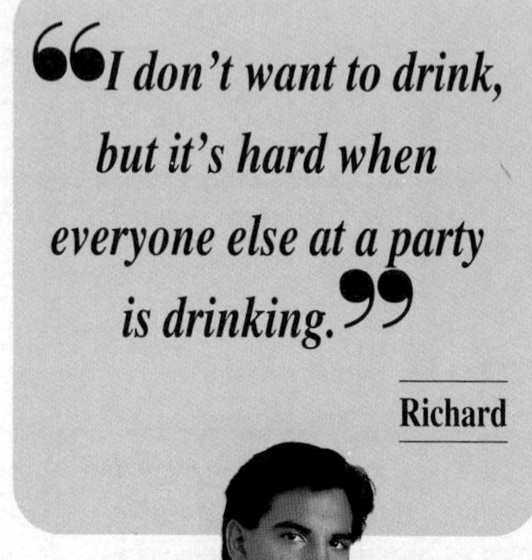

Richard knows that Options 1 and 3 are not compatible with his values because they might lead to drinking. Option 2, to stay home, *is* compatible with his values. But it doesn't have as many benefits as Option 4, to persuade the girls to go to a movie instead of the party.

Option 4 has more benefits than any of the other options, does not have many negative consequences, and is consistent with his values. It has now become clear to Richard that Option 4 is the best option for him.

He has made a responsible decision.

Step 6. Act It may seem that things should be smooth sailing after you finally make a decision. You just *do* it, right? In reality, it takes some thought and planning to ensure that you will act on your decision. Richard made the following list of actions he would take to implement his decision:

1. I will find out ahead of time which movies will be showing the night of the party and make a note of several that sound good.
2. I will make sure I can get the car that night so I can drive everyone to the theater.
3. I will tell Nicole and Selena about all the good movies showing in town and ask them if they would like to go to one of them instead of going to the party.
4. I will be prepared to tell them the truth if they ask me why I don't want to go to the party.

Step 7. Evaluate the Results Once the decision is made and you have acted on the decision, you should evaluate the results.

Ask yourself the following questions. How well did the decision work out? How well did you identify the potential benefits and negative consequences of the option you chose? How can you improve the way you make decisions in the future?

As it turned out, Nicole and Selena went along with his idea to go to the movie. Nicole was a little reluctant because she had been looking forward to the party, but Selena was happy to avoid the pressure to drink. No one quizzed Richard about why he didn't want to go to the party. All three had a good time at the movie, and Richard got to know Selena better. When Richard evaluated the results, he felt he had made the best decision possible.

But what if the situation had turned out differently? What if the girls had refused to go with him and had made fun of him? It wouldn't mean that he had made the wrong decision. It would mean that no matter how good his decision was, he couldn't control other people's behavior. All Richard could control was his *own* behavior. A good decision is not necessarily one that works out well, but one that is made responsibly.

What Would You Do ?

Making Responsible Decisions

A Friend Needs Your Help

You've seen Richard use the decision-making steps to work through his problem and make a responsible choice. Now practice using those same steps by making a decision about what you would do if faced with the following dilemma.

You know your friend Juliette has been depressed lately, but every time you ask her what's wrong, she changes the subject. Then one day you notice a bruise on her face that she's tried to cover with makeup. At first she tells you that she got hit in the face with a softball, but then, leaning against her locker and crying, she admits that her stepfather beat her up. "He knocks me around every time he has a bad day at work," Juliette says. "Mom doesn't even know about it because she gets home from work after he does."

"Why don't you tell your mother about it?" you ask. But Juliette shakes her head. "I don't want to break up Mom's marriage. She's happier now than she's been in a long time."

That night you keep thinking about Juliette. You want to help your friend, but you don't want to make her situation worse. What would you do?

Remember to use the decision-making steps:

1. **State the Problem.**
2. **List the Options.**
3. **Imagine the Benefits and Consequences.**
4. **Consider Your Values.**
5. **Weigh the Options and Decide.**
6. **Act.**
7. **Evaluate the Results.**

What Would You Do ?

Answers will vary. Accept any answers that demonstrate students' abilities to comprehend and apply the decision-making model to a chosen dilemma.

Review Answers

1. (1) state the problem, (2) list the options, (3) imagine the benefits and consequences of each option, (4) consider your values, (5) weigh the options and decide, (6) act, (7) evaluate the results.

2. Values are important when making a decision because values enable people to choose between good and bad and between right and wrong. Also, if people go against their values when making a decision, they are likely to feel bad about themselves.

3. Accept any answer that shows an understanding of the decision-making model.

4. Students may answer honesty, trustworthiness, responsibility to oneself and others, self-control, and social justice. Answers, however, will vary. Accept any reasonable response.

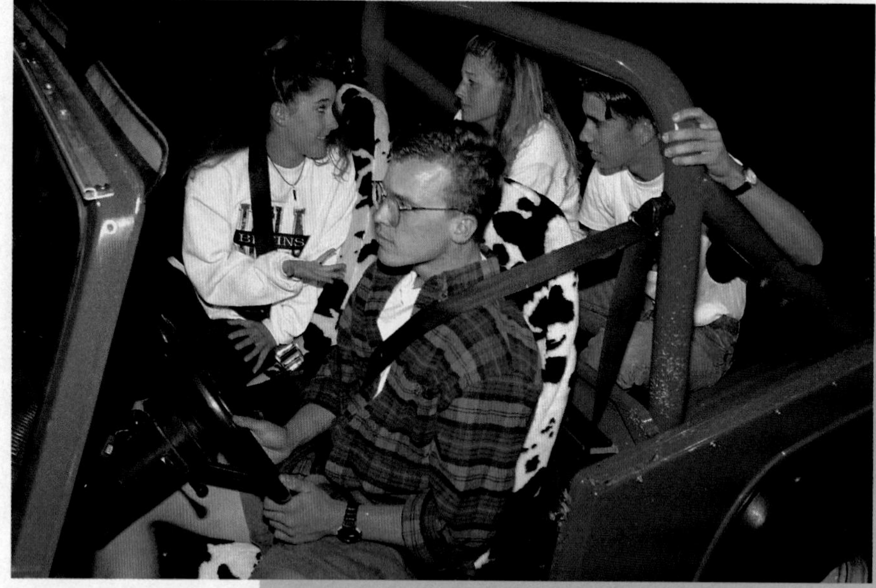

(FIGURE 2-6) **What if you're riding around in a car with friends and you have to make a quick decision about whether to go to a party? When under this kind of pressure, consider your values first.**

What Happens When You Have to Make a Quick Decision? Because Richard had plenty of time before the night of the party, he was able to systematically follow the decision-making steps. He was lucky that time. But let's say Richard was riding around in a car with some friends who wanted to go to a beer party right then. He wouldn't be able to whip out his notebook and pencil and make lists of the options, benefits, and consequences. He would have to respond immediately.

When under pressure, it is best to consider your values first. It also helps if you have practiced the decision-making steps many times before. Then the process would come almost naturally. The ''What Would You Do?'' activity on the previous page will give you an opportunity to sharpen your decision-making skills in preparation for the times when you have to make quick decisions.

Review

1. *Name the steps of the decision-making model presented in this chapter.*
2. *Why are values important in making responsible decisions?*
3. ***LIFE SKILLS: Making Responsible Decisions*** *Here is your dilemma: You are very attracted to someone in your school named Kris, but a friend recently told you that Kris uses a lot of drugs. Decide whether you should pursue your interest in Kris, using the steps of the decision-making model.*
4. ***Critical Thinking*** *Name three values that are very important to you.*

ASSESS

Section Review

Have students answer the Section Review questions.

Alternative Assessment

Evaluating a Decision

Have students use the decision-making model to write an evaluation for a decision that they may have personally made or that they studied in this section. The evaluation should state the problem, describe the action taken and the consequences of the action, and explain whether or not the results were satisfactory.

Closure

Taking Responsibility

In the Student Journal, have students make a list of things people do or say to deny responsibility for poor decisions or negative actions. (Starter examples might include statements such as the following: "____ made me do it." "Everybody does that." "It wasn't my fault.") Then have them write in their journals specific ways in which using a decision-making model could help them take more responsibility for their actions.

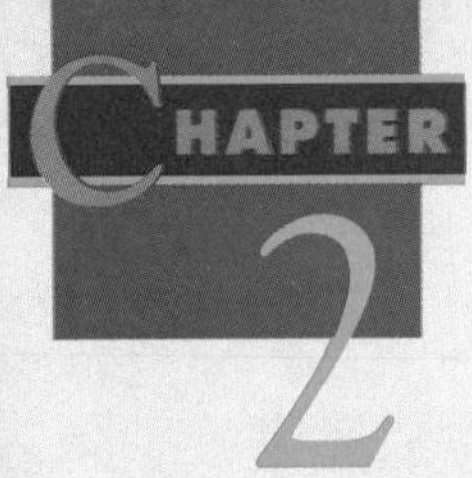

Highlights

Summary

- People who are able to make responsible decisions have a great deal of control over their own lives.
- The top three causes of death among Americans between the ages of 15 and 24 are accidental injury, homicide, and suicide. Each of these can directly result from the choices a person makes.
- The top three causes of death for Americans between the ages of 55 and 64 are cancer, heart disease, and stroke. Each of these can result from choices made early in life, such as smoking.
- A person who has a high quality of life leads a life that is full of enrichment and reward.
- There is a series of steps you can learn that will help you make responsible decisions.
- Talking to someone whose opinions you trust can help you make a good decision. Be sure, though, that you are not persuaded to make a decision to do something that is bad for you.
- A person's values, or strong beliefs and ideals, can be influenced by family, culture, and religious and spiritual leaders.
- Whenever you are under pressure to make a quick decision, make sure you consider your own values first.
- The most important values include honesty, trustworthiness, responsibility to oneself and others, self-control, and social justice.

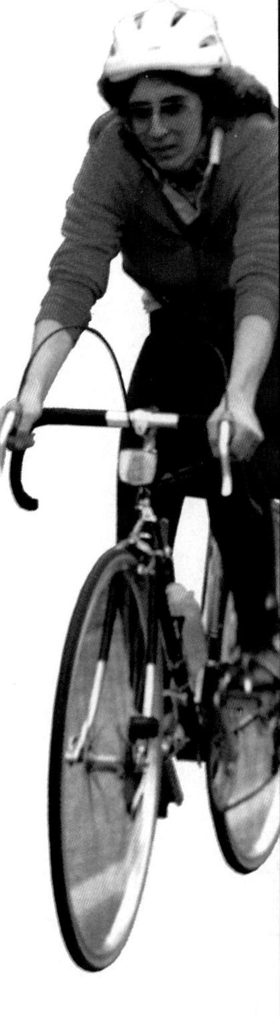

Vocabulary

life expectancy the number of years a person can reasonably be expected to live.

quality of life the degree to which a person lives life to its fullest capacity with enjoyment and reward.

decision-making model a series of steps that helps a person make a responsible decision.

values a person's strong beliefs and ideals.

Chapter 2 Highlights Strategies

Summary

Have students read the summary to reinforce the concepts they have learned in Chapter 2.

Vocabulary

Have students create a poster that features an illustrated formula for wise decision making. They should use all of the vocabulary terms in the formula. The following is an example:

Responsible use of the decision-making model
+
Consideration of values
=
Longer life expectancy
+
Higher quality of life

Extension

Have students create a collage, painting, or other visual work that communicates their view about a lifestyle decision that is important to them. The work should clearly show the decision made, suggest the values that helped them decide, and show how their quality of life has been or will be affected.

CHAPTER 2 ASSESSMENT

CHAPTER REVIEW

Concept Review

1. accidental injury, homicide, suicide
2. cancer, heart disease, stroke
3. alcohol, drugs
4. 76
5. emphysema
6. quality of life
7. state the problem
8. values
9. beliefs, ideals
10. evaluate the results

Expressing Your Views

Sample responses:

1. Eating nutritious snacks, a well-balanced diet; exercising; not smoking; not using illegal drugs; not drinking alcohol; wearing protective items or devices when necessary.
2. Research has proven that over the long term, cigarette smoking increases a person's chance of developing not only lung cancer but other cancers, as well as other lung diseases such as emphysema, chronic bronchitis, and heart disease.
3. Tell the friend that you care about her and then tell the friend that her drinking has you concerned. If the friend continues to drink, a short-term consequence may be an accident or the friend may experience long-term consequences such as becoming addicted to alcohol.

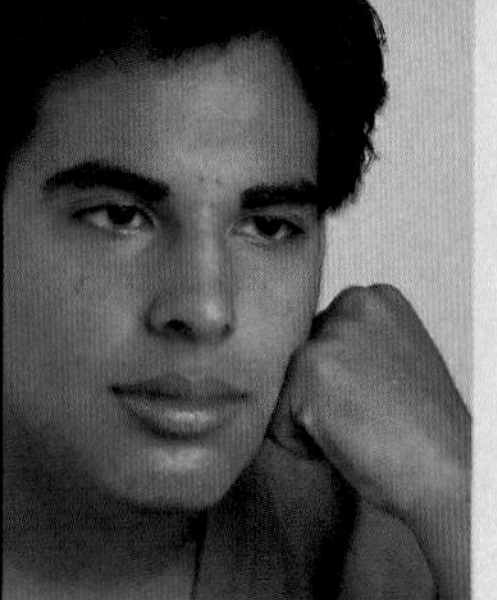

Chapter Review

Concept Review

1. The top three causes of death of people ages 15–24 are ________, ________, and ________.
2. The top three causes of death of people ages 55–64 are ________, ________, and ________.
3. It has been shown that the use of ________ and ________ greatly increases the chances that a person will experience serious injury, be involved in violence, or commit suicide.
4. A person born in the United States today has a life expectancy of ________ years.
5. If you choose to smoke, you are more likely to get lung cancer or ________________, a lung disease.
6. The degree to which a person lives life to its fullest capacity with enjoyment and reward is known as ________________.
7. The first step in making a decision is to ________________.
8. Your ________ allows you to choose between right and wrong and show the kind of person you are.
9. If you have trouble deciding between two options that seem equally desirable, choose the one that better reflects your strong ________ and ________.
10. Once a decision is made and you have acted on the decision, the next step in the decision-making process is to ________________.

Expressing Your Views

1. What are some changes you could make in your lifestyle to improve your quality of life in later years?
2. You have a friend who smokes cigarettes and is reluctant to quit. He says smoking has never made him feel sick, and that it's not going to harm him.
   What would you tell him?
3. Your best friend got drunk again at the party Saturday. You know that she has been getting drunk pretty often lately, but you're not sure whether you should say something to her about it. What do you think you should do? What are some long- and short-term consequences for her health?

Life Skills Check

Sample responses:

1. Answers may include using the steps of the decision-making model to decide what to do in this situation.
2. Students should list each step of the decision-making model and record their thoughts, feelings, decisions, and/or behaviors at each step.

Life Skills Check

1. **Making Responsible Decisions** Terry is someone you've always wanted to be friends with, so you're pretty happy the two of you have started to do stuff together. Unfortunately, one thing Terry really likes to do most is skip class and go to the park. You haven't done it yet, but Terry wants the two of you to cut math class Friday. You don't want to miss the class; you have a quiz the next week, and you'd feel really funny about cutting a class anyway. But you also don't want to lose Terry's friendship. What would you do?
2. **Making Responsible Decisions** Some close friends of yours have started using drugs and alcohol on a regular basis. Using the steps of the decision-making model, decide whether you want to continue associating with this group of friends.

Projects

1. Design a bulletin board that displays the leading causes of death for Americans between the ages of 15 and 24, and for those between the ages of 55 and 64. Suggest ways to reduce the number of deaths from these causes.
2. Work with a group of students to come up with a list of problems for which the decision-making model might be useful. What issues would not be suitable for the model?
3. Write a short essay about how a person's values are important in a friendship. Include how your own values may have changed over the years.
4. Work with a partner to find magazine pictures that show people attempting to improve their quality of life. Create a collage on a poster board using the pictures you have found. Next to the collage, list the ways the people in the pictures are striving for a more satisfying life.

Plan for Action

Health involves many decisions. Think of some choices you can face through the use of the decision-making model.

Projects

Have students plan and carry out the projects for responsible decision making.

Plan for Action

Discuss with students decisions they will be making in the near future and how the decision-making model described in this chapter can be used to assist them. Have each student think of a decision that is coming up. Have the class suggest considerations for each step of the decision-making process. Ask the student how well the model fits his or her particular situation.

ASSESSMENT OPTIONS

Chapter Test
Have students take the Chapter 2 Test.

Alternative Assessment
Have students do the Alternative Assessment activity for Chapter 2.

Test Generator
The Test Generator (Macintosh® or IBM® format) contains an additional 50 assessment items for this chapter.

Issues in Health

EVALUATING MEDIA MESSAGES

What Is a Media Message?

Have students read the Evaluating Media Messages feature. Discuss with students their responses to the situation described: Have they ever felt they wanted something because of the image presented in an advertisement? Have they bought something based on media persuasion? Were they pleased with the decision? Or, have there been times when their best interests were not the same as those of the seller? If so, how could they be better prepared the next time they have such a decision to make?

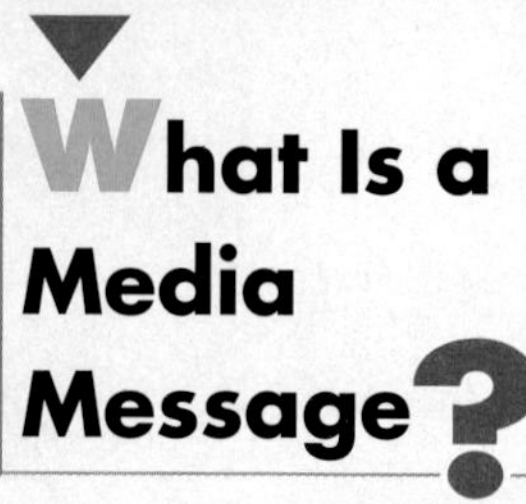

What Is a Media Message?

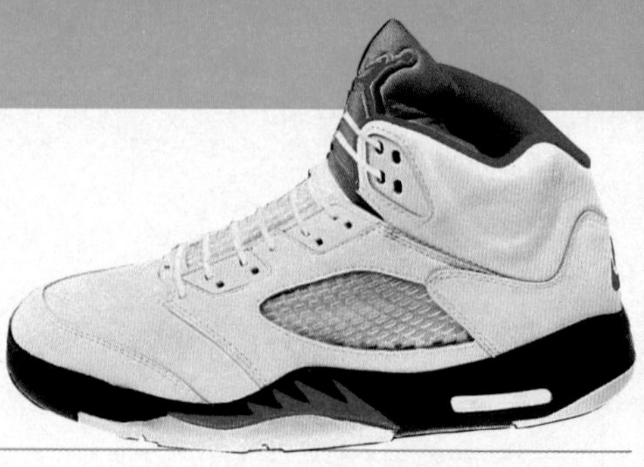

Mike needs some new athletic shoes. Like many of his friends, Mike wants a popular name brand endorsed by famous athletes. He loves to think that wearing those particular shoes will impress his friends and make him more popular at school. Unfortunately, the shoes cost three times as much money as Mike has to spend. When Mike asks his father if he will help with the purchase, his father says no.

''Come on, Dad,'' Mike says. ''All the NBA stars are wearing these shoes. They're the best!''

''That may be, Mike,'' his father replies, ''but they are not the best choice for you. They're just too expensive. Before you make a decision based only on the influence of a media message, why don't you do a little research on several kinds of shoes.''

''Okay, Dad,'' Mike agrees. ''But what's a media message, anyway?''

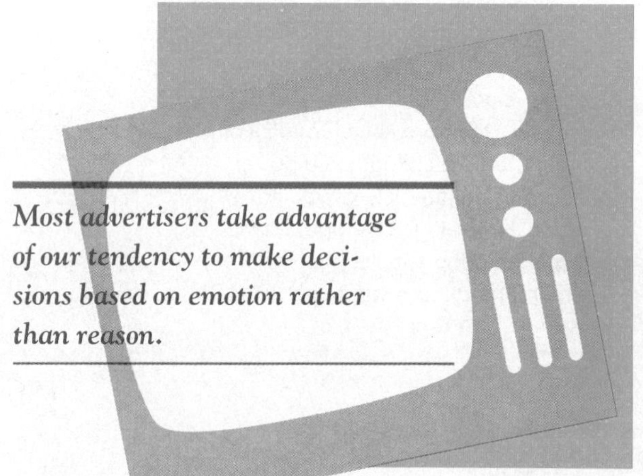

Most advertisers take advantage of our tendency to make decisions based on emotion rather than reason.

As Mike's father explained, media messages are the information conveyed by television, radio, magazines, newspapers, and other types of mass media (forms of communication that reach large numbers of people). They are found primarily in advertisements, television programs, and movies, but are also found in news stories, art, literature, and even rock music lyrics.

Media messages not only contain information but also express social values and persuade people to make judgments and to take certain actions. Because such messages reach so many people, they greatly affect people's opinions of what is normal, attractive, successful, and even healthy. Often, the forms of persuasion used in media messages encourage people to make decisions based on emotion rather than reason. Consequently, the purpose, source, and nature of any media message should be carefully evaluated before making a decision based on the message.

The ads that make Mike feel he must have a certain type of athletic shoes are examples of media messages designed to persuade. Some of the ads mention comfort, foot support, durability, and endorsements by medical experts, which are all logical reasons for buying a particular shoe. But many ads rely on visual images of athletes wearing that brand of athletic shoes. The athletes project an image of attractiveness and success that is emotionally appealing. By association, whatever the athlete is wearing, eating, or doing may be perceived as contributing to the athlete's attractiveness and success. This is why Mike feels that if he wears the same athletic shoes, he too will be attractive and successful.

All of us have a tendency to make decisions based on emotion rather than reason. Most advertisers take advantage of this tendency. When evaluating media messages like athletic-shoe ads, it is important to remember the purpose of the ads—to sell shoes and make money for the shoe companies. The athletes also make money by doing the ads. Such interests may conflict with the best interests of buyers.

Once Mike understood how and why he came to desire the expensive athletic shoes, he realized that he would rather base his decision on his own best interests. After making a list of several types of athletic shoes and their features, Mike talked to some of the coaches at school about how the different brands compare in terms of performance and durability. By applying the decision-making model he learned in health class, Mike finally chose a style that is more comfortable, lasts longer, and costs a lot less money than the brand he wanted originally.

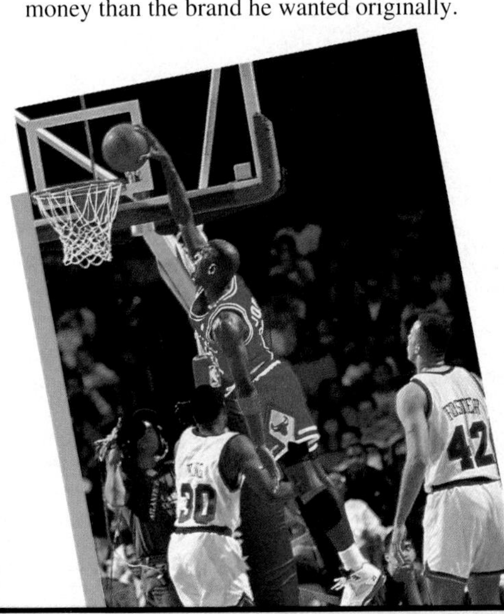

It also provides good foot support and looks great. Even though Mike's choice still costs more money than he has, it is clearly his best choice overall. And his father agreed to help with the purchase after all.

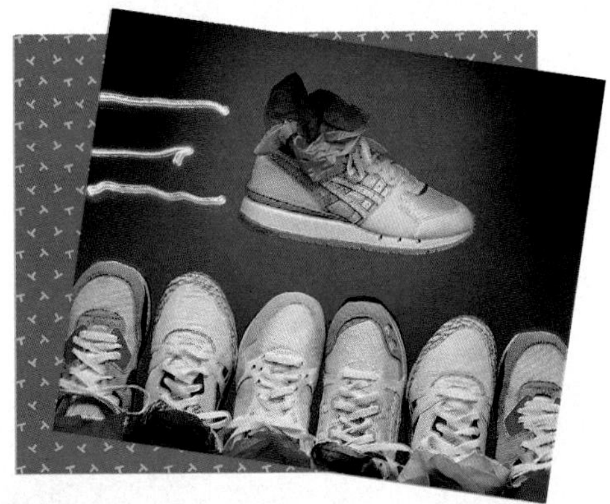

Critical Thinking

1. Find several ads for a common item such as a type of clothing, a toy, a kid's cereal, a type of sporting equipment, or an automobile. Analyze the ads for the media messages they convey.

- What information is given upfront?
- What information is unspoken or in the background?
- What type of media—print, radio, or television—does each ad use? Which do you think is the most effective?
- Does the ad appeal to your emotions or your sense of reason?
- Choose what you think is the best ad upon which to base a decision to buy.

2. For each ad you analyzed for item 1, ask yourself the following questions.

- How will I benefit if I buy what the ad is trying to sell?
- How will the advertiser benefit if I buy what the ad is trying to sell?

UNIT 2

Health and Your Body

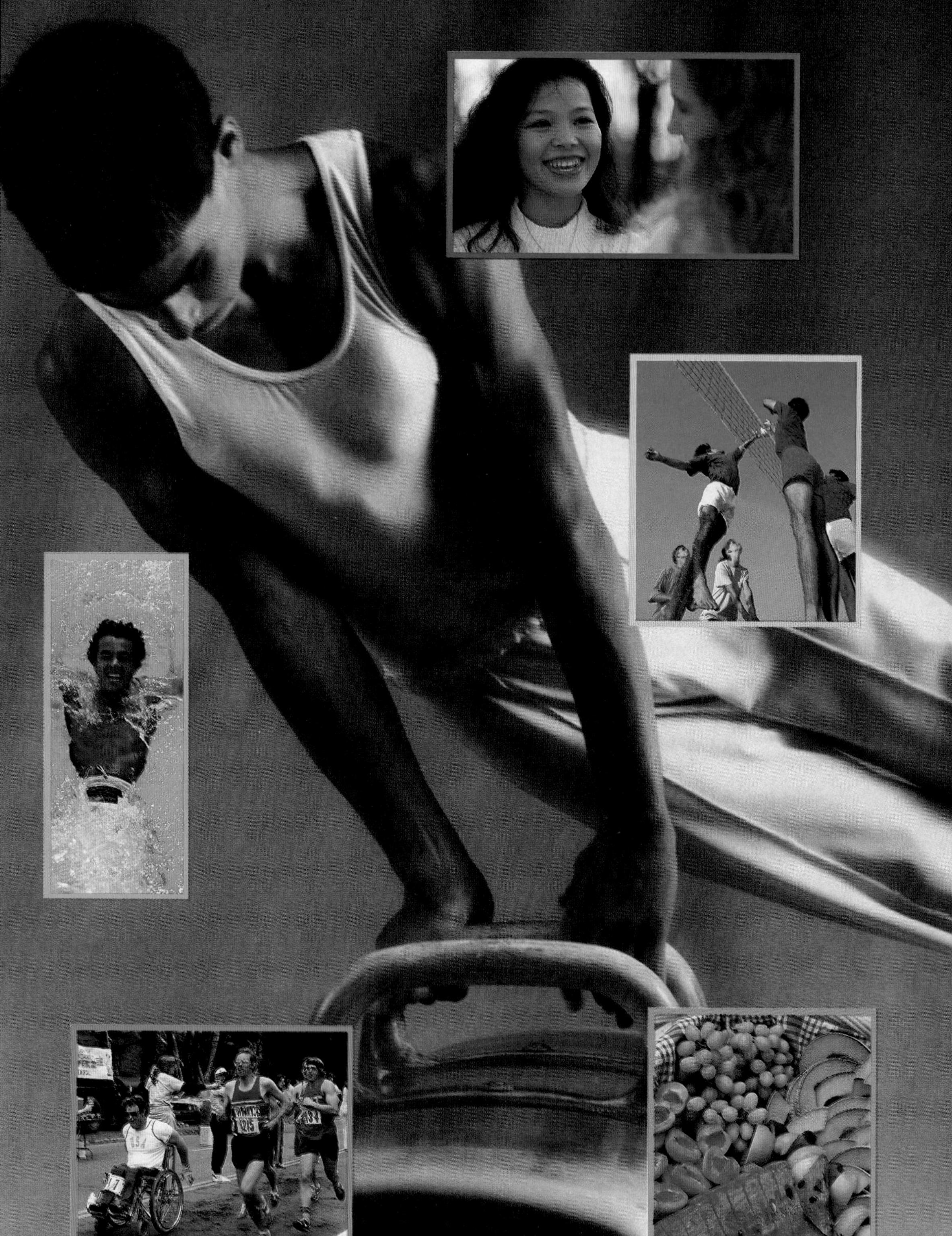

CHAPTER OVERVIEWS

CHAPTER 3

PHYSICAL FITNESS

This chapter explains the mental and physical benefits of exercise and describes the four categories of physical fitness. It explores ways to improve fitness and provides tests for judging it. The differences between aerobic and anaerobic exercise are explained, and examples are given. Students learn about the dangers of steroid abuse, how to avoid injury while exercising, and how to determine target heart rate. The chapter helps students set exercise goals and design an exercise schedule. It emphasizes the importance of sleep in maintaining fitness, explains the two categories of sleep, and provides suggestions for coping with insomnia.

CHAPTER 4

NUTRITION PRINCIPLES

The chapter opens with a discussion of how hunger, appetite, and environment affect food choices. This is followed by a thorough presentation of the functions of the essential nutrients and the problems that nutrient deficiencies can cause. Students learn to define their nutritional needs, classify foods into appropriate groups, and interpret food labels. This prepares them to apply guidelines in order to make healthy food choices and to understand the special nutritional needs of selected populations.

CHAPTER 5

WEIGHT MANAGEMENT AND EATING DISORDERS

Basic information about maintaining a healthy weight is presented in this chapter. Students learn how the body uses energy, how body composition helps to determine ideal weight, and how to lose or gain weight sensibly. Then they learn how to recognize eating disorders and avoid developing them. Next, students learn about disorders that affect the digestive system, ways to treat them, and the differences between food allergies and food intolerances.

CHAPTER 6

PERSONAL CARE AND APPEARANCE

Personal hygiene is important to self-esteem and to health. In this chapter, students learn to care for their skin, hair, nails, teeth, and gums. They also learn about the structure of the skin, hair, and teeth, and how to recognize and deal with skin, hair, and dental problems. In addition, students learn to choose a dentist and make a dental appointment.

UNIT TWO

HEALTH AND YOUR BODY

Chapter 3

Physical Fitness

Chapter 4

Nutrition Principles

Chapter 5

Weight Management and Eating Disorders

Chapter 6

Personal Care and Appearance

Unit Preview

The information presented in this unit will help students make good choices in exercise, eating, and personal care. They learn the components of physical fitness, the elements of a nutritious diet, how to determine an ideal weight, and how to care for their skin, hair, nails, teeth, and gums. Students also learn how to identify problems and are given suggestions for dealing with them. The five major health themes are emphasized throughout the unit, as indicated in the chart below.

Themes Trace

	WELLNESS	BUILDING SELF-ESTEEM	DECISION MAKING	DEVELOPING LIFE-MANAGEMENT SKILLS	ACCEPTANCE OF DIVERSITY AMONG PEOPLE
Chapter 3	p. 43		p. 53	pp. 44–45, 49, 61–62	pp. 40, 43
Chapter 4				pp. 68, 90–91, 94–100	pp. 69, 92–93
Chapter 5	p. 113	pp. 115–117	p. 116	pp. 109–112	p. 107
Chapter 6	p. 124	p. 135		pp. 128, 131–132, 134–135, 138–142	p. 125

PHYSICAL FITNESS

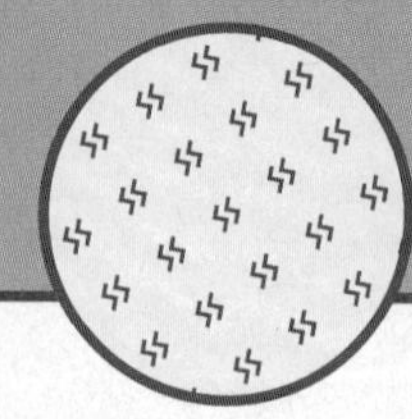

PLANNING GUIDE

TEXT SECTIONS	OBJECTIVES	TEXT FEATURES	OUTSIDE RESOURCES	NOTES
3.1 **Why Exercise?** pp. 39-43 2 periods	• Name three physical benefits of exercise. • Name two mental benefits of exercise. • Name the four categories of physical fitness.	**ASSESSMENT** • Section Review, p. 43	**TEACHER'S RESOURCE BINDER** • Lesson Plan 3.1 • Personal Health Inventory • Journal Entries 3A, 3B, 3C • Section Review Worksheet 3.1 • Section Quiz 3.1 • Reteaching Worksheet 3.1 **OTHER RESOURCES** • Transparency 3A • English/Spanish Audiocassette 2	
3.2 **How Physically Fit Are You?** pp. 44-45 2 periods	■ Know the ways to test physical fitness.	**ASSESSMENT** • Section Review, p. 45	**TEACHER'S RESOURCE BINDER** • Lesson Plan 3.2 • Journal Entries 3D, 3E • Section Review Worksheet 3.2 • Section Quiz 3.2 • Reteaching Worksheet 3.2	
3.3 **About Exercise** pp. 46-53 2 periods	• Know the difference between aerobic and nonaerobic exercise. • Name three examples of aerobic exercise. • Name three effects of steroid abuse. • Know what to do to avoid basic injuries. ■ Know the range of your target heart rate.	■ LIFE SKILLS: Assessing Your Health, p. 49 **ASSESSMENT** • Section Review, p. 53	**TEACHER'S RESOURCE BINDER** • Lesson Plan 3.3 • Journal Entries 3F, 3G, 3H, 3I, 3J • Life Skills 3A, 3B • Section Review Worksheet 3.3 • Section Quiz 3.3 • Reteaching Worksheet 3.3 **OTHER RESOURCES** • Making a Choice 3A, 3B	
3.4 **Getting Started** pp. 54-59 2 periods	• Set your exercise goals. • Design your own exercise schedule.	**ASSESSMENT** • Section Review, p. 59	**TEACHER'S RESOURCE BINDER** • Lesson Plan 3.4 • Journal Entries 3K, 3L • Section Review Worksheet 3.4 • Section Quiz 3.4 • Reteaching Worksheet 3.4 **OTHER RESOURCES** • Transparencies 3B, 3C	
3.5 **Sleep** pp. 60-62 2 periods	• Know the two different categories of sleep. • Describe what happens during each phase of the sleep cycle. • Name two ways to cope with insomnia. ■ Know how much sleep you need each night.	**ASSESSMENT** • Section Review, p. 62	**TEACHER'S RESOURCE BINDER** • Lesson Plan 3.5 • Journal Entries 3M, 3N • Section Review Worksheet 3.5 • Section Quiz 3.5 • Reteaching Worksheet 3.5	

■ Denotes LIFE SKILLS objectives

• Items in blue are also part of the *Holt Health Activity Book.*

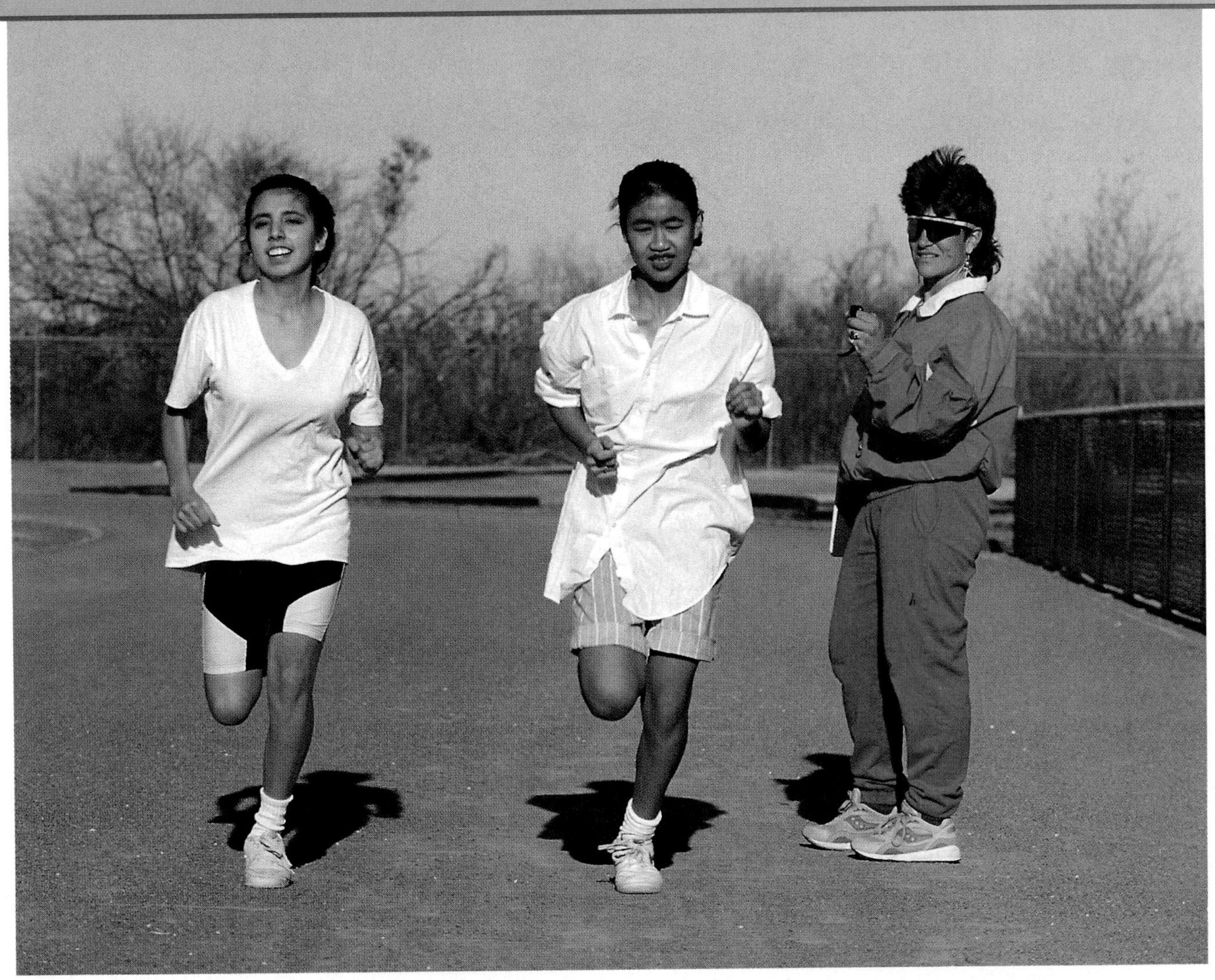

CONTENT BACKGROUND

Exercise and Adolescents

DURING THE 1988–89 SCHOOL YEAR, 4,050 of 9,000 young people aged 5 to 16 were able to pass four of the seven physical fitness tests that measured endurance, strength, and flexibility. The Amateur Athletic Union Youth Fitness Study of 12,000 teenagers in 1989 yielded similar statistics.

Some health and fitness experts who view these results as unsatisfactory blame excessive amounts of television—an average of 24 to 26 hours per week—viewed by children and adolescents. Others, however, fault "the system."

- **As many as one-third of all physical education instructors in the United States do not hold current certification in physical education. And because of budget constraints, most schools are not hiring physical education specialists.**
- **Studies by the U.S. Department of Health and Human Services have found that many elementary and middle schools in the United States are inappropriately substituting recess for physical education classes.**
- **Because of budget constraints, only about half of all the fifth- through twelfth-graders in the United States have physical education classes at least three days a week.**
- **Among students who have adequate facilities and equipment,**

fewer than half actively perform the 20 minutes of daily aerobic activity recommended by the American College of Sports Medicine.

- **The major reason for adolescent disinterest in sports and regular exercise, according to many teenagers, is that they don't enjoy activities in which too much emphasis is placed on winning and competing.**

The consensus among experts seems to be that we cannot expect our school systems to be the sole providers of exercise for children and adolescents today. Many communities are working with health and fitness experts to improve the quality of physical education in the schools and to help students discover and participate in extracurricular exercises and sports.

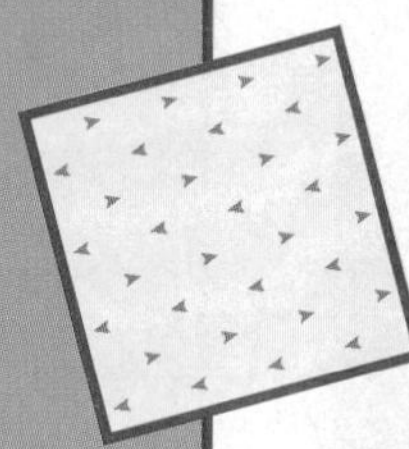

PLANNING FOR INSTRUCTION

KEY FACTS

- **Exercise benefits the body by providing more energy, creating a well-rested feeling, strengthening the bones, decreasing the level of cholesterol, lowering blood pressure, and reducing excess body fat.**
- **Exercise benefits the mind by reducing anxiety and depression. It causes an increase in the production of endorphins, which affect an individual's moods.**
- **Unlike anaerobic exercises that can be done for no more than a few minutes, aerobic exercises can be continued for a much longer time. Aerobic exercises help improve the respiratory and circulatory systems.**
- **Rules to remember when exercising: F stands for frequency—three or four times a week; I for intensity—at or slightly above the target heart rate; T for time—at least 30 minutes of continuous exercise, preceded by warming up and followed by cooling down.**
- **To treat basic injuries, follow the five simple actions known as PRICE: P (physician), R (rest), I (ice), C (compression), E (elevation).**
- **Anabolic steroids are illegal drugs that increase muscle size and body weight. They are dangerous because they cause several physical and behavioral problems.**
- **Sleep can be divided into two categories: NREM (nonrapid eye movement) sleep and REM (rapid eye movement) sleep. The more a person exercises, the more time he or she spends in stages III and IV of NREM sleep, during which more resting and restoring of the body occurs.**

MYTHS AND MISCONCEPTIONS

MYTH: There is no such thing as exercising too much.

Too much exercise can be harmful. People can become so addicted to exercise that it dominates their lives.

MYTH: If there is no pain while exercising, there is no gain in fitness.

Exercise can be effective without causing pain. Jogging, walking, and cycling improve fitness without causing pain.

MYTH: Just 10 minutes of aerobic exercise a day can help you become fit.

You must spend 20 to 30 minutes doing aerobic exercises to become fit.

MYTH: Muscle turns to fat when a person stops working out.

Muscle cannot turn to fat, because these are different kinds of tissue. Muscle can, on the other hand, lose its tone, which can make it look flabby.

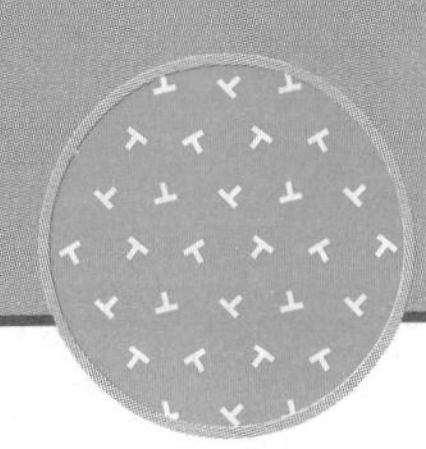

MYTH: Exercise alone can help you lose weight.
You must also reduce the amount of fattening food you consume in order to lose weight.

MYTH: A person can't be too thin.
Being underweight can be dangerous to a person's health when it is carried to an extreme, as in anorexia.

VOCABULARY

Essential: The following vocabulary terms appear in boldface type:

blood vessels
cholesterol
blood pressure
aerobic exercise
anaerobic exercise
anabolic steroid
brain waves
REM
insomnia

Secondary: Be aware that the following terms may come up during class discussion:

endorphins
physical fitness
aerobic fitness
flexibility
body composition

FOR STUDENTS WITH SPECIAL NEEDS

Visual Learners: Use aerobic fitness videos to demonstrate the typical exercises that will help students become fit. Make the videos available before or after class—if this complies with school policy—to students who may wish to work with others to achieve aerobic fitness. Find out which fitness videos are available at the library. Preview them to make sure they meet safety standards for the general public.

Auditory Learners: Invite members of a school team, preferably a male and a female athlete, to discuss their physical fitness tips with students. Ask students to prepare questions about fitness that they would like answered.

Kinetic Learners: Give students index cards with situations related to physical fitness that would lend themselves to role-playing or skits. Index cards might include a student who hates sports but knows that he or she needs physical exercise; a student who spends three hours a day watching television and gets no exercise; a friend who is discouraged because he diets but can't seem to lose weight.

ENRICHMENT

- Invite a fitness advocate who is not a well-known athlete but who can inspire students to make physical fitness a lifetime goal. You may want to invite a panel of people of various ages. Students may be able to suggest someone admired for his or her interest in fitness.
- Have students collect magazine articles about physical fitness. Have folders entitled "Being Fit," "Aerobic Exercises," and "Sleep and Dreams." Display the folders with the articles where students can read them. You may also wish to add a test question that allows students to discuss an item they read from the folders.

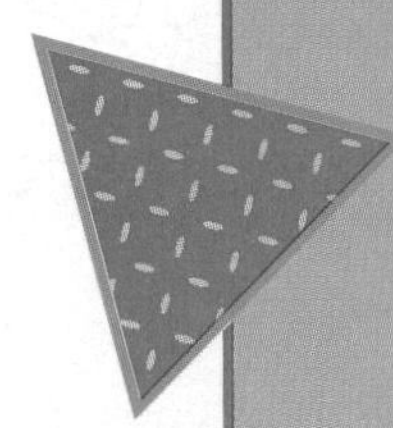

CHAPTER 3
CHAPTER OPENER

GETTING STARTED

Using the Chapter Photograph

Ask students if they think the basketball player in the picture is physically fit. Have them name the traits a physically fit person has. Ask them to discuss how the basketball player is an example of someone with desirable fitness traits. Tell them that the chapter will help them determine if they are physically fit. It will also help them improve their fitness skills, while at the same time bringing to light some of the misconceptions people have about keeping fit.

Question Box

Have students write out any questions they have about being physically fit and put them in the Question Box. The Question Box provides students with an opportunity to ask questions anonymously. To ensure that students with questions are not embarrassed to be seen writing, have students who do not have questions write something they already know about physical fitness on the paper instead.

Preview the questions and then answer them at appropriate points in the chapter. You may wish to allow students to write additional anonymous questions as they go through the chapter.

Personal Issues *ALERT*

When dealing with issues related to physical fitness, be aware of the feelings of students who are overweight and not physically fit. Although this section will deal with being fit, every care should be taken not to draw attention to someone who does not measure up to what is thought to be optimally fit. Students who are physically and mentally impaired may find a chapter on physical fitness particularly disturbing. Finally, some students may find it economically impossible to meet the equipment requirements for some physical activities. Try to discuss the value of activities that are within everyone's means.

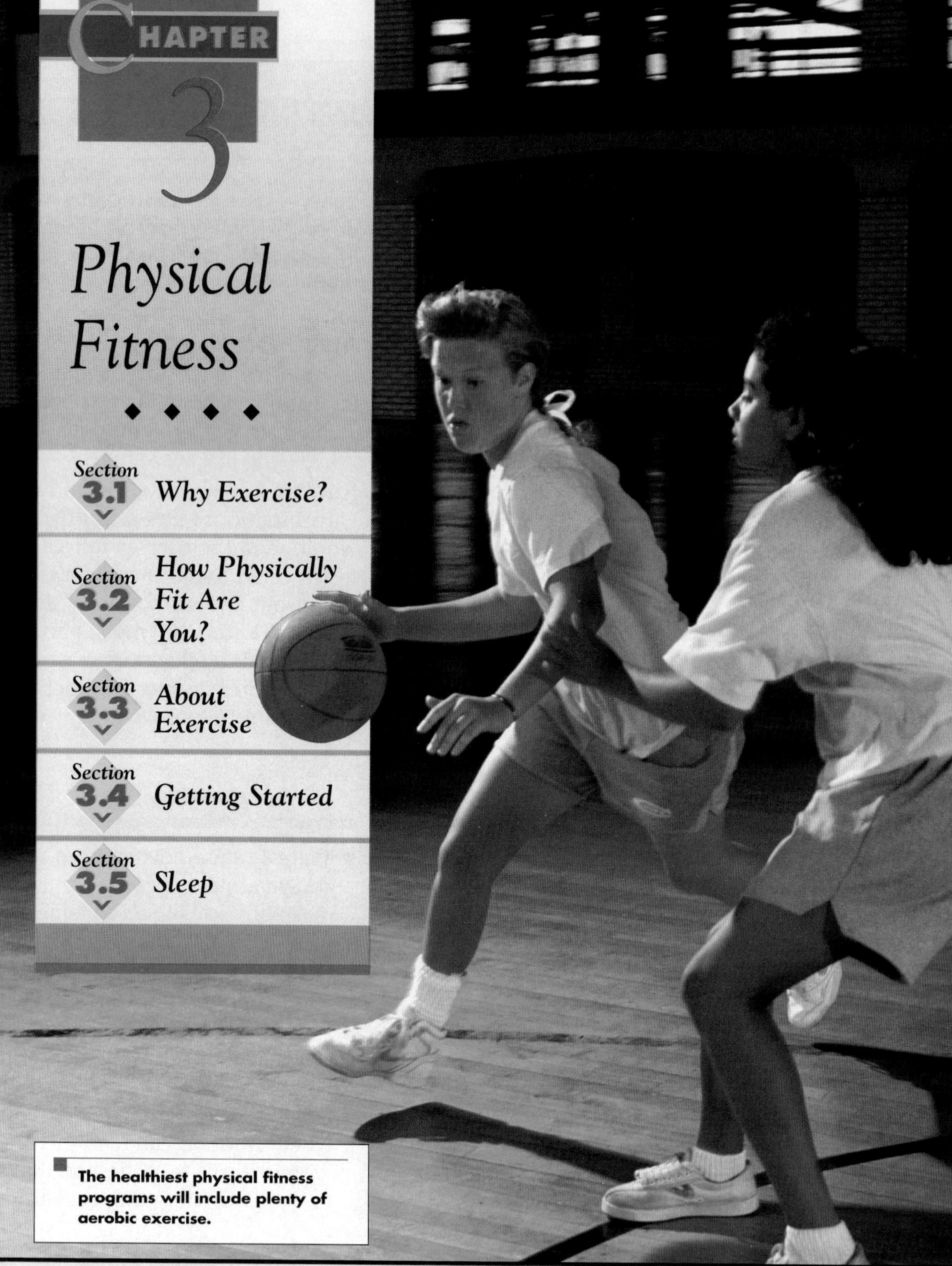

CHAPTER 3

Physical Fitness

The healthiest physical fitness programs will include plenty of aerobic exercise.

Christine can't seem to stay awake anymore. She has to drag herself out of bed every morning, and at school she sits bleary-eyed in class, counting seconds until the bell rings. After staring into space at her after-school job, she barely begins her homework before nodding off, at around 8 P.M. Her friends, family, and teachers have noticed that she's been acting strange lately, and Christine herself is concerned about her lack of energy.

She's also worried about the layer of fat that she has recently noticed on her stomach and the back of her arms. Christine knows that having some body fat is perfectly normal, but she also realizes that she has been eating too many sweets between meals. She wonders whether her busy, stressful life has something to do with her constant exhaustion and huge appetite. Then one day it dawns on her that she can't remember the last time she got any exercise.

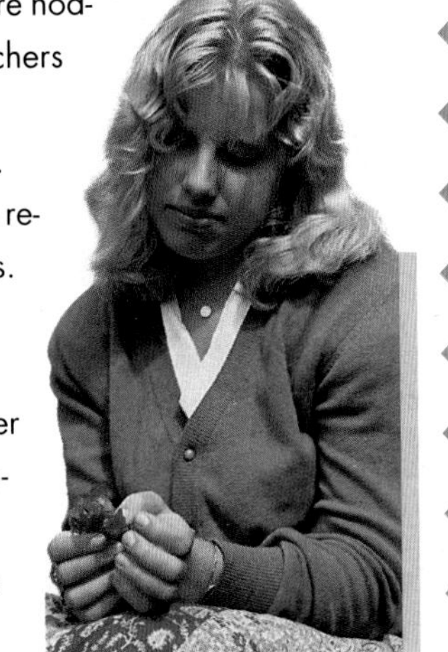

Section 3.1 Why Exercise?

Objectives

- *Name three physical benefits of exercise.*
- *Name two mental benefits of exercise.*
- *Name the four categories of physical fitness.*

You've probably heard all about how good exercise is for you. You know that it can help you develop muscles and lose weight. What you may not realize is that regular exercise helps you cope better with the stress and anxiety you probably face every day, and that it greatly increases your energy level. It can even help you avoid some serious diseases later on in life.

Some people like to exercise more than others. If you're the wide receiver on your school football team, you will have an easier time figuring out how to be physically active than if you hate the thought of lacing up a pair of sneakers. But exercising regularly does not have to mean competing against the best athletes in your class or taking a swimming lesson when it's freezing outside. Walking for half an hour before supper, or biking to school instead of taking the bus, is often enough to give your body the exercise it needs.

Background

The Medical Benefits of Exercise

Exercise is credited by research teams for preventing and sometimes curing several diseases and conditions of the body. Osteoporosis is one such disease. It is caused by a loss of minerals in the bones and results in brittle bones that break easily. Bones need physical exercise to keep them strong. Exercise increases bone mass, as evidenced by a study of the bones of athletes. This effect of exercise may offset the damaging results of osteoporosis.

Research seems to indicate that some kinds of cancer may be prevented by exercise. A study followed graduates of Harvard University over 20 years. Those who led sedentary lives were more likely to die of cancer than those who were active. This may be attributed to smaller amounts of body fat in those who exercised. Since body fat is related to the development of some cancers, this may be why those who exercise are not as likely to grow cancerous tissue.

Section 3.1 Lesson Plan

MOTIVATE

Journal 3A
Am I Physically Fit?

This may be done as a warm-up activity. Encourage students to write in the Student Journal in the Student Activity Book their feelings about becoming involved in a physical fitness program and about whether they think they are already physically fit.

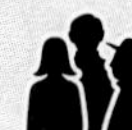

Cooperative Learning
Feeling Tired

Have students form small groups to discuss Christine's problem of being tired all the time. Ask them to discuss the following questions: How would you categorize Christine's condition? Have you ever felt as she does? What do you think was the basic cause of Christine's problem? What might happen if she continues in this way for a long period of time? What could she do to improve her condition? What experiences have you had that prove that exercise can help you feel less tired?

TEACH

Class Discussion
Benefits of Physical Fitness

Write on the chalkboard: Becoming more physically fit can improve your quality of life. Ask: **What are some examples that support this statement?** *[When a person is alert and feeling ener-*

Background
Endorphins

Exercise induces the brain to increase its release of endorphins into the bloodstream. Intense activity is necessary to trigger the release of these chemicals. When an activity uses 60 percent of the maximum possible intake of oxygen, it causes significant elevations in endorphins. With similar exercise, comparable increases in endorphins occur in both males and females. The response is similar at any age.

Endorphins are neuropeptides that seem to regulate emotional responses in the brain. They act both as neurotransmitters and as hormones and are known to decrease the sensation of pain. The fact that the brain releases additional endorphins as the result of physical exertion may explain why people feel better when they exercise.

The Benefits of Exercise

Christine bought an exercise tape and started working out four times a week. It surprised her how quickly she started feeling better. Her energy level bounced back to normal, and she found it hard to believe that at one time she could barely stay conscious until early evening. By combining physical workouts with a new diet of nutritious, low-fat foods, she began to lose the extra weight.

In addition, Christine forgot that her days were once filled with depression and anxiety. Her dark moods lifted, and she no longer woke up in the morning with a sense of dread in the pit of her stomach. Her exercise routine became a part of her day-to-day life, so she no longer had to force herself to do the activities that improved her physical and mental well-being so dramatically.

Not everyone will get the same benefits from exercise as Christine. It could be that your body will not respond as easily or as quickly to physical activity. In addition, many teenagers are depressed or anxious—not because they haven't exercised, but because something is happening at school or at home that may be troubling them. If you are feeling sad or stressed out, and you don't think it has anything to do with the amount of exercise you've been getting, you may want to talk to someone, like a teacher, a coach, or a counselor. See Chapter 7, Mental and Emotional Health, for more information on this.

For more information on where to seek help for anxiety and depression, see Chapter 7.

Physical Benefits Many people who suddenly decide to exercise regularly do so because they want to lose weight. They have heard that exercise burns calories, and many of them think if they exercise enough, they can eat what they want and still lose weight healthfully. They're partly correct. Exercise does burn calories, and it shrinks the size of your fat cells. Even so, the healthiest way to lose weight is to eat a nutritious diet as well as get plenty of exercise. If you combine regular exercise with sound nutrition, as Christine did, not only will you lose excess body fat, but you'll add muscle weight, and become stronger. Dieting without exercise can help you lose weight, but you may risk losing muscle tissue as well as fat tissue. Before you decide on the need to lose weight, however, keep in mind that it's perfectly normal to gain a few pounds during this time of your life. In fact, it would be unusual and even a bit strange if you didn't. All healthy adults have some fat on their bodies, particularly around the hips and abdomen. In addition, some people are heavier than others as a result of genetic, or inherited, factors, and may not lose weight easily even with regular exercise and a low-fat diet.

Regular exercise gives you more energy. It may seem strange that doing strenuous activities would actually make you *less* tired, but exercise tends to make changes in your body that help your heart, lungs, and muscles work more efficiently. When you exercise, your blood vessels expand, which helps your blood circulate more freely. In addition, your heart grows larger and stronger, and your resting heart rate slows down. Even though your heart is pumping more slowly, you're still getting the same amount of blood to the muscles, because with each stroke your heart is now pumping more blood than it was previously.

Because your heart does not have to work as hard as it did before, and because your blood is circulating more freely, your body does not get as tired as it would if you were not exercising regularly. You also don't have to breathe as often, because like your heart, your lung volume gets bigger and it can do the job of transferring oxygen into the body much more efficiently when you exercise. As a result, you'll feel not only more energetic, but more calm as well.

• • • TEACH continued

getic, he or she can think better and respond better to other people. An energetic person can learn with less effort in school and can be more cooperative at home and at work.] Record student contributions on the chalkboard. Ask students to suggest activities they enjoy that give them a beneficial physical workout. Discuss the effects of exercise on Christine—how she felt after she began using the exercise tape.

Have students distinguish between the physical and psychological benefits of exercise. Point out that not all psychological problems are due to lack of exercise but that exercise might be a help if they cannot decide what is making them feel depressed.

Cooperative Learning
What Makes an Athlete Great?

After students read about the physical benefits of exercise, ask them to discuss what surprised them most about the effects of exercise. Have them share any personal experiences that document how beneficial exercise can be.

Teaching Transparency 3A
Percentage of Fat in Physically Fit Bodies

Use the "Percentage of Fat in Physically Fit Bodies" transparency to complete the material on losing weight as a benefit of exercising and dieting. It shows the percentage of males' and females' body weight that should be fat. Have students calculate the amount of fat in

Exercise can do more for your body. Doing regular exercises like walking, jogging, running, and most other sports activities can help your bones get bigger, stronger, and less likely to break or fracture. There are also body changes that you can't see or feel. For example, exercise can lower your **cholesterol** level. Cholesterol is a waxy substance found in the body's cells. High levels of blood cholesterol can cause plaque, or particles of fat, to form on the inside of your artery walls, which can clog up your blood vessels and lead to a heart attack. Plaque can begin to build up in your blood while you're still young. But if you exercise and eat right, you can slow down this buildup.

Regular physical activity can also help lower blood pressure, or the force with which the blood pushes against the inside of the blood vessels. If left untreated, **high blood pressure** can lead to heart failure.

Finally, the more exercise you get, the lower your chances are of having conditions such as osteoporosis (a loss of bone mass), which often occur during the aging process.

cholesterol: *a waxy, fatlike substance that can block the arteries and cause heart disease.*

high blood pressure: *a condition in which the blood pushes harder than normal against the inside of the blood vessels.*

Myths and Facts About Exercise

MYTH	FACT
No pain, no gain.	Exercise doesn't have to hurt in order to be effective. Jogging, walking, or cycling at a pace that allows you to carry on a normal conversation, for example, will improve your aerobic fitness without pain.
Just 10 minutes of aerobic exercise a day can help you get fit.	You must spend at least 20 to 30 minutes doing a given aerobic activity if you want it to be effective.
When you stop working out, your muscle will turn to fat.	It is impossible for muscle to turn into fat, because muscle and fat are two different kinds of tissue.
There is no such thing as exercising too much.	Too much exercise can be unhealthy. Make sure that exercise is part of your life, but don't let it dominate every thought. Believe it or not, people have become addicted to exercise.
You can't be too thin.	Being underweight is possible, and can be very dangerous. If you do think you need to lose weight, set limits for yourself. Remember that you're dieting and exercising for your health. Overdoing either one can defeat this purpose.

(FIGURE 3-1) **Not everything you hear about exercise is true. Here are some examples of some popular but untrue statements.**

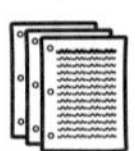

Personal Health Inventory

Have students complete the Personal Health Inventory for this chapter. The inventory helps them assess their physical fitness and safety awareness.

Section Review Worksheet 3.1

Assign Section Review Worksheet 3.1, which requires students to recognize the physical and mental benefits of exercise and also the four categories of physical fitness.

Section Quiz 3.1

Have students take Section Quiz 3.1.

a 150-pound male and in a 115-pound female. Suggest that students calculate the weight of fat in their own bodies.

Demonstration
Exercise and Your Lungs

Give students a new balloon to blow up. Most will find that at first the balloon resists being blown up. After several attempts, blowing up the balloon becomes very easy. Ask students to compare a new balloon to the lungs of someone not used to exercise. Have them compare the lungs of someone who exercises regularly to the balloons that were blown up again and again. Lung volume increases with exercise, and oxygen is transferred into the body more efficiently.

Journal 3B
Coping With the Blues

Have students write in the Student Journal what they usually do to try to get over a bad mood or feeling depressed. Ask them to describe how successful their method is and how long it takes to work.

Role-Playing
Dealing With Stress

Have students role-play a situation in which one member of the group is upset after an argument with a friend or relative. It is the afternoon before final exams and the upset person is unable to concentrate on studying. Other members of the group offer suggestions on how to help calm down the person who is upset. They should emphasize what they have learned about

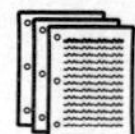

Reteaching Worksheet 3.1

Students who have difficulty with the material may complete Reteaching Worksheet 3.1, which requires the students to complete a concept map showing the physical and mental benefits of exercise. It also requires them to recognize the four categories of physical fitness.

endorphin: *a substance that is produced inside the brain and has pleasurable effects. Exercise can stimulate the production of endorphins.*

physical fitness: *the ability to perform daily tasks vigorously and to perform physical activities while avoiding diseases related to a lack of activity.*

Mental Benefits Studies have shown that aerobic exercise helps people with emotional problems control their mood swings. So it makes some sense that doing physical activity can help everyone cope with everyday anxiety and occasional, mild forms of depression. Exercise is good for your mental well-being for several reasons. First of all, knowing that you are doing something healthy for your body is very satisfying. Second, studies show that exercise improves your mood. According to research, certain types of physical activity may cause your brain to manufacture hormones called **endorphins**, which are natural substances that make you feel good. Vigorous physical activity helps your body produce greater amounts of endorphins, which may be part of the reason why people who get exercise on a regular basis are often more emotionally stable and more confident than those who don't.

People who are physically fit also tend to be less nervous and less stressed. Exercise relaxes your muscles and eases anxiety, which not only helps you cope with tensions during the day but also lets you put them aside at night, when you're trying to sleep. This is one reason why people who exercise regularly sleep better than those who don't. Another is that they are more tired. Physical activity may give you more energy during the day, but it makes you more tired at the right time—at night. You'll learn more about sleep later on in this chapter.

What's Physical Fitness?

Ask a few experts what **"physical fitness"** means, and you may very well get a few different answers. Most experts do agree that people who are physically fit (1) perform their day-to-day tasks with energy and vigor and (2) can participate in a variety of physical activities. They can do these while staying relatively clear of diseases related to a lack of exercise. Physical fitness can be divided into four categories:

- aerobic fitness
- muscular strength and endurance
- flexibility
- body composition

Aerobic Fitness Aerobic fitness refers to your body's ability to endure 10 minutes or more of continuous exercise. By definition, aerobic exercises are actions that increase the heart rate and supply oxygen to the muscles. They range from solitary activities such as walking or jogging to competitive sports such as basketball and soccer.

Muscular Strength and Endurance Muscular strength refers to the amount of force you can generate at one time; muscular endurance is the amount of force you can generate repeatedly for an extended period. Attempting to lift a 300-pound sofa alone requires tremendous muscular strength; unloading four hundred, 50-pound bags of potatoes takes great muscular endurance. Exercises that force the muscles to push against a force heavier than they normally meet can easily develop both of these.

Flexibility Flexibility refers to your body's ability to extend and flex its major joints. Young people are usually more flexible than adults, but it's a good idea to include stretching in your exercise program regardless of your age. Having a high level of flexibility will not give you bigger muscles or better endurance. It *can*, however, help prevent injury—as important a factor as anything else when it comes to exercise.

Body Composition Body composition refers to the proportion of fat and muscle mass in your body, which changes according to your eating and exercise habits. Of course, the more you exercise, the more muscle and less fat you will have.

• • • TEACH continued

the role of exercise on the production of endorphins. After each role-playing skit, you may want students to discuss how the advice given during the role-play would work for them when they are upset.

Journal 3C
What Is Physical Fitness?

Ask students to write in the Student Journal what they think physical fitness means. Have them list any categories that they think physical fitness would include.

Game
Name the Category

Try this game after students have read about the four categories of physical fitness. Divide the class into groups and provide each group with a stack of cards. On each card list one of the four categories of physical fitness or an activity that helps a person achieve a particular category of physical fitness. Each team member selects a card. If the card has the name of a category, the player must name an activity that achieves that category of fitness. If the card has the name of an activity, the player must name the category of physical fitness the activity will foster.

Extension
Promoting Physical Fitness in Gym

Encourage students to discuss with their physical education teacher what activities he or she uses in class to promote proficiency in each of the four categories of physical fitness.

Another way to think of physical fitness is to consider it in terms of your own needs and goals. If you are in good physical condition, you should be able to perform your everyday tasks without getting too tired to function. If you find that, like Christine, you're yawning at your desk a lot, you have trouble relaxing, and even low levels of exertion exhaust you, your physical fitness level may be lower than it should be. What about mood swings? Do you get depressed or anxious easily? These may also be symptoms of a lack of physical fitness, and they can disappear quickly if treated with a program of regular exercise.

Physical Fitness and Physical Disabilities

Have you ever tried pushing yourself in a wheelchair for 26 miles? Or sprinting for 100 meters with one real leg? How about pitching to major-league hitters when you have only one hand? Chances are you haven't. But think for a moment of how difficult these activities are, and then ask yourself: Can having a physical disability prevent a person from being physically fit?

Sharon Hedrick, Dennis Oehler, and Jim Abbott know the answer to that question. Hedrick, a double-amputee, used tremendous arm and shoulder strength to push her wheelchair to victory in an exhibition marathon race at the 1988 Olympics in Seoul, South Korea. Oehler, who lost his right leg in an automobile accident, wears a prosthesis, or an artificial leg. His time of 12.01 seconds in the 100-meter dash is a world record for athletes with disabilities, and is only 2 seconds slower than that of two-time Olympic champion Carl Lewis, who has two legs. Being born without a right hand did not stop Abbott, who is able both to throw and catch with his left hand, from winning 18 games for the California Angels in 1991.

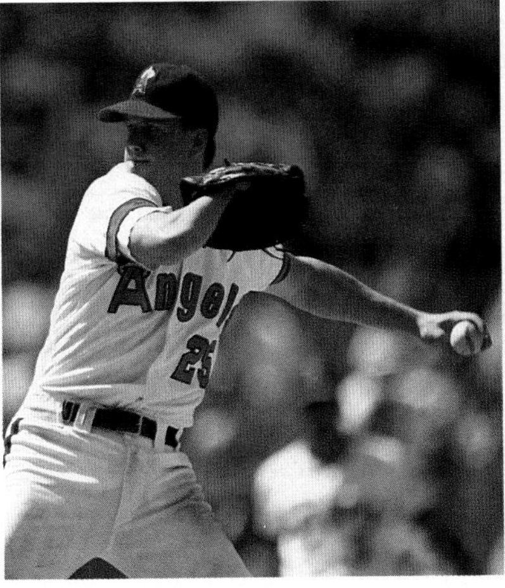

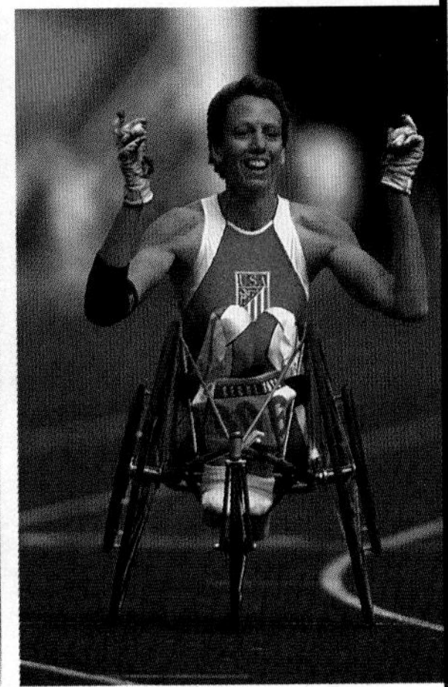

(FIGURE 3-2) **Jim Abbott (left), who is missing a right hand, is a major-league pitcher. Double-amputee Sharon Hedrick (right) is a champion wheelchair marathoner.**

Of course, you don't have to perform athletic miracles in order to be in good physical condition. Most people who are physically fit could not win 18 games in the Major Leagues, but they do know how to keep themselves healthy. And just as physical disabilities do not stop world-class athletes from achieving greatness, they do not block people who want to be in good physical condition from doing so. Most important, the state of wellness—of being physically, emotionally, and spiritually healthy—is a realistic, reachable goal every person is capable of achieving. People with physical disabilities have as much chance as anyone does of leading long, full, healthy, and happy lives.

Review

1. *Name two physical benefits and two mental benefits of exercise.*
2. *What are the four categories of physical fitness?*
3. ***Critical Thinking*** *Why is it important to be physically fit?*

Review Answers

1. Physical benefits include increase in energy level; weight loss; more efficient heart, lungs, and muscles; better circulation; increase in heart size and strength; decrease in resting heart rate; increase in bone strength; increase in muscle size and strength; lower blood cholesterol levels; and lower blood pressure. Mental benefits include ability to cope better with stress and anxiety; better control of mood swings; improvement in overall mood; more emotionally stable and confident; and better able to sleep.

2. Aerobic fitness, muscular strength and endurance, flexibility, body composition

3. Answers will vary. Accept any answer that shows an understanding of the benefits of being physically fit. The students may answer that being physically fit improves overall physical health, helps control weight, improves mental health and well-being, helps control stress and anxieties, increases energy levels during the day, and enables one to sleep better at night.

ASSESS

Section Review

Have students answer the Section Review questions.

Alternative Assessment

Why Be Fit?

Ask students to explain in their own words what it means to be physically fit. Have them list the disadvantages of being unfit.

Closure

Giving Yourself Good Advice

Have students write letters to themselves from the point of view of a friend who wants to encourage them to join a fitness group. Tell them the letters should include advice on how they could become more physically fit.

Background
Body Composition

Body composition refers to the ratio of muscle tissue to fat tissue. Body composition affects health, longevity, and quality of life. It is improved by aerobic and anaerobic activities, since exercise develops muscle tissue and reduces fat tissue. Research indicates that body composition may be closely related to one's susceptibility to life-threatening diseases.

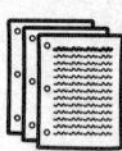

Section Review Worksheet 3.2

Assign Section Review Worksheet 3.2, which requires students to complete a form that contains directions for assessing physical fitness.

Section Quiz 3.2

Have students take Section Quiz 3.2.

Section 3.2 How Physically Fit Are You?

Objectives

- *Know the ways to test physical fitness.*
  - ***LIFE SKILLS: Assessing Your Health***

Before you plan your exercise program, take some time to figure out whether you're physically fit. Here are some simple tests you can do to determine at what level of exercise you need to begin.

aerobic fitness: *the ability to endure at least 10 minutes of strenuous activity.*

Aerobic Fitness

Next time you're on your school track, run or walk one mile as quickly as you can. Then check your results against Figure 3-3, Aerobic Fitness Standards.

After you have finished the exercise, place the middle and index fingers of your right hand on your wrist, just below the base of your left thumb. Can you feel your pulse? Using the second hand on a watch, count the beats for 15 seconds. Now multiply that number by four to determine your beats per minute. Normal rates generally range between 100 and 140.

muscular strength and endurance: *the muscles' ability to push against a very heavy force over a short period of time (strength) or to apply force over a sustained period (endurance).*

Muscular Strength and Endurance

Lie on your back, keeping your knees bent at a 90-degree angle and your feet flat on the floor. Place your left hand on your right shoulder, and your right hand on your left shoulder. Sit up until your shoulders are off the ground. As you are lifting your shoulders, bring your knees in toward your elbows. Now lie down until your shoulders

Aerobic Fitness Test Standards: One-Mile Walk/Run

Check the time it takes you to walk or run one mile against these standards to determine your aerobic fitness.

Age	Minimum Standard for Boys	Minimum Standard for Girls
12	10 minutes	12 minutes
13	9 minutes, 30 seconds	11 minutes, 30 seconds
14-16	8 minutes, 30 seconds	10 minutes, 30 seconds
17-19	8 minutes	9 minutes, 30 seconds

(FIGURE 3-3) **Check the time it takes you to walk or run one mile against these standards to determine your aerobic fitness.**

Section 3.2 Lesson Plan

MOTIVATE

Journal 3D
Counting Heartbeats

This may be done as a warm-up activity. Have students find their pulse by placing three fingers on their wrist. Tell them to count and record in the Student Journal the number of their heartbeats in 30 seconds. They should multiply the result by two to find their heart rate per minute. Tell students that they will be recording their heart rate from time to time for comparison, since it may change as they follow a fitness plan.

TEACH

Cooperative Learning
Test Yourself

Test for muscular endurance: Have volunteers demonstrate the proper method for doing the bent-knee sit-up. Let students work in pairs to test themselves on their muscular endurance while their partners hold their feet. Have them record their number of sit-ups in the Student Journal.

Test for flexibility: Have volunteers demonstrate the test, and then allow students to work in pairs when taking the test. Have them record in the Student Journal the number of inches they can reach.

Test for body composition: Have students do this test on themselves.

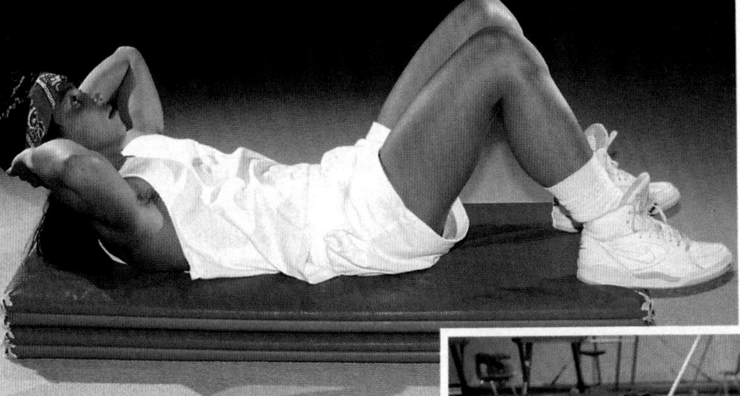

(FIGURE 3-4) **In order to test your muscular strength and endurance, see how many sit-ups you can complete in one minute.**

(FIGURE 3-5) **The more flexible you are, the farther you can reach your arms beyond your feet in this "box test."**

touch the floor. You've just completed one sit-up. Girls should be able to do between 33 and 35, and boys between 40 and 44, sit-ups in one minute.

To test your upper-body strength and endurance, grasp a horizontal bar, keeping your arms and legs straight and your palms facing outward. The bar should be high enough so that your feet don't touch the floor. Now use your arms to raise your body until your chin is above the bar. Girls should be able to do one pull-up, and boys three to five, without stopping.

Flexibility

Before testing your **flexibility**, take some time to stretch your lower-back and hamstring muscles to keep yourself from getting injured. Now sit on the floor with your legs straight in front of you and your feet flat against a box. Bend forward from your waist, and stretch your arms as far out as you can. If you're flexible, you should be able to stretch your hands between 1 and 4 inches past your feet in this "box test."

Body Composition

Grasp a fold of skin from your abdomen with your thumb and forefinger. Now test the flesh on your upper arm, your thigh, and the back of your lower leg. If you can pinch more than an inch in any of these areas, you may want to change your diet and also get more exercise.

Review

1. ***LIFE SKILLS: Assessing Your Health*** *What are four ways to test physical fitness?*
2. *What areas of fitness do you need to improve?*
3. ***Critical Thinking*** *Why is it a good idea to test your level of physical fitness before you begin an exercise program?*

flexibility: *the ability to move muscles and joints through their full range of motion.*

body composition: *the division of the total body weight into fat weight and muscle weight.*

Reteaching Worksheet 3.2

Students who have difficulty with the material may complete Reteaching Worksheet 3.2, which requires students to write directions for measuring pulse rate and body fat.

Review Answers

1. Aerobic—check the time it takes you to run or walk one mile; muscular strength and endurance—see how many sit-ups and/or pull-ups you can complete in one minute; flexibility—see how far you can reach your arms beyond your feet in the box test; body composition—check to see if you can pinch more than an inch in the pinch-an-inch test
2. Answers will vary according to each individual student's level of fitness.
3. Answers will vary. Accept any reasonable answer. Some answers might include that by knowing your level of fitness you will know at what level to start and how to better structure an exercise program to improve the areas of weakness.

Extension
Your Mental Outlook

Invite a fitness instructor to speak on the subject of exercise and its relationship to one's appearance and to one's mental outlook.

ASSESS

Section Review

Have students answer the Section Review questions.

Alternative Assessment
What's Wrong With Sitting Still?

Ask students to write an article entitled "Inactivity Is Hazardous to Your Health" for the school newspaper.

Closure
Setting Goals

Ask students to write in the Student Journal their feelings about their own physical fitness and how they think they can improve.

Background
Health Effects of Aerobic Exercises

Kenneth Cooper has studied the effects of aerobic exercise on health and has written extensively about his experiments. See Cooper, Kenneth H., *The Aerobics Program for Total Well-Being* (New York: M. Evans & Co., 1982). Cooper has identified 31 different aerobic exercises, giving them point values and charting them according to age categories, while differentiating between goals for men and women.

Background
Potential and Performance

Although aerobic potential is set by heredity, aerobic performance can continue to improve with training. The reason for this seeming contradiction is that training allows a higher percentage of a person's aerobic capacity to be maintained for a longer period of time. Capacity does not change after one's potential has been reached, but physiological adaptations permit the body to function closer and closer to its maximum capability.

Section 3.3 About Exercise

Objectives

- *Know the difference between aerobic and anaerobic exercise.*
- *Name three examples of aerobic exercise.*
- *Name three effects of steroid abuse.*
- *Know what to do to avoid basic injuries.*
- *Know the range of your target heart rate.*
  - ***LIFE SKILLS: Assessing Your Health***

You have just found out that physical fitness is divided into four categories. You should also know that exercise has different subsets as well:

- **aerobic exercises** are physical activities that continue for more than 10 minutes.
- **anaerobic exercises** are intense, all-out actions that last from a few seconds to a few minutes.

Aerobic Exercises

aerobic exercise: *physical activity that increases the heart rate and supply of oxygen to the muscles, and that can be continued for a period of time without resting.*

Aerobic exercise is the most important, most healthy thing you can do for your body. Every time you run, walk, bike, or do any kind of aerobic activity for an extended amount of time, you breathe rapidly and your heartbeat temporarily increases. When this happens your lungs transfer more oxygen to your bloodstream. But most important, aerobic activity lowers your heart rate and increases your breathing rate, which can help your respiratory and circulatory systems stay healthy. For these reasons, you should make sure you include at least one of the following aerobic exercises in your exercise schedule, no matter what your ultimate physical fitness goal is.

Walking Walking may seem too easy to be really good for you, but walking a mile or two every day burns calories and may stimulate the production of endorphins. These are a few reasons why walking regularly can make you feel so good. Another reason is that because this type of exercise does not take much mental power, it allows you time

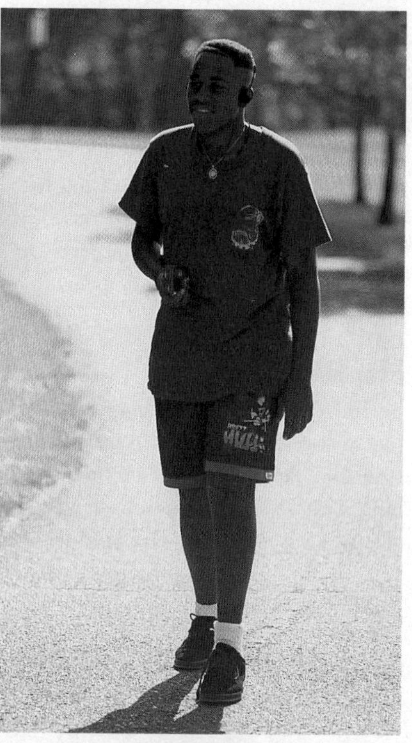

(FIGURE 3-6) **Walking for an hour or so is a good way to exercise your muscles and relax your mind.**

Section 3.3 Lesson Plan

MOTIVATE

Journal 3F
Starting Points

This may be done as a warm-up activity. Ask students to use the Student Journal to record how they would feel about starting an exercise program if they were (1) in poor physical shape, (2) in fairly good shape, (3) on the varsity basketball team, or (4) physically impaired. Have them write how they would motivate someone in each of the groups to begin exercising.

TEACH

Class Discussion
Benefits of Aerobic Exercise

Write on the chalkboard: *Aerobic exercise is the most healthy thing you can do for your body.* Make a fish-bone map to record the reasons students offer to explain why this statement is true.

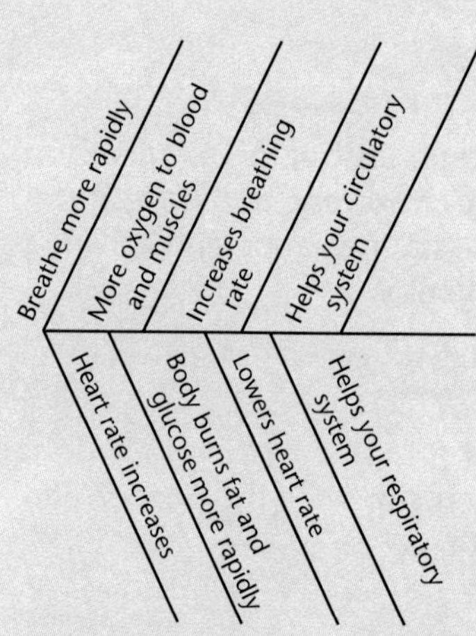

to think about things that may be bothering you or causing you anxiety. Next time you have a bad day, try taking a long walk. Take along a radio and headphones if you feel like listening to music, and check your mood after about an hour—chances are you'll be feeling much better.

Running Running is harder to do than walking, but you may find that the things it can do for you make the extra effort worthwhile. Studies show that running causes your brain to produce endorphins, and it burns calories at a faster pace than walking does. In addition, running causes you to breathe more rapidly, which, as you learned earlier, allows more oxygen into your system. This extra oxygen eventually increases your lung capacity. If you find that you're breathing very heavily after you've run a mile today, try running the same distance three times a week for a month. At that point you may very well laugh when you think about how tired and breathless it once made you.

Swimming and Biking Swimming and biking can give you the same benefits as running, but they may not be as convenient, because they require equipment that can be expensive. If you have a bike, you may find that you prefer cycling to running, or that it provides a good change of pace. Swimming is an excellent aerobic activity because it exercises not only your legs but also your arms and torso. If your school doesn't have a pool, try calling your neighborhood YMCA. These organizations often have good pools (as well as other exercise programs) at a fair price.

Aerobic Exercise to Music Aerobic exercise to music is one of the best ways to develop physical fitness. Like swimming, aerobic exercise uses the entire body, and like running and biking, it can increase your lung capacity and burn calories. Finding an aerobic exercise class should not be especially difficult. If your school doesn't offer one, check your city's yellow pages. You should be able to find a class at a reasonable price. Make sure the class you choose is on the right fitness level for you: You may find that you prefer a high-impact class that stresses jumping, or that you're more comfortable doing low-impact exercises that concentrate more on stretching. Be equally careful if you have a VCR and want to buy an aerobic tape. Before you buy anything, ask your friends what tape (if any) they use, and whether they like it—you don't want to be stuck with a tape you hate.

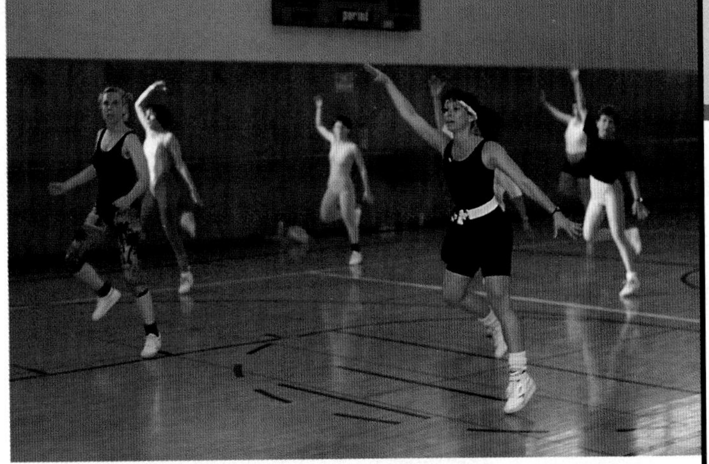

(FIGURE 3-7) **Aerobic exercise to music is a great workout for just about every muscle in the body. If you want to do this type of exercise, make sure you find a class that is on the right level for you.**

Team Sports Team sports such as basketball, hockey, and soccer can not only give you many of the same benefits as other aerobic exercise, but they can become great social events, because they are activities you can do with friends. If you like playing team sports more than any of your friends do, find out if your neighborhood has pickup games you can join. You may also want to call the YMCA in your neighborhood, which may be able to set you up with a team that matches your skills and ability.

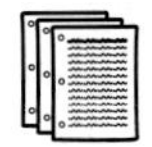

Life Skills Worksheet 3A

Using Community Resources

Assign the Using Community Resources Life Skills Worksheet, which the students, through interviewing a coach, will extract information about a particular school sport.

Role-Playing
Getting Started

Have students role-play how someone might be motivated to perform aerobic exercise on a regular basis if he or she belonged to one of the following categories: (1) poor physical condition, (2) good physical condition, (3) varsity basketball player, (4) physically impaired. Follow up the role-playing with a discussion of which motivation would work for each category.

Journal 3G
Choosing an Exercise

Have students write in the Student Journal the aerobic exercises covered in the text that they would select for their exercise program. Tell them to explain why they think these exercises would work best for them. Have them include what they dislike about exercise.

Class Discussion
Benefits of a Brisk Walk

Ask: **What are the physical benefits of aerobic exercise?** *[Helps control weight, helps your respiratory and circulatory systems stay healthy, lowers blood pressure and heart rate]* Have students discuss the mental and social benefits of aerobic exercise. Tell them to recall the effect of a long walk alone or with a friend.

Making a Choice 3A

Reasons for Exercising

Assign the Reasons for Exercising card. The card requires students to work in groups to brainstorm for excuses they have heard for not exercising and then to role-play these excuses.

Making a Choice 3B

Sport Safety

Assign the Sport Safety card. The card requires the students to list safety rules to follow when participating in various sports and to recognize high-injury sports.

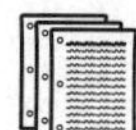

Life Skills Worksheet 3B

Resisting Pressure

Assign the Resisting Pressure Life Skills Worksheet, which asks students to think of positive ways of refusing offers of illegal drugs.

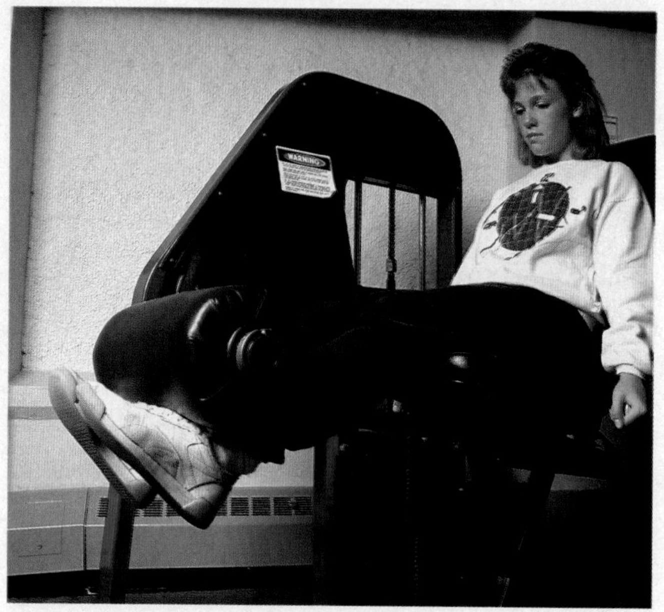

(FIGURE 3-8) **Anaerobic exercises develop muscular strength and endurance. They also use up oxygen as quickly as the body can supply it, which is why they can't be continued for more than a few minutes without interruption.**

anaerobic exercise:

physical activity that increases muscle size and endurance, and that cannot be continued for a long period of time without resting.

Anaerobic Exercises

Because **anaerobic exercises** take so much immediate energy and effort, they make you breathe even more rapidly than aerobic activities. But at the same time, the exercises you are doing need the oxygen you are supplying right away. This type of exercise does not necessarily help the body's respiratory and circulatory systems, and it does not burn calories as effectively as aerobic exercises do. But it will improve your muscular strength and endurance. Sprinting, weight lifting, and gymnastics are three examples of anaerobic activities.

Some Basic Rules

No matter how enjoyable an activity is, it's never much fun to memorize its rules. But they are a very important part of exercising safely, and you're going to have to know them before you can start your own exercise program. So take some time to learn them now.

Make Sure You Exercise Often Enough, Long Enough, and at the Right Intensity Your exercise program should allow time for exercise at least three or four days a week. Of course, those exercises won't do you too much good if they are either too easy or too difficult for you. In other words, you should make sure your program is at the right intensity for you. In order to do this, you will need to know what your target heart rate range is. Find out what yours is by reading the Life Skills feature on page 49.

Jot these numbers down in your notebook. Next time you exercise, check your pulse to see whether it falls within the range you had written down. If it's too low, you need to make your workouts more difficult (unless you are just beginning your exercise program, in which case you will want your pulse to be on the low side). It's okay if your pulse is slightly above the upper limit of your range, but if it's more than five beats per minute higher, you need to make your workouts less intense. Another way to test your program's intensity is to follow the "can you talk" guideline. If the intensity of your program is correct, you should be perspiring slightly, but still be able to carry on a conversation. If you're having trouble speaking after exercising, your program is too intense.

Finally, each time you do an aerobic activity, count on spending at least 30 minutes exercising. Aerobic exercises can do wonders for your physical fitness, but they won't count for much if you don't spend enough time doing them. Anaerobic exercises do not take very long to complete, but they alone will not improve your overall physical fitness.

• • • TEACH continued

Role-Playing
Convincing a Friend

Have students role-play a situation in which one student hates to do aerobic exercise. A friend tries to convince the reluctant student of the need to do aerobic exercise, perhaps linking some of the student's problems in school or at home to a lack of exercise. The friend should think of ways to coax the student to change his or her attitude toward exercise.

Journal 3H
Feelings About Sports

Have students use the Student Journal to describe their feelings about playing sports. Ask them to write down their positive and negative feelings about sports. If they have negative feelings, have them list a sport they might enjoy playing with others of their same level of proficiency.

Cooperative Learning
Favorite Forms of Exercise

Have students work in groups to survey the types of aerobic exercise enjoyed by other members of the class. Along with stating the exercise of their choice, students should also explain why they find the exercise worthwhile. Each group should record its findings. Then have the groups share their data with the rest of the class by means of a class exercise preference chart. Ask

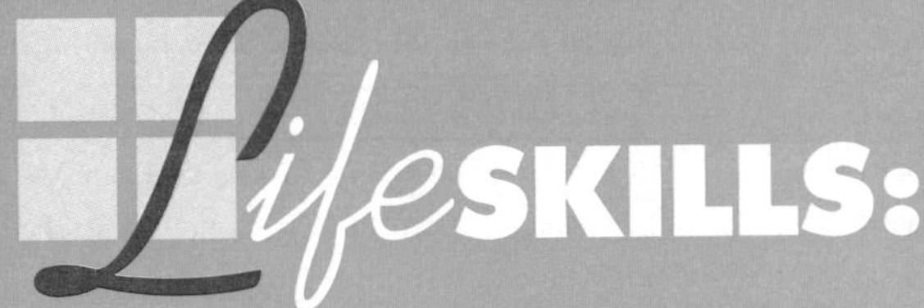

Determining Your Target Heart Rate Range

In order to find out your target heart rate range, you must know your maximum heart rate (MHR), which is the fastest your heart can possibly beat. If you happened to take your pulse the last time physical activity left you so worn-out that your heart pounded and you were completely breathless, you may know what your MHR is. If you didn't, you can find out your MHR by subtracting your age from 220.

Your target heart rate, or the pace you want your heart to beat when you exercise, should be between 60 percent and 80 percent of your maximum heart rate. In order to find your target heart rate range, multiply your MHR first by .6 to determine the lower end of the range, and then by .8 to determine the upper end of the range.

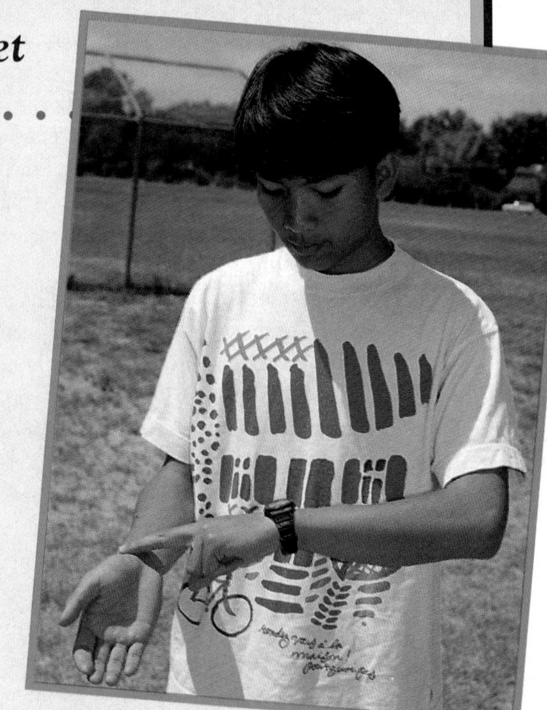

You can find your MHR and your target heart rate range by checking this chart:

Age	Maximum Heart Rate	Target Heart Rate Range
13	207	124-166
14	206	123-165
15	205	123-164
16	204	122-163
17	203	122-162
18	202	121-162

LifeSKILLS

Determining Your Target Heart Rate Range

Have students practice finding their maximum heart rate and their target heart rate range. Tell them to follow the steps and perform the calculations in order to figure out these rates even when they do not have a chart available. Give each student an index card on which to record the information they need. Tell them to exercise and check their heart rate following the exercise, some time before the next class period.

students to discuss whether knowing the preferences of their peers will influence their selection of one form of exercise over another.

Writing
Someone to Admire

Have students write a paragraph describing someone who is their ideal in the area of physical fitness. Tell them the person does not have to be a sports figure. The person may be someone their own age who is concerned about physical fitness, or it may be a friend or family member.

Class Discussion
Aerobic vs. Anaerobic Exercise

Ask students to explain the difference between aerobic and anaerobic exercises. Ask for examples of both kinds of exercise. Encourage students to suggest characteristics or effects of each type of exercise through a series of questions such as the following: What effect does aerobic exercise have on the circulatory and respiratory systems? What effect does anaerobic exercise have on these systems?

Remind students that the value of aerobic exercise is that it can be continued for longer periods of time, providing the exerciser with enhanced respiratory and cardiovascular activity.

Journal 3I
Measuring Your Heart Rate

Have students write in the Student Journal how their exercising heart rate

Background
Reasons for Warming Up and Cooling Down

Warm-up involves a general body warming plus a specific warming related to the skills to be performed in a particular exercise. Studies show that proper warm-up lessens the possibility of injury because the process stretches and lengthens the muscles, putting less tension on any one part of the muscle. No more than 15 minutes should elapse between warm-up and the aerobic exercise. Cooling down properly decreases lactic acid levels in the blood and muscles. Lactic acid is a product of metabolism and results from the incomplete breakdown of sugar in the muscle cells. A buildup of lactic acid causes the muscles to feel tired and sore.

A good way to remember all this information is to think of the word FIT:

- F stands for frequency, which should be three to four times per week.
- I stands for intensity, which should be at or slightly above your target heart rate.
- T stands for time, which should be at least 30 minutes of continuous exercise.

Warm Up and Cool Down Every athlete talks about how important it is to warm up before doing any strenuous physical activity. It is a good rule of thumb to spend a few minutes walking or jogging, and then do some mild stretching to warm up your muscles and raise your body temperature before you begin exercising.

It's also important to cool down *after* you finish exercising. If you don't, you may get dizzy or feel nauseated, and your muscles can become sore and cramped. Don't stop moving immediately after a strenuous exercise. Slow down, but continue walking or moving for another five minutes or so, to cool down your muscles in the same way that you warmed them up.

Start Slowly No matter how impatient you are to get your body into top physical shape, don't begin your exercise program by doing too much too soon. If your goal is to run 5 miles without stopping, but you haven't run in a while, pushing yourself beyond your current limitations can hurt you both physically and mentally. You may find yourself nursing cramped muscles, struggling for breath, and figuring that you would rather do just about anything rather than set foot on a track again.

Here's another example. Let's say you're in a weight-training program, and your goal is to lift a certain amount of weight that seems impossibly heavy right now. The best way to reach your goal is to choose a program that forces you to lift slightly more weight each workout. This is called using the progressive resistance principle, and it can and should be used in any type of exercise program you choose.

Vary Your Workout Just as you can get sick of hearing your favorite song too often, doing one exercise all the time can become boring. It can also injure your muscular and skeletal systems. Try to include a variety of aerobic exercises—called cross training—in your schedule. If you run one day, cycle another, and play tennis a third, you can both cut down on your chances of injury and keep yourself interested in each activity. This will help you receive the full benefit from each workout.

In addition, place some limits on the amount of exercise you do each week. Don't exercise intensely more than three or four times a week, and try to arrange your schedule so that you have a day to rest between each workout.

Avoiding Injuries

Even if you follow every exercise rule perfectly, you still run a small risk of injury when you exercise. The more physically fit you are, the lower this risk will be. But to be on the safe side, even if you are in terrific physical condition (and especially if you're not), read the following suggestions carefully and follow basic safety rules so you can keep your chances of getting hurt at a minimum.

Listen to Your Body Signals Make sure you pay close attention to the way your body is feeling. Minor aches and breathlessness are a normal part of exercise, but anything more serious than that—a sharp pain, for instance—probably means something is wrong and should not be ignored.

Even when everything seems fine, take time after each workout to let your body analyze things for you. Are you sweating?

• • • TEACH continued

compares with the range in the Life Skills feature. Tell them to compare rates again after they have been exercising for some time.

Class Discussion
Frequency, Intensity, and Time

Write the letters F, I, and T on the chalkboard. Ask students what the initials stand for. Remind them that frequency, intensity, and time are important parts of their exercise program. Ask why warming up and cooling down are important in any exercise program.

Journal 3J
Changing Ideas

Have students write in the Student Journal whether their ideas about exercising have changed while reading this chapter. If they have changed, tell them to explain why this happened. If their ideas about exercising have not changed, ask them to explain why.

Cooperative Learning
Getting the Word Out

Have students form small groups to advertise one of the basic rules of exercising. The groups may advertise by means of a poster, a slogan, a rap song, or any other method that would convey their message. Encourage students to be creative and to include reasons for the rule in their advertisements. Let them share their advertisements in class.

If you're not, the workout was probably too light. If you're out of breath, are you still that way after 10 minutes of rest? If so, you may have exercised too hard. Of course it's normal to feel tired after exercising, but exhaustion that lasts for more than 24 hours is definitely a signal of some sort. Do you feel nauseated or dizzy? Next time you exercise, wait two minutes after the end of your workout, and then check your heart rate. If your pulse is more than five beats quicker than the upper limit of your target heartbeat range—and especially if you are experiencing these other symptoms as well—you must lighten your workouts.

When you're feeling ill, don't make things worse by exercising. It won't make you feel any less sick, and you'll be much better off if you rest instead. When you're completely well again, work out lightly for a few days before returning to your full exercise schedule, just to be on the safe side.

Dress for the Weather Don't let the fact that exercise increases your body temperature fool you into thinking that it's perfectly fine to exercise outdoors on extremely cold days without dressing properly. The best thing you can do when it's freezing outside is to exercise indoors. If you do insist on being outside, make sure you're dressed for it. Put on two or three layers of clothing instead of one heavy outfit. Wear a hat to keep your head warm, and make sure your ears, fingers, nose, and toes are covered properly. Keep your clothing as dry as possible, and take extra time warming up before you begin your workout.

Be even more careful on hot, humid days. Again, you're best off staying in a cool gymnasium when the weather's hitting 90 degrees, but if you do go out, wear light-colored, lightweight clothing. Never wear rubberized suits or try to lose weight by sweating. This could seriously overheat your body. Most important, drink lots of water before, during, and after your workouts. The water will keep you from becoming dehydrated, and it will help you sweat so you can stay cooler.

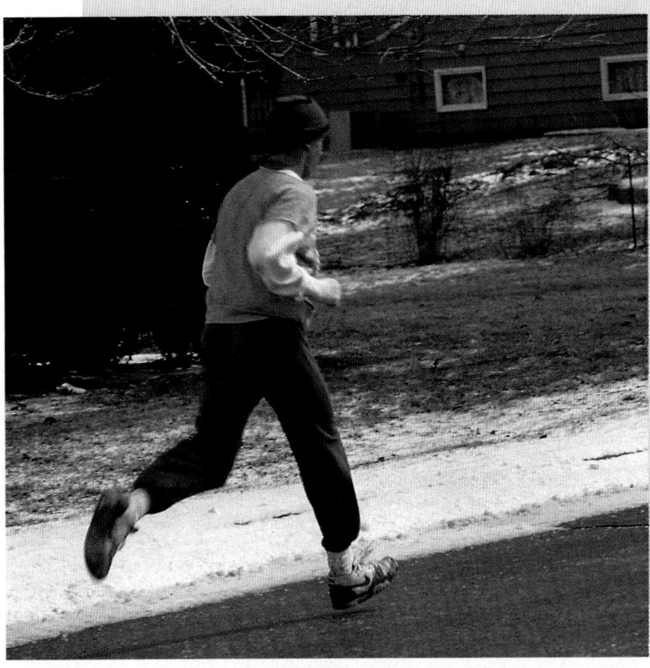

(FIGURE 3-9) **If you must exercise outdoors when it's cold outside, remember to dress properly. Wearing layers of clothing will keep you warmer than just a heavy jacket.**

Don't Be Just a Weekend Exerciser

It's always easier to find time to exercise on a Saturday or Sunday than it is during the week, especially during the school year. Unfortunately, exercising only on the weekends can be risky. People who rely on weekend activity to improve their aerobic fitness can overdo it, and they often find themselves nursing sprained ankles and sore knees after they have burned up the tennis court or running track. In addition, exercising only once a week will do little for your overall fitness level.

Section Review Worksheet 3.3

Assign Section Review Worksheet 3.3, which requires the students to verify facts concerning aerobic and anaerobic exercises, to explain how following rules keeps you safe when exercising, and to identify the effects of steroid abuse.

Section Quiz 3.3

Have students take Section Quiz 3.3.

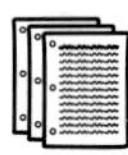

Reteaching Worksheet 3.3

Students who have difficulty with the material may complete Reteaching Worksheet 3.3, which requires students to identify examples of aerobic and anaerobic exercises and to list benefits of each kind of exercise.

Debate the Issue

Testing for Steroids

Let students debate the topic: Should student athletes be tested for steroids? Tell students to research the dangers of steroids and the violations that have been uncovered in the past. The teams should prepare arguments for their side of the debate. Remind them that for the sake of debate they can defend a position in which they do not believe. After presentations and rebuttals, the audience can question the debaters.

Extension

Interview

Suggest that students research one type of aerobic exercise—such as swimming, cycling, running, walking, or aerobic dancing—to determine how the time or distance covered in each exercise session should be increased over a period of several weeks. Students may wish to interview a coach to see how he or she increases player workouts.

Background
Injuries
Continuous application of a cold pack on an injured part of the body can cause tissue damage. To avoid this, an ice pack should be applied for 20 minutes every hour for a period of 1 to 72 hours, depending on the extent of the injury. Compression on an injured part decreases swelling and avoids hemorrhage.

If you can exercise only on weekends, make sure that you warm up thoroughly before each activity and that you take frequent breaks. If at all possible, try to find time for a short workout at least once during the week. By following these suggestions, you will make your weekend sports routine less hazardous to your health.

anabolic steroid: *an artificially made, complex substance that can temporarily increase muscle size.*

How to Treat Basic Injuries

No matter how careful you are, accidents and injuries can happen. In case one happens to you, keep in mind the five simple actions—known as PRICE—involved in the emergency treatment of injuries:

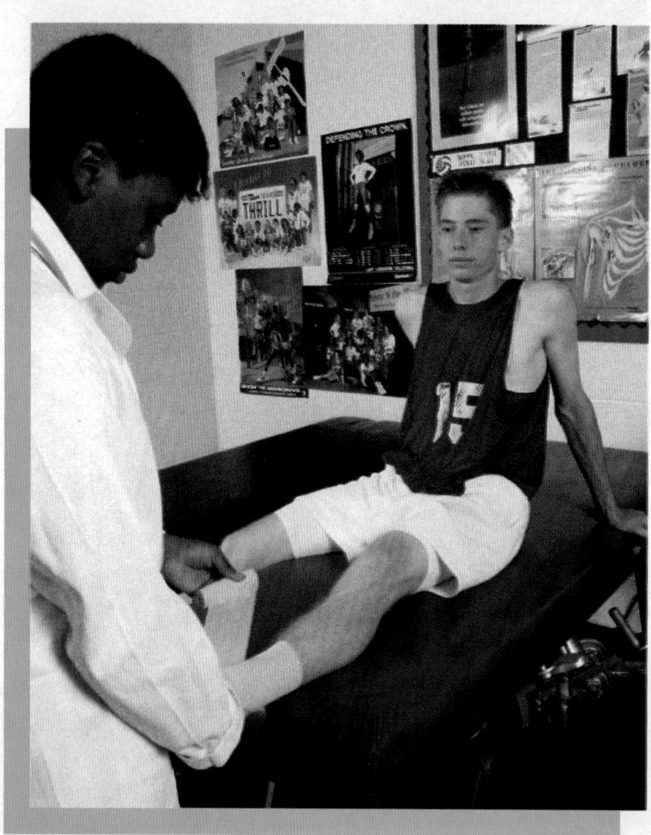

(FIGURE 3-10) **If you think you've seriously injured yourself exercising, seek medical attention immediately.**

- P (physician): decide whether you need to see a doctor immediately, or whether it's safe to wait a few days.
- R (rest): stop exercising immediately, and stay off the body part you've injured. If you've hurt a leg, ankle, or foot, use crutches if you have them.
- I (ice): to keep swelling to a minimum, put ice on your injury as soon as possible.
- C (compression): wrapping a towel or bandage firmly around the ice also helps limit swelling.
- E (elevation): keep your injured limb raised above your heart level. This will drain extra fluid from the injury.

If you decide that you're not hurt badly enough to see a doctor—and make this decision very carefully—begin treating your injury as soon as you can. Apply ice, in periods of 15 to 20 minutes, until the swelling goes down. At that point, remove the ice and use moist-heat compresses instead. Depending on how severe your injury is, you can start exercising again in four or five days. Be very careful when you do this—take extra care to warm up properly and to follow the other basic safety rules. You don't want to reinjure yourself and start the treatment process all over again.

Anabolic Steroids

Even if you're not a big sports fan, you may remember what happened to Canadian runner Ben Johnson, who was stripped of his gold medal after breaking the Olympic and World records in the 100-meter dash at the 1988 Olympics. Johnson, it turned out, had taken **anabolic steroids**, an illegal drug some athletes use to make them stronger and faster.

Steroids, which are made from a hormone called testosterone, do have some medical value. Doctors prescribe them to treat people with a blood condition called anemia, to help patients recovering from surgery, and also to replace a missing hormone in people who have not grown properly. But steroids have also become very popular illegal drugs, because they can increase muscle size and body weight. Famous athletes are not the only ones known to use steroids—thousands of high school students have taken them as well.

Not only are steroids illegal, but they're also very dangerous. They can cause high blood pressure, liver damage, cancer, damage to the reproductive system, and facial deformities, as well as violent behavior and other psychiatric problems.

It's not always easy to know if someone is taking steroids, but some common symptoms of this type of drug abuse include the following:

- noticeable change in muscle mass
- dramatic increase in ability to lift heavy weights
- aggressive behavior
- dramatic amounts of acne

It may seem as though steroids have their advantages. After all, they can make you stronger and faster without your having to work too hard. Even so, they're not worth the risk. A lot of the damage they cause may be permanent. Why ruin your life over some extra muscle? And anyway, depending on steroids to make you look good robs you of the pleasure of achievement. It doesn't count for much if you're strong just because you took a drug. Finally, you don't need steroids to make you stronger and faster. By combining weight training with a healthy diet and a program of regular aerobic exercise, you can help your body produce natural hormones to make your muscles grow. For additional information on gaining body weight, read the Gaining Weight Safely section in Chapter 5. For more information on steroid abuse, see Chapter 15.

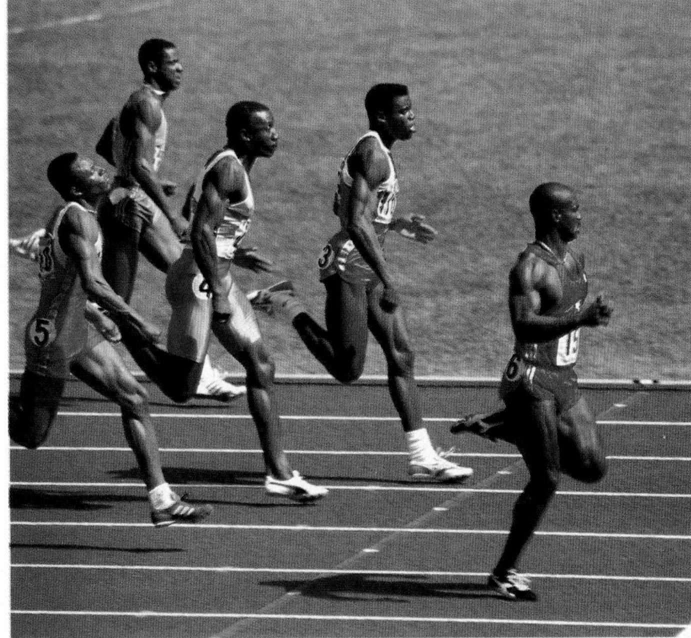

(FIGURE 3-11) **Ben Johnson (right) was stripped of his gold medal at the 1988 Olympic games when traces of anabolic steroids were found in his blood.**

Review

1. *Describe the difference between aerobic and anaerobic exercise.*
2. *Name two examples of aerobic exercises, and two examples of anaerobic exercise.*
3. ***LIFE SKILLS: Assessing Your Health** Your workouts are making you tired, and you wonder whether they may be too intense for you. What's a good way to find this out?*
4. ***Critical Thinking** Which is more important to overall physical fitness: aerobic exercise, or anaerobic exercise? Why?*

For more information on how to gain weight safely, see Chapter 5.

Anabolic Steroids are also discussed in Chapter 15.

Review Answers

1. Aerobic exercises are physical activities that continue for more than 20 minutes. Anaerobic exercises are intensive actions that last no more than a few minutes.
2. Accept any correct answer. Examples of aerobic exercises include walking, running, cycling, swimming, and team sports. Examples of anaerobic exercises include sprinting, weight lifting, and gymnastics.
3. You could check your target heart rate.
4. Aerobic exercise is more important because it helps improve circulation, burns calories, produces energy, lowers blood pressure and heart rate, and increases your breathing rate. Aerobic exercise helps a person lose or control weight and helps a person's respiratory and circulatory systems stay healthy.

ASSESS

Section Review

Have students answer the Section Review questions.

Alternative Assessment

Defending Physical Education

Have students plan a mock school board meeting where the budget is being considered. Some board members are suggesting that the only way to balance the budget is to limit physical education classes. The physical education teacher has asked students and their parents to express their opinions before the school board. Have students meet in cooperative groups to plan their appeal to the school board. Let each group share their response with the class.

Closure

It Pays to Follow the Rules

Ask students why exercisers must follow the basic rules of exercise. *(To get the most out of exercising and to prevent injuries.)*

Background

The Need to Stay Active

Just a few weeks of being confined to bed or to a wheelchair produces muscle atrophy, bone demineralization, and decreased aerobic capacity. An effort should be made, with the approval of a physician, to work on a limited exercise program even when a person is recovering from an injury or accident. The body was made for strenuous physical activity. Modern people are much more sedentary than their ancestors. Effort must be made to meet the needs of an active body.

Section 3.4 Getting Started

Objectives

- *Set your exercise goals.*
- *Design your own exercise schedule.*

Now that you've read through all the rules and regulations of physical activity, not to mention the benefits of being physically fit, it's time to sit down and figure out what your exercise goals are. Then you can design a program that can help you meet them. Remember that your main ambition does not have to be to play basketball like Michael Jordan or tennis like Jennifer Capriati. It could be that you're looking to lose weight, or that you want to have more energy, or that you just want to stay healthy.

Your exercise schedule should reflect your personal goals, and may for that reason be very different from those of your close friends. That's why it's so important that you take plenty of time to design your own program.

Your Goals and How to Achieve Them

By now you most likely have some idea of what you want from your exercise program. In case you don't, here's a list and brief description of goals you may want to strive for. When you've decided what's best for you, look at Figure 3-13 to find out what type of exercises you should do.

Aerobic Fitness Earlier in this chapter you learned that when you are aerobically

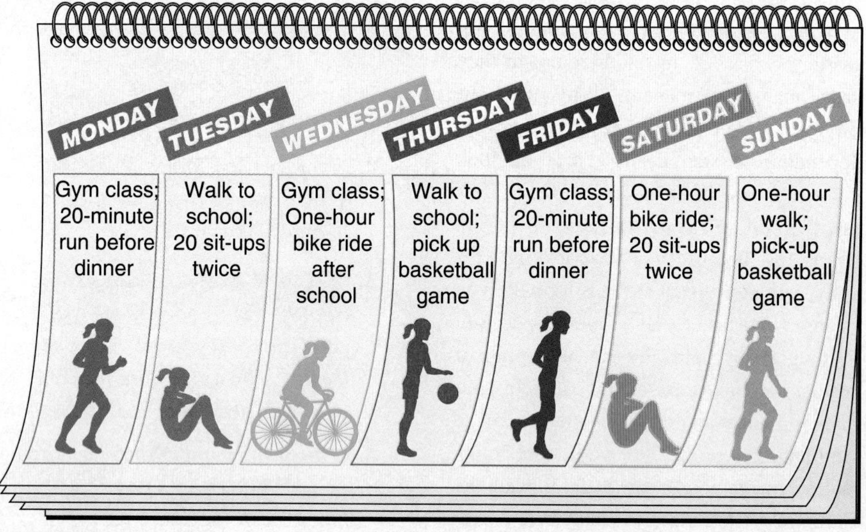

(FIGURE 3-12) **Good exercise schedules leave time for some sort of physical activity every day of the week.**

Section 3.4 Lesson Plan

MOTIVATE

Journal 3K

Plans for Exercise

This may be done as a warm-up activity. Encourage students to write in the Student Journal their promise about starting a personal exercise program. They do not have to be specific as to which exercises they will do. A simple affirmation of their intention to start on a program they can stay with for a long time is sufficient at this time.

TEACH

Cooperative Learning

An Exercise Schedule

Have students discuss in groups the "Sample of an Exercise Schedule" in Figure 3-12. Ask them to express their opinions of the sample schedule in terms of developing a long-term exercise program. (Students may like the variety of activities. They may find it less boring than only one type of exercise. Some students may not like the kinds of exercise suggested.) Have them make suggestions to improve the sample schedule. Have each group share their revisions of the sample schedule with the class.

Your Exercise Goals, and How to Achieve Them

Goal	Type of Exercise	How, and How Often
Weight Loss, Good Body Composition, Flexibility	*Aerobics*	*30 to 60 minutes, four or five times a week*
Aerobic Fitness	*Aerobics*	*Three or four times a week, at or above your target heart rate*
Muscular Strength	*Weight Training*	*Two or three times a week. Use weights that are up to 90% of the heaviest weight you can lift.*
Muscular Endurance	*Aerobics plus Weight Training*	*Three or four times a week. For weight training, use weights that are no more than 70% of the heaviest weight you can lift.*

(FIGURE 3-13) **Remember when you design your exercise program to keep your goals simple. Too much exercise too soon can do more harm than good.**

fit, not only is your body able to undergo 10 minutes or more of continuous exercise, but your circulatory and respiratory systems are in top working order. This is the most important part of physical fitness. Even so, chances are that your goal right now is not to improve your circulation and respiration. But remember that aerobic fitness is essential no matter what your exercise goals are, and that you must include aerobic exercises in your schedule even if you couldn't care less how fast your heart is beating. If you don't, your other exercises will be a waste of time. Remember that if you start taking care of your circulatory and respiratory system *now*, you can reduce your chances of getting certain diseases later on.

Weight Control Exercise is a valuable part of every weight-loss program. Consider the following:

- Exercise can decrease your appetite.
- Exercise burns calories.
- Exercise helps you lose fat without losing muscle.

SECTION 3.4

Section Review Worksheet 3.4

Assign Section Review Worksheet 3.4, which requires the students to design an exercise schedule to meet certain exercise goals.

Section Quiz 3.4

Have students take Section Quiz 3.4.

Teaching Transparency 3B
"Your Exercise Goals"

Ask students to study the transparency of the table "Your Exercise Goals and How to Achieve Them" (Figure 3-13). Ask: What are the goals listed in the chart? What type of exercise would you use to obtain the goal of weight loss? What type of exercise would help you attain muscular strength? How is the type of exercise used to gain muscular strength different from exercise used to gain muscular endurance?

Writing
Charting Exercise Goals

Encourage students to list their specific goals in one column and the type of exercise they will do to achieve their goals in a second column. Students should list how, and how often, they will do these exercises in a third column. They can base their table on the one in Figure 3-13.

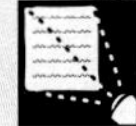

Teaching Transparency 3C
Burning Calories

Have students examine the transparency of the table "Various Aerobic Activities and the Calories They Burn" (Figure 3-14). Ask: Which activities burn the fewest number of calories? Which activities burn the greatest number of calories? Discuss which activities would be most helpful for someone interested in weight loss and a change in body composition.

Background
Muscular Endurance

Muscular endurance involves the ability to contract the muscles repeatedly. After many repetitions, the muscle becomes tired and will not contract when a person wishes it to. An exercise program helps increase the possible number of contractions a muscle can make. The amount of force exerted in a single contraction indicates the strength of a muscle. Any muscle in the body becomes stronger with use.

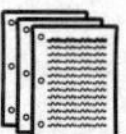

Reteaching Worksheet 3.4

Students who have difficulty with the material may complete Reteaching Worksheet 3.4, which requires the students to identify the exercise goals that can be achieved by following a specific exercise schedule.

Various Aerobic Activities and the Calories They Burn

Activity	Approximate Calories Burned (per hour)
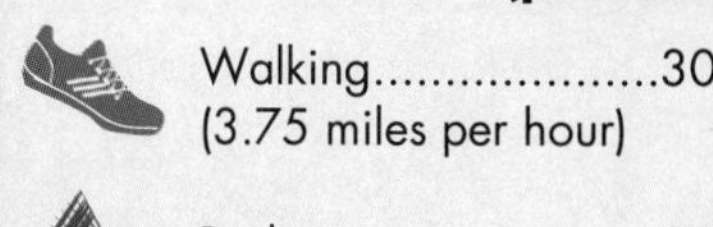 Walking (3.75 miles per hour)	300
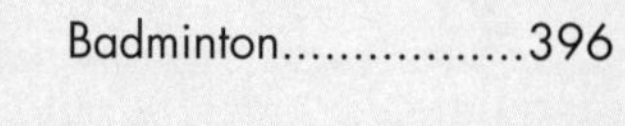 Badminton	396
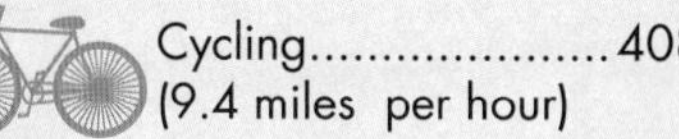 Cycling (9.4 miles per hour)	408
Tennis (singles)	450
Swimming	500
Fencing	539
Field Hockey	546
Basketball	564
Skiing	791
Wrestling	791
Handball	864
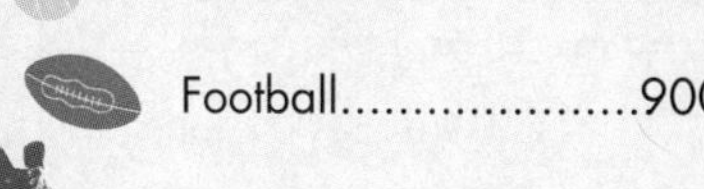 Football	900
Ice Hockey	930
Walking Up Stairs	1100
Running:	
5.8 miles per hour	570
8.0 miles per hour	760
10.0 miles per hour	900
11.4 miles per hour	1300
13.2 miles per hour	2330
14.8 miles per hour	2880
15.8 miles per hour	3910
17.2 miles per hour	4740
18.6 miles per hour	7790

A word of warning: Contrary to what you may hear, there is such a thing as being too thin. There is also such a thing as exercising too much. Remember that the only thing wrong with being overfat is that sooner or later it can cause health problems. Having some body fat is not only perfectly normal, but is absolutely critical to normal development. If you become addicted to dieting and exercising, you can easily become underweight—a condition every bit as unhealthy as being overweight.

The best weight-loss exercises are the aerobic ones, because they require more time, and often more energy, to complete. But if you are interested, as many teenagers are, in activities that strengthen the muscles in your abdomen, there are some specific exercises you can do. Check Figure 3-15 for some suggestions.

Strength and Muscle Development

The principle behind building your strength is to push your muscles against a strong resistance. This eventually causes your muscles to adapt by getting bigger and stronger. If this is your chosen goal, take special care to use the progressive resistance component of fitness described on page 50.

The best strategies for muscle development vary according to what goals you have in mind. If you're trying to gain muscle strength, you'll want to lift moderate weights. If, on the other hand, you want to increase your muscle mass or bulk, you may be advised to lift heavier weights. Talk to an experienced trainer before attempting any of these exercises.

(FIGURE 3-14) **Although some aerobic activities burn more calories than others, pure numbers can sometimes be misleading. It is impossible, for example, to run at an 18-mile-an-hour pace for a full hour.**

• • • TEACH continued

Journal 3L
Refining an Exercise Plan

Encourage students to write in the Student Journal the activities that they could realistically engage in on a regular basis and the number of calories burned by those activities in an hour.

Demonstration
Abdominal Exercises

Ask for student volunteers to demonstrate the exercises in Figure 3-15, "Exercises for the Upper and Lower Abdomen." Have students point out what the demonstrator has to bear in mind to achieve the goal for doing a particular exercise. Ask students: **What can be achieved by exercising for weight control?** *[Exercise can decrease appetite, burn calories, and help you lose fat without losing muscle.]*

Class Discussion
Flexibility Exercises

Have students study Figure 3-16, "Flexibility Stretching Exercises." You may want to have student volunteers demonstrate the exercises. Ask students to state the purpose of flexibility exercises. Have them explain why these exercises prevent sports injuries.

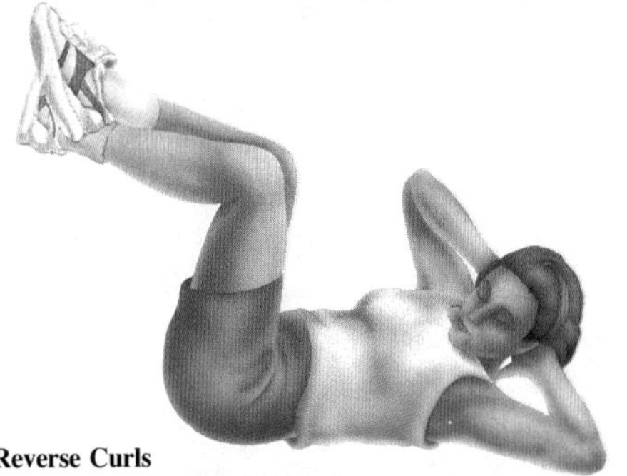

LOWER ABDOMINALS

Reverse Curls

Lie on the floor with fingers locked behind your head. Knees are bent. Contract your lower abs to curl hips off the ground about 3 to 5 inches bringing knees towards chest. Slowly return to the floor. Do not "whip" your legs. Let the abs do the work. Remember to press your lower back into floor throughout the exercise.

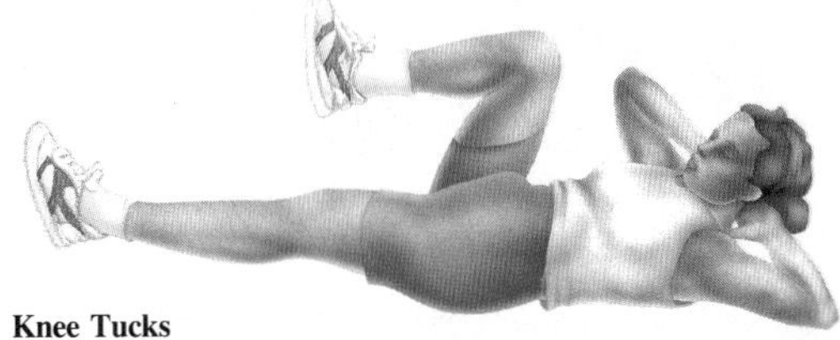

Knee Tucks

Lie on your back with hands supporting your head. Tuck one knee to your chest and extend the other straight a few inches off the floor. Hold 2 counts and switch legs. Some hip flexor work is involved, but keeping the low back pressed to the floor will work the lower abs isometrically.

INTERNAL EXTERNAL/OBLIQUES

Oblique Twisters

Lie on your back, bend your knees, and point both knees to the left. Extend your arms over your right hip. Slowly curl shoulders and upper back off the floor to a half-upright position. Reverse the curl to return to the floor. Repeat with the opposite side.

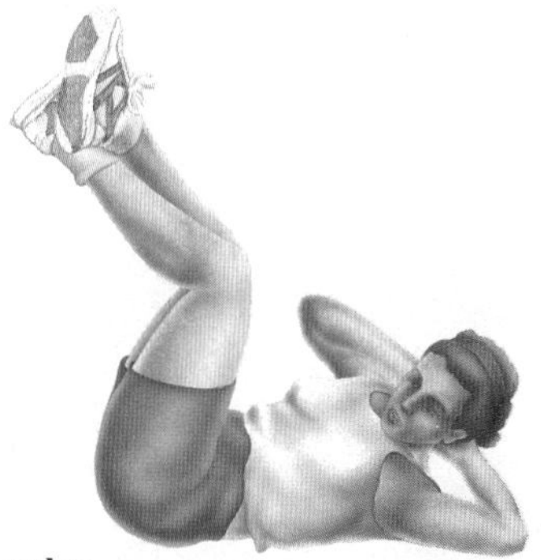

Twisting Crunches

Lie on your back with knees bent, ankles crossed and fixed. Contract abdominals to lift shoulder and upper back off floor. Twist trunk, bringing left elbow to right knee. Repeat to opposite side.

UPPER ABDOMINALS

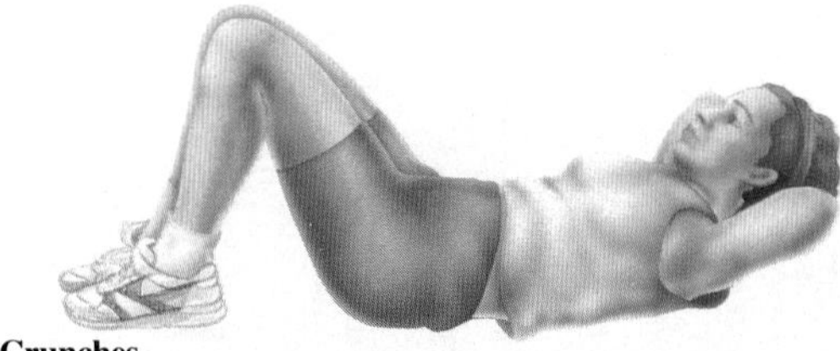

Crunches

Lie on your back with knees bent, feet flat on the floor. Hands support your head. Look at the ceiling and contract the abs to lift the shoulders and upper back off the floor. Lift one knee and bring it in toward your elbow. Press the low back to the floor, hold briefly, then return to floor.

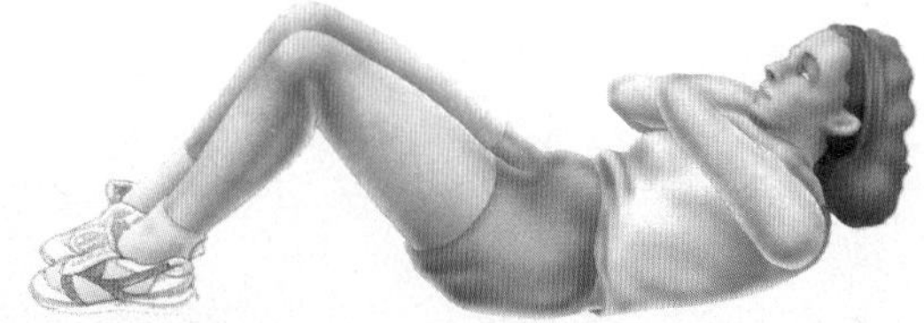

Gravityfighters

Start with knees bent, feet flat and body rounded to a position 45 degrees off the floor. Arms are crossed over the chest, chin is tucked. The body is gradually lowered until the shoulder blades touch the floor. Reverse the movement to starting position.

(FIGURE 3-15) **These exercises can strengthen your abdominal muscles, but they can also cause injury if not done correctly. Check with your coach to make sure you're doing them properly.**

Case Study

Physical Fitness and the Physically Impaired

Discuss the achievements of Sharon Hedrick, Dennis Oehler, and Jim Abbott, who were mentioned in Section 3.1. Call attention to the fact that these young athletes have won the respect of athletes and spectators alike. Tell students that when they begin to lose motivation in their own physical fitness program it might be a good idea to recall the odds these achievers had to overcome.

Extension

Research Report

Suggest that students visit the library to familiarize themselves with books on physical fitness. Tell them to write a report on one aspect of physical fitness that interests them.

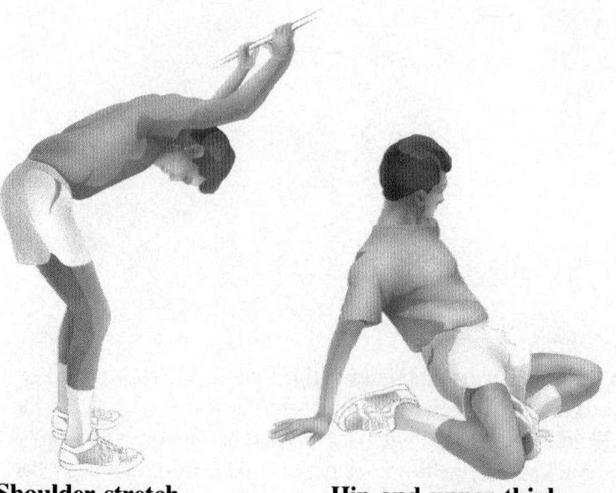

Shoulder stretch
Hold onto an object about shoulder height. With hands on the support, relax and keep arms straight and chest moving downward, feet under hips, and knees slightly bent.

Hip and upper thigh
Tighten the left side of the buttocks as the hip is turned in that direction for five to ten seconds. Relax the buttocks, and repeat the exercise on the right side.

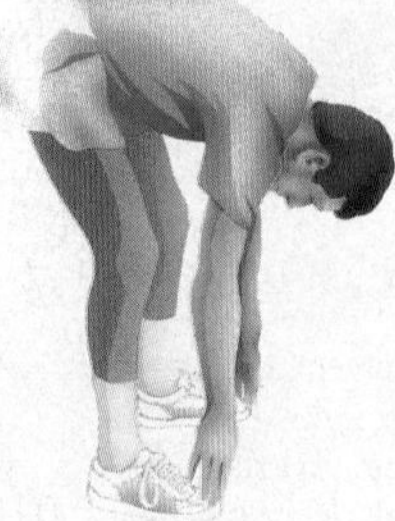

Hamstring (a)
With knees slightly bent, slowly bend forward from the hips until you feel a stretch in the back of your legs.

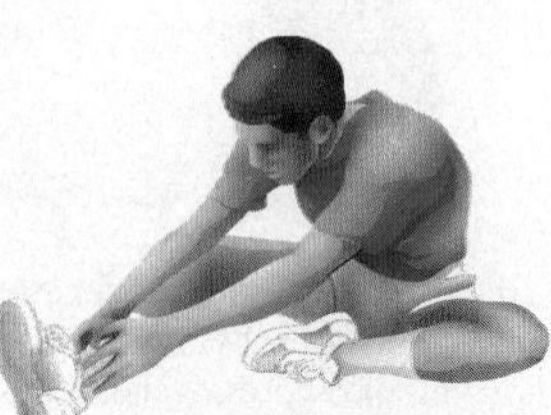

Hamstrings (b)
Keep only a slight bend in the front leg, with the other foot next to the inside of the leg. Bend forward at the hips until you feel slight pressure.

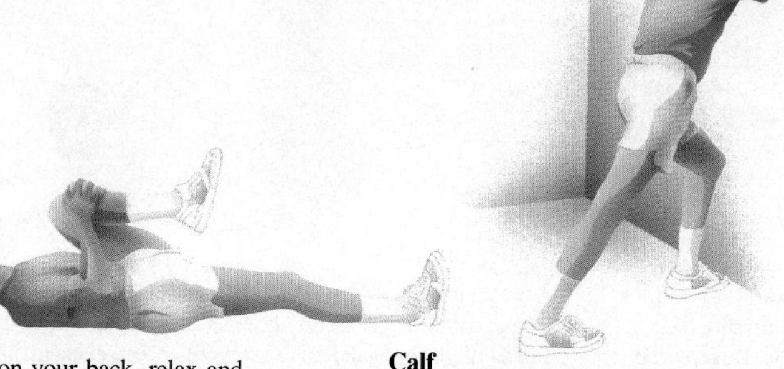

Hip
Lying on your back, relax and straighten both legs. Pull the left foot toward the chest. Repeat using the right foot.

Calf
Stand slightly away from a wall and lean forward with the lead leg bent and the rear leg extended. Move the hips forward with the heel of the straight leg on the ground until you feel a stretch in the calf.

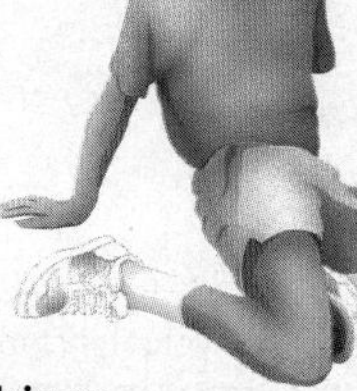

Quadriceps
Sit with right leg bent and the heel just to the outside of the right hip. Bend the left leg, with the sole next to the inside of the upper right leg.
Lean back until you feel an easy stretch.

Archillies tendon and soleus
Bend the back knee slightly with the heel flat. Lean forward as in the calf stretch.

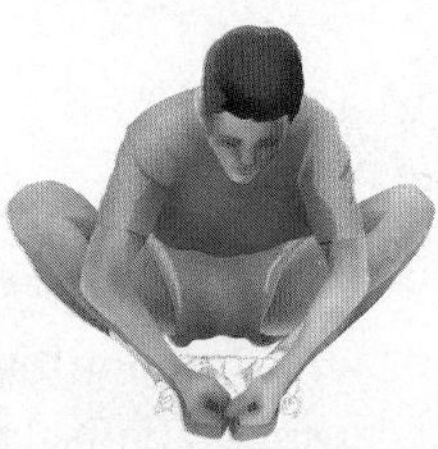

Groin (a)
With soles of the feet together, place hands around the feet and pull yourself forward.

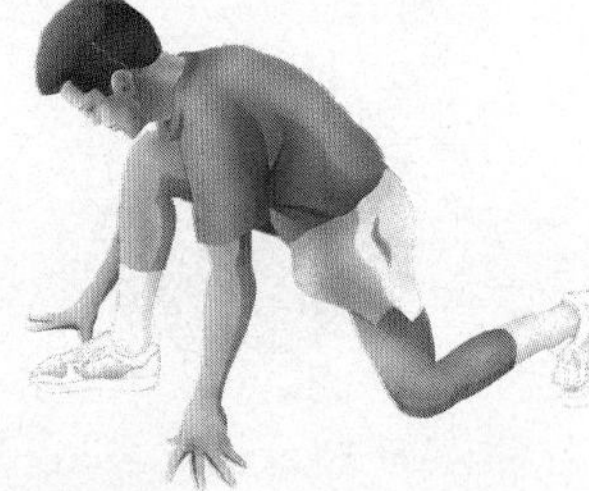

Groin (b)
Move one leg forward until the knee is directly over the ankle. The back knee rests on the floor. Lean forward and hold.

(FIGURE 3-16) **Stretching exercises not only increase flexibility, but also decrease your chances of injury. Take time to stretch before doing any vigorous physical activity.**

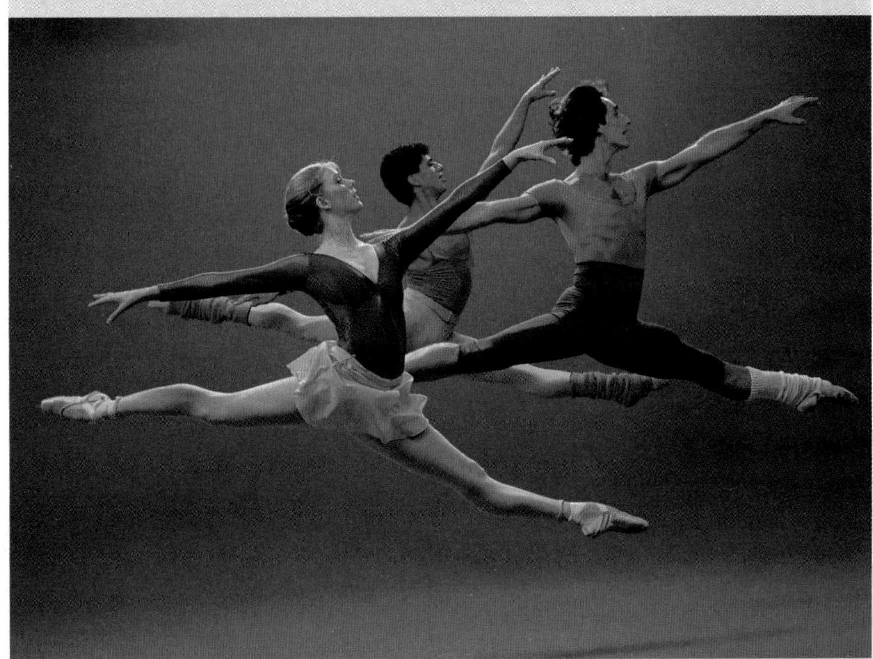

(FIGURE 3-17) **Having good flexibility is an important requirement for dancers and gymnasts.**

Flexibility and Body Composition Unless you're a gymnast or a dancer, flexibility is not likely to be an ultimate exercise goal for you. But doing stretching exercises, as suggested in Figure 3-16, is an important part of warming up for—and cooling down from—your regular exercise routine. Also, good flexibility helps prevent sports injuries. Body composition may very well be near the top of your list of challenges. Having a high percentage of lean muscle tissue will certainly help keep you healthy in the long run, and it is good to keep this in mind as you exercise. But becoming too obsessed with losing fat or becoming muscular can lead to extremely dangerous behavior, such as starvation or steroid abuse. Remember that having some body fat is perfectly normal. The best program for healthy body composition will include plenty of aerobic exercise and eating a healthy diet.

Review

1. *What are your exercise goals?*
2. *Write out a realistic exercise schedule.*
3. ***Critical Thinking*** *You and your friend want to work out together, but you have completely different exercise goals. What should you do?*

Review Answers

1. Students may answer aerobic fitness, weight control, strength and muscle development, flexibility, and body composition.
2. Answers will vary. Accept any exercise schedule that shows an understanding of the relationship among exercise goals, type of exercise, and how often the exercise is performed.
3. Answers will vary. Accept any reasonable response. Students may suggest that they and their friends may do warm-up exercises together, as well as flexibility stretching exercises. And perhaps they can work out together during the aerobic part of their exercise schedule.

ASSESS

Section Review

Have students answer the Section Review questions.

Alternative Assessment

Expectations for Exercise

Have students write a letter to a friend describing their physical exercise program and what they expect it will do for them. Perhaps they could encourage their friend to join them in becoming more physically fit.

Closure

Results of Planning

Have students sum up in a brief paragraph what they feel planning their own exercise program has done for their mental outlook.

Background
REM Sleep

The recognition that REM sleep is correlated with dreaming is credited to Eugene Aserinsky, Nathaniel Kleitman, and William Dement. Research has shown that the brain stem is responsible for sleep and dreaming. The studies of many researchers have made dreams physically diagnosable. Some interesting hypotheses attempt to explain dreaming: (1) dreams help the dreamer to get rid of redundant or useless information, (2) dreaming prepares the dreamer for survival mechanisms that may be necessary in the future, (3) infants dream to prepare their reflexes, and (4) dreaming may not so much rest the brain as help to organize information.

Section 3.5 Sleep

Objectives

- *Know the two different categories of sleep.*
- *Describe what happens during each phase of the sleep cycle.*
- *Name two ways to cope with insomnia.*
- *Know how much sleep you need each night.*

LIFE SKILLS: Solving Problems

brain waves: *electrical patterns produced by the brain that fluctuate greatly during the sleep cycle.*

There is another aspect to physical fitness. No matter how strong, flexible, lean, and aerobically healthy you are, you're not going to feel or function well if you don't get enough sleep. Most high school students need about eight or nine hours of sleep, but you may find that you do fine with seven, or that you can't stay alert unless you've gotten ten. Whatever your personal requirements are, try to stick to them, because it is while you are asleep that your body recovers from the activities of the day that has just ended, and prepares itself for the new day ahead.

What Happens When You Sleep?

It may seem as though your body shuts off completely while you're asleep. This is not totally off the track, because your breathing and heart rate do slow down, and your blood pressure and body temperature drop slightly. But at the same time, your brain continues to recognize outside information, so it remains about as active, in a different way, as it is when you're awake. It exhibits this activity in the form of **brain waves**, or electrical changes that take place in the brain. By studying these brain waves, scientists have been able to recognize the different stages of sleep, and what goes on in the brain during each phase.

The Sleep Cycle

Sleep can be divided into two categories. The first of these, called nonrapid eye movement sleep, or **NREM**, has four stages of its own. If you're like most teenagers, you spend only a short amount of time in stage I, which ends as soon as you have fallen asleep. When this happens, you enter stage II, in which your brain waves slow down. Those brain waves are at their slowest in stages III and IV, the phases of deepest sleep. Evidence indicates that the more you exercise, the more time you spend in stages

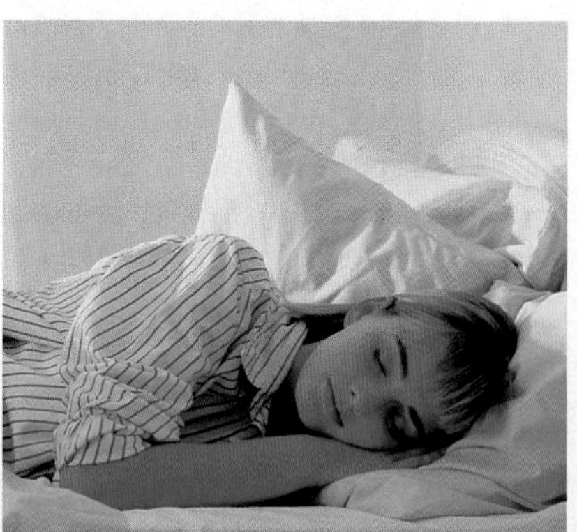

(FIGURE 3-18) **Your brain remains active and continues to process information when you are asleep.**

Section 3.5 Lesson Plan

MOTIVATE

Journal 3M
How Do You Sleep?

This may be done as a warm-up activity. Have students use the Student Journal to write down the answers to these questions. How many hours of sleep do you generally get? How often do you have trouble sleeping at night? Write down a dream you remember having recently.

TEACH

Class Discussion
Sleep Stages

Draw two squares on the chalkboard. Ask students to name two categories of sleep. Write NREM in the first square and REM in the second square. Beneath NREM draw four spokes to represent each of the four stages, and label each one. Have students state what happens in each of the four stages of NREM and what happens during REM. Use arrows to show how a sleeper returns in the sleep cycle to the earlier stages, and then returns to the REM stage.

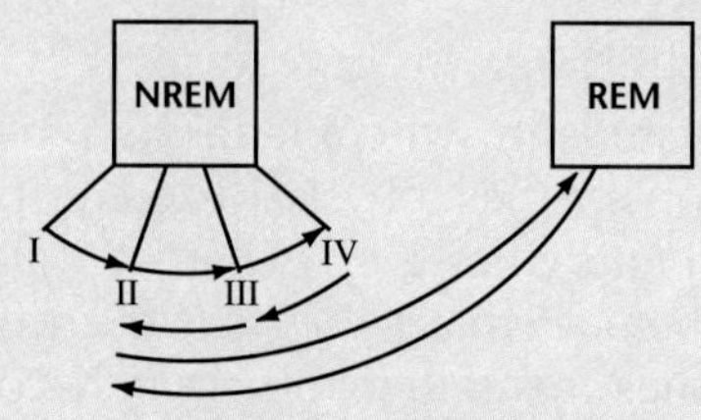

III and IV. These stages are believed to be the phases at which the body does most of its resting and restoring. Even so, most teenagers pass through these first four stages less than two hours after they have fallen asleep.

When stage IV ends, the cycle reverses, and you travel back through stages III and II. At this point, you enter the second category of sleep: rapid eye movement, or **REM**. It is during REM, studies show, that you do your dreaming, because during this stage your brain waves are at their most active, and move very rapidly. The first REM stage usually lasts no longer than 15 minutes, but it extends to about 30 minutes when it is entered again. Most high school students spend about a fourth of their sleeping time in the REM phase.

When this final stage ends, the cycle will begin again. During the course of your night's sleep, you will enter each stage of the cycle (except the first, which you left for good when you fell asleep) four or five times.

Insomnia

Everyone has **insomnia**, or trouble sleeping, from time to time. You may find it hard to get to sleep when you've got a big exam the next day, for instance, or when you've eaten too much at dinner. Maybe it's hot outside, and you find your room stuffy even with the windows open. In general, these are temporary situations. When they disappear, your insomnia should too. But if you have had trouble sleeping over the course of a few months, it could be more serious.

Long-term insomnia can cause moodiness and concentration lapses. It can also wear down your immune system, making you more vulnerable to illness. If you have had trouble sleeping for a long period of time, it could be that you're not getting enough exercise. You know now that exercise helps the sleeping process because it makes you more tired at the right time. If you are exercising regularly and still have trouble sleeping, you may want to see a doctor.

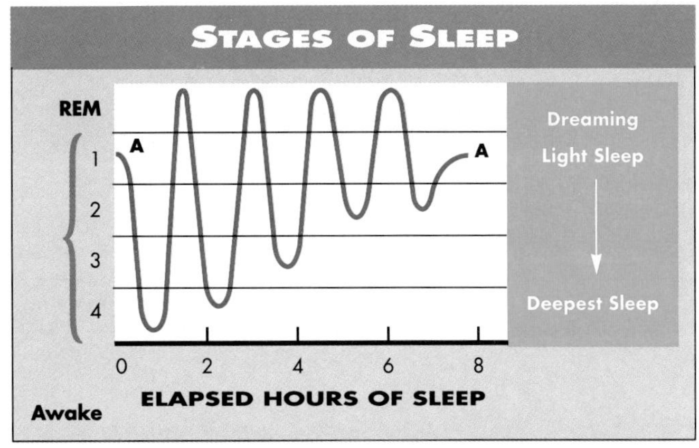

(FIGURE 3-19) **During a typical night you may pass through each stage of sleep four or five times.**

Tips for Sound Sleeping

If not everyone needs the same amount of sleep, how can you tell whether you're getting enough? You're the only one who can answer that question, so be honest about it. Recognize that you may need more sleep if you're feeling irritable, having trouble concentrating, or if you're just plain tired. It doesn't prove anything to stay up until 11:30 when you secretly felt like going to sleep at 10:00.

If you decide that you do need to get more sleep, or if you're suffering from insomnia, here are some ways to get back on track:

1. Keep a regular sleep schedule. Try to set a regular bedtime, so that you're ''programmed'' to get tired when it's time to turn in.
2. Go to bed when you're tired. It's pointless to stay up when you can't. If it's a little earlier than usual, enjoy the extra sleep you'll be getting.

REM:

(rapid eye movement) the dreaming part of the sleep cycle, in which the eyes move back and forth rapidly under the eyelids.

insomnia:

temporary or continuing loss of sleep.

SECTION 3.5

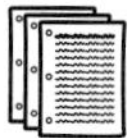

Section Review Worksheet 3.5

Assign Section Review Worksheet 3.5, which requires students to complete a diagram illustrating the sleep cycle and to answer questions concerning the categories and stages of sleep.

Section Quiz 3.5

Have students take Section Quiz 3.5.

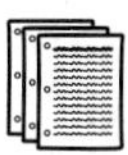

Reteaching Worksheet 3.5

Students who have difficulty with the material may complete Reteaching Worksheet 3.5, which requires students to compare the characteristics of the two categories of sleep by means of a charting process.

Ask: What physiological changes take place while you are sleeping?

Class Discussion
The Need for Sleep

Write on the chalkboard: *If sleep does not serve an absolutely vital function, then it is the biggest mistake the evolutionary plan has made.* Have students discuss this statement made by a prominent researcher on sleep, Dr. Allan Rechtschaffen. This topic will give students the opportunity to compare their own need for a certain amount of sleep with the needs of other members of the animal kingdom. It will also allow students to hypothesize as to the actual purpose of sleep. Students may wish to research the problem of the effect of sleep loss over a long period of time.

Journal 3N
Sleep Habits

Have students write in the Student Journal how they view their sleeping habits: How could they improve their sleeping habits? How would better sleep improve the quality of their lives?

Extension
Sleep Deprivation

Have students do research on sleep deprivation. Sometimes individuals are deprived of sleep for research. Sleep deprivation has also been used in brainwashing techniques. Have students find out why sleep deprivation can effectively be used in brainwashing.

Review Answers

1. NREM (nonrapid eye movement) and REM (rapid eye movement)
2. NREM: Stage I—ends when you have fallen asleep; Stage II—brain waves slow down; Stages III and IV—brain waves are at their slowest; this is the phase of deepest sleep when the body does most of its resting and restoring.
REM: dreaming and brain waves are the most active
3. Students may answer: keep a regular sleep schedule, go to bed when you are tired, finish your exercise program at least three hours before bedtime, keep your room dark and quiet, don't lie in bed if you can't sleep, don't use alcohol or tobacco, don't drink caffeine after about six at night, don't eat too late, don't rely on over-the-counter sleep medication.
4. Students might answer that they should go to sleep and set their alarm to get up an hour earlier in order to finish studying for the test.
5. Scientists have been able to recognize the different stages of sleep and what goes on in the brain during each stage.

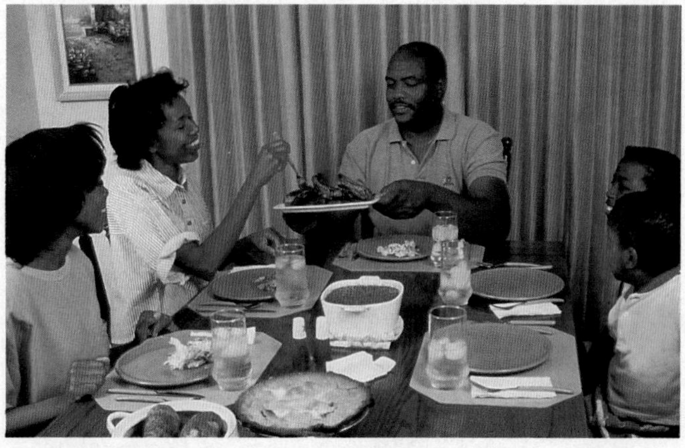

(FIGURE 3-20) **If at all possible, eat dinner early in the evening. A too-full stomach can keep you awake at night.**

3. Finish your exercise program at least three hours before bedtime. It's not a great idea to do anything too physically trying right before going to sleep. Instead, do some reading, listen to music, or watch a little television, to get your mind off your day.
4. Keep your room dark and quiet. You may love to listen to the radio, but if you're having trouble getting to sleep, it may be keeping you up. Try doing without it.
5. Don't lie in bed if you can't sleep. In general, tossing and turning won't help you fall asleep. Get out of bed and try reading. A warm bath or shower sometimes helps too.
6. Don't use alcohol or tobacco. Alcohol may cause drowsiness, but it does not help insomnia. Besides being addictive and dangerous, tobacco contains ingredients that stimulate your mind and body, and is therefore the worst thing to take late at night.
7. Don't drink caffeine, which is also a stimulant, after about 6 P.M. If you do drink soda at night, be sure that it's decaffeinated.
8. Don't eat too late. Indigestion or a too-full stomach can cost you precious hours of sleep. If at all possible, eat dinner before 6 P.M., and avoid snacking right before going to bed.
9. Don't rely on over-the-counter sleep medications. They may help you sleep for a night, but they often leave you groggy in the morning. And if they do work once, you may start to depend on them to get to sleep.

If you find that none of these help you get the sleep you need, see a doctor. Long-term insomnia can be caused by a number of things, from mental depression to poor eating habits. A health professional can determine what the problem is, and can often help you sleep well again in no time. Getting the sleep you need is probably the easiest part of any physical fitness program, and is well worth the time you put into it.

Review

1. *Name the two categories of sleep.*
2. *Describe what happens during each phase of the sleep cycle.*
3. *Name two things you can do to help yourself sleep better.*
4. ***LIFE SKILLS: Solving Problems*** *You have a big test in the morning, and you know you haven't finished studying for it. But it's late, and you're getting really tired. What should you do?*
5. ***Critical Thinking*** *How does studying brain waves help scientists figure out what happens while we sleep?*

ASSESS

Section Review

Have students answer the Section Review questions.

Alternative Assessment

Why Do We Need Sleep?

Ask students to write one or two paragraphs about why they think all mammals need sleep.

Closure

Sleep Record

Ask students how much sleep they usually get each night. Ask them how they know they are getting an adequate amount.

CHAPTER 3

Highlights

Summary

- Exercise offers benefits in four broad areas: aerobic fitness, muscle strength and endurance, body composition, and flexibility.
- Aerobic exercises such as walking, running, biking, and swimming can help your circulatory and respiratory systems stay healthy.
- Anaerobic exercises such as sprinting and weight lifting increase your muscle strength and muscle endurance.
- Exercise should be done often enough, long enough, and at the right intensity.
- You can avoid many exercise injuries if you warm up correctly before your workout, and if you exercise regularly without pushing yourself.
- Becoming addicted to dieting and exercise can cause you to become underweight, which is as unhealthy as being overweight.
- The sleep cycle consists of four stages of NREM sleep and a period of REM sleep.

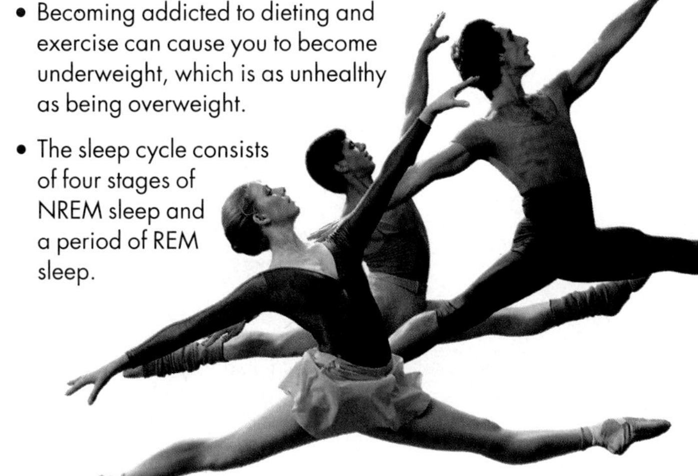

Vocabulary

cholesterol a waxy substance that can block the arteries and cause heart disease.

high blood pressure a condition in which the blood pushes harder than normal against the inside of the blood vessels.

endorphin a substance that is produced inside the brain and has pleasurable effects.

flexibility the ability to move muscles and joints through their full range of motion.

body composition the division of the total body weight into fat weight and muscle weight.

aerobic exercise physical activity that increases the heart rate and supplies oxygen to the muscles, and that can be continued for a period of time without resting.

anaerobic exercise physical activity that increases muscle size and muscle endurance, and that cannot be continued for a long period of time without resting.

brain waves electrical patterns produced by the brain that fluctuate greatly during the sleep cycle.

REM (rapid eye movement) the dreaming part of the sleep cycle, in which the eyes move back and forth rapidly under the eyelids.

CHAPTER 3 HIGHLIGHTS STRATEGIES

SUMMARY

Have students read the summary to reinforce the concepts they have learned in Chapter 3.

VOCABULARY

Have students work in groups to make up games that can be used to review vocabulary words. Have each group demonstrate its game to the class.

EXTENSION

Ask students to create posters that will stimulate the class (and perhaps the entire student body) to become more physically fit. The posters should use slogans to stimulate interest and convey the message of physical fitness.

Chapter 3 Assessment

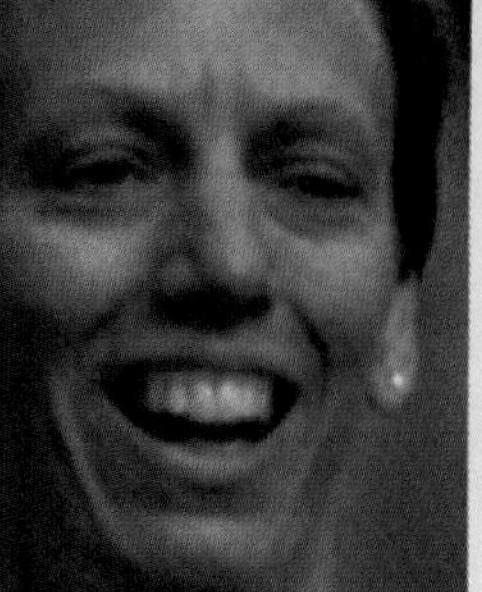

Chapter Review

Concept Review

1. What are some physical changes brought on by exercise that you can't see or feel?
2. What effect do endorphins have on your body?
3. Aerobic exercise causes you to breathe more rapidly. How does your body adjust to this increased need for oxygen?
4. What are the three basic rules to know before you start your exercise program? (clue: FIT)
5. What are three ways to avoid injuries when exercising?
6. If an accident or injury happens, what are the five simple actions involved in emergency treatment?
7. Name three effects of steroid abuse.
8. Describe what happens to your body while you sleep.
9. How do you know if you are getting enough sleep?

Expressing Your Views

1. Do you think Americans are more physically fit today than a century ago? Why or why not?
2. You've noticed that the football team begins every practice session with stretching exercises and ends every session jogging around the track. Why do you think the coach has the players do this?
3. Tim is 15 years old and wants big muscles. What type of exercise would be helpful for him? Sophia is 14 years old and wants to help her heart and lungs stay healthy. She doesn't enjoy exercising alone. What type of exercise would be suitable for her?
4. When planning an exercise program for yourself, do you think it is important to include a variety of activities? Do different exercises contribute different benefits?

Chapter Review

Concept Review

1. Exercise helps your body manage blood fats such as cholesterol more effectively. It can also lower blood pressure and lower your chances of having osteoporosis.

2. They produce a sense of pleasure and make you feel good.

3. Your lungs transfer more oxygen to your bloodstream and then to your muscles.

4. Exercise frequently, three to four times a week; exercise at an intensity which should be at or slightly above your target heart rate; exercise for a least 30 consecutive minutes

5. Listen to your body signals, stop if you feel something is wrong, don't exercise if you are feeling ill, dress for the weather, don't be just a weekend athlete, warm up and cool down when exercising

6. Decide whether you need to see a doctor immediately, stay off of (and rest) the body part you have injured, put ice on your injury, compress the injury by wrapping a bandage around it and the ice, elevate an injured limb above heart level

7. High blood pressure, liver damage, cancer, damage to the reproductive system, facial deformities, violent and/or aggressive behavior, increase in acne, psychiatric problems

8. Your breathing and heart rate slow down, and your blood pressure and body temperature drop slightly.

9. You may need more sleep if you feel irritable, are having trouble concentrating, or if you feel tired.

Expressing Your Views

Sample responses:

1. No. Most Americans have sedentary jobs and they also commute to work by car, train, or bus instead of walking or riding a bicycle. Many American children watch television instead of exercising.

2. To warm and stretch the muscles before vigorous exercise in order to avoid injury; to cool down the muscles and to prevent them from becoming sore and cramped, as well as to prevent dizziness or nausea

3. Anaerobic such as weight lifting; team sports that require aerobic exercise, such as basketball or soccer

Chapter 3 Assessment

Life Skills Check

1. Testing Physical Fitness
   You would like to start an exercise program but you are not sure at what level you need to begin. What can you do to test your physical fitness?
2. Sleeping Well
   Your friend has been having trouble sleeping at night. Often he is late to school or cancels weekend plans in order to catch up on sleep. What advice could you give your friend?
3. Determining Your Heart Rate
   Work with a partner to identify each other's target pulse rates. One at a time, run in place for two or three minutes and take your pulse to find your MHR. Then determine your target pulse rate by using the directions on p. 47. What is your target pulse rate? Do you think this rate changes according to how fit you are?

Projects

1. Work with a group of students to find out what exercise, health, or sports facilities are available in or near your community. Are there swimming pools, tennis courts, jogging or biking trails, aerobics classes, basketball courts, or volleyball sand pits? If you live in a large city, each group might investigate one recreational area.
2. Design a survey to find out why people exercise. Think of four questions to ask, then work in a small group to collect and combine responses. Analyze the results to determine whether physical or psychological benefits were more motivating.
3. Write to the President's Council on Physical Fitness and request suitable programs or fitness norms for your age group. The address is
   202 Pennsylvania Avenue NW
   Suite 250
   Washington DC 20004

Plan for Action

Plan a balanced weekly exercise program to fit you own personal needs.

4. Yes, because different types of exercises contribute different benefits

Life Skills Check

Sample responses:

1. You can do some simple tests to determine at what level you need to begin: aerobic, muscular strength and endurance, flexibility, and body composition.

2. Students should name three of the Tips for Sound Sleeping listed in Section 3.5.

3. Answers for target heart rate will vary with each student. No, the rate doesn't change, but how quickly you reach that rate will change. The more fit you are, the longer or more vigorously you must exercise to reach your target heart rate.

Projects

Have the students plan and carry out projects for physical fitness education.

Plan for Action

Have students describe plans for their own physical exercise program. Ask students how their personal plans fulfill their exercise goals and have them respond to the plans of other students.

Assessment Options

Chapter Test

Have students take the Chapter 3 Test.

Alternative Assessment

Have students do the Alternative Assessment activity for Chapter 3.

Test Generator

The Test Generator (Macintosh® or IBM® format) contains an additional 50 assessment items for this chapter.

NUTRITION PRINCIPLES

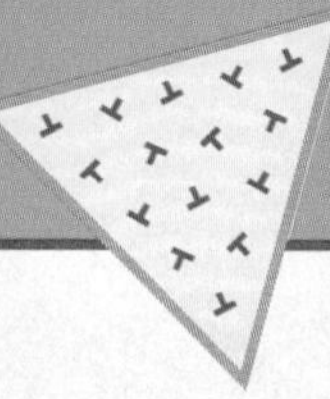

PLANNING GUIDE

TEXT SECTIONS	OBJECTIVES	TEXT FEATURES	OUTSIDE RESOURCES	NOTES
4.1 Influences on Food Choices pp. 67-69 1 period	• Describe the difference between hunger and appetite. ■ Describe how different factors affect your food choices. • List the short-term consequences of making poor nutritional choices.	• Check Up, p. 68 **ASSESSMENT** • Section Review, p. 69	**TEACHER'S RESOURCE BINDER** • Lesson Plan 4.1 • Personal Health Inventory • Journal Entries 4A, 4B • Section Review Worksheet 4.1 • Section Quiz 4.1 • Reteaching Worksheet 4.1 • **OTHER RESOURCES** • English/Spanish Audiocassette 2	
4.2 Nutritional Components of Food pp. 70-81 2 periods	• Describe the roles and functions of the six classes of dietary nutrients. • Identify problems that can occur from inadequate amounts of certain nutrients. • List recommended dietary levels for various nutrients. • Describe the differences among the various types of cholesterol.	**ASSESSMENT** • Section Review, p. 81	**TEACHER'S RESOURCE BINDER** • Lesson Plan 4.2 • Journal Entry 4C • Section Review Worksheet 4.2 • Section Quiz 4.2 • Reteaching Worksheet 4.2 • **OTHER RESOURCES** • Making a Choice 4A	
4.3 Analyzing Your Nutritional Needs pp. 82-100 3 periods	• Define the nutritional requirements for healthy teens as described by the U.S. Dietary Goals. • Classify foods into the appropriate food groups. • Interpret food labeling to analyze nutritional breakdown. ■ Make food selections that satisfy nutritional requirements. • Identify special nutritional needs of selected populations.	• Check Up, p. 84 ■ LIFE SKILLS: Practicing Self-Care, pp. 94-95 **ASSESSMENT** • Section Review, p. 100	**TEACHER'S RESOURCE BINDER** • Lesson Plan 4.3 • Journal Entry 4D • Life Skills 4A, 4B, 4C, 4D • Section Review Worksheet 4.3 • Section Quiz 4.3 • Reteaching Worksheet 4.3 • **OTHER RESOURCES** • Making a Choice 4B • Transparency 4A, 4B	
End of Chapter pp. 101-103		**ASSESSMENT** • Chapter Review, pp. 102-103	**TEACHER'S RESOURCE BINDER** • Chapter Test • Alternative Assessment • **OTHER RESOURCES** • Test Generator	

■ Denotes LIFE SKILLS objectives

• Items in blue are also part of the *Holt Health Activity Book*.

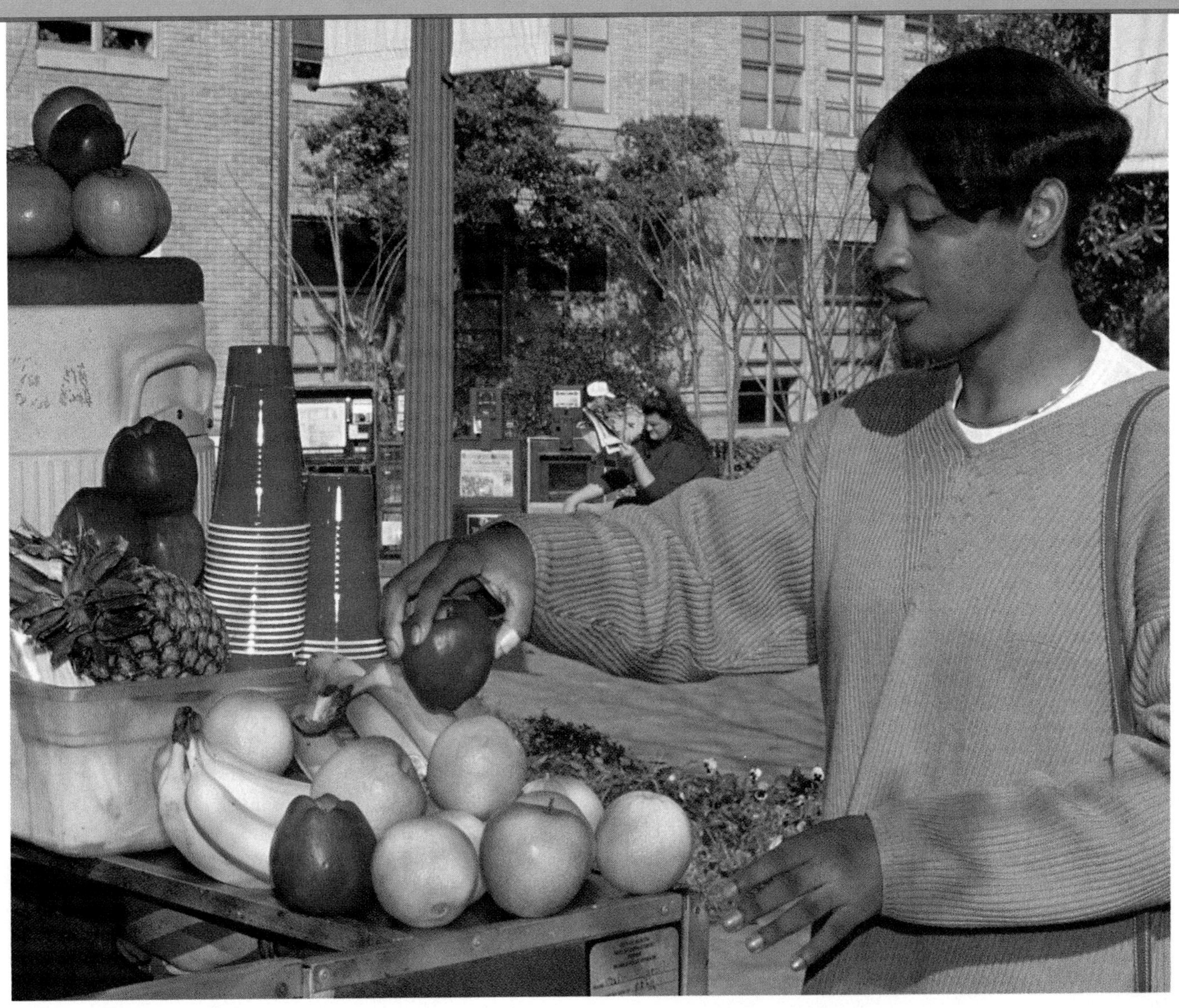

CONTENT BACKGROUND The American Diet

DESPITE AMERICA'S OBSESSION WITH thinness, there has been a 54 percent increase in the number of obese children between the ages of 6 and 11 in the past two decades, according to a study conducted by Harvard University. While the lack of physical activity is partly to blame, many experts cite poor nutritional choices—either out of ignorance or convenience—as the reasons for this dramatic increase. For example, in many families, both parents work outside the home. Snacks and meals are often prepared by the children. According to one national survey, approximately 62 percent of American children under the age of 13 prepare at least one meal per week on their own. Often the meal is high-calorie, prepackaged food or fast food. Also, many families today eat out at least once or twice a week and often consume more high-calorie foods at restaurants than they might prepare at home.

Most Americans are aware of the need for a well-balanced diet, but too few actually put this knowledge into practice. For example, the National Cancer Institute and other major health organizations suggest five or more servings per day of fruits and vegetables. Yet recent dietary studies reveal that only about 9 percent of us eat as many as five servings. Almost half of all Americans eat no fruit, and nearly 25 percent eat no vegetables on a given day. About 10 percent eat neither fruits nor vegetables daily. When the Produce for Better Health Foundation asked 3,000 people why they ate so few fruits and vegetables, most cited lack of availability. The second most frequent response was cost. Convenience was the third most frequently cited reason for not eating these foods; about 750 respondents said that fruits and vegetables took too much time to prepare. Interestingly, most people said they really liked fruits (over 80 percent) and vegetables (over 70 percent).

Another reason for many of our poor nutritional choices seems to be persistent myths about the nutritional value of certain foods and nutrients. For example, most Americans believe that a large portion of protein should be consumed at every meal. And in fact, Americans eat about twice the recommended amount of this essential nutrient. But according to the most recent nutritional guidelines, too much protein causes weight gain. The United States Department of Agriculture suggests consuming only two to three servings—between about 40 and 60 grams—of protein per day.

Another common myth is that breads, pastas, and potatoes are fattening. But according to the USDA guidelines, 6 to 11 servings from this group should be consumed each day. Whole-grain choices are very nutritious and contain needed fiber. Furthermore, these foods contain fewer calories per gram than their fat and protein counterparts; one gram of carbohydrate provides four calories while one gram of fat provides nine.

Suggestions for changing and improving the American diet include teaching the consumer how to read and understand food labels and how to choose and prepare nutritious meals. The majority of nutritionists and dietitians insist that these habits must be developed early in life, with parents or guardians as role models.

According to pediatricians, most healthy children will, when provided with nutritious choices at each meal, get the necessary nutrients they need over the course of several meals. Parents and guardians should not be alarmed if a healthy child eats little at one meal and heavily at the next. Also, snacking makes an important nutritional contribution to the diets of infants and children. Snacks should provide about 20 to 25 percent of a growing child's daily food intake. They should be offered well before meals and should include fresh fruits and vegetables, whole-grain breads and crackers, low-fat dairy products, and other foods low in both sugars and fats.

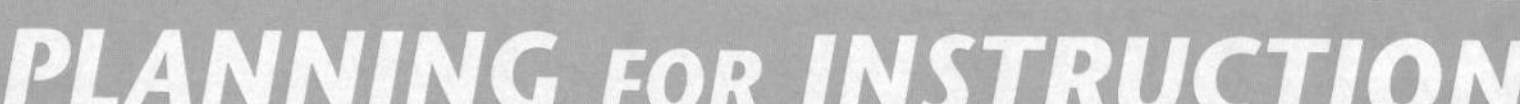

PLANNING FOR INSTRUCTION

KEY FACTS

- **Healthy eating habits include eating to satisfy hunger (a physical need) rather than just to appease appetite (the desire for food). Many factors, ranging from culture to personality and education, affect eating habits.**
- **Adequate nutrition requires the intake of six essential nutrients in correct amounts. Carbohydrates, fats, and protein provide energy, while vitamins, minerals, and water allow the body to use other nutrients properly.**
- **Excessive intake of fats and cholesterol by many Americans has increased the incidence of heart disease and cancer.**
- **Lack of vitamins can lead to deficiency diseases; lack of calcium can weaken and damage bones; and too much sodium may contribute to high blood pressure. Consuming too little water is dangerous and can be life-threatening.**
- **Recommended Dietary Allowances (RDAs) of nutrients are tailored to age, gender, activity, and other factors.**
- **To achieve both variety and balance in your diet, it is helpful to categorize foods into these food groupings and eat the recommended number of servings from each one daily: vegetables and fruits (4 servings), breads and cereals (4 servings), dairy products (4 servings), and meats, poultry, fish,**

and beans (2 servings). Fats and sweets should be avoided or used in moderation.

- Young people should try to consume less sugar and fat and more complex carbohydrates. They should also learn to analyze food labeling terms to better meet their nutritional needs.

MYTHS AND MISCONCEPTIONS

MYTH: Drinking 10 cups of any fluid fulfills the daily requirement for water.

While many fluids contain a lot of water, they are not all water. Drinks that contain caffeine and alcohol actually act as diuretics, which cause your body to eliminate water rapidly and increase the body's demand for fluid.

MYTH: Athletes need extra protein, so they should consume lots of meat and protein supplements.

The average athlete's protein needs are not increased. What is important is that the athlete take in adequate nutrition to replace the extra calories expended. This does not mean extra protein, but more calories; the percentages of nutrients in relation to each other remain the same.

MYTH: Eating right means cutting out snacks.

A number of nutritionists recommend eating several small meals and snacks throughout the day. Healthful snacks are fine.

VOCABULARY

Essential: The following vocabulary terms appear in boldface type.

hunger
appetite
essential nutrients
calorie
carbohydrates
complex carbohydrates
HDL
LDL
proteins
essential amino acids
complete protein
incomplete protein
dietary fiber
fats
saturated fats
unsaturated fats
cholesterol
vitamins
minerals
dehydration
carbohydrate loading

Secondary: Be aware that the following terms may come up during class discussion.

kilocalorie (C)
glucose
sucrose
glycogen
lipids
adipose cells
macrominerals
trace minerals
electrolytes
lactating
RDAs
U.S. RDAs

FOR STUDENTS WITH SPECIAL NEEDS

Kinesthetic: Have students bring to class an assortment of food items and supplement them as necessary to represent the four food groups. Ask small groups to select a variety of foods that would provide a balanced diet for one day. Rate students' selections for nutritional balance and adequacy, using tables that give RDA values.

Auditory Learners: Have students interview a nutritionist or prepare questions for a nutritionist guest speaker and take notes on the answers they receive. Suggest that each student focus on one area, such as nutrients, menu planning, or evaluating diets.

ENRICHMENT

- Have students keep a log of television commercials about food for a week, noting the type of food promoted. They may analyze the data, make graphs to show food groups represented, and write critiques of the ads from a nutritionist's point of view.

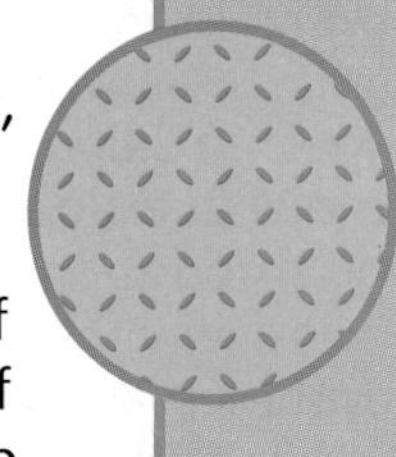

- Have groups of students study food customs of various cultures and prepare a display and brief demonstration of food preparation. Each group might produce a summary of dietary strengths and weaknesses of the culture they studied.

Chapter 4 Chapter Opener

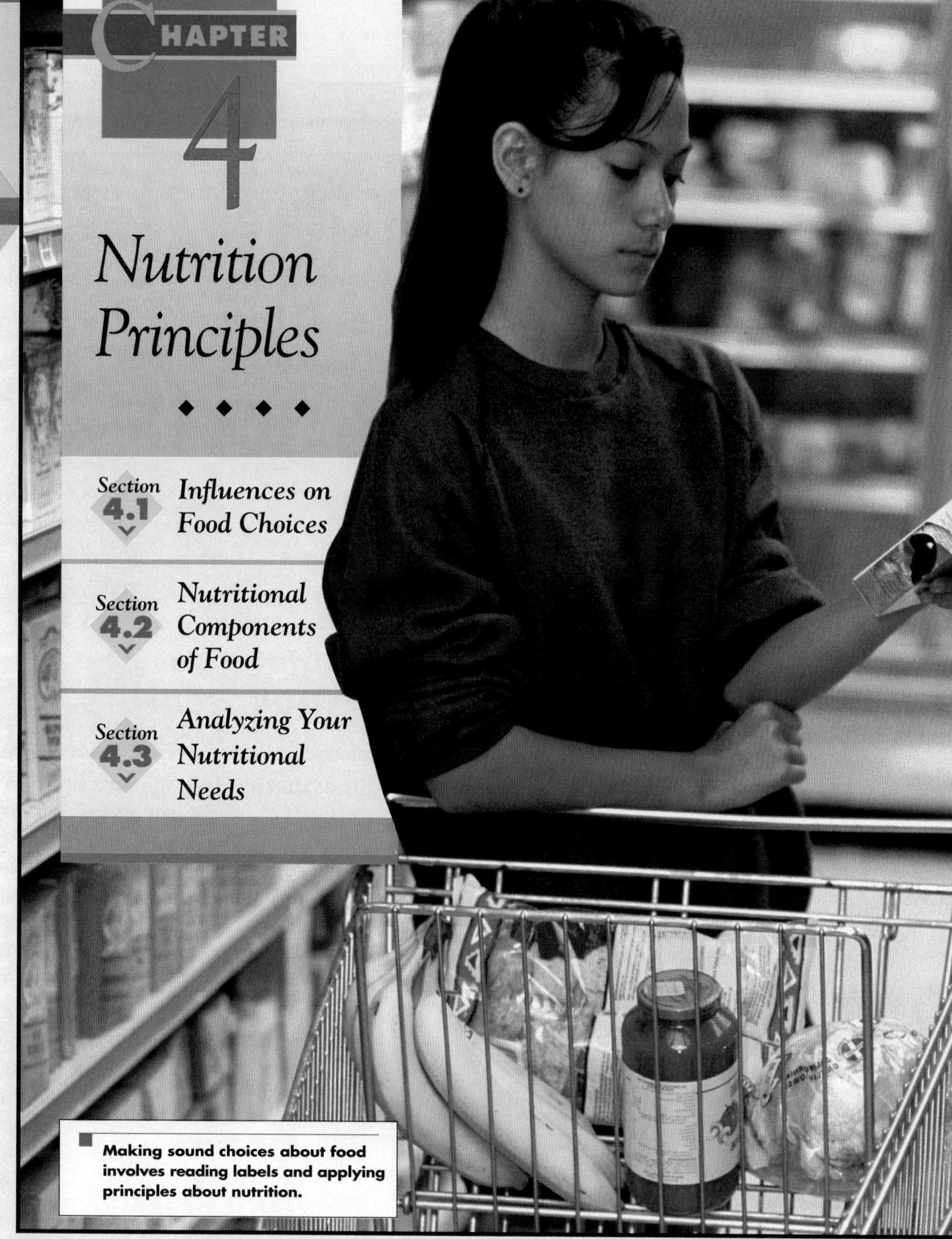

Making sound choices about food involves reading labels and applying principles about nutrition.

Getting Started

Using the Chapter Photograph

Ask students to describe the two photographs. Which person is in a better position to make a healthy food choice? Discuss what nutrition information appears on package labels. How does the information help you make good choices? Are any healthy snacks likely to be found in a vending machine? Which ones do you think are best?

Question Box

Have students anonymously write any questions they have about nutrition or diet and put them in the Question Box. To ensure that students with questions are not embarrassed to be seen writing, have students who do not have questions write something else—such as what they already know about essential nutrients or proper food selection for a balanced diet—on the paper instead. You may wish to allow students to write additional anonymous questions as they go through the chapter.

Preview the questions and then answer them at appropriate points in the chapter. You may wish to allow students to write additional anonymous questions as they go through the chapter.

Personal Issues *ALERT*

Students who are seriously overweight or underweight may be reluctant to discuss eating habits. Be aware that some students may be reluctant to discuss diet because of religious or ethnic food customs practiced at home. The privacy of such students should be respected; allow them to volunteer information.

Mary Anne is really hungry and tired. She's got two more classes and then band practice. A snack would be great right about now. Standing in front of the vending machine, she wonders what to pick—chips, candy, gum, pretzels, or cookies. The candy bar looks really good, especially since Mary Anne feels she needs energy to stay awake through her next two classes and get through the band workout. A half-hour after eating the candy bar, she feels terrible. Could Mary Anne have made a better snack choice from the machine to satisfy her hunger and give her a boost of energy?

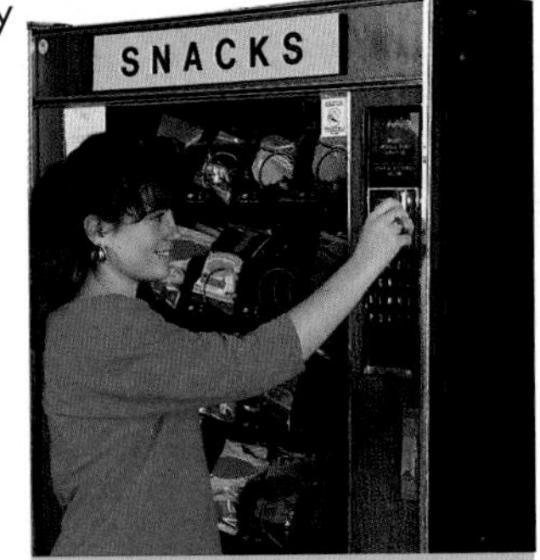

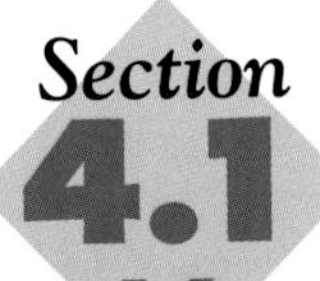

Section 4.1 Influences on Food Choices

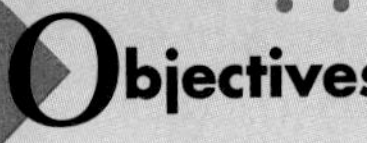

Objectives

- Describe the difference between hunger and appetite.
- Describe how different factors affect your food choices.
  LIFE SKILLS: Assessing Your Health
- List the short-term consequences of making poor nutritional choices.

Picture yourself in this scene. Your best friend says she is hungry and wants a snack. You are not really hungry, but you decide to join her and eat anyway.

Hunger Selecting snacks and eating when you are not hungry are two situations that may be common in making choices about what and when you eat. To understand some important issues regarding food, you need to think about why you eat. There are two important terms that are related to eating: hunger and appetite. **Hunger** is the body's physical response to the need for fuel. Your body uses food as the fuel to power the many chemical reactions that keep you alive and functioning. Hunger is a feeling you are born with. Symptoms of hunger include hunger pangs, weakness, dizziness, nausea, and a loss of concentration. Symptoms of hunger are relieved by eating. So how much should you eat? That is a question you will explore in detail in this chapter and the next one. For now, it is enough to say that you should eat until you feel full. The feeling of fullness you feel after eating is called *satiety*.

hunger: *the body's physical response to the need for food.*

Appetite Hunger differs from appetite. **Appetite** describes your desire to eat based on the pleasure you get from eating certain foods. When you are dealing with appetite, you might ask, What do I want to eat? There are a number of factors that influence your appetite, such as the taste, texture, or aroma of certain foods. Your physical health can affect your appetite. If you are

appetite: *the desire to eat based on the pleasure derived from eating.*

SECTION 4.1

Background
Effects of Poor Nutrition
Nutrition directly affects growth and development, tooth decay, and obesity in adolescents. In addition, poor diet contributes to the development of many chronic diseases that afflict American adults. Five of the ten leading causes of death in the United States have been related to poor or unbalanced diet: coronary heart disease, various cancers, stroke, noninsulin-dependent diabetes mellitus, and atherosclerosis.

Background
Patterns of Diet Inadequacy
Nutritional deficiencies were once prevalent in the United States; this pattern has given way to overeating and imbalance of dietary components needed for proper nutrition. However, undernutrition remains a problem for the isolated and the poor.

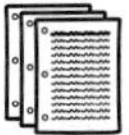

Personal Health Inventory
Have students complete the Personal Health Inventory for this chapter. The inventory helps them assess their eating habits.

Section 4.1 Lesson Plan

MOTIVATE

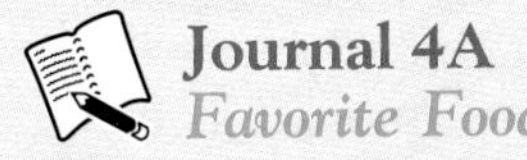

Journal 4A
Favorite Foods
This may be done as a warm-up activity. Ask students to think of a food that has always been a favorite of theirs, and why it is a favorite. Have them write in the Student Journal in the Student Activity Book about their memories associated with this food.

Class Discussion
Snack Choices
Ask students to name factors they think influenced Mary Anne's snack choice. *(Preference, belief that it was the best source of energy, advertising, possible sugar and/or chocolate addiction)* Have volunteers suggest why the candy bar was a poor choice. *(Sugar and chocolate supply a spurt of energy and stimulation, but low energy and a depressant effect follow immediately.)*

TEACH

Journal 4B
Motivations for Eating
Have students silently recall times when they have eaten but were not hungry or continued eating after they were full. They should record in the Student Journal in the Student Activity Book what factors they think caused them to behave this way.

Check Up

Have students hand in their Check Up answers anonymously and tally results of several (such as 1, 3, 6, and 8) on the chalkboard. Encourage students to note trends and decide which factors seem most influential for them.

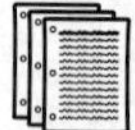

Section Review Worksheet 4.1

Assign Section Review Worksheet 4.1, which requires students to distinguish between hunger and appetite, identify consequences of poor nutrition, and list factors that affect food choices.

Section Quiz 4.1

Have students take Section Quiz 4.1.

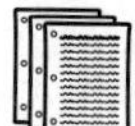

Reteaching Worksheet 4.1

Students who have difficulty with the material may complete Reteaching Worksheet 4.1, which has them classify symptoms of hunger and appetite and identify consequences of poor nutrition.

Check Up

Charting Your Appetite

Answer the following questions related to hunger and appetite on a separate sheet of paper.

1. When is your desire to eat strongest?
2. When is your desire to eat weakest?
3. What moods cause an increase in your appetite?
4. What moods reduce your appetite?
5. What people affect your appetite?
6. What places cause an increase in your appetite?
7. What times of day do you notice an increase in your appetite?
8. At what times of day or in what situations do you eat, even if you aren't hungry? Why?

Now look at your responses. Do you have food habits that can lead to overeating? What changes can you make to have better control over your appetite?

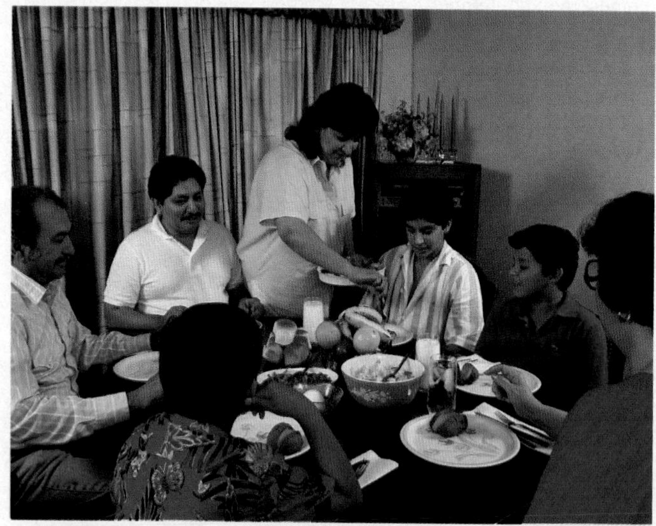

(FIGURE 4-1) **Eating can be a highly social activity, causing you to eat even when you are not hungry.**

sick, you generally don't feel like eating. If you become very active, your appetite can increase dramatically. The weather can affect your appetite. Some people lose their appetites when it is very hot outside, or they will only eat cold foods. Your culture and religion can have a major effect on your appetite. You may derive a lot of pleasure from eating certain foods that you grew up eating. You may also lose your appetite when presented with foods from another culture that appear unappealing to you.

Appetite refers to a desire for food. Hunger is your body telling you to eat. When hunger and appetite work together, you have a nice balance. But if you let appetite drive your eating behavior, you eat even when you are not hungry. When some people are depressed, they eat because they think they will feel better. Other people refuse to eat when they are depressed. Some people eat out of habit. They eat dinner at 5 P.M. whether they are hungry or not. All these reasons for eating help explain why so many people have trouble managing their weight. To strike the right balance between hunger and appetite, you need to understand when and why you eat.

What you should learn from this chapter is to make your selections based on sound nutritional practices. Selecting foods in this way will help maintain your physical and emotional well-being. Figure 4-2 lists major health problems related to poor nutrition. For young people, there is another special issue related to diet. Young people who are overweight are more likely to become obese adults than are young people of normal weight.

Environmental Factors There are several factors that influence the foods you choose and how much of them you eat. Perhaps most important among these factors are the social influences. The kinds of food you select are often determined by such

• • • TEACH continued

Class Discussion
Eating Habits and Health

Have students name all the factors they can think of that affect where, when, and how often a person eats. Write the list on the chalkboard and have volunteers identify factors that they think contribute to poor nutrition in America.

Role-Playing
Broadening Tastes in Food

If you have several students who are knowledgeable about the food of another region or country, pair them with students who are not familiar with the foods of those places. Then have them role-play ordering a meal in a restaurant in that country or region. The waiter can describe several dishes, and the customer can make a selection.

Extension
Ethnic Foods in Your Area

Encourage students to contact the local chamber of commerce and learn about ethnic restaurants in the area. Some students may prepare a graph showing how different cultures are represented. Others may contact selected restaurants to learn about foods they serve.

Selected Health Problems Related to Diet

Short Term Conditions

Fatigue
Bad moods
Depression

Long Term Conditions

Obesity
Heart disease
Stroke
Adult-onset diabetes
High blood pressure
Cirrhosis of the liver
Tooth decay
Cancer (some types)
Birth of low birth weight babies with poor mental and physical development
Dietary deficiency diseases (such as scurvy)

(FIGURE 4-2)

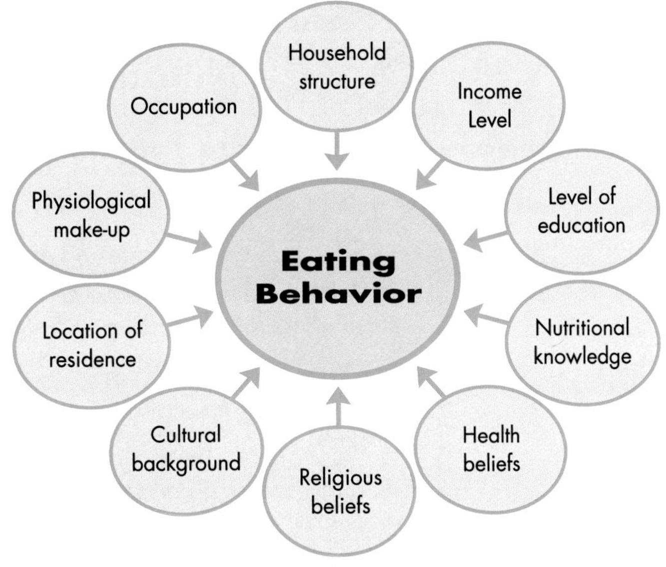

(FIGURE 4-3) **What you eat and when you eat is influenced by many factors. Describe how each of these factors affects your own food selections.**

things as your own family experiences, cultural heritage, cost, and other factors shown in Figure 4-3. For example, if you have grown up in the southwestern United States, you probably have eaten a lot of Mexican food even if it was not part of your ethnic background. Growing up on the East Coast, you might have eaten more seafood than someone who grew up in the Midwest Farm Belt. Your personality can also influence your food selections. Some people are very adventuresome about food and like to try new things. Other people feel very uncomfortable when faced with the thought of trying something new.

Review

1. *How does hunger differ from appetite? Should you eat to satisfy hunger or to satisfy your appetite?*
2. ***LIFE SKILLS: Assessing Your Health*** *List two ways in which your ethnic background may affect the types of food you eat.*
3. *Describe two consequences of poor nutrition that could affect you as an adult.*
4. ***Critical Thinking*** *How do you know when you are hungry? How do you know when your appetite is at work?*

Review Answers

1. Hunger is your body telling you to eat; appetite is your desire to have food. You should eat to satisfy your hunger.

2. Students may answer that some foods may be more appealing than others because of familiar ethnic dishes or spices. Ethnic holidays may influence the types of foods eaten and how they are prepared.

3. Answers may include fatigue, bad moods, depression, obesity, heart disease, diabetes, high blood pressure, tooth decay, cancer, and dietary deficiency diseases.

4. Signs of hunger include hunger pangs, weakness, dizziness, nausea, and a loss of concentration. Your appetite is at work when you are eating for reasons other than being hungry.

ASSESS

Section Review

Have students answer the Section Review questions.

Alternative Assessment

Psychology of Eating

Have students explain in their own words why many decisions to eat are based on psychological or emotional reasons rather than physical reasons.

Closure

Persuading People Into Good Health

Have students write a brief paragraph persuading readers to follow a healthy diet in order to avoid health problems.

Background
Teen Nutrition Savvy
Most teens know that eating too much fat, sugar, and salt puts them at risk, yet many do not know which common foods are loaded with these things. A national adolescent student health survey showed that 73 percent know that eating foods high in saturated fat can cause heart disease. Yet 45 percent of this same sample did not know that a ham sandwich contains more fat than a turkey sandwich, and about 40 percent eat fried foods at least four times a week.

Section 4.2 Nutritional Components of Food

Objectives

- *Describe the roles and functions of the six classes of dietary nutrients.*
- *Identify problems that can occur from inadequate amounts of certain nutrients.*
- *List recommended dietary levels for various nutrients.*
- *Describe the differences among the various types of cholesterol.*

essential nutrients: *six categories of substances from food that nourish the body: carbohydrates, fats, proteins, vitamins, minerals, water.*

calorie: *a unit of measurement for energy. 1 nutrition calorie = 1 kilocalorie.*

carbohydrates: *a class of nutrients containing starches, simple sugars, glycogen, and dietary fiber.*

Nutrition refers to the study of the way in which the substances in food affect our health. Over the last 100 years, the American diet has changed drastically. It was not uncommon for a person's diet 100 years ago to reflect a heavy dependence on grains, fruits, and vegetables. While there is far more attention paid today to health and nutrition, the typical American diet is not as nutritionally balanced as that of our grandparents. Analyzing your eating patterns is very important because diet is related to six of the ten leading causes of death in the United States. Diet also plays a role in infant death, tooth decay, and being overweight, as shown in Figure 4-3.

A recent national survey of 10th graders indicates most students know that too much fat, sugar, and salt are unhealthy. They know these substances increase the chance of getting chronic diseases such as heart disease and cancer. But most students cannot choose between foods based on their fat, sugar, salt, and fiber content. It is also clear that the eating patterns of students frequently include many fried foods and snack foods, and beverages that have added sugar and salt. In this section you will learn about the basic nutrients. In the next section you will apply this knowledge to choose foods that provide energy, taste good, and keep you healthy.

Basic Principles of Nutrition

Foods contain substances needed for growth and development. The substances are classified into six groups called **essential nutrients,** which are necessary for the maintenance of health. There are six categories of essential nutrients: *carbohydrates, fats, proteins, vitamins, minerals, and water.* Of these six groups, carbohydrates, fats, and protein provide energy for the body in the form of **calories** *. The remaining three nutrients—vitamins, minerals, and water—are essential for the body to use these other nutrients properly.

Carbohydrates The term *carbohydrate* comes from the names of the three chemical elements in carbohydrates: carbon, oxygen, and hydrogen. In fact, the oxygen and hydrogen in carbohydrates are in the same proportions as found in water. Therefore, we get the name carbo (carbon) and hydrate (water).

Sugars and starches are **carbohydrates.** They are the main source of energy

*The nutrition calorie is actually a kilocalorie of energy (abbreviated kcal). There are 1000 calories in a nutrition calorie (sometimes spelled with a capital C).

Section 4.2 Lesson Plan

MOTIVATE

Cooperative Learning
Nose for Nutrition News
Make available a number of food sections from assorted newspapers and magazines. Have small groups of students scan the articles to find nutrition subjects they want to know more about and questions they would like to find answers for as they complete this section of the chapter. Have students write their questions and subjects on 3″ x 5″ cards and post them on a bulletin board. The cards can be regrouped under headings for the six nutrients and discussed as students learn about them.

TEACH

Class Discussion
Nutrient Knowledge Challenge
List the six groups of essential nutrients on the board as column headings. Have volunteers write one fact about each nutrient. Then have students challenge information they believe is misplaced or wrong. Tell students they will learn about the different types of nutrients in this section.

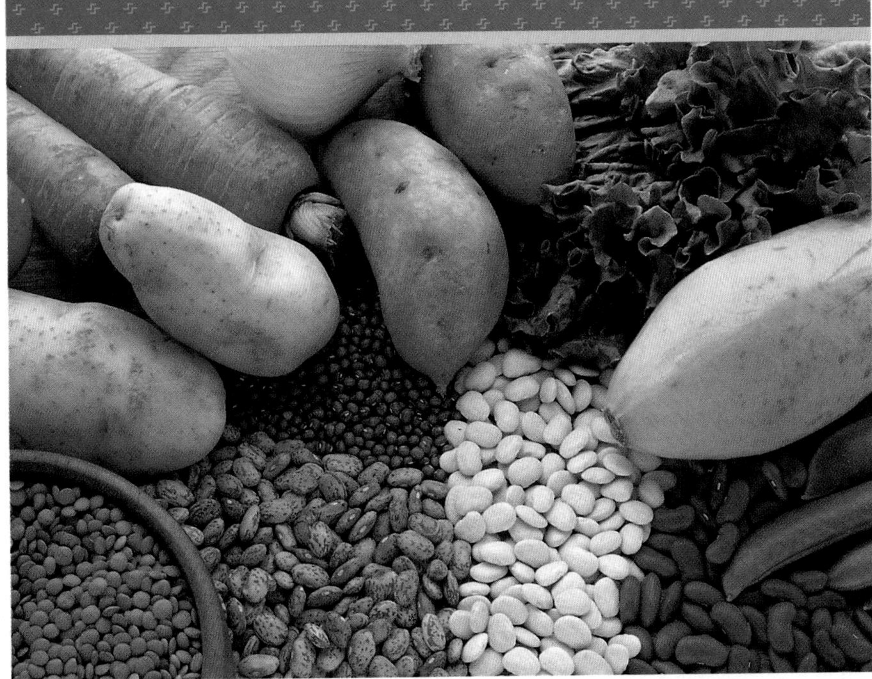

(FIGURE 4-4) **Complex carbohydrates have the added value of providing dietary fiber.**

upon which we depend. Each gram of carbohydrate provides four calories of energy. Carbohydrates provide the same number of calories per gram as protein and less than half the calories of fat, which provides 9 calories per gram.

There are generally two categories of carbohydrates: simple and complex. Simple carbohydrates are sometimes called *simple sugars.* Simple sugars are found in fruits, milk, and vegetables. Glucose is perhaps the most important simple sugar, because it is the major source of energy for the body. The process of digestion eventually breaks down all foods to this simple sugar. Glucose is used for energy and for repair of tissues in the body. The sugar you get from the sugar bowl is sucrose. Sucrose is made up, in part, of glucose.

The most common **complex carbohydrates** are starch, glycogen, and dietary fiber. These carbohydrates are called complex because they consist of three or more simple sugars attached to form long chain molecules. Starches come from plant products such as vegetables, potatoes, rice, and beans. Rich sources of complex carbohydrates include grains such as wheat, corn, and oats, and foods made from them (such as bread, cereal, and pasta). Almost all these sources of complex carbohydrates are low in fat and rich sources of vitamins, minerals, fiber, and proteins. Therefore, foods containing complex carbohydrates should be included in your daily diet.

Some excess glucose is stored as glycogen in the liver and in some muscle tissues. Glycogen can be broken down into glucose when the body needs energy. The remainder of excess glucose is stored in fatty tissue.

Dietary fiber is a complex carbohydrate, but unlike sugars it is not digested. Fiber helps increase the speed at which food

complex carbohydrates:

a subclass of carbohydrates that includes starches, dietary fiber, and glycogen.

dietary fiber:

a subclass of complex carbohydrates with a high ratio of plant material that is not absorbed by the body.

Background

America's Sweet Tooth

Americans as a group consume enormous quantities of sugar, much of it hidden in prepared foods heavily sweetened to appeal to our sweet tooth. In the late 1980s, data showed that the average American eats 120 pounds of sugar a year. When you consider that a 12-ounce soft drink contains 9 teaspoons of sugar, and some cereals are 90 percent sugar, it isn't surprising. Teens should become label readers and take note of the types and amounts of sugars in foods before purchasing them. Sugar has various names, such as sucrose, dextrose, maltose, and corn syrup.

Class Discussion

Fiber Rich, Calorie Poor

Why should you eat fiber-rich foods, since fiber isn't digested and provides no energy? *[Fiber is essential to healthy functioning of the digestive tract. Americans tend to take in too many calories. Eating foods high in fiber helps reduce the number of calories taken in; at the same time, it tends to increase intake of complex carbohydrates, vitamins, and minerals, for fiber-rich foods tend to be high in these nutrients, too.]*

Cooperative Learning

An Apple a Day

Have students work in small groups to list as many reasons as possible why an apple is a better snack than a candy bar. Suggest that they include both the positives of the fruit and the negatives of the candy.

Demonstration

Fat in Snack Foods

Display a number of popular snack foods. For each, provide a craft stick marked off in tenths. Ask students to guess the percent of total calories that are fat. Then color in the portion of the stick that indicates the actual percentage of fat content. (Use product labels and this information to calculate: there are 252 calories in an ounce of fat and an ounce of fat is equal to 28.3 grams.)

Making a Choice 4A

Party Refreshments

Assign the Party Refreshments card. The card asks students to plan healthy refreshments for a party.

fats:

a term used to describe a class of compounds in foods called lipids. Fats are energy storage molecules and supply more energy per gram than carbohydrates or proteins.

saturated fats:

fats that contain single bonds between carbon atoms and the maximum number of hydrogen atoms bonded to carbon.

moves through the digestive tract. Fiber is therefore a factor in preventing constipation. There is some evidence that dietary fiber probably plays a role in reducing the risk of certain diseases such as colon cancer. Fruits, vegetables, and grains are good sources of dietary fiber. Carbohydrates should make up more than 50 percent of the calories in your daily diet.

Fats The energy source that provides the most calories per ounce is **fats**. There are 252 calories in one ounce of fat. Carbohydrates contain only 112 calories per ounce. You can see that fats contain far more calories per ounce than carbohydrates.

Fats are also called lipids. Like carbohydrates, fats consist of carbon, hydrogen, and oxygen, but they are arranged differently. Like glycogen, fats are stored in adipose (fat) cells. Fats, perhaps even more than sugars, help make food tasty.

Functions of Fats in the Body

1. They store energy in a form that can be used when the body needs it.
2. They pad and protect organs.
3. They insulate the body from cold.
4. They are an important ingredient of several hormones.
5. They are necessary for the storage and transport of certain vitamins throughout the body.

Even though fats are important, most experts agree that most people eat far more fats than are necessary. It is recommended that less than 30 percent of the calories in your diet should come from fat. And of this 30 percent, no more than 10 percent should be the saturated kind.

Animal fats are generally **saturated fats,** which in chemical terms means saturated with hydrogen atoms. Saturated fats

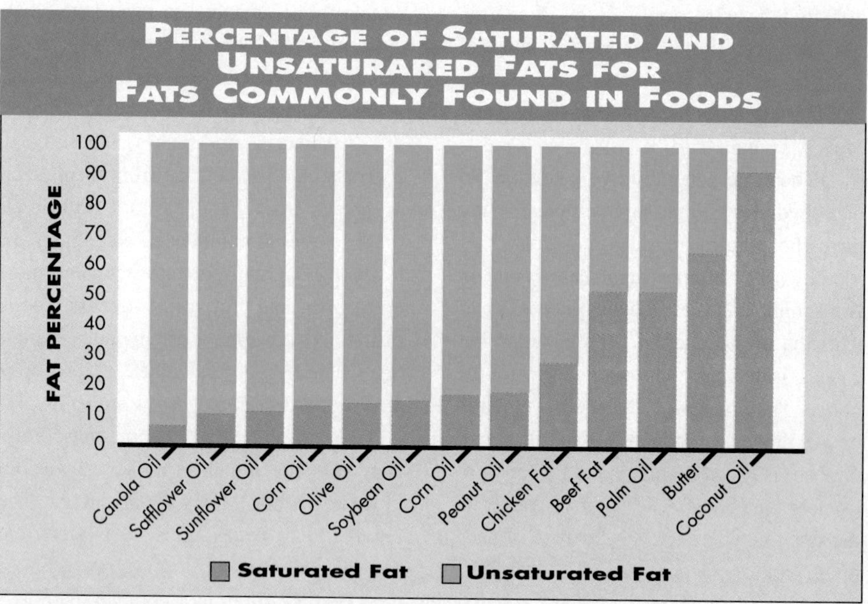

(FIGURE 4-5) **Avoid foods with ingredients that have high percentages of saturated fats.**

• • • TEACH continued

Reinforcement

There's Fat and There's FAT

Stress to students the importance of distinguishing between saturated fat and unsaturated fat. Have them study Figure 4-5 and name the types of oil or fat that contain more saturated fat than is healthful. *(Chicken fat, beef fat, butter, palm oil, and coconut oil)*

Provide several snack food labels and ask students to determine (1) the grams of fat per serving, and (2) the amount of saturated fat compared with unsaturated fat. Students can then rate each food according to a "health rating scale" they invent. You might include snack foods such as potato chips, crackers, pretzels, cookies, and doughnuts.

Class Discussion

Favorite Foods and Fat

Refer students to Figure 4-6 to discover other favorite foods that are high in fat. Ask: Which foods that you eat often should you eat less of?

Reinforcement

Cholesterol Confusion

Students need to understand that cholesterol is not the same as fat. Write on the chalkboard:

CHOLESTEROL ≠ FAT

Stress the fact that eating foods that contain no cholesterol is not a guarantee that you will have a low cholesterol blood serum level. In addition, foods with no cholesterol are not necessarily

PERCENTAGE OF CALORIES FROM FATS

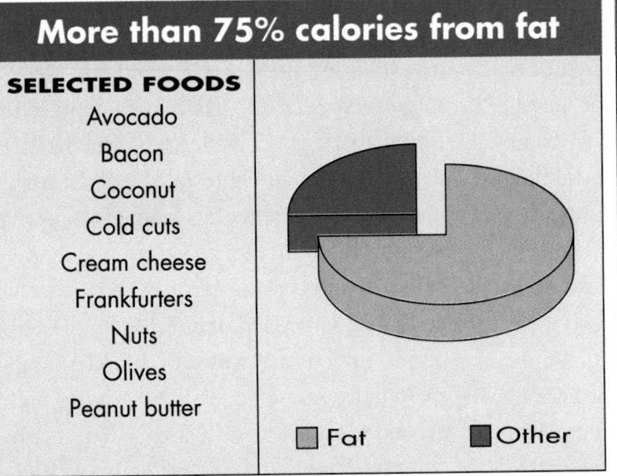

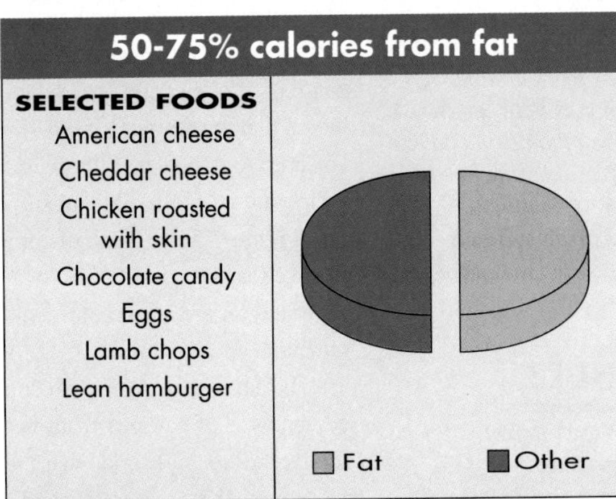

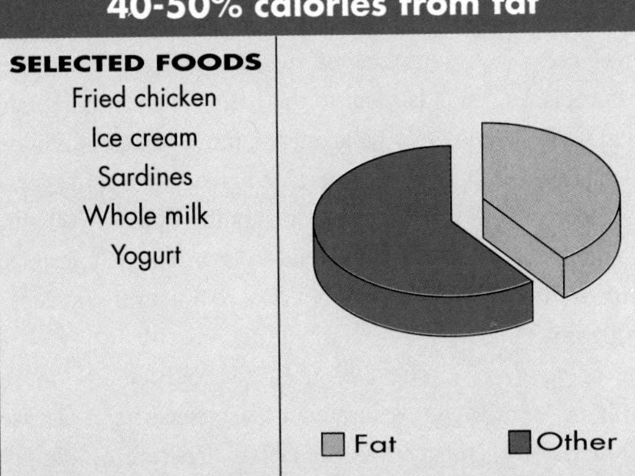

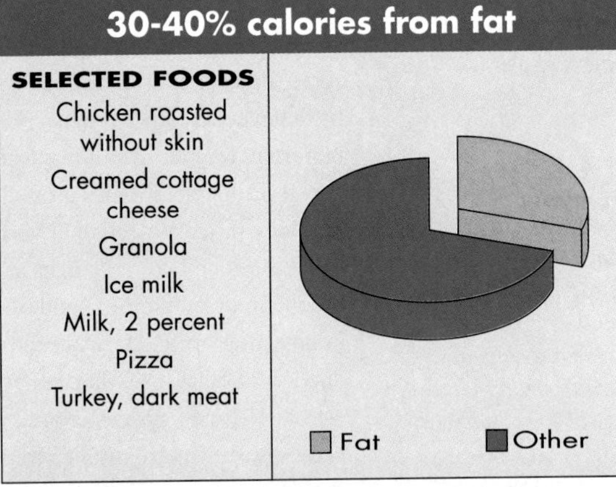

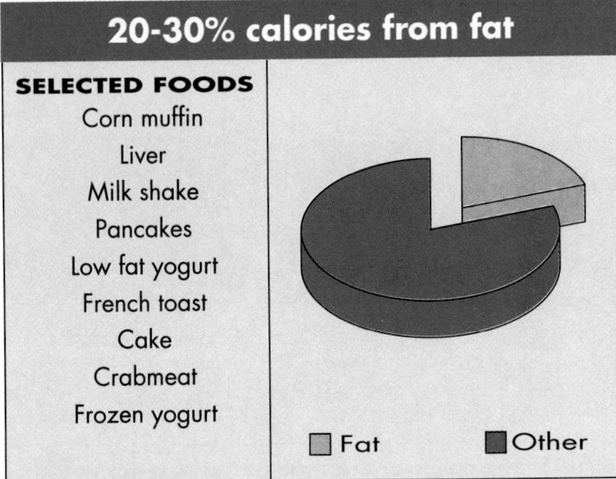

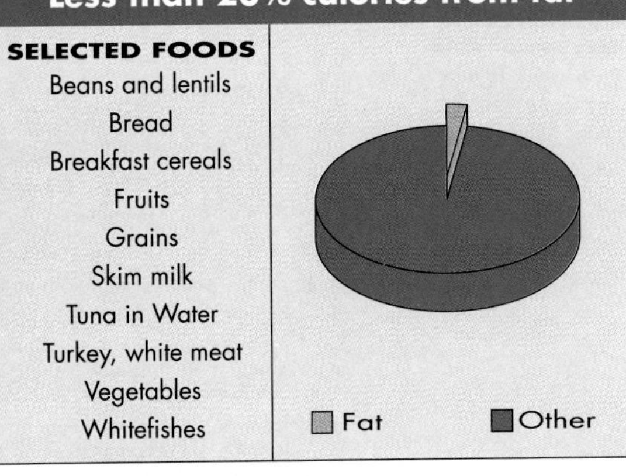

(FIGURE 4-6) **You might be surprised at the amount of fat some foods contain. Learn how to determine these percentages later in this chapter.**

low in fat. Have students refer again to snack food labels and compare cholesterol with fat content.

Many factors influence the level and types of cholesterol circulating in the blood. Also write on the board:

CHOLESTEROL INTAKE ≠ CHOLESTEROL IN BLOOD

For example, eating foods high in saturated fats can increase cholesterol level. When saturated fats are digested, they circulate in the bloodstream as forerunners of the components of LDL ("bad cholesterol"). The body can then use these components to build LDL.

Class Discussion
Limiting Cholesterol

If cholesterol is essential, why should you worry about how much you eat? *[The body makes cholesterol to fill its needs. Ingesting great amounts of cholesterol and saturated fats can lead to a buildup of the fatlike substance in the artery walls, which ultimately can lead to heart disease. In addition, high cholesterol is linked to some kinds of cancer.]*

Demonstration
Clinical Bloodwork to Show Serum Cholesterol Levels

To help students differentiate HDL from LDL, ask a medical lab or a doctor's office for a facsimile of a lab form for bloodwork, showing hypothetical results for a patient's levels of cholesterol in general and broken down into

unsaturated fats:

fats that contain one or more double bonds between carbon atoms and have less than the maximum number of hydrogen atoms bonded to carbon.

HDL:

"high-density lipoproteins" that remove cholesterol from the blood and transport it back to the liver.

LDL:

"low-density lipoproteins" are composed mostly of cholesterol and provide a means of transporting cholesterol to cells for cell processes.

cholesterol:

a fatlike substance that is part of all animal cells and is needed for the production of some hormones and fat digestion.

are generally solid at room temperature. The exception is palm and coconut oils, which are liquid at room temperature. **Unsaturated fats** generally come from plant sources. They contain fewer hydrogen atoms than a saturated fat of similar length. Unsaturated fats are often liquid at room temperature. Corn oil is mostly unsaturated fat. Figure 4-5 is a graph of commonly used fats. Those fats or oils with over 20 percent saturated fat are not recommended for good nutrition.

Figure 4-6 provides information on the percentages of calories from fat for various foods. Almost all foods that are sources of fat contain both saturated and unsaturated fats.

Cholesterol is a fatlike substance in some foods of animal origin. It is produced by the liver and other organs. Cholesterol is important to your health in several ways. It is part of the membranes around cells and it provides some protective covering to nerve fibers in your body. It is essential for the production of vitamin D and bile salts used in digestion of fat. It is needed for the production of certain sex hormones (androgen, estrogen, and progesterone). Although cholesterol is an important part of the diet, it is not a nutrient. The body makes all it needs. Cholesterol is a factor in the development of heart disease and stroke—two major killers of Americans.

You may have heard about two different terms relating to cholesterol, *high-density lipoproteins (HDL)* and *low-density lipoproteins (LDL)*. **HDL** is sometimes referred to as good cholesterol and **LDL** is described as bad cholesterol. LDL carries cholesterol and other fats from the digestive system through the blood to the body's cells. If more cholesterol is carried to the cells than is needed, the excess cholesterol builds up on the walls of blood vessels. Eventually, these deposits or plaques build up and clog arteries. Clogged arteries restrict the supply of oxygenated blood to the heart, resulting in a heart attack. The reason HDL is sometimes referred to as good is because it carries cholesterol from the bloodstream to the liver, where it is broken down to be used or removed from the body. It is now generally agreed that cholesterol levels in the blood should be below 200 milligrams per deciliter (mg/dL). Cholesterol intake should not exceed 300 milligrams per day.

Diets high in fat, particularly those high in saturated fat, can cause heart disease and certain cancers. Therefore, dietary guidelines suggest reducing intake of foods high in saturated fat and cholesterol.

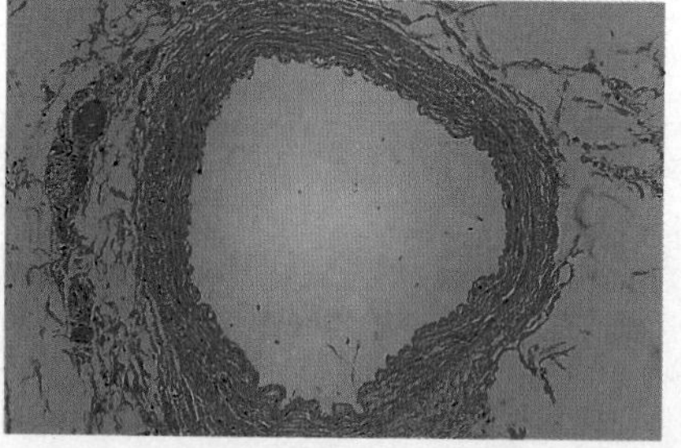

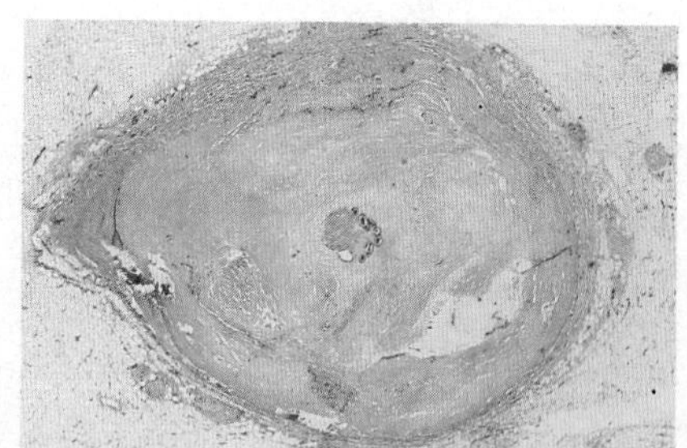

(FIGURE 4-7) **Heart disease resulting from clogged arteries can be the long-term effect of a diet that is high in cholesterol. The artery on the right is completely blocked with plaque, which contains high levels of cholesterol. Start now to monitor cholesterol levels throughout your life.**

• • • TEACH continued

HDL and LDL levels. Or, you may prefer to use the following example.

TEST NAME	RESULT	UNITS	NORMAL RANGE
Cholesterol	190	MG/DL	120 – 200
LDL	170*	MG/DL	130 – 160
HDL	20**	MG/DL	30 – 90

*High level may mean higher risk; desirable LDL = 130 MG/DL or less; 130–159 MG/DL = borderline level.

**Low level may mean higher risk; HDL should be above 35 MG/DL.

Copy the form for viewing on the overhead projector or chalkboard and help students read and interpret the data. The example included here shows that a normal range cholesterol level may, when further broken down to show HDL and LDL, reveal a high level of LDL, or "bad cholesterol."

Cooperative Learning

Picturing Plenty of Protein

Have small groups of students locate and clip pictures of foods that are good sources of protein. They should divide the pictures into foods that provide complete or incomplete proteins, and select several that would provide adequate protein for a day.

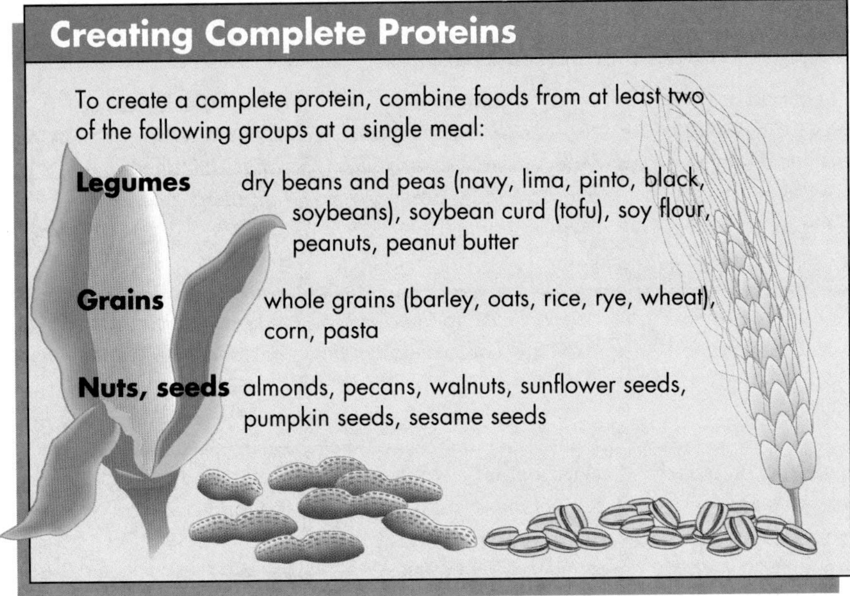

(FIGURE 4-8) **When selecting nuts and seeds to create complete proteins, limit the amount you eat because they are high in fat.**

Proteins Like carbohydrates and fats, **proteins** are made of carbon, hydrogen, and oxygen, but they also contain nitrogen. Proteins play a unique role in the growth and repair of body tissues. All cells contain some protein. It is also found in antibodies and some hormones. Enzymes that speed up the rate of chemical reactions in the body are proteins.

All proteins are made of amino acids. There are 20 amino acids; 11 of them can be made in the body and 9 others must be supplied by food. The 9 amino acids that cannot be produced in the body are called **essential amino acids.**

Because proteins perform so many necessary functions, you can see that the foods you select should include good sources of protein. However, the proteins found in the human body are not supplied directly from food. During digestion, proteins in food are broken down to their amino acids. These amino acids are the building blocks of new proteins for growth and tissue repair.

The proteins in food are sometimes classified as complete or incomplete proteins. A **complete protein** is one that contains all nine essential amino acids; an **incomplete protein** contains only some of these nine amino acids. Generally, foods that come from animal products (meat, poultry, fish, and milk products) contain complete proteins. Most proteins that come from plant sources are incomplete. It is possible, however, to get the proper amount of complete proteins from plant sources by selecting various protein sources so that all essential amino acids are supplied. Figure 4-8 contains a recommendation on how to select from a mix plant foods to achieve a diet that has complete proteins. Proteins should make up about 15 percent of your daily caloric intake for adequate nutrition.

proteins:

class of nutrients consisting of long chains of amino acids, which are the basic components of body tissue and provide energy.

complete protein:

a protein that contains all nine essential amino acids.

incomplete protein:

a protein that lacks one or more of the essential amino acids.

essential amino acids:

a group of nine amino acids that cannot be manufactured by the body and must be supplied by food.

Class Discussion
Complete vs. Incomplete

Help students see that proteins supplied by plants are not inferior because they are incomplete. **How is it possible to provide your body with all essential amino acids if you eat incomplete proteins in plant food?** *[Eating certain combinations of plant proteins provides all the essential amino acids.]* **What would be an advantage of getting most of your protein from plant sources?** *[If you provided enough of the right kinds of amino acids, you would at the same time boost your intake of vitamins, minerals, fiber, and complex carbohydrates, which are all more likely to be lacking than protein in the American diet.]*

Class Discussion
Some Things Bear Repeating

Have students explain why it's a good idea to eat foods rich in vitamins C and B every day. Ask them to respond to the following scenario:

Suppose a healthy person who has had an adequate diet is shipwrecked. She finds water on the island but no food. She is rescued one week later. **What vitamin(s) will she need most?** *[B and C]* **Why?** *[The body can't store them, but must replenish them daily.]*

Game
Vitamin Spin

Make a wheel with the 13 vitamins listed on it, and a spinner. A student team spins the wheel and must de-

Fat Soluble Vitamins

Vitamin	Function	Sources	Deficiency
A	*Maintains healthy eyes, skin, bones, teeth, keeps lining of Digestive tract resistant to infection*	*Milk products, liver, yellow and dark leafy green fruits and vegetables*	*Night blindness, impaired growth*
D	*Promotes normal growth, assists with calcium and phosphorus use in building bones and teeth*	*Fish-liver oils, fortified milk, liver, egg yolk, salmon, tuna*	*Rickets (inadequate growth of bones and teeth)*
E	*Prevents destruction of red blood cells; needed for certain enzymes to work*	*Wheat germ, vegetable oils, legumes, nuts, dark green vegetables*	*Red blood cell rupture causing anemia*
K	*Assists with blood clotting*	*Green, leafy vegetables and vegetable oils, tomatoes, potatoes*	*Slow clotting of blood, hemorrhage*

(FIGURE 4-9) **Fat-soluble vitamins can be stored in the body, while water-soluble vitamins (shown on the next page) cannot. It is best to obtain vitamins from food sources rather than from vitamin supplements.**

vitamins:

organic substances that assist in the chemical reactions that occur in the body.

Vitamins **Vitamins** are compounds that help regulate certain chemical reactions in the body. Though vitamins do not supply energy, they are essential for good health. The only vitamins the body can make are vitamins D and K.

Vitamins are grouped into two different categories: those that are fat soluble and those that are water soluble. *Fat soluble* means that the substance dissolves in fat. Fat-soluble vitamins include vitamins A, D, E, and K. Because they dissolve in fat, these vitamins can be stored in body fat. A balanced diet, which you will learn about in the next section, provides the right levels of fat-soluble vitamins and the fats needed to store these vitamins. If a person takes in high levels of fat-soluble vitamins from taking too many vitamin pills, the excess amounts of these vitamins are stored in the body. The excess can be harmful. Figure 4-9 contains a listing of the fat-soluble vitamins, their sources, and their importance to health.

Water-soluble vitamins like B and C are not stored in body tissue. Because water-soluble vitamins dissolve in water, any excess vitamins are excreted in urine. Therefore, you must have regular sources of water-soluble vitamins to prevent deficiency diseases. If you supplement your diet far beyond your dietary needs, you will excrete the excess. Figure 4-9 also contains a listing of the water-soluble vitamins, their

• • • TEACH continued

scribe a function, one source, and a deficiency related to the vitamin landed on. The majority of team members must agree with the answers provided by the spokesperson. For each correct answer, the team wins 5 points. If all three answers are correct, the team spins again. A vitamin may be used more than once, but answers should not be duplicated.

Debate the Issue
Vitamin Pills

Have two teams of students debate the question: Should teens take vitamin pills? Each team will need time to collect information and organize presentations. After both sides of the issue have been presented and rebuttals given, have the rest of the class tell which arguments were most convincing, and why.

Class Discussion
Vitamin Megadoses

Students should be aware of the negative effects of large doses of vitamin supplements. Ask what might happen if they took megadoses of vitamin A or E. *(The body would use what it needs. Then it would store these fat-soluble vitamins, even to a toxic level.)* What are the effects of megadoses of vitamin C? *(The body will excrete the excess, wasting the vitamins.)*

Water Soluble Vitamins

Vitamin	Function	Sources	Deficiency
B1 Thiamine	*Assists with conversion of carbohydrates to energy, normal appetite and digestion, nervous system function*	*Pork products, liver, legumes, enriched and whole grain breads, cereals, nuts*	*Beriberi (inflamed nerves, muscle weakness, heart problems)*
B2 Riboflavin	*Assists with nerve cell function, healthy appetite and release of energy from carbohydrates, protein, and fats*	*Milk, eggs, whole grain products, green leafy vegetables, dried beans, enriched breads, cereals, and pasta*	*Cheilosis (skin sores on nose and lips, sensitive eyes)*
B3 Niacin	*Maintenance of normal metabolism, digestion, nerve function, energy release*	*Red Meats, organ meats, fish, enriched breads and cereals, green vegetables*	*Pellagra (soreness on mouth, diarrhea, irritability, depression)*
B6 Pyridoxine	*Necessary for normal carbohydrate, protein and fat metabolism*	*Whole grain products, fish, bananas, green leafy vegetables*	*Anemia, dermatitis*
B12	*Necessary for formation of red blood cells; normal cell function*	*Lean meats, liver, egg products, milk, cheese*	*Pernicious anemia, stinted growth*
Folacin	*Necessary for formation of hemoglobin in red blood cells; necessary for production of genetic material*	*Green vegetables, liver, whole grain products, legumes*	*Anemia, diarrhea*
Pantothenic Acid	*Assists with energy release from carbohydrates, protein, and fats; used to produce some hormones*	*Whole grain cereals, liver green vegetables, eggs, nuts*	*None noted*
Biotin	*Necessary for normal metabolism of carbohydrates and some other B vitamins*	*Organ meats, egg yolks, green vegetables*	*Skin disorders, hair loss*
C Ascorbic Acid	*Needed for normal development of connective tissue, including those holding teeth; wound healing; use of iron*	*Citrus fruits, melons, green vegetables, potatoes*	*Scurvy (slow healing of wounds, bleeding gums and loose teeth)*

Class Discussion
Minerals Stand Alone

How do minerals differ from other nutrients? *(They are not produced by organisms.)* Do you need macrominerals more than you need trace minerals? *(No. You need macrominerals in larger doses than trace minerals, but both types are essential.)*

Class Discussion
Minerals Up Close and Personal

Have students refer to Figure 4-10 and identify the macrominerals and the trace minerals. Ask them to assess their diets and note any deficiencies they may have. Encourage students to discuss reasons why calcium and sodium intake should be kept at recommended doses. *(Calcium deficiency leads to bone weakness and osteoporosis; excess sodium intake is thought to be related to heart disease and high blood pressure.)*

Class Discussion
Salt Without Shakers

How can a person who uses no table salt be getting adequate sodium in his or her diet? *(Various foods contain sodium; sodium intake comes from other forms than sodium chloride—e.g., MSG, sodium nitrate.)*

Background
Getting Enough Calcium

Recent research shows that women in general and teens in particular don't get enough calcium. Adolescent and young adult women particularly need to increase their food calcium consumption. A recent study showed that only 15 percent of the girls and 53 percent of the boys ages 12 to 16 consume the RDA of 1,200 mg of calcium.

About 55 percent of the calcium in U.S. diets comes from dairy products; the rest, comes from such foods as canned fish, vegetables and legumes, and seeds and nuts.

sources, and their importance to health. A well-balanced diet provides enough of each of these necessary vitamins without the need to add vitamin pills.

minerals: *inorganic substances that are generally absorbed to form structural components of the body.*

Minerals **Minerals** are naturally occurring substances that contribute to the normal functioning of the body. Unlike vitamins that are produced and found in living materials, minerals are not produced by living organisms. More than 20 minerals have been found that are needed for healthy functioning. Figure 4-10 contains a summary of some of the most important minerals.

Sometimes minerals are divided into two different categories: *macrominerals*, which include calcium, chlorine, magnesium, phosphorus, potassium, sodium, and sulfur; and *trace minerals*, which include fluorine, copper, iodine, iron, manganese, and zinc. Macrominerals are needed in large amounts by the body, and trace minerals are needed in smaller doses. There have been a number of important health issues raised recently regarding several of these minerals, most particularly regarding sodium (in table salt) and calcium.

Sodium is one of the electrolytes. An electrolyte is an electrically charged particle. Proper electrolyte balance is needed to keep the body's internal environment stable. Many chemical reactions in the body require a certain electrolyte balance. A major source of sodium in the diet is salt. If you take in too much salt, you get thirsty. Too much sodium outside of your body cells causes your cells to lose water in response to the high sodium concentration. Because your body is losing water, you feel thirsty. In most cases, the body has special systems to keep a normal water balance even when you eat salty foods. However, a diet high in sodium exceeds the body's capacity to maintain stability. When there is an imbalance, other health problems can occur.

The amount of sodium you take in each day is thought to be related to high blood pressure. High blood pressure (also hypertension) is thought to result in stroke, coronary artery disease, congestive heart failure, and kidney failure. There is some controversy regarding the relationship between sodium and these diseases. So far, there appears to be no evidence that sodium causes high blood pressure in healthy, normal individuals. However, people who have other risk factors for these diseases, such as a family history of heart attacks or stroke, should try to reduce sodium intake. This can be done by not adding salt to food during cooking or at the table, and by reading food labels to determine the amount of sodium in processed foods. Sodium appears in foods as various compounds, such as monosodium glutamate (MSG), sodium bicarbonate, sodium nitrite, sodium benzoate, sodium propionate, and sodium citrate. In choosing foods, look for these compounds on the ingredient label. A balanced diet should include foods that together provide no more than 3 grams (3000 milligrams) of sodium per day.

Calcium is the most abundant mineral in the body. Most calcium in the body is found in bones and teeth. It is an important mineral because of its presumed role in preventing osteoporosis. Osteoporosis is a degenerative disease in which bones weaken with age because they become less dense. Weakened bones break easily, which becomes a common problem for the elderly. Women are affected more than men by osteoporosis. Calcium supplements add calcium to the diet to help maintain bone density. However, experts agree that calcium pills are not as effective in providing calcium for bone growth as are foods containing calcium. Osteoporosis is a complex disease and other factors such as exercise may be just as important in preventing it.

• • • TEACH continued

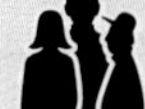

Cooperative Learning
Bone Builders

Have students bring to class labels from calcium-rich foods and work in groups to determine several ways to supply the 1,200 mg of calcium they need every day. Suggest they use a form like the one at right to record their data.

Food	Serving size	mg calcium serving	No. of servings needed

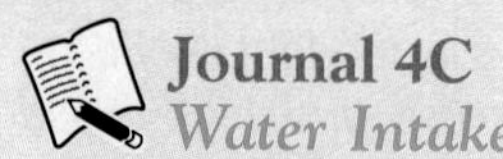

Journal 4C
Water Intake

Have students note in the Student Journal how much water they drink in a day. Suggest that they list times during the day when it would be convenient to have a drink of water.

Class Discussion
Importance of Water

Why might water be considered the most important of the six nutrients? *[It makes up the greatest part of the body; it provides a medium for essential body reactions and keeps levels of other nutrients in balance; water regulates temperature and allows passage of gases, nutrients, and wastes.]*

Listing of Important Minerals and Their Function

Mineral	Function	Sources
Calcium	*Necessary for normal growth of bones and teeth, transmission of nerve cell impulses, Muscle contract*	*Milk and dairy products, dark leafy green vegetables*
Chlorine	*Maintenance of water balance*	*Table salt, high salt meats (ham), some cheese, crackers*
Copper	*Needed for normal production of hemoglobin, bone, and melanin (involved in skin color)*	*Liver, shellfish, legumes, nuts, whole-grain products*
Iodine	*Essential for production of thyroid hormone*	*Iodized salt, seafood*
Iron	*Found in hemoglobin; needed for some enzymes*	*Organ meats, red meat, whole grains, dark green vegetables, legumes*
Magnesium	*Needed for chemical reactions during metabolism*	*Milk, dairy products, green leafy vegetables*
Manganese	*Used in enzymes for synthesis of cholesterol, formation of urea, normal function of nervous tissue*	*Whole grain products, leafy green vegetables, fruits, legumes, nuts*
Phosphorus	*Necessary for normal structure of bones and teeth, and plays a role in normal metabolism*	*Meats, poultry, fish, cheese, whole grain products, legumes and nuts*
Potassium	*Helps maintain normal metabolism, nerve and muscle function*	*Meats, poultry, fish, fruits, vegetables*
Sodium	*Essential for proper water balance in cells and tissues; nerve cell conduction*	*Table salt, high salt meats (ham), cheeses, crackers*
Sulfur	*Found in several amino acids*	*Meats, milk, eggs, legumes, nuts*
Zinc	*Needed for several digestive enzymes; plays a role in respiration, bone and liver metabolism, and healing of wounds*	*Seafood, meats, milk, poultry*

(FIGURE 4-10) **The amount of minerals you need to consume each day measures out to about a tablespoon. You need greater amounts of minerals than vitamins.**

Section Review Worksheet 4.2

Assign Section Review Worksheet 4.2, which asks students to list functions of six classes of nutrients, identify symptoms of calcium deficiency, specify recommended dietary levels for various nutrients, and distinguish between the two types of cholesterol.

Section Quiz 4.2

Have students take Section Quiz 4.2

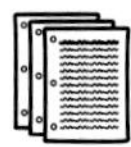

Reteaching Worksheet 4.2

Students who have difficulty with the material may complete Reteaching Worksheet 4.2, which asks them to classify nutrients and complete a graph showing recommended dietary levels of three nutrients.

Demonstration
Thirsty Cells

You can model the process that stimulates thirst: excess sodium in the blood causes water to move out of cells and into the blood. In other words, water diffuses across cell membranes to equalize the concentration of solutions. This can be illustrated with a small clear cup containing colored water (representing the cell) and a clear glass container of salt water (representing the fluid around the cell). Cover the cup of colored water with a piece of cheesecloth, held on with a rubber band. Lower it carefully into the container of salt water. Over time, colored water should diffuse through the fabric "cell membrane" into the surrounding salt water. Explain that water leaves the cells to try to correct the imbalance of sodium concentration in the blood. This triggers a signal to the brain, resulting in a feeling of thirst.

Reinforcement
Who Needs Water?

Most Americans fail to drink enough water. Remind students of the following.

1. Body processes and cell maintenance cannot proceed normally without adequate water intake. Dehydration doesn't just make you feel bad; it *is* bad for your body!

2. Some things people think they can substitute for water actually cause their bodies to lose water. For example, al-

Your diet should supply about 1200 milligrams of calcium per day for good health. This level is also sufficient for pregnant women and women who are breastfeeding (lactating). The elderly need more, because calcium is not as readily absorbed as you get older. Figure 4-19 shows some excellent natural sources of calcium.

Water Water is an essential compound in your diet. About two-thirds of your body weight is water (65 to 70 percent in males, 55 to 65 percent in females). The percentage of water in the body depends on the amount of body fat a person has. People with high percentages of body fat have lower percentages of body water than normal. Much of this water is found inside your cells. The remaining water is found in the spaces surrounding cells, and in your bloodstream. Most body fluids, such as blood and digestive juices, are 80 percent water. If a 16-year-old male weighs 150 pounds, as much as 105 pounds of that weight is water. Similarly for a 16-year-old female weighing 120 pounds, as much as 78 pounds of that weight is water. The importance of water in the diet becomes obvious when you look at all the ways the body uses water to maintain its stability.

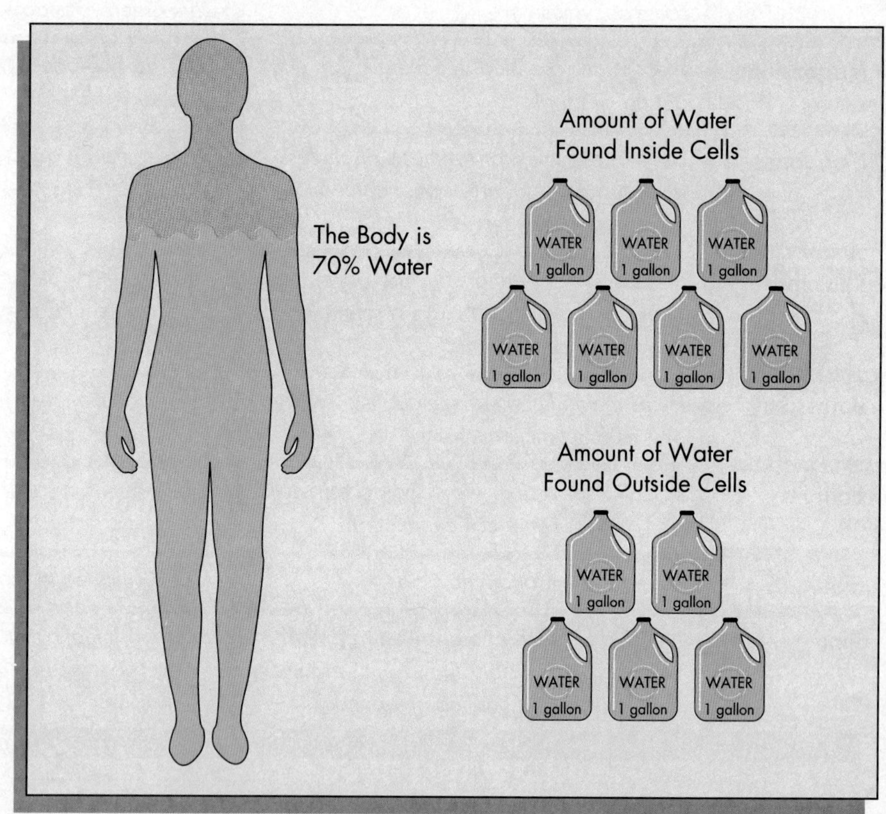

(FIGURE 4-11) **Since the body is mostly water, maintaining proper fluid balance is critical for good health.**

• • • TEACH continued

cohol and drinks containing caffeine (like many soft drinks) act as diuretics; that is, they cause water to be pumped out of the body.

Extension

Salt Watch

Have students interview adults who are monitoring their sodium intake, to learn what methods they use to reduce their salt consumption.

Functions of Water in the Body

1. All body functions are the result of chemical reactions. Most chemical reactions in the body can occur only in a water medium because substances dissolve in water.
2. The speed at which some of these chemical reactions occur is affected by how acidic body fluids are. Water helps maintain acidity at the proper levels.
3. Water is a product of the chemical reactions that supply energy to drive your body processes.
4. Water in body fluids provides a medium to transport gases, nutrients, and waste products throughout the body.
5. Water helps regulate body temperature. Water loss through perspiration helps cool the body.

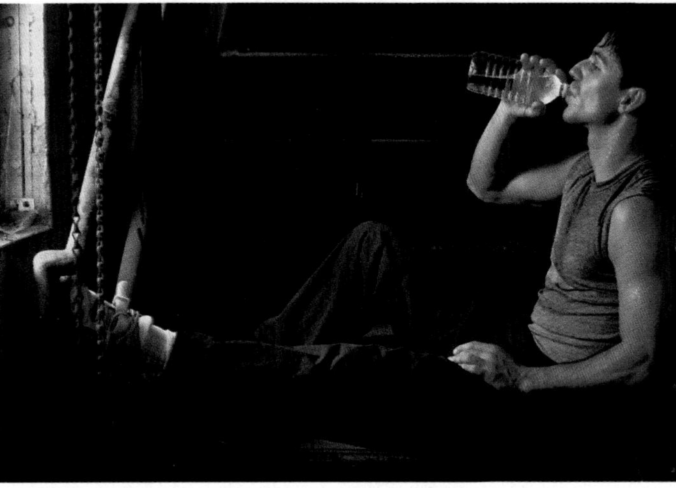

(FIGURE 4-12) **Drinking water after heavy activity replaces fluids lost from sweating.**

Water is so vital that it is rare to live for more than 10 days without water, even though you could live several weeks without food. When the amount of water excreted exceeds the amount of water taken in, you are in a state of **dehydration**. A prolonged state of dehydration can lead to kidney failure and death. Dehydration can occur as a result of heavy physical activity or an illness that includes throwing up, diarrhea, or fever. Drinking too much alcohol or eating a high-protein diet can also cause dehydration.

We ingest water by drinking fluids and by eating. Many foods contain large amounts of water. Some fruits and vegetables, such as potatoes, apples, lettuce, and watermelon, are almost 80 percent water. You need to consume at least 8 to 10 cups of water per day. If you are very active or live in a very hot climate, you will need more to keep your body functioning properly.

dehydration:

a state in which the body has lost more water than has been taken in.

Review

1. *Describe the importance of complex carbohydrates in the diet.*
2. *Which nutrient supplies the most calories per ounce?*
3. *How does a low calcium intake affect the body?*
4. *Why should you limit the amount of sodium in your diet?*
5. *Why are saturated fats to be avoided in making food selections?*
6. *How much of your daily caloric intake should come from carbohydrates, fats, and proteins?*
7. *Why do you need to have some fat in your diet?*
8. ***Critical Thinking*** *Why is it misleading to label peanut butter as having "no cholesterol"?*

Review Answers

1. Complex carbohydrates supply the body with energy as well as vitamins, minerals, proteins, and fiber.
2. fat
3. It can lead to osteoporosis, or weakened bones that break easily.
4. High levels of sodium may cause high blood pressure in some people.
5. Saturated fats contain large amounts of low-density lipoproteins (LDL), which have been associated with coronary artery disease. High fat intake has also been associated with certain cancers.
6. 50 percent carbohydrates; 30 percent fats; 15 percent proteins
7. Fat is a source of stored energy and is needed for storage and transport of certain vitamins throughout the body. Fats in the body help protect vital organs and also insulate the body from cold. They are also an important ingredient of several hormones.
8. Peanut butter never has had cholesterol. Cholesterol is found in foods of animal origin only.

ASSESS

Section Review

Have students answer the Section Review questions.

Alternative Assessment

Good Food Salesmanship

Have students bring in fresh foods to "sell" to the class. Each must persuade other students of the food's value in promoting good health by explaining its nutrients.

Closure

Importance of Fats

Have students explain the pros and cons of fats—why we need fats in the diet—but not too many.

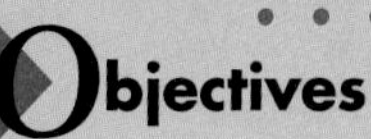

Section 4.3 Analyzing Your Nutritional Needs

Objectives

- *Define the nutritional requirements for healthy teens.*
- *Classify foods into the appropriate food groups.*
- *Interpret food labeling to analyze nutritional breakdown.*
- *Make food selections that satisfy nutritional requirements using the Food Pyramid and Dietary Guidelines.*
  LIFE SKILLS: Making Responsible Decisions
- *Identify special nutritional needs of selected populations.*

In the last section you studied the nutrients that are part of your diet. In this section you will learn how to use this information in selecting foods that provide a nutritionally balanced diet. There are some specific sources of information available to judge a person's dietary needs, including the Recommended Dietary Allowances (RDAs), the U.S. RDAs, and the Dietary Guidelines for Americans. Let's take a brief look at each.

1. ***Recommended Dietary Allowances (RDAs)*** are based on a number of personal characteristics such as age, gender, height, weight, and activity level. There are also specific guidelines for women who are pregnant or breast-feeding an infant. RDAs provide some general guidelines for the intake of nutrients for which the requirements are known (protein; vitamins A, D, E, K, C, B_1, B_2, B_3, B_6, B_{12}; folic acid; calcium; phosphorus; zinc; iron; magnesium; iodide; and selenium).

   Figure 4-14 contains an overview of the RDAs for young adults. RDAs are set high to cover the nutritional

Recomended Dietary Allowances (RDAs) for Teenagers

Category	Age (years)	Weight (pounds)	Height (inches)	Food Energy (calories)	Protein (grams)	Calcium (milligrams)
Males	11-14	99	62	2,700	45	1,200
	15-18	145	69	2,800	59	1,200
Females	11-14	101	62	2,200	46	1,200
	15-18	120	64	2,100	44	1,200

Section 4.3 Lesson Plan

MOTIVATE

Class Discussion
May I Take Your Order?

Display (or make a transparency of) a menu from a local restaurant and ask students to select items they would order for breakfast, lunch, or dinner. Encourage the class to discuss reasons for their choices and speculate about which choices are healthiest.

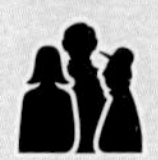

Cooperative Learning
Unwelcome Surprises in Packaged Foods

Provide small groups with labels saved from prepared food products. Have students analyze them for amount of sodium (or salt), fat (saturated versus unsaturated), and sugar (in its various forms). Have them pick out the three biggest "surprises"—foods that were unexpectedly high in these three nutrients. Stimulate discussion about reasons why Americans have trouble limiting their intake of fat, salt, and sugar.

TEACH

Class Discussion
RDAs and U.S. RDAs

Why were RDAs and U.S. RDAs developed? *[To provide guidelines for monitoring nutritional adequacy of diet.]* **How do the two measures differ and why are U.S. RDAs given on food labeling?** *[RDAs are tailored to certain*

Food Labeling/Dietary Information

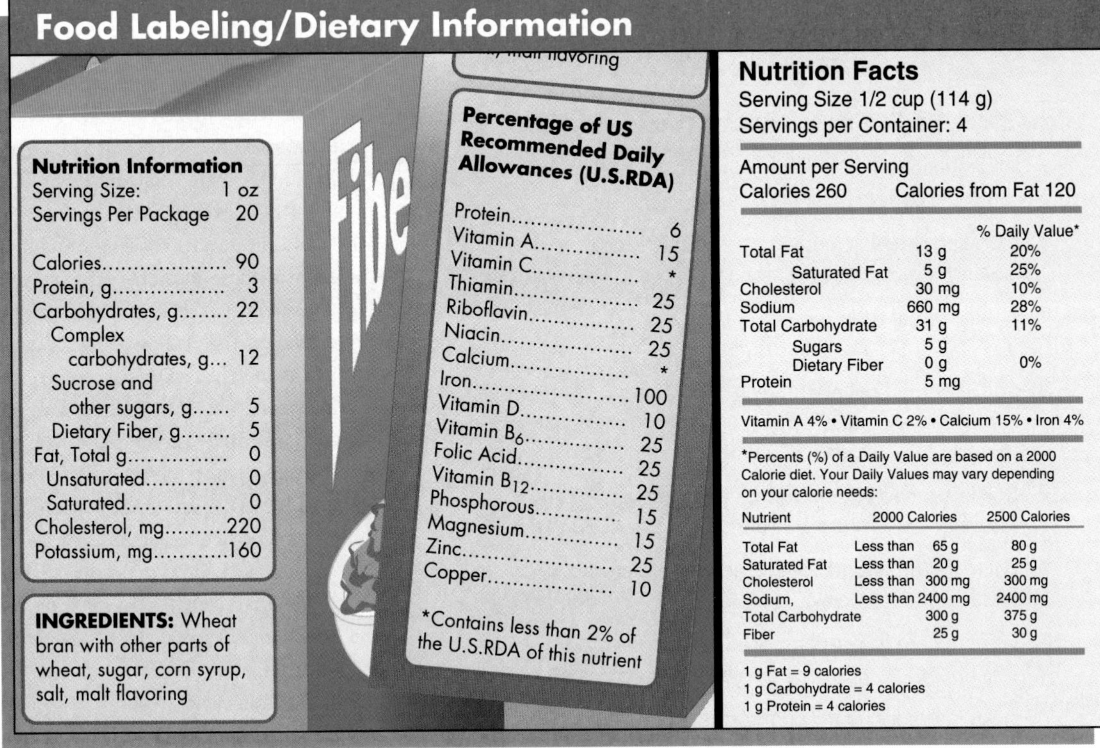

(FIGURE 4-13) **U.S. RDAs were once the basis for providing nutritional information on packaged foods. The food label, on the left, is based on U.S. RDAs. The Nutrition Facts food label, on the right, is based on the Dietary Guidelines for Americans. In what ways is the new labeling system better?**

(FIGURE 4-14)

Phosphorus (mg)	Iron (mg)	Viamin A (international units)	Thiamin (mg)	Riboflavin (mg)	Niacin (mg)	Ascorbic Acid (vitamin C)(mg)
1,200	*12*	*1,000*	*1.3*	*1.5*	*17*	*50*
1,200	*12*	*1,000*	*1.5*	*1.8*	*20*	*60*
1,200	*15*	*800*	*1.1*	*1.3*	*15*	*50*
1,200	*15*	*800*	*1.1*	*1.3*	*15*	*60*

personal characteristics, such as age, gender, height, weight, and level of activity. U.S. RDAs simply use the highest RDA value for a nutrient. Food labels must provide information about adequate levels to the whole population. Using a median number would underestimate the needs of many people.]

Class Discussion
Determining Your RDAs

Have students study Figure 4-14 to find out their RDAs according to age, gender, height, and weight. Have them note nutrient requirements that differ for males and females.

Cooperative Learning
Assessing Nutrient Values

In small groups, have students evaluate the nutrition of the cereal in Figure 4-13, using the guidelines in Figures 4-14 and 4-15. Require that students determine the following:

- how the cereal fits within guidelines for fat, cholesterol, protein, carbohydrate, and sodium intake
- what percentage of the RDA for calories for a 16-year-old male is supplied by one serving
- how many milligrams or grams of vitamins, minerals, and protein are supplied in a serving.

Class Discussion
Rounding Out Breakfast

After students have analyzed the nutrition of the cereal described in Figure 4-13, have them suggest other foods

Check Up

How Much Do You Know About Food Selection?

Have students turn in their choices for the 10 items and tally the answers on the board. Discuss the answers to items many students got wrong.

Check Up

How Much Do You Know About Food Selection?

From the statements listed below, choose the best answer. Then check the correct answers below.

1. Cooking practice that increases fat in foods
   baking broiling frying don't know
2. Boiling vegetables reduces vitamins
   yes no don't know
3. Salt in peanut butter-and-jelly sandwich compared with a hot dog
   less salt more same don't know
4. Salt in canned vegetables compared with frozen
   less salt more same don't know
5. Fat in frozen yogurt compared with ice cream
   less fat more same don't know
6. Fiber in corn flakes compared with bran cereal
   less fiber more same don't know
7. Fiber in baked beans compared with baked potato
   less fiber more same don't know
8. Eating fatty foods may cause
   cavities stomach cancer
   heart disease don't know
9. Eating too little fiber may cause
   colon cancer high blood pressure
   heart disease don't know
10. Eating sugar may cause
    heart disease low blood pressure
    cavities don't know
11. Amount of iron needed by females compared with males
    less iron more same don't know
12. Amount of calcium needed by teenagers compared to middle-aged women
    less calcium more same don't know

1) frying; 2) yes; 3) less salt; 4) more salt; 5) less fat; 6) less fiber; 7) more fiber; 8) heart disease; 9) colon cancer; 10) cavities; 11) more iron; 12) more calcium.

needs of almost all healthy people in a particular age group.

2. ***United States Recommended Daily Allowances (U.S. RDAs)*** are the recommendations of the Food and Drug Administration. For each nutrient, the highest RDA level is taken as the U.S. RDA and the result is a single number for each of these nutrients. When you look at a nutrition label, the percentage of the recommended allowances for each nutrient is the U.S. RDA percentage for that nutrient. The U.S. RDA is one set of standards for everyone. However, since these values represent averages, some U.S. RDAs are higher than required for a particular person.

   Figure 4-13 shows a nutrition label from a breakfast cereal. The label shows the cereal has 25 percent of the U.S. RDA for thiamin, riboflavin, niacin, vitamin B_6, folic acid, vitamin B_{12}, and zinc. In this case, the 25 percent value is the same for everyone. There is no adjustment for age or gender. This points up the principal difference between RDAs and U.S. RDAs. RDAs are unique for groupings of people, while U.S. RDAs provide nutritional requirements for everyone.

3. ***Dietary Guidelines for Americans*** were established by the American Heart Association in an attempt to reduce the rate of several chronic diseases in the United States: cardiovascular disease, cancer, hypertension, stroke, diabetes, and cirrhosis of the liver. Along this line, other groups have proposed dietary guidelines, including the U.S. Senate Select Committee on Nutrition and Human Needs, the American Cancer Society, and the National Cancer Institute. Figure 4-15 is the American Heart Association guidelines.

• • • TEACH continued

that could be added to make a well-rounded breakfast. *(Students may suggest milk, citrus fruit or berries, whole-wheat toast with margarine.)*

Writing

Correcting Your Nutritional Deficits

After students have interpreted Figure 4-14 on RDAs, have them estimate whether their diet contains any deficiencies (for example, calcium or vitamin C) or excesses (for example, calories). Suggest that students list three steps they will take to correct this deficiency or excess.

Cooperative Learning

Ranking Products That Get Media Blitz

Ask students to bring to class a product (or packaging from a product) that they see advertised often on television. Divide the class into small groups to study the ingredients list and classify the ingredients into food groups. They will find that many popular products represent multiple food groups, and often contain items from the "Foods to Avoid" lists in their label. Have them rank their products according to nutritional value and explain their ranking to the class.

Class Discussion

The Shape of Balanced Nutrition

Why is the pyramid a good shape to illustrate the needs for various food groups? *[We need a broad base of*

Sample Dietary Guidelines for Healthy Americans

Saturated fats should provide less than 10 percent of calories consumed.
Total fat intake should provide no more than 30 percent of the total calories consumed.
Cholesterol intake should not exceed 300 milligrams per day.
Protein should provide approximately 15 percent of total calories consumed.
Carbohydrates should provide between 50 to 55 percent of total calories consumed, and there should be an emphasis on foods containing complex carbohydrates.
Sodium intake should not exceed 3 grams (3000 milligrams) per day.
Total calories consumed should be sufficient to maintain a person at an appropriate body weight.
A person's diet should include a wide variety of food.

(FIGURE 4-15) **These guidelines reflect the thinking of groups such as the American Heart Association and the American Cancer Society.**

Categorizing Foods—The Food Pyramid

You should know by now that the best nutritional strategies include eating a variety of foods. When you choose a variety of foods, your diet can supply all your daily requirements. One way to select from a variety of foods is by grouping them. The idea of four basic food groups was once used to group foods for nutritional purposes. You probably learned about the four food groups in elementary school. However, in May 1992, the U.S. Department of Agriculture provided a new way of categorizing foods called the Food Pyramid, shown in Figure 4-16 on the next page.

Let's look at how the Food Pyramid should be used in planning your diet. The pyramid organizes foods into groups based on the Dietary Guidelines. Notice that the bread, cereal, rice, and pasta group is on the bottom. This placement indicates that foods from this group should be the largest part of your diet. Each day, you should have 6 to 11 servings from this group for good health. Figure 4-17 shows some foods that are part of this group.

As you move up the pyramid, you see that you need fewer servings from the remaining groups to be healthy. For example, you need 3 to 5 servings daily from the vegetable group and 2 to 4 servings from the fruit group. You need only 2 to 3 servings from the milk, yogurt, and cheese group, and the same number of servings from the meat, poultry, fish, dry beans, eggs, and nuts group. Finally, at the top of the pyramid you find fats, oils, and sweets. Foods in this category are not part of a food group. These foods should be used only in small amounts.

SECTION 4.3

Background

More Guidelines on Adequate Diet

Dieting can have unexpected bad side effects if calories are reduced too drastically. In general, a diet that includes less than 1,000–1,200 calories a day (1,500 for a large person) stresses the body. The restricted intake has long-term implications. It triggers a survival mechanism, causing the dieter to lose muscle mass, the metabolism to slow down, and the percent of body fat to increase. The body converts mass to fat because it requires fewer calories to be maintained. Result: the body needs fewer calories than before the diet. After the diet, a return to normal food intake causes weight gain because of the body's changed method of handling energy supplies.

breads, cereals, rice, and pasta, which fits the broad base of the pyramid structure. Lesser (but still substantial) requirements for vegetables and fruits fit on the next layer of the pyramid. Still fewer servings of milk and meat groups fit on the next layer. The small triangle at the top represents the few fats and sweets needed.]

Reinforcement

Americans' Upside Down Food Triangle

Emphasize to students the relative area of the food triangle given to each food group. Far too often, young people's eating habits reverse these proportions. Many people still mistakenly believe that the bread-cereal group is fattening and curtail their intake when dieting, so that they get too few complex carbohydrates. Sweets and fats, which should be discouraged, are actively encouraged by advertising.

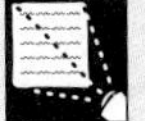

Teaching Transparency 4A

Nutrients in Food

Use this transparency to relate the information in the food pyramid to the six classes of nutrients discussed in Section 4.2.

Bread, Cereal, Rice, and Pasta Group

Foods from this group are made from whole grains and grain products. The term ''cereal'' is used to describe the food crops—rice, wheat, and corn. These grains supply more than half of the energy humans use daily. Foods derived from these cereal crops are good sources of complex carbohydrates and dietary fiber. They are generally low in fat and high in B vitamins. ''Generally low in fat'' means you should look at labels to determine if the food selection from this group is low in fat. Recommended serving sizes from this group include one slice of bread, one-half cup of cereal, or one-half cup of pasta.

Foods to Limit: Foods containing a lot of butter or eggs should be limited. For example, the following could be very high in fat, cholesterol, and calories: butter rolls, croissants, cheese breads, egg breads, store-bought donuts, muffins, sweet rolls, and

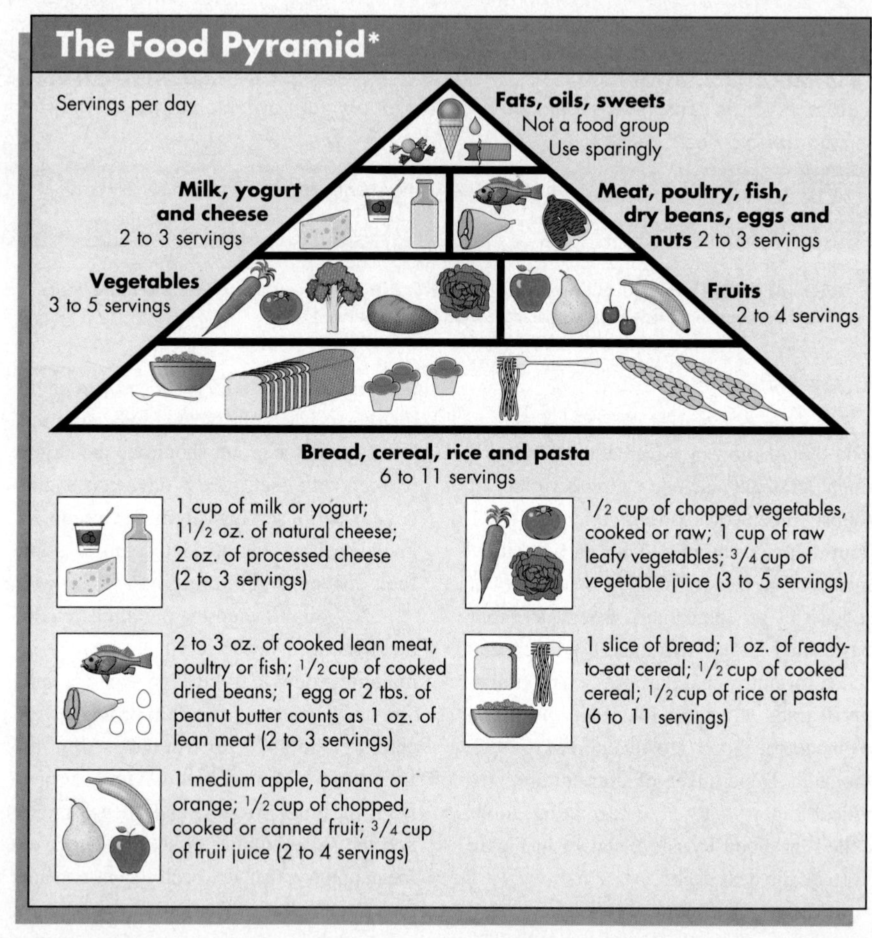

*Source: U.S. Department of Agriculture and Department of Health and Human Services

(FIGURE 4-16) **The Food Pyramid replaces the four food groups concept.**

• • • TEACH continued

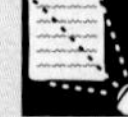

Teaching Transparency 4B
Dietary Guidelines

Use this transparency to review with the students the dietary guidelines for healthy Americans.

Class Discussion
Don't Butter Me Up

How can some baked and cereal products be undesirable, since everyone needs a high percentage of complex carbohydrates? *[If they are made with butter, lard, vegetable shortening, or eggs, baked goods can be high in saturated fat and cholesterol.]* **Considering the need to know the nutritional content of foods, what is a disadvantage of buying fresh bakery goods?** *[They are generally not labeled in the way grocery store baked goods are; it is not possible to tell what sorts of fats are included, or in what amounts.]* **What is an advantage?** *[These goods usually do not contain additives and preservatives.]*

Demonstration
Your Fruit and Veggie IQ

Challenge students to bring in samples of fruits and vegetables they think many students may not have tried. (Some possibilities include kale, kohlrabi, artichoke, mango, ugli fruit, spaghetti squash, plantain, papaya, kiwi.) Students should have nutritional information about each item they bring (vitamin and mineral content).

Place each item at a separate station and have students rotate through all

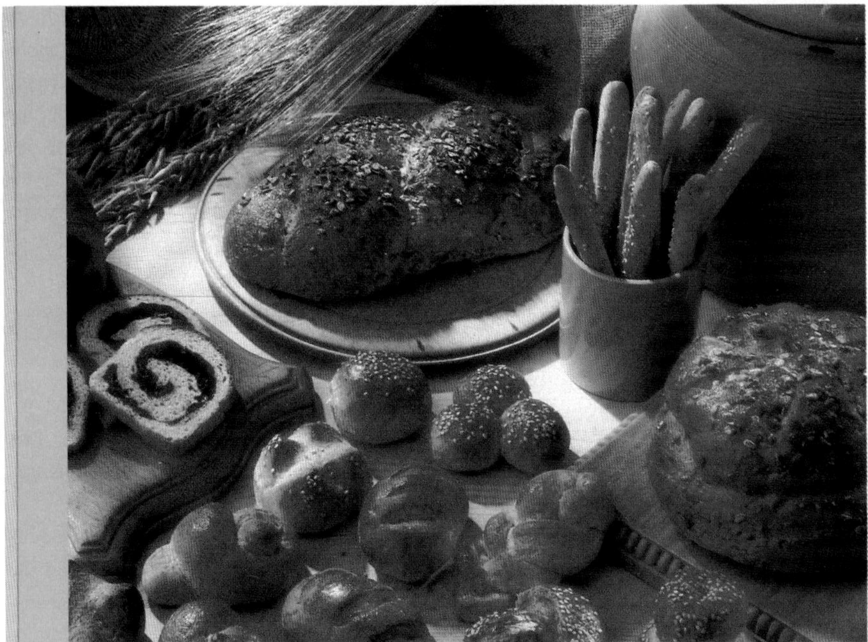

(FIGURE 4-17) **You should have 6 to 11 servings daily from foods in the bread, cereal, rice, and pasta group. Limit sweet bakery in favor of low-sugar, complex carbohydrates.**

biscuits. Buttered popcorn (including microwave products), products made with coconut or palm oil, soups made with cream, and high-fat meats should also be limited.

Vegetable Group Foods from this group are high in vitamins, minerals, and carbohydrates and very low in fat. All vegetables are part of this group. Vegetables are generally good sources of dietary fiber. Foods from this group generally supply the best nutrition for the fewest calories. The size of a serving is a half-cup of cooked or raw vegetables, a cup of raw leafy vegetables, or three-fourths cup of vegetable juice. Try to select a vegetable or fruit that is high in vitamin C at least once a day. Select vegetables and fruits that are high in vitamin A several times a week.

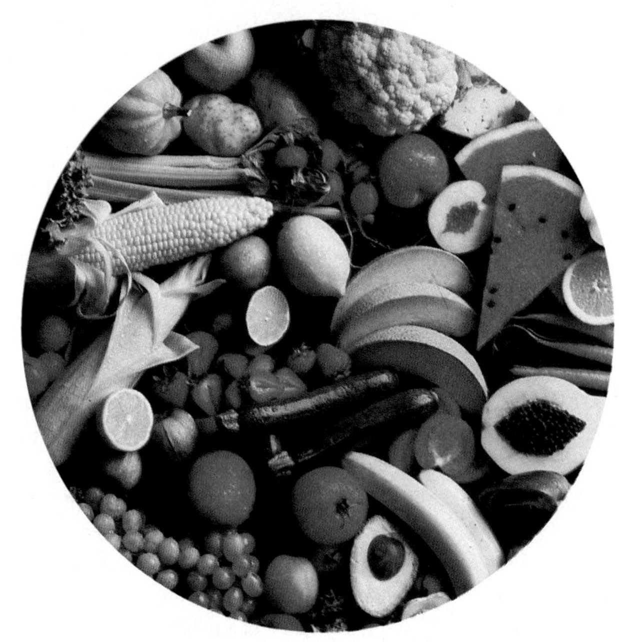

(FIGURE 4-18) **You should have 5 to 9 servings daily of fruits and vegetables. Both of these groups provide good sources of dietary fiber.**

the stations to examine the fruits and vegetables. They can complete a chart, giving the name and nutritional information about each food they know. Then students can request information from the students who brought in the food about the items they don't know.

Writing

Produce Trek: The New Generation

Ask students to write a plan to shop for and try one or more new vegetables or fruits each week. Have them create a chart to show their progress and leave space for notes on their reactions to different foods.

Class Discussion

Diets: How Do You Know What to Cut?

Health concerns such as high blood pressure, heart attacks, or a family history of high cancer incidence cause some people to restrict their diets. **Why are limitations placed on foods in the dairy and meat-related groups? Why are restrictions placed on foods in the fruits and vegetables group?** *[The former are relatively high in fat and protein, which are connected with the most pressing health problems of our society; the latter have very little fat and are generally high in fiber, minerals, vitamins, water, and complex carbohydrates, which are linked with low incidence of cancer and heart disease.]*

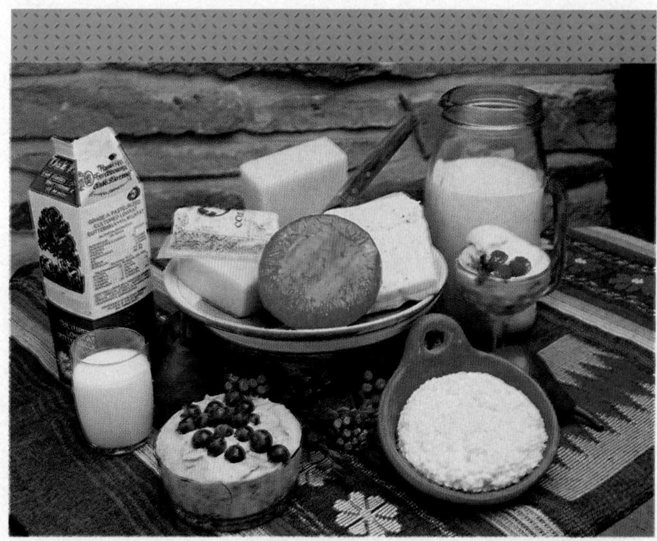

(FIGURE 4-19) **You should have two to three servings daily from foods in the milk, yogurt, and cheese group. Limit cheese and milk products with high fat content. Those items shown are good low-fat selections.**

Vitamin C-rich vegetables: asparagus, broccoli, brussel sprouts, cabbage, greens (mustard, kale, collard, beet), green pepper, potatoes, spinach, and tomatoes.

Vitamin A-rich vegetables: broccoli, carrots, greens, pumpkin, romaine lettuce, spinach, sweet potatoes, tomatoes (cooked), and winter squash.

Foods to Limit: Though most fruits and vegetables are low in fat, avocados and olives should be limited, as they are high in fat and therefore high in calories.

Fruit Group Foods from this group are also high in vitamins and minerals while being low in fat. Like vegetables, fruits are also good sources of dietary fiber. The fiber content of raw fruit or dried fruit is much higher than that of fruit juices. If you prefer fruit juice, drink 100 percent juice. Fruit drinks do not have the same nutritional value as juices. If you eat canned or frozen fruits, select those packed in light syrups or natural juices.

The size of a serving is one medium-sized piece of fresh fruit, such as an apple, banana, or orange; one-half cup of chopped, cooked, or canned fruit; or three-fourths cup of fruit juice. In making selections in this group, you should also look for good sources of vitamins A and C.

Vitamin C-rich fruits: cantaloupe, grapefruit, oranges, and tangerines.

Vitamin A-rich fruits: apricots, cantaloupe, mango, papaya, and peaches.

Milk, Yogurt, and Cheese Group All dairy products are found in this group. This group provides the best sources of calcium, good sources of protein, vitamins A and D, and some minerals. Teens and young adults are still building their bones and need the calcium supplied by five servings a day from this group. One cup of milk or yogurt, one and one-half ounces of cheese, or two ounces of processed cheese are recommended serving sizes.

Foods to Limit: Milk products with more than 1 percent fat should be limited. This includes buttermilk and yogurt made from whole milk, condensed milk, evaporated milk, all types of cream, nondairy cream substitutes, and any sour cream substitutes with palm oil. Also limit cheeses with more than 2 grams of fat per ounce of cheese, such as cream cheese, creamed cottage cheese, and most processed cheeses.

Meat, Poultry, Fish, Dry Beans, Eggs, and Nuts Group These foods are high in protein and B vitamins, and are also good sources of certain minerals. Foods from this group can be very high in fat and cholesterol. Good choices are the leanest possible cuts of any meat. Skinless poultry and fish are preferred selections over red meat. The new turkey-based products, such as turkey hot dogs, cold cuts, and sausages are the food industry's way of providing foods with less fat than the pork or beef versions. The

• • • TEACH continued

Demonstration
The Meaning of Lean

The differences in fat content of various grades of ground beef can be dramatically illustrated. Cook equal portions of 75 percent, 80 percent, and 90 percent lean ground beef. Pour off and measure the fat from each cooked portion and ask students to estimate how much more fat is consumed when a hamburger is made from 75 percent lean beef, compared to 90 percent lean beef. To dramatize the fact that this animal fat is saturated, allow it to congeal before discarding.

Debate the Issue
How Much Fast Food?

Have students debate the issue: Teenagers should limit their fast-food meals to no more than three a week. Allow time for students to gather information from fast-food restaurants, periodicals, and books. Be sure students consider factors such as the needs of today's families, knowledge of teen consumers, broadening of fast-food menus, nutritional content of fast foods, and peer pressure.

serving size for this group would be 2 to 3 ounces of cooked lean meat, poultry, or fish. One egg or 2 tablespoons of peanut butter count as 1 ounce of lean meat.

Foods to Limit: Select low-fat meats with no more than 2 grams of fat per ounce of meat. Limit bacon, sausage, corned beef, pastrami, ribs, regular ground meat, goose, duck, and organ meats. Though liver is high in cholesterol, it is very rich in iron and vitamins. Liver provides important nutrients and should be eaten in moderation. Peanut butter and most nuts are high in fat and should be eaten sparingly.

(FIGURE 4-21) **There are standards set to define the meaning of low-fat, but not for foods labeled "light" or "lite." Look carefully at the nutritional analysis label to be sure that the item is not really part of the fats-sweets category (having a high percentage of calories from fat).**

(FIGURE 4-20) **You should select two to three servings daily from foods in this group. Select low-fat ways to prepare meats, fish, eggs, and poultry. Note that nuts and beans are also part of this group.**

Fats-Sweets (use sparingly/occasionally) The top of the pyramid contains foods that are high in calories and fats, but low in nutrients. It also contains beverages such as soft drinks, coffee, tea, and alcohol that provide little or no nutrition other than providing water. High-fat diets have been associated with increased risk of heart disease and certain kinds of cancer. If you choose foods from this category the key word should be moderation.

Background
What's for Dessert?—Sugar and Fat

Western societies consume a diet very high in sugar and fat. Sweet desserts combine these two nutrients in great amounts; for example, in chocolate products, sugar and fat typically account for 80 to 90 percent of total calories. The combination of sugar and fat make them uniquely tasty, but studies show that this combination is also uniquely fattening. Data from studies indicate that eating sugar/fat mixtures leads to the deposit of more body fat than does eating an equal amount of sugar and fat at different times of the day.

Role-Playing
Break the Burger Habit

Ask for volunteers to role-play a group of friends ordering dinner at a fast-food restaurant. One student should try to convince the others to change the standard order (burger, fries, and cola drink); others demonstrate peer pressure to eat unhealthy foods. Have others in the class comment on the realism of the dialogue and suggest additional arguments that might have been used.

Game
Calorie Countdown

Create a number of food cards to represent typical choices for breakfast, lunch, and dinner. Glue food pictures on one side of a 4" x 6" card and write "calories per serving" on the opposite side. One team is to select foods that provide the day's needed calories for a teenage male or female. If the choices they make come within 200 calories of the 2,800 or 2,100 needed, they win 50 points and a chance to compile another day's menu. If they miss by more than 200 calories, the other team takes its turn. The first team to reach 200 points wins.

Journal 4D
Plan for Improving Your Diet

Have students write in the Student Journals a plan for improving their food selections. Suggest that they select several actions from the "Guide-

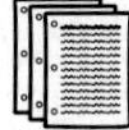

Life Skills Worksheet 4A

Evaluating Your Diet

Assign the Evaluating Your Diet Life Skills Worksheet, which requires students to evaluate their diet, using information from the text and other sources.

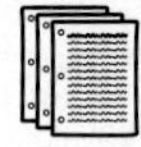

Life Skills Worksheet 4B

Planning a Menu

Assign the Planning a Menu Life Skills Worksheet, which requires students to plan a daily menu, using information from the text and other sources.

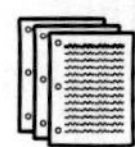

Life Skills Worksheet 4C

Examining Food Labels

Assign the Examining Food Labels Life Skills Worksheet, which requires students to search for food labels that list various forms of sugar, fat, or sodium.

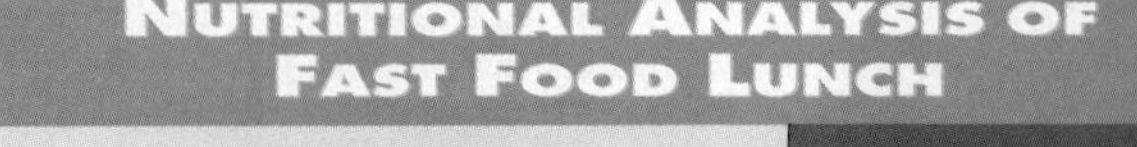

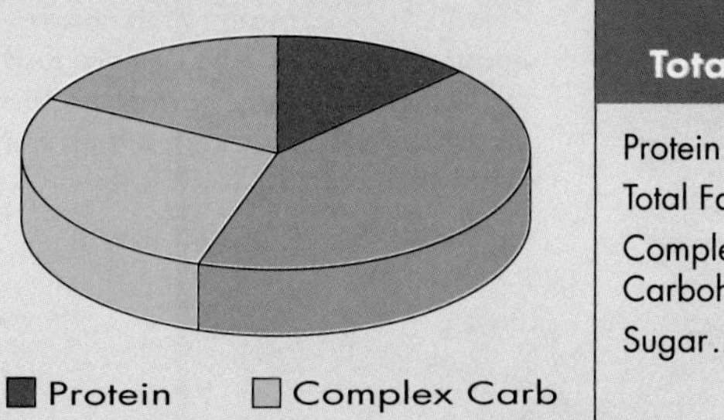

933 Total Calories

Protein.............13%
Total Fats 42%
Complex Carbohydrates ..28%
Sugar..............16%

(FIGURE 4-22) **The fast-food diet is high in calories and fat. Compare these values to the guidelines in Figure 4-15.**

Analyzing the Typical American Diet

How does the typical American diet compare with recommended dietary guidelines? Let's take a look at one meal that is fairly standard for teenagers: a fast-food hamburger, a large order of french-fried potatoes, and a cola drink. According to the RDAs and dietary guidelines, males should consume 2800 calories daily of which 56 grams should be protein. Females should consume 2100 calories and 46 grams of protein. In a day, no more than 30 percent of your total calories should come from fats, 15 percent from proteins, and 55 percent from carbohydrates. Figure 4-22 is a summary of the nutritional content of this fast food.

As you can see, this one meal provides more than 40 percent of a teenage girl's daily caloric intake and more than one-third of a teenage boy's. This meal contains an appropriate amount of protein, but far too much fat and far too few complex carbohydrates.

Guidelines for Improving Your Food Selections

Now that you have read about basic nutrition principles, you can use the following points to guide you in making nutritious food selections.

1. Sugars

To reduce the amount of refined sugars in your diet you can

a. reduce the number of soft drinks you have each day.

b. eat fresh fruit for dessert instead of baked goods.

c. read food labels and reduce your intake of foods high in sugar.

d. reduce the amount of sugar you add to foods.

• • • TEACH continued

lines for Improving Your Food Selections" and explain how they will implement them in their diets. Further suggest that students review their progress on each action during the next few weeks.

Reinforcement

More Than the Price Is Wrong

Not only are processed foods generally more expensive, ounce for ounce, than fresh foods, but they also are generally likely to contain saturated fats. Saturated fats are often added to processed foods in order to enhance their palatability and shelf life. Encourage students to read labels on the processed foods they buy, to become aware of these "hidden" fat calories they consume.

Role-Playing

Shopping at the Grocery Store

Have pairs of students take turns role-playing shoppers in a grocery store. One student can criticize the other's choice of snack, breakfast, or other food. The other must defend his or her choice by providing proof from the package label and facts about sound nutrition. Have others in the class comment about how convincing the actors were and whether they would make the purchase or not.

2. **Complex Carbohydrates**
   To increase the percentage of complex carbohydrates in your diet you can
   a. eat more fruits, vegetables, cereals, breads, and legumes at each meal.
   b. eat fresh fruits as snacks.
   c. increase the number of whole-grain products you eat (such as whole-wheat bread rather than white bread).
   d. eat more pasta, noodles, and rice.
3. **Fats**
   To reduce the amount of fat in your diet to match the recommended level, you can
   a. substitute complex carbohydrates for foods high in fat.
   b. reduce the amount of high-fat meats you eat (for example, regular hamburger, ribs, sausages, and hot dogs).
   c. eat lean meats (for example, white chicken meat roasted without the skin).
   d. increase the amount of fish in your diet as a substitute for meats.
   e. reduce the amount of nuts, peanuts, and peanut butter in your diet.
   f. trim fat from meat before cooking.
   g. limit fried foods.
   h. bake, broil, or cook meats so that fat will drain away from food as it is cooked.
   i. substitute skim or low-fat milk for whole milk.
   j. use low-fat salad dressings.
   k. reduce the amount of butter or margarine you use.
   l. reduce your use of eggs.

Eating Right Is Not Expensive Many people believe that eating nutritiously is expensive because fresh fruits and vegetables appear to be more costly than processed foods. But that notion is not true. For example, a large bag of potato chips costs about as much as a bag of apples. Using prepackaged and frozen dinners can be far more expensive than preparing the same meals from scratch. Prepackaged foods can have a lot of preservatives and be high in sodium and fat. Preparing foods from scratch allows you to better control the amounts and types of fats you eat. In buying meats, chicken and turkey are good values that are better for you and less costly than most cuts of beef and pork. You can also save by watching for sales on fresh food items, by using coupons, and by planning menus in advance.

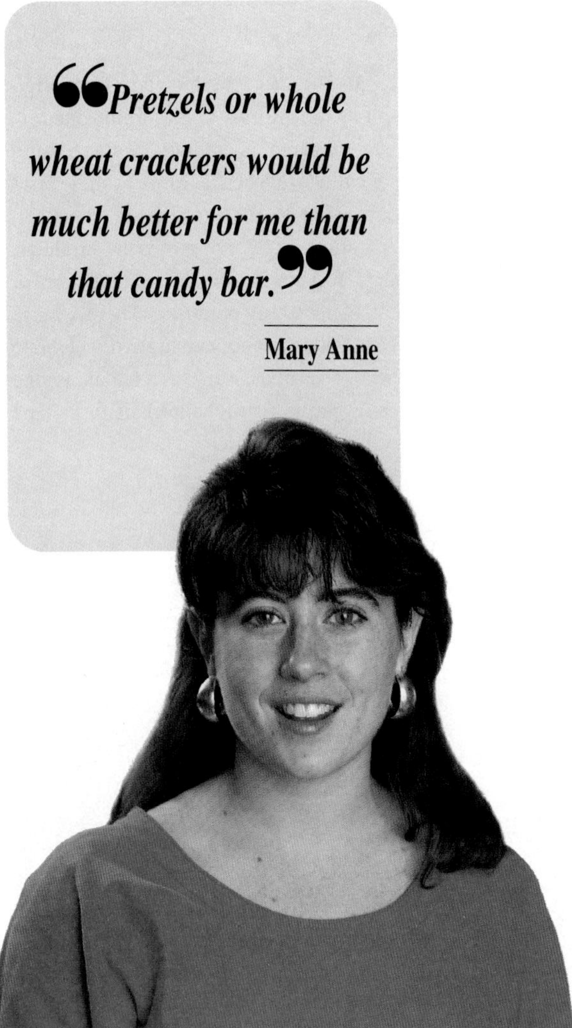

Section 4.3

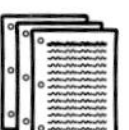

Life Skills Worksheet 4D

More for Your Money
Assign the More for Your Money Life Skills Worksheet, which requires students to compare the cost of prepared foods and fresh foods.

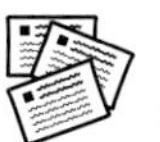

Making a Choice 4B

Eating Away from Home
Assign the Eating Away from Home card. The card asks students to plan a healthy diet for people who are away from home, and assess the availability of healthy food options in the community.

Cooperative Learning
Fresh vs. Processed Foods

Have students bring in food ads from local newspapers. They should work in groups to compare the costs of buying fresh foods and processed ones in preparing a day's meals and snacks. You may wish to give each group a budget for their group and have them see if they can stay within the budget in purchasing food for the day.

Class Discussion
Strategies for Lowering Sugar and Fat Intake

After students have read the guidelines for improving food selection, ask them to suggest realistic substitutes for soft drinks that are lower in sugar. (Club soda, specialty waters, fruit juices and fruit juice blends, milk, herbal tea, and water may be mentioned.) Then have them review the 12 guidelines for reducing dietary fat, keeping in mind their food habits and the reasons for them. (For example, if most students eat fast food often, why do they? If they simply have developed bad habits, how might they change them?) Ask the class to vote on their "top five"—the five guidelines for reducing fat intake that can most realistically be implemented.

Background

Chinese Diets Healthier

Studies suggest that the Chinese diet is much healthier than the American standard. The Chinese consume a third of the fat Americans do, but twice as much starch. Their plant-rich diet includes three times as much dietary fiber as ours typically does. Only 7 percent of protein in the Chinese diet comes from animal sources, whereas 70 percent of Americans' protein comes from animals. The study showed very low incidence of osteoporosis and anemia (resulting from calcium and iron deficiency respectively); there is a higher incidence of these problems in societies whose diets are focused on animal products.

Cultural DIVERSITY

Dietary Patterns and Food Selection Tips

Although most Americans eat many of the same kinds of foods, people have some distinct dietary patterns based on their cultural backgrounds.

Jewish Foods Jewish dietary laws originated as the "Rules of Kashruth," and all foods prepared according to these rules were called "kosher." Most of these laws today apply to the methods of slaughter, preparation, and serving of meat products, and to restrictions on the combination of meat, fish, and egg products. There are also special foods to commemorate or celebrate special occasions, such as challah (white bread), gefilte fish (chopped fish), matzoh (unleavened bread), and potato latkes (fried grated potatoes).

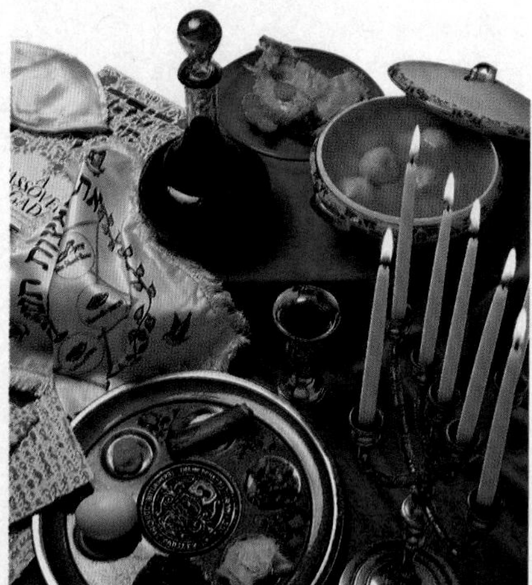

African-American Foods The African-American diet includes nutritious items, such as collard greens, sweet potatoes, corn bread, rice, black-eyed peas, lima beans, kidney beans, navy beans, and pinto beans. This selection of foods provides good sources of vitamins A and C, protein, and complex carbohydrates. Fish and chicken are commonly used instead of red meat. Salt, butter, fatback, and salt pork are used in flavoring foods. Limiting items high in salt and fat provides an African-American diet with the nutrients for good health.

Mexican Foods Today's Mexican food customs represent a blend of the food habits of early Spanish settlers in this country and Native-American tribes from the southwest. With this mixing of customs, three foods emerged as important: dried beans, chiles (chili peppers), and corn. Corn is the basic grain for breads and cereals. Masa is a dough made from dried corn that is soaked in water and lime, boiled, then ground into a paste-like dough. This dough is made into tortillas.

Puerto Rican Foods Although Puerto Rico shares a common heritage with Mexico, Puerto Rican foods include many fruits and vegetables not available in Mexico, such as viandas (starchy fruits and vegetables: yams, sweet potatoes, green bananas, and cassava). A typical day's menu might include coffee for breakfast, viandas and codfish for lunch, and rice, beans, and viandas for dinner.

• • • TEACH continued

Writing
Adventures in International Cuisine

Ask students to select a distinctive cultural cuisine they think they would like to try. Have them write about several opportunities they might create to try these foods: purchase the items from a specialty grocery store or the ethnic foods aisle of supermarket; borrow a cookbook from library; ask a friend, relative, or neighbor who is an expert; or go to an ethnic restaurant. After they have tried the food, students can write a description of the experience.

Writing
A Menu With Cosmopolitan Flair

Students who are familiar with the foods of another culture can imagine they are opening a restaurant specializing in the foods of that culture. Have them write food descriptions for their menus. Their object is to entice the restaurant customer to try a variety of healthy foods from that culture.

Cooperative Learning
Cooking Up Good Health—International Style

Assemble a collection of cookbooks of other countries—library offerings may be supplemented by books brought from home. Set up a small group to represent each cuisine. Within each group, allow students time to explore

Chinese Foods Chinese cooking is based on enhancing the natural flavor of foods and preserving their color and texture. Chinese prefer to cook fresh foods quickly, stir-frying them. Vegetables are cooked slightly to retain crispness, flavor, and vitamins.

Japanese Foods The Japanese diet contains far more seafood, particularly raw fish, than does the Chinese diet. A traditional Japanese meal might begin with unsweetened tea, followed by tofu or soybean cake served with raw fish (sashimi) or radish (komono), followed by broiled fish, vegetables, steamed rice, fruits, soup, and more tea.

Selecting Foods from Other Cultures

Italian Pasta is a good choice for carbohydrates. Select vegetable sauces without cream, and dishes without a lot of high-fat cheese and meat. Italian ices are good, low-calorie choices for desserts.

Oriental Choose steamed, broiled, or stir-fried dishes rather than deep-fried. Limit your use of soy sauce, which is high in sodium. Select noodle dishes with soft noodles rather than hard noodles, which are fried. Dishes with tofu are high in protein and low in calories.

French Avoid foods with rich sauces like hollandaise and bechamel that are very high in fat and cholesterol. Select foods prepared in wine sauces and ask how the sauce is prepared, to assure that it is low in fat and calories. Foods from southern France are generally prepared with olive oil and with lots of vegetables, which would provide more nutrition with fewer calories.

Greek Select Greek salads, but use the cheese, anchovies, and olives sparingly, as they are high in fat and sodium. Select fish dishes or broiled shish kebab. Avoid dishes with phyllo dough because they are generally made with lots of butter.

Eastern Indian Foods from this culture are generally low in saturated fat and cholesterol. Look for seekh kabob, marinated lamb or chicken, and fish cooked in clay pots. Avoid foods cooked in coconut milk or cream, as they are high in saturated fat.

Mexican Limit tortillas that are fried with lard. Select shrimp or chicken tostadas made with corn tortillas that are baked. Look for dishes without cheese or ask for the cheese on the side. Rice and beans are good choices because they are low in fat and provide complete protein. Limit refried beans as they are often cooked in lard.

Middle Eastern Select dishes made with vegetables, grains, and spices, like couscous or steamed bulgur, topped with vegetables or chicken. Shish kebab is also a good choice as long as it is not basted in butter. Fresh fruits such as melons, figs, and grapes are excellent choices for dessert.

Southeast Asian Limit deep-fried foods and cream soups. Select stir-fried dishes with fresh vegetables and small portions of meat or fish. Grilled meat dishes and hot-and-sour soup are also good low-fat choices.

the ingredients and preparation methods for typical foods of the culture. Their goal is to prepare a 3 to 5 minute presentation describing the healthfulness and balance of ingredients of several recipes.

Class Discussion
Special Nutritional Needs and Risks

Stress the risks teens take when they fail to eat a balanced diet, especially pregnant teens. A diagram such as the one at right might be placed on the chalkboard as students provide causes of poor teen nutrition and list possible results.

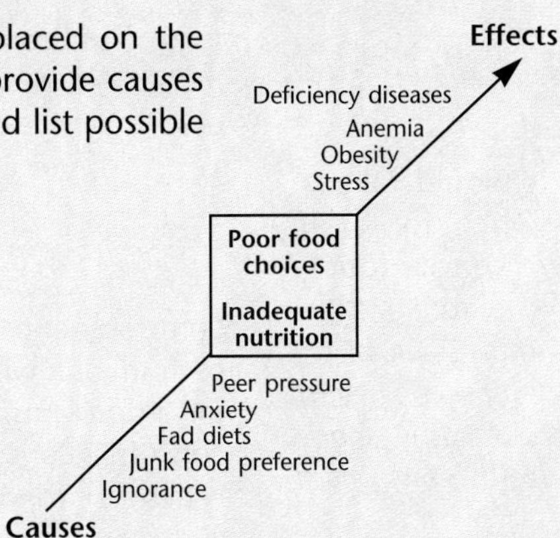

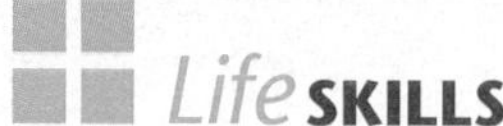

New Labeling System for Foods

Have students study the food label to find the four items specified on the label. Ask them to calculate the percentage of total calories provided by fats and by carbohydrates.

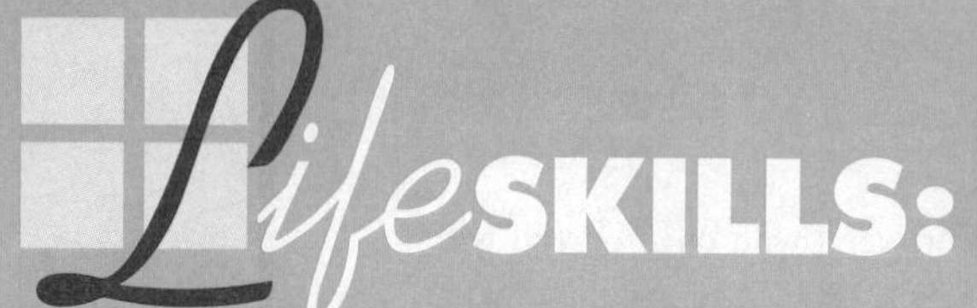

Practicing Self-Care

New Labeling System for Foods

The Food and Drug Administration has changed its food labeling requirements to help you analyze the nutrient values of foods. These new labeling requirements are more in line with the Dietary Guidelines for Healthy Americans. The Nutrition Facts portion of a food label will now contain much more thorough information. Though the new type of labeling shown on the right might look complicated, it is really very easy to understand. Let's look at this new labeling system in detail using the label on the right.

Part 1: Serving Size Information

The serving portion is listed in both English and metric measurements. The number of servings in each package is also given. These figures are very important, because all the information that follows applies to the serving size stated.

Part 2: Calorie Information

This section provides the number of calories per serving and the total number of fat calories in that serving. Fat calories are figured by multiplying the total number of grams of fat in the food (found in Part 3) by the following conversion.

1 gram fat = 9 calories

Part 3: Selected Nutrient Information

In this section, you will find the number of grams for each component. The Daily Value percentages are based on a 2000 calorie per day diet. Therefore, if a serving of food contains 13 grams of fat, it provides 20% of your fat calorie intake for the day. The 30 mg of cholesterol in this serving provides 10% of your daily cholesterol intake if you are on a 2000 calorie per day diet. This same reasoning applies to the percentages given for sodium, carbohydrates, and protein.

The 2000 calorie per day diet is more than adequate for children, women, and some men.

Part 4: Vitamin and Mineral Information

This section gives the percentage daily requirements for certain vitamins and

• • • TEACH continued

Class Discussion

What's the Motivation?

What do you think it would take to convince teens to switch from unhealthy to healthy snack foods? *[There should be a wide range of responses, but students may think of the need for education, a desire to be healthier, a conviction that unhealthy snacks really do harm their health now, advertising of healthy snacks, and the need to make healthy snacks more readily available for on-the-go teens.]*

Extension

Surveying Improved Food Selection

Some students might conduct a survey to find out which of the "Guidelines for Improving Your Food Selections" consumers are already following. They will need to design a response form with places for "Always," "Often," "Seldom," and "Never" answers.

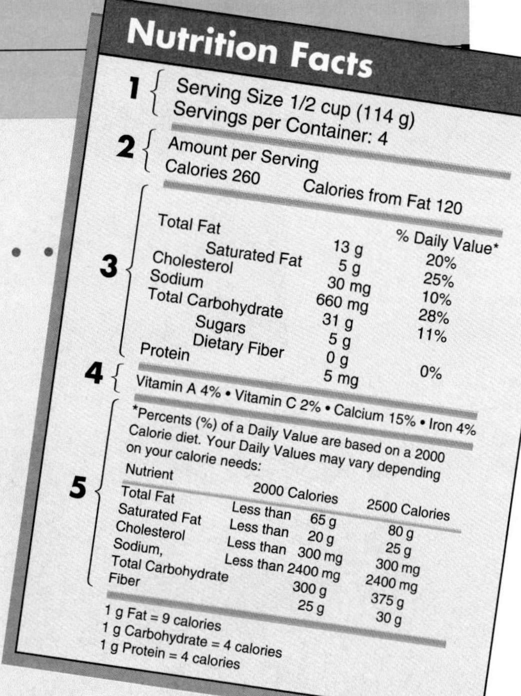

minerals in the food. Daily Value percentages are also based on a 2000 calorie per day diet. One serving of this food supplies 4% of the daily requirement for vitamin A and 2% of the daily requirement for vitamin C. Minerals are listed in the same way.

Part 5: Reference Amounts

In this section, you look at the total daily recommended intake of various nutrients using 2000 and 2500 calorie per day diets. These figures are used to calculate the percentages you see in Part 3. Thirteen grams of fat was listed as 20% of the Daily Value. A 2000 calorie diet specifies no more that 65 grams of fat per day. The calculation to get 20% is

$$\frac{13 \text{ grams}}{65 \text{ grams}} \times 100 = 20\%$$

The same reasoning applies in using the reference guides to calculate the other Daily Value percentages in Part 3. Notice that calorie conversions for fats, carbohydrates, and proteins are given.

The 2500 calorie per day diet is included in this section to accommodate those that need a higher daily caloric intake (some men, highly active individuals, and some pregnant women). In Chapter 5, you will learn how to calculate your daily caloric needs based on your activity level.

The new labeling system may look technical, but the information it now provides can make your selection of nutritious low-fat foods much easier.

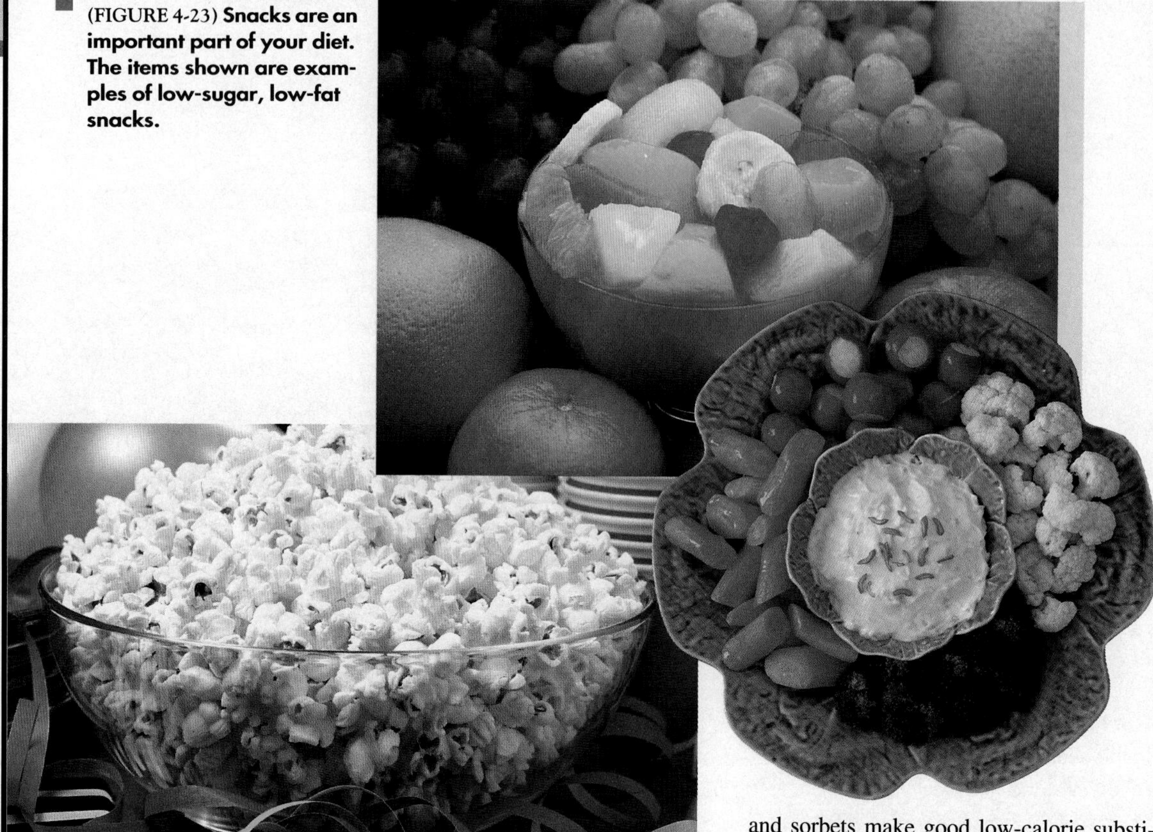

(FIGURE 4-23) **Snacks are an important part of your diet. The items shown are examples of low-sugar, low-fat snacks.**

Snacks

Snacking is a large part of the American diet. Snacking, in and of itself, is not a bad habit. Some nutritionists actually recommend small meals and snacks rather than three large meals per day. Most weight loss programs include snacks as part of the meal plan. How can you incorporate nutritious snacks into your diet? Let's look at Mary Anne's decision in the beginning of the chapter to select a candy bar. What better choice could she have made?

Fruits Fresh fruits, dried fruits, or canned fruits without added sugar provide vitamins and are a quick energy source. Fruit ices and sorbets make good low-calorie substitutes for ice cream.

Vegetables Fresh vegetables are low in fat and low in calories.

Grains Baked tortilla chips, low-fat snack chips (read the labels), pretzels, unbuttered popcorn, whole-grain homemade baked goods (using low-fat ingredients), gingersnaps, newtons, and angel food cake can be low in fat and calories.

Milk products Low-fat or nonfat yogurts and cheeses make excellent snacks.

Foods to Limit: The following are high in sugar or fat and provide little nutrition: all types of candy, store-bought cookies, pies, cakes, coconut, deep-fried chips, desserts with cream or cream cheese, specialty ice creams, and milk shakes made with whole milk and ice cream.

Selecting Foods When Eating Out

There are healthful choices in almost any restaurant, if you take the time to look and give some thought to your choices. Remember the nutritional principles that guide your choices in other settings. Order your meal by selecting a variety of foods from several food groups in the pyramid, and try not to overeat. If you watch what you eat for most of the week, one meal—even one that is high in calories, fat, and sodium—will not cause a problem if you are a healthy person. Rather than avoiding certain things when you eat out, take positive steps.

- If you want salad dressings, toppings, gravies, or other high-fat additions to food, ask for them to be brought ''on the side,'' and use only small amounts.
- When possible, choose low-fat alternatives, such as fish, pasta with vegetables, chicken with its skin removed, low-fat milk or cheese, and baked potatoes instead of fried potatoes.
- Even most fast-food restaurants now offer alternative menus. When possible, choose broiled or baked foods rather than fried foods.
- Choose whole-grain breads or bagels rather than biscuits.

The fast-food menus in Figure 4-24 contain some common choices available in fast-food restaurants. Examine the fat content closely; there are some surprises.

Teenage Nutritional Needs

All the guidelines we have discussed until now are designed for healthy, average adult Americans. The onset of puberty brings many bodily changes. During the teenage years maturation speeds up, creating greater demands on body processes. The hormonal changes that control the development of sex characteristics have an important influence on growth and development.

Both boys and girls experience increased demands for energy, protein, vitamins, and minerals to deal with developmental changes. When you snack to get energy, select snacks with nutritional value rather than candy bars or high-fat desserts. You really need protein for muscle growth, along with calcium and iron for other developmental changes. Teens tend to stop drinking milk as they get older. Carbonated beverages do not provide the calcium you need to increase your bone density. Girls must take care to select foods high in iron, since they begin to lose iron when menstruation begins. This iron loss results in fatigue and iron-deficiency anemia. You need to select foods high in vitamins and minerals.

What Influences Your Food Choices

Your food choices are influenced by what your friends eat.

- Lifestyles are such that you may be eating a lot of fast food for convenience. A steady diet of fast food can be a junk diet if you don't watch what you select. Figure 4-24 shows that a ''salad'' is not always the best fast-food choice.
- The social pressure to be ''thin'' can cause teens to make inappropriate and often dangerous choices that lead to eating disorders (covered in Chapter 5). Poor nutrition can make you thin and sickly, which is not attractive.

To summarize, the most common dietary deficiencies seen among teenagers involve a lack of vitamins and minerals such as B, C, A, iron, and calcium.

Background

A Teen's Eye View of Nutrition

Young people are likely to regard advice to eat a healthy diet to prevent chronic disease and health problems as something that applies to middle-aged and elderly people—not to them. However, poor eating habits and poor nutrition harm them now, even in terms of their long-term health. The heart disease, cancer, and diabetes that afflict many elderly people in American society began much earlier in their lives; prevention requires changing habits at a younger age. In addition, autopsies of young accident victims have shown early signs of plaque buildup in arteries. The best time to start a healthy diet for life is now.

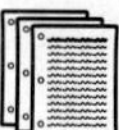

Section Review Worksheet 4.3

Assign Section Review Worksheet 4.3, which requires students to classify foods and complete a food pyramid.

Section Quiz 4.3

Have students take Section Quiz 4.3.

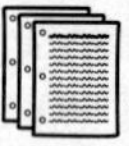

Reteaching Worksheet 4.3

Students who have difficulty with the material may complete Reteaching Worksheet 4.3, which asks them to create and interpret an ingredients label and to evaluate the nutritional needs of teenagers.

Fast Food Menu Comparisons

Item	Amount	Calories	% Fat
Roy Rogers	**Meal 1**		
Bacon cheeseburger	one sandwich	581	61
French fries	one large serving	357	46
Chocolate shake	one serving	359	26
Total Calories		**1297**	
Roy Rogers	**Meal 2**		
Roast beef sandwich	one	317	29
Hot popped potato, plain	one potato	211	0
Diet cola, caffeine free	12 ounces	1	0
Total Calories		**529**	
McDonald's	**Meal 1**		
Big Mac	one	562	52
French fries	one serving	312	47
Chocolate milkshake	one serving	388	24
Total Calories		**1262**	
McDonald's	**Meal 2**		
Chicken salad oriental	one serving	141	22
Lite viniagrette dressing	one tablespoon	15	27
Diet Cole, caffeine free	12 ounces	1	0
Total Calories		**157**	
Taco Bell	**Meal 1**		
Soft Taco Supreme	one serving	272	53
Cinnamon Twist	one serving	171	42
Cola	12 ounces	151	29
Tatal Calories		**594**	
Taco Bell	**Meal 2**		
Bean Burrito	one serving	387	33
Diet cola, caffeine free	12 ounces	1	0
Total Calories		**388**	
Taco Bell	**Meal 3**		
Taco Salad	one serving	905	61
Iced tea, unsweetened	12 ounces	1	0
Total Calories		**906**	

(FIGURE 4-24) **The calorie value for the taco salad is a real surprise. Look back at the dietary guidelines to see which menus fit.**

Nutritional Needs of Pregnant Women As with the teenage years, pregnancy carries with it increased demands for nutrients. The development of the fetus is a period of rapid physical growth from the fertilized egg to a full-term baby. Good nutrition during this time is a major factor in determining the baby's overall health. Pregnant women need to increase the number of calories they consume to meet energy demands and to increase the amount of protein to make tissues. For example, protein is necessary for growth of the placenta, growth of breast and uterine tissue, formation of amniotic fluids, and increased blood volume, all of which provide the right environment for the growing fetus.

To deal with these demands, there must be adequate attention to protein-rich foods, calcium, iron, and B vitamins. The protein RDA for pregnant women is 60 grams per day. The calcium requirement is 1200 milligrams. The iron requirement is 30 milligrams. Compare these values to those found in Figure 4-14 which gives your U.S. RDA for calcium, protein, and iron.

Vegetarian Diets

Vegetarians choose not to eat meat and meat products. Some also avoid dairy products. The number of vegetarians in this country appears to be increasing each year, and contrary to what many believe, a vegetarian diet can be healthful. However, because plant products do not contain complete proteins, it is important for vegetarians to be aware of protein requirements. Vegetarians must eat a variety of foods to get a mix of proteins that will supply all of the essential amino acids. Since vitamin B_{12} is found only in animals, vegetarians must take a B_{12} supplement if no dairy or meat products are eaten. Because the risk of inadequate nutrition is so great, you should seek the guidance of a qualified dietitian before becoming vegetarian.

Nutrition and Athletes

Athletes have specific nutritional needs for their training and performance requirements. The number of calories an athlete needs depends on the sport and level of competition. Some competitive speed skaters and bicyclists consume 10,000 calories per day or more and still maintain their weight. Those involved in endurance sports, like marathon running, should be aware of carbohydrate loading. **Carbohydrate loading** involves eating large quantities of complex carbohydrates to increase the amount of glycogen stored in the liver and muscle tissues. This increased amount of glycogen allows for longer peak performance periods. Pasta dishes, potatoes, and pancakes are commonly selected for carbohydrate loading before competition. This practice occurs over a seven-day period of heavy and light workouts before the competition. It takes this amount of time, combined with varying levels of physical activity, to increase the amount of glycogen stored in muscles.

The notion of eating a steak dinner before a game to improve performance is a myth. We now know that protein is not digested quickly enough to supply any energy to a player during a game. Protein supplements will not enhance performance, either.

Replacing fluids lost through sweating, during and after competition or heavy exercise is essential. Water or drinks with less than 10 percent sugar are your best choice for quenching thirst and supplying the fluid needed to avoid dehydration.

carbohydrate loading:

consuming large quantities of complex carbohydrates over a seven-day period to provide energy for endurance sports.

Review Answers

1. Answers may include reduce the number of soft drinks you have each day, reduce your intake of foods high in sugar, reduce the amount of high-fat meals you eat, avoid fried foods, eat lean meats, substitute skim milk for whole or 2 percent milk, eat more fruits and vegetables, increase the number of whole-grain products you eat.
2. **a.** bread-cereal
   b. bread-cereal
   c. fish-beans
   d. vegetable-fruit
   e. fish-beans
   f. fish-beans
   g. vegetable-fruit
   h. bread-cereal
   i. vegetable-fruit

Answers to Questions 1 and 2 are on p. 99.

3. a. 50 mg for males and females ages 11–14, 60 mg for males and females ages 15–18
   b. 9 calories
4. a. bran cereal with skim milk (less fat and cholesterol, more complex carbohydrates and fiber)
   b. vegetable soup and salad with whole-wheat roll (more vegetables, less fat)
   c. broiled chicken with rice and salad (leaner meat, less fat)
   d. pretzels (less fat)
5. Increase need for energy or carbohydrates, proteins, minerals (especially calcium and iron for girls), and vitamins (especially vitamins B, C, and A)
6. 21 grams of fat at 9 calories per gram equals 189 calories from fat. 189/430 x 100 = 44%. Sixty-five percent of a beef burrito's calories come from fat. This is too much fat from one source of food. Fat should make up about 30 percent of total calories.

Elderly Nutritional Needs

Nutritional needs of the elderly are similar in many ways to that of the general population. As you age, you should continue to eat a variety of foods to reduce the likelihood of missing important nutrients. Many elderly people find they lose their sense of thirst and must remember to drink liquids to prevent dehydration. Because many elderly people are also taking medications, they must be aware of any side effects that can change the way some nutrients are absorbed by the body. Anyone taking medications must read labels carefully and discuss any changes in dietary needs with a doctor.

As you age, you will need fewer calories. Your daily caloric needs will depend heavily on how much you exercise. If, as you age, you do not decrease your caloric intake, you will gain weight.

Review

1. *List eight dietary goals for healthy teens.*
2. *Place the following foods into the correct food groups.*
   a. *tortilla*
   b. *rice*
   c. *bean sprouts*
   d. *olives*
   e. *peanut butter*
   f. *salmon*
   g. *salsa*
   h. *tabouleh*
   i. *potato chips*
3. *Look at Figures 4-13 and 4-14 to answer the following.*
   a. *How much vitamin C do you need per day?*
   b. *How many calories are supplied by a gram of fat?*
4. ***LIFE SKILLS: Making Responsible Decisions** Which of the following in each pair is the most nutritious food choice for each meal? State reasons for your answers.*
   a. **Breakfast**
      scrambled eggs and bacon
      or
      bran cereal with skim milk
   b. **Lunch**
      hot dog on whole-wheat bun with potato chips
      or
      vegetable soup and salad with whole-wheat roll
   c. **Dinner**
      broiled chicken with rice and salad
      or
      grilled steak with french fries and salad
   d. **Snack**
      peanuts or pretzels
5. *Describe the special nutritional needs of teenagers.*
6. ***Critical Thinking** A beef burrito weighs 206 grams. The burrito supplies 430 calories and has 21 grams of fat. What percentage of the burrito's total calories is due to fat? How does this value compare with the dietary guidelines for fats?*

ASSESS

Section Review

Have students answer the Section Review questions.

Alternative Assessment

Using the Food Pyramid

Have students draw a food pyramid with the food groups represented and write a healthful day's menu around it, drawing arrows from each item to its food group and totalling the numbers of servings for each group for the day.

Closure

Evaluating Food Labels

Provide each student with a food label to study. Ask that students write a paragraph evaluating the food's fat, sugar, and sodium contents, calories per serving, and percentages of U.S. RDAs.

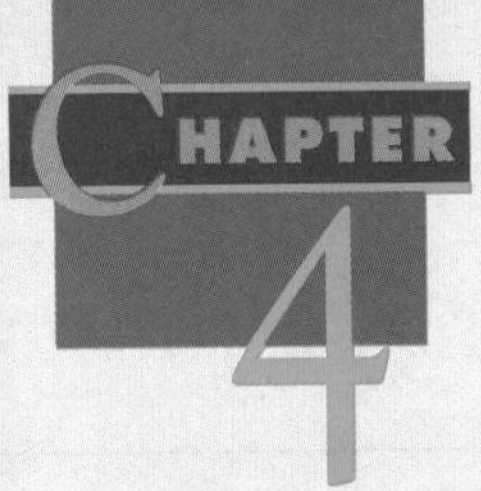

Highlights

Summary

- Appetite refers to a desire to eat food. Hunger is your body telling you to eat. To get a good balance, appetite and hunger should work together.
- Diet is related to six of the ten leading causes of death in the U.S.
- The six categories of essential nutrients are carbohydrates, fats, proteins, vitamins, minerals, and water.
- The body's primary sources of energy are carbohydrates and fats.
- High-density lipoproteins (HDL) are referred to as good cholesterol, and low-density lipoproteins (LDL) are referred to as bad cholesterol.
- Water is needed for all body processes, for carrying nutrients to cells and waste to the kidneys, and for temperature regulation.
- The Food Pyramid organizes foods into five categories based on daily nutritional needs.
- The Food Pyramid and the U.S. Dietary Guidelines are guides for a healthful, well-balanced diet.

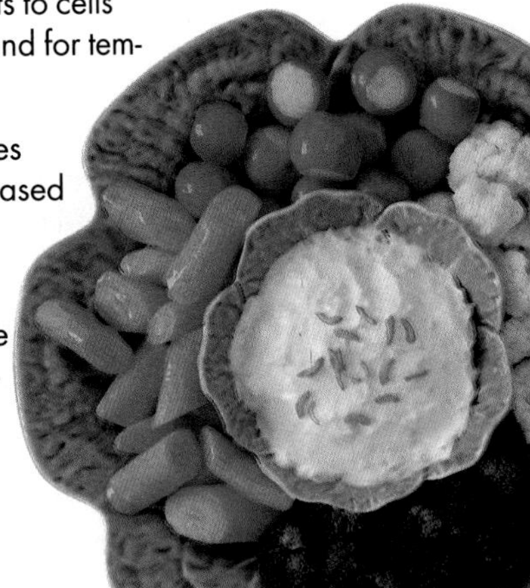

Vocabulary

carbohydrates a class of nutrients containing simple sugars, starches, glycogen, and dietary fiber.

saturated fats fats that contain single bonds between carbon atoms and the maximum number of hydrogen atoms bonded to carbon.

unsaturated fats fats that contain one or more double bonds between carbon atoms and have less than the maximum number of hydrogen atoms bonded to carbon.

cholesterol a fatlike substance that is part of all animal cells and is necessary for the production of some hormones and fat digestion.

proteins class of nutrients consisting of long chains of amino acids, which provide energy and are the basic components of body tissue.

vitamins organic substances that assist in the chemical reactions that occur in the body.

minerals inorganic substances that are generally absorbed to build structural components of the body.

Chapter 4 Highlights Strategies

Summary

Have students read the summary to reinforce the concepts they learned in Chapter 4.

Vocabulary

Have students write a letter to the editor of a newspaper persuading teens to change their diet habits. They should use at least 10 of the vocabulary words.

Extension

Have small groups of students work together to compile a Survivor's Handbook for Fast-Food Nutrition. The pamphlet could list specific menu items for different fast-food restaurants and tell why they are nutritionally sound.

Chapter Review

Concept Review

1. family experiences, cultural heritage, your personality, and cost
2. Carbohydrates are the main source of energy; pasta. Fats provide energy; butter. Proteins play a role in growth and repair of body tissues; meat. Vitamins and minerals are essential for good health; fruits. Water is needed for the body to function and to maintain its stability.
3. Simple carbohydrates are foods that contain simple sugars—sugars that are quickly broken down into glucose. Simple carbohydrates, especially sucrose, have little nutritional value and should be limited. Complex carbohydrates are complex because they contain three or more simple sugars attached to form long chain molecules.
4. Saturated fats generally come from animals and often are solid at room temperature. Unsaturated fats generally come from plant sources and often are liquid at room temperature.
5. Cholesterol is a fat-like substance that is found in some foods that come from animals. It is also produced by the liver and small intestine. Too much cholesterol is a factor in the development of heart disease and stroke.
6. You could develop a deficiency disease.

Chapter 4 Assessment

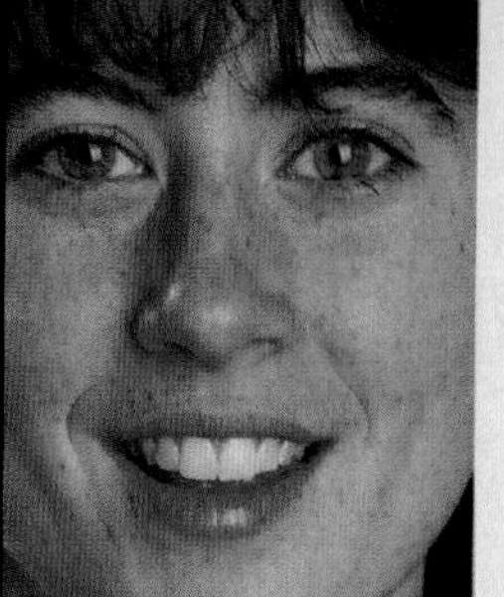

Chapter Review

Content Review

1. List four factors that influence the foods you choose.
2. List the six nutrients, then describe what each one does for the body. Name a food source for each nutrient.
3. What is the difference between simple carbohydrates and complex carbohydrates?
4. What is the difference between saturated fats and unsaturated fats?
5. What is cholesterol and how can it affect your health?
6. What can happen to your body if your diet is deficient in vitamins and minerals?
7. Why is water an important nutrient?
8. Identify the five food categories on the food pyramid and list two foods from each group.
9. Explain the organization of the food pyramid.
10. Name four ways to reduce the amount of fat in your diet.
11. What can you do to help prevent osteoporosis?
12. Why do protein requirements increase during pregnancy?
13. List the daily dietary guidelines for fats, cholesterol, carbohydrates, and sodium.

Expressing Your Views

1. Studies have shown that many teenagers in the United States do not make nutritious food choices. Why do you think this is so?
2. Your younger brother loves sweets. He will often eat only a dessert at meal time and you have noticed that he eats sweet snacks all day. He says not to worry because he eats plenty of carbohydrates and they are a source of energy. However, you are concerned that his diet is not adequate. What advice could you give him?
3. Why is making food selections based on calories alone not a good method for planning your diet?
4. Why is it so important to drink 8 glasses of water each day?

Answers to Questions 1-6 are on p. 101.

7. Most chemical reactions in the body can occur only in a water medium; water helps maintain acidity at proper levels; water in body fluids provides a medium to transport gases, nutrients, and waste; and water helps to regulate body temperature.
8. Bread, cereal, rice, and pasta; bread, cereal. Vegetables; beets or carrots. Fruit; pears or apples. Milk, yogurt, and cheese; butter or cheese. Meat, poultry, fish, dry beans, eggs, and nuts; chicken or pecans.
9. The foods at the bottom should be the largest part of your diet. As you move up the pyramid, the food groups should make up a smaller part of your diet. At the very top are fats, oils, and sweets, which should be used only in small amounts.
10. Trim fat from meat before cooking, avoid fried foods, reduce the amount of butter or margarine you use, and substitute skim milk for whole milk.
11. Increase the amount of calcium-rich foods in your diet and exercise.
12. The mother needs extra protein to meet the demands of growth of the placenta, breast, and uterine tissue; formation of amniotic fluids; and increased blood volume.
13. Students should list the guidelines in Figure 4-15.

Expressing Your Views

1. Food choices are often influenced by peers; social pressure to be thin can cause teens to make inappropriate choices.
2. I would tell him that although he is eating foods high in carbohydrates, they are simple carbohydrates that contain little vitamins and minerals. I would suggest that he eat more balanced meals and save the sweets for last.
3. Many calories are "empty," that is, calories that are not accompanied by nutrients that the body needs.
4. Your body needs a lot of water to maintain its stability. It also loses water through perspiring. This water must be replaced.

Life Skills Check

1. Italian—avoid cream sauces or a lot of high-fat cheese and meat; Oriental—avoid deep-fried food and avoid the use of soy sauce; French—avoid rich sauces; Greek—avoid dishes with high-fat cheese,

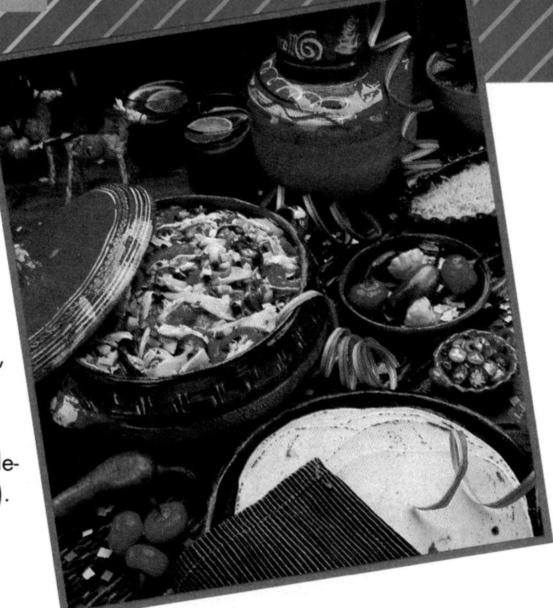

Life Skills Check

1. Practicing Self-Care
You enjoy eating food from other cultures. You want make healthful choices when selecting food at restaurants specializing in these dishes. Make a list of foods to avoid when you eat at each of the following restaurants: Italian, Oriental, French, Greek, Mexican, Middle Eastern, and Southeast Asian.

2. Practicing Self-Care
Calculate the percentage of calories from fat for 1 tablespoon of blue cheese salad dressing (about 14 grams). The tablespoon of salad dressing is 77 calories with 8 grams of fat.

Projects

1. List all the foods you eat for three days. Then evaluate your diet using a booklet of food values. Did you eat the correct number of servings from the food groups each day? Does your diet match the guidelines for fat, calories, and salt? What changes if any, do you need to make?
2. Work with a group to obtain nutritional information from various fast-food restaurants (perhaps by asking for a menu). Analyze this information and decide which foods are the healthiest and most nutritious in each type of restaurant.
3. Bring to class a recipe for a cake, a pie, cookies, or some other dessert. Discuss ways to make substitutions in the recipes to reduce the fat, sugar, and salt. After making these substitutions, develop a "healthy dessert" recipe file with the class. Compile all of your recipes into a pamphlet and distribute the pamphlets throughout the school.

Plan for Action

The foods you eat every day have an effect on your overall health. Do you choose healthful foods every day? List five changes you will make in your food selections in order to achieve a more healthful diet.

anchovies, and olives, as well as those made with phyllo dough; Mexican—avoid white-flour tortillas, deep-fried foods, and refried beans; Middle Eastern—avoid fried foods and those basted with butter; Southeast Asian—avoid deep-fried foods and cream soups.
2. Eight grams of fat equal 72 calories (9 calories per gram). Therefore, fat provides 93.5 percent of the total calories in each tablespoon.
72 calories/77 calories x 100 = 93.5%

Projects
Have students plan and carry out the projects on nutrition.

Plan for Action
Have students discuss ways to improve public awareness of the importance of good nutrition. Ask them to plan a nationwide television campaign, deciding which concepts from the chapter are most vital and how they will communicate them.

ASSESSMENT OPTIONS

Chapter Test
Have students take the Chapter 4 Test.

Alternative Assessment
Have students do the Alternative Assessment activity for Chapter 4.

Test Generator
The Test Generator (Macintosh® or IBM® format) contains an additional 50 assessment items for this chapter.

WEIGHT MANAGEMENT AND EATING DISORDERS

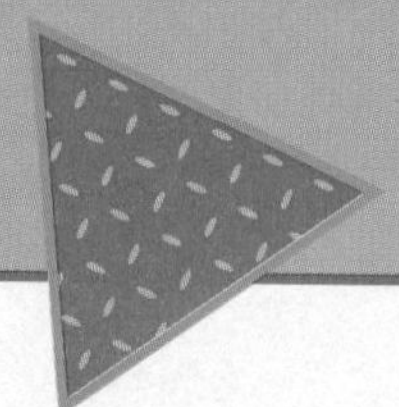

PLANNING GUIDE

TEXT SECTIONS	OBJECTIVES	TEXT FEATURES	OUTSIDE RESOURCES	NOTES
5.1 Metabolism and Ideal Weight pp. 105-112 4 periods	■ Describe how to determine your daily calorie expenditure. • List the factors that should be used to determine your ideal weight. • Identify the characteristics of fad diets. • Identify the characteristics of healthy weight-loss and weight-gain plans.	■ LIFE SKILLS: Assessing Your Health, p. 109 **ASSESSMENT** • Section Review, p. 112	**TEACHER'S RESOURCE BINDER** • Lesson Plan 5.1 • Personal Health Inventory • Journal Entries 5A, 5B, 5C • Life Skills 5A • Section Review Worksheet 5.1 • Section Quiz 5.1 • Reteaching Worksheet 5.1 **OTHER RESOURCES** • Transparency 5A • Making a Choice 5A • Parent Discussion Guide • English/Spanish Audiocassette 2	
5.2 Eating Disorders pp. 113-117 2 periods	• List the health hazards of anorexia, bulimia, and pica. • Describe the characteristics of individuals most at risk for anorexia or bulimia. • Explain how you can avoid eating disorders.	• Check Up, p. 114 • What Would You Do?, p. 116 **ASSESSMENT** • Section Review, p. 117	**TEACHER'S RESOURCE BINDER** • Lesson Plan 5.2 • Journal Entries 5D, 5E, 5F • Section Review Worksheet 5.2 • Section Quiz 5.2 • Reteaching Worksheet 5.2	
5.3 Disorders Affecting the Digestive System pp. 118-120 2 periods	• List the most common digestive disorders. • Describe ways to treat constipation and diarrhea. • Describe the differences between food allergies and food intolerances.	**ASSESSMENT** • Section Review, p. 120	**TEACHER'S RESOURCE BINDER** • Lesson Plan 5.3 • Journal Entries 5G, 5H • Media Worksheet • Section Review Worksheet 5.3 • Section Quiz 5.3 • Reteaching Worksheet 5.3 **OTHER RESOURCES** • Making a Choice 5B	
End of Chapter pp. 121-123		**ASSESSMENT** • Chapter Review, pp. 122-123	**TEACHER'S RESOURCE BINDER** • Chapter Test • Alternative Assessment • Personal Pledge **OTHER RESOURCES** • Test Generator	

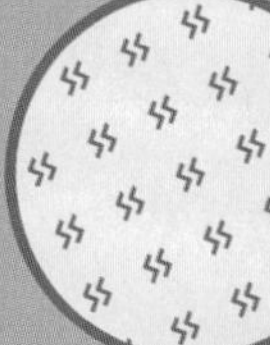

■ Denotes LIFE SKILLS objectives

• Items in blue are also part of the *Holt Health Activity Book*.

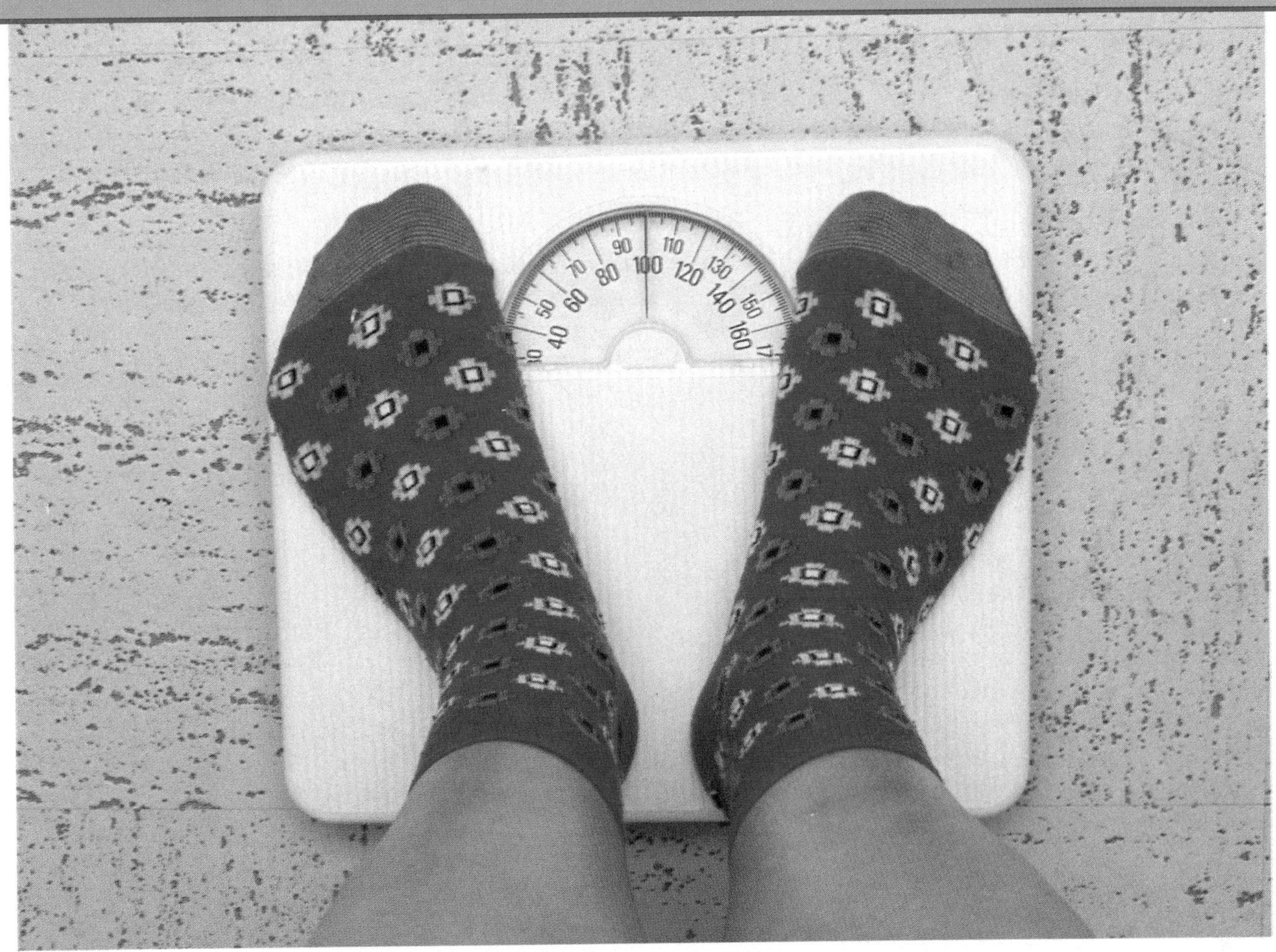

CONTENT BACKGROUND

Two Common Eating Disorders—Anorexia Nervosa and Bulimia

ANOREXIA NERVOSA

Until the late 1980s, eating disorders such as anorexia nervosa and bulimia were thought to be phases that many adolescents, particularly girls, passed through. Now both are considered psychiatric conditions. According to the USDA's Nutrition Information Center, 0.5 to 1.0 percent of all teenage girls develop anorexia nervosa. These girls tend to do well in school, are generally good friends to their peers, and are considered good family members. They do, however, generally suffer from low self-esteem.

People who are anorexics restrict their food intake because they have an intense fear of gaining weight. They have unrealistic images of their bodies and are subject to severe mood changes. Anorexics diet and exercise to extremes.

Anorexia nervosa can cause many health problems. They include digestive problems, dry hair and skin, cessation of menstruation, hormonal and electrolyte imbalances, mood changes, impairment of kidney function, osteoporosis, and cardiac ailments. It is estimated that about 10 percent of all anorexics die from this disorder.

Although the causes of anorexia are not known, researchers at Concordia College in Minnesota found that frequent negative or critical remarks made by parents or guardians correlate

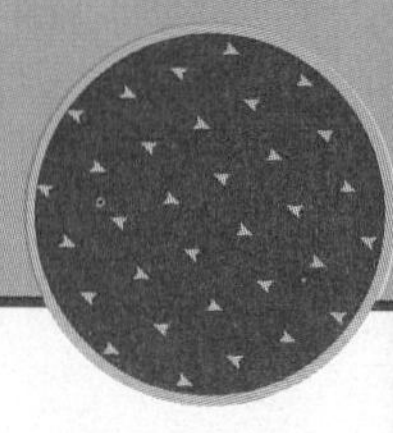

highly with the development of character traits associated with eating disorders.

BULIMIA

Bulimia tends to develop a little later in life than anorexia nervosa. The average bulimic is a white female between the ages of 17 and 36. In fact, according to the United States Department of Agriculture's Nutrition Information Center, from 5 to 20 percent of college-age females suffer from bulimia. Those afflicted overeat and then eliminate the food from their bodies by vomiting, taking laxatives, or using diuretics once, twice, or many times a day.

Bulimics, like anorexics, strive to be people pleasers and often have difficulties expressing their feelings. They tend to come from families with fathers who are strict, logical, intelligent, successful, and hard-working, but who often overlook the needs of their children. The mothers of bulimics tend to be responsible child rearers who often are overwhelmed by having to raise the children by themselves. Both parents expect their children to be competitive and high achievers. Even though the children often succeed at attaining the parent-imposed goals, they lack self-esteem.

Bulimics, too, may have health problems. Teeth, gums, and the esophagus become damaged by the excessive amounts of acid with which they come in contact during vomiting. Some other common problems associated with bulimia are depression, electrolyte imbalances, alkalosis, malnutrition, and dehydration. Even more serious is the fact that this eating disorder and the drugs that may be used to induce vomiting can interfere with the function of the heart muscle and can cause irregular heart rhythms. This can lead to heart failure and ultimately death.

Like other problems that may be linked to social pressures, family influences, and childhood experiences, bulimia can sometimes be successfully treated with psychotherapy. Many bulimics have stopped the binge-purge cycle after participating in group therapy.

PLANNING FOR INSTRUCTION

KEY FACTS

- **Weight management involves balancing the body's energy requirements and the calories consumed in food.**
- **The body's daily energy usage is the sum of the energy required to keep the body functioning at rest—the basal metabolic rate—plus energy expended in activities.**
- **The ratio of fat to lean muscle mass, called body composition, is a key factor in determining whether one's weight is ideal.**
- **Fad diets are seldom effective in long-term weight control and may have serious effects on one's health.**
- **Anorexia nervosa and bulimia are both eating disorders. They seem to be psychological in nature and medical treatment plus therapy are required to cure them.**
- **Disorders of the digestive system, such as constipation and diarrhea, are sometimes the result of personal behavior.**
- **Some people experience allergic reactions—which are, in rare cases, life-threatening—to particular foods.**
- **Some people experience digestive upset—often caused by a food additive—after consuming certain foods.**

MYTHS AND MISCONCEPTIONS

MYTH: You can never be too thin.

Statistics indicate that individuals who are below normal weight have a shorter life expectancy than those who maintain a normal weight.

MYTH: As long as my weight is within the range shown in a weight table, I don't need to worry about it.

The amount of fat compared to the amount of protein, or muscle mass, is a factor in determining a healthy weight. It is possible to be within a specified weight range but have too much fat in the body.

MYTH: A person with anorexia simply refuses to listen to those who want to help.

A person with anorexia is incapable of recognizing the reality of what is happening to them. Medical intervention, emotional counseling, and family support are required in order to help people with this disorder.

MYTH: Diarrhea is nothing more than an annoying and unpleasant condition.

Diarrhea can be a serious disorder, particularly in infants in countries where sanitation and nutrition are deficient. When a person has diarrhea for an extended period of time, the loss of water can be very dangerous to health.

VOCABULARY

Essential: The following terms appear in boldface type.

basal metabolic rate (BMR)
energy-balance equation
lean mass
essential fat
storage fat
overweight
obesity
fad diet
anorexia nervosa
bulimia
pica
constipation
diarrhea
food intolerance

Secondary: Be aware that the following terms may come up during class discussion.

metabolism
body composition
binge
purge
food allergies
food additives
anaphylactic shock

FOR STUDENTS WITH SPECIAL NEEDS

Visual Learners: Show students a selection of books and advertisements dealing with diets and plans for losing weight. Students can make a bulletin-board display of such items and then a chart listing the points in a balanced plan for losing weight.

At-Risk Students: For these students, use an exercise video to stress the popularity of such items in weight control plans. Allow students to critique the video. They may wish to learn some of the routines and put on a demonstration for the rest of the class.

ENRICHMENT

- Many communities have clinics that primarily treat people with eating disorders. Have a person who works at such a clinic, preferably a therapist, speak to the class about the difficulties faced by a person with a serious eating disorder.
- Have interested students do a survey on the number of weight control plans and products that they see advertised on television during the time that this topic is being studied. They might graph their findings to show the number of times they were exposed to such advertising each day. Have them report their findings to the class and lead a discussion of the implications. How heavily are weight control plans and products advertised?

Chapter 5
Chapter Opener

GETTING STARTED

Using the Chapter Photograph

Have students describe the girls in the photographs. What are they doing? Do they appear to have unusual or dangerous eating patterns? What, if anything, can you tell from the way they look? Discuss the importance placed on weight and personal appearance in our society, and the effects this may have on an individual's behavior.

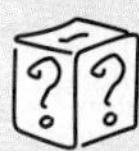

Question Box

Weight and weight control are topics of concern to many teenagers. Have students write out anonymously any questions that they have about ideal weight, weight control, and eating disorders. To ensure that students with questions are not embarrassed to be seen writing, have those who do not have questions write down some factors that affect weight.

Preview the questions and then answer them at appropriate points in the chapter. You may wish to allow students to write additional questions as they go through the chapter.

Chapter 5
Weight Management and Eating Disorders

◆ ◆ ◆ ◆

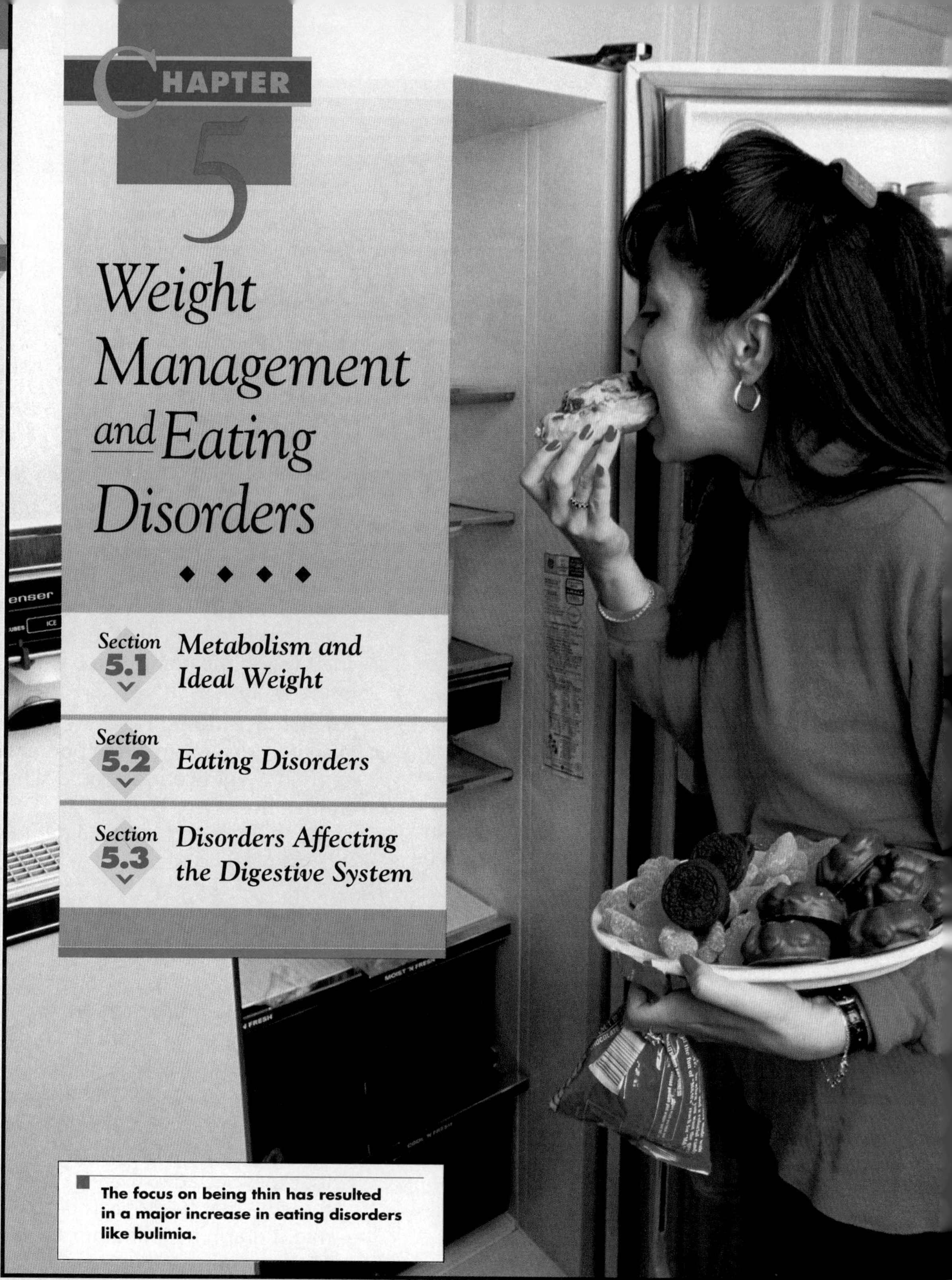

The focus on being thin has resulted in a major increase in eating disorders like bulimia.

Personal Issues *ALERT*

Discussions about weight and how to control it may cause embarrassment for some students. Those who are overweight or underweight are likely to be sensitive about these topics. Care must be exercised to avoid having students feel that they are to blame for not having an "ideal" appearance and weight. Encourage the class to be sensitive to the feelings of others when discussing these topics.

Members of the class may know relatives or friends who have some of the eating disorders discussed in this chapter. Students themselves may experience such disorders. Since eating disorders are personal medical matters, privacy must be respected. Encouraging students to reveal personal problems is not recommended.

Margaret and her best friend, Dale, are 15 years old. Yesterday, Dale was rushed to the local hospital and almost died. When she was admitted to the hospital Dale weighed only 80 pounds. Margaret knew Dale had been dieting for a long time to "get thin." She tried to convince Dale that she was already thin and that she was "starving herself to death." But Dale would not listen. Every time Dale looked in the mirror, she complained about being fat. No one else saw her that way. Dale and her mother argued constantly about eating. It seemed that as Dale got thinner, she ate even less. She exercised all the time. Margaret didn't know how Dale found the strength. What was happening to Dale? Margaret wondered what was causing Dale to feel she had to be so thin, even when she was beginning to lose her health? Why couldn't Dale see that she was already thin? Why was she being so stubborn about eating? What could Margaret have done differently to help Dale? What can Margaret do now to help Dale recover? What can Dale's mother do?

Metabolism and Ideal Weight

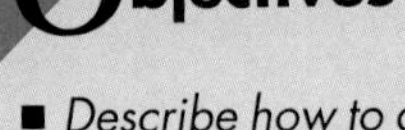

- *Describe how to determine your daily calorie expenditure.*

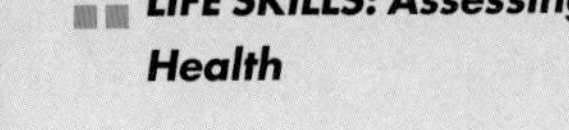

- *List the factors that should be used to determine your ideal weight.*
- *Identify the characteristics of fad diets.*
- *Identify the characteristics of healthy weight-loss and weight-gain plans.*

Weight Management Concepts

There isn't a day that goes by that you don't hear something about weight control or dieting. The TV is filled with weight-loss ads. The stores are filled with diet products. Yet many Americans are dangerously overweight. The chances of being overweight at some point during your life are high. Therefore, in this chapter you will study basic information about how your body uses calories and what you can do to maintain a weight that's good for your health. You can control your weight by knowing when and why you eat, and some-

Background

New Weight Tables

Many weight tables show desirable weight ranges for adults based on height and, often, body frame. Such tables also give separate ranges for men and women. However, they often do not take age into consideration. New tables based on more recent data now provide desirable weight ranges that take age into account. In general, persons over 35 years of age have a wider range of desirable weight for a given height. Like the older tables, the newer tables are based on life expectancy data gathered by insurance companies.

Section 5.1 Lesson Plan

MOTIVATE

Journal 5A
Concerns About Weight

This may be done as a warm-up activity. Encourage students to describe any concerns they may have about their weight in their Student Journal in the Student Activity Book.

Role-Playing
The Diet Message

Have four or five students act as ad writers planning a commercial for a new diet pill. Have them suggest reasons why consumers should use the pill. Then have them compare their message with actual advertisements they have heard for diet pills. Ask students to discuss whether or not the reasons listed are the most important reasons for trying to lose weight.

TEACH

Class Discussion
BMR

To help students grasp the concept of basal metabolic rate, compare it to energy use by a car that is in neutral with the motor running. Point out that even though the car is not moving, it is using energy—and that this is the minimal amount of energy required when the motor is running. **How would the**

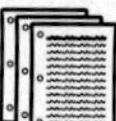

Personal Health Inventory

Have students complete the Personal Health Inventory for this chapter. The inventory helps them assess their own behavior with respect to weight management.

basal metabolic rate:

energy needed to fuel the body's ongoing processes while the body is at complete rest.

energy-balance equation:

eating the same number of calories that you burn each day.

thing about your body's composition. Look back at the Check Up you answered on page 68. Are there times when you eat or overeat that are not related to hunger?

How Your Body Uses Food Energy

Metabolism describes all the chemical reactions that occur in the body to break down food and build new materials. The body breaks down food so it can be used for energy and other purposes. But how much food do you need? The amount of calories you should consume is determined by two factors: basal metabolism rate and your level of activity. In Chapter 3 you learned how physical activity affects the amount of energy you expend each day. **Basal metabolic rate (BMR)** refers to the amount of energy it takes to keep your body functioning normally when you are at rest. These functions include breathing, circulating blood throughout the body, and providing energy to run cells and build tissues. BMR does not include the energy needed to digest food. BMR changes as you age, differs between men and women, and differs depending on your body type. A fit, lean individual will have a higher BMR than someone who weighs the same but has less muscle mass.

If you add your BMR to the energy required for all your activities during a 24-hour period, and to the energy needed to digest the food you have eaten, you end up with the energy your body needs. For example, if your BMR was 1000 calories, and your activity level required another 800 calories per day, your body would need approximately 180 calories to digest food. Your total energy requirement per day to maintain your current body weight is 1980 calories. This concept is called the **energy-balance equation** and is covered in the Life Skills on page 109. You can maintain your current body weight if you balance the number of calories you eat with the number of calories you burn.

Standard Body Weights

Based on Life Insurance Data*

Height	Standard Body Weight, pounds: Women	Standard Body Weight, pounds: Men
4 feet 9 inches	94–106	
4 10	97–109	
4 11	100–112	
5 0	103–115	
5 1	106–118	111–122
5 2	109–122	114–126
5 3	112–126	117–129
5 4	116–131	120–132
5 5	120–135	123–136
5 6	124–139	127–140
5 7	128–143	131–145
5 8	132–147	135–149
5 9	136–151	139–153
5 10	140–155	143–158
5 11	144–159	147–163
6 0		151–168
6 1		155–173
6 2		160–178
6 3		165–183

*Weight of insured persons in the United States and Canada with the longest life expectancy. Values listed are for persons with medium frame and aged 25 years and over. Heights and weights are measured without shoes or other clothing.[6]

(FIGURE 5-1) **Height and weight tables do not define ideal body weights.**

Body Composition

The body is made of several kinds of tissue, including fat and **lean mass.** You learned in the last chapter that your diet must include some fat to maintain important body functions. For example, some vitamins can only be used by the body if they are dissolved in fat. The amount of fat that you need for normal functioning is called **essential fat.** Fat intake beyond essential fat is considered excess **storage fat.** Ordinarily, essential fat makes up no more than 3 percent of total

• • • TEACH continued

minimal amount of energy differ in a car with a larger motor? *[It is likely that more energy would be used.]* Point out that, like cars, people differ in their minimum energy requirements, or BMR. Have students discuss how the car in motion is similar to a person engaged in physical activity.

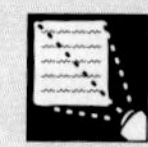

Teaching Transparency 5A
Adolescent Dieting Practices

Use this transparency to acquaint students with safe and unsafe dieting practices for adolescents.

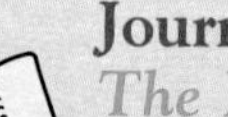

Journal 5B
The Energy Balance Equation

Have students copy the calculation of their own caloric needs into their Student Journal in the Student Activity Book. They can use the data to help determine what adjustments, if any, they need to make in their eating and activity habits to help them gain or lose weight.

Class Discussion
Weight Tables

Have students look at the tables in Figure 5-1. **On what are the weights listed in the table based?** *[The weights of insured persons who have the longest life expectancy]* **Why is that a good basis for standard weights?**

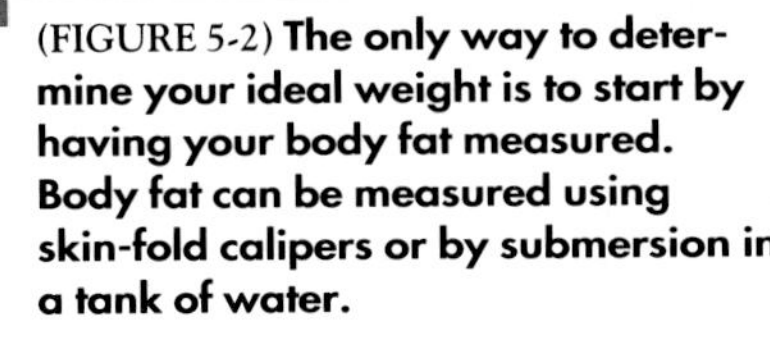

(FIGURE 5-2) **The only way to determine your ideal weight is to start by having your body fat measured. Body fat can be measured using skin-fold calipers or by submersion in a tank of water.**

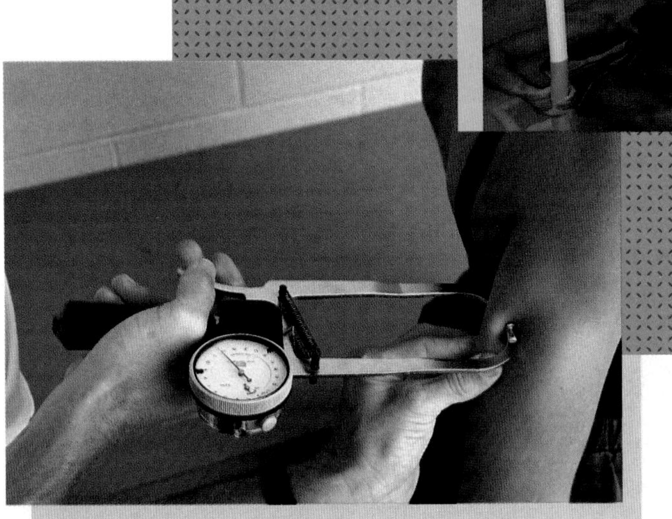

body weight for men, and 10 to 12 percent for women. Desirable total body fat levels for teens are about 15 percent for males and about 21 percent for females. The higher fat content for females is related to different hormonal needs for the reproductive system. A big percentage of your body weight is made of lean muscle, bone, and body fluids.

Figure 5-1 is a summary of recommended weights based on height for men and women. This table is a guide, not a specific target for body weight. There is no fixed ideal body weight for each person. Each person is different, and ideal body weight is based on what feels and looks comfortable for a person. Height and weight charts are guidelines. Rather than using height and weight charts, you should examine your body composition (the relationship between fat and lean mass) as a better method of determining your ideal (or rather, healthy) weight.

You store a pound of body fat when you eat 3500 calories more than you need. If you weigh 10 percent more than your ideal recommended weight, then you are considered **overweight**. The term **obesity** is used to describe a condition in which one weighs more than 20 percent over an ideal body weight. Being overweight is unhealthy, but being obese is a substantial risk to health and life.

Nathan is 18 years old, 5 feet 8 inches tall and weighs 170 pounds. His close friend Rico is also 18 and the same height, but weighs 180 pounds. Some height/weight charts suggest that both Nathan and Rico should weigh about 155 pounds. Nathan and Rico agree to be weighed in an

lean mass:

total body weight minus the weight due to fat.

essential fat:

the amount of fat needed for certain metabolic processes to occur.

storage fat:

excess fat stored in the body.

overweight:

weighing 10 percent more than one's recommended weight.

obesity:

a condition in which one weighs 20 percent more than the recommended weight.

SECTION 5.1

Life Skills Worksheet 5A

Being a Wise Consumer

Assign the Using Community Resources Life Skills Worksheet, which requires students to compare different weight control services by conducting a telephone survey.

Making a Choice 5A

Weight Control Practices

Assign the Weight Control Practices card. The card requires students to generate, discuss, and illustrate ways of controlling weight.

[Because it links standard weights to health] **What are the limitations of this system?** *[It is for people of medium frame over 25 years old; it does not take into account the proportion of fat and lean in body composition.]*

Reinforcement

Body Fat and Weight

Use the discussion that compares Nathan and Rico in terms of weight to stress the limited value of weight tables in determining what the healthy weight for a particular individual is. Point out that the amount of body fat is a significant factor in health—regardless of what the person's weight is.

Demonstration

Snacks and Calories

Have students list the kinds of snacks they favor. Then have them find out how many calories are in each of these snacks. (Students can check labels or they may have to look up calorie tables if the foods are unpackaged.) Students can calculate how many snack calories they consume on an average day.

Journal 5C

Personal Dieting

Encourage students to record information in the Student Journal about diets that they have tried when attempting to lose weight. Did the diet include pills, did it stress eating certain foods, did it recommend avoiding particular foods, or did it stress changes in eating habits? Students who have not tried a diet can describe the diets of someone they know.

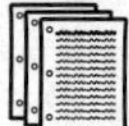

Section Review Worksheet 5.1

Assign Section Review Worksheet 5.1, which requires students to recognize characteristics of fad diets and guidelines for weight loss and weight gain.

Section Quiz 5.1

Have students take Section Quiz 5.1.

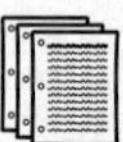

Reteaching Worksheet 5.1

Students who have difficulty with the material may complete Reteaching Worksheet 5.1, which requires them to recognize good weight control practices.

underwater tank to determine their percentage of body fat. Nathan finds that 19 percent of his body weight is fat, while Rico measures 12 percent body fat. What do these measurements mean? To find out, you need to do some math to find Nathan's and Rico's actual body fat. Nineteen percent of 170 pounds is 32.3 pounds for Nathan, and 12 percent of 180 pounds is 21.6 pounds for Rico. Nathan has much more body fat than Rico, even though he weighs 10 pounds less. Now you see why height/weight charts may not be very useful. A person can have too much fat from overeating and lack of exercise, and still not be overweight according to a weight chart. Weight charts do not consider body composition, and body composition is a better predictor of health than height/weight ratios. Rather than losing weight, Nathan could lose fat by improving his nutritional choices and becoming more active. He might actually gain five pounds while reducing his percentage of body fat. Nathan would be healthier even though he would weigh more.

Weight Gain Can Occur Slowly

There are many ways you can put on weight without realizing it. Suppose your total energy expenditure is 1800 calories per day. Eating that level of calories you would maintain your present weight. Now imagine that you develop a habit of buying a package of pretzels after school and eating them on your way home. The label on the package tells you that this is a relatively low-fat snack with about 100 calories. Eating the pretzels adds 100 calories more each day than you need. Not much? Well, if you do not increase your exercise to compensate for these pretzels each day, by the end of the first week you will have eaten 500 calories more than you needed. In seven weeks this becomes 3500 calories and you gain a pound. By the end of the school year you have eaten enough (just one bag of pretzels a day) to add seven to eight pounds of body fat. Gaining weight over long periods of time does not always mean eating lots of food all at once. Being overweight or obese increases your risks of high blood pressure, diabetes, and elevated cholesterol. When someone is obese, the risk of death from coronary heart disease, cancer, diabetes, and stroke is substantial.

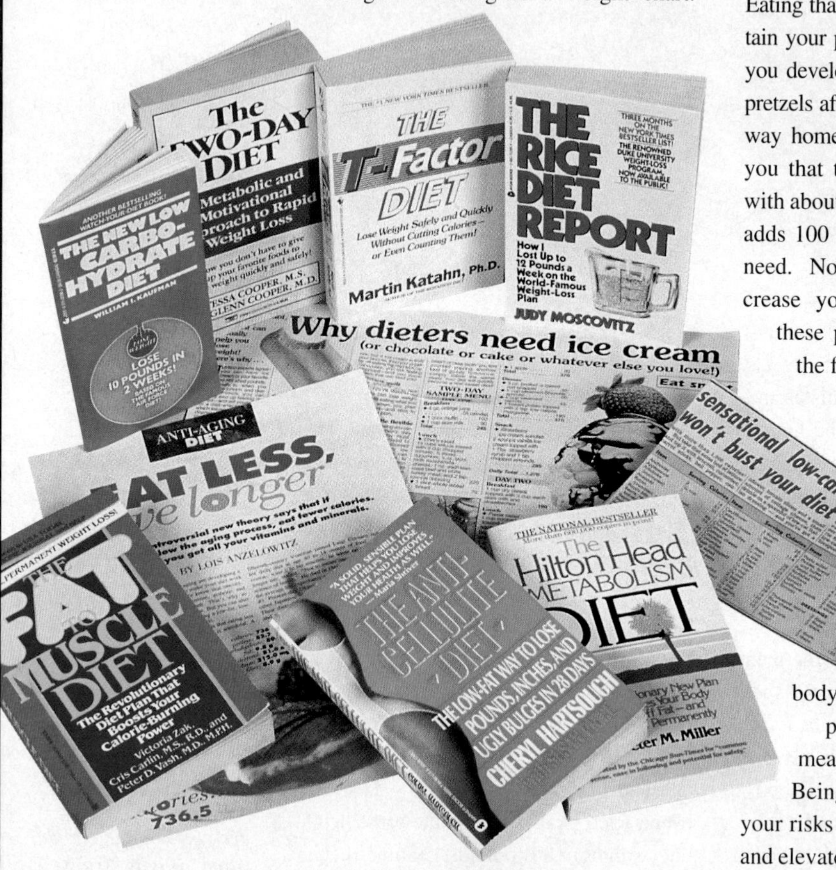

(FIGURE 5-3) **While there is a wealth of information available on losing weight, the guidelines are actually very simple. Avoid programs that promise unrealistic results.**

• • • TEACH continued

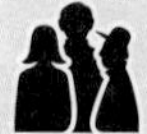

Cooperative Learning
Designing a Diet

Form small groups. Have students review the advice on losing weight safely, then prepare a sample day's diet and exercise program. They should suggest reasonable foods for breakfast, lunch, dinner, and snacks; recommend activities that keep the person active and away from food; and suggest exercises. Each group can post its plan for others to review.

Class Discussion
Family Meals and Being Overweight

Have students discuss whether the foods selected and served in a family are a significant factor in whether a person is overweight. Do cultural factors play a role?

Debate the Issue
Discrimination Based on Weight

Have students debate the topic: Should individuals who are overweight or underweight be protected from discrimination in the workplace? Encourage students to view discrimination in a broad sense—not just from a legal perspective.

Class Discussion
Gaining or Losing Weight

Have students compare the recommendations for losing weight with

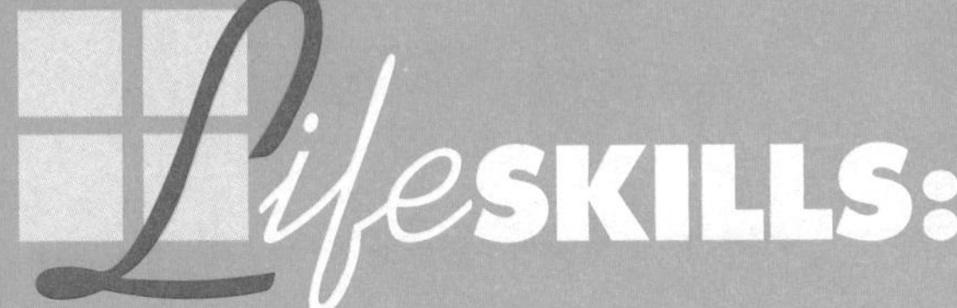

Assessing Your Health

Calculating Your Caloric Needs

Your total caloric needs for the day depend on your BMR, your activity level, and the number of calories you need to digest food. The actual measurement of a BMR is very expensive. The formulas given here will give you rough estimates.

1. Calculating BMR Calories

Females
body weight (pounds) × 10 = BMR Calories

Males
body weight (pounds) × 11 = BMR Calories

2. Calculating Activity Levels

Activity Level	% BMR Calories	Multiply by
inactive	30	0.30
average activity	50	0.50
very active (some strenuous activity)	75	0.75

3. Calculating Calories Needed to Digest Food

(BMR Calories + Activity Calories) (0.1) = Digestion Calories

4. Total Calories needed = Step 1 + 2 + 3

Example
Marianne weighs 130 lb. Her activity level is average. Marianne needs 2145 calories to maintain her weight.

130 lb × 10 = 1300 BMR Calories
0.50 × 1300 = 650 Activity Calories
1950 × 0.1 = 195 Digestion Calories
2145 Total Calories

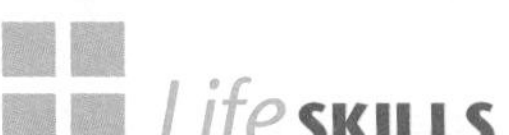

Calculating Your Caloric Needs
Have students do the Life Skills activity in the text to determine their daily caloric needs. Point out that the calculation is an approximation.

those for gaining weight. **What are the similarities between the two sets of advice?** *[Both involve an analysis of one's eating and exercise habits.]*

Reinforcement
Safe Dieting

Whether attempting to gain or lose weight, a person must keep some important factors in mind.

1. Dieting is best done under a doctor's supervision.

2. Regular exercise is an important part of any diet.

3. Well-balanced meals are important, no matter what the weight goal.

4. Restricting the amount of fat in the diet is essential for weight loss. The reverse is true for weight gain.

Extension
Fads in Dieting

Have students, or groups of students, investigate the kinds of fad diets that are currently advertised and popular. Ask them to gather information on the requirements of the diet, the weight loss (or gain) that is promised, and who, in particular, seems to be targeted by the advertisements (teenagers, women). You might also ask students to gather information on how the diets are advertised.

Background

Diet Centers and Diet Pills

Weight loss plans are extremely popular. Two popular approaches to losing weight are taking over-the-counter diet pills and joining weight control programs. Diet pills may contain mild stimulants that tend to increase metabolic activity. In some cases, the pills contain an appetite suppressant. Weight loss achieved through pills is frequently temporary, since the pills are not supposed to be taken over a long period of time and they don't teach new eating habits.

Weight control programs often involve dietary restrictions coupled with group meetings that can include exercises. Staying with such programs becomes an obstacle for many people.

(FIGURE 5-4) **Long-term weight loss involves exercise and a nutritious eating plan that includes healthy snacks.**

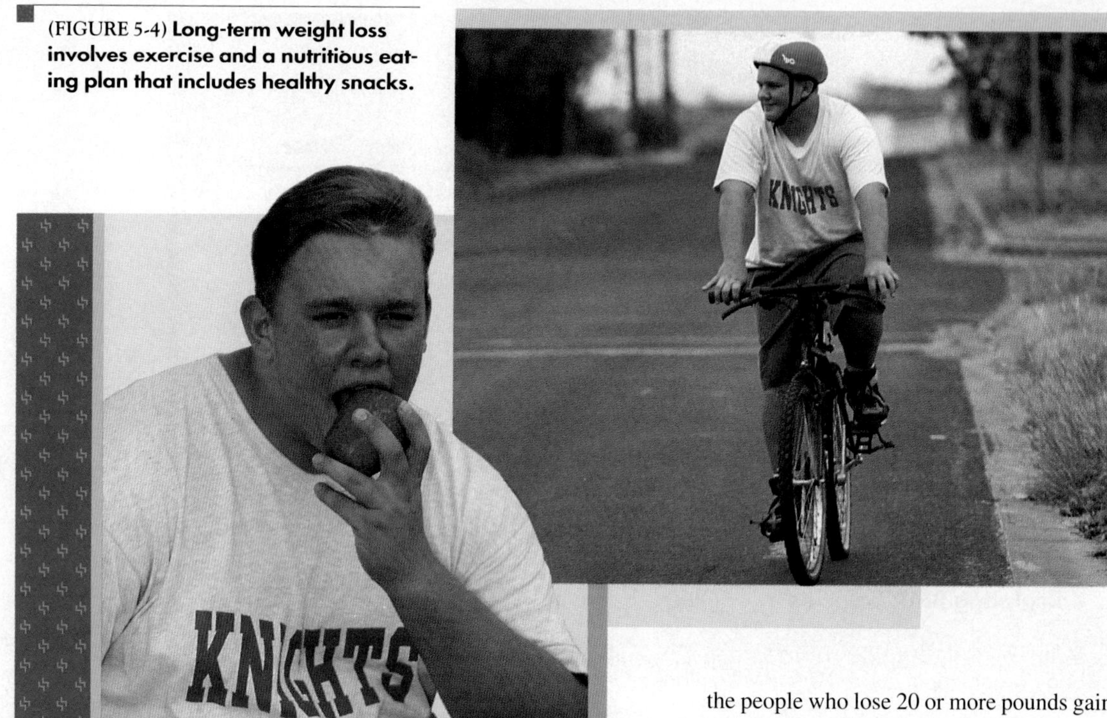

Losing Weight Sensibly

If you determine that you need to lose weight, you should visit your doctor to help you develop a sensible weight loss plan. Your doctor will probably suggest you lose weight by reducing the number of calories you eat and increasing the number of calories that you burn. Your doctor may also tell you that it is possible to lose weight *too* rapidly and may refer you to a registered dietician. Losing more than one or two pounds per week can be dangerous to your health. That is because during weight loss, stored fats are used for energy. As these fats are transported through the bloodstream to be metabolized, they can clog arteries.

Each year a large number of people try to lose weight. Those who go on diets are rarely successful. As many as 90 percent of the people who lose 20 or more pounds gain them back. However, it is possible to lose weight and keep it off. Here are guidelines that can help you manage your weight.

1. Establish a reasonable weight goal and strategy for reaching that goal. Recognize that losing weight is a long-term project. It takes time and effort.
2. Recognize that weight control is a long-term commitment to healthy choices in your diet, not something that you do only until you lose a few pounds. Look back at Figure 4-15 for food guidelines. In reducing the number of calories you eat, you want to maintain a similar percentage for fats, proteins, and carbohydrates. Reducing your fat consumption will generally mean you are eating less.
3. The most successful weight-loss and maintenance programs involve a change in diet along with an increase in exercise. Seek the advice of a dietician who can give you accurate and reliable information about diet and health.

4. When you want a snack, choose fruits, vegetables, or other low-fat snacks rather than high-calorie or high-fat foods.
5. Do not eat when you are not hungry, and don't eat just because food is available.
6. You may find that keeping a diary of what you eat is helpful. Analyze the diary to learn how and why you make certain food choices. Keep track of the times you eat and where you are when eating. Then briefly describe what you were thinking and feeling.

Gaining Weight Safely

Many teenagers are unhappy with the way they look. Very thin teenagers may find that they are the focus of jokes from their friends or family members. For these teens, being too thin can be stressful and emotional. They may be slow to develop, and a metabolic disorder may prevent them from gaining weight. Being too thin and wanting to gain weight can be just as frustrating as being too heavy and wanting to lose weight. The best strategies for overly thin teenagers are much the same as those for obese individuals. For example, one should check with a doctor or registered dietician for safe weight-gain strategies.

Refer to the points listed for weight control. Modify them slightly to get a reasonable plan for weight gain. Add the following points.

1. Examine your eating patterns. Try to avoid skipping meals. If you have trouble eating three large meals a day, try eating six smaller meals spaced over the full day. Do you tend to eat the same foods all the time? Be willing to try new foods. A well-balanced diet is easier to achieve when you eat a variety of foods.
2. Examine your snacking patterns. Do you snack close to mealtime? Snacking increases blood sugar levels, which reduces hunger and appetite. If you wish to snack, do so at least two hours before a meal.
3. If you are sedentary, start to exercise. If you are exercising, increase your activity level. Exercise can increase your metabolism and you will feel less tired.
4. No single food will help you gain weight safely. Eating a variety of foods is best. Look for nutritious foods (such as nuts and dried fruits) that are high in calories. Try to eat more of these foods.

Remember that it takes an extra 3500 calories to gain one pound. If you can increase your caloric intake by 500 calories above what you burn each day, you should be able to gain about one pound a week.

Fad Diets

There are some people who would do just about anything to lose or gain weight. Because losing weight takes time and careful planning, many people turn to fad diets for the promise of quick and easy results. A **fad diet** is one that promises results that are not possible. In our society thin people seem to have greater popularity. Obese people are subject to health risks and are often the butt of jokes and other kinds of ridicule. These are some of the reasons why fad diets are so popular. Fad diets take advantage of people's emotions and give them false hopes. These diets promise a quick fix for obesity, or weight loss with little effort. Unfortunately, advertisements for fad diets are everywhere. They appear in most newspapers and magazines, and on television and radio.

The problem with fad diets is that they do not deliver the desired results, but also that they can be dangerous to your health. Fad diets can require food selections that do

fad diet:
a weight-loss plan that promises unrealistic results.

SECTION 5.1

Background

The Dangers in Dieting

Diet programs and books promoting numerous types of weight loss diets continue to appear on the market. They have included low carbohydate diets, low protein diets, grapefruit diets, water diets, and many others. In some cases, the diets have proven to be unsafe, and the health of the dieters has been impaired. Congressional committees have investigated the dieting industry, hearing testimony from individuals whose health has been adversely affected by diet programs. The hearings could result in new regulations concerning diet products and programs, and dietary claims made about these diets.

Review Answers

1. Answers will vary depending on students' BMR and level of activity. Students should follow the steps in the Life Skills feature.

2. Body composition and the weight that feels and looks comfortable for a person

3. Fad diets can be dangerous to one's health. They often do not provide adequate nutrition and can sometimes lead to death. Also, it is difficult to maintain weight loss with a fad diet.

4. Lose weight gradually; change your diet to reduce the number of calories and the percentage of fats, proteins, and carbohydrates; increase exercise; eat only when hungry; choose snacks that are low in fat and also nutritious, such as fruits and vegetables

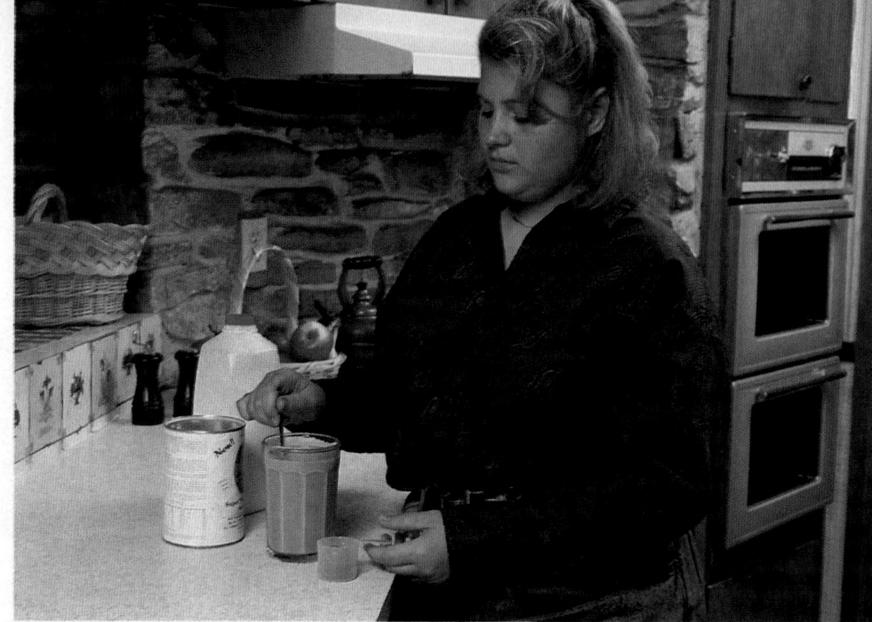

(FIGURE 5-5) **Fad diets can appear to be sound programs for weight loss. Don't be fooled. People have died from lack of nutrition from some fad diets. Follow a doctor's or dietician's instructions for a weight-loss plan.**

not provide adequate nutrition. Altering nutritional requirements should only be done with a doctor's supervision. There have been numerous deaths related to fad diets. Empty promises are not worth the risk. No weight-loss plan that is dependent on pills or other medications should be tried without *your own* doctor's advice and supervision. If the diet promises quick weight loss with no effort, avoid it. Before starting on any diet, ask yourself the following questions.

1. Does the diet represent sound, well-balanced choices from a variety of foods?
2. Does the diet follow the guidelines of dietary recommendations described earlier in Chapter 4?
3. Does the diet represent a pattern of eating that you would be comfortable following for the rest of your life? If you answer "no" to any of these questions, do not use the diet.

There is one additional note about dieting. There is evidence to indicate that a constant on-and-off cycle of dieting actually makes you fatter. Your body responds to periods of semistarvation by storing fat. When you go back to your old eating habits your body stores more fat in anticipation of a fasting or starvation period. As a result, you don't process fat, and you gain weight.

Review

1. Calculate your daily caloric need.
2. What factors should be considered in assessing your ideal weight?
3. What are the drawbacks of fad diets?
4. What are the characteristics of a healthy weight-loss plan?

ASSESS

Section Review

Have students answer the Section Review questions.

Alternative Assessment

Weighty Advice

Have students write a paragraph describing the advice they would give to a friend who wanted to lose weight in order to become more popular.

Closure

Weight and Health

What are the health risks associated with being obese? What are the health risks associated with fad diets? Have students express their opinions about steering a course in between.

Section 5.2 Eating Disorders

Objectives

- *List the health hazards of anorexia, bulimia, and pica.*
- *Describe the characteristics of individuals most at risk for anorexia or bulimia.*
- *Explain how eating disorders can be avoided.*

Dale has carried weight control and dieting too far. She's become attached to a body image that is unreasonable. The only way to achieve that image involves endangering her health.

Think about the body image you would like to have. Does it suit you or is it the image of someone else? Your mind can be flooded with images of young, thin beautiful models as the ideal. As a result, you may feel you are too heavy or unattractive even when you are not.

It is far more important to visualize yourself as a fit, healthy person. Being fit and engaging in healthful behaviors should provide a body image that is right for you. The heavy emphasis on body image in today's society has produced a dramatic increase in the number of people suffering from eating disorders. In this section we want you to explore the emotional and physical effects of these disorders. Let's start by looking at how they come about in the first place. While eating disorders are not new diseases (there is evidence that they date back to the Middle Ages), it appears that the percentage of people affected by these disorders is increasing. An estimated one million teenagers are affected by eating disorders. As many as 90 percent of all people with these disorders are female.

There are many reasons why females are more likely to have these disorders. One of the major reasons is that thinness appears to be associated with femininity and sensuality in females. Another reason is that women often think thinness is a factor in being popular.

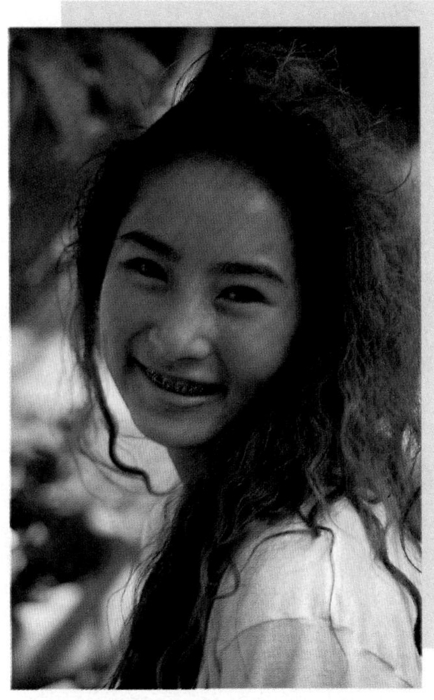

(FIGURE 5-6) **It is better to see yourself as a fit, healthy person than to try to look like a fashion model.**

Background
Diet Survey

A study of diet practices conducted as part of the National Adolescent Student Health Survey confirms that females are more likely to diet and engage in other dietary practices than are males. Over 60 percent of tenth-grade females surveyed reported dieting within the past year. By contrast, less than 30 percent of males in the same grade reported dieting. Vomiting after eating, a practice associated with bulimia and sometimes with anorexia nervosa, was practiced by almost 10 percent of the females but by less than 3 percent of the males.

Section 5.2 Lesson Plan

MOTIVATE

Journal 5D
Concerns About Eating Disorders

This may be done as a warm-up activity. Encourage students who have concerns about eating disorders to record their concerns in the Student Journal. Students could also record their feelings concerning Dale and her trouble.

Cooperative Learning
Dale's Dieting Problem

Have students form small groups to discuss the kinds of pressure, including peer pressure, that might be contributing to Dale's disorder. Students should also consider ways in which an individual can be helped to resist such pressure.

TEACH

Class Discussion
Body Image vs. Self-Esteem

Elicit from students what they think society views as the ideal body image. Students might give examples of celebrities that exhibit such an image. Ask students how the ideal image differs in males and in females. Then have them suggest definitions of the term self-esteem. Discuss the relationship

Check Up

Have students turn in anonymously their answers to the Check Up. Tally the results and discuss them. Encourage students to identify the areas in which students in the class are at risk. Challenge them to find patterns in the way people in the class eat.

Background

Factors in Anorexia Nervosa

Anorexia nervosa is a complex disorder; its cause, or causes, are speculative. Onset is typically in the adolescent years. Some researchers believe that fear of one's developing sexuality is a contributing cause. Many anorexics are described as being obsessive, hardworking, and overachievers. The family structure is characterized as rigid and overprotective. Anorexia may involve the need to be in control of one's body. The possibility that chemical/neurological imbalances are involved has not been ruled out.

Check Up

Are You at Risk for an Eating Disorder?

People with eating disorders will respond with a "yes" to most of the following questions.

1. Do you prefer to eat alone?
2. Are you terrified of being overweight?
3. Do you constantly think about food?
4. Do you "binge" (overeat drastically) occasionally?
5. Are you highly knowledgeable about the calorie content of all the foods you eat?
6. Do you always feel "stuffed" after meals?
7. Are you constantly weighing yourself?
8. Do you eat a lot of "diet" foods?
9. Do you over-exercise to burn all the calories you eat?
10. Do you take a long time to eat meals?
11. Are you frequently constipated?
12. Do you feel guilty when you eat sweet or fattening foods?
13. Do you feel the urge to throw up after eating?
14. Do you feel your life is controlled by food and eating?

If your responses suggest that you may be at risk for an eating disorder, it is suggested that you discuss your situation with an adult or doctor.

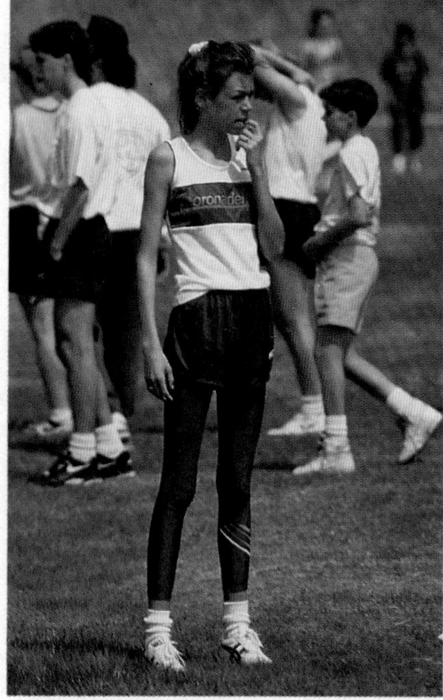

(FIGURE 5-7) **One sign of anorexia is excessive exercise.**

anorexia nervosa:

an eating disorder in which the person refuses to eat because of a fear of weight gain.

Anorexia Nervosa

Anorexia nervosa is a condition in which a person is constantly dieting and carrying this dieting to an extreme. The anorexic, like Dale in the story, is in a state of starvation. Someone who diets to lose much more weight than is necessary may be anorexic. Dale feels she is overweight. She cannot be convinced to stop dieting because she sees herself as fat. The anorexic is obsessed with becoming thin and doesn't recognize when she becomes dangerously thin. She may exercise excessively and will appear to have no appetite. Signs of hunger and appetite are there, but the anorexic does not respond to them.

In dealing with the anorexic, parents and friends may attempt to force the victim to eat. These attempts will generally make the problem worse. The anorexic becomes more determined not to eat. However, on occasion, the anorexic will eat to avoid the hassles of dealing with family or friends. Unfortunately, it is likely that the anorexic will then go to a private place and throw up to get rid of the food.

Anorexia occurs as a result of emotional problems. The anorexic is generally described as the "perfect" child. The victim is generally popular, does well in school, and is obedient and respectful. Par-

• • • TEACH continued

between having low self-esteem and wanting to have an ideal body image.

Case Study

Karen Carpenter

Talent, popularity, and success are not a shield against anorexia nervosa. Karen Carpenter was a recording star with all of these things in her favor. Still, she developed anorexia nervosa. Although the disorder was recognized, treatment was ineffective and Karen Carpenter died, a victim of this disorder. Use this case study to emphasize that anorexia nervosa is an emotional disorder that requires professional help to overcome.

Role-Playing

I Need to Diet

Select two students, one to play the role of an anorexic and the other to play the role of a sympathetic friend. (Use care in selecting students.) Instruct the student acting as the anorexic to resist evidence from her friend that she is not overweight and is, in fact, too thin. In addition, have students show how futile it is to persuade an anorexic to eat and how the persuasion itself can aggravate the problem.

Reinforcement

Anorexia Is Life-Threatening

Emphasize that anorexia nervosa is a life-threatening disorder and not simply a phase that some individuals go through. Summarize for students some

ents or guardians of anorexics may unknowingly be very domineering and have unreasonably high expectations of their child. Controlling eating behavior may be the only area where the anorexic feels she has firm control. Part of the therapy often involves helping the anorexic gain independence.

Effects of Anorexia Nervosa The anorexic experiences other physical effects related to the excessive weight loss. Heart rate, BMR, and body temperature all drop to low levels. Because the fat stored in the body is used up, the body begins breaking down muscle tissue for energy. Loss of muscle tissue can cause permanent heart damage. When this disorder occurs during puberty, sexual maturity and growth will stop. Sometimes a girl feels threatened by sexual maturity and will use dieting and weight loss to avoid changes that come with growing up.

The anorexic has low self-esteem, which is generally the cause of the disorder. The state of starvation results in frequent depression. Relationships among family and friends can be strained as the anorexic becomes more and more obsessed with not eating.

Treatment As many as 10 percent of anorexics die of starvation without treatment. Treatment requires a team of professionals—physicians, nurses, psychiatrists, family psychologists, and dieticians—working together. Psychotherapy is required to successfully treat the disorder. A treatment plan is developed that deals with the physical effects of the disorder and the emotional reasons for its occurrence. Early treatment is essential to prevent permanent damage to one's health. Treatment may sometimes involve forced feeding on a temporary basis. The first priority of treatment is aimed at meeting nutritional deficiencies to prevent long-term medical problems.

Bulimia

Bulimia is a disorder in which a person binges on food. A binge involves eating large amounts of food over a very short period of time. This *bingeing* is then followed by *purging* (either throwing up or using laxatives). Bulimia generally appears from the teen years through adulthood. Bulimia is far more common in teenage girls than is anorexia. Bulimics are threatened by being overweight, but derive a lot of pleasure from going on a binge. However, feelings of guilt and fear of weight gain set in and the need to purge themselves of the binge foods takes over.

Effects of Bulimia A bulimic may throw up daily to purge. Throwing up causes the enamel on the teeth to dissolve from exposure to acid from the stomach. The teeth are more prone to decay. The salivary glands become large from overproducing saliva to prevent dehydration. Frequent throwing up

bulimia:

an eating disorder based on a cycle of bingeing and purging food.

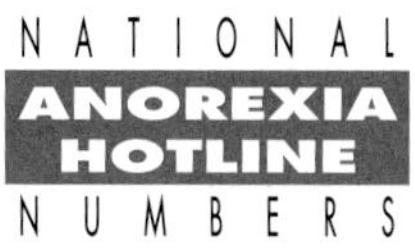

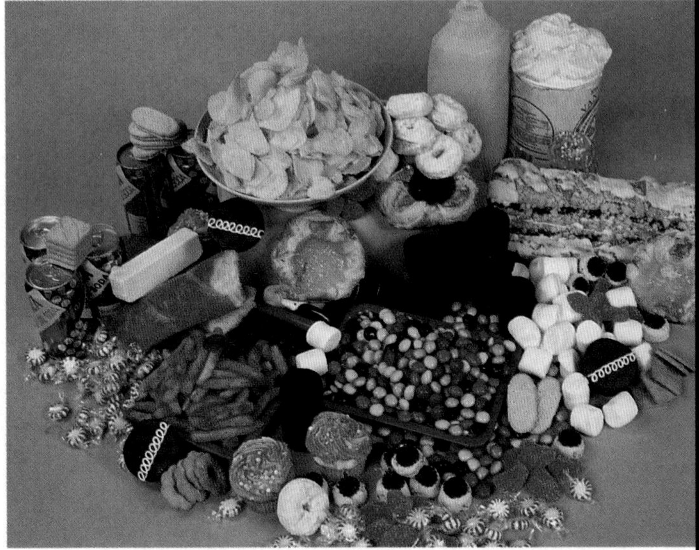

(FIGURE 5-8) **These are some of the items a bulimic might eat and purge over a two-day binge. There are reports of bulimics consuming more than 30,000 calories in a day of binge-purge eating.**

Background

Understanding Bulimia

Bulimia and anorexia nervosa are related disorders. The same set of factors—personality type, family structure, socioeconomic class—are common to both. Unlike an anorexic, a person with bulimia may appear healthy. However, there are some warning signs. These include depression, inability to sleep well, talking about suicide, fear of appearing fat, and purchasing large quantities of food. As with anorexia, both medical treatment and psychological therapy are needed to cure the disorder.

of its physical effects:

- Drop in metabolic rate, with associated drop in heart rate and body temperature
- Utilization of muscle tissue as an energy source
- Damage to the heart muscle, which can be irreversible
- Associated mental disorders—particularly depression

Journal 5E

An Anorexic Friend

Have students record in the Student Journal how they might feel toward, and react to, a friend who has anorexia nervosa. Ask them to consider whether they might be sympathetic or unsympathetic to the friend.

Class Discussion

Anorexia and Bulimia

Have students discuss the similarities and differences between the disorders anorexia nervosa and bulimia. Elicit from students that both are emotional disorders in which low self-esteem is a factor. Both involve body image perceptions. Have students distinguish the constant dieting of the anorexic from the binge-purge cycle of the bulimic.

Cooperative Learning

Bulimia: A Serious Disorder

Have students work in small groups to think of ways in which bulimics and

What Would You Do ?

Pam Is in Trouble

Have students read about Pam's situation and think about how they would try to help her as a friend. Remind them to use the seven decision-making steps to help them come to a conclusion about the best course of action.

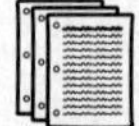

Section Review Worksheet 5.2

Assign Section Review Worksheet 5.2, which requires students to identify common eating disorders.

Section Quiz 5.2

Have students take Section Quiz 5.2.

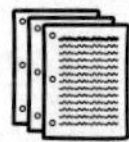

Reteaching Worksheet 5.2

Students who have difficulty with the material may complete Reteaching Worksheet 5.2, which asks students to recognize characteristics and consequences of eating disorders.

What Would You Do

Making Responsible Decisions

Pam Is in Trouble

Imagine that your best friend, Pam, has been starving herself on a diet for a long time and you think she has gone too far. Every time you say something to her, she tells you that she is too fat. She says everyone makes fun of her because she is too fat and that if you were a real friend you would be supportive of what she is doing.

You have a feeling there is a problem. You have heard about anorexia nervosa. You think Pam is becoming anorexic. Pam gets very angry when you try to talk to her about her weight. It's obvious that your friendship is in trouble. What do you do?

Remember to use the decision-making steps:

1. **State the Problem.**
2. **List the Options.**
3. **Imagine the Benefits and Consequences.**
4. **Consider Your Values.**
5. **Weigh the Options and Decide.**
6. **Act.**
7. **Evaluate the Results.**

can disturb the electrolyte balance in the body and can result in mineral deficiencies. Bulimics may also use laxatives, which do not rid the body of the calories consumed. Weight loss caused by using laxatives is water loss from the body. Excessive use of laxatives disturbs the normal bowel function. The bulimic may find that she has to continue taking the laxatives for the bowels to function at all. The use of diuretics can also alter the electrolyte balance of the body. Excessive use of diuretics can also cause high blood pressure.

The binge-purge cycle begins to dominate the bulimic's life. Depression is very common. The enormous food habit can be very expensive. A bulimic might engage in the same behaviors as a drug addict to obtain the money needed to support a food habit.

Treatment Bulimia can be hard to diagnose because its victims appear to be of normal weight. The disorder becomes apparent only after the person has had the disorder for a long time.

There is some evidence to indicate that bulimia may be related to a metabolic condition. Some people with bulimia can't recognize when they are "full." The signals the body gives for fullness may only appear in very low amounts in people who have bulimia. Like anorexia, the emotional basis of this disorder lies in the victim's low self-esteem. Therapy involves training in appropriate, nutritional eating habits, along with activities that develop confidence and build self-esteem.

Anorexia and Bulimia in Combination

About 30 to 50 percent of anorexics also go through binge-purge cycles. Throwing up is one way anorexics maintain their low calorie consumption and keep weight low. Having both disorders just increases the health risks you've read about for each disorder. Professional counseling would almost always be required to successfully treat someone with both disorders.

What Should You Do?

Recognize that eating disorders result from placing too much emphasis on body shape and weight. Because thinness is highly valued in the United States culture, these disorders occur more frequently here than in

• • • TEACH continued

anorexics might be helped by peer group counseling. Have them role-play group sessions in which a person pretending to have an eating disorder reveals that fact and the others try to help.

Debate the Issue

Advertisements and Body Image

Have a panel of students debate the issue: Advertisements that stress a particular body image as being necessary for a happy life contribute to eating disorders and should be censored. Have students point out the relationship between advertisement messages that focus on body image and the increase in the number of people with eating disorders. Encourage students to consider in the debate whether censoring harmful ad messages is unwarranted interference with free speech.

Journal 5F

Am I at Risk?

Have students record in the Student Journal whether or not they think that they are at risk for anorexia or bulimia. If they think they are at risk, encourage them to identify the risk factors and to consider talking to someone who can help. Students should be encouraged to use the Check Up list in determining their risk.

other parts of the world. The focus on thinness, an obsession with food, and a domineering family situation are prime factors in the cause of these disorders.

Being fit and eating nutritiously will automatically make you feel good about yourself. If you feel good about yourself, it is unlikely that you will do things that could damage your health. Learn to be comfortable with your body and realize that there is only so much you can do to change it. In trying to be popular, remember that it is your personality that makes a relationship last.

If you have, or are at high risk for, an eating disorder, seek help now. Talk to an adult you trust. Figure 11-8 on page 235 gives a list of some of the people in your life with whom you could discuss your problem. A visit to the doctor and a complete physical would help you know where to start, if treatment is needed. There are now numerous eating disorder clinics throughout the country. Check the *Hospital* listing in your phone book for places you can call for help.

Treating these disorders is generally a long, slow process. These risky behaviors do not go away overnight and require professional treatment.

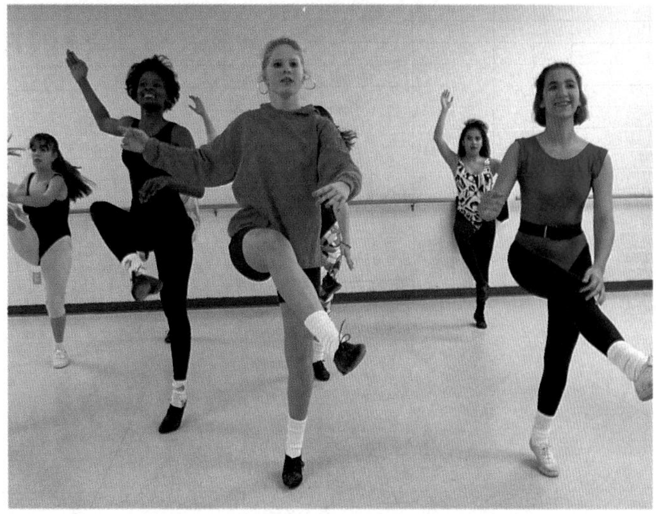

(FIGURE 5-9) **Setting a goal to be fit will help boost your self-esteem. When you feel good about yourself, you are less likely to do things that damage your health.**

Pica

Pica is a little-known eating disorder that involves eating substances not normally considered as food. People experiencing pica have cravings for such things as clay, soil, or laundry starch. This disorder generally occurs among pregnant women. Most pica is reported among pregnant African-American women living in rural areas of the southern United States. The disorder is also found in certain groups living in Australia and Africa. There is some evidence to suggest that pica results from cultural beliefs related to pregnancy, along with changes in food preferences among pregnant women.

The health dangers of pica result from eating harmful bacteria that could be present in clay, soil, or laundry starch. Eating these substances can change the way minerals are absorbed by the body, and mineral deficiencies can result. Eating large quantities of clay can also block the intestines.

pica: *an eating disorder in which the person eats nonfood substances like starch, clay, or soil.*

Review

1. What are the health risks of bulimia?
2. You think your best friend is bulimic. What signs do you look for to know for sure?
3. How is self-esteem related to some eating disorders?

Review Answers

1. Tooth decay, enlarged salivary glands, disruption of the body's electrolyte balance, mineral deficiencies, dehydration and disruption of normal bowel functions, high blood pressure, behaviors similar to drug addicts
2. Answers may include eating binges, purging, concern about being overweight, low self-esteem.
3. When self-esteem is based upon weight, the person may become obsessed with being thin in order to avoid rejection or seek approval from others.

Cooperative Learning
A Plan for Fitness

Have students meet in groups to formulate a nutrition and exercise plan that they feel would have a positive effect on an individual's overall health and self-esteem. Have several groups of students present their plans to the class.

Extension
Eating Disorder Clinics

Have a speaker from a nearby clinic speak to the class about how eating disorders are diagnosed and treated.

ASSESS

Section Review

Have students answer the Section Review questions.

Alternative Assessment
The Nature of Anorexia Nervosa

Ask students to write a clinical report on a fictitious person who has anorexia nervosa. The report should be in three parts: personal background, symptoms, recommended treatment.

Closure
Eating Disorders

Define anorexia nervosa and bulimia on the chalkboard. Have students differentiate between the two.

Background
A Deadly Disease
In developing countries, diarrhea is a leading cause of death among infants and young children. Death results from the rapid and severe dehydration and the loss of electrolytes. The disorder is often caused by bacteria or viruses transmitted by contaminated food and water. Even in the United States it is not uncommon for infants to be hospitalized for treatment of the disorder.

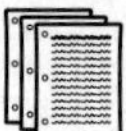
Evaluating the Media Worksheet
How In Is Thin?
Have students complete the How In Is Thin? Evaluating the Media worksheet for Unit 2.

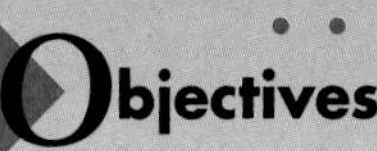

Section 5.3 Disorders Affecting the Digestive System

Objectives

- *List the most common digestive disorders.*
- *Describe ways to treat constipation and diarrhea.*
- *Describe the differences between food allergies and food intolerances.*

diarrhea:
loose bowel movements that occur when food moves too quickly through the digestive system.

As with many other health-related issues, disorders of the digestive system are frequently related to personal choices, like eating behaviors. Overeating and eating foods that the body has difficulty digesting most frequently cause digestive problems. But digestive problems can also be the result of a specific disease. The most common signs and symptoms of digestive disorders include such things as pain in the chest and abdomen, nausea and vomiting, and constipation and diarrhea.

constipation:
a condition in which bowel movements are infrequent or difficult.

Constipation

Constipation refers to a condition in which a person has difficult or infrequent bowel movements. It usually results when too much water is removed from waste products in the large intestine. This loss causes difficulty in moving waste material through to the rectum. There are many reasons why constipation may occur, including such things as a low-fiber diet, not drinking enough fluids, lack of exercise, stress, or some disease process. To prevent constipation, your diet should include plenty of fluids, foods high in fiber, and regular exercise. You should try to limit the number of high-fat foods you eat. These foods take longer to travel through your digestive system. If you have a problem with frequent constipation, you should see a physician to rule out the possibility of serious illness.

Diarrhea

Diarrhea occurs when food moves through the digestive system too quickly and there is not enough time for water to be removed. When this happens, the stools are loose and watery, and bowel movements may occur quite often. Usually diarrhea lasts for only a short period of time and can be easily cured. Even though the stools are watery, a person with diarrhea should drink plenty of liquids. The water that is normally removed from digested food in the large intestine is an important source of nutrients for the body. During diarrhea there is a loss of nutrients, and dehydration can occur. When a person has diarrhea for an extended period of time, the large loss of water can be very dangerous to health, or even fatal.

The electrolytes sodium, potassium, and chloride can also be lost during bouts of extended diarrhea—or through any large fluid loss (like heavy perspiration). The proper balance of electrolytes prevents problems resulting from dehydration, such as cramping, heat exhaustion, and heat stroke. Therefore, if diarrhea lasts for more than two days, a physician should always be consulted.

Section 5.3 Lesson Plan

MOTIVATE

Journal 5G
Food Preferences
This can be done as a warm-up activity. Suggest to students that they record in the Student Journal foods that they like very much and foods that they dislike. Then tell them to review their lists and identify any foods that seem to cause digestive upset or allergic reactions.

TEACH

Class Discussion
Digestive Disorders
Most members of the class, if not all, will have experienced the common digestive disorders discussed here—constipation and diarrhea. Stress that these disorders sometimes indicate the presence of a serious condition. Point out that chronic constipation can lead to laxative dependence. Students should also be made aware that diarrhea can be a very serious condition, particularly in infants, because they dehydrate very rapidly.

Journal 5H
Emotions and Digestive Disorders
Have students record in the Student Journal personal evidence linking anxiety to disorders of the digestive system. Encourage them to consider whether,

Food Allergies

Allergies brought about by food can cause reactions such as diarrhea, rashes, congestion, sneezing, and itchy, watery eyes. Food allergies are the result of the body's immune system responding to the food as if it were a disease-causing organism. The most common food allergies involve cow's milk, eggs, peanuts, wheat products, shellfish, and fish. The allergic responses are the result of the body's reaction to the foreign proteins in these foods. The most severe food allergy reaction is called anaphylactic shock. The victim of anaphylactic shock experiences severe itching, hives, sweating, tightness in the throat, and difficulty in breathing, followed by low blood pressure, unconsciousness, and eventually death. If you are diagnosed as having a specific food allergy (diagnosis should come from an allergist), you must avoid the food that produces the reaction. This means looking carefully at labels to determine if combination foods are made with substances you are allergic to.

Many allergies begin in infancy and are thought to result from introducing solid foods too early in the infant's diet. It is recommended that cow's milk not be given to infants until they are at least six months of age. Other common allergic foods should not be given to infants until they are past their first birthday. Certain chemical additives in foods (such as dyes) can also cause allergic reactions.

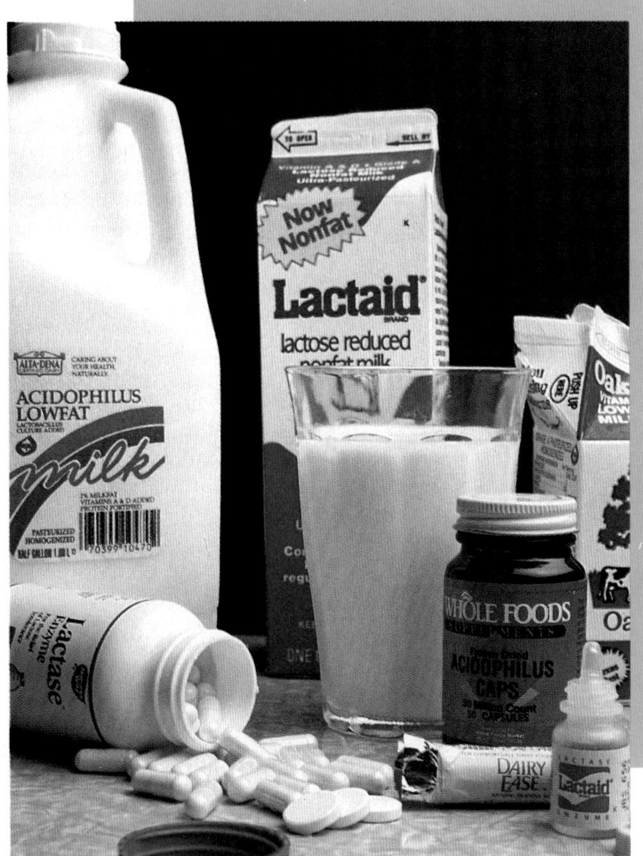

(FIGURE 5-10) **Lactose intolerance can produce some very uncomfortable symptoms. Fortunately, there are products to eliminate these discomforts when consuming milk products.**

Food Intolerances

Negative reactions to specific foods that do not involve the body's immune system are called **food intolerances.** Lactose intolerance is one of the most common of these reactions. People with lactose intolerance cannot tolerate milk and milk products. Their bodies do not produce lactase, the enzyme that breaks down lactose in milk. Lactose intolerance is high among Asians, Africans, Native Americans, and African-Americans. Drinking milk if you don't produce lactase will cause you to experience bloating, diarrhea, gas, and severe cramps. Fortunately, people who have lactose intolerance can purchase milk already treated with lactase, or add special lactase drops to milk. Lactase tablets can also be used with meals that include milk products. If you have lactose intolerance, you need to be sure you still get an adequate supply of calcium in your diet.

food intolerance:

a negative reaction to food which is not brought about by the immune system.

Background
What Are Additives?

Although there are many reasons why additives are put into food, most often they are used for one of four purposes—to add flavor, color, or texture to food, or to preserve food. Spices, natural flavors, and artificial flavors are added to enhance the taste of food. Coloring agents are used to make food look more appealing. Texturing additives are used to thicken food or to stabilize it, that is, to keep it from separating. Preservatives are added to prevent food from spoiling.

Other reasons for using food additives are to increase the nutritional quality, to help certain foods remain moist, and to prevent foods from becoming acidic or alkaline.

Making a Choice 5B

Lactose-Free Foods

Assign the Lactose-Free Foods card. The card requires students to consider ways of using lactose-free foods as substitutes for dairy products.

for themselves, anxiety is more important than other causes, such as eating the wrong foods, in triggering digestive upset.

Role-Playing
Food Allergies

Have a student play the role of someone who is seriously allergic to a particular food. Have a second student play the role of a friend trying to convince the person with the allergy to sample some of the forbidden food that he or she has prepared.

Case Study
Lactose Intolerance

Ask for a volunteer who knows that he or she has a lactose intolerance to describe how he or she came to realize that the condition was present, how long it took to realize it, and how he or she handles the condition, with respect to diet.

Debate the Issue
Eliminate Food Additives

Have teams debate the topic: Should food additives be banned because they cause serious health problems for some individuals? Have students propose measures to deal with the health problems created by food additives.

Extension
What's in Food?

Have students use library sources to investigate the kinds of foods in which additives are used. Have them read food labels to identify some foods that contain one or more additives. Have

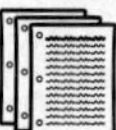

Section Review Worksheet 5.3

Assign Section Review Worksheet 5.3, which requires students to complete sentences about digestive system disorders.

Section Quiz 5.3

Have students take Section Quiz 5.3.

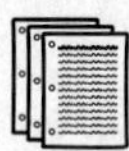

Reteaching Worksheet 5.3

Students who have difficulty with the material may complete Reteaching Worksheet 5.3, which requires students to complete a network describing digestive system disorders.

Review Answers

1. Answers may include chest and abdomen pain, cramping, nausea, vomiting, constipation, diarrhea, gas, and bloating.

2. Liquids prevent dehydration that occurs during diarrhea.

3. Food allergies, unlike food intolerances, involve the body's immune system. The immune system responds to the food as if it were an invading organism or germ.

Common Food Additives and Environmental Contaminants

Additive	Source	Side Effects
MSG	*Oriental foods, processed meats*	*Chest pain, headache, sweating, burning feeling*
Coloring agents	*Beverages*	*Allergic reactions: rash, digestive problems*
Sodium nitrite	*Smoked meats: ham, bacon, sausage, cold cuts*	*Possible link to cancer*
Sulfites (sulfur dioxide)	*Potatoes, packaged foods, wine*	*Allergic reactions including anaphylactic shock*
Estrogen	*Meats*	*Possible link to cancer*
Lead	*Calcium supplements from dolomite*	*Lead poisoning*
Mercury	*Contaminated fish*	*Mercury poisoning*

(FIGURE 5-11)

Other common intolerances include the inability to adequately digest substances such as prunes, blueberries, corn, and MSG (monosodium glutamate). MSG can produce a reaction often called "Chinese-restaurant syndrome" (MSG is commonly used in Chinese foods). MSG is an additive in many foods. Reactions to MSG include chest pain, headache, sweating, and a burning feeling.

Figure 5-11 shows some other additives commonly used in foods that can cause the body to react negatively. If you have a food intolerance you will need to check food labels carefully. When eating out, be sure to ask questions about the ingredients used in preparing the food.

Review

1. List the symptoms of a digestive disorder.
2. Why are liquids so important in treating diarrhea?
3. How does a food allergy differ from a food intolerance?

• • • TEACH continued

them catalog the possible side effects from eating each type of food.

ASSESS

Section Review

Have students answer the Section Review questions.

Alternative Assessment

Digestive Disorders

On the chalkboard create a reference table on digestive disorders while students provide the information. The table should contain four columns: Disorder, Causes, Symptoms, Treatment/Prevention.

Closure

Treating Digestive Problems

Ask students to explain how constipation can be prevented, and then to explain why diarrhea can be dangerous.

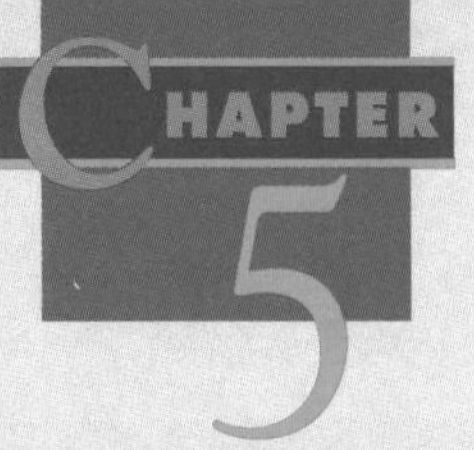

Highlights

Summary

- The number of calories you should consume is determined by basal metabolism rate and your level of activity.
- The body is made of several kinds of tissue, including fat and lean mass. Females have a higher fat content than males.
- A person's ideal weight should be determined by the ratio of fat to lean mass.
- Obesity has serious health risks, including heart disease, cancer, diabetes, and stroke.
- Fad diets are rarely effective and can be dangerous to your health.
- Anorexia nervosa is a starvation eating disorder that can result in depression, permanent heart damage, and even death.
- Bulimia can cause harmful changes in body organs.
- Some common digestive disorders are constipation, diarrhea, food allergies, and food intolerances.

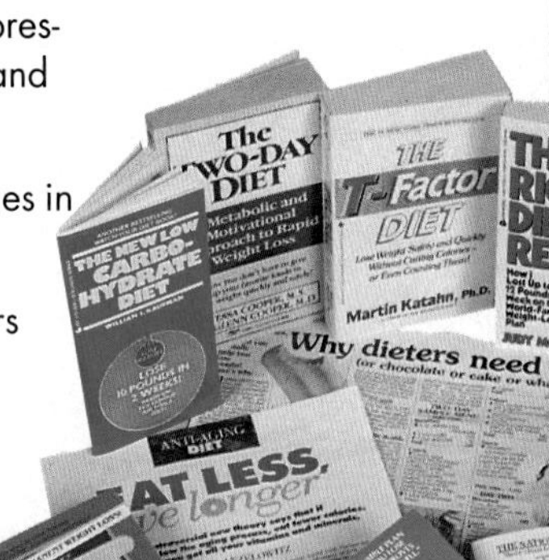

Vocabulary

basal metabolic rate energy needed to fuel the body's on-going processes while the body is at complete rest.

energy-balance equation eating the same number of calories that you burn each day.

lean mass also known as the lean muscle mass portion of your body. It is your total body weight minus the weight due to fat.

essential fat the amount of fat needed for certain metabolic processes to occur.

storage fat excess fat stored in the body.

overweight weighing 10 percent more than one's recommended weight.

anorexia nervosa an eating disorder in which the person refuses to eat because of a fear of weight gain.

bulimia an eating disorder based on a cycle of binging and purging food.

pica an eating disorder in which the person eats nonfood substances like starch, clay, or soil.

constipation a condition in which bowel movements are infrequent or difficult.

diarrhea loose bowel movements that occur when food moves too quickly through the digestive system.

food intolerance a condition in which a reaction occurs to food that is not brought about by the immune system.

Chapter 5 Highlights Strategies

Summary

Have students read the summary to reinforce the concepts they learned in Chapter 5.

Vocabulary

Have students write a paragraph for a student newspaper using as many of the vocabulary terms as they can.

Extension

Have students visit a grocery store or supermarket, paying attention to the locations on shelves, locations in the store, and size of displays devoted to foods that are high in fat.

CHAPTER 5 ASSESSMENT

CHAPTER REVIEW

Concept Review

1. basal metabolic rate (BMR)
2. body composition
3. diabetes, blood pressure, cholesterol
4. eat, burn
5. nutrition
6. bulimia
7. anorexia nervosa
8. fluids, fiber, exercise
9. diarrhea
10. lactose intolerance

Expressing Your Views

Sample responses:

1. I would tell Patricia that diets promising fast weight loss are not healthy, as they do not provide adequate nutrition. I would also tell her that height and weight charts are only a guide, not a specific target for body weight. There is no fixed ideal body weight for each person. Since each person is different, a person's ideal body weight should be based on what feels and looks comfortable for that person. Patricia would be better off using body composition rather than height and weight charts as a method of determining her ideal weight.

2. Thinness appears to be associated with femininity and sensuality in women, and most women think that thinness is a factor in being popular.

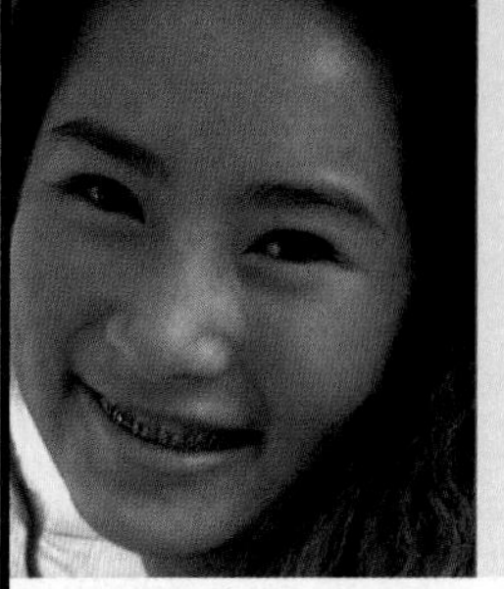

Chapter Review

Concept Review

1. Your ________ refers to how fast your body burns calories.
2. Rather than using height and weight charts, you should examine your ________ as a better method of determining your ideal weight.
3. Being overweight or obese increases your health risks of ________, high ________, and elevated ________.
4. A simple rule for healthy weight control is to ________ fewer calories than you ________.
5. Fad diets can be dangerous to your health because they require food selections that do not provide adequate ________.
6. A condition called ________ can lead to tooth decay and mineral deficiencies from repeated vomiting.
7. ________ is a condition in which a person is obsessed with becoming thin.
8. To prevent constipation, your diet should include plenty of ________, foods high in ________, and plenty of ________.
9. When a person has ________ for an extended period of time, the large loss of water can be very dangerous to your health.
10. A common negative reaction to milk and milk products is called ________.

Expressing Your Views

1. Patricia is 5′5″ and weighs 140 pounds. She was surprised when she saw a height/weight chart at the doctor's office that gave her ideal weight as no more than 135 pounds. She is now looking for a diet that promises fast results. What would you advise her? What could you tell her about height/weight charts?
2. Anorexia nervosa and bulimia appear more often in girls than in boys. Why do you think this is true?
3. Daniel has lactose intolerance. How can he be sure his body gets enough calcium?
4. Calculate your daily caloric needs using the formulas on page 109.

3. Daniel can drink milk in which the lactose has already been broken down by lactase. This type of milk is available for purchase or Daniel can add special lactase drops to regular milk. Daniel can also use lactase tablets with meals that include milk products containing lactose. Daniel can be sure to get an adequate supply of calcium in his diet by eating calcium-rich foods that do not contain lactose, such as sardines.

4. Answers will vary depending on a person's weight, sex, and activity level.

CHAPTER 5 ASSESSMENT

Life Skills Check

1. **Assessing Your Health**
   You will be traveling next summer on a long road trip. Most of your day will be spent riding in the car. Calculate your total calorie needs for the day. Then design a plan for protecting yourself against digestive disorders and for maintaining your weight in a healthy way during the trip.

2. **Making Responsible Decisions**
   Your friend Charlene eats a huge amount of food every day at lunch, but never seems to gain weight. She leaves the lunch room for a few minutes as soon as she finishes eating and occasionally you have seen her taking laxatives. You suspect she is purging and you are worried about her health. What should you do?

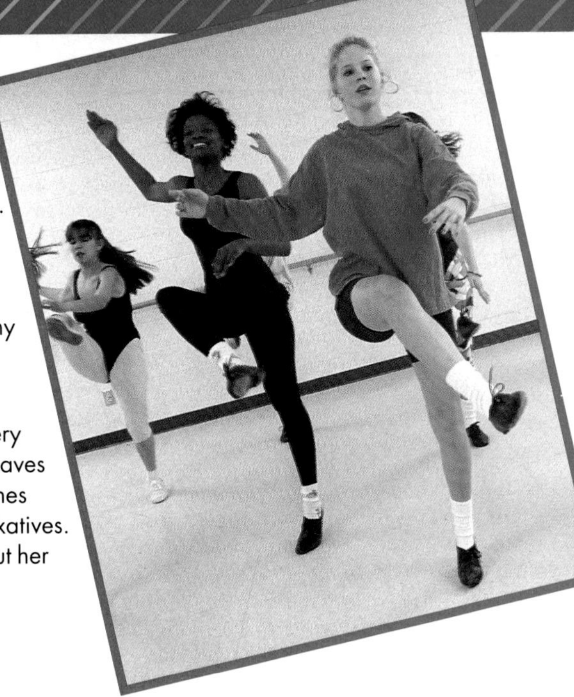

Projects

1. Starvation can be self-induced as in anorexia nervosa or can be caused by poverty, drought, overpopulation, political upheaval, and other factors. To find out how problems of world hunger compare to problems related to anorexia nervosa, work with a group and choose an area of the world where people are starving. Research the causes, health consequences, and aid provided to the victims. Then list ways to help alleviate world hunger.

2. Call a local fitness center to find out about their body building and weight loss programs. What does the center provide in the way of therapy or group support, education, or professional staff members? Summarize your findings in writing.

Plan for Action

Eating patterns and food selection directly affect weight control. List four strategies you will use to help you gain, lose, or maintain your present weight depending on your individual needs.

Life Skills Check

Sample responses:

1. Total calorie needs will vary with each student. Students should protect themselves from constipation by drinking plenty of fluids; by including foods high in fiber in their diet; and, when driving, stopping every couple of hours at a rest stop to get out of the car, stretch, and walk about. They could also stay at motels that have pools and increase their level of exercise by swimming. To maintain their weight on their trip, they could eat more fruits and vegetables and less high-calorie, high-fat foods.

2. I would use the decision-making steps to assess the situation and decide how best to help Charlene.

Projects

Have students complete the projects on weight management and eating disorders.

Plan for Action

Ask students to discuss the role that weight control can play in a person's life and what role they would like it to play in their lives.

Personal Pledge

Have students read and sign the personal pledge for Chapter 5.

ASSESSMENT OPTIONS

Chapter Test

Have students take the Chapter 5 Test.

Alternate Assessment

Have students do the Alternative Assessment activity for Chapter 5.

Test Generator

The Test Generator (Macintosh® or IBM® format) contains an additional 50 assessment items for this chapter.

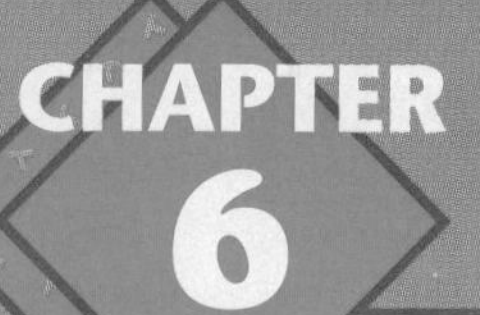

Personal Care and Appearance

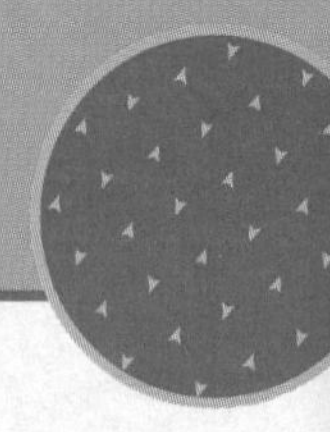

PLANNING GUIDE

TEXT SECTIONS	OBJECTIVES	TEXT FEATURES	OUTSIDE RESOURCES	NOTES
6.1 Skin Care pp. 125-132 1 period	• Name the two main layers of the skin. • Recognize skin problems. ■ Explain how you can improve the condition of your skin if you have acne. ■ Explain how you can avoid sun damage to your skin.	**ASSESSMENT** • Check Up, p. 126 • Section Review, p. 132	**TEACHER'S RESOURCE BINDER** • Lesson Plan 6.1 • Personal Health Inventory • Journal Entries 6A, 6B, 6C • Section Review Worksheet 6.1 • Section Quiz 6.1 • Reteaching Worksheet 6.1 **OTHER RESOURCES** • Transparency 6A	
6.2 Hair and Nail Care pp. 133-135 1 period	• Describe three common hair and scalp problems. ■ Explain how to care for your hair. ■ Explain how to care for your nails.	**ASSESSMENT** • Section Review, p. 135	**TEACHER'S RESOURCE BINDER** • Lesson Plan 6.2 • Journal Entries 6D • Life Skills 6A • Section Review 6.2 • Section Quiz 6.2 • Reteaching 6.2 **OTHER RESOURCES** • Making a Choice 6A	
6.3 Teeth and Gum Care pp. 136-142 1 period	• Explain how dental cavities develop. ■ Explain how to care for your teeth and gums. ■ Be able to make an appointment with a dentist.	• LIFE SKILLS: Being a Wise Consumer, p. 141 **ASSESSMENT** • Section Review, p. 142	**TEACHER'S RESOURCE BINDER** • Lesson Plan 6.3 • Journal Entries 6E, 6F, 6G • Life Skills 6B, 6C • Section Review 6.3 • Section Quiz 6.3 • Reteaching 6.3 **OTHER RESOURCES** • Making a Choice 6B • Transparency 6B	
End of Chapter pp. 143-145		• Chapter Review, pp. 144-145	**TEACHER'S RESOURCE BINDER** **OTHER RESOURCES** • Chapter Test • Alternative Assessment • Test Generator	

■ Denotes LIFE SKILLS objectives

• Items in blue are also part of the *Holt Health Activity Book.*

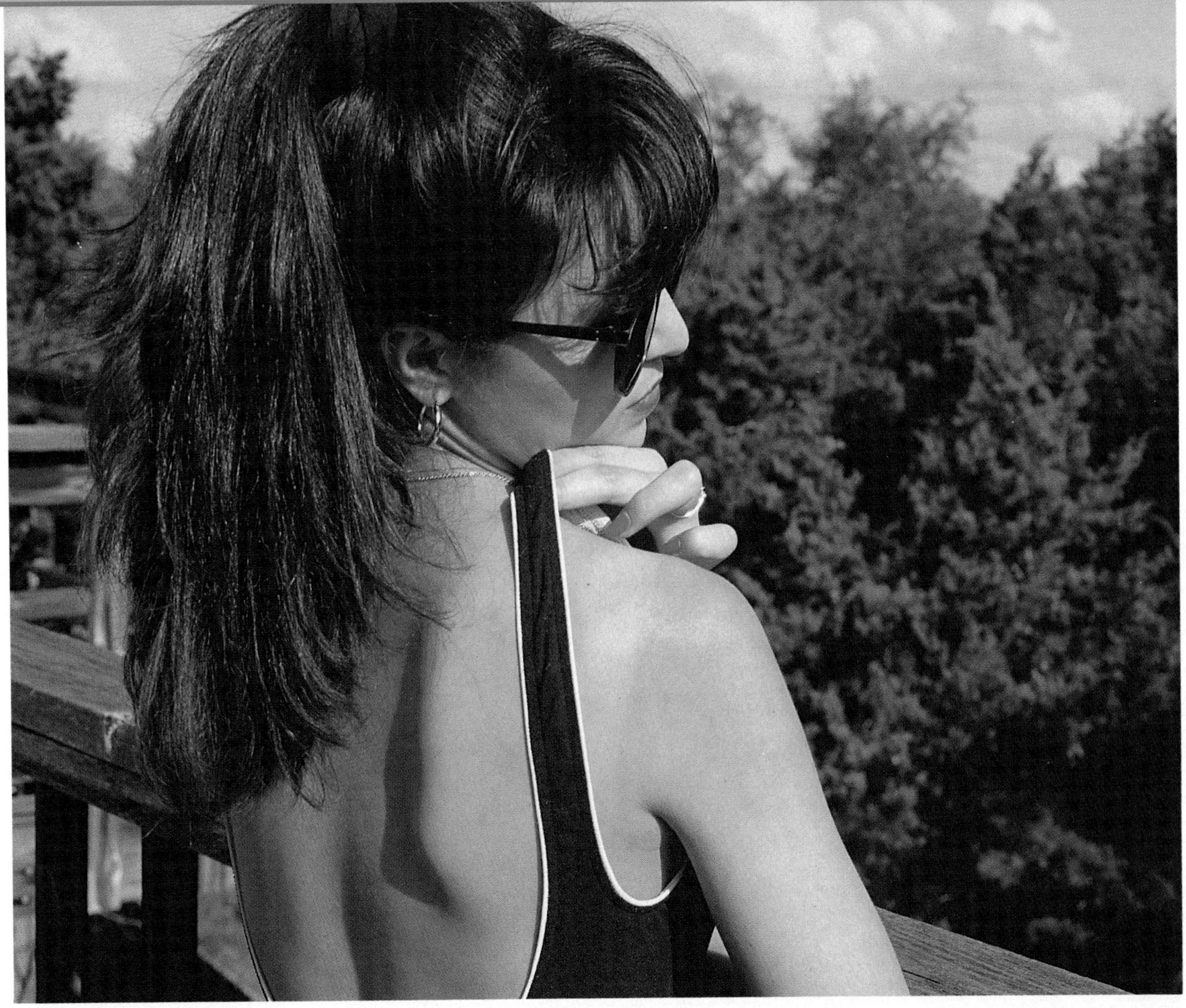

CONTENT BACKGROUND Skin and Dental Care

MANY SKIN-CARE EXPERTS AGREE THAT the three most damaging activities to human skin are sunbathing, smoking, and daily cleansing. Too many people in the United States, including the majority of adolescents, are injuring their skin cells simply by performing their daily hygienic regimes. Most dermatologists recommend using a washcloth to gently wash the skin on the face once a day with warm water and a mild soap. In areas with high levels of air pollutants, a cotton ball moistened with a toner containing no alcohol can be rubbed over facial skin.

Showering or bathing should be done in tepid water. Again, gently whisking the skin with a washcloth and mild soap for a few minutes is sufficient to cleanse skin. Skin should be patted dry with a towel. Moisturizers can be applied to the skin once it is dry. To ensure healthy skin, a person also needs to drink plenty of water (at least eight 8-ounce glasses per day), exercise daily, and use a sunscreen with a sun protection factor (SPF) of 15 anytime skin is exposed to the sun.

According to most dermatologists, if people were not exposed to sunlight, skin wouldn't start to age until midlife. More serious than the problems associated with aging, however, is skin cancer. It is occurring in record high numbers in the United States, killing nearly 9,000 people each year. There are three basic kinds of skin cancer:

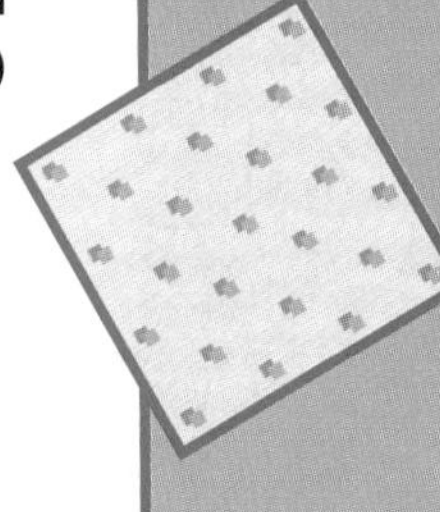

basal cell carcinoma, squamous cell carcinoma, and melanoma. Melanoma is the most serious type. Each year, about 32,000 Americans get the disease and about 6,700 die of it. When caught early, melanoma can be treated and cured. One person in fifty who has had the disease, however, will have a recurrence.

Because nearly 60 percent of the people living in the United States drink fluoridated water, over half of all school children have excellent dental health as opposed to only about 20 percent 10 years ago. A 1988 study by the National Institute of Dental Research indicates that about 50 percent of the children between the ages of 5 and 17 are cavity-free. Tooth decay in this age group has decreased 36 percent since 1980.

The greatest danger to teeth today is periodontal or gum disease. These bacterial infections cause an estimated 70 percent of the tooth loss in adults. And interestingly, although most teenagers and adults know that regular brushing and flossing are critical to dental care, most don't carry out these activities on a regular basis or do not perform them correctly.

Most dentists recommend using a soft nylon toothbrush having rounded bristles and a relatively small head that is effective in cleaning all surfaces of each tooth. The bristles should also be used to gently massage the gums as well as to remove any accumulated debris between teeth. Toothbrushes should be allowed to air-dry and should be replaced every few months and after an illness. Waxed and unwaxed floss are equally effective in removing plaque between teeth.

Research has shown that in addition to regular dental care and treatment, diet greatly affects dental health. Research has indicated that the acids in apple and orange juices and colas—both regular and diet—erode enamel and expose underlying tissue. This exposure makes teeth more susceptible to decay.

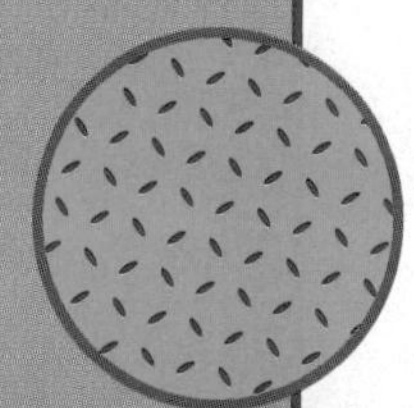

PLANNING FOR INSTRUCTION

KEY FACTS

- **The skin protects the body from germs, regulates body temperature, transmits sensations, and acts as a waterproof cover to hold the body together.**
- **The top layer of skin is the epidermis; skin oil and sweat are carried in pores to the surface of the epidermis.**
- **The dermis is the layer of skin beneath the epidermis. The dermis contains nerves, oil glands, sweat glands, and the roots of thousands of hairs.**
- **Changes in moles should be reported to a doctor as they could indicate skin cancer.**
- **Sunlight contains ultraviolet rays, which are responsible for sunburn, wrinkles, and skin cancer. Sunscreen can block harmful ultraviolet rays and help prevent skin damage.**
- **Hair should be washed regularly. Inexpensive shampoos work just as well as expensive ones.**
- **Brushing stimulates the scalp and brings oils to the scalp surface, whereas blow drying and using electric curlers dries hair out.**
- **Plaque forms when food particles combine with saliva and bacteria; plaque produces an acid that eats through tooth enamel.**
- **Cavities form when acid reaches below the enamel of a tooth and infects it.**
- **Gum disease, the leading cause of tooth loss in adults, can be prevented.**
- **Good dental care involves eating nutritious foods, brushing and flossing teeth regularly, and having regular dental checkups.**

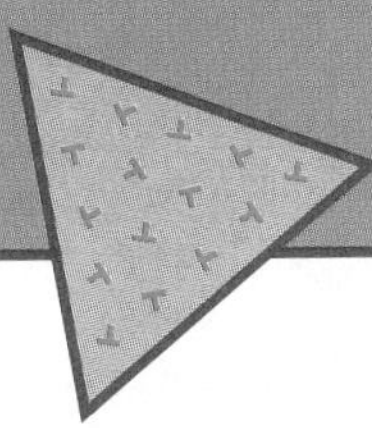

Myths and Misconceptions

MYTH: Beach umbrellas provide adequate protection against sunburn.

Beach umbrellas provide little protection against sunburn because ultraviolet rays reflected from sand and water can strike a person sitting in the shade of the umbrella.

MYTH: Sunburn cannot occur on foggy, overcast, or hazy days.

Ultraviolet rays are scattered by these atmospheric conditions and produce severe sunburn even if the sun isn't visible.

MYTH: Cocoa butter, baby oil, and mineral oil are effective sunscreens.

These products provide lubrication to minimize the sun's drying effects but do not protect against sunburn.

MYTH: Shaving makes hair grow faster.

Hair roots, where hair growth begins, are located in the dermis and are unaffected by the shaving of the hair shafts on the surface of the skin.

Vocabulary

Essential: The following vocabulary terms appear in bold face:

epidermis	enamel
dermis	plaque
acne	calculus
sunscreen	dental floss

Secondary: In addition, the following terms may require early attention:

melanin	fungi
hormones	allergic reaction
antiperspirants	malignant melanoma

For Students with Special Needs

Visual Learners: Demonstrate to students that perspiration passes through the skin to the outside. The demonstration illustrates the cooling mechanism of sweat production and reinforces the necessity for good hygiene. Have a student place a large, clear plastic bag over one hand and have another student secure the bag with a string. Make sure the bag is tight enough to prevent air from escaping but not tight enough to cut off circulation. After 10 minutes, have students examine the bag. They should notice water droplets—perspiration—inside it.

Kinesthetic Learners: Invite a dental hygienist, dentist, or school nurse to demonstrate the correct teeth-cleaning technique. Allow students to handle the models and equipment used and to practice the techniques demonstrated.

Enrichment

Have students research different types and brands of sunscreen. Ask them to compare the products on the market as to price and ingredients. Have them prepare a brief report to the class about their findings.

CHAPTER 6
CHAPTER OPENER

GETTING STARTED

Using the Chapter Photograph

Ask students to name some of the ways the people in the photograph take care of themselves. Have them discuss how taking care of themselves makes them feel and look better. Tell them that the chapter will discuss skin, hair, and dental concerns and care.

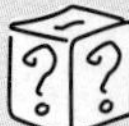 **Question Box**

Encourage students to write questions about any aspect of personal care and put them in the Question Box. The Question Box provides them with an opportunity to ask questions anonymously. To ensure that students with questions are not embarrassed to be seen writing, have those who do not have questions write something else—such as something they already know about acne or skin care—instead.

Preview the questions and then answer them at appropriate points in the chapter. You may wish to allow students to write additional anonymous questions as they go through the chapter.

CHAPTER 6

Personal Care and Appearance

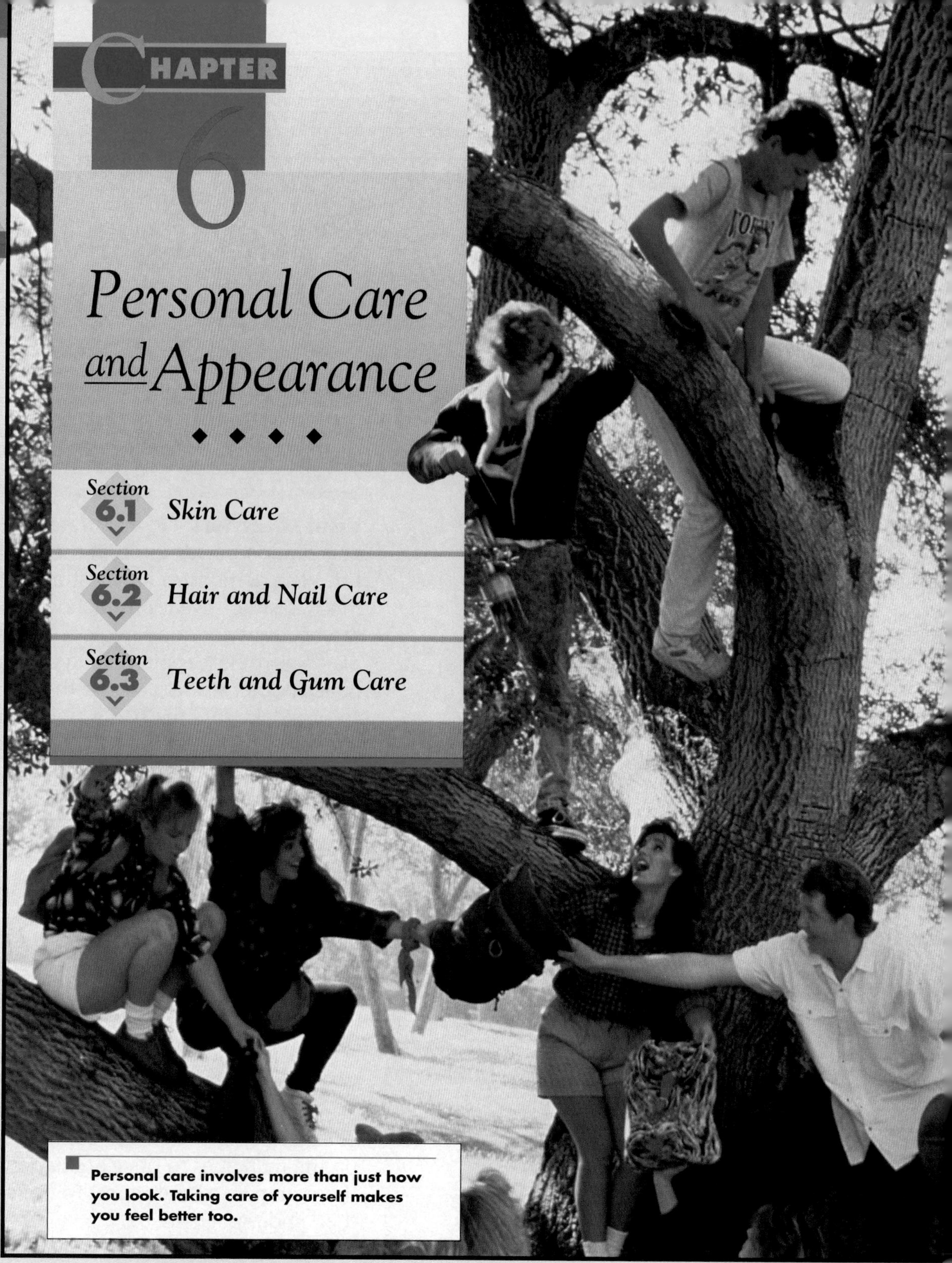

Personal care involves more than just how you look. Taking care of yourself makes you feel better too.

Personal Issues *ALERT*

Several issues in this chapter may be sensitive to some students. Prepare students to be respectful and tolerant toward their classmates. Some students may be self-conscious about the condition of their skin and may be uncomfortable during the discussion of acne. If students in the class are of predominantly one race, students of a different race may feel self-conscious during the discussion of sunburn and skin color. Some students may be self-conscious about their hair, especially if it is thinning or if it cannot conform to the latest styles. Some students who have braces may be self-conscious about their orthodontia. Others who are in need of orthodontia work but are unable to have it may also be self-conscious.

The day at the beach was perfect. David and Elena had a great time, swimming and listening to music and watching the waves. When they got home, though, David was red and sunburned all over. Elena told him he looked like a giant tomato. She was teasing, but it wasn't funny. When Elena touched his arm, it felt like a lit match on his skin.

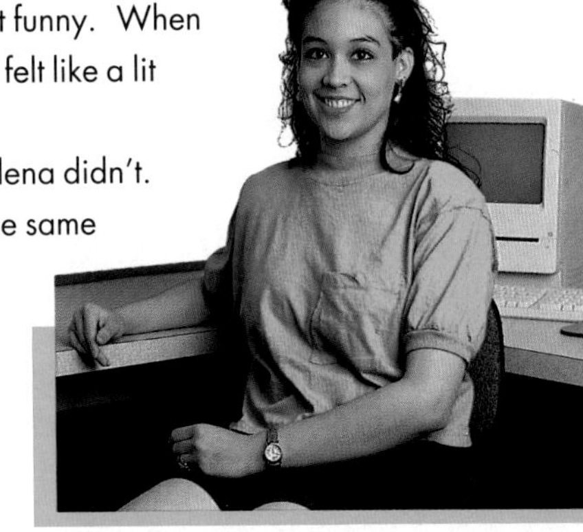

David couldn't understand why he got sunburned and Elena didn't. They both used the same suntan lotion. They put it on at the same time. They were in the sun exactly the same amount of time—from 10:00 A.M. till 4:00 P.M. They both swam for the same length of time. Why did they have such different reactions to the sun?

Section 6.1 Skin Care

Objectives

- *Name the two main layers of the skin.*
- *Recognize skin problems.*
- *Explain how you can reduce your chances of getting acne.*
  LIFE SKILLS: Practicing Self-Care
- *Explain how you can avoid sun damage to your skin.*
  LIFE SKILLS: Practicing Self-Care

David discovered the reason for their different reactions to the sun when he talked with a pharmacist. The pharmacist explained that differences in tanning are due to a substance called melanin in the skin. The more melanin people have in their skin, the darker their skin is and the less likely they are to get sunburned. David is blond, blue-eyed, and fair complexioned, so he sunburned easily. Elena has dark eyes, black hair, and brown skin, so she tanned instead.

In this chapter, you'll learn to protect your skin from the sun and other hazards. You'll also learn how to take good care of your hair, nails, and teeth. And you'll learn that good grooming helps you stay healthy and improves your personal appearance.

Skin Care and How You Look

Care of the skin is an important part of your appearance. This is particularly true during the teen years. Your body has more chemicals called hormones now than when you were a child. Hormones affect your skin and how it looks. Why is it that one day you

Section 6.1 Lesson Plan

MOTIVATE

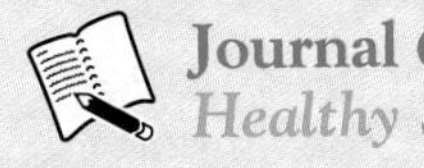

Journal 6A
Healthy Skin

This may be done as a warm-up activity. Encourage students to write in the Student Journal in the Student Activity Book how they think healthy skin can be a key factor in self-confidence and social acceptance.

Class Discussion
A Common Problem

Ask students whether they have read or heard of famous people, real or fictional, who suffered from acne. Help them reach the conclusion that acne is a common problem and has been so for thousands of years. For example, tell students about Tutankhamen, a pharaoh in ancient Egypt. Archeologists believe Tutankhamen had a problem with pimples because in his tomb they discovered medications to treat acne in his afterlife.

TEACH

Class Discussion
Sunburn

Have students look at the photograph of David and Elena and speculate which one of the pair will sunburn more easily. Ask them to explain their thinking. Have them discuss their own experiences with sunburn. Find out whether any students have ever sunburned on foggy, hazy, or overcast days, or on a

Check Up

Have students turn in their answers to the Check Up questions anonymously and then discuss the responses with the class. As these topics are quite personal in nature, there will probably be differences of opinion about what constitutes proper care.

Check Up

How Well Do You Take Care of Yourself?

Which of the following actions do you take to improve your appearance and health?

- Wash skin regularly with soap and water
- Use a sunscreen of at least 15 SPF when outdoors
- Watch any moles for changes in their appearance
- Wash hair regularly
- Limit the use of electric hair dryers and curlers
- Brush teeth at least twice a day
- Floss teeth once a day

have a clear complexion and the next day it's full of pimples? It's because of hormones. You can't do anything to change the hormones in your body, but you *can* improve the look of your skin.

Functions of the Skin

The skin is the largest organ in the body—bigger than your lungs or heart. In an adult, the skin may weigh seven pounds and cover 20 square feet. That's about half the size of a sheet that fits a twin bed, or the size of 20 sheets of notebook paper taped together.

The skin has four important functions:

1. to protect the body from germs
2. to regulate body temperature
3. to transmit sensations such as pain
4. to act as a waterproof cover to hold the body together.

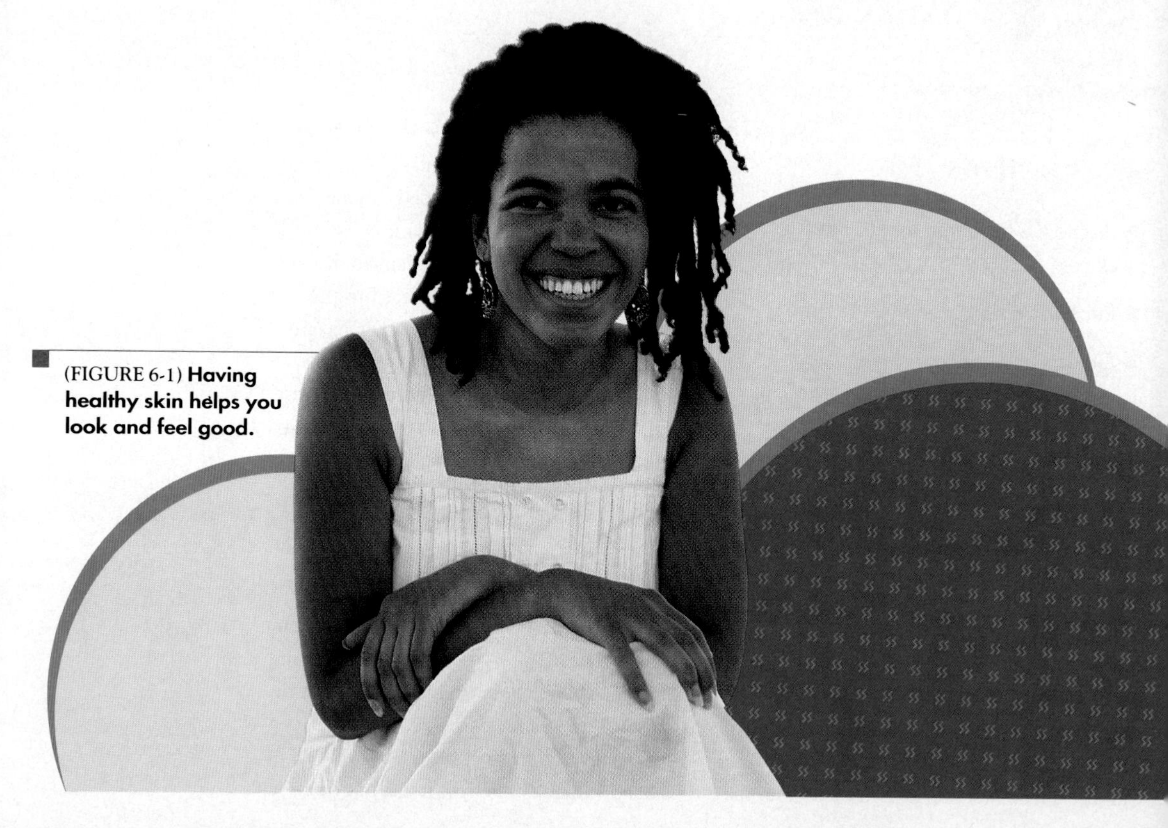

(FIGURE 6-1) **Having healthy skin helps you look and feel good.**

• • • TEACH continued

sunny day while sitting beneath a beach umbrella. Ask students to name some remedies they have used to lessen the discomfort from sunburn. Point out that a serious sunburn needs to be treated by a physician.

Demonstration

The Weight and Size of Skin

To demonstrate the possible weight and size of the skin of an adult, provide students with a gallon of milk or a 7-pound weight to lift, and have them use a yardstick to determine the amount of space covered by a 20-square-foot area.

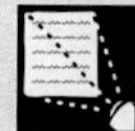

Teaching Transparency 6A

Structure of the Skin

Show the diagram of the structure of the skin (Figure 6-2). Point to various parts that make up the structure—such as a sweat gland, oil gland, and hair root—and ask students to identify each structure. Ask a volunteer to locate the epidermis and dermis layers.

Reinforcement

Functions of Skin

Review the functions of the skin. Point out that excretion is another important skin function. In the form of sweat, the skin excretes water, salt, and *urea* (nitrogen wastes). After perspiration, wastes remaining on the skin surface may make the skin feel sticky.

Structure of the Skin

As you can see in Figure 6-2, the skin has two main layers—the **epidermis** and the **dermis**. Under these two layers is a layer of fatty tissue called the subcutaneous layer. The subcutaneous layer insulates the body from temperature changes and connects the skin to the body.

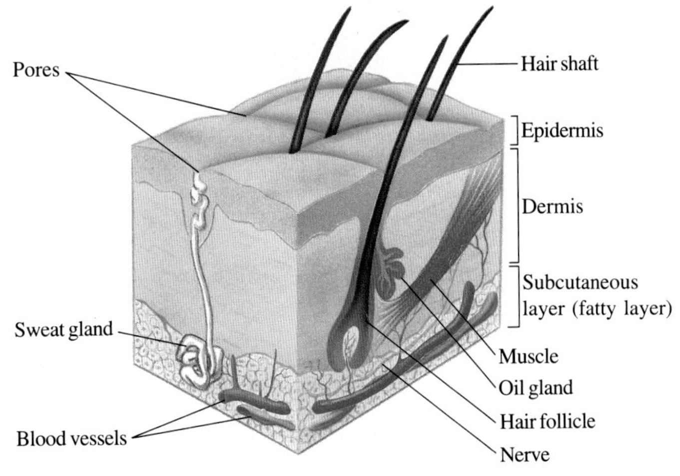

(FIGURE 6-2) **The two main layers of the skin are the epidermis and the dermis. The epidermis is the layer you can see from the outside. The dermis is beneath the epidermis and contains the oil glands.**

The Epidermis The epidermis is the top layer of the skin. This is the part of the skin that you see. It is made up of cells that are replaced once a month, which means that none of the skin you see is over a month old.

The epidermis has small openings called pores. These pores are like little pipes that lead to the surface of the body from below the epidermis. Skin oil and sweat are carried in these pores up to the surface of the skin.

Melanin, the substance that causes suntans, is found in the epidermis. Melanin protects the skin from the sun's rays and is produced whenever the skin is exposed to the sun. But melanin does not give complete protection from the sun—everyone can get a sunburn. Melanin is also the substance that produces freckles.

The Dermis The dermis, which is the layer of skin just below the epidermis, carries heat and nutrients to the surface of the skin. The dermis has thousands of tiny hairs in it. Each hair has a root that is surrounded by oil glands. The oil travels along the hair until it reaches the surface of the skin. That is what makes a person's skin feel oily sometimes. The oil is very valuable for the body, because it helps keep the skin moist, soft, and waterproof.

The dermis also has thousands of tiny sweat glands, which produce sweat. Have you ever wondered how the body usually manages to stay about the same temperature? It has a lot to do with the skin. On hot days, the body produces more sweat, which cools off the skin. On cold days, the body doesn't perspire much, so it doesn't lose heat when it needs it.

Another important part of the dermis is nerves. When we touch something, the nerves in the dermis send a message to the brain about what we touched. The nerves are like telephone lines to the brain. Then the brain sends a message back, telling the body what to do. Without the nerves in the dermis, we would never be aware that we touched anything.

Skin Problems

One of the first things people see when they look at you is your skin, so it is especially frustrating when you have skin problems. Some skin problems, like acne, are common during the teen years. Other problems may occur at any time. The following are some of the most common problems.

Acne **Acne** results when pores in the skin become clogged with oil. Acne is parti-

epidermis:
the very thin outer layer of the skin.

dermis:
the second layer of skin; the dermis contains the most important structures of the skin.

acne:
a condition in which the pores of the skin become clogged with oil: acne can take the form of blackheads, whiteheads, or pimples.

Background
Accutaine

Accutaine, a medication for severe acne, has proved to be effective in 90 percent of the patients who have used it. However, it may cause side effects such as peeling of the skin, headaches, nausea, and nosebleeds, among other serious problems. Accutaine can also cause miscarriages and serious birth defects when taken by pregnant women. The drug is sold with warnings about the potential danger to unborn children.

Demonstration
Nerve Endings in Skin

Have students determine whether all areas of the skin contain the same number of nerve endings. Have a student hold two toothpicks together and gently poke the arm of a blindfolded volunteer until the volunteer feels the pressure and identifies how many toothpicks he or she feels. Have the first student move the toothpicks slightly apart and repeat the procedure. Continue until the blindfolded volunteer feels the touch of two toothpicks. Measure and record the distance between the toothpicks. Test other parts of the body such as the cheek, shin, and fingertip. Students should find the nerve endings are closest in the fingertips.

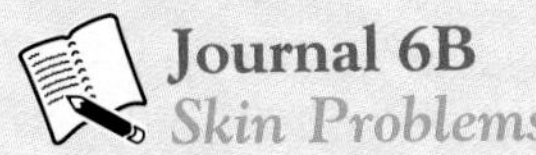

Journal 6B
Skin Problems

Ask students to use the Student Journal in the Student Activity Book to describe a skin problem they may have had and how they felt about it.

Class Discussion
Causes of Acne

Where on the body does acne commonly occur? *[The face and neck are the most usual sites, but acne often occurs on the back, shoulders, and chest, too.]* Point out that acne is most common in teenagers but that many adults get it for the first time in their twenties and thirties, or even their forties and fifties. Explain that the cause of acne is not known. Some doctors believe that

Background
Athlete's Foot

Athlete's foot can be caused by several different kinds of fungus and can vary in appearance. Warm, moist skin provides ideal growing conditions for fungus. For that reason prevention of athlete's foot includes complete drying of feet after bathing or swimming, especially between the toes, and paying attention to foot gear. Socks should be changed often and should be made of 100 percent cotton, and shoes should be made of leather or canvas. Because athlete's foot is slightly contagious, it is recommended that family members and friends not share towels or use the same bath mat as the infected person.

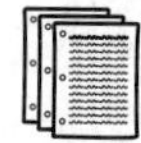

Personal Health Inventory

Have students complete the Personal Health Inventory for this chapter. The inventory helps them assess their personal care and appearance.

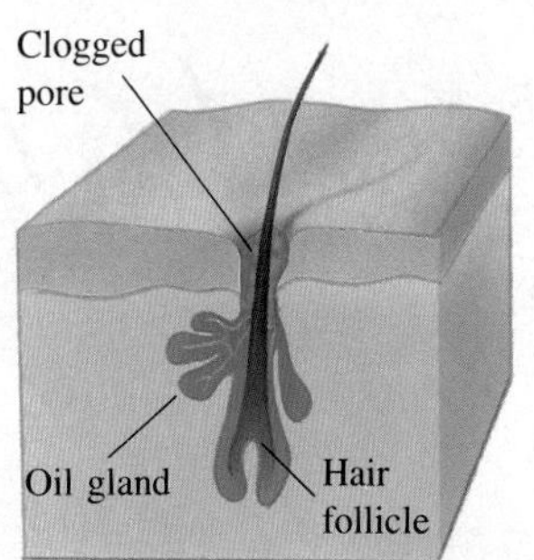

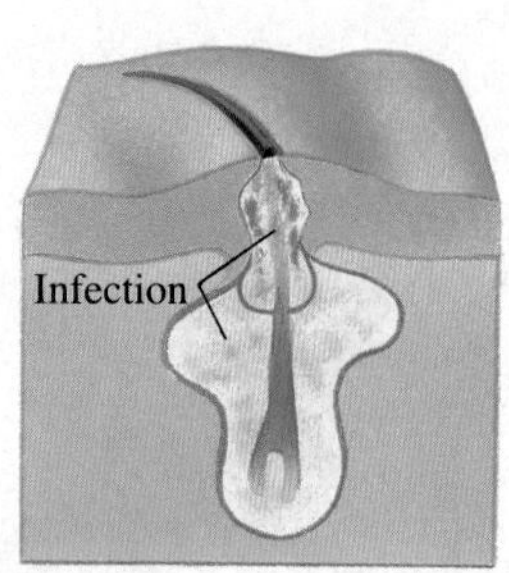

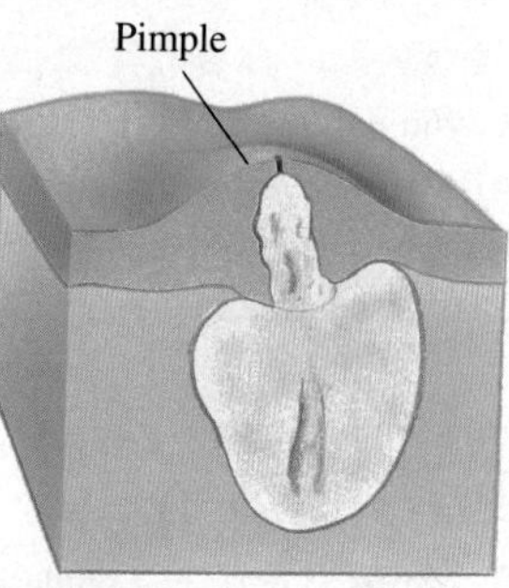

(FIGURE 6-3) **A pimple develops when bacteria infect a pore that is already clogged with oil.**

cularly common among teenagers because teenage skin tends to produce a lot of oil.

There are three main forms of acne: blackheads, whiteheads, and pimples. Blackheads occur when a pore becomes clogged with excess oil and dead skin cells. The combination of oil and dead skin cells turns black when exposed to air. Whiteheads result when the clogged pore is not exposed to air, because it is covered by the epidermis. Pimples occur when a clogged pore becomes infected with bacteria.

Acne cannot be totally prevented or cured, but you can reduce your chances of having it if you follow the steps listed in Figure 6-4.

What If You Have Acne?

Wash your face several times a day with a gentle soap to reduce the amount of oil and bacteria on your face.

If you use makeup on your skin, use products that are labeled "water-based." Oily cosmetics can clog the pores.

Do not squeeze or pick at pimples. Squeezing and picking can cause infection and scarring.

If you have mild acne, an over-the-counter medication that contains benzoyl peroxide may help.

If you have severe acne, see a dermatologist — a doctor who specializes in disorders of the skin. He or she may prescribe medications that can improve your skin's condition.

(FIGURE 6-4)

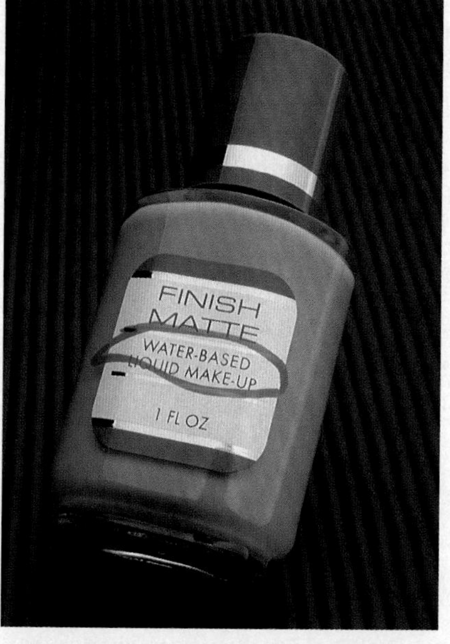

(FIGURE 6-5) **If you have acne, but want to wear makeup on your skin, be sure to buy products that are labeled "water-based." Oil-based products can make acne worse.**

• • • TEACH continued

heredity may be a major factor in whether acne will strike an individual and how severe the case will be. Many doctors believe that cosmetics are the leading cause of acne in adult women. They think oily moisturizers and foundations can clog pores.

Cooperative Learning
Controlling Body Odor

Divide the class into small groups and ask them to provide tips for controlling body odor. These tips may come from their own experience, from other people, or from the media. After the groups have generated their lists, have them create a master list and copy it on the chalkboard. Their tips may include

1. bathing frequently
2. changing clothes daily and laundering them frequently
3. using an underarm deodorant or antiperspirant to control odor
4. wearing fabrics such as cotton that allow moisture to escape
5. using underarm shields to protect clothing from perspiration

Reinforcement
Signs of Skin Cancer

Stress the importance of reporting to physicians any changes in moles, as the changes may be symptoms of malignant melanoma, the most serious type of skin cancer.

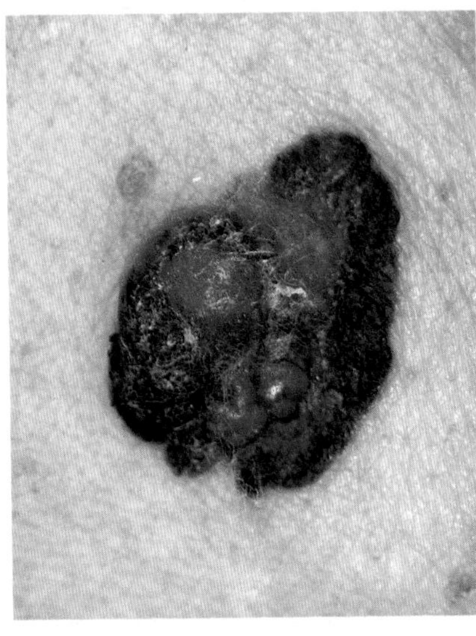

(FIGURE 6-6) **If you notice any changes in a mole, report it immediately to a doctor. A mole can become a malignant melanoma (shown above), a very serious cancer.**

Body Odor When people perspire, the sweat on the surface of the skin is attacked by bacteria. This is what causes body odor to develop. Either deodorants or antiperspirants may be used to control body odor. The difference between them is that deodorants *conceal* body odor, while antiperspirants actually reduce the amount of perspiration. Many products contain both a deodorant and an antiperspirant.

Foot Odor Foot odor can become offensive when the feet perspire heavily. To combat foot odor, be sure to wash your feet thoroughly every day. Wearing cotton socks and open-weave shoes will help reduce foot perspiration, and dusting the feet with plain talc will help absorb moisture. It is also a good idea to alternate pairs of shoes so they can dry out between wearings.

Moles A mole is a small round dark area on the skin. Most moles are not harmful; in fact, they are sometimes called "beauty marks." But just to be safe, report any changes in the size, color, or condition of the mole to a doctor, because these changes may indicate skin cancer.

Warts A wart is a small growth caused by a virus. Although there is no cure for warts, they are usually harmless. Often several warts will appear in the same area. The best treatment for warts is to have them removed by a doctor. If you use an over-the-counter product for wart removal, be very careful. Wart-removal products contain acid that may harm the surrounding skin if they are not applied carefully.

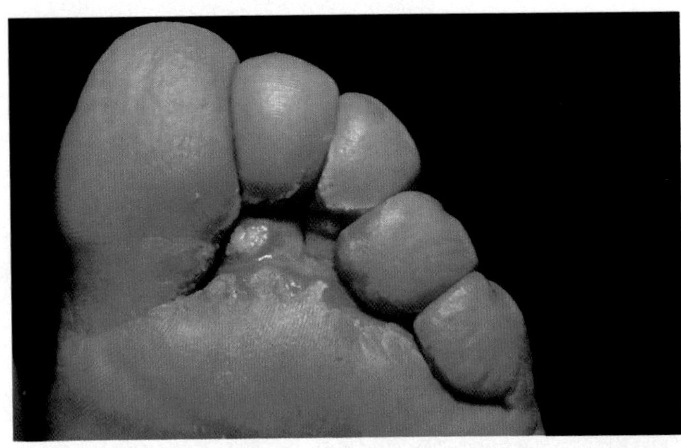

(FIGURE 6-7) **Athlete's foot is caused by a fungus. The symptoms are redness and itching.**

Athlete's Foot and Jock Itch Athlete's foot and jock itch are both caused by microscopic fungi. Athlete's foot does occur on the foot, but a person doesn't have to be an athlete to get it. Jock itch occurs around the genitals. Symptoms of both conditions are redness and itching. The best way to prevent these fungal infections is to keep the skin in these areas as dry as possible. Since athlete's foot and jock itch are difficult to cure with over-the-counter medications, you may want to visit a doctor for treatment.

Background
Moles

At birth, most moles are present under the skin. When exposed to sunlight, they grow larger, become darker, and raise up above the normal surrounding skin. Moles are also found in areas covered by clothing but they are usually not as dark. Most moles are harmless, but changes in a mole should be reported to a physician, especially if it spreads, changes color, develops a black edge, bleeds, or becomes itchy. These may be symptoms of malignant melanoma, the most serious type of skin cancer. A new mole that develops after adolescence may be a symptom of malignant melanoma, too.

Background
Warts

Warts are caused by viral infections of the epidermis. The virus invades skin cells and makes them reproduce rapidly. They can spread to other body parts if they are picked, scratched, or touched, because viral infections are contagious. A wart usually disappears in a few months to 1 or 2 years.

Reinforcement
Warts

Point out that warts are contagious—they can be spread from one part of the body to another, or from one person to another. Warts that grow in the mucous membranes of the penis or vagina are much like other warts but are considered to be a venereal disease (even if they were spread from a person's own fingers) because they can be spread by sexual contact. They should be treated by a physician.

Journal 6C
Skin Diseases

Ask students to record in the Student Journal how they feel when they see people with impetigo, psoriasis, or other skin ailments. Ask them to write how they would feel if they contracted one of these conditions.

Reinforcement
Poison Ivy Exposure

The following are some additional suggestions for dealing with exposure to poison ivy:

1. Change clothes as soon as possible.
2. After washing the exposed area with soap and water, apply rubbing alcohol.
3. Wash your clothes.
4. If your dog rubs against poison ivy, avoid skin contact with his fur and wash him using rubber gloves.

Class Discussion
Sunburn and Time of Day

Does time of day have an impact on sunburn when sunbathing? *[The sun*

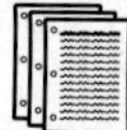

Section Review Worksheet 6.1

Assign Section Review Worksheet 6.1, which requires students to complete a concept map showing the structure of skin and disorders of the skin.

Section Quiz 6.1

Have students take Section Quiz 6.1.

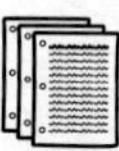

Reteaching Worksheet 6.1

Students who have difficulty with the material may complete Reteaching Worksheet 6.1, which requires them to recognize causes and treatments for common skin problems.

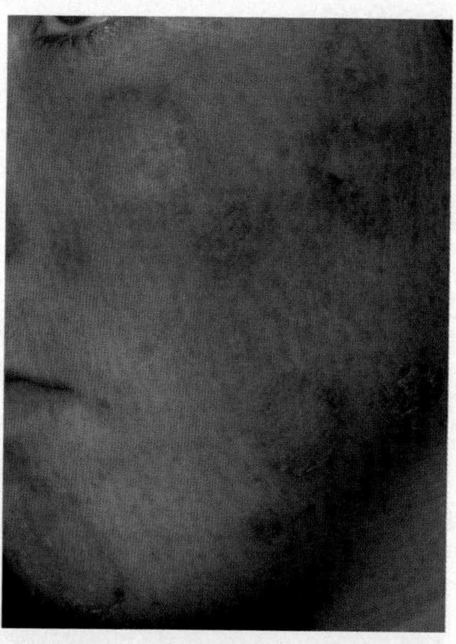

(FIGURE 6-8) **Impetigo is a bacterial infection that causes sores with crusts.**

Impetigo Impetigo is a common infection caused by bacteria, which causes sores with crusts on the skin. It begins in moist areas of the body, in areas where there is friction, and in cuts. Impetigo is most common in children, but may also occur in teenagers and adults. A photograph of impetigo is shown in Figure 6-8. If you think you have impetigo, it is best to seek medical attention.

Poison Ivy, Poison Oak, and Poison Sumac Many people have an allergic reaction to poison ivy, poison oak, or poison sumac. Touching these plants can cause redness, blisters, and severe itching. Each type of plant is shown in Figure 6-9. Memorize how they look so you can be sure to avoid them. Take the following precautions if you touch any of the three plants:

- Immediately wash the skin that came into contact with the plant.

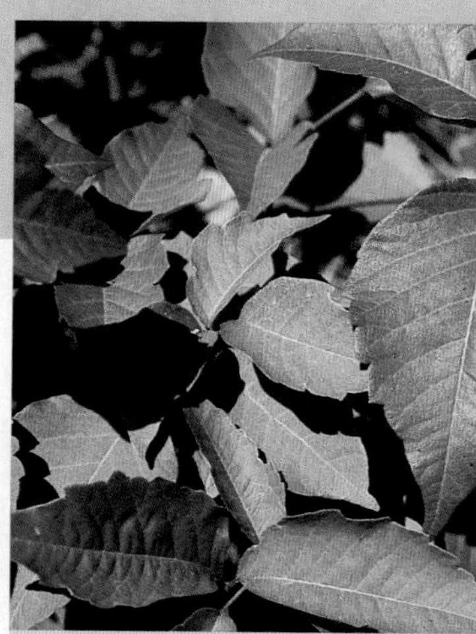

Poison ivy

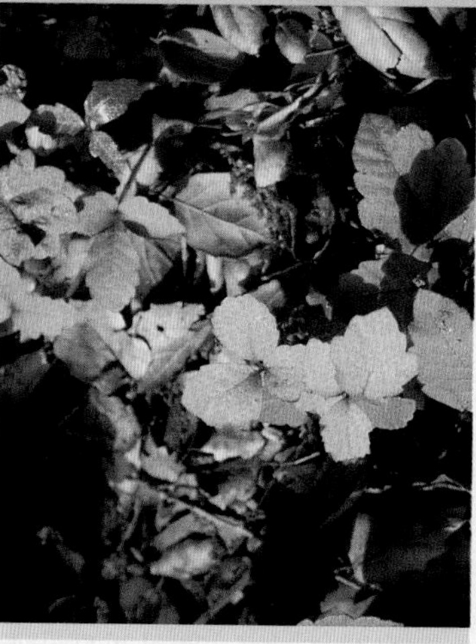

Poison oak

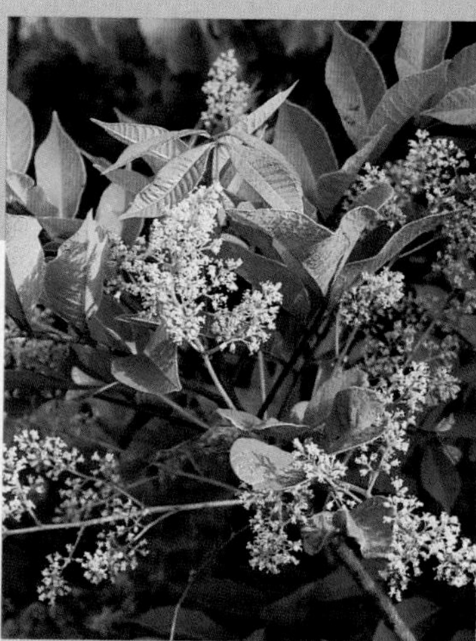

Poison sumac

(FIGURE 6-9) **Touching these plants can cause a painful allergic rash.**

• • • TEACH continued

is strongest at midday because sunlight travels its shortest and most vertical route through the atmosphere.]

Reinforcement
SPF 15

Discuss Figure 6-11 with students and then review methods to reduce the risk of sunburn.

1. Try to avoid the sun between 10 A.M. and 2 P.M. standard time.
2. Spend only 20 to 30 minutes your first time sunbathing in a season. Increase this by 30 minutes a day.
3. Use sunscreen. Read the directions on the sunscreen container carefully.
4. If you have a problem with acne, use an alcohol-based sunscreen.
5. After sunbathing, bathe and then apply a soothing lotion to your skin.
6. Use sunscreen on your face when skiing, as ultraviolet rays reflected from snow can cause sunburn.

Extension
Accutane

Ask students to find out more about Accutane, a controversial drug that some doctors prescribe for the worst cases of acne, which cannot be helped by other treatments.

- If you have a mild allergic reaction, obtain a cream for it from a pharmacy.
- If you have a severe allergic reaction, see a doctor immediately.

Psoriasis Psoriasis is a condition in which red, raised patches appear on the skin. Later the skin becomes dry and flakes off. Areas most commonly affected are the elbows, knees, and scalp. See a doctor for treatment if you have this condition.

Skin and the Sun

Lots of people want to get a suntan because they think it will make them look more attractive. But the sun can be very dangerous, causing damage to your skin now and in the future. Some of the dangers of exposure to the sun include sunburn, wrinkles, and skin cancer.

Sunburn The sun has particular light rays—called ultraviolet rays—that cause sunburn. Ultraviolet rays are strongest around midday. David and Elena were at the beach during this period, so they were exposed to the sun while its rays were at their most intense.

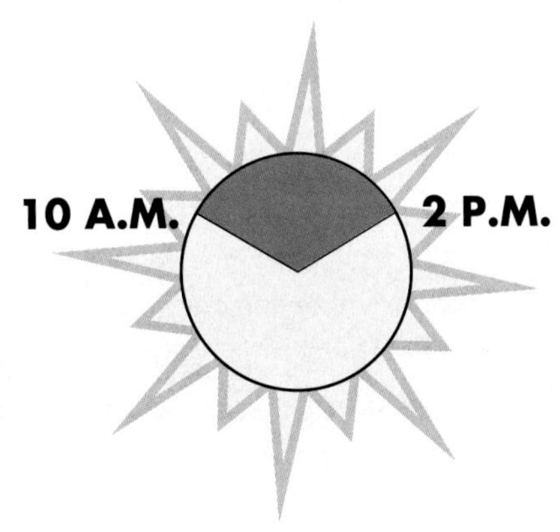

(FIGURE 6-10) **Ultraviolet rays are at their most intense around midday. This is when you are most likely to get sunburned.**

It usually takes about four to six hours before you can feel the full effects of a sunburn. So even if you feel fine while you are out in the sun, remember that a sunburn won't show up until hours later.

People often have confused ideas about sunburn. Some people think you can get sunburned only on clear days. They don't realize that ultraviolet rays are also present on foggy and cloudy days. In addition, many people think that sunburning is limited to people with light skin. In fact, African-Americans and others with dark skin can also get sunburned.

Wrinkles The skin of people who spend a lot of time in the sun tends to age faster than others. They get wrinkles earlier, and they get more wrinkles as time goes on.

Skin Cancer People who spend a lot of time in the sun without protection or who had severe sunburns during youth are at a higher risk for getting skin cancer. Most skin cancers are easily treatable, but one type called malignant melanoma is very serious. Malignant melanomas are cancers of the cells that produce melanin. If you notice any change in a mole, you should see a physician immediately to make sure you don't have a melanoma.

More information about skin cancer can be found in Chapter 24.

Skin cancer is also discussed in Chapter 24.

How to Protect Yourself From the Sun Using a **sunscreen** is one of the most important actions you can take to protect your skin from the sun. A sunscreen is a substance that blocks the harmful ultraviolet rays of the sun.

sunscreen: *a substance that blocks the harmful ultraviolet rays of the sun.*

Sunscreens can be purchased at a drugstore or supermarket. You can tell which suntan products have a sunscreen because they have an SPF number on the label. SPF stands for "sun protection factor." The higher the number, the stronger the

SECTION 6.1

Background

Photosensitivity

Certain foods, cosmetics, and medications contain substances that cause photosensitivity in people, making them susceptible to severe sunburn with relatively short exposure to the sun. Common photosynthesizers include celery, figs, parsnips, many blue dyes, iodine, Tetracycline, and some antihistamines. Products that may include photosynthesizers are perfumes, after-shave lotions, detergents, shampoos, and hair conditioners. The dyes in tattoos can cause extreme photosensitivity in skin adjacent to the tattoo.

Review Answers

1. epidermis and dermis
2. See a doctor and describe to him any changes in the size, color, and condition of the mole.
3. It helps reduce the amount of oil and bacteria on the skin's surface.
4. by avoiding being out in the sun during midday, because this is when the sun's rays are the most intense; by applying and reapplying a sunscreen of SPF 15 or higher to all areas exposed to the sun
5. Both are caused by fungi and thrive in warm, moist areas.

(FIGURE 6-11) **Anyone who spends time in the sun should use a sunscreen with an SPF of at least 15. Unprotected sun exposure can lead to sunburn, wrinkling, and skin cancer.**

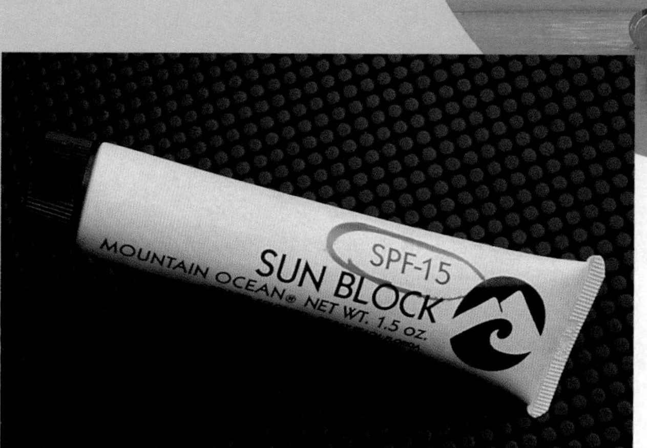

sunscreen. This means that a rating of 2 offers very little protection, while a rating of 15 offers almost complete protection. You should use a sunscreen with an SPF of at least 15. Some sunscreens wash off easily, so when you go swimming you might need to put it on again after going into the water.

If you do get a sunburn, you can relieve the pain by applying wet, cool cloths to your burned skin and taking aspirin or acetaminophen. If the sunburn causes blisters or problems with your vision, you should get medical attention.

Review

1. *Name the two main layers of the skin.*
2. *If you had a mole that changed color, what would you do?*
3. ***LIFE SKILLS: Practicing Self-Care*** *Why does washing the face with soap several times a day reduce a person's chances of getting acne?*
4. ***LIFE SKILLS: Practicing Self-Care*** *Explain how you can avoid sun damage to your skin.*
5. ***Critical Thinking*** *What causes the similarity in symptoms between athlete's foot and jock itch?*

ASSESS

Section Review

Have students answer the Section Review questions.

Alternative Assessment

Maintaining Healthy Skin

Ask students to describe ways to keep their skin healthy.

Closure

Time in the Sun

Ask students what they would think of someone who sunbathes often and maintains a deep tan during the warm months. Would they try to change the person's mind? If this person asked them to join in marathon sunbathing sessions, would they?

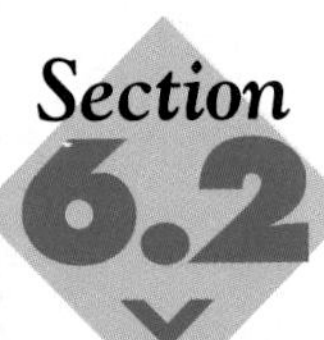

Section 6.2 Hair and Nail Care

Objectives

- *Describe three common hair and scalp problems.*
- *Explain how to care for your hair.*
  LIFE SKILLS: Practicing Self-Care
- *Explain how to care for your nails.*
  LIFE SKILLS: Practicing Self-Care

Hair is important to not only our appearance but also our health. In the winter, we depend on hair to keep our heads warm. Throughout the year, we rely on the hair in our noses and ears to keep dust out of the body. And every time we blink, our eyelashes, which are specialized hair, protect the eyes.

Structure of Hair

The roots of the hair are in the dermis, where the hair starts growing. But hair cells die when they leave the dermis. That's why it doesn't hurt to have your hair cut—the hair is already dead.

Hair on the head grows for two to six years, then rests for several months. Lots of hair falls out after the rest period, but this is normal and should not cause any concern. It is typical to lose up to a hundred hairs a day, which isn't very many when you consider that most people have 100,000 to 200,000 hairs on their heads.

The part of the hair that we can see is called the hair shaft. The shape of the hair shaft determines whether hair will be straight, curly, or wavy.

Hair color is inherited. It is determined by the kind and amount of melanin in your hair. The melanin in hair decreases as people get older, causing their hair to turn gray and then white. The age at which hair turns gray is determined by heredity.

Thinning of the hair or baldness is an inherited condition affecting mainly men. It occurs with age, but can also result from illness. When hair loss is a result of illness, it is usually only a temporary loss.

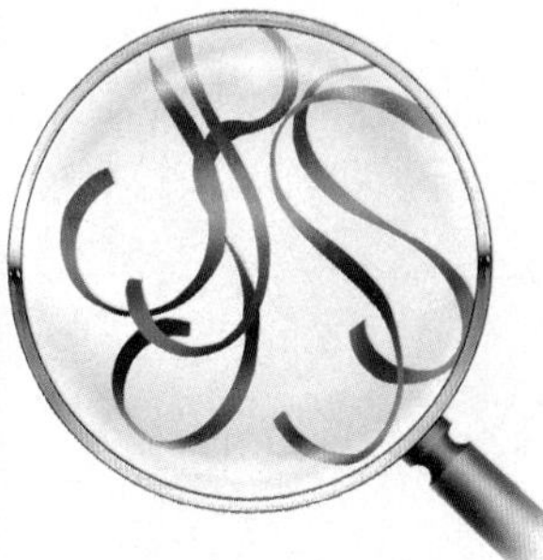

Flat hair shafts = curly hair

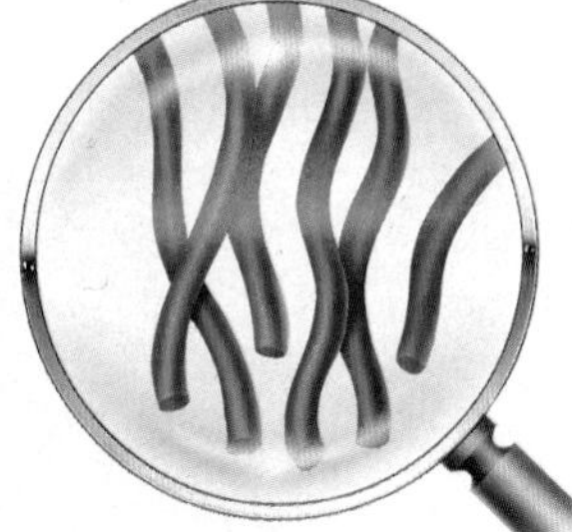

Oval hair shafts = wavy hair

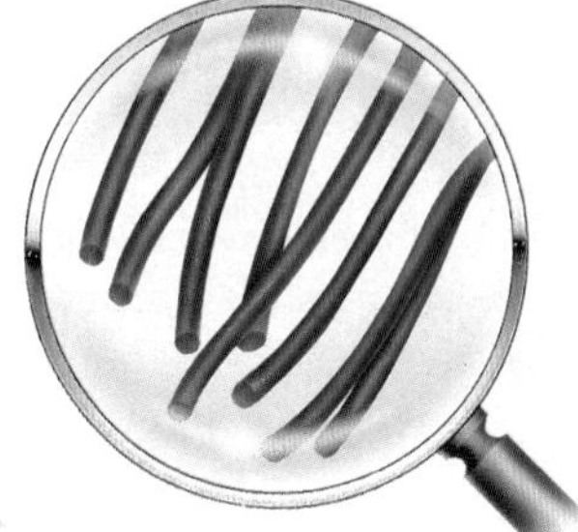

Round hair shafts = straight hair

(FIGURE 6-12) **The shape of the hair shaft determines whether hair will be curly, wavy, or straight.**

Background

Head Lice

Head lice are tiny wingless insects that do not jump or fly. They live on the scalp and can usually be found behind the ears and at the back of the head of an infected person. Using six pairs of hooks in their mouths, they attach themselves to hair shafts. Head lice are difficult to see, but one sign of them is a persistent itching of the scalp. Close inspection of the hair will disclose nits—small silvery eggs attached to individual strands of hair. Personal cleanliness is not a total safeguard against head lice. They are transmitted from one infected person to another through the use of items such as combs, brushes, hats, hair decorations, towels, bedding, coats, even the headrests of airline, bus, and train seats.

Making a Choice 6A

Hair Care

Assign the Hair Care Card. The card requires students to discuss proper hair care for a specific condition.

Section 6.2 Lesson Plan

MOTIVATE

Journal 6D
On Hair

This may be done as a warm-up activity. Encourage students to write in the Student Journal about how they feel about their hair. What do they like best? What do they dislike?

TEACH

Demonstration
Close Look at a Hair

Provide students with microscopes or powerful magnifying glasses. Ask them to pluck a hair from their head and examine it.

Class Discussion
Healthy Hair

Ask students to describe the effects on hair of excessive blow-drying, bleaching, perming, and exposure to sun. **What role does heredity play in relation to hair?** *[It determines color, curliness, thinning or baldness, and the age at which it turns gray.]*

Debate the Issue
Rules About Hair

Tell students that many schools, organizations, and businesses dictate the standards for hair length and style for students and employees. Ask them to

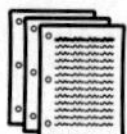

Life Skills Worksheet 6A

Comparing Shampoos

Assign the Comparing Shampoos Life Skills Worksheet, which requires students to compare brands of shampoos and to examine recommendations.

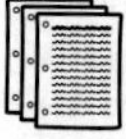

Section Review Worksheet 6.2

Assign Section Review Worksheet 6.2, which requires students to complete sentences and to describe hair care in given situations.

Section Quiz 6.2

Have students take Section Quiz 6.2.

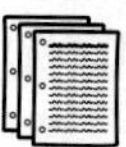

Reteaching Worksheet 6.2

Students who have difficulty with the material may complete Reteaching Worksheet 6.2, which requires them to identify problems of the hair and scalp, their causes, and their prevention and treatment.

Hair Care Tips

Get a good haircut that fits your lifestyle. Swimmers, for example, may want a short cut that doesn't require much styling.

Brush your hair to get the oil to the ends of the hair. Brushing also stimulates the scalp. It is best to brush with a natural bristle brush and to brush gently. If your hair gets tangled, don't yank at it. Instead, untangle it slowly.

Wash your hair regularly. Washing is good for both the hair and the scalp.

Rather than using a blow-dryer, let your hair dry naturally. Repeated use of blow-dryers can dry out hair. Electric curlers can also dry out hair.

Limit the number of perms you get, since they can damage the hair and scalp. Hair dyes and bleaches can also damage your hair.

(FIGURE 6-13)

Hair Care and Appearance

Taking care of your hair will keep it healthy and looking good. Some tips for keeping your hair in good condition are shown in Figure 6-13.

Keep in mind that you don't need to spend lots of money to have clean hair. Tests of a variety of shampoos have shown that inexpensive shampoos work just as well as the more expensive ones.

Hair and Scalp Problems

The most common problems that affect the hair and scalp can be prevented by good grooming practices. It is most important to shampoo regularly and to avoid sharing combs or brushes.

Dandruff Dandruff is dead skin that flakes off the scalp. If you have dandruff, take the following steps:

- Wash your hair regularly; this will usually clear it up.
- Use a dandruff shampoo if regular washing with other shampoos doesn't eliminate the dandruff.
- Make sure your scalp doesn't get too dry from blow-drying your hair too often.

Head Lice Head lice, which are parasites that live in the scalp and hair, are shown in Figure 6-14. You will know if you get head lice because they cause almost unbearable itching. Head lice are often spread by the comb or brush of someone who is infected. If you have head lice, ask your doctor or pharmacist about medications that remove the lice. Thoroughly wash or discard clothing and bedding that has come into contact with your head. Do not share combs, brushes, or clothing with others, because this practice could spread the infection to other people.

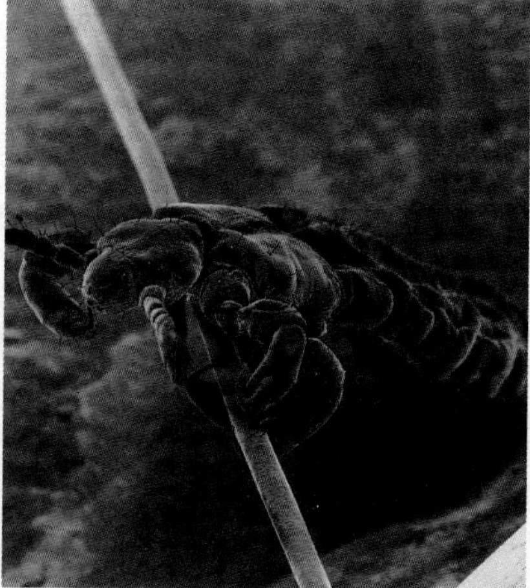

(FIGURE 6-14) **Head lice are easy to control with the right medication.**

• • • TEACH continued

debate whether these standards violate individual freedom of expression.

Reinforcement

Dandruff

Review the causes and remedies of dandruff. Point out that sometimes shampoo left over in the hair forms a scaly, dandruff-like residue. Rinsing shampoo completely out of the hair will eliminate the problem.

Reinforcement

Shaving Tips

The following shaving tips might be helpful for males who have acne:

1. Shave as infrequently as possible.
2. Use an electric razor. If you prefer to use a blade razor, use a new blade each time. Wash your face with soap and hot water to soften the beard. Lather shaving cream on your beard and leave it there for at least a minute before shaving.
3. When finished, rinse first with hot water, then with cold. An astringent can be used to remove excess oil and tighten the skin.
4. If shaving is intolerable, grow a beard.

Extension

History of Personal Care

Assign students to find out how personal care varied at any of these times in history: during the time of the Roman Empire, during the Middle Ages, during the American colonial period. Have them tell about their findings.

Ringworm Ringworm is caused by a fungus that forms a whitish ring on the skin. It is usually found on the scalp but can also appear on other parts of the body. Ringworm is easily spread to other people by the towels, combs, and brushes of a person who has it. A picture of a ringworm infection is shown in Figure 6-15. If you think you might have ringworm, see a doctor.

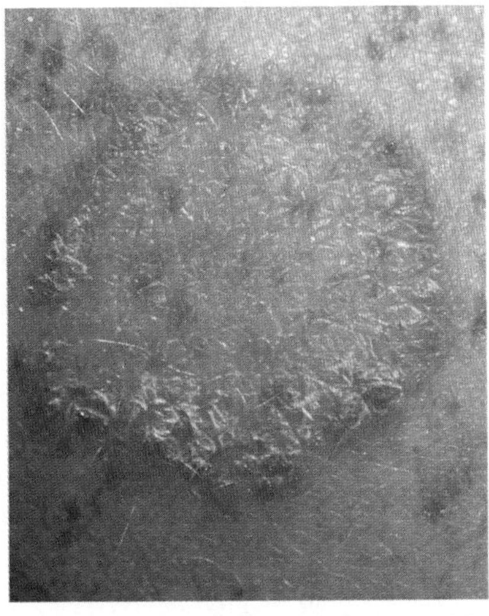

(FIGURE 6-15) **Ringworm is spread by sharing towels, combs, and brushes.**

Removing Unwanted Hair

The most common way to remove unwanted hair is to shave it off with a razor. The skin must first be moistened with water and soap or shaving cream. Otherwise the skin can dry out and is also more vulnerable to cuts and sores. Waxing is another hair-removal method, in which a wax is heated and applied to the skin. When the wax has cooled and hardened, it is stripped off, along with the hair. The effects are longer lasting than those of shaving, but waxing can be a bit painful. The only permanent method of hair removal is electrolysis. During electrolysis, an electrical current is sent into each hair follicle. Like waxing, electrolysis can be painful, and it is also expensive.

Nail Care Tips

Trim fingernails so they are slightly rounded.

Always file nails in one direction.

Push the skin around the nail (the cuticle) back and clip loose pieces with a nail clipper.

Clip toenails straight across. Do not cut them too short.

(FIGURE 6-16)

Nails

Nails that are well cared for can help make a good impression when you meet someone. This is especially true for important events like job interviews. But just as valuable, nice nails can make you feel well groomed, which will add to your self-confidence. Tips for caring for your nails are shown in Figure 6-16.

Review

1. *Describe three common hair and scalp problems.*
2. ***LIFE SKILLS: Practicing Self-Care*** *Explain how to care for your hair.*
3. ***LIFE SKILLS: Practicing Self-Care*** *Explain how to care for your nails.*
4. ***Critical Thinking*** *Can a person live in the same house with someone who has ringworm and not get this condition? Explain your answer.*

Review Answers

1. Dandruff is dead skin that flakes off the scalp. Head lice are parasites that live on the scalp and hair. Ringworm is characterized by whitish rings on the scalp and skin. Ringworm is caused by a fungus.

2. Get a haircut that fits my lifestyle; brush the hair to get oil to the ends of the hair; wash the hair regularly; don't overuse blow dryers and electric curlers; limit the number of times the hair is permed or dyed.

3. Trim fingernails so they are slightly rounded; always file nails in one direction; push the cuticle back and clip loose pieces with a nail clipper; clip toenails straight across.

4. Answers will vary. It is possible, but unlikely. Ringworm is very contagious and can be passed from shared towels, combs, brushes, bed linens, and clothing.

ASSESS

Section Review

Have students answer the Section Review questions.

Alternative Assessment

Hair Analysis

Do we make assumptions about people based on their hair? Collect examples of these assumptions from students and list them on the chalkboard under the headings *beard, mustache, hair color, length,* and *style.* Have students write a paragraph about the accuracy of the assumptions.

Closure

Hair and Scalp Problems

Have students identify common hair and scalp problems and their remedies.

Background
Why Orthodontics Is Needed

Ideally, teeth should be straight and spaced regularly, with no overlap or gaps, and they should be the right size for the jaw. However, few people have perfect teeth. Because traits are inherited from both parents, a person may inherit teeth and jaws that don't match. For example, a person could have large teeth in a small jaw, or small teeth in a large jaw.

Orthodontics is the dental specialty that deals with malocclusions—abnormal relationships between the teeth in the upper jaw and the teeth opposite them in the lower jaw. Uncorrected malocclusions can lead to deformities in the face and jaw.

Section 6.3 Teeth and Gum Care

Objectives

- *Explain how dental cavities develop.*
- *Explain how to care for your teeth and gums.*
  LIFE SKILLS: Practicing Self-Care
- *Be able to make an appointment with a dentist.*
  LIFE SKILLS: Being a Wise Consumer

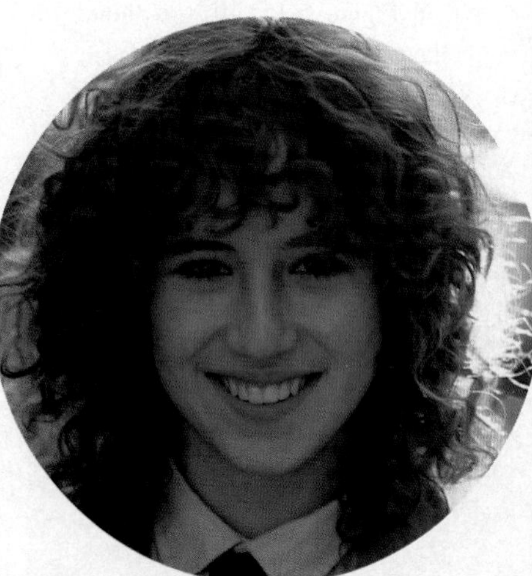

(FIGURE 6-18) **Having healthy teeth makes it easy to smile.**

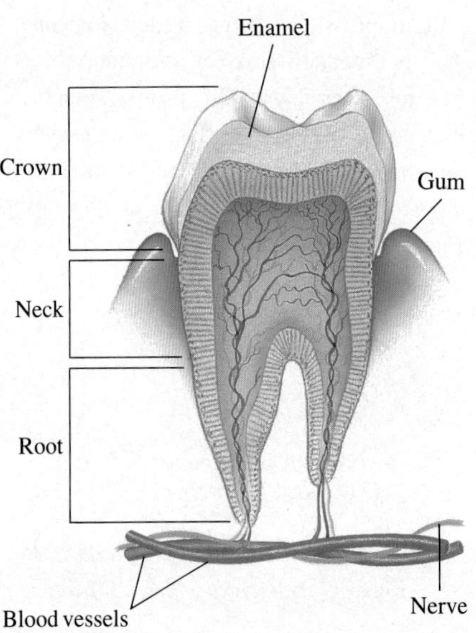

(FIGURE 6-17) **The three main parts of the tooth are the crown, the neck, and the root. The crown is the part that is visible above the gums. Covering the crown is a substance called enamel, the hardest substance in the body.**

Have you ever noticed the teeth of people on TV? They almost always look perfect and shiny white. In truth, most of us don't have perfect teeth. In fact, people on TV often have cosmetic dental work done to make their teeth appear whiter and straighter than normal. All of us, however, can have clean teeth that are well cared for. It is simply a matter of good dental care.

Structure of a Tooth

The tooth is divided into three parts, which are shown in Figure 6-17. The crown is the visible part of the tooth above the gum. The neck is just below the gum line where the crown and root come together. The root is the part of the tooth below the gum line.

Section 6.3 Lesson Plan

MOTIVATE

Journal 6E
Feelings About Teeth

This may be done as a warm-up activity. Ask students to write in the Student Journal how they feel about their smile. Do they like how their teeth look? Are they embarrassed about their teeth? Is there something they would like to change?

TEACH

Reinforcement
Anatomy of a Tooth

Ask a student to draw on the chalkboard the parts of a tooth and label them. Point out that enamel, unlike other body tissues, cannot repair itself once it is damaged or worn down.

Journal 6F
Losing Primary Teeth

Ask students to record in the Student Journal their memories of losing their primary teeth. Do they remember how they felt when their first tooth fell out? Do they remember the feeling of having a loose tooth? Do they remember what it was like to eat with their front teeth missing?

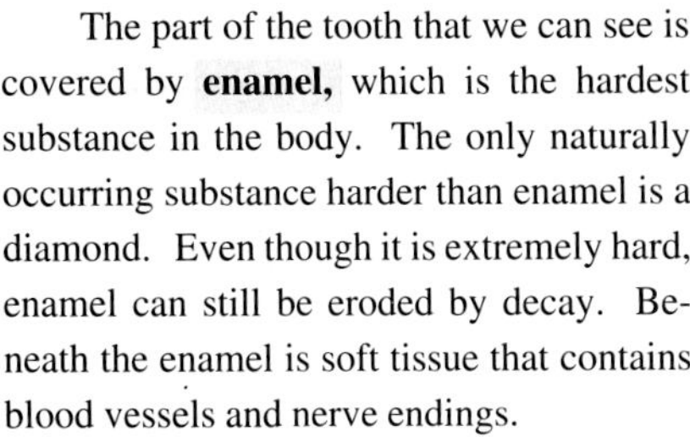

The part of the tooth that we can see is covered by **enamel,** which is the hardest substance in the body. The only naturally occurring substance harder than enamel is a diamond. Even though it is extremely hard, enamel can still be eroded by decay. Beneath the enamel is soft tissue that contains blood vessels and nerve endings.

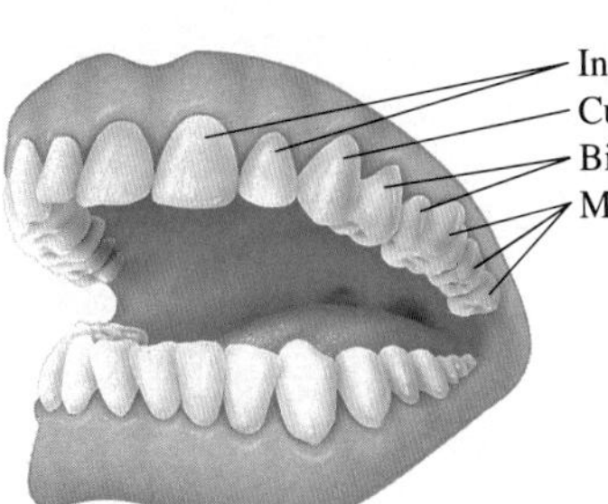

(FIGURE 6-19) **Each of the four types of permanent teeth has a different function in breaking up food before it is swallowed.**

enamel: *the substance covering the crown of the tooth; hardest substance in the body.*

Types of Teeth

People have two sets of teeth during their life. First, they have 20 primary teeth—also called baby teeth—that are usually in by age three. These fall out, and permanent teeth start developing around the age of six. By the time people are grown, they have 32 permanent teeth. The four types of permanent teeth and their functions are shown in Figure 6-19.

Dental Problems

Have you ever had a toothache? Have you ever had to go to the dentist and have a cavity filled? Sometimes these dental problems can be avoided. Taking good care of your teeth can prevent cavities and gum diseases from developing.

Dental Cavity Figure 6-20 shows how a dental cavity develops. A dental cavity results from tooth decay. The decay begins when food is eaten and tiny food particles remain in the mouth. The food particles combine with bacteria and saliva to form

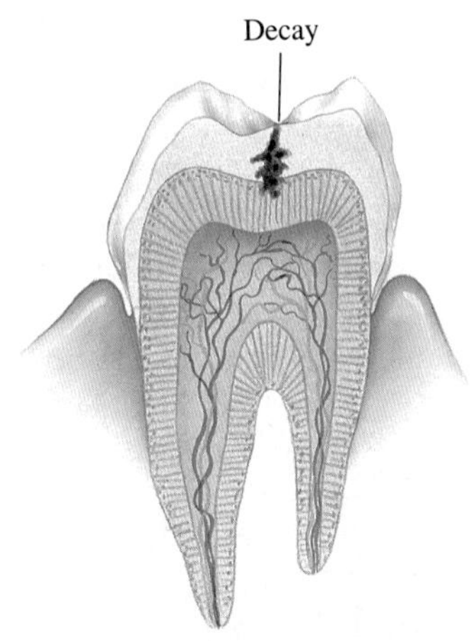

1. Acid eats through the enamel of a tooth.

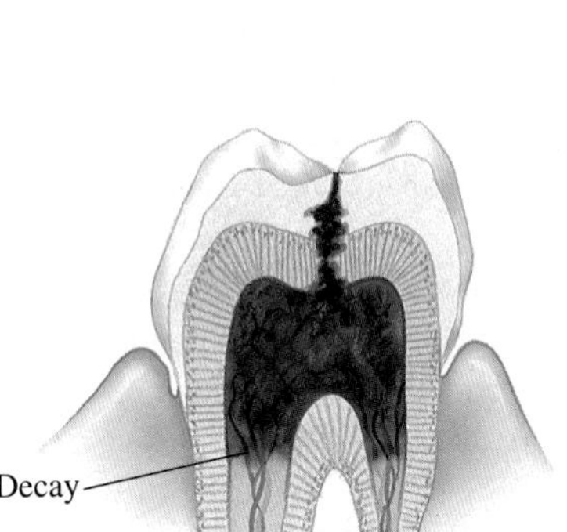

2. Acid reaches the tissue below the enamel and causes infection.

(FIGURE 6-20) **Bacteria produce acids that eat away tooth enamel, eventually causing dental cavities.**

SECTION 6.3

Making a Choice 6B

Personal Care

Assign the Personal Care Card. The card requires students to review personal hygiene in game or discussion activities.

Life Skills Worksheet 6B

Resisting Peer Pressure

Assign the Resisting Peer Pressure Life Skills Worksheet, which requires students to examine strategies for resisting peer pressure in a variety of given situations.

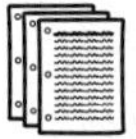

Life Skills Worksheet 6C

Toothbrush Choices

Assign the Toothbrush Choices Life Skills Worksheet, which requires students to investigate claims and evaluations for types of toothbrushes and additives to toothpaste and mouthwashes.

Reinforcement

Sequence of Cavity Formation

Copy the sequence below for cavity formation and ask students to put the steps in the proper order.

Acid attacks tooth enamel. (5)

Infection spreads to bone socket and tooth becomes abscessed. (8)

When saliva and food particles combine, plaque forms and coats the teeth. (3)

Tiny food particles remain between the teeth. (2)

Bacteria in plaque produce acid. (4)

Food is eaten. (1)

Acid eats through enamel and reaches tissue beneath it. (6)

Tissue becomes infected, forming a cavity. (7)

Class Discussion

Braces

Students who are now wearing braces or who have had braces may wish to share their experiences with the class. They may want to bring a "before" photograph to class.

Demonstration

Brushing and Flossing

Ask a dentist or dental hygienist to bring dental models to class and demonstrate proper brushing and flossing techniques. If this is not feasible, perhaps your school nurse could demonstrate these techniques.

Background
Gum Disease

Gum disease is the major cause of tooth loss for adults over 40, but it can occur in children, too. Gum disease is caused by the buildup of plaque and calculus on the teeth. It can result in severe inflammation. The first stage of gum disease, called gingivitis, is typified by bleeding gums. If left untreated, gum disease can cause the destruction of the supporting tissues around the teeth. Pyorrhea or periodontitis is advanced gum disease. The gums begin to separate from the teeth and the space between them fills up with tartar, bacteria, and plaque. The teeth loosen and can fall out. Eventually, gum disease attacks and destroys the bone in which the teeth are anchored. Fortunately, gum disease will not cause permanent damage if treated early.

calculus: *hardened plaque.*

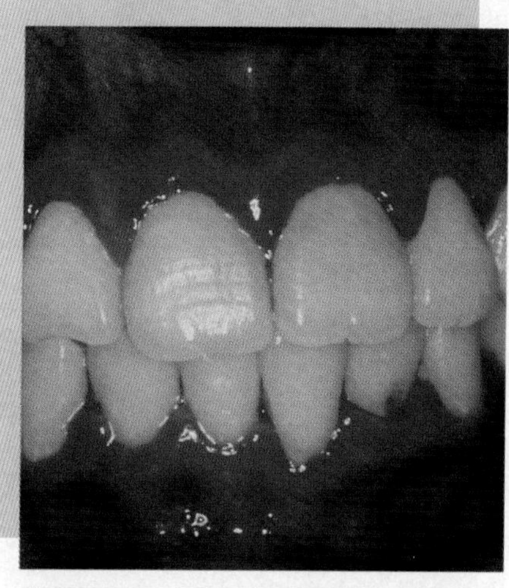

(FIGURE 6-21) **Gum disease is often caused by a buildup of calculus (tartar) on the teeth. If not treated by a dentist, gum disease can cause teeth to fall out.**

plaque: *a film of food particles, saliva, and bacteria on teeth.*

plaque, which coats the teeth with a very thin film. The bacteria in plaque produce an acid that eats through the enamel of teeth. If the teeth are not cleaned properly, more plaque is formed and more enamel gets eaten away. Finally, the acid reaches the tissue beneath the enamel of a tooth and infects it. The tooth now has a cavity. Cavities that are very small are not always easy to detect without an x-ray, because they are not painful. If the cavity isn't taken care of at this point, however, the infection spreads down to the bone socket and the tooth becomes abscessed.

If you have a dental cavity, see a dentist immediately. Your tooth will only get worse until it is treated. You'll find out later in this section how to prevent cavities.

Bad Breath Most bad breath is the result of plaque, decayed teeth, and gum and throat infections. Mouthwashes may provide fresh breath for a little while, but it will not be lasting. In addition, mouthwashes usually contain alcohol, which can worsen a throat or tooth infection. Sometimes bad breath results from eating strong-smelling foods—garlic, for example. A coated tongue may also cause bad breath. Most dentists recommend cleaning the tongue by brushing it with a toothbrush.

Gum Disease Gum disease is the leading cause of tooth loss in adults. It begins when a material called **calculus** builds up near the gums. Calculus, which is also known as tartar, is simply plaque that has become hardened. Calculus must be removed at a dentist's office.

The first sign of gum disease is bleeding when the teeth are brushed. Later, the gums pull back from the teeth and form pockets that may fill with pus. The teeth may then loosen and fall out. Although more common in adults, gum disease can also occur during the teenage years. If treated early, it usually will not cause permanent damage or tooth loss. See a dentist if you think you might have gum disease.

Poor Alignment Usually the top teeth fit exactly over the bottom teeth. When they don't fit correctly, there is an alignment problem. Poor alignment may make it difficult to eat or speak or clean the teeth adequately. People whose teeth don't align properly are born that way; it is not caused by anything they do. If your teeth are poorly aligned, you may need braces to correct the alignment. If the problem is serious, surgery may be required.

Dental Care

Good dental care involves more than just brushing your teeth. The behaviors that are most important to good dental care are: eating nutritious foods, brushing teeth, flossing teeth, and having regular dental checkups.

• • • TEACH continued

Reinforcement
Dental Care

Share the following suggestions for good dental care with students.

1. If you must have sweets, eat them during meals. Finishing a meal with cheese is a good idea, as cheese is effective in neutralizing acid formation.
2. Use disclosing tablets. They contain a dye that stains plaque and makes it visible. Brushing and flossing removes the plaque and the stain.
3. Use floss to remove plaque, never toothpicks. Toothpicks can damage your gums.
4. Use a toothpaste with fluoride. Fluoride hardens the surface of the tooth and makes it more bacteria-resistant.
5. Cigarette smoking stains teeth and fouls breath.

Journal 6G
My Own Dental Care

Ask students to record in the Student Journal how frequently they go for dental checkups. If they have had their teeth cleaned by a dentist or dental hygienist, have them describe it.

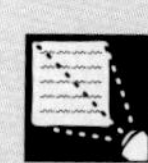

Teaching Transparency 6B
Personal Care and Appearance

Use this transparency to review the problems, precautions, and treatments

Eating Nutritious Foods A balanced diet will help you have healthy gums. And not eating lots of sugary foods will cut down on cavities and gum disease.

Brushing Teeth When you learned to brush your teeth as a child, you might have been instructed to scrub them as completely as possible. But dentists have since discovered that scrubbing the teeth may tear the gums and remove enamel from the teeth. A new, safer way to brush your teeth is shown in Figure 6-22. You should brush your teeth at least twice a day, immediately after you eat if possible.

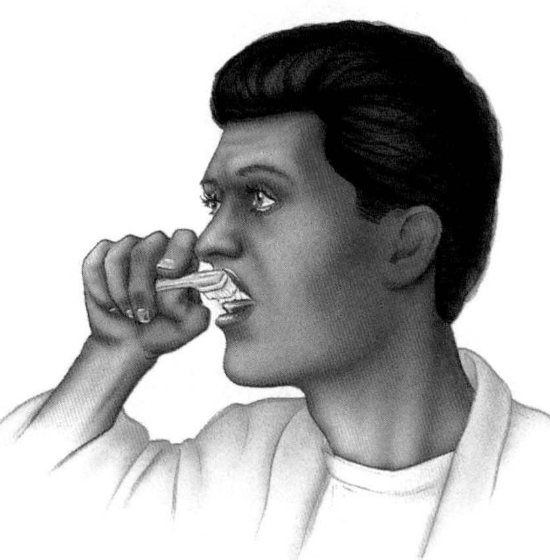

1. Hold the toothbrush at a 45-degree angle to the gums.

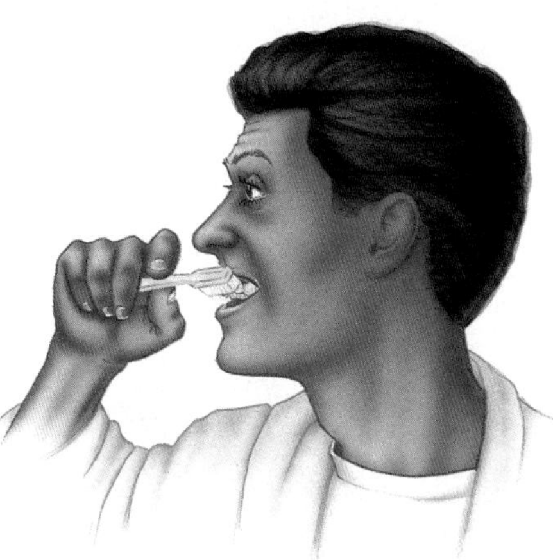

2. Move the brush gently in a circular motion on two teeth at a time. Don't brush hard! Gentle brushing will remove plaque without hurting your teeth.

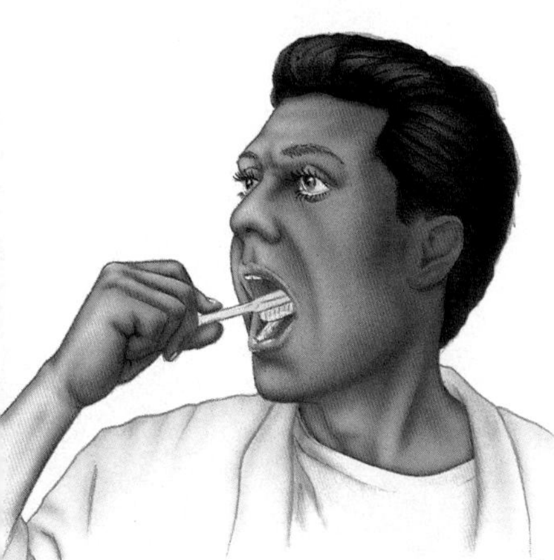

3. Brush all the surfaces of your teeth, including the backs of teeth.

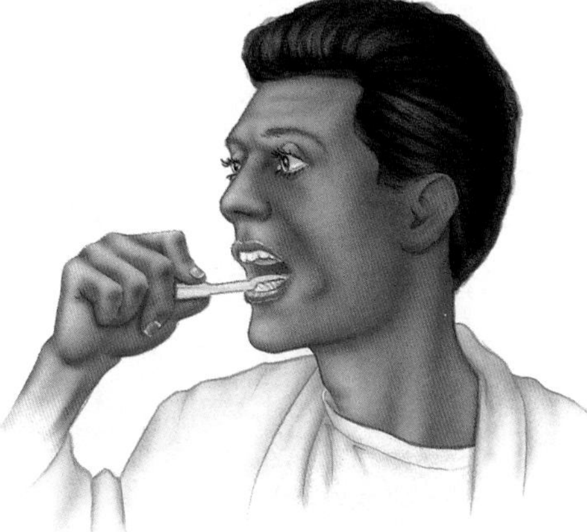

4. Continue until you have brushed all your teeth.

(FIGURE 6-22) **Brush your teeth at least twice a day, immediately after you eat if possible. Use a soft, flat brush that can reach all your teeth.**

relating to personal care and appearance described in the text.

Extension

Topics of Interest

Have individual students find information on one of the following topics and present brief reports on them to the class: use of the laser beam in dentistry, danger of mercury-type fillings, dentistry in the barbershop, and the technique of dental implants.

dental floss:

a special string that removes plaque from the teeth.

Flossing Teeth **Dental floss** is a special string sold at most supermarkets and drugstores. Flossing once a day will remove most plaque. Flossing is shown in Figure 6-23.

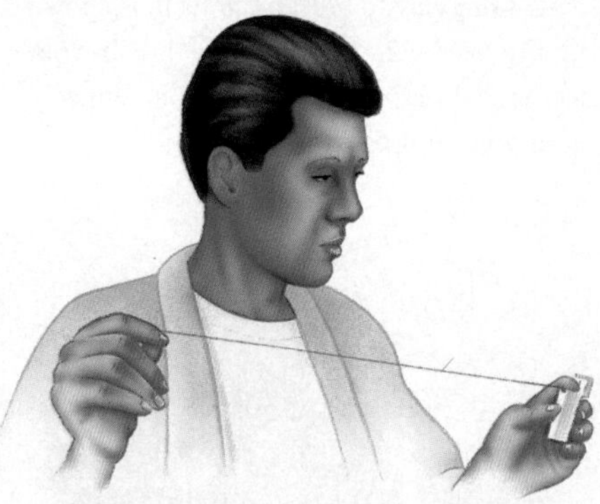

1. Cut off a piece of dental floss about 18 inches long.

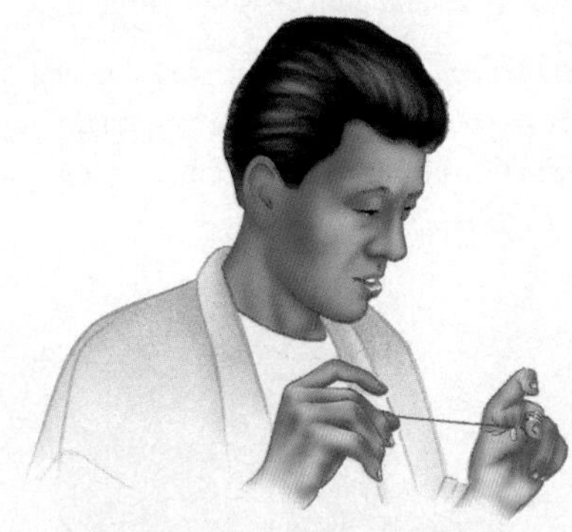

2. Wrap the ends of the floss around your middle fingers.

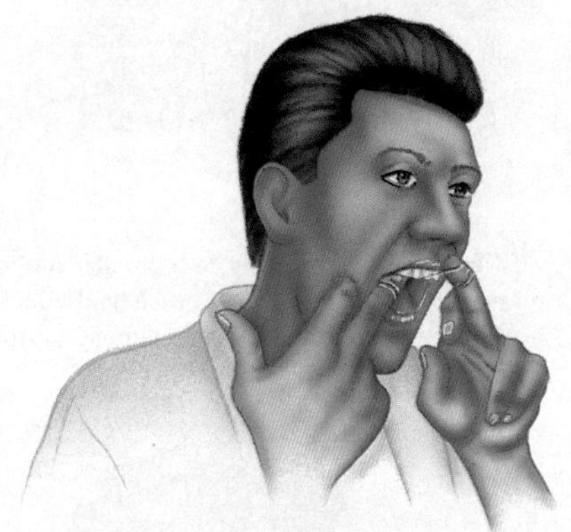

3. Very gently push the floss between two teeth.

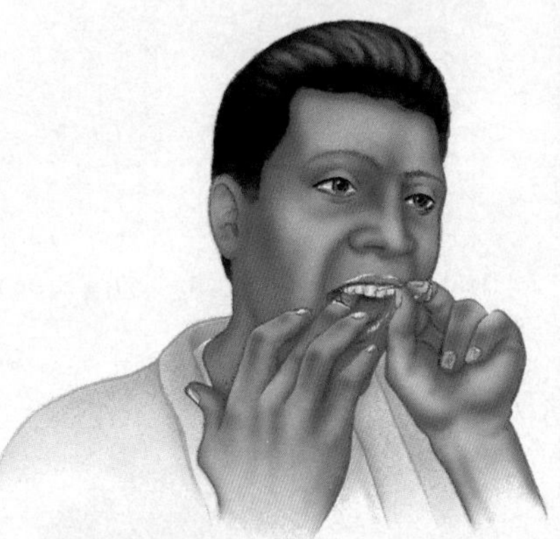

4. Pull the floss around one of the teeth to make a horseshoe shape with the floss. Gently move the floss up and down to clean the sides of that tooth.

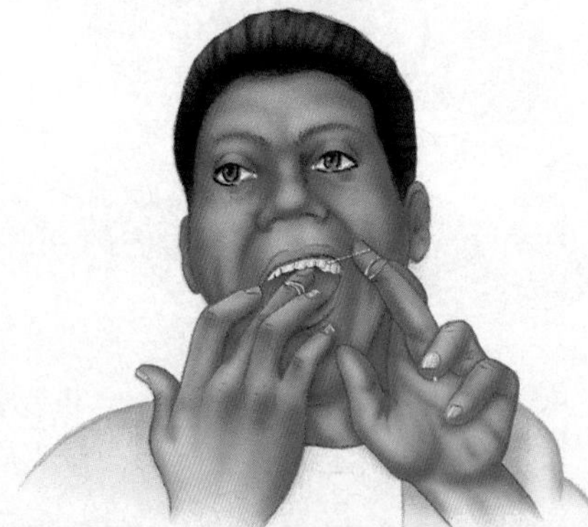

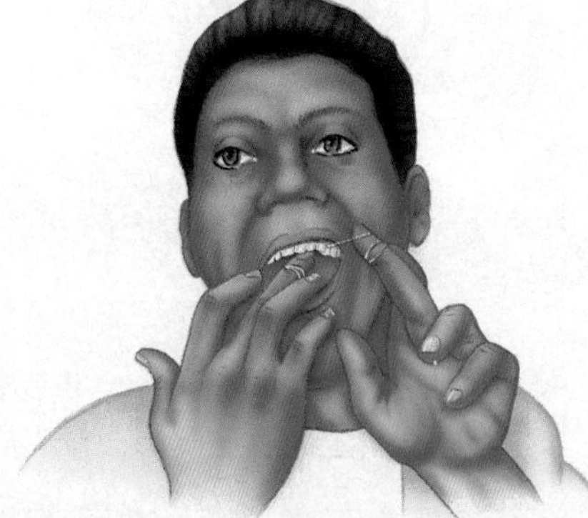

5. Continue until you have flossed all your teeth. Use a clean section of floss on each tooth.

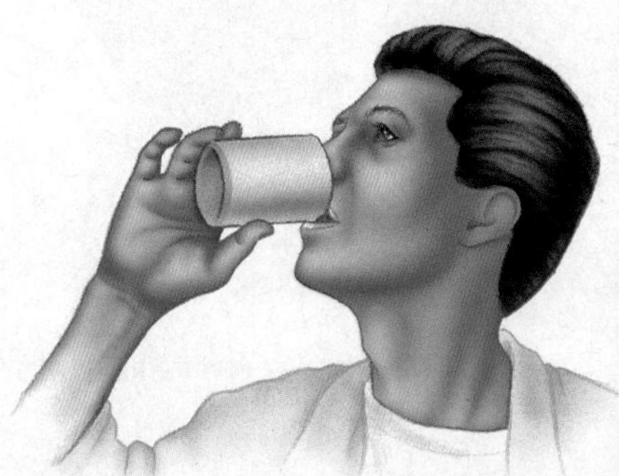

6. Rinse your mouth with water.

(FIGURE 6-23)
Flossing removes the plaque between the teeth. You should floss your teeth every day.

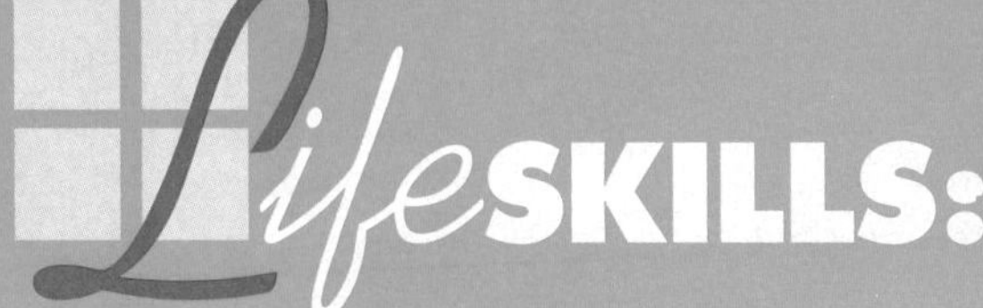

Being a Wise Consumer

Making a Dental Appointment

Making a dental appointment is something most teenagers haven't had any practice doing. It's actually quite easy to compare dentists and choose the one who suits your needs. You may already have a dentist or know of one you want to see. If not, follow these steps to choose a dentist and make an appointment.

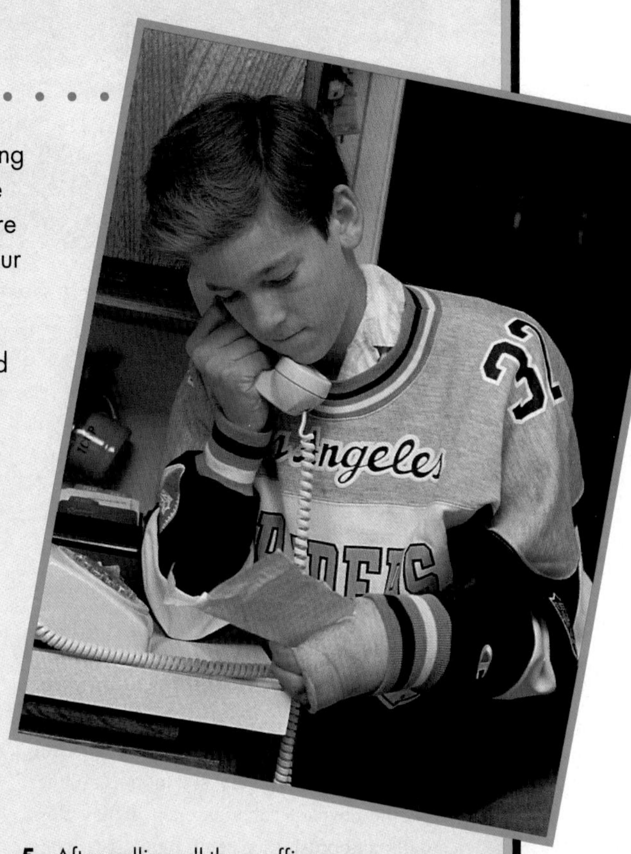

1. Look in the yellow pages of the phone book under "Dentists" and find three dentists who are close to where you live or go to school.
2. Write down their phone numbers and call them.
3. Tell the receptionist who answers that you are just trying to get some information right now—you're not making an appointment. Ask how much an initial visit would cost to examine your teeth and clean them. This price will probably include X-rays of your teeth.
4. Ask when the office would be able to see you. Some dentists have a long waiting period, while others can see people quickly.
5. After calling all three offices, compare the costs of the dentists. Also compare the length of time you would need to wait before seeing each dentist.
6. Now you're ready to make an appointment with the dentist that you have chosen.

Life SKILLS

Making a Dental Appointment

Have students do the Life Skills activity in the text, writing notes on paper as they complete the steps.

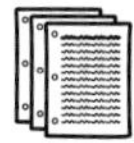

Section Review Worksheet 6.3

Assign Section Review Worksheet Section 6.3. It requires students to classify causes of gum and dental disease and to answer questions about them.

Section Quiz 6.3

Have students take Section Quiz 6.3.

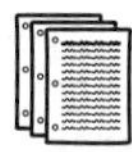

Reteaching Worksheet 6.3

Students who have difficulty with the material may complete Reteaching Worksheet 6.3, which requires them to label the parts of the tooth and identify the steps necessary to prevent or correct dental disease.

Review Answers

1. Bacteria in plaque produce an acid. This acid eats through the enamel of teeth. When the enamel gets eaten away and the tissue below the enamel becomes exposed, a cavity has formed.

2. Brush twice daily, floss once a day, eat nutritious foods, and see a dentist for regular checkups.

3. Students should state the description given in Figure 6-23.

4. In the Yellow Pages, find the names of three dentists near where you live. Write down their names and phone numbers. Call their office to find out their fees and how soon the dentist could see you. Compare the information gathered and then choose a dentist. Call that dentist back to make an appointment.

5. Answers will vary. Students might answer that enamel protects the living tissue of the tooth. Enamel is hard so that it does not wear away over the years as people use their teeth to chew food.

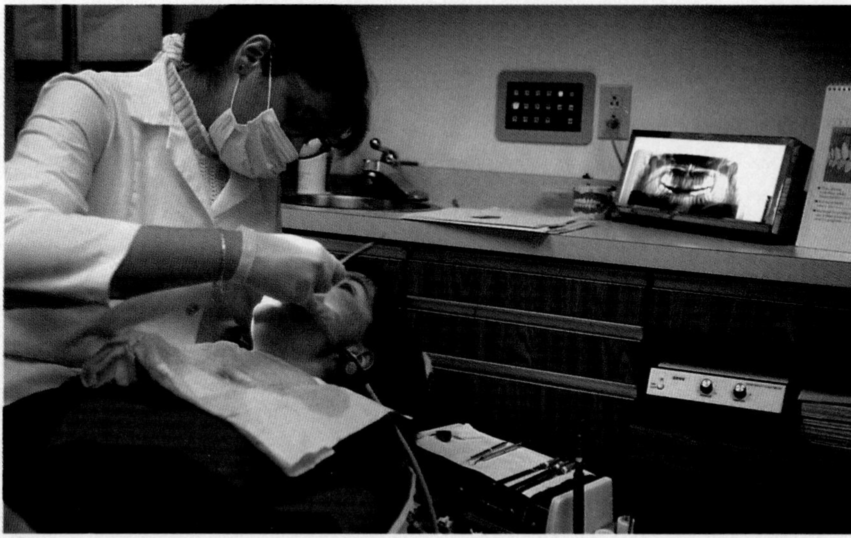

(FIGURE 6-24) **Dentists usually wear a mask and gloves to protect themselves and their patients from infection.**

Dental Checkups How often do you think a person should see a dentist for a checkup?

- Every three months?
- Every six months?
- Every year?
- Every two years?

The answer depends on the person. Some people don't develop cavities or gum disease easily and may not need a checkup more often than every six months. Other people develop calculus even if they floss daily and brush their teeth regularly. They may need to have their teeth cleaned every three months. Most people do not need checkups more often than every six months.

Dentists and dental hygienists clean teeth with tools that look a little like pencils with scrapers on the end. They use these to scrape the calculus off the teeth and polish them. Most people experience very little discomfort with this process and are pleased with the result—nice, clean, polished teeth. When teeth are flossed and brushed regularly, they usually stay nice-looking during the period between cleanings.

Review

1. *Explain how dental cavities develop.*
2. *What are four things you can do to have healthy teeth?*
3. ***LIFE SKILLS: Practicing Self-Care*** *Describe how to floss the teeth.*
4. ***LIFE SKILLS: Being a Wise Consumer*** *Describe one method of choosing a dentist.*
5. ***Critical Thinking*** *What purpose do you think the enamel of teeth serves?*

ASSESS

Section Review

Have students answer the Section Review questions.

Alternative Assessment

Healthy Teeth and Gums

Ask students to write a paragraph describing how to keep their teeth and gums healthy.

Closure

Overcoming Fear in the Dentist's Chair

Discuss the fears many people have of dentists. Ask students to suggest ways that people could get over their fears.

Chapter 6 Highlights

Summary

- The skin functions to protect the body from germs, to regulate body temperature, to transmit sensations such as pain, and as a waterproof cover that holds the body together.
- The epidermis and the dermis are the two main layers of the skin. The dermis contains oil and sweat glands as well as nerves.
- Acne, a common skin problem for teens, results when pores in the skin become clogged with oil. It usually can be controlled by washing frequently with soap and water.
- Other skin problems include moles, warts, athlete's foot and jock itch, impetigo, poison ivy, poison oak, poison sumac, and psoriasis.
- Changes in the size, color, or condition of a mole should be reported to a doctor because the changes may indicate skin cancer.
- Exposure to the sun can cause sunburn, wrinkles, and skin cancer. Use of a sunscreen is the most important action you can take to protect your skin from the sun.
- Hair insulates the head from heat and cold. Eyelashes and eyebrows protect the eyes from foreign matter. Hair in the nose and ears keeps foreign matter out of the nose and ears.
- A tooth is made up of a crown, a neck, and a root. The part of the tooth we see is covered by enamel.
- The bacteria in plaque produce acid, which eats through the enamel of teeth and causes decay.
- Good dental care includes brushing and flossing teeth, eating nutritious foods, and having regular checkups.

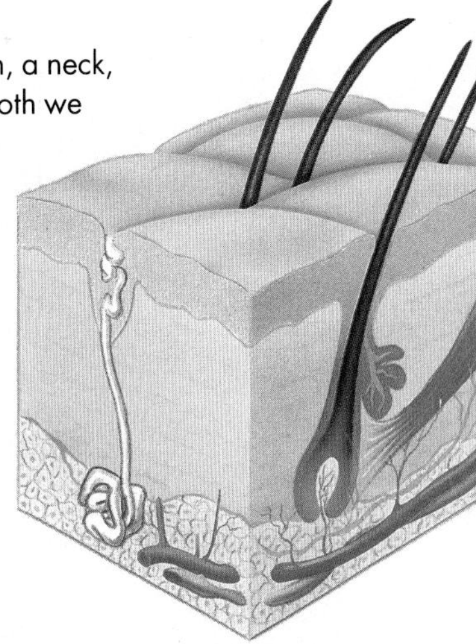

Vocabulary

epidermis the very thin outer layer of the skin.

dermis the second layer of skin; contains the most important skin structures.

acne a condition in which the pores of the skin become clogged with oil; acne can take the form of blackheads, whiteheads, or pimples.

enamel the substance covering the crown of the tooth; hardest substance in the body.

plaque a film of food particles, saliva, and bacteria on teeth.

dental floss a special string that removes plaque from the teeth.

Chapter 6 Highlights Strategies

Summary

Have students read the summary to reinforce the concepts they have learned in Chapter 6.

Vocabulary

Ask students to use each of the vocabulary words in a sentence having to do with personal care.

Extension

Have students investigate what problems homeless people face in keeping clean and caring for their teeth and gums. What provisions do homeless shelters make for them? Are there sources of supply in your community for toothpaste, soap, shampoo, and so on? Are there ways students could help collect or distribute supplies? In some schools, students collect free samples—which travelers bring home from hotels and resorts—for this purpose.

CHAPTER 6 ASSESSMENT

CHAPTER REVIEW

Concept Review

1. To protect the body from germs, to regulate body temperature, to transmit sensations such as pain, and to act as a waterproof cover to hold the body together

2. The epidermis is made up of cells and contains pores. It also contains melanin. The dermis contains hair and oil and sweat glands, as well as nerves.

3. Fungus—athlete's foot, jock itch; bacteria—impetigo; virus—wart

4. When there is a change in size, color, or condition because these changes could indicate skin cancer

5. To protect the skin from ultraviolet rays which can cause sunburn, skin cancer, and wrinkles. The higher the SPF number, the more protection the sunscreen provides in blocking ultraviolet rays.

6. Hair insulates the head from heat and cold. Eyelashes and eyebrows protect the eyes from foreign matter. Hair in the nose and ears keeps foreign matter out of the body.

7. Dandruff appears because the scalp gets too dry. You can control dandruff by washing your hair regularly, using a dandruff shampoo, and making sure your scalp doesn't get too dry.

8. Head lice are parasites. To get rid of head lice, ask your doctor or pharmacist to recommend a medication to remove them. You should also wash or discard clothing and bedding that have come in contact with your head. You should also not share combs, brushes, or clothing with others.

9. Well-cared-for nails make a good impression and add to your self-confidence.

10. Crown, neck, root; crown and neck

11. Plaque is a film of bacteria on teeth. By removing plaque you are removing the bacteria that produce the destructive acid which causes tooth decay.

12. Plaque, decayed teeth, and gum and throat infections

13. Adults. Gum disease is caused by a buildup of hardened plaque, or calculus. Gum disease can be controlled through regular brushing, flossing, and cleaning at the dentist's office.

Expressing Your Views

Sample responses:

1. It can cause infection and scarring. I would tell Julie to wash her face several

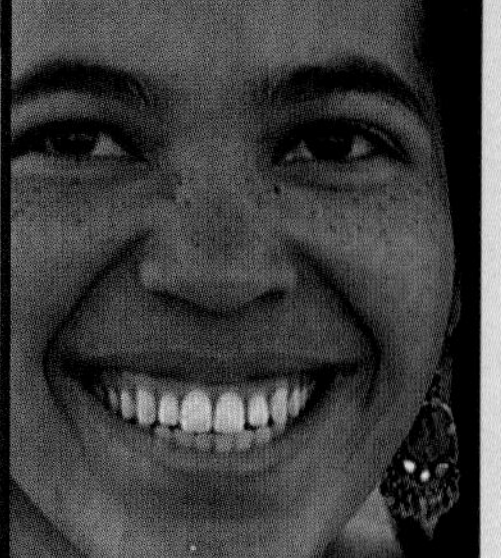

Chapter Review

Concept Review

1. What are three important functions of the skin?
2. Name two things found in each of the two layers of the skin.
3. Name a skin condition caused by fungus; by bacteria; by a virus.
4. When should a mole be checked by a doctor? Why?
5. Why is it important to use a sunscreen? What do the SPF numbers mean on suntan products?
6. How is hair important to our health?
7. Why does dandruff appear? What can you do to control it?
8. Head lice live in the scalp and hair. What are they and what should you do if you become infected with them?
9. Why is it important to take good care of your nails?
10. Name the three parts of a tooth. Which part(s) is above the gum line?
11. What is plaque? How can plaque removal help prevent cavities?
12. What are three things that can cause bad breath?
13. Who usually suffers from gum disease? What causes it and how can it be controlled?

Expressing Your Views

1. Julie has a mild case of acne. You notice that she wears heavy makeup to cover the pimples, and you often see her picking at her face. How will her behavior damage her skin? How would you advise her?
2. You are embarrassed to remove your shoes in public because when you do you have a very offensive foot odor. What could you do to relieve this problem?
3. You brush your teeth twice a day but lately you have noticed a few dark spots on your teeth that are beginning to hurt. What should you do to keep your teeth healthier?
4. Your friend is bothered by unwanted hair on her face. She doesn't want to shave it off because it might make her skin rough and unattractive. What else can she do to get rid of the hair?

CHAPTER 6 ASSESSMENT

Life Skills Check

1. Practicing Self-Care
You took a summer job as a lifeguard at a nearby pool. You have fair skin and you know you will be spending six hours a day in the sun. Should you take extra care to protect your skin from the sun? Why?

2. Being a Wise Consumer
Lamar has just moved to your community and needs to visit a dentist. He doesn't know any of the dentists in town, and he is not familiar with the streets. Explain how you would help him choose a dentist and make an appointment.

3. Practicing Self-Care
Your friend just made the diving team and is concerned about caring for her hair, since she will spend a lot of time in the water. Her shoulder-length hair appears dry and damaged. What advice can you give her?

Projects

1. Work with a group to create a poster illustrating tips for proper health care. Each group will be assigned one of the following categories of personal care: hair, skin, nail, and dental. Display your group's poster in the classroom.
2. Borrow two or three microscopes from the science department to examine the different shapes of hair shafts from you and your classmates. Take turns viewing the different hair structures, then draw and label what you see.
3. Interview a dermatologist or dentist to find out the most common problems he or she encounters with teens. You might ask them what the main causes of the problems are and how they might be prevented. Summarize the information and present it to the class.

Plan for Action

A person's physical appearance reflects a person's health. List five improvements you can make regarding your grooming habits.

times a day with a gentle soap, to wear only water-base make-up, and not to pick at pimples. She may try over-the-counter medications containing benzoyl peroxide.
2. Wash my feet every day, wear cotton socks, dust my feet with talc, and alternate pairs of shoes
3. See my dentist as soon as possible and follow his or her advice.
4. Waxing or electrolysis

Life Skills Check

Sample responses:
1. Yes, to protect your skin from wrinkles and skin cancer.
2. Look in the Yellow Pages to find three dentists near where he lives. Call to find out their fees and how soon the dentist could see him. Compare the information and choose a dentist.
3. Cut her hair shorter, wear a swim cap, wash her hair after swimming, let her hair air dry, don't use electric curlers or a curling iron

Projects

Have students plan and carry out the projects on hair, skin, nail, and dental care.

Plan for Action

Divide the chalkboard into five sections: Early Morning, Noontime, Afternoon, Evening, and Bedtime. Invite students to come up one at a time to fill in one activity involving hair and skin care, dental care, and personal hygiene that they might routinely do in one time slot. Have the class discuss the resulting schedule.

ASSESSMENT OPTIONS

Chapter Test

Have students take the Chapter 6 Test.

Alternative Assessment

Have students do the Alternative Assessment activity for Chapter 6.

Test Generator

The Test Generator (Macintosh® or IBM® format) contains an additional 50 assessment items for this chapter.

Issues in Health

EVALUATING MEDIA MESSAGES

How In Is Thin?
Have students read the Evaluating Media Messages feature. Then ask them to think of a person they know and like who does not fit the ideal body type as conveyed in the media. Have them suggest aloud, or list for themselves, attractive personality characteristics of that person. Then ask: In what way are the physical characteristics of the person important to you? Do they limit your relationship with the person? *[Encourage honest responses, which may include an admission that physical features are very important.]* **Do the other attractive features of the person seem as important, more important, or less important than the physical features? Have you ever found that a person you didn't think of as particularly attractive became attractive once you got to know the person?**

Evaluating Media Messages

How In Is Thin?

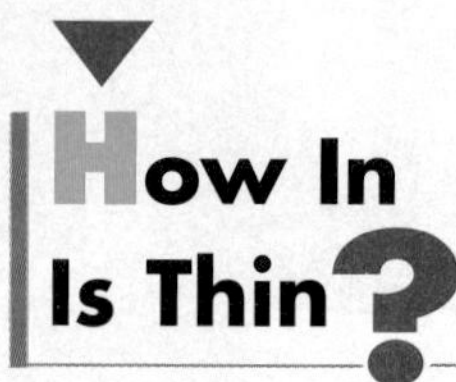

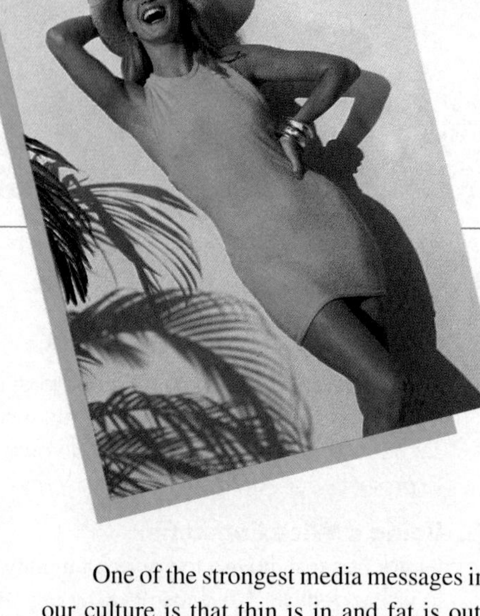

When Cara told Jennifer, "I love this dress, but it makes me look so fat!" Jennifer just stared at her friend. She wanted to say, "Cara, I hate it when you complain about being fat. You know I'm a lot bigger than you, and when you talk like that, it makes me feel huge!" Jennifer also wanted to tell her friend that she had started to worry about how thin Cara was getting and about what Cara was doing to get even thinner.

Does this sound familiar? Recent studies have shown that very few teenage girls are happy with their appearance, especially their weight. An alarming percentage of these girls report being overweight, even when their weight is healthy by medical standards. One source of such attitudes is the media messages about what is attractive that are found in advertisements, television programs, and movies.

The message to be thin can be both good and bad. Healthy people come in all shapes and sizes.

One of the strongest media messages in our culture is that thin is in and fat is out. Because marketing studies have shown that women's clothes sell better when pictured on thin models, girls get the strongest message to be thin. However, boys are also affected by media stereotypes. For males, attractiveness is usually associated with a muscular, athletic build. While this is a healthy model, a boy can also be healthy and fit without being muscular or athletic. Remember that the primary objective of most media messages is to sell something and that you do not have to look like a media stereotype to be healthy and happy.

When questioned about what they consider attractive, many teenagers automatically agree with the media stereotypes—the ultrathin girl and superjock boy—but only at first. As they continue to express their true attitudes and feelings, they tend to emphasize other, more important qualities:

"What I like most about Chad is that he's never boring. He has a great sense of humor and relates to people really well."

"What I love about Mai is that she knows what she wants out of life and really goes for it."

''Jerry is really sensitive and sweet. He wants his own band someday, but he works real hard in school, too, so he'll have more options.''

When you evaluate your attitudes toward personal appearance, be aware of how media messages influence you. Think about what the messages actually say and why they say what they do. Are they eroding your self-esteem? Are they causing you to engage in potentially harmful behavior? Also be aware of mixed messages. An example of a mixed message is a magazine article about proper nutrition and health that is surrounded by ads featuring extremely thin models. Ask yourself which of these messages is encouraging you to make realistic decisions that are truly in your best interest.

The message to be thin or athletic can be good or bad from a health standpoint. Naturally thin or athletic-looking people can be very healthy. However, these body types are not in the majority. Furthermore, healthy people come in all shapes and sizes. Too often, naturally full-figured people try to achieve the unrealistic goal of a fashion model's thin figure or athletic build by resorting to unhealthy behaviors.

Recently, many well-known personalities, including actors, fashion models, and athletes, have admitted that they engaged in unhealthy eating habits and took dangerous medications to maintain their weight and build. Several of these individuals now promote healthier lifestyles. One very moving appeal for a healthier lifestyle came from Lyle Alzado, a former NFL football player who died of cancer in 1992. Before he died, Mr. Alzado used the media to campaign against the use of steroids by athletes who want to increase their size and weight. He believed that the steroids he took were the cause of his cancer.

Persuasive messages are a fact of life in our society. We can't eliminate them, but we can guard against being manipulated by them. With a clear understanding of your values and a strong sense of self-esteem, you can evaluate media messages and use them to your best advantage by using effective decision-making skills.

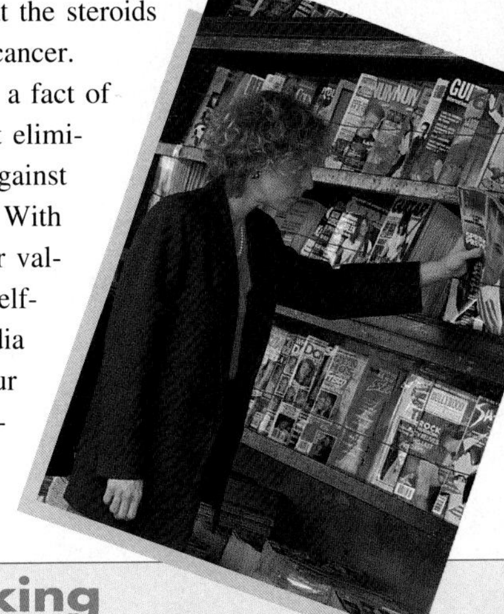

Critical Thinking

1. Find in a magazine a picture of someone you think is really attractive, or watch a favorite actor or actress. Ask yourself:

   - Do I really want to look like this person? Why?
   - Does someone have to look like this person for me to be able to be friends with him or her?
   - Why do I feel like this? Does this really match my values?
   - If someone I cared for gained a lot of weight, would that change my feelings for that person? If *I* gained a lot of weight, would I understand if a friend tried to break off our friendship?
   - Are my personal appearance and fitness goals realistic and healthy?
   - What will I gain by attaining this goal? (Will I get a boyfriend/girlfriend if I lose five pounds?)
   - What do I have to do to attain this goal? Is the effort worth it?

2. See if you can find an example of a mixed message in an advertisement, television program, or movie.

3. Name a movie or television program that contains characters who are attractive without fitting the stereotypical models of ''attractiveness.''

UNIT 3
HEALTH AND YOUR MIND

CHAPTER OVERVIEWS

CHAPTER 7

MENTAL AND EMOTIONAL HEALTH

This chapter describes the characteristics of a mentally healthy person. It defines emotions and explains their role in mental health. It offers suggestions for managing negative emotions and describes and evaluates defense mechanisms. Students are shown how to develop definitions of their self-concept and self-ideal and how to relate Maslow's hierarchy of needs to these definitions. The chapter then describes categories of mental and emotional disorders. Students learn to recognize the signs of mental and emotional problems and the kinds of therapy that are available to help people deal with them.

CHAPTER 8

BUILDING SELF-ESTEEM

A definition of self-esteem opens the chapter. Then students learn how self-esteem develops and how to assess their own self-esteem. The chapter ends by offering students suggestions for raising self-esteem.

CHAPTER 9

MANAGING STRESS

Students learn that stress results from a combination of a stressor and a stress response, and that it may cause physical or mental disorders. A stress model is presented and ways to manage stressors on a daily basis are suggested. Strategies for managing stress over a lifetime complete the chapter.

CHAPTER 10

COPING WITH DEATH

This chapter offers information to help students cope with death and help a person who is dying. The five stages of adjustment to dying are described. The chapter also helps students deal with their grief and that of others.

CHAPTER 11

PREVENTING SUICIDE

Factors that may be responsible for the increase in teen suicides are presented. Students learn to distinguish between myth and fact regarding suicide and to recognize the warning signs. Intervention strategies for dealing with someone who is suicidal are suggested. Finally, students learn what to do if they feel suicidal.

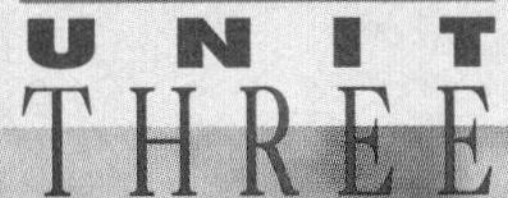

HEALTH AND YOUR MIND

UNIT PREVIEW

This unit deals with the role that emotions play in determining wellness. It helps students understand mental health and offers strategies for coping with emotional problems. Students learn that improving self-esteem is an important way to avoid self-destructive behaviors; they learn ways by which they might raise their own self-esteem. Students also receive suggestions for dealing with stress and for coping with death and grief. Finally, students learn to recognize the warning signs of suicide in others and how to cope with their own suicidal feelings. The five major health themes are emphasized throughout the unit, as indicated in the chart below.

THEMES TRACE

	WELLNESS	BUILDING SELF-ESTEEM	DECISION MAKING	DEVELOPING LIFE-MANAGEMENT SKILLS	ACCEPTANCE OF DIVERSITY AMONG PEOPLE
Chapter 7	p. 162	pp. 158–161	p. 170	pp. 152–158, 161, 168–169	pp. 164–165
Chapter 8		pp. 176–186	pp. 178, 182, 186	pp. 180–186	pp. 179, 185
Chapter 9	pp. 206, 208	p. 192		pp. 197–208	
Chapter 10			p. 216	pp. 214–216, 219–221	
Chapter 11			pp. 231, 235	pp. 232–236	

Mental and Emotional Health

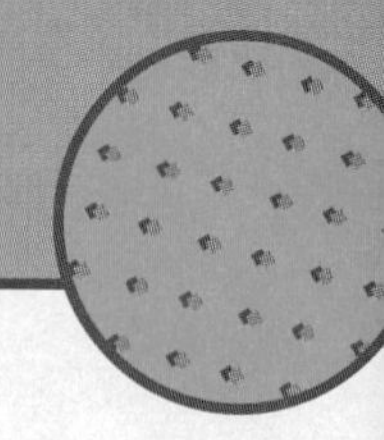

PLANNING GUIDE

TEXT SECTIONS	OBJECTIVES	TEXT FEATURES	OUTSIDE RESOURCES	
7.1 Understanding Mental Health and Emotions pp. 151-158 1 period	• List the characteristics of a mentally healthy person. ■ List qualities that can lead to happiness. ■ List ways to manage negative emotions.	• Check Up, p. 153 • Check Up, p. 157 ■ LIFE SKILLS: Coping, p. 155 **ASSESSMENT** • Section Review, p. 158	**TEACHER'S RESOURCE BINDER** • Lesson Plan 7.1 • Personal Health Inventory • Journal Entries 7A, 7B, 7C • Life Skills 7A • Section Review Worksheet 7.1 • Section Quiz 7.1 • Reteaching Worksheet 7.1	
7.2 Defense Mechanisms and Positive Strategies pp. 159-162 1 period	• Describe the purpose of defense mechanisms and how they can be helpful. ■ Define your self-concept and self-ideal. • Relate Maslow's hierarchy of needs to self-esteem and self-ideal.	**ASSESSMENT** • Section Review, p. 162	**TEACHER'S RESOURCE BINDER** • Lesson Plan 7.2 • Life Skills 7B • Section Review Worksheet 7.2 • Section Quiz 7.2 • Reteaching Worksheet 7.2	
7.3 Types of Mental and Emotional Disorders pp. 163-167 1 period	• Describe the differences among eating, organic, personality, somatoform, mood, and dissociative disorders.	**ASSESSMENT** • Section Review, p. 167	**TEACHER'S RESOURCE BINDER** • Lesson Plan 7.3 • Section Review Worksheet 7.3 • Section Quiz 7.3 • Reteaching Worksheet 7.3	
7.4 Seeking Help pp. 168-172 1 period	• Describe the signs of mental and emotional health problems. ■ List community resources that help with mental and emotional problems. • Differentiate among types of treatment for mental and emotional problems.	■ LIFE SKILLS: Using Community Resources, p. 170 **ASSESSMENT** • Section Review, p. 172	**TEACHER'S RESOURCE BINDER** • Lesson Plan 7.4 • Journal Entry 7D • Life Skills 7C, 7D • Section Review Worksheet 7.4 • Section Quiz 7.4 • Reteaching Worksheet 7.4 **OTHER RESOURCES** • Transparency 7A • Making a Choice 7A, 7B	
End of Chapter pp. 173-175		**ASSESSMENT** • Chapter Review, pp. 174-175	**TEACHER'S RESOURCE BINDER** • Chapter Test • Alternative Assessment **OTHER RESOURCES** • Test Generator	

■ Denotes LIFE SKILLS objectives

• Items in blue are also part of the *Holt Health Activity Book.*

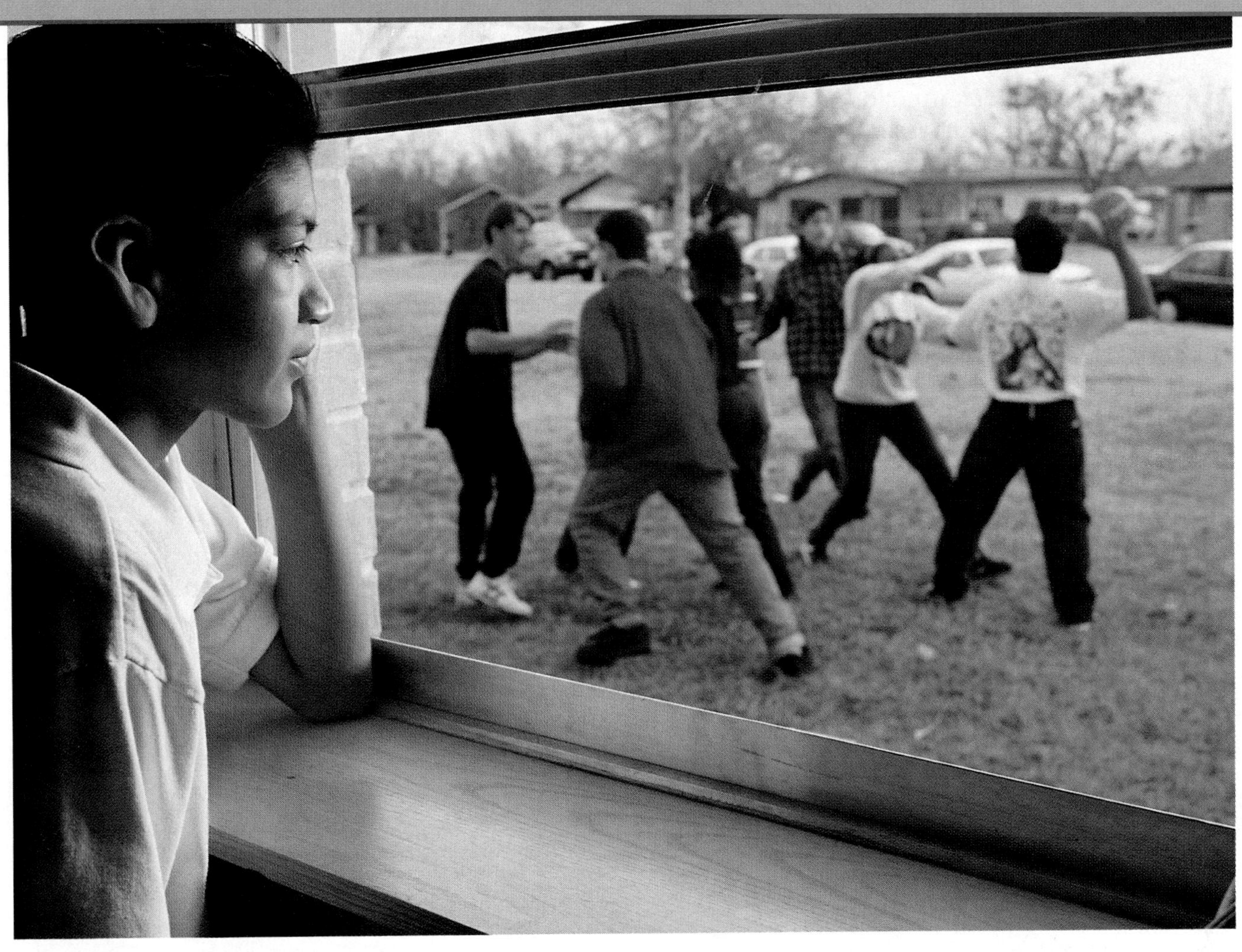

Content Background: Loneliness

When youths reach adolescence and leave the environment of elementary school, they are no longer in an environment that focuses on social interaction as a central part of the curriculum. The environment becomes more academic, and the social aspects of the young person's life are left to his or her own responsibility. Adolescents who have difficulty making friends experience a forced loneliness. Because they have not chosen this state, it is a sad experience. Furthermore, loneliness is linked to physical illness, depression, suicide, mental disorders, alcoholism, drug abuse, and marijuana use. It occurs more frequently and is more intense among adolescents than among any other age group.

Several factors contribute to loneliness in students. Students may be feeling loss and grief as a result of a divorce in the family, a serious illness, the loss of a family member, or even the loss of a pet. Teenagers who have moved recently may feel lonely if they haven't made new friends. In addition, some adolescents may have habits or personality traits that are difficult for their peers to accept but that are difficult to change.

You may recognize lonely students among those who are aggressive—sometimes inappropriate or disruptive in behavior—or withdrawn and shy. Lonely students may not be given positive attention by their peers. This is not because there is something inherently wrong with them; instead, the emotion they feel sets them apart and may isolate them. It is difficult for them to break through socially to other students—so you may see awkward attempts that either push too hard or not hard enough. It is a situation that may get worse without attention, because the isolation can become habitual. The lonely student may respond very well to therapy.

A prominent identifier of loneliness is alcoholism. Women in late adolescence are more likely than women in any other age group to turn to alcohol. Alcoholism risk is high for male adolescents as well. Conclusions drawn from a study conducted from 1985 to 1987 in the southwestern United States suggest "reduction and prevention of loneliness in adolescence and adulthood can be effective in the treatment and prevention of alcohol abuse." Some research suggests that intervening efforts to combat loneliness could reduce adolescent health risk behavior.

Once loneliness is identified in a student by a responsible adult and the student acknowledges the loneliness, what can be done? Few models of intervention exist. We lack applied research and evaluation studies on the subject. Recognition of loss and grief issues and of loneliness as a cause of other common teenage problems is one step. The withdrawn student, the "quiet kid," merits as much attention as the actively disruptive child. If the serious consequences of loneliness—illness, depression, suicide, and so on—are treated without the loneliness being alleviated, these problems will remain chronic.

Teachers can observe students who do not fit in for one reason or another and can establish dialogue with them. They can help the students make connections with other teachers, an advisor or counselor, clergy, or other trusted adults. They can also encourage group interactions. Several efforts could be directed at a single, important goal—to get the lonely student talking.

PLANNING FOR INSTRUCTION

KEY FACTS

- **A mentally healthy person feels good about himself or herself, relates well to others, and is generally able to work through problems.**
- **All people experience both pleasant and unpleasant emotions; learning to manage and express these emotions in positive ways is a key to good mental health.**
- **A healthy lifestyle, a sense of some control in life, meaningful work and relationships, and adaptability can bring happiness.**
- **Negative emotions can be managed. Positive self-talk and sensible planning of the environment can help to reduce fears.**
- **Defense mechanisms are means of coping and avoiding hurt; however, if used consistently, they merely put off facing an issue.**
- **Self-actualization is possible once physical, security, and emotional needs are met.**
- **Mental and emotional disorders may be categorized as organic (stemming from physical causes) or functional (due to internal struggles and related to surroundings).**
- **They may also be categorized as anxiety disorders (phobias), dissociative disorders (amnesia), mood disorders (depression), personality disorders (antisocial), or somatoform disorders (schizophrenia).**
- **Signs that someone is suffering an emotional or mental disorder may include prolonged depression, intense fears, sleeplessness, and out-of-control, self-destructive behaviors.**
- **Mental health agencies and hotlines, therapists, and certain drugs help in the treatment of mental disorders.**

MYTHS AND MISCONCEPTIONS

MYTH: Mentally ill people are dangerous.
People suffering from mental illness are no more dangerous than those who suffer from any other serious illness. In fact, many are so afraid of the world that they are more likely to withdraw from others than to accost them. Personality, not physical or mental health, is the key to violent reactions.

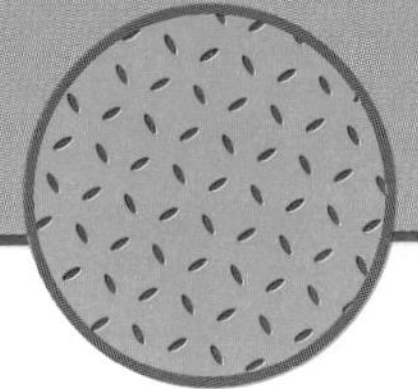

MYTH: Mentally ill people act crazy all the time and remain ill for life.

People who suffer from the most severe mental illnesses generally experience episodes of psychotic behavior; however, they are in touch with reality most of the time. Most mental illness responds well to treatment; up to 80 percent of those who get appropriate treatment can return to normal, productive lives. Medications and various forms of therapy have proven quite effective.

MYTH: Emotional troubles should be kept to yourself; you should be able to handle them.

Mental illness needs treatment as much as physical illness does. Americans have traditionally hidden away emotional problems, feeling that they show a shameful weakness. As a result, millions have led miserable, self-destructive lives. Because mental illness is so treatable, it is important to change this attitude in order to permit sufferers to have normal, productive lives.

VOCABULARY

Essential: The following vocabulary terms appear in boldface type:

- **mental health**
- **defense mechanisms**
- **self-concept**
- **self-ideal**
- **organic disorder**
- **functional disorder**
- **anxiety disorder**
- **dissociative disorder**
- **mood disorder**
- **personality disorder**
- **somatoform disorder**

Secondary: Be aware that the following terms may come up during class discussion:

- external locus of control
- internal locus of control
- obsessive-compulsive disorder
- panic disorder
- phobia
- amnesia
- multiple personality disorder
- mania
- manic-depressive disorder
- passive-aggressive personality disorder
- hypochondria
- schizophrenia
- psychoanalysis
- behavior therapy
- group therapy
- chemotherapy

FOR STUDENTS WITH SPECIAL NEEDS

LEP Students: To help students connect the names of common defense mechanisms with the behaviors these mechanisms describe, have them draw and label cartoons illustrating defense mechanisms. You might wish to display the cartoons on a bulletin board.

Visual Learners: Show the American Psychiatric Association film *Faces of Anxiety,* and have students tell how the film has changed their ideas about people who suffer from anxiety disorders.

ENRICHMENT

- Have students read and report on a famous person (living or historical) who suffered mental illness. The report should explain how the person's illness contributed to fame and achievement or to the ruin of a life. Some possibilities include Friedrich Nietzsche, Caligula, Vincent Van Gogh, Sylvia Plath, Adolf Hitler, Vivien Leigh, Robert Schumann.
- Students might wish to research the physiological changes that take place during a fight-or-flight response. Suggest that they summarize their findings in the form of a poster.
- Encourage students who have access to a video camera to create a brief film about a teen who learns to manage loneliness, anger, jealousy, or fear in a positive way.

Chapter 7 Chapter Opener

GETTING STARTED

Using the Chapter Photograph

Ask students to describe the feelings expressed in the photographs. Are they pleasant or unpleasant emotions? Are they expressed appropriately? Discuss ways in which unpleasant feelings can be handled well and how pleasant feelings enhance a sense of well-being.

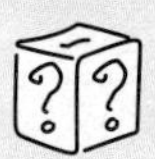

Question Box

The Question Box provides students with an opportunity to ask questions anonymously. To ensure that students with questions are not embarrassed to be seen writing, have those who do not have questions write something else—such as what they already know about emotions or mental disorders—on the paper instead. You may wish to allow students to write additional anonymous questions as they go through the chapter.

Personal Issues *ALERT*

Most teens are experiencing an emotional roller coaster because of rapid physical and hormonal changes. They may need reassurance that their range and intensity of emotions are normal and that most mental disorders are rare. Many gay and lesbian teens suffer extreme isolation and are continually vulnerable to verbal and physical violence; the discussion of emotional expression allows a chance to sensitize students to the rights of homosexuals. You also may have a student or two who has a mental disorder or a family member with a mental disorder. These students may withdraw from discussion or be angry and defensive. Keep the classroom tone open, and be understanding.

Chapter 7

Mental and Emotional Health

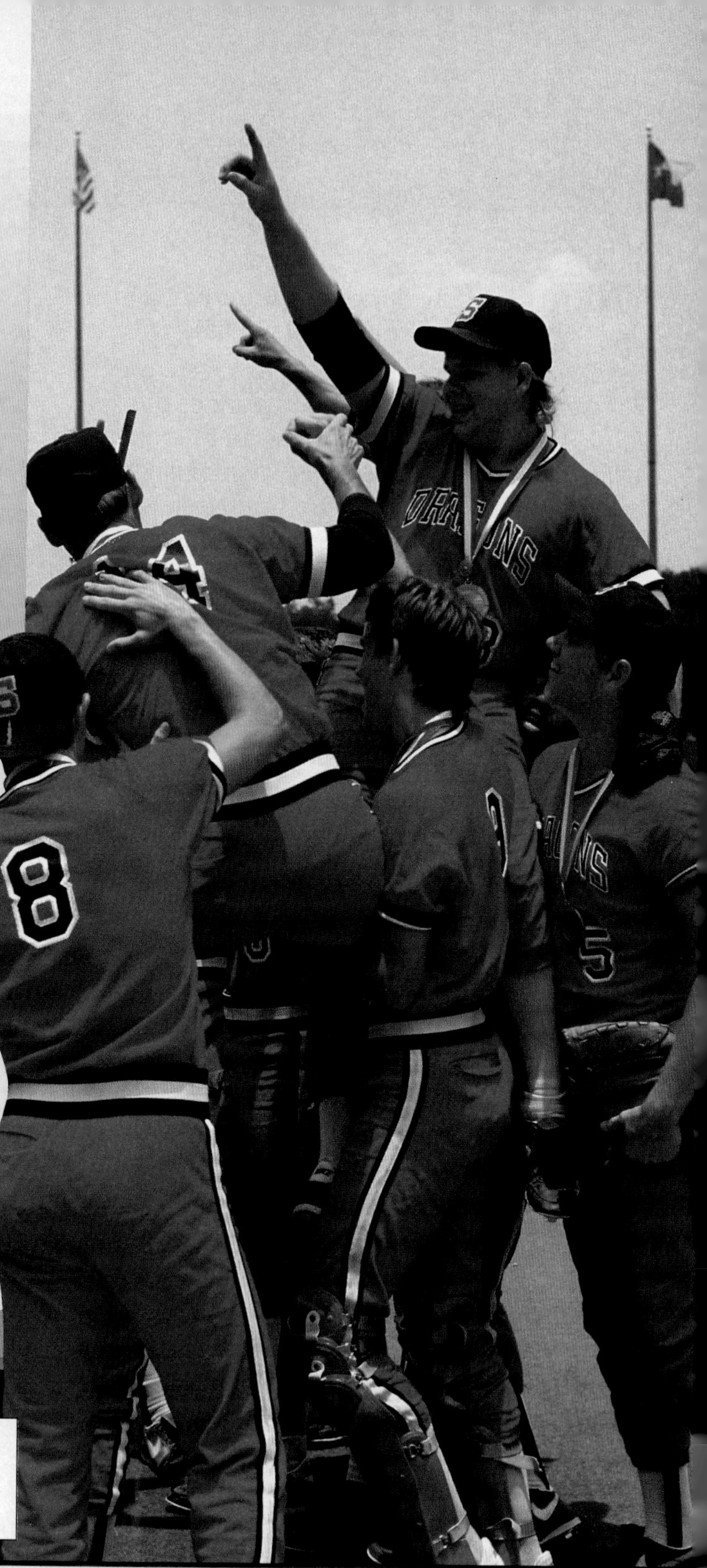

Emotionally healthy people feel a range of emotions and know how to express them in the right way.

Gena was really scared this time. Kevin had been so angry she was really afraid he would hurt her. Why was this happening? Why was he so mad? She thought about when they first met and started going together. He had been so nice. Lately though, Kevin was really possessive. He didn't like it when Gena talked to any other guys, and now he was beginning to be resentful of her girlfriends.

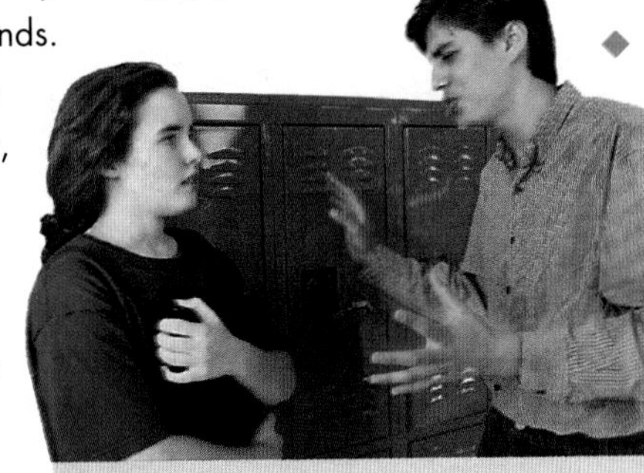

This last argument seemed so stupid. Gena was talking to Mr. Estrada, her history teacher, when Kevin walked up. That afternoon he told her he didn't want to see her talking to Mr. Estrada again. Gena couldn't believe it. When she tried to explain, he flew into a rage and pushed her against the wall. What was she going to do?

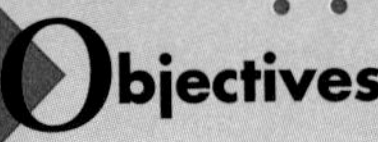

Section 7.1 Understanding Mental Health and Emotions

Objectives

- *List the characteristics of a mentally healthy person.*
- *List qualities that can lead to happiness.*
  LIFE SKILLS: Setting Goals
- *List ways to manage negative emotions.*
  LIFE SKILLS: Coping

People once thought of *mental health* as the absence of mental illness. Now it is defined in much more positive terms. **Mental health** refers to how you use the various aspects of health to achieve positive feelings about yourself and improve your ability to deal with problems. Do you feel good about yourself and the things you do? Can you cope with problems effectively? Do you have close friendships? Can you work through problems with your friends? If you can answer yes most of the time, you are probably mentally healthy.

It is important to recognize that there will be times when you will not feel good about yourself and times when you will have difficulty resolving problems. While having problems is normal, you can develop skills that will enable you to be more effective in dealing with problems.

The National Association for Mental Health describes someone with good mental health as having the following characteristics:

- feels comfortable with himself or herself
- has good relationships with others
- meets the demands of life

mental health: *the feelings you have about yourself and your abilities to deal with problems.*

Section 7.1 Lesson Plan

MOTIVATE

Journal 7A
Concerns About Emotions

This may be done as a warm-up activity. After students have read the chapter opener, have them write their concerns about their negative emotions, such as anger, in the Student Journal in the Student Activity Book.

Class Discussion
Gena's Choices

Discuss with students what Gena should do about Kevin's intense behavior. Why is she fearful? What are her options? What might be the result of each action?

TEACH

Journal 7B
Defining Mental Health and Mental Illness

Ask students to complete these statements in the Student Journal in the Student Activity Book:

Mental (and emotional) health is __________.

Mental illness is __________.

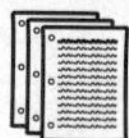

Personal Health Inventory

Have students complete the Personal Health Inventory for this chapter. The inventory helps them assess their own behavior with respect to expressing their emotions.

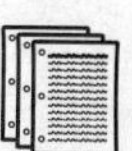

Life Skills Worksheet 7A

Making Friends

Assign the Making Friends Life Skills Worksheet, which asks students to formulate a strategy for making new friends.

Emotions Are Normal

Emotions are feelings in response to an activity or an experience. Understanding emotions and expressing them effectively are important parts of having positive mental health.

Everyone has emotions, and they make you feel good or bad. Emotions themselves aren't good or bad, but the way you express emotions or feelings can be positive or negative. For example, feeling angry is okay, but expressing your anger by hitting someone is not.

You may feel happy one minute and depressed the next. This range of feelings is normal, too. Your body is changing rapidly, and substances in your body can cause dramatic changes in emotions and mood swings. Scientists are studying the relationships between diet and moods. Drugs and other substances can have a profound effect on moods. For example, some people can be very irritable if they consume too much caffeine.

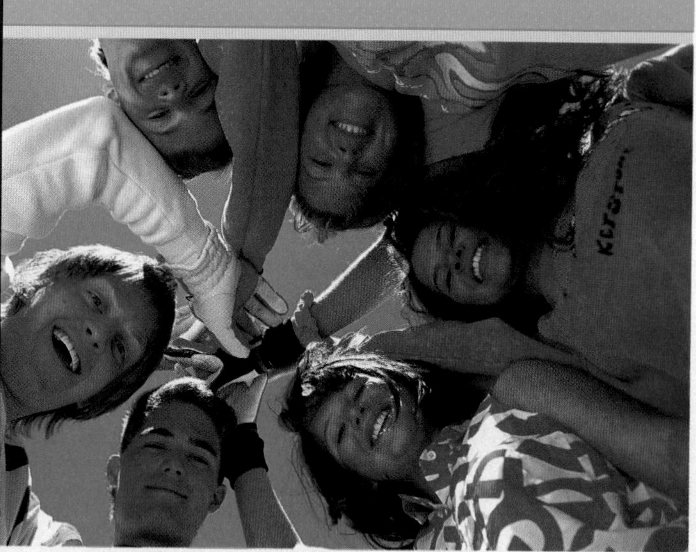

(FIGURE 7-1) **Laughter makes you feel good. Keeping a sense of humor helps you deal with stress effectively.**

Expressing Emotions

You learn to express emotions based on past experiences. These experiences include what you learn from your interactions and from seeing how others react. You *model* your reactions on the reactions of someone else. It is important to recognize how to express your emotions in a positive way. Learning how to do this is a continual process. Instead of hitting someone when you're angry, you learn it is better to hit a pillow, or do some strenuous exercise, or tell someone you're angry. One valuable skill in expressing emotions positively is to think of a particular emotion and rehearse what you will do when it occurs.

Kinds of Emotions

We have the ability to feel a wide variety of emotions, from extreme happiness and joy to sadness and misery.

Love Love is the feeling of strong affection or caring for another person. Love can be a very strong emotion that grows deeper and stronger with time. We all have the need to love, and the need to be loved by others.

There are different types of love. You may feel love for the members of your family. You may also feel love for another person. That might be in the form of caring and loyalty to a friend, or in the form of romantic love. Romantic love is different from other forms of love because of the way you feel. Your heart beats faster when you think of the person you love, and you can't stand to be apart. Yet, sometimes it is hard to tell the difference between attraction and love.

Happiness Happiness is a feeling of joy and well-being or contentment. While happiness is an emotion, it is also a goal that drives people. Bookstores are filled with

• • • TEACH continued

Class Discussion

Dimensions of Emotions

Any emotion has two dimensions that can be represented on a set of continuums: 1) amount of excitement and 2) degree of pleasing sensation. Draw the continuums on the chalkboard and have students place each emotion discussed in the section on both continuums. Help students understand that emotions can be both physical *and* mental stressors, and to recognize the physiological effects of emotions.

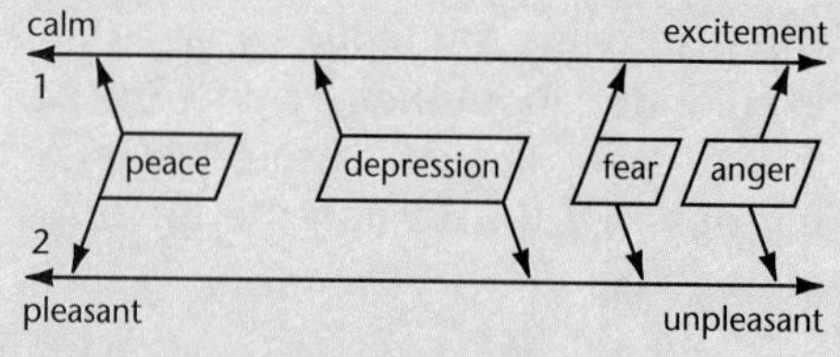

Writing

Expressing Love

Have students write on the chalkboard a list of different kinds of love. Then have them write a second list of the feelings and actions that show love, or caring, for someone. Ask each student to focus on one type of love and write a poem, letter, or brief essay about how that love is expressed.

Journal 7C

Achieving Happiness

Have students choose, from the list on page 153, two things they could do to be happy. Have them list in the Student Journal three specific steps they could take to accomplish each goal.

books on how to achieve happiness—how to feel happy. The first step toward achieving this state is to recognize that you have some control over your life. Your attitude about life and how you react to situations are decisions only you make. Adopting a healthy lifestyle by following the guidelines you'll read about throughout this book will put you on the road to happiness. Here are some other things you can do to be happy.

- Establish close relationships with others.
- Work hard at tasks you find meaningful.
- Have a positive attitude.
- Think about what makes you happy and make time for those activities.
- Take good care of your body.
- Be organized, but flexible, so you can adapt to changes as they occur in your life.

Optimism Feeling optimistic means feeling that life experiences will be positive. It means realistically balancing the ups and downs of life and attempting to keep a positive attitude. Optimism is a healthy emotion that in turn affects your physical well-being. Is optimism part of your range of emotions? Do the following to find out.

Write down all the positive things you expect will happen to you in the future. Then list any of the bad things that you think could happen in the future as well. Now look at your lists. Have you described more positive things or more negative things? How could you revise your lists to look at each negative event with optimism?

Humor Humor provides a way of expressing some negative emotions in a more positive way. Laughing and finding humor in a stressful situation is a very healthy way of coping. Medical research has found that laughter can increase the effectiveness of your immune system in fighting disease.

Check Up

Assessing Your Mental Health

Answer the following questions and count the characteristics of good mental health that you possess.

1. Are you willing to assume responsibilities appropriate for your age?
2. Do you participate in activities appropriate to your stage of life?
3. Do you accept your responsibilities?
4. Do you attack problems rather than evade them?
5. Do you make decisions with a minimum of worry?
6. Do you stick with a choice you make until new factors surface?
7. Are you satisfied with your accomplishments?
8. Do you recognize that thinking about a problem is taking action?
9. Do you learn from failures or defeats?
10. Do you keep successes in perspective?
11. Do you enjoy working and enjoy playing?
12. Do you say no to negative situations even though they may provide temporary pleasure?
13. Do you say yes to situations that will be positive even though there may be some momentary displeasure?
14. Can you show anger?
15. Can you show affection?
16. Can you endure frustration when the source cannot be changed or eliminated?
17. Can you make compromises in dealing with difficulties?
18. Can you concentrate and work at a single goal?
19. Do you recognize the challenges of life?
20. Can you develop and maintain family and intimate relationships?

Check Up

Discuss the questions with students before they answer them, having students provide suitable examples. You may want to collect students' anonymous answers and tally results for an overall perspective of the group's self-concepts.

Reinforcement
Laughter is Good Medicine

The act of laughing, even forcing laughter, has a positive impact on attitude and sense of well-being. Try having students monitor their state of mind and how they feel, then have them laugh for a full minute and note any changes. Experiment by beginning each class with this exercise. After a week, ask students to evaluate the value of laughter.

Class Discussion
Fear: Enemy or Friend?

Illustrate the usefulness of fear by asking students to describe incidents when being afraid helped them. **Why is it necessary for people to feel fear?** *[Fear heightens physical ability and quickens response time and can save your life.]* **When is fear harmful?** *[When it prevents you from living a normal life]* Have students list fears that are not helpful or reasonable.

Role-Playing
Acting on Emotions

Divide the class into six groups and have each group create a role-playing situation illustrating anger, guilt, depression, jealousy, loneliness, or shyness. The scene should show what caused the emotion as well as how it was expressed. After each presentation, the class can evaluate the healthfulness of the expression of emotion or suggest other ways it might have been expressed.

Background
Fight-or-Flight Response and Evolution

Fear and its physiological effects were great survival tools of the earliest humans. Dangers were everywhere and constant; to live, a human had to be able to respond quickly by fighting or running away. Fear increases adrenalin production and provides energy to the major muscle groups, making an individual temporarily stronger, faster, and fiercer. It is not hard to see why natural selection favored this genetic trait. As humans evolved, this valuable characteristic was retained. Today, we don't face the same hazards as early humans, but we still possess this fight-or-flight response. The fear you feel, for example, as you wait to present a speech is the body gearing up for a situation it perceives as dangerous.

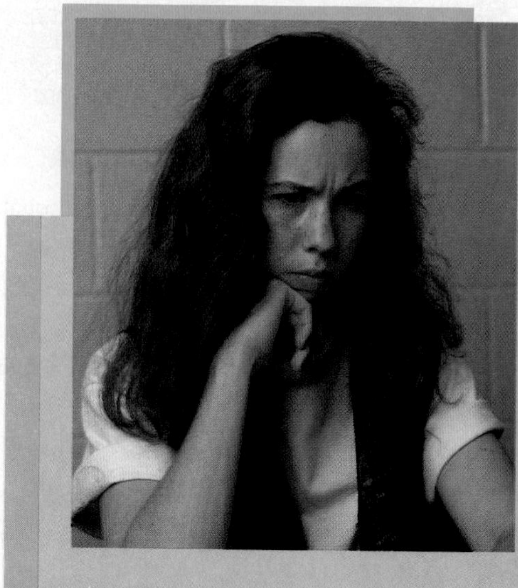

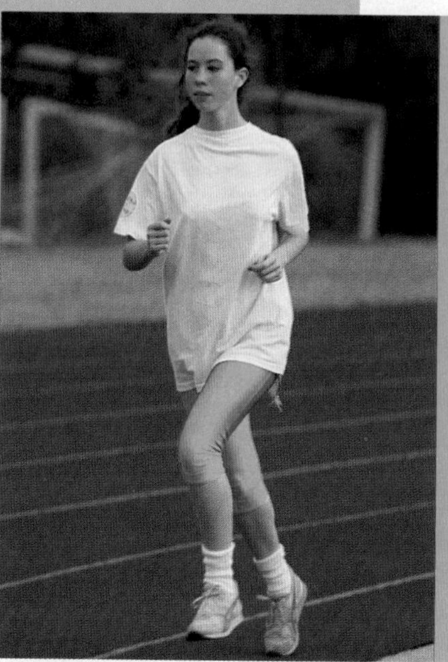

(FIGURE 7-2) **It is normal to feel anger over an irritating situation. Exercise can provide a good outlet to relieve anger or it can just help you manage anger better.**

Fear Fear is the feeling of danger. When you are afraid, your heart beats faster to supply more blood to muscles. Your muscles become tense and your senses become more alert. All these reactions prepare your body to deal with danger. Your body returns to normal once you have dealt with the situation that caused the fear. It is important to work through fears so that the body doesn't stay in this state of alarm for an extended time.

Fears are often learned from experiences that you had when you were young. If you fell off a horse when you were nine years old, you might now be afraid to go riding. Fears also may be learned from other people, particularly your family. If your mother was robbed, you might be afraid to be alone at night. Some of these fears may be valid, while others may not be. For example, your parents probably told you never to accept rides from strangers when you were young. As a result, you may have developed a fear of strangers as a child that is still useful as you get older. However, as a child you may have been told not to go outside after dark. If you developed a fear of the dark as a consequence, that is not useful. Fears related to things that are risky and can cause you harm are healthy fears.

Managing Fears There are some very effective ways to manage fears. Two of these are self-talk and environmental planning. *Self-talk* is saying things to yourself to view the fear more realistically. For example, if you have become afraid of the dark you might make the following self-talk statements.

1. I've never been hurt in the dark before. I probably won't be hurt in the dark now.
2. I sleep in a dark room every night and nothing bad ever happens to me.

• • • TEACH continued

Reinforcement
Chapter Cross-Reference

Depression, as a mood, generally refers to normal feelings of discouragement and sadness. It becomes a symptom of physical or mental illness when it is so severe as to hinder or halt normal functioning. Depression as a mental disorder is discussed later in this chapter, and is discussed as a contributing factor to suicide, in Chapter 11.

Class Discussion
Building Confidence

Have students rate the self-help tips for overcoming shyness from most helpful to least helpful, explaining why they think as they do. **How might each tip help build self-esteem? Why might forcing yourself to be with people and to try new things help build confidence?** *[Students may say these actions will allay fears and make the shy person confident, if the strategies succeed.]*

Cooperative Learning
The Shy and the Lonely

Shyness, loneliness, depression, and lack of confidence often go together. Discuss reasons why a person might feel all these emotions. Then have students work in groups to create a diagram showing how they are related. They could make one poster of their diagram and another showing or listing actions that can help a person overcome these negatives.

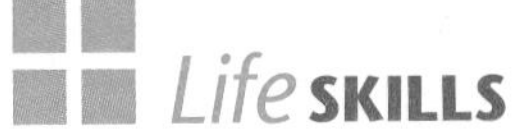

3. It doesn't matter whether it's dark or light. It's whether the place or people are dangerous, and since they aren't in this place, there is nothing to fear.

Environmental planning involves rearranging the environment to reduce your fear. For example, if you are afraid to fly on an airplane you could employ the following environmental planning strategies.

1. Travel with a friend or relative who can comfort you.
2. Bring something to read on the plane to take your mind off the fear.
3. Meditate or engage in some other form of relaxation exercise while flying.

Anger Anger is a strong feeling of irritation. Everyone feels angry at some time. The important thing is how you deal with the anger.

LifeSKILLS: Coping

Managing Fears

Think about something that makes you afraid. With that situation in mind, answer the following questions.

1. What can you say to yourself to be less fearful in that situation?
   a. ____________
   b ____________
   c. ____________
   d. ____________
   e. ____________
2. How can you adjust your environment to be less fearful in that situation?
   a. ____________
   b ____________
   c. ____________
   d. ____________
   e. ____________

Are you prepared to actually use this plan? If you use it, you'll be less afraid.

Americans' Top Ten Fears

Fear	%
1. Speaking to a group	41%
2. Heights	32%
3. Insects/bugs	22%
4. Financial problems	22%
5. Deep water	22%
6. Sickness	19%
7. Death	19%
8. Flying	18%
9. Loneliness	14%
10. Dogs	11%

Life SKILLS
Managing Fears

Review Americans' Top Ten Fears before students complete the exercise. Students should write suggestions independently, but they should share responses. You might break the class into groups that address the same or similar fears to make the sharing easier.

Extension
Helping Yourself to Happiness

Encourage students to search libraries, bookstores, and their own homes for self-help books on becoming happier, becoming more positive in outlook, or overcoming destructive emotions. Display the books, and ask volunteers to read and review several for the class.

Background
Anger as a Coverup of Fear

Fear can be an underlying cause of anger, which in turn masks the fear. Because for many it is difficult to express vulnerability, individuals may—consciously or unconsciously—express or manifest that fear as anger. For example, a parent may lash out angrily at a teen for coming home late, when the primary emotion was fear that the teen had been hurt in an accident. In the story, Kevin's fear that he is losing Gena is expressed as anger. Many people are not aware that they are expressing fear as anger.

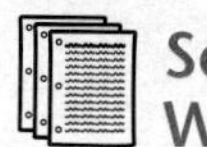

Section Review Worksheet 7.1

Assign Section Review Worksheet 7.1, which requires students to identify characteristics of a mentally healthy person, ways of being happy, and strategies for dealing with negative emotions.

Anger is not only experienced in your mind. A physical reaction accompanies anger. This reaction is varied but may include an increased heart rate and higher blood pressure, headaches, and nausea. It is important to find a positive release for these reactions. That is why exercise is recommended as a way to alleviate angry feelings.

Anger is negative if it is expressed in a violent form. Unfortunately, anger sometimes results in child abuse or spouse abuse. Too often, it also is expressed through aggressive behavior, such as fighting. In the introductory story, Kevin used violence to express his anger at Gena. If such behavior continues unchecked, Kevin will need professional help.

Managing Anger It is important to channel emotions appropriately so that anger can be expressed in a positive way. It is helpful to recognize your feelings and the source of the anger. Once you do this, you may wish to talk to the person with whom you are angry. You are likely to have the most positive results from the talk if you do not blame the other person. Keep in mind that other people do not make you angry. You choose to allow yourself to be angered. Recognizing this simple fact gives you the opportunity to choose whether you will be angry. You decide how you will react.

If you are not able to talk with the person to resolve the problem, do something physical to release your anger and relieve some of the physical symptoms. Remember that it is not helpful to keep your feelings pent up inside.

Guilt Guilt is the feeling that you have done something wrong or are responsible for something bad happening. You may feel guilty after you have had an argument with someone you love. Or you may feel guilty if you have done something unintentionally, that caused something bad to happen.

Guilt can be your cue to resolve a problem. Guilt may also drive you to do the right thing in a situation. You may be nice to someone you really don't like because you feel guilty if you're mean.

Managing Guilt If you feel guilty about something you've done, think about the source of your guilt. Have you done something wrong or are you responding to how others see the situation? For example, if you have stood up to others during a conflict, have you allowed a parent or guardian to make you feel guilty for being assertive? Try not to be critical of yourself. If you've made a mistake, correct it and then move on. If you find guilt over an issue or problem to be overwhelming, seek professional help so you can work through the problem.

Depression Depression is a feeling of sadness, loneliness, and despair. Depressed people feel tired throughout the day and sleep many more hours than usual. Everyone feels depressed occasionally. However, extended periods of depression may indicate a serious mental disorder that requires professional help. Serious depression can lead to suicide. Depression in relation to suicide is covered in Chapter 11.

There are several factors that are linked to developing depression.

- *Family History* The tendency for depression appears to be hereditary. This is especially true of serious forms of depression. The majority of patients suffering from depression have family members who also are depressed.
- *Major Life Stresses* Personal trauma often precedes depression. Children may experience depression as a result of neglect, abuse, or separation from a parent. Women seem more likely to suffer from

depression as a result of a personal relationship. Men are more likely to be depressed due to job-related problems. Depressed people often delay seeking help for the problem. The depressed person may have difficulty identifying the stressor as a problem, or may be overwhelmed by feelings of guilt because he or she cannot cope.

- *Physical Illness* People with physical illnesses are more likely to be depressed.
- *Substance Abuse* Alcoholics and drug abusers have higher rates of depression.
- *Gender* Depression is more likely to occur in women.

Managing Depression When you feel depressed, try to identify why you feel that way. Once you do that, put things in perspective to see if they are really that bad. Focus on the positive things in your life to keep you from dwelling on the things that aren't going so well. Talk to a trusted friend to help you with your perspective.

Get some exercise. When you get a workout your body produces chemicals that make you feel good. Exercise is a natural way to improve your outlook.

Jealousy Jealousy is the feeling of wanting something that someone else has or of losing something that you have. For example, Mary's parents don't have much money. Mary works after school, but most of her money goes to help pay the family's expenses. Mary sees girls who don't have to work, but have lots of nice clothes. Mary is jealous because they have things she would like, but can't have.

The situation with Kevin in the introductory story shows an example of jealousy that results from the possibility of losing something. Kevin and Gena have been dating for six months. Gena has started tutoring Jordan after school. Kevin is jealous of Jordan because he has Gena's time and attention.

Managing Jealousy If you are jealous of someone, you should discuss these feelings with the other person involved. Remember that people don't own other people, so they can't "lose" them. Jealousy is an emotion that can be very destructive if it is not controlled. In the introductory story, Kevin's jealousy was driving him to anger. That anger was expressed in a violent way. The jealousy is Kevin's problem, not Gena's. Gena's best course of action would be to stop seeing Kevin until he can get his emotions under control.

Check Up

Are You at Risk for Depression?

Depression occurs in people of all ages. Among teens, 4.7 percent are clinically depressed. If feelings of depression last more than two weeks, help should be sought. To determine whether you (or a friend) are experiencing depression, answer the following questions.

1. Do you have problems concentrating or making decisions?
2. Are you almost always tired, or do you have problems sitting still because you are so upset?
3. Do you sleep well? Are you sleeping much more or much less than usual?
4. Have you gained or lost a significant amount of weight?
5. Do you find that you no longer enjoy things that used to make you happy?
6. Do you feel worthless most of the time?
7. Do you have thoughts of death?

If you (or your friend) answered YES to four or more of these questions, speak with a mental health specialist.

Check Up

You may want to discuss some questions to be sure students put them in the appropriate context. For example, a change in diet or exercise patterns could be an alternative explanation for weight loss in some teens. Sleep pattern disturbances due to a busy schedule of practices, rehearsals, or work are not necessarily serious.

Students should complete the activity independently, but should be urged to talk to a trusted adult if they feel they are at risk. Students who acknowledge frequent thoughts of death or suicide are especially at risk.

Section Quiz 7.1

Have students take Section Quiz 7.1.

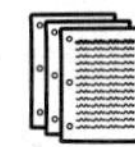

Reteaching Worksheet 7.1

Students who have difficulty with the material may complete Reteaching Worksheet 7.1, which has them classify emotions and describe strategies for dealing with fear.

Review Answers

1. Answers may include I feel good about myself; I feel good about the things I do; I can deal with problems effectively; I have close friends; and I have good relationships with friends and members of my family.

2. Answers will vary but may include find close relationships with others; work hard at tasks you find meaningful; have a positive attitude; think about what makes you happy and make time for those activities; take good care of your body; be organized and flexible.

3. Answers may include talk with the person with whom you are angry; do something physical, such as exercise, to relieve some of the physical symptoms of anger; do not keep angry feelings pent up inside.

4. Answers may include call friends, join groups, and get involved in volunteer work.

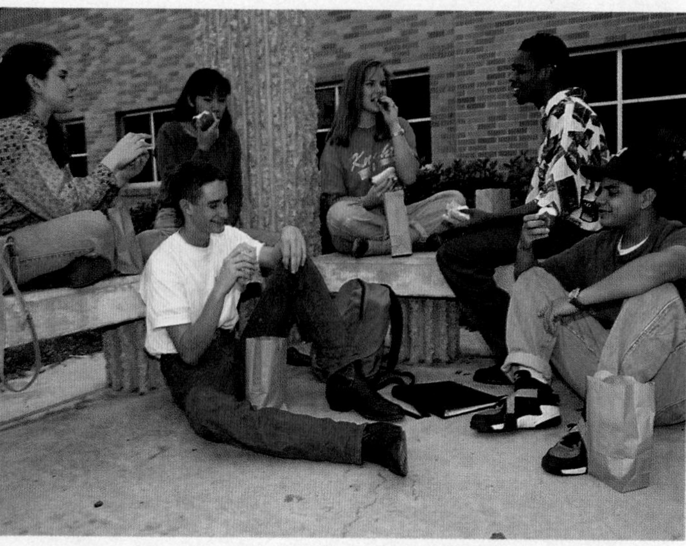

(FIGURE 7-3) **Loneliness is a feeling that you can manage by taking some action. Look for ways to interact with people.**

Loneliness Loneliness is a feeling of isolation or alienation. It is not the same as being alone. Being able to enjoy time by yourself is a part of good mental health. Loneliness can be a particular problem for teens, because in trying to become independent, teens sometimes alienate one another.

Managing Loneliness Engage in activities that will make you part of a group. Don't wait to be asked to join in. Take charge of your loneliness. Make the effort to contact your old friends. Get involved in volunteer work as an interest and way of meeting new people. There are times in life when you will be alone. Therefore it is a good idea to start now in being comfortable by yourself.

Shyness Shyness is the feeling of being timid or bashful. Shy people can appear to be less friendly or open. What often happens is that shy people are thought to be snobs or stuck up. Working to improve self-esteem will help in making shyness less of a problem. People who are confident are less controlled by feelings of shyness. Shyness is something that everyone feels at times.

Managing Shyness/Improving Self-Esteem If you are shy, you might try the following.

1. Make a list of your strengths and positive traits.
2. Never say things about yourself such as "What a dummy," or "Boy, am I stupid." These things make you feel inferior.
3. Purposely put yourself in situations with lots of people. As you do, you'll become more confident.
4. Do not spend time with people who make you feel badly about yourself. People who are always putting you down should be avoided. If the person putting you down is a family member and can't really be avoided, keep remembering your strengths and positive traits.
5. Don't be afraid to try new things or be afraid to fail. Failure teaches you lessons that help you grow as a person, and may lead to other opportunities that are successful.

Review

1. *How would you know if you are mentally healthy?*
2. *List four goals you can set for yourself to achieve happiness.*
3. *Describe some positive strategies for managing anger.*
4. ***Critical Thinking*** *List three things you can do to keep from feeling lonely.*

ASSESS

Section Review

Have students answer the Section Review questions.

Alternative Assessment

Good Humor Prescription

Ask students to write a paragraph describing a situation in which they could use humor to relieve an emotionally stressful incident. They should identify the emotion that needs management and explain how laughter would prevent the destructive expression of emotion and promote a healthier atmosphere.

Closure

Picture Your Emotions

Have each student select an emotion that is potentially harmful to mental health and draw a picture illustrating the expression of that emotion. Beneath the illustration, have students write two or three sentences explaining how the emotion can be healthfully channeled or managed.

Section 7.2 Defense Mechanisms and Positive Strategies

Objectives

- *Describe the purpose of defense mechanisms and how they can be helpful.*
- *Define your self-concept and self-ideal.*
  LIFE SKILLS: Assessing Your Health
- *Relate Maslow's hierarchy of needs to self-esteem and self-ideal.*

Defense mechanisms are techniques you use to protect yourself from being hurt. They provide a way to deal with problems and maintain self-esteem. However, too much reliance on defense mechanisms is not healthy if they are used consistently to avoid facing an issue. Figure 7-4 is a listing of common defense mechanisms. Look through the list and think of one way to use each mechanism that would be helpful and one way that would be harmful.

defense mechanisms: *techniques people use to protect themselves from being hurt.*

Promoting Positive Mental and Emotional Health

Each day you are faced with problems or situations that affect your mental health. While it is easy to let your problems get you down, there are things you can do to stay mentally healthy. The road to good mental health starts with feeling positive about yourself which means getting to know yourself thoroughly.

Self-Esteem Having high self-esteem is very important in developing and maintaining good mental health. Self-esteem is feeling good about yourself and the things you do. These feelings give you a sense of confidence. Take a moment to consider the positive things about yourself and the things you do well. Make a list of these. Pay particular attention to these positive aspects when you are feeling down. Chapter 8 will give you a number of strategies for building your self-esteem.

Sense of Control Another important factor for staying mentally healthy is acquiring a sense of control. High self-esteem gives you a sense of control. People with low self-esteem feel that events affecting their lives are beyond their control. These people have an *external locus of control.* Others believe they can control at least some aspects of their lives. These people have an *internal locus of control.* If you believe you are in control of a situation, you will do what you need to do to stay in control. If you think what you do influences your grades, you'll find out from your teacher how to do better. If you think you have no control over your grades, you won't bother. The reality is that you always have some control over your life. You need to work out the ways you can influence your future. You cannot solve problems by blaming others and bad luck for your situation.

As a teen, there are certain limits to the control you have. If you want to go to college and you don't have the money, that is a limitation. However, you can set college as a goal and begin to explore possible options

Background

Defense Mechanisms—Coping or Compounding Trouble?

Many teens are unaware that they use defense mechanisms. They may rely on them in part because they have not yet had the time and experience to integrate their emotions with their thought processes and reactions. In mature responses, a feeling is consciously understood and acted upon. For example, you may understand that you are frustrated by a situation and realize that you should talk it over and find some way to resolve the feeling. A teen may instead daydream to escape the feeling of frustration—a temporary relief that changes nothing. Simply by learning about defense mechanisms, students may begin to be aware of behaviors they carried out unconsciously.

Section 7.2 Lesson Plan

MOTIVATE

Class Discussion
Putting Off Dealing With Emotions

Have students think of a time when they did not express how they felt about a situation. **Why did they put off expressing the feelings?** *[They may suggest wanting to think over a response, sort out the feelings, fear of rejection or violence, feeling the emotion was unacceptable]* Ask students whether it is healthy or unhealthy to delay or avoid expressing emotions.

TEACH

Role-Playing
Defense Mechanisms

Have students work in pairs or individually to role-play typical defense mechanisms. Have the rest of the class identify the mechanism being portrayed. Examples include lying to a friend about your feelings because you think the friend can't handle the truth (rationalization), blaming your best friend for keeping you out too late last night (projection), being rude to someone you think would never respect you (reaction formation), whining when the library closes before you've finished your work (regression), and eating a giant ice cream sundae when you're feeling sad about a lost opportunity (substitution).

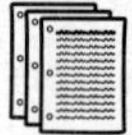

Life Skills Worksheet 7B

Defense Mechanisms

Assign the Defense Mechanisms Life Skills Worksheet, which asks students to evaluate the positive and counterproductive uses of defense mechanisms.

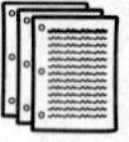

Section Review Worksheet 7.2

Assign Section Review Worksheet 7.2, which requires students to complete a drawing of Maslow's hierarchy of needs and identify defense mechanisms.

Common Defense Mechanisms

Mechanism	Description	Examples
Compensation	*covering a weakness by over-achieving in another area*	*focusing all your attention on sports because you think you are a better athlete than student*
Daydreaming	*escaping from an unpleasant situation by using your imagination*	*in the dentist's chair you focus on the fun you'll have over the weekend with friends, because you hate being at the dentist*
Denial	*failure to accept reality*	*refusing to accept the death of a close friend or relative; refusing to accept that your relationship with a romantic friend is over*
Displacement	*the transfer of negative feelings about someone to someone else*	*you are very angry with your mother and you take out that anger in dealing with your sister or best friend*
Projection	*putting (projecting) negative feelings on someone else*	*blaming your teacher for failing a test when you did not study*
Rationalization	*justifying when you behave irrationally*	*not doing your homework one evening because you feel you've spent too much of your time on schoolwork*
Reaction formation	*expressing emotions that are the exact opposite of what you feel*	*acting like a clown in a group to hide your shyness*
Regression	*using childlike ways of expressing emotions like anger or disappointment*	*throwing a tantrum when you don't get to watch your favorite TV program*
Repression	*blocking out unpleasant memories*	*forgetting when you were in the hospital*
Sublimation	*redirecting bad or unacceptable behavior into positive behavior*	*channeling your aggression into an athletic sport where aggressive behavior is accepted*
Substitution	*replacing an unattainable goal with an attainable goal to relieve disappointment*	*not getting a summer job at the hospital so you sign up for volunteer work instead*

(FIGURE 7-4)

• • • TEACH continued

Class Discussion
Defining Locus of Control

Ask students to list aspects of their lives over which they have some control and a second list of aspects over which they have no control. List these in two columns on the chalkboard with space between them. Which aspects fall into a gray area in between? As students argue about placement, point out that often perception of control is a matter of perception of self. A self-confident person more actively looks for ways to positively affect his or her future.

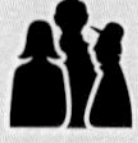

Cooperative Learning
Self-Ideal

Have students work in small groups to distinguish cultural and individual factors that go into self-ideals. Each group should come up with a description (and sketch) of the ideal man and ideal woman, as defined in their social community. Then they should discuss how they see their own self-ideals as differing from the culturally defined one. Does the cultural ideal fit *anyone*? What kinds of differences do healthy individuals inject?

Class Discussion
Sliding Up and Down Maslow's Hierarchy

Have a volunteer define *hierarchy*. *(a system of things arranged in order of rank)* Refer students to Maslow's hierarchy, stressing that it builds upward as more basic needs are met. Which needs relate directly to survival? Which

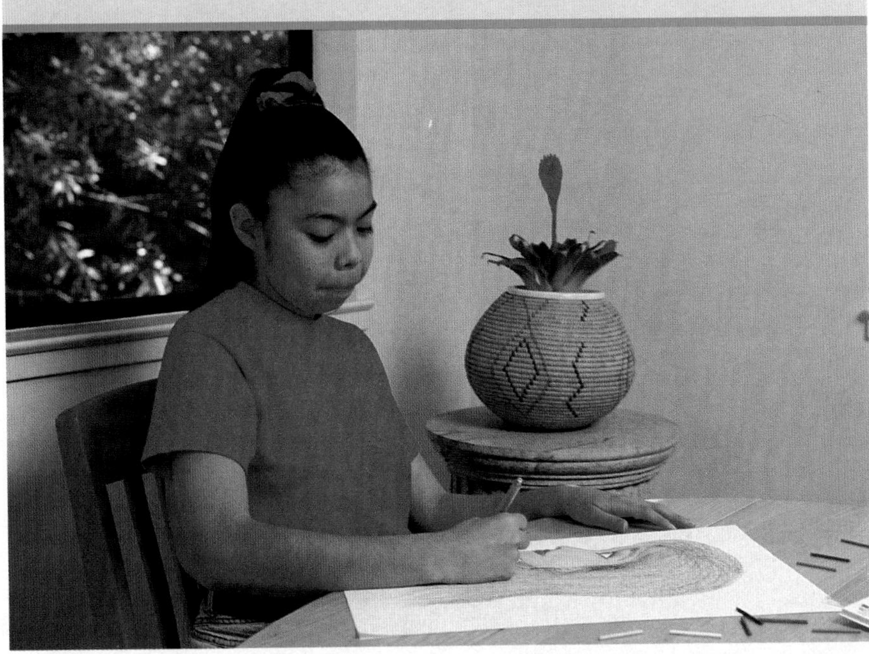

(FIGURE 7-5) **How closely does your self-concept match how you look and feel? What could you do to improve how you see yourself?**

for getting there. You may be able to seek financial aid or apply for scholarships. To look for ways to take charge of and solve a problem is to be mentally healthy. To give up and run away from your problems is to be unhealthy. If you focus on the negative, you'll be unhappy. If you focus on the positive, you'll be happier. Having a positive outlook will help improve and maintain your mental health.

Self-Concept Rating your level of self-esteem requires a thorough analysis of your **self-concept**, or self-image as it is sometimes called. It means looking realistically at how you see yourself.

Take out a piece of paper and draw a picture of yourself. Now look at the picture. Are you satisfied with the picture you've drawn? What kinds of things can you learn about how you feel about yourself by looking at the picture you've drawn? Do you see yourself as big or small? Did you draw yourself as happy or sad? Does your picture fill up the whole paper or is it off in a corner? Does your picture reflect a positive view of yourself?

Now think about what you would like your picture to look like. This image represents your **self-ideal**. Your self-ideal can be an image to strive for, as long as it is realistic. For example, if you are short you can't expect to achieve a goal of being tall. If you are sad, you can work at being happy. Your self-ideal should represent your feelings about yourself. Your self-ideal should be based on what you think, not on what your parents think, your friends think, or your teachers think.

Once you have a realistic self-ideal you can set reasonable goals for moving your self-concept closer to your self-ideal.

self-ideal:
your mental image of what you would like to be.

self-concept:
your current mental image of yourself.

Background
Abraham Maslow (1908–1970)

Abraham Maslow, best known for his theory of self-actualization, distinguished himself from psychologists in other schools of thought by focusing on well-adjusted people rather than on troubled patients. Whereas behaviorists saw people as controlled by instincts and environment, and psychoanalysts saw them as controlled by unconscious drives, Maslow and other humanistic psychologists saw people as motivated by a hierarchy of needs and controlled by their own values and choices. He saw integration of the self as the primary goal of psychotherapy.

Section Quiz 7.2
Have students take Section Quiz 7.2.

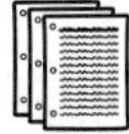

Reteaching Worksheet 7.2
Students who have difficulty with the material may complete Reteaching Worksheet 7.2, which requires them to match defense mechanisms with their descriptions.

needs relate to emotional survival? How are these needs met for a small child? for a teen? for an adult? Point out that a person may progress up the pyramid and slide back down it numerous times. Also, few people achieve true self-actualization. Maslow himself felt that only one person in a hundred achieves self-actualization, or true fulfillment of potential.

Extension
Comic Strip Defense Mechanisms

Have students clip comic strips from the newspaper (or draw their own) to illustrate various defense mechanisms in action. Encourage them to create clever headings or sayings to label their comics and display them on a bulletin board.

Review Answers

1. Defense mechanisms are used to protect a person from being emotionally hurt and to provide a way for the person to deal with problems and maintain self-esteem. Defense mechanisms can be misused when they are consistently used to avoid facing an issue.

2. Maslow's hierarchy includes basic physical needs, safety-security, love and affection, self-esteem, and self-actualization. Self-esteem enables a person to know what he or she does well. People with high self-esteem will be able to set reasonable goals for moving closer to their self-ideal.

3. Answers will vary. Students may answer work on ways to increase happiness, take control over your life, focus on the positive, and believe in yourself.

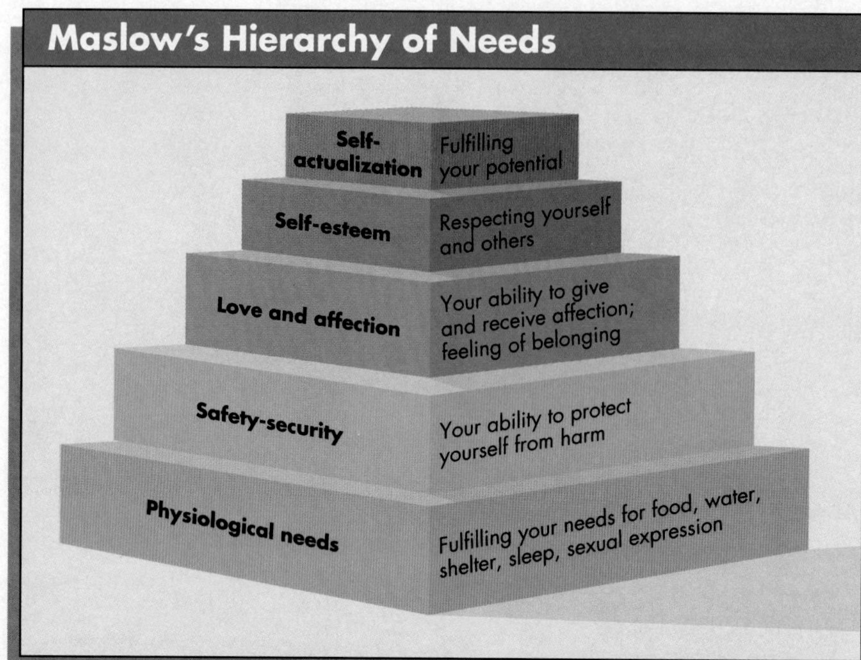

(FIGURE 7-6) **According to Maslow, you cannot reach a state of fulfillment without satisfying your basic physiological needs first. Each step in the pyramid requires that the needs in the section below have been met.**

Maslow's Hierarchy of Needs

Focusing on the positive aspects of human behavior was the subject of Abraham Maslow's work on emotional development. Maslow organized human needs by priority in achieving a state of wellness. Maslow's Hierarchy is shown in Figure 7-6. People grow emotionally when they can satisfy their needs from bottom to top of the hierarchy. Reaching the top of the scale represents the fulfillment of one's potential. This stage represents a state of wellness. Self-actualization and fulfillment may be your self-ideal. However, to reach this goal your self-esteem needs must be satisfied. You cannot grow emotionally without self-esteem.

Review

1. *Why do people use defense mechanisms? When are defense mechanisms misused?*
2. *List the phases in Maslow's hierarchy. How is your self-esteem related to self-ideal?*
3. ***Critical Thinking*** *List four things you can do to bring your self-concept closer to your self-ideal.*

ASSESS

Section Review

Have students answer the Section Review questions.

Alternative Assessment

Problem-Solving and Feeling in Control

Ask students to explain how a person's defense mechanisms and problem-solving strategies relate to his or her feeling of being in control. They should point out that defense mechanisms delay problem solving; the ability to resolve emotional issues strengthens an internal locus of control, and vice versa.

Closure

The Real "Me"

Have students describe the differences they perceive in their own private, public, and ideal selves.

Section 7.3 Types of Mental and Emotional Disorders

Objectives

- *Describe the differences among eating, organic, personality, somatoform, mood, and dissociative disorders.*

Everyone faces a variety of challenges. It may be the challenge of moving to a new town and making friends. Or it may be the challenge of rejection when you learn that the person you have a crush on doesn't feel the same about you. Most of the time, we are able to face challenges, learn from them, and move forward. Sometimes we are bogged down by them for a time. In these cases, our capacity to cope is exceeded, and the challenge interferes with our ability to function day to day. The inability to function for an extended period of time may be indicative of a mental or emotional disorder. The American Psychiatric Association has categorized mental and emotional disorders according to specific behaviors that people demonstrate. These mental and emotional disorder categories include the information in Figure 7-7. The diagnosis of a mental or emotional disorder should be made by a qualified doctor. People should never attempt to diagnose themselves or others just by reading a short description of a disorder in a textbook. If you are having difficulty, talk to a trusted adult. Counseling may help you deal with your problems. There is nothing wrong with seeking counseling. Seeking help for emotional problems is no different than seeking help for physical problems.

Organic Disorders

Mental and emotional disorders resulting from a *physical* cause are called **organic disorders**. There is evidence that some organic disorders are genetic. Other evidence indicates that these disorders develop as a response to various life experiences. Organic disorders may be caused by a physical illness, injury, or chemical imbalance. Because they involve the body as well as the mind, organic disorders are usually more serious than other types of mental and emotional problems.

organic disorders: *mental and emotional disorders resulting from a physical cause.*

An example of a physical illness causing an organic disorder is a brain tumor. A brain tumor can affect mood, speech, and comprehension. These won't improve until the tumor is removed. An example of an injury causing an organic disorder is a severe blow to the head. Brain cells may be destroyed during the injury and the functioning of the brain can be affected.

A chemical imbalance can also cause an organic disorder. For example, drinking alcohol or using other drugs may destroy brain cells, which in turn causes a chemical imbalance. The result can be an organic disorder. Brain cells may also be destroyed by lack of oxygen, such as when someone almost drowns. Chemicals help your brain send messages to your body. An imbalance in chemicals can affect the way you feel and act.

Eating Disorders

In Chapter 5, you learned about the characteristics of the two major eating disorders—anorexia and bulimia. The refusal to eat,

Background

Films Available

A series of three films is available through Modern Talking Pictures Service, 1-800-243-MTPS. They are *Depression: The Storm Within (1991), Faces of Anxiety (1990),* and *The Panic Prison (1989).* This series is produced by the American Psychiatric Association in videocassette format. Each film is 29 minutes long and features a psychiatrist interacting with patients, documentary style. Each portrays symptoms, effects of the specific illness, treatment options, course of action taken, and recovery. There is no charge for rental.

Section 7.3 Lesson Plan

MOTIVATE

Class Discussion

Mental Disorders in the Media

Ask students to recall movies or programs that included a mentally ill character. (Students may mention *The Fisher King, Three Faces of Eve, One Flew Over the Cuckoo's Nest, I Never Promised You a Rose Garden, Ordinary People, Sybil, Prince of Tides, What About Bob?*) What caused the character's crisis? What behaviors show that the person has lost the ability to function normally in society? What impression of mental illness is given in each film?

TEACH

Class Discussion

Organic and Functional Disorders

What is the difference between functional disorders and organic disorders? *[Functional disorders arise from internal struggles; organic disorders from physical causes.]* **Which kind of disorder is a neurosis?** *[Functional]* **Which kind is psychosis?** *[Functional]* **A brain tumor is which kind of disorder?** *[Organic]* **What are three possible causes of organic disorders?** *[Physical diseases, injury, chemical imbalance]* **Can a person's behavior bring about an organic disorder?** *[Yes, drug and alcohol use can impair brain cells, causing a chemical imbalance.]*

anxiety disorder: *a condition in which fear or anxiety prevents one from enjoying life and completing everyday tasks.*

that is characteristic of anorexia, or the binge eating that is characteristic of bulimia are not the actual disorders. Anorexia and bulimia describe behaviors that are the result of deep emotional problems related to self-image and self-esteem.

Eating disorders are included again in this chapter because of their increasing frequency among teens. They are also included here because the cure for these disorders requires psychiatric treatment. The goal of therapy is to find the underlying cause of one's obsession with body image and weight. In some cases, family therapy is needed to provide insights into why the patient has a negative image of herself. In other cases, the eating disorder may have been caused by severe depression, or the result of some form of sexual abuse.

Anxiety Disorders

You learned in Section 7.1 that fear is a protective emotion that helps you recognize and prepare for danger. It can be beneficial to you on occasions when you should feel afraid. For example, if you are contemplating doing something that is illegal, the fear of getting caught might prevent you from doing the wrong thing. In this case, the fear is helpful.

However, to be constantly afraid of things you should not fear is not normal.

Cultural DIVERSITY

Social Support and African-American Churches

You read at the beginning of this chapter that having good relationships with others—having social support—is an important part of being mentally healthy. Different people find this support in different ways. For many African-Americans, churches serve as an important base of social support.

In fact, African-American churches have a long history of providing support and a sense of community to their members. Almost from the beginning, the churches served as community centers where African-Americans could gather to socialize. In the segregated past, their churches were often the *only* public buildings where they could have large gatherings.

People still come together at churches for services, weddings, baptisms, concerts, suppers, socials, plays, parties, meetings, discussion groups, educational programs, and sports like basketball and softball. Most African-American churches are open at least four nights a week to accommodate all these events.

At times, the support African-American churches give is more than social; families in financial trouble often go to their churches for housing, clothing, and money. Recently, some churches have even begun addressing their members' health-care needs.

• • • TEACH continued

Class Discussion
When Fears Are Out of Control

What are some biological purposes of fear? *[In the evolution of humans, it served the useful purpose of preparing a person to fight or flee from danger; it heightens alertness and enhances physical prowess.]* **How do anxiety disorders differ from healthy fears?** *[They do not help you avoid danger but prevent you from living normally or enjoying life; they interfere with day-to-day function.]* Have volunteers point out ways in which each anxiety disorder expresses abnormal fear.

Reinforcement
Dissociative Disorders in Film and Fiction

Most students have read stories or seen movies about people suffering from amnesia or multiple personality disorder. Stress that these disorders are rare. Amnesia is not usually as intense, dramatic, or long lasting as it is portrayed.

Role-Playing
Mental Disorders

Divide the class into small groups and assign each group a mental disorder. Have students in the group role-play a situation that represents this disorder. Have the class identify and discuss the disorder afterward.

Case Study
Patty Duke Astin—Breaking the Manic-Depressive Cycle

In 1992, Patty Duke Astin went public with her story of two decades of suffer-

Constant fear prevents you from participating in many aspects of a normal life. It can also damage you physically, because your body experiences a number of changes when you are afraid. Your heart rate speeds up, you perspire, and your blood pressure rises. If these changes occur most every day, they can be harmful and become the symptoms of an **anxiety disorder**. Phobias are the most well-known anxiety disorders. A fear of flying in a plane, of riding in an elevator, or of even leaving the house is a very real fear to someone with an anxiety disorder.

Anxiety disorders are the most common mental and emotional disorders. They affect over 7 percent of the population. For some reason, more women are affected (9.7 percent) than men (4.7 percent). Anxiety disorders cause, or are a contributing factor in, 20 percent of all medical conditions for which Americans seek care.

Dissociative Disorders

A condition in which someone's personality changes dramatically is called a **dissociative disorder**. A person afflicted with a dissociative disorder believes he or she is really someone else. People with dissociative disorders separate themselves from their real personality.

dissociative disorder: *a condition in which someone's personality changes to the point that the person believes he or she is someone else.*

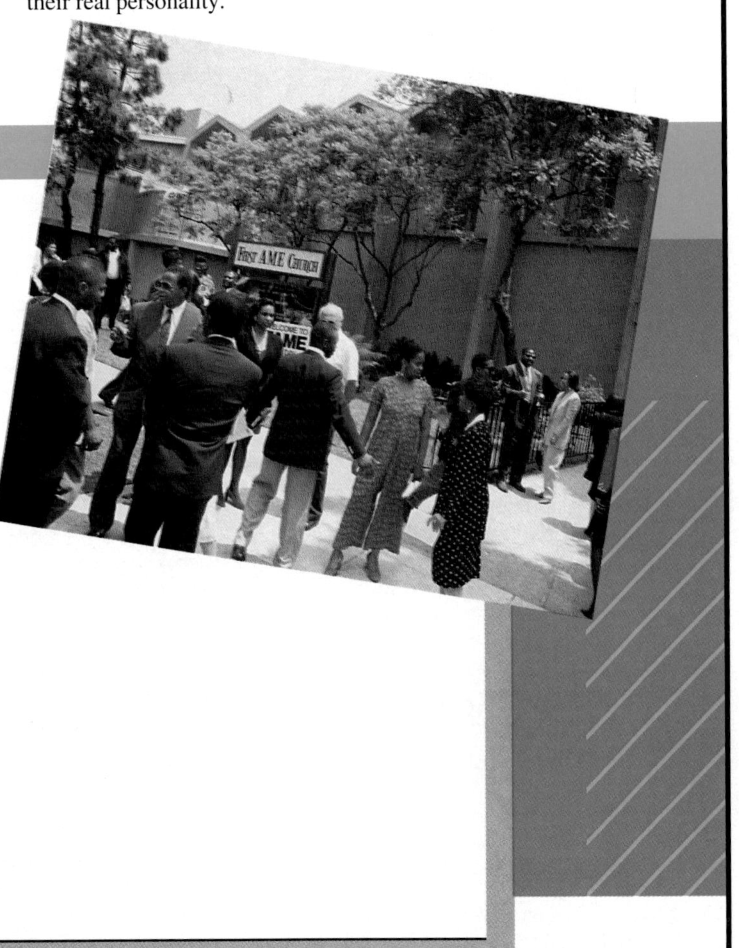

In addition, churches have played a crucial role in the ongoing battle against racial discrimination. In the 1800s, African-American churches were active in the movement to abolish slavery. They were also part of the "underground railroad" that helped escaped slaves find their way to freedom.

Later, black religious institutions furnished much of the leadership for the civil rights movement. Two of the most important leaders of that time, Martin Luther King, Jr., and Malcolm X, began their civil rights work as religious leaders. King was a Baptist minister and Malcolm X was a speaker for the Nation of Islam. Today, African-American churches continue to work for social justice.

ing with manic-depressive disorder. Like most manic-depressives, she spent long periods in bed, battling severe depression that led to frequent suicide attempts. Finally diagnosed correctly, she received medical treatment and therapy that turned her life around. By telling her experience, Astin hopes to promote public awareness and understanding of the disorder, which is treatable in 90 percent of all cases.

Extension

Understanding Mental Disorders

Have students explore the library and community mental health clinics for books, articles, and pamphlets on specific mental disorders that interest them. They may work alone or in pairs to prepare a report, poster, or display that will educate the public about a mental disorder.

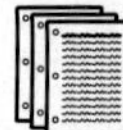

Section Review Worksheet 7.3

Assign Section Review Worksheet 7.3, which requires students to complete sentences that describe mental and emotional disorders discussed in the section.

Section Quiz 7.3

Have students take Section Quiz 7.3.

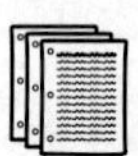

Reteaching Worksheet 7.3

Students who have difficulty with the material may complete Reteaching Worksheet 7.3, which requires them to classify and compare mental and emotional disorders.

Background

"Split Personality"

Schizophrenia has historically been commonly called "split personality." It is not a personality disorder. Logical thought processes are split, resulting in bizarre behaviors, distortions of reality, misperceptions—even delusions and hallucinations.

Some Mental and Emotional Disorders

Type of Disorder		Characteristics
Eating Disorders	*Anorexia*	*excessive dieting resulting in a state of self-starvation*
	Bulimia	*binging on food then purging to avoid weight gain*
Anxiety Disorders	*General Anxiety*	*constant feeling of anxiety and fear with physical symptoms like increased heart rate, shortness of breath, perspiration, shaking, and diarrhea*
	Obsessive-Compulsive	*persistent recurring thoughts accompanied with the need to repeatedly perform some action, such as repeatedly washing one's hands*
	Panic	*intense feelings of terror that occur suddenly without cause*
	Phobia	*persistent fear of something; Hydrophobia–fear of water, claustrophobia–fear of small, enclosed spaces; agoraphobia–fear of public places*
Dissociative Disorders	*Multiple Personality*	*having two or more distinct personalities which can show different physical conditions and are often the exact opposite of each other*
	Amnesia	*loss of memory*
Mood Disorders	*Depression*	*experiencing feelings of sadness, loneliness, and hopelessness for an extended period of time*
	Manic-Depressive	*experiencing exaggerated feelings of euphoria, irritability, depression; exaggerated mood swings; displaying reckless behavior*
Personality Disorders	*Antisocial*	*showing a preference to remain distant from others*
	Paranoid	*consistent mistrust of others*
	Passive-Aggressive	*behavior that displays an inner conflict between being dependent and being assertive which results in erratic moods*
Somatoform Disorders	*Hypochondria*	*believing and showing signs of serious illness without any physical cause*
	Schizophrenia	*impaired perceptions, thinking processes, emotional health, and physical activity*

(FIGURE 7-7)

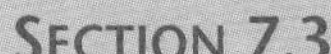

Review Answers

1. Eating disorders are the result of deep emotional problems related to self-image and self-esteem. A personality disorder is an emotional condition in which a person's pattern of behavior negatively affects the person's ability to get along with others.

2. Anxiety disorders

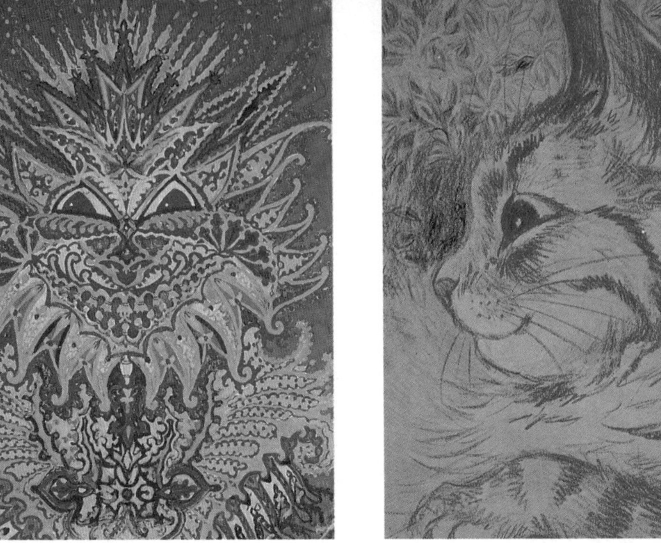

(FIGURE 7-8) **These drawings made by an artist with diagnosed schizophrenia show how perception has been impaired.**

Dissociative disorders occur infrequently. They are usually the result of a traumatic experience. For example, they may result from severe sexual, physical, or emotional abuse in childhood. These disorders may be the mind's way of avoiding the pain associated with a very unpleasant experience. Amnesia and multiple personality disorder are examples of dissociative disorders.

Mood Disorders

A **mood disorder** occurs when one mood, which is often an unhappy mood, is experienced almost to the exclusion of other feelings. Just over 5 percent of Americans suffer from mood disorders: 6.6 percent of women and 3.5 percent of men. A mood disorder usually lasts a long time and interrupts the ability to complete daily activities.

Personality Disorders

Traits that negatively affect a person's ability to get along with others are called **personality disorders**. These traits may affect a person's work, relationships, and sense of satisfaction with life. Most personality disorders are very difficult to treat, since one's personality is difficult to change.

Somatoform Disorders

People with physical symptoms caused by emotional problems are said to have **somatoform disorders**. However, a person with a somatoform disorder has no actual physical illness. Only 1 in 1,000 Americans experiences this type of disorder. Hypochondria is an example of a somatoform disorder. Hypochondriacs believe they are ill even though they have no real illness.

Review

1. *How do eating disorders differ from personality disorders?*
2. *What disorders are related primarily to fears?*

somatoform disorder:
an emotional condition in which there are physical symptoms but no identifiable disease or injury. The physical symptoms are caused by psychological factors.

mood disorder:
a condition in which one mood is experienced almost to the exclusion of other feelings.

personality disorder:
an emotional condition in which a person's patterns of behavior negatively affect that person's ability to get along with others.

ASSESS

Section Review

Have students answer the Section Review questions.

Alternative Assessment

Dissociative and Personality Disorders

Have students write a paragraph explaining differences between dissociative and personality disorders, citing specific behaviors.

Closure

Anxiety and Mood Disorders

Have students take turns describing specific behaviors for others to classify as representative of mood disorders or anxiety disorders.

Section 7.4 Seeking Help

Objectives

- *Describe the signs of mental and emotional health problems.*
- *List community resources that help with mental and emotional problems.*
  - ***LIFE SKILLS: Using Community Resources***
- *Differentiate among types of treatment for mental and emotional problems.*

Most times you can work through difficult times without outside help. Sometimes, though, you may need to ask for help from friends, parents, or relatives. Still, there may be times when your problems are so disturbing that it is important to seek professional help. That is when you need the assistance of a mental health specialist.

Background

Dorothea Lynde Dix (1802–1887)

Before the mid-1800s, mentally ill people were treated no better than animals. Usually they were brutally treated, housed with criminals, and often denied basic human needs such as proper food, clothing, and blankets. Dorothea Lynde Dix became aware of the dismal conditions of prisons and almshouses in which the mentally ill were housed in the 1840s. She fought for legislation to improve these institutions. Her activities resulted in the construction or improvement of over 30 mental hospitals in the United States and Canada. She was also responsible for the reform of some of the deplorable conditions in these institutions.

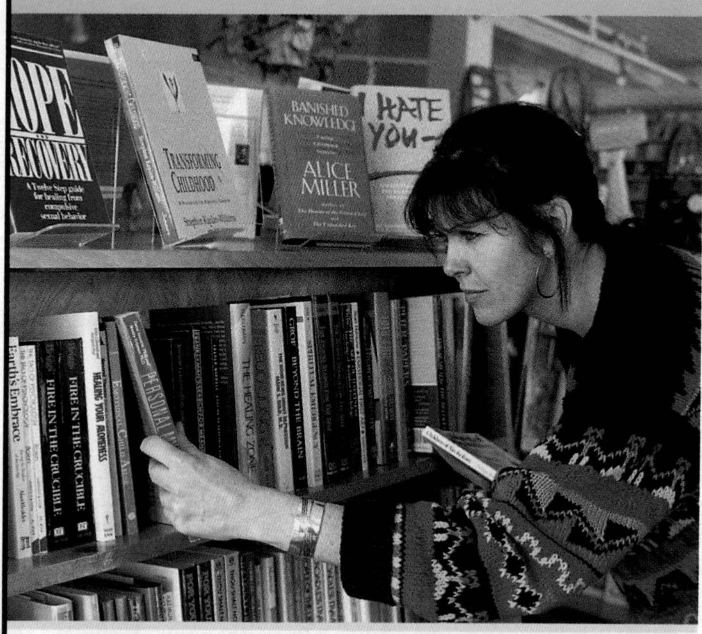

(FIGURE 7-9) **There are many books written by qualified medical and health professionals that can be of help in trying to deal with an emotional problem.**

When to Seek Help for Mental and Emotional Health Problems

You may need to obtain professional help with your problems if you experience any of the following characteristics.

- a prolonged feeling of depression and hopelessness
- a feeling that life is out of control
- the inability to concentrate and make decisions
- difficulty getting along with family and friends
- intense fears
- persistent difficulty sleeping
- emotional problems coping with a physical illness
- inability to stop destructive behaviors like drinking, overeating, and abusing drugs

Mental and Emotional Health Services

If you need help or if someone you know needs help, contact a person you trust. That may be a parent, a teacher, a school counselor, a doctor, or a member of the clergy. Don't wait, thinking that the problems will clear up. Deep problems can only clear up if *you* take some action.

Section 7.4 Lesson Plan

MOTIVATE

Journal 7D
Attitudes Toward Mental Illness

As a warm-up activity, talk with students about their attitudes toward emotional illness and the mentally ill. Would they avoid, talk to, or try to help a mentally ill person? Most people misunderstand and fear mental illness, adding to the false mystique of shame and secrecy that surrounds it. How do students think this attitude can be changed? Have students turn to the Student Journal and complete this statement: "If my friend were mentally ill, I'd ______."

TEACH

Role-Playing
Recognizing Signs of Mental Illness

Have students work in small groups to come up with skits in which one student exhibits several of the signs of mental illness, and others play friends or family members. The audience can make notes telling what signs they saw and when family or friends should have been alerted.

Most communities provide mental and emotional health services. These services may be offered through community mental health centers, local hospitals, and numerous other agencies. Agencies like these in your community are listed in your local telephone book. Look in the phone book under *hospitals, psychologists, psychotherapists, mental health information, and treatment centers.*

In addition, hotline phone services are available in many communities. Where these exist, information and counseling are provided over the phone.

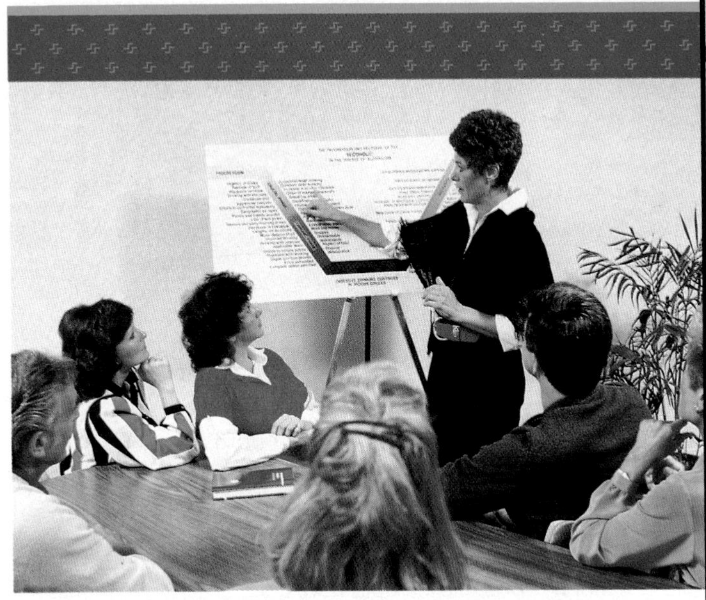

(FIGURE 7-10) **Support groups such as Al-Anon, Alateen, Alcoholics Anonymous, and many others can provide the support needed to work through specific emotional problems. The Yellow Pages of your phone book can provide information for contacting various support groups in your community.**

Mental and Emotional Health Therapies

Mental health specialists help people with mental and emotional health problems. For a description of the various types of mental health specialists, see the Career Appendix. The goal of therapy is to help a person work

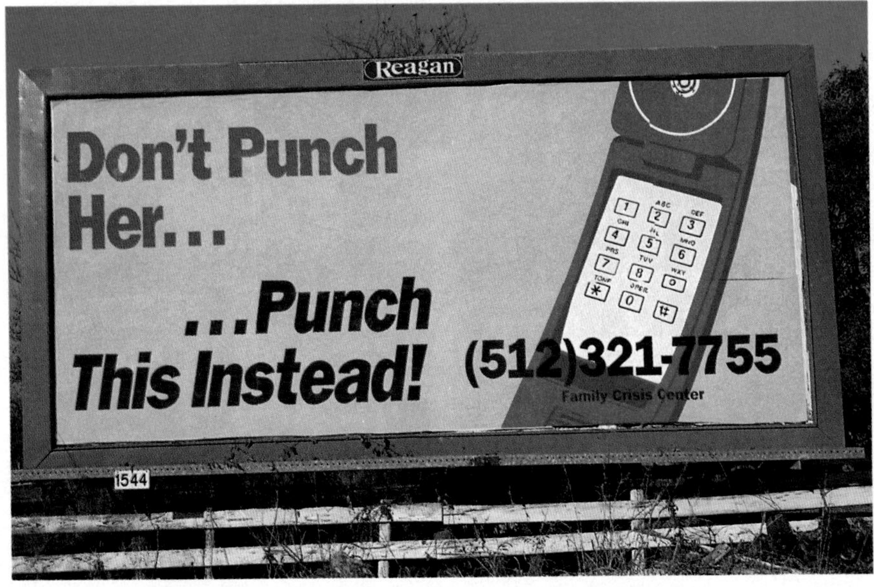

(FIGURE 7-11) **There are many sources of help in your community for emotional problems.**

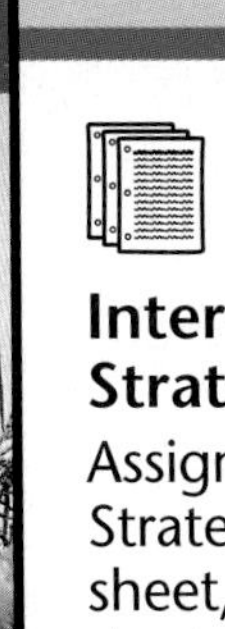

Life Skills Worksheet 7C

Intervention Strategies

Assign the Intervention Strategies Life Skills Worksheet, which asks students to identify the need for counseling and consider strategies for persuading someone to seek help.

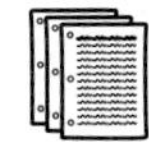

Life Skills Worksheet 7D

Help in Your Community

Assign the Help in Your Community Life Skills Worksheet, which asks students to assess community resources for obtaining therapy.

Making a Choice 7A

Coping With Mental and Emotional Disorders

Assign the Coping With Mental and Emotional Disorders card. The card asks students to discuss coping strategies for living with a family member who is mentally ill.

Class Discussion
Mental Illness—Helping Yourself and Others

Ask students to name actions they could take if they believed a friend or relative were mentally ill. Allow students to argue the pros and cons of actions described and list the most valuable of these on the chalkboard. *(Some possible actions might include notifying a responsible adult, not leaving the person alone, remaining calm and nonjudgmental.)* Stress that it takes a trained mental health professional to diagnose and treat mental illness. However, students should be aware of behaviors that indicate mental illness and should have thought of positive actions they can take.

Debate the Issue
Mental Health Checkups

Have students debate the issue: Employers and schools should offer preventive insurance for periodic mental health checkups for employees and students.

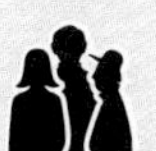

Cooperative Learning
Community Mental Health Resources

Divide the class into small groups to gather information about mental health services. Supply a phone book to each group for locating local telephone numbers and addresses. You may also suggest that groups contact a national or state organization, such as the following, for free materials.

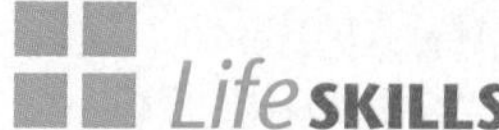

Choosing a Therapist
Discuss the guidelines with students. If possible, ask a therapist to visit the class and discuss these issues of choice and treatment.

Making a Choice 7B

Assessing Attitudes
Assign the Assessing Attitudes card. The card asks students to examine prevailing attitudes about therapy.

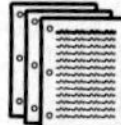

Section Review Worksheet 7.4
Assign Section Review Worksheet 7.4, which requires students to identify types of therapy, to describe behaviors that suggest a need for professional help, and to list resources for finding professional help.

Section Quiz 7.4
Have students take Section Quiz 7.4.

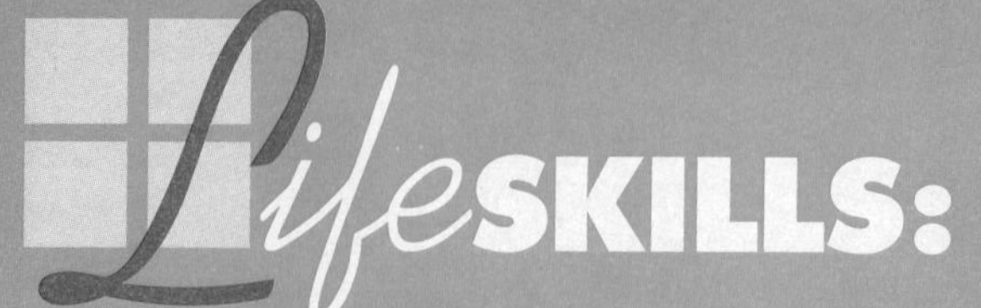

Using Community Resources

Choosing a Therapist

At some time during your life, you or someone close to you will feel the need to seek professional counseling. In choosing a therapist, consider the following guidelines.

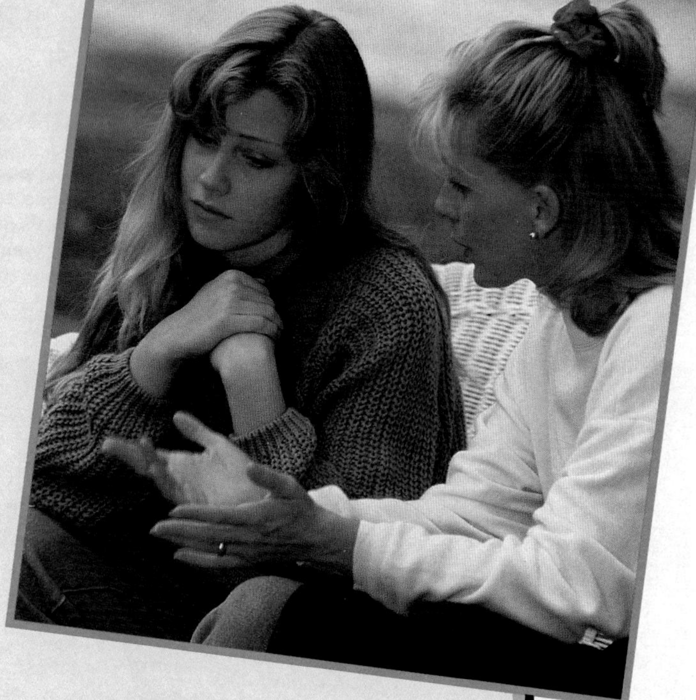

1. Check the background certification, experience, and credentials of the therapist. Does the therapist have a state license?
2. Find out how often you would see the therapist. Do you feel it is frequent enough to meet your needs?
3. Find out if the therapist has experience dealing with problems similar to yours.
4. Use an introductory session to determine whether you feel comfortable with the setting and how the therapist plans to work with you.
5. Look for signs that you are being treated with respect. Do you feel the therapist is concerned about your situation? Do you feel the therapist can be trusted with very personal information about your life? If you are not being treated in an appropriate manner, find another therapist. Do not ever feel you must continue with someone who makes you continually uncomfortable.
6. If during treatment you start to feel very uncomfortable, or if you do not feel you are making any progress, discuss the situation with your therapist. If you cannot resolve the issues, you should feel no obligation to continue with this therapist.

• • • TEACH continued

- National Mental Health Association, 1021 Prince St., Alexandria, VA 22314-2971 (703) 684-7722
- National Institute of Mental Health, 5600 Fishers Ln. 15C-105, Rockville, MD 20857 (301) 443-3673

Have groups compare lists to avoid duplication. Students within a group can divide their lists and call or write to various services and agencies to find out details of their operation—what is their principal role, what sorts of problems do they treat, what sorts of therapy do they offer, who is eligible, how expensive is therapy, what community outreach is available, how do they educate the public?

Class Discussion
Benefits of Group Therapy

How might group therapy be beneficial to a person dealing with a specific crisis? *[It dispels the myth that one is alone with his or her problem; promotes social and communication skills; provides sounding boards and support for trying out new behaviors.]*

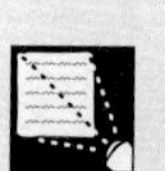

Teaching Transparency 7A
Mental and Emotional Health

Use the transparency to summarize the information in this chapter.

Extension
History of Treatment of Mentally Ill Patients

Until fairly recently in history, the mentally ill were treated as less than human.

through difficulties so that he or she can return to normal activities and be more capable of dealing with challenges. Different therapies may be used.

Psychoanalysis Psychoanalysis is a form of therapy used to examine unresolved conflicts from the past. For example, Clancy earns extra money by doing odd jobs for people. But he tries to avoid anything that involves climbing over 5 ft. high on a ladder. He could make lots more money if he were not afraid of heights so he decided to undergo psychoanalysis. Clancy discovered during treatment that he had been stranded in a treehouse as a child when the ladder to the treehouse fell down. Although he had forgotten the incident, the fear of the experience made him terrified of heights. The psychoanalyst helped him discover the source of his fear, which may in turn help Clancy overcome his fear of heights.

The process of psychoanalysis was developed by Sigmund Freud. He believed that unresolved conflicts surface as problems later in life. The person examines experiences to improve awareness. The intent is that awareness helps the person understand and resolve the problems.

Behavioral Therapy Behavioral therapy focuses on the patient's behavior, rather than on the underlying causes of problems. The therapist rewards desirable behavior

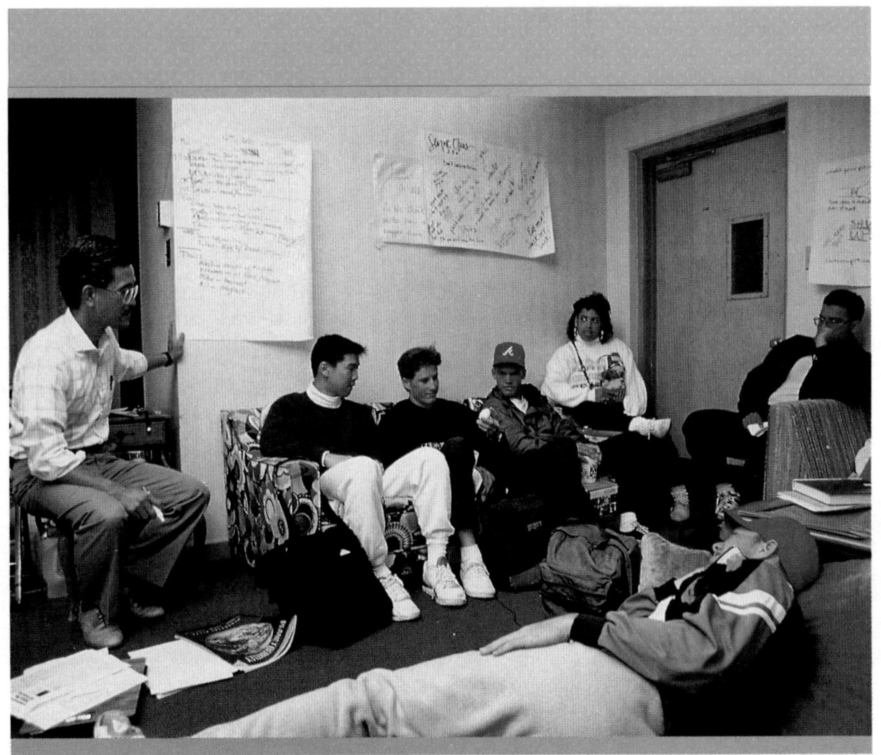

(FIGURE 7-12) **Group therapy can provide a supportive environment and a broader view for dealing with problems.**

Section 7.4

Reteaching Worksheet 7.4

Students who have difficulty with the material may complete Reteaching worksheet 7.4, which requires them to identify behaviors that signal a need for professional help, classify types of therapy, and list questions they might ask a therapist.

Review Answers

1. The person might be depressed, feel that his or her life is out of control, be unable to concentrate and make decisions, have difficulty getting along with others, have intense fears, be unable to sleep, have emotional problems coping with illness, or be unable to stop destructive behaviors.

2. Students should list a community hospital, agency, or mental health center where psychiatrists, psychologists, psychotherapists, or social workers are available.

Have students research and report on ways different societies in different ages have treated the mentally ill. Some students may prefer to learn about the work of people who pioneered in mental health reform, such as Phillipe Pinel, Dorothea Lynde Dix, and Clifford Whittingham Beers.

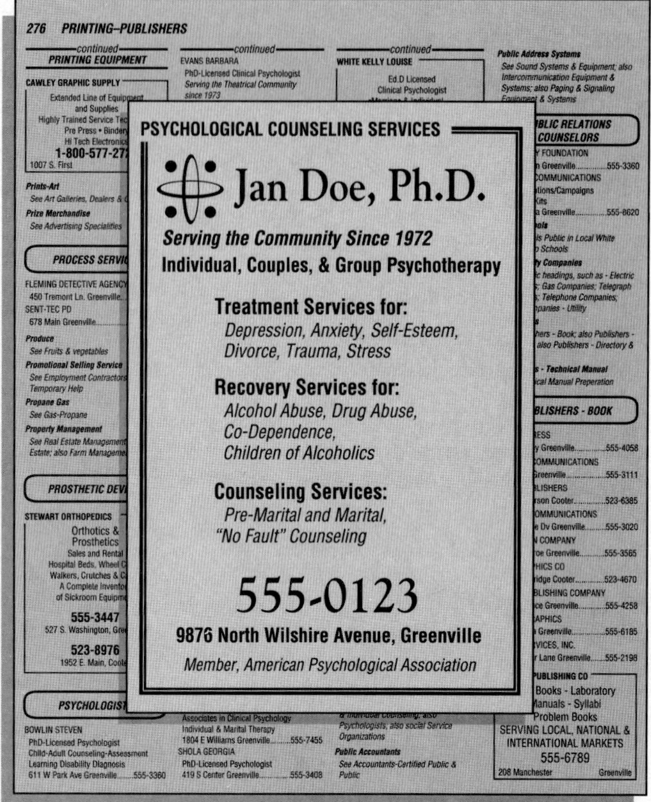

(FIGURE 7-13) **This advertisement is representative of the kind of mental health services provided by counselors.**

and punishes undesirable behavior. This process is called **behavior modification**. Behavior modification programs help patients learn new ways to respond to situations, ways more effective than the ones they were using.

Group Therapy Group therapy involves meetings of people with similar problems. They meet with a therapist to discuss their problems, and the therapist and group suggest solutions. Group therapy suggests that more heads are better than one. Hearing ideas or analyses from a group of people will have a greater effect on the patient than hearing one perspective.

Chemical Therapy Chemical therapy is the use of drugs to treat mental and emotional disorders. Drugs are prescribed to help control some symptoms of a disorder, such as aggressiveness or to correct an imbalance of chemicals in the brain that can cause disorders like depression. Though drugs can bring some conditions under control, it is important to note that there can be serious side effects to their use. For example, the antidepressant *Prozac* works very well in controlling depression for some patients. In other patients, it appears to cause violent or suicidal behavior. As with any perscription medication, the use of these drugs should be closely monitored for possible serious side effects.

Review

1. *How would you know if your best friend or someone in your family needed counseling?*
2. *List the places in your community where you could go if you were having an emotional problem. List one place you could go if you had an eating disorder. List two places you could go if there was a problem in your family that required counseling.*
3. *Make a list of four questions you would ask if you were choosing a therapist.*
4. *How does group therapy differ from behavior modification?*
5. ***Critical Thinking*** *If you were suffering from a mental or emotional problem, who would you go to for advice?*

Answers to Questions 1 and 2 are on p. 171.

3. Answers may include: What type of certification do you have? Do you have experience dealing with my type of problem? What degree do you hold? Do you have a state license? What are your fees? What are your hours? How often would I need to see you?

4. Behavior modification deals with an individual. It uses techniques that reward desirable behavior and ignore or punish undesirable behavior. Group therapy involves meeting with several people who have the same problem. The therapist and group members will often suggest solutions for other members' problems, as well as provide support.

5. Students might respond that they would seek the advice of a parent, teacher, coach, school counselor, school nurse, school social worker, or member of the clergy. Students may even call a hotline number for mental and emotional problems.

ASSESS

Section Review

Have students answer the Section Review questions.

Alternative Assessment

Giving Advice

Ask students to imagine they are advice columnists who have received a letter from a young girl. She is frightened by the way her mother has been acting lately and describes symptoms and behaviors indicative of manic-depressive disorder. Have each student write the girl's letter and a reply to it.

Closure

Qualifications of a Mental Health Specialist

With the class, compile a list of skills and personal qualities students think are important in a mental health professional. Write the ideas on the chalkboard. Students should be ready to explain why each characteristic they suggested is important.

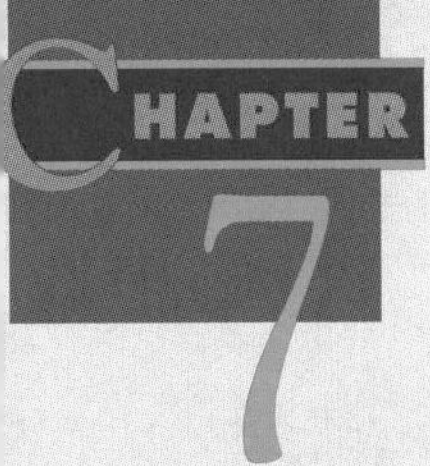

Highlights

Summary

- According to the National Association for Mental Health, someone with good mental health feels comfortable with himself or herself, has good relationships with others, and meets the demands of life.
- It is important to express emotions in a positive way.
- Defense mechanisms provide a way to deal with problems and maintain self-esteem. Overuse of these mechanisms is not healthy.
- Maslow believed that all individuals can achieve self-actualization or a state of fulfillment if their basic physiological needs are met first.
- It is just as important to seek help for emotional problems as it is to seek help for physical problems.
- Most difficult times can be worked through without outside help. Sometimes, however, you may need to ask for help from friends, parents, or mental health specialists.
- Some therapies that certain specialists practice are psychoanalysis, behavioral therapy, group therapy, and chemotherapy.

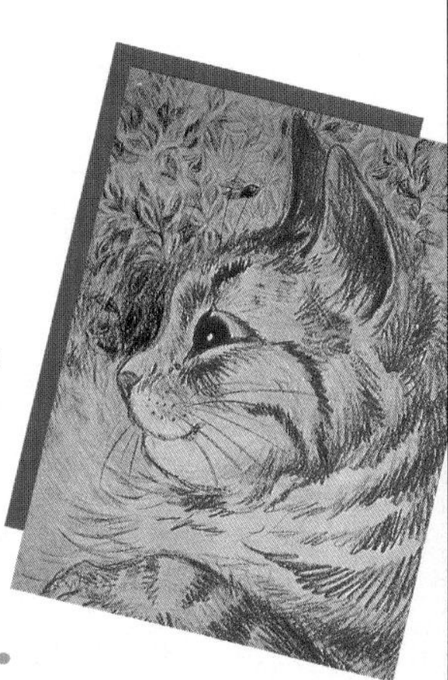

Vocabulary

self-concept the current mental image you have of yourself.

self-ideal your mental image of what you would like to be.

organic disorders mental and emotional disorders resulting from a physical cause.

eating disorders compulsive eating behaviors caused by emotional problems and an obsession with body weight.

anxiety disorder a condition in which fear or anxiety prevents one from enjoying life and completing everyday tasks.

dissociative disorder a condition in which someone's personality changes to the point that the person believes he or she is someone else.

mood disorder a condition in which one mood is experienced almost to the exclusion of other feelings.

personality disorder an emotional condition in which a person's patterns of behavior negatively affect that person's ability to get along with others.

somatoform disorder an emotional condition in which there are physical symptoms but no identifiable disease or injury. The physical symptoms are caused by psychological factors.

Chapter 7 Highlights Strategies

Summary

Have students read the summary to reinforce the concepts they learned in Chapter 7.

Vocabulary

Have students write a paragraph about mental and emotional health that uses a minimum of eight of the chapter's vocabulary words correctly.

Extension

Have students write true-false or multiple choice items for a mental illness awareness quiz. Go over these in class and have students select 10 items that they think would best educate the general public about mental illness. Suggest that students make posters that convey some of the items selected. Display the posters in the school or, if possible, in a public place such as the local library or community center.

Chapter 7 Assessment

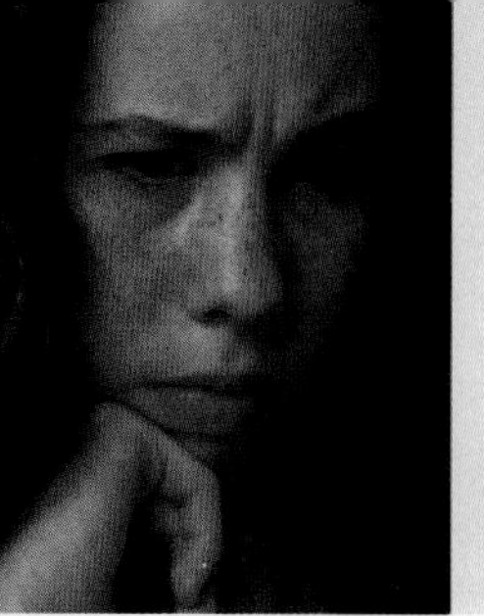

Chapter Review

Concept Review

1. Which of the following characteristics define good mental health?
   - fears new experiences
   - has good relationships with others
   - avoids responsibility
   - has a negative attitude
   - meets the demands of life

   Add one characteristic of your own.
2. Identify and describe four emotions most people experience.
3. Why is loneliness a particular problem for teens?
4. In what way can guilt be a positive emotion?
5. Why should you avoid using defense mechanisms too frequently?
6. According to Maslow, when do people grow emotionally? What does reaching the top of the scale represent?
7. Name three possible causes of organic disorders. Are organic disorders more or less serious than other types of mental and emotional problems? Why?
8. Panic attacks and phobias are examples of what kind of disorder?
9. List three factors that are linked to developing depression.
10. Describe four treatments for mental disorders.

Expressing Your Views

1. Your text states that eating disorders are most often caused by parents. Do you agree? Why or why not?
2. Martin's grandmother died recently. He has been very depressed, so he decided to go to a therapist. His friends have been very critical and told him that anyone who seeks counseling is weak. How should Martin respond to these people?
3. Every time Ruth fails at something she rationalizes her failure. Why do you think she does this? How could this behavior be harmful?

Chapter Review

Concept Review

1. Has good relationships; meets the demands of life; feels comfortable with himself or herself

2. Love—a strong feeling of affection for someone; happiness—feeling of joy or contentment; optimism—feeling that life experiences will be positive; humor—finding something funny in a situation; fear—feeling of danger; anger—strong feeling of irritation; guilt—feeling that you have done something wrong or are responsible for some mishap; depression—feelings of sadness and despair; jealousy—feeling of wanting something someone else has or of losing something you have; loneliness—feeling of isolation or alienation; shyness—feeling of being timid or bashful

3. As teens try to become independent they can alienate one another and feel lonely.

4. Feeling guilty can be a clue that you need to resolve a problem. Guilt may also drive you to do the right thing.

5. Defense mechanisms are often used to avoid facing an issue. If the issue is never resolved, it may become a bigger problem.

6. When they can satisfy their needs from the bottom to the top of the hierarchy; reaching one's potential

7. Genetic; response to various life experiences; physical illness, injury, or chemical imbalance. Usually they are more serious because they involve the body as well as the mind.

8. Anxiety disorders

9. Family history, major life stresses, physical illness, substance abuse, and gender

10. Psychoanalysis is a form of therapy used to examine unresolved conflicts from the past. Behavioral therapy focuses on the patient's behavior rather than on the underlying causes of problems. Group therapy involves meetings of people with similar problems. Chemotherapy is the use of drugs to treat mental and emotional disorders.

Expressing Your Views

1. Yes. Functional disorders are not caused by any physical problems, therefore, they must be caused by the environment.

Chapter 7 Assessment

Life Skills Check

1. Coping
You are angry because one of your friends borrowed your car and burned a hole in the seat. Now your friend refuses to help pay for the damage. How could you handle your anger in a positive way?

2. Using Community Resources
Your sister has been acting strangely for the past few months. You are worried about her and think she probably needs help. What advice would you give her? Where could she go for help?

3. Using Community Resources
Find out what 12-step programs are and make a list of those in your area. Include information on how these programs are connected to spiritual health.

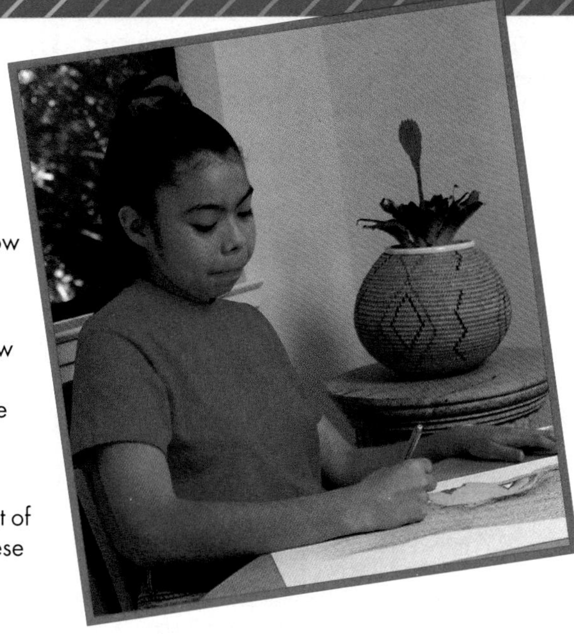

Projects

1. Maslow thought Abraham Lincoln, Eleanor Roosevelt, and Thomas Jefferson were self-actualized people. Name someone you would add to Maslow's list and write a one-page essay describing your reasons for choosing this person.
2. Read *One Flew Over the Cuckoo's Nest* by Ken Kesey and note the mental disorders of the characters.
3. Work with a group to compile a list of activities in your school or community that promote good mental health. Suggest other activities that could be offered.
4. Why do you think some music is called the blues? Visit the library to find out the history of the blues. Prepare a brief report and presentation that includes some examples of blues music.

Plan for Action

The things people say about themselves often indicate how they feel about themselves. Write 10 statements about yourself in order to evaluate your self-concept, and, if necessary, devise a plan for improvement.

2. He should remember that feeling depressed is a normal part of the grieving process. He should keep in mind that he is a stronger person for seeking help when he finds that he cannot cope with these feelings on his own.
3. Ruth is using the defense mechanism of rationalization. Ruth is using rationalization to avoid facing an issue. This can be harmful because Ruth is not taking responsibility for her failure.

Life Skills Check

1. I could do something physical to release my anger, such as exercise.
2. I would advise that she talk with a person she could trust, such as a teacher, a school counselor, a school nurse, her parents, myself, or a religious leader.
3. Answers will vary, but lists should include the necessary information.

Projects

Have students complete the projects on mental health.

Plan for Action

Have students plan a mental illness awareness campaign. Various group assignments could include the following:

- creating a logo and visuals for posters, flyers, advertisements, or bumper stickers.
- writing public service announcements and columns that provide facts, and getting them broadcast.
- finding mental health specialists and inviting them to speak to health classes or an all-school assembly.

Assessment Options

Chapter Test

Have students take the Chapter 7 Test.

Alternative Assessment

Have students do the Alternative Assessment activity for Chapter 7.

Test Generator

The Test Generator (Macintosh® or IBM® format) contains an additional 50 assessment items for this chapter.

BUILDING SELF-ESTEEM

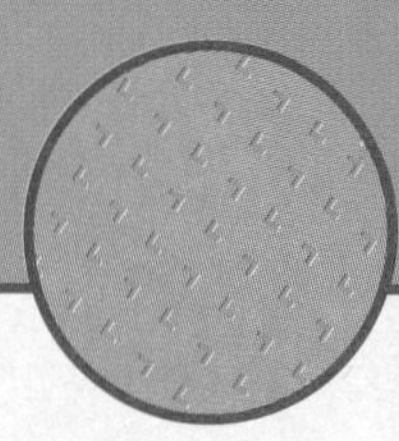

PLANNING GUIDE

TEXT SECTIONS	OBJECTIVES	TEXT FEATURES	OUTSIDE RESOURCES	NOTES
8.1 The Importance of Self-Esteem pp. 177-181 1 period	• Define self-esteem • Describe how self-esteem develops. • Explain how media messages can affect one's self-esteem. ■ Assess your own self-esteem.	■ LIFE SKILLS, Assessing Your Health, pp. 180-181 **ASSESSMENT** • Section Review, p. 179	**TEACHER'S RESOURCE BINDER** • Lesson Plan 8.1 • Personal Health Inventory • Journal Entries 8A, 8B • Section Review Worksheet 8.1 • Section Quiz 8.1 • Reteaching Worksheet 8.1 **OTHER RESOURCES** • Making a Choice 8A, 8B • Parent Discussion Guide • English/Spanish Audiocassette 3	
8.2 How to Build Your Self-Esteem pp. 182-186 2 periods	• Name the most important way of raising your self-esteem. • Name at least three other ways of raising your self-esteem. ■ Make a plan to raise your own self-esteem. ■ Use a self-esteem scale to assess your health.	**ASSESSMENT** • Section Review, p. 186	**TEACHER'S RESOURCE BINDER** • Lesson Plan 8.2 • Journal Entries 8C, 8D • Life Skills 8A, 8B, 8C, 8D • Section Review Worksheet 8.2 • Section Quiz 8.2 • Reteaching Worksheet 8.2 **OTHER RESOURCES** • Transparency 8A, 8B • Making a Choice 8B	
End of Chapter pp. 187-189		**ASSESSMENT** • Chapter Review pp. 188-189	**TEACHER'S RESOURCE BINDER** **OTHER RESOURCES** • Chapter Test • Alternative Assessment • Test Generator	

■ Denotes LIFE SKILLS objectives

• Items in blue are also part of the *Holt Health Activity Book.*

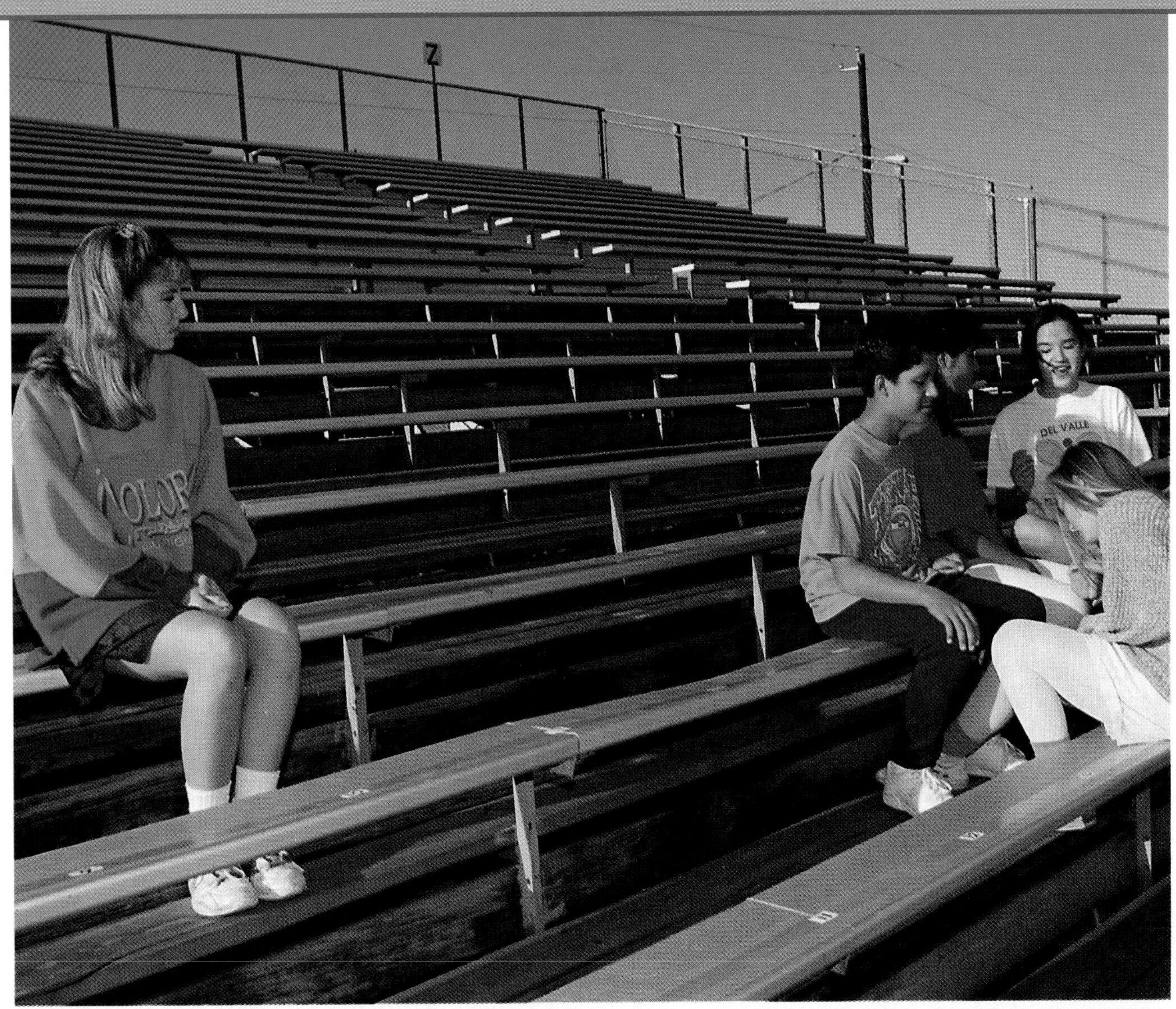

CONTENT BACKGROUND

Self-Esteem Among Adolescent Boys and Girls

RECENT STUDIES HAVE FOUND THERE IS an alarming drop in self-esteem among girls as they reach adolescence. There is a much smaller—but still significant—decline in boys' self-esteem during the same years. The Harvard Project on the Psychology of Women and the Development of Girls found that girls up to about age 10 are essentially self-confident, not much different from boys of the same age. Similarly, in a 1990 survey, the American Association of University Women (AAUW) found that 60 percent of girls studied in the elementary grades strongly agreed with the statement, "I'm happy the way I am." Sixty-seven percent of the 600 boys polled responded the same. However, by the time students reached middle school, only 56 percent of the boys and 37 percent of the girls strongly agreed with the statement. By high school, 46 percent of males still felt the same about their self-esteem, but the percentage of females who strongly agreed with the statement had dropped to 29. Among boys, 20 percent shifted from high self-esteem into a lower category; among girls the number was 31 percent.

Social scientists disagree on the reasons for this abrupt decline in self-esteem among girls. The

AAUW argues that the two most influential groups of adults in a child's life—parents and teachers—encourage different behavior in boys than in girls, to the detriment of girls. A study of 40 fathers and their daughters by the Harvard Couples and Family Center at Cambridge Hospital found that fathers seem to be more concerned than mothers that their children behave according to our society's sex-role stereotypes. Of the 40 girls in the study, those whose fathers offered verbal encouragement when they had problems putting together a jigsaw puzzle, had higher self-esteem than those whose fathers physically assisted in assembling the puzzle.

The AAUW further argues that schools "tailor instructional techniques to the learning style of boys." Researchers in the education department at American University in Washington, D.C., found that male students of all ages get more feedback than their female counterparts. These researchers contend that teachers work more closely with boys toward a solution to a problem than with girls. If a girl appears to be having difficulty with a question or a problem, most teachers are apt to solve it for her rather than encourage her to think critically.

Other researchers cite the change from the somewhat small, intimate environment of a middle school or junior high school to the larger, "impersonal" high school as another factor in the falling self-esteem of girls.

The biological changes that accompany puberty are also cited. Because girls can experience these bodily changes up to a year and a half earlier than most boys, girls may suffer more pronounced changes in self-confidence and self-esteem sooner than boys. And in a society that emphasizes the "perfect" body, teenage females with negative images of their bodies often succumb to eating disorders such as anorexia nervosa and bulimia.

Teachers and parents, made aware of their differential behavior toward girls and boys, can change the way they contribute to self-esteem problems among teenage girls. And the decline in self-esteem may gradually reverse for students who find close friends in high school.

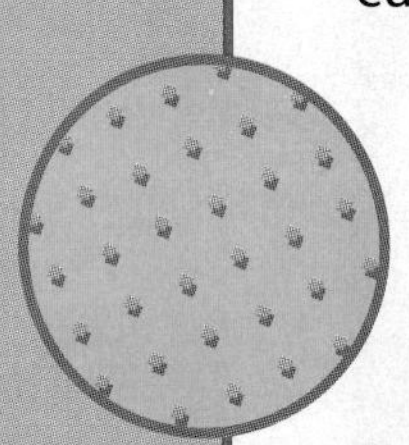

PLANNING FOR INSTRUCTION

KEY FACTS

- **Self-esteem is one's feeling of personal worth and acceptance. The level of self-esteem is directly related to ability to sustain relationships and cope with life.**
- **Parents play a vital role in developing self-esteem in their children.**
- **It is possible, but not simple, to change your level of self-esteem.**
- **A healthy, realistic view of your body is part of self-esteem.**
- **The most important part of raising self-esteem is accepting yourself.**
- **An important element of high self-esteem is appreciation of the worth of others and the ability to treat them with respect and compassion.**

MYTHS AND MISCONCEPTIONS

MYTH: Nobody likes to be around people who say good things about themselves.

People react most positively to those who recognize their good qualities and are self-confident without being overbearing.

MYTH: Modesty is the best policy; saying nothing about, or even belittling, yourself makes people like you more.

Failure to talk and think positively about yourself leads to a negative self-image which can quickly become self-fulfilling. People tend to see you as you see yourself.

MYTH: Copying the mannerisms of someone in the "in crowd" in order to be accepted causes you to lose your own personality.

One basic way of learning is through imitation. The teenage years are an important time for imitating different mannerisms and roles, and for experimenting with many aspects of self-expression. However, honesty is important; if a teen is trying on qualities he or she really doesn't like for reasons he or she doesn't like, it's time for reevaluation.

MYTH: People who are good looking always have a good self-image and high self-esteem.

People who don't feel good about their inner selves tend to have an unrealistic, critical body image, regardless of their looks. Their inner feelings of self-doubt extend to their outer appearance.

VOCABULARY

Essential: The following vocabulary terms appear in boldface type:

self-esteem
body image
positive self-talk
support group
self-disclosure

Secondary: Be aware that the following terms may come up during class discussion:

devalue
ethnicities
cultivate
distortions
transferring responsibility
generalization

FOR STUDENTS WITH SPECIAL NEEDS

Auditory Learners: Students who learn best by listening and speaking can spend several days making notes on comments they hear that signal how people value themselves. They can then analyze these comments and the contexts in which they occurred. For each negative comment, ask that they recreate the context and act out the scene, replacing the negative with a positive "I" statement.

Kinetic Learners: The body image projected by an individual depends on posture, gesture, manner of moving, and so on. For kinetic learners, suggest a three-day period in which they observe others and themselves. Ask them to isolate and demonstrate five elements of body language that communicate low self-esteem, and then suggest and show replacement behaviors that project a positive self-image.

At-Risk Students: Assist students in creating personal profiles of their self-esteem. Formats can be individualized, and headings might include "Who I Am" (likes, dislikes, strengths, weaknesses), "Starring Me!" (things I do well), "A Change Artist" (negatives I can do something about and a plan for changing them), and "The Feel-Good Gang" (people in my support group, or who I want in my support group).

ENRICHMENT

- Challenge students to write brief science fiction stories that illustrate the arbitrary way society assigns value to physical characteristics. Ask them to create characters exhibiting different levels of self-acceptance. For instance, in a society that especially values long necks, most long-necked people could have high self-esteem. One character, though short-necked, could have developed high self-esteem through positive experiences with parents and teachers who were not bound by social prejudices.
- Encourage students interested in art to study how artists have represented the ideal man and woman through the ages. Have them describe how the body images projected in paintings vary with different times in history.
- Ask students to compile a class history book of men and women who succeeded against great odds despite physical, social, or intellectual handicaps. Have them read biographies to discover the level of self-esteem the person showed at each stage: Did high self-esteem help a disadvantaged person to succeed? Or, did success contribute to increased self-esteem? What patterns do students see?

CHAPTER 8 CHAPTER OPENER

CHAPTER 8

Building Self-Esteem

◆ ◆ ◆ ◆

Everyone does something well. If you make the most of whatever it is you do well, you will build your self-esteem.

GETTING STARTED

Using the Chapter Photograph

Ask: **What are these kids doing? Why do you think they are doing this?** *[Showing one another dance steps; seeing who is the best dancer; showing off their dancing skills. They might do it to entertain each other, to feel good about themselves, to get feedback about how well they have learned the steps, and so on.]* Have students brainstorm for skills and qualities that they have or would like to have. Encourage a wide variety of responses. Write the responses on the chalkboard. Discuss why people need to feel that they do something well or that they have admirable qualities.

Question Box

Have students write out any questions they have about self-esteem and how to acquire it and put them in the Question Box. The Question Box gives students an opportunity to ask questions anonymously. To ensure that students with questions are not embarrassed to be seen writing, have students who do not have questions write something else—such as something they already know about self-acceptance and body image—on the paper instead.

Preview the questions and then answer them at appropriate points in the chapter. You may wish to allow the students to write additional anonymous questions as they go through the chapter.

Personal Issues *ALERT*

The teenage years are a uniquely difficult time for building and maintaining self-esteem. Teens fear rejection by their peers, for this is the group whose opinions matter most to them. The fear of rejection is even stronger in students with low self-esteem, who may not have close relationships with peers. Watch for feedback that may alert you to students who are more sensitive than most to rejection. This chapter provides some unique opportunities for individuals to assess their ability to overcome negative self-image and shyness. However, students should not be forced, and right to privacy must be respected.

Lindsey feels ugly and unlikable. She compares herself with the models in the fashion magazines and wishes she could be as thin. When she looks in the mirror, she sees a chubby girl. Yet Lindsey is 5'3" tall and weighs only 105 lbs. She isn't really chubby at all. She constantly fantasizes about being popular, but feels that she doesn't have a chance. She is very shy and doesn't often talk to other students because she is afraid they won't like her.

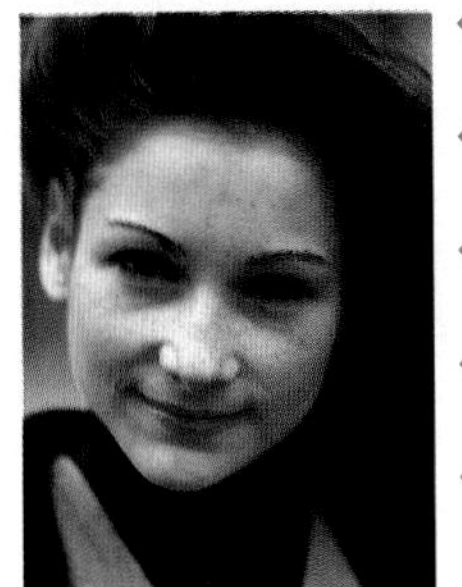

Lindsey realizes that many people her age feel the way she does. However, she has made a silent promise to herself to find ways to feel better about herself and her life.

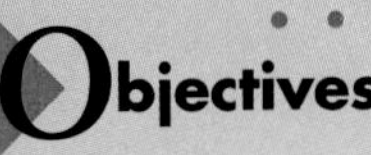

Section 8.1 The Importance of Self-Esteem

Objectives

- *Define self-esteem.*
- *Describe how self-esteem develops.*
- *Explain how media messages can affect one's self-esteem.*
- *Assess your own self-esteem.*
  - ***LIFE SKILLS: Assessing Your Health***

Self-esteem is your pride in and acceptance of yourself. It is your sense of personal worth. When you feel worthwhile, you are able to make good decisions, experience acceptance from others, and give and receive love.

Lindsey has decided to improve her self-esteem. To do so, she must learn to respect herself, consider herself worthy, and avoid comparing herself with others.

Your self-esteem influences your relationships with your family, friends, teachers, and bosses. It affects how you do in school and at work. Low self-esteem can be very damaging, and has been linked to serious problems such as alcohol and drug abuse, eating disorders, suicide, and other self-destructive behaviors.

How Self-Esteem Develops

The development of self-esteem begins at birth. Early on, our feelings about ourselves tend to be a reflection of how we are treated by the people most important in our lives—usually our parents or guardians. We learn to see ourselves as we think they see us.

Most parents love their children and wouldn't knowingly do anything to damage their child's self-esteem. But parents are only human. Sometimes they don't say exactly what they mean. For example, a

self-esteem:

pride in and acceptance of yourself; your sense of personal worth.

Background
Shaping Young Lives

Teacher expectations play a vital role in young students' success. One study of grade-school students and teachers involved an intelligence test. Teachers were told, following the test, which students ranked in the top 20 percent of the class. (Actually, the tests were not scored, and the names were picked at random.) Most of the students said to be at the top of the class had previously been considered average by the teachers. Nonetheless, teachers' attitudes toward these students now changed: they became more respectful and confident of the students' success; and their body language toward the students was more positive (smiling, eye contact, leaning toward student, nodding). In a follow-up, this 20 percent of the students tested significantly higher than other classmates on the IQ test. The superior performance was attributed solely to change in teacher attitude.

Section 8.1 Lesson Plan

MOTIVATE

Journal 8A
Lindsey's Decision

This may be done as a warm-up activity. Ask students to study the photograph of Lindsey after they read about her problem. Encourage them to write down their reactions to Lindsey's feelings about herself in the Student Journal in the Student Activity Book.

Class Discussion
A Teenager's Self-Image

To start students thinking about how teenagers form perceptions of themselves, ask: Why do you think Lindsey believes she is overweight? What might be some reasons she feels unlikable? Do you think her fears and concerns are grounded in a realistic view of herself? Why or why not?

TEACH

Class Discussion
Feeling Good About Yourself

Have students personalize a definition of self-esteem by brainstorming for words that describe feelings associated with high self-esteem. (Students might suggest the following adjectives: confident, likable, valuable, content, capable, lovable, self-accepting, secure.) Next, have them do the same for

Background

Tips for Building Self-Esteem

Here are some ways of nurturing self-esteem in youth.

1. Give plenty of praise.
2. Praise effort, not just accomplishment.
3. Help the young person set realistic goals.
4. Avoid comparing the young person's efforts with others'.
5. Take responsibility for your own negative feelings. (Use "I" messages rather than blaming.)
6. Give real responsibility.
7. Show you care.

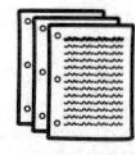

Personal Health Inventory

Have students complete the Personal Health Inventory for this chapter. The inventory helps them assess their self-esteem.

parent might say, "I don't like you very much when you fight with your brother." The child may think the parent means, "I don't like you." It would be better if the parent said, "I get scared and nervous when you and your brother fight." That way, the parent makes it very clear that it is the behavior that is being criticized, not the worth of the child.

But parents aren't psychologists. The odds are that most parents aren't even aware that their words are so harsh. Most parents honestly want to support and encourage their children and help them feel loved. They try, but they don't always do everything perfectly.

A more serious situation exists when parents neglect or abuse their children. Jonathan, for example, grew up without the care and attention he needed. He was a neglected child. His mom suffered from depression, and Jonathan remembers many days when his mother spent the entire day in bed. Since Jonathan's dad worked long hours, he wasn't around much. It seemed that the only time his parents paid any attention to him was when he did something wrong. By the time he got to high school, Jonathan had very low self-esteem.

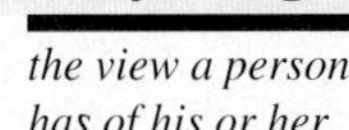

body image: *the view a person has of his or her body.*

At some point during the first years of life, we make a "decision" about our own worth, based on how we think others see us. The decision is not a conscious one, but it is a decision nevertheless. After a while, it seems to be reality. You look at your feelings and behaviors and think, That's the way I am.

Because self-esteem is a decision, a person can make a new decision later in life. You can decide, like Lindsey, to raise your self-esteem.

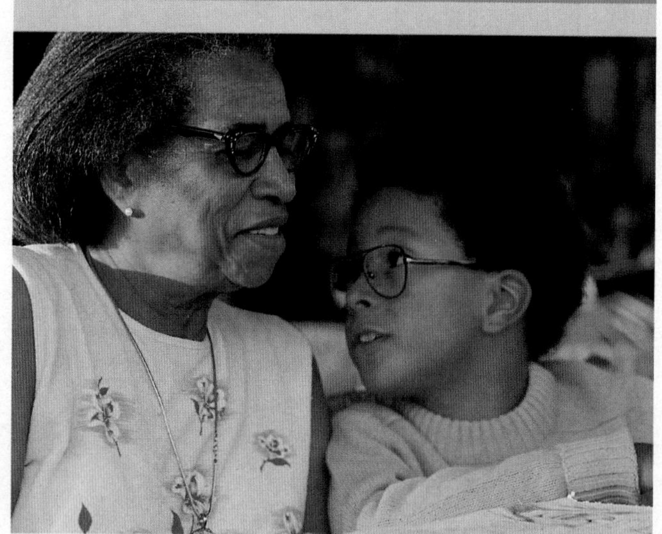

(FIGURE 8-1) **We make a "decision" about our own worth early in life, based on how we think other people view us.**

Body Image, Media Messages, and Self-Esteem

Your **body image** is your view of your body—how you see your appearance, your fitness, and your health. It is sometimes difficult for teenagers to maintain a positive body image, because during the teen years so many natural physical changes are taking place.

Teenage girls have an especially hard time, because of media messages that say girls and women must look a certain way in order to be considered attractive. Lindsey has a negative body image, because she compares herself with very thin models in advertisements.

People are constantly bombarded with magazine and television advertisements that show "perfect" faces and bodies. This can cause us to devalue ourselves because we look different, which lowers our self-esteem. Lindsey looks at the ads showing extremely thin women, and without realizing it, she chooses these women as the standard by which she must judge herself.

• • • TEACH continued

words associated with low self-esteem. (Students might name the following descriptives: unwanted, dissatisfied, unassertive, weak, useless, inferior, withdrawn, frustrated.)

Cooperative Learning

Guiding Children Without Criticism

Working in small groups, students can invent situations in which a parent must react to correct a child or keep the child safe from harm. For each situation, the group should write a command or comment that seems critical of the child and that might damage self-esteem. They should then write a second command that will correct the problem without undermining the child's feelings of worth.

Class Discussion

Society's Body Image

Have several magazines in which students can search for advertisements projecting "desirable" body images. Allow students to react to them and to discuss their feelings about the standards society seems to set for them. **What is the perfect body? face? personality? Who decides what is perfect? Why would anyone want or need to be perfect?**

Point out to students that no one's body is as perfect as those in the pictures. The pictures of the models are often altered in some other way to remove blemishes, shadows, or add or change colors.

(FIGURE 8-2) **Standards of beauty change. In the 1950s, women with curves were considered attractive. A decade later, extremely thin women were fashionable. There is nothing wrong with any body type, but there *is* something wrong with media messages that encourage people to feel bad about their bodies.**

The funny thing about advertising is that the "perfect" face and body change over time. Thin bodies for women may be fashionable at one time, and curvaceous bodies may be fashionable at another. Women who would be considered beautiful in one time might be thought unattractive in another. If you look at ads from earlier periods, you see how our ideal of beauty has changed. However, people cannot very well change their bodies with the fashion.

An important thing for Lindsey to learn is that there is nothing wrong with her body type. But there *is* something wrong with the advertisements that make her feel bad about her body.

If Lindsey looked around her, she would see that success comes in all kinds of "packages." Success comes to people of both sexes, of all ethnicities, and of various body types, from fat to very thin. It comes to plain people, good-looking people, tall people, short people, and people with physical disabilities. Lindsey could think of a well-known person in each of these categories who has developed unique gifts and become a star in his or her field.

Review

1. *Define self-esteem.*
2. *Describe how a person's self-esteem develops.*
3. *Explain how media messages can affect a person's self-esteem.*
4. ***LIFE SKILLS: Assessing Your Health*** *Describe what you have learned about your own self-esteem.*
5. ***Critical Thinking*** *How do you think poverty could contribute to low self-esteem?*

Review Answers

1. Pride in, and acceptance of, oneself; a person's sense of personal worth
2. Self-esteem begins at birth and develops as a person reflects on and internalizes messages about herself or himself from important people in her or his life. These people include parents or guardians, other family members, peers, and teachers.
3. The media can have a negative effect on a person's self-esteem if that person does not have a body image that matches the "perfect" body that the media promote.
4. Answers will vary depending on the students' individual evaluations of self-esteem.
5. Answers will vary. The students may answer that the media, as well as society, portray poverty as undesirable. In this way, the media and society could negatively affect a person's self-esteem. Inability to buy clothes and other material items that the media or peers deem necessary could lower a person's self-esteem.

Have students look at Figure 8–2, and ask: **What contradiction do you see in these two images of "beauty"?** *[They represent different physical types, yet at different times each was considered beautiful.]* **What danger do you see in letting media images dictate the kind of physical traits that are desirable?** *[Dissatisfaction with self because of an arbitrary, unreal standard; seeking to conform to image by unhealthy dieting or even surgery; inability to accept self]*

Cooperative Learning

Comparing Your Positives and Negatives

You may suggest that students do this activity with a group of family members or friends. First, an individual should list his or her best and worst physical features in two columns on a sheet of paper. Next, the individual should ask six others to write a positive comment about his or her physical appearance on a slip of paper and compare these comments with the personal list. The comparison should reveal any positive features the individual has but did not notice about himself or herself.

Demonstration

Communicating Self-Image Through Body Language

Demonstrate for the class various postures, gestures, poses, and styles of movement that communicate positive self-image and acceptance of others

Making a Choice 18A

Body Image

Assign the Body Image Card to the students. It asks them to examine changing cultural values with respect to body language.

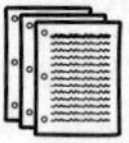

Section Review Worksheet 18.1

Assign Section Review Worksheet 8.1, which requires students to complete a concept map showing the definition and development of self-esteem.

Section Quiz 18.1

Have students take Section Quiz 8.1.

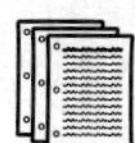

Reteaching Worksheet 18.1

Students who have difficulty with the material may complete Reteaching Worksheet 8.1, which asks students to classify components of self-esteem.

LifeSKILLS: Assessing Your Health

Self-Esteem Scale

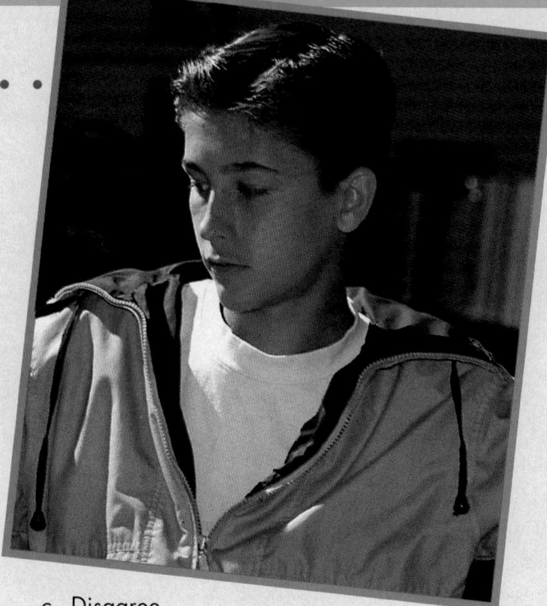

On a separate sheet of paper, write the letter that most accurately describes how you feel:

1. I feel that I'm a person of worth, at least equal to others.
 a. Strongly agree
 b. Agree
 c. Disagree
 d. Strongly disagree

2. I feel that I have a number of good qualities.
 a. Strongly agree
 b. Agree
 c. Disagree
 d. Strongly disagree

3. All in all, I am inclined to feel that I am a failure.
 a. Strongly agree
 b. Agree
 c. Disagree
 d. Strongly disagree

4. I am able to do things as well as most other people.
 a. Strongly agree
 b. Agree
 c. Disagree
 d. Strongly disagree

5. I feel I do not have much to be proud of.
 a. Strongly agree
 b. Agree
 c. Disagree
 d. Strongly disagree

6. I take a positive attitude toward myself.
 a. Strongly agree
 b. Agree
 c. Disagree
 d. Strongly disagree

• • • TEACH continued

(erect but relaxed posture, energetic walk, firm handshake, sitting forward with hands open and maintaining eye contact, and so on). Contrast these with body language that communicates lack of confidence and rejection of others (slouching, scuffing floor with each step, averting eyes, stiffness, sitting back with arms and legs crossed, and so on).

Case History

On Dave Dravecky

Dave Dravecky "had it all"—good looks, money, athletic skill, a loving family, and a brilliant career in pro baseball. However, in 1989 a cancerous tumor reappeared in his arm, and the entire arm and shoulder had to be removed in order to save his life. The story of his recovery and return to productive life is a lesson in self-acceptance and the real source of self-esteem. Ask students to locate articles about Dravecky's experience. Suggest that they prepare a brief report and be ready to explain how they think Dravecky conquered his fears and negative feelings.

Journal 8B

Self-Esteem Scale

Have students write in the Student Journal their reaction to the self-esteem score they tallied. Was the result a surprise? Would they like to improve their self-esteem? Then, suggest that they write a brief contract stating

Life **SKILLS**

Self-Esteem Scale

Have students complete the self-esteem scale, placing their answers on a separate sheet of paper. Then ask them to score their responses and evaluate their self-esteem as positive or negative.

7. On the whole, I am satisfied with myself.

a. Strongly agree

b. Agree

c. Disagree

d. Strongly disagree

8. I wish I could have more respect for myself.

a. Strongly agree

b. Agree

c. Disagree

d. Strongly disagree

9. I certainly feel useless at times.

a. Strongly agree

b. Agree

c. Disagree

d. Strongly disagree

10. At times I think I am no good at all.

a. Strongly agree

b. Agree

c. Disagree

d. Strongly disagree

Scoring. To score the scale and derive a measure of your self-esteem, follow these instructions.

1. The positive responses for questions 1–3 are:
question 1: (a) or (b)
question 2: (a) or (b)
question 3: (c) or (d)

If you answered two or three of these questions positively, give yourself 1 point.

2. The positive responses for questions 4 and 5 are:
question 4: (a) or (b)
question 5: (c) or (d)

If you answered either one or both of these questions positively, give yourself 1 point.

3. If your answer to question 6 was (a) or (b), give yourself 1 point.

4. If your answer to question 7 was (a) or (b), give yourself 1 point.

5. If your answer to question 8 was (c) or (d), give yourself 1 point.

6. If your answer to question 9 or 10 or both was (c) or (d), give yourself 1 point.

Add up all the points you gave yourself.

The range of scores on this self-esteem scale is 0–6. The higher the score, the more positive your self-esteem.

their intent to take responsibility for their attitudes toward themselves and change them if they feel they should.

Extension

Beauty of the Past

Have students locate and prepare copies of ideals of physical attractiveness for both men and women in an earlier time, such as the 1920s or the 1700s. Then have students work together to prepare a time-line display showing how viewpoints have changed through the years.

ASSESS

Section Review

Have students answer the Section Review questions.

Alternative Assessment

Self-Esteem Indicators

Have students make sketches of two people, one with high self-esteem and one with low self-esteem. It should show expression, posture, and other self-esteem indicators.

Closure

Letter to Yourself

Have students write a letter to themselves explaining why the teenage years are the most difficult in which to maintain high self-esteem, and making suggestions for ways to avoid feeling unlovable or worthless.

Background
Cognitive Therapists
Cognitive therapists are trained to help people learn the skill of positive self-talk. They teach clients to talk to themselves in order to change the way they think about things and to affirm that their feelings are OK. They also help clients break problems down into manageable parts and work on one aspect at a time to avoid seeing the problem as a catastrophe and as something that cannot be overcome.

Section 8.2 How to Build Your Self-Esteem

Objectives

- *Name the most important way of raising your self-esteem.*
- *Name at least three other ways of raising your self-esteem.*
- *Make a plan to raise your own self-esteem.*
  LIFE SKILLS: Building Self-Esteem

As you read earlier, self-esteem is a decision we make about our worth as people. The first self-esteem decision is made in childhood and is based on how we think about ourselves in relation to the "big people" around us.

If you have low self-esteem, you can make a new, more accurate, and more positive decision about yourself. You can acknowledge the influence of your past, but resolve to move on. Your self-esteem is now your responsibility. It isn't easy to raise low self-esteem, but it can be done. By deciding to take responsibility for yourself and your own self-esteem, you can make big changes in the way you see yourself. You will be delighted when you discover how much more fun and rewarding your life can be when you feel good about yourself.

Accept Yourself

Accepting yourself is the most important part of raising your self-esteem. This means learning to appreciate yourself and believing in your worth as a unique and special person.

How can you learn to accept yourself? First, realistically assess your strengths and weaknesses. Don't be modest. No one needs to know what you think your strengths are except you.

Second, try not to judge yourself by unrealistic standards. Don't, for example, compare your looks to the actors or actresses you see on television shows and in the movies.

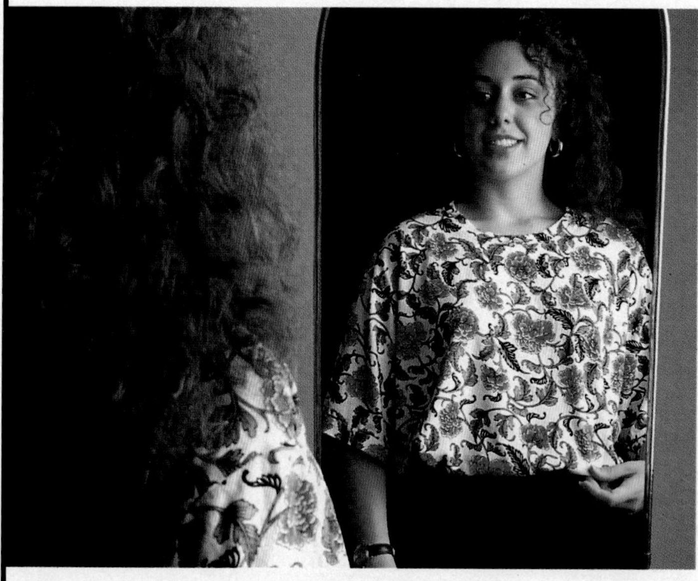

(FIGURE 8-3) **Accepting yourself just as you are is the most important part of raising your self-esteem. Though you aren't perfect, you are a unique and valuable person.**

Section 8.2 Lesson Plan

MOTIVATE

Journal 8C
Expectations of Yourself

This may be done as a warm-up activity. Most teenagers feel dissatisfied with themselves to some degree, often because of unreasonable expectations they place on themselves. Encourage students to write in the Student Journal, completing this statement: "I would feel really good about myself if I ___." Then ask that they explain to themselves whether they think this expectation is reasonable, and why.

TEACH

Reinforcement
Fighting Low Self-Esteem

Taking responsibility for how they view themselves may be hard for students with low self-esteem and intense feelings of helplessness and hopelessness. Stress that past events in their lives and their effects need to be acknowledged but that they do not control the future. Discussion of elements over which people do have control may be helpful to such students.

Class Discussion
Learning to Accept Yourself

Have students discuss which of the steps in learning to accept oneself would be most difficult for them. Then ask: **What phrases or statements can you think of that might help you**

Third, decide that you are o.k. as you are, even though there are things about yourself you would like to change. Remember that even though you aren't perfect, you are a unique person with value. No one else is exactly like you. No one else has exactly the same gifts to offer the world. There isn't a single person anywhere who is perfect, and it certainly isn't necessary that *you* be perfect.

Finally, expend energy on changing only the things about yourself that you *can* change. You can't change your height, for instance, so don't spend time worrying about it.

The more you accept and like yourself, the more others will accept and like you. If you project to others that you like yourself, they are less likely to judge you or to pressure you to conform to their ideals. And even if they do, you are less likely to cave in to their pressure.

Use Positive Self-Talk

We are constantly talking to ourselves—not necessarily out loud, but internally. Often this talk is negative. "I'm such an idiot," you might say to yourself. "Why did I do such a stupid thing?" Talking negatively like this can damage your self-esteem.

When you use **positive self-talk,** on the other hand, you can raise your self-esteem. Positive self-talk is talking in a positive way about yourself to yourself. An example of positive self-talk might be: "I did a great job on this project. I'm really good at this."

Lindsey usually feels nervous and uncomfortable around other students. "They think I'm no fun," she says to herself. "Why can't I ever think of anything interesting to say?" Because she feels this way and talks to herself this way, Lindsey appears to be awkward and shy.

Now suppose that Lindsey decides to use positive self-talk. She might say to herself, "I'm sometimes shy, but I can also be pretty funny, and people usually enjoy my company." As she talks to herself this way and begins to believe what she says, Lindsey will be more likely to converse with other students. As they begin to respond to her more positively, Lindsey's confidence will grow. She will become more comfortable with other people, and her self-esteem will improve.

Be Good at Something

Everyone has something he or she does well. Make the most of whatever it is *you* do well. It might be playing guitar, making up dance steps, playing basketball, telling stories, writing essays, making other people laugh, being a good friend—the possibilities are endless. Even if it's something as seemingly trivial as being good at bicycle stunts, you'll develop more confidence in yourself if you cultivate your natural ability. Being very good at one thing will also make it easier for you to try out new skills and take positive risks. You *know* that you're good at bicycle stunts, so if you try playing basketball and aren't so good at it, you won't feel too bad.

Use "I" Statements

If you take responsibility for your feelings and words by using "I" statements, you will build self-esteem. People with low self-esteem are often afraid to do this because they fear criticism.

For instance, when Lindsey says, "It is really hard to make friends," she is making a generalization that may not be true for other people. By beginning her statement with the impersonal pronoun "it," she is not taking responsibility for her feelings.

positive self-talk: *talking in a positive way to yourself about yourself.*

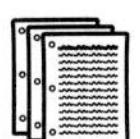

Life Skills Worksheet 8A

Wise Self-Disclosure

Assign the Wise Self-Disclosure Life Skills Worksheet, which requires students to evaluate the wisdom of self-disclosure to specific individuals.

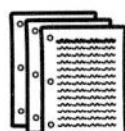

Life Skills Worksheet 8B

Finding Support Groups

Assign the Finding Support Groups Life Skills Worksheet, which requires students to locate support groups serving a variety of needs.

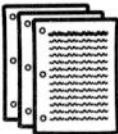

Life Skills Worksheet 8C

Choosing Supportive Relationships

Assign the Choosing Supportive Relationships Life Skills Worksheet, which requires students to evaluate the effect that other people have on a person's self-esteem.

carry out these positive steps? *[Possibilities include: "I'm good at ____," "Nobody's perfect," "You can't believe everything on TV," "I'm as good as anybody else," and "I'm trying to change the things I can about myself. The things I can't change, I accept."]* Suggest that students write several such statements on 3" x 5" cards and post them in their rooms or lockers, where they will see them often.

Role Playing

Practicing Positive Self-Talk

Positive self-talk is a habit that can be learned. Assign pairs of students to role-play the positive, optimistic side of a hypothetical personality and the negative, pessimistic side. Have each actor pretend to be another person and respond to various situations with suitable statements. Be sure students switch roles so that both experience positive self-talk.

A possible example follows.

Situation: *Joining a group at lunch*

Negative: What am I doing? They don't want me with them! I'll probably say something stupid and they won't like me.

Positive: They look friendly, and there's space at their table. This is a great opportunity to find out about their interests. I'll bet we have a lot of things in common.

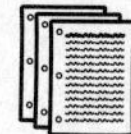

Life Skills Worksheet 8D

Self-Esteem Strategies

Assign the Self-Esteem Strategies Life Skills Worksheet, which requires students to classify the behaviors that build or lower self-esteem.

Making a Choice 8B

Self-Image Crutches

Assign the Self-Image Crutches Card. It requires students to examine the use of material items as crutches for self-esteem.

15 Ways to Boost Your Self-Esteem

FIGURE 8-4

1. *Make a list of your good qualities and keep it with you at all times. Place extra copies on your mirror, in your school desk, or other places you will see it. Read over the list on a regular basis and at any time when you experience negative thoughts.*
2. *Avoid wasting time thinking about your negatives.*
3. *Seek new challenges in your life. Don't be afraid to try new things. Mastering a new task or ability can build self-esteem.*
4. *Avoid putting yourself down to others or to yourself. Accept compliments with a "thank you" and a smile.*
5. *Find something that you do very well and work to improve that skill.*
6. *Reward yourself when you accomplish a task or finish a project.*
7. *Accept the fact that neither you nor anyone else is perfect. Avoid dwelling on mistakes; laugh them off and continue with the positive.*
8. *Take a moment to look at yourself in the mirror each day and give yourself a verbal compliment.*
9. *Keep yourself well groomed, maintain a positive attitude, and develop a sense of humor to handle the difficult situations.*
10. *Join at least one activity that involves other people. Volunteer for service with an organization or group in your school or community.*
11. *Associate with other positive thinkers in your school and community. Create your own support group of friends who are a positive influence on you and your self-esteem.*
12. *Don't fight a fact; deal with it. Try to avoid thinking that people and things in your life that are out of your control should be different. They aren't, and that is the reality.*
13. *Accept that life does not have to be perfect for you to be happy. Happiness is a way of thinking; a content feeling, not a constant euphoria.*
14. *Remember that sometimes bad things happen that are not within your control. Expect this and try not to let it set you back too much. Do the best you can to change what you can, and avoid dwelling on what you cannot change.*
15. *Remind yourself that each of us is important and valuable. Try to be the best "you" can be. Remember, you're the best one for the job.*

• • • TEACH continued

Reinforcement

Mirror Talking

Suggest the following exercise for students to try at home in front of a mirror. Tell them the exercise may sound silly and may be hard to do at first, but that it really is effective if continued long enough. It amounts to reprogramming the way one looks at oneself. The exercise consists of looking at yourself in the mirror and saying aloud, "I really am a great person."

When this routine becomes comfortable, students should add a positive statement about themselves, such as, "I like the way I look today," or "I look great." Choose a statement that calls attention to an attribute that you have trouble accepting.

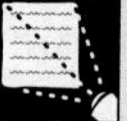

Teaching Transparency 8A
Building Self-Esteem

Use the Building Self-Esteem transparency to discuss the process of developing a positive self-image.

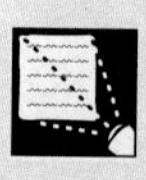

Teaching Transparency 8B
"15 Ways to Boost Your Self-Esteem"

Use this transparency to discuss with students the various ways to build your own self-esteem.

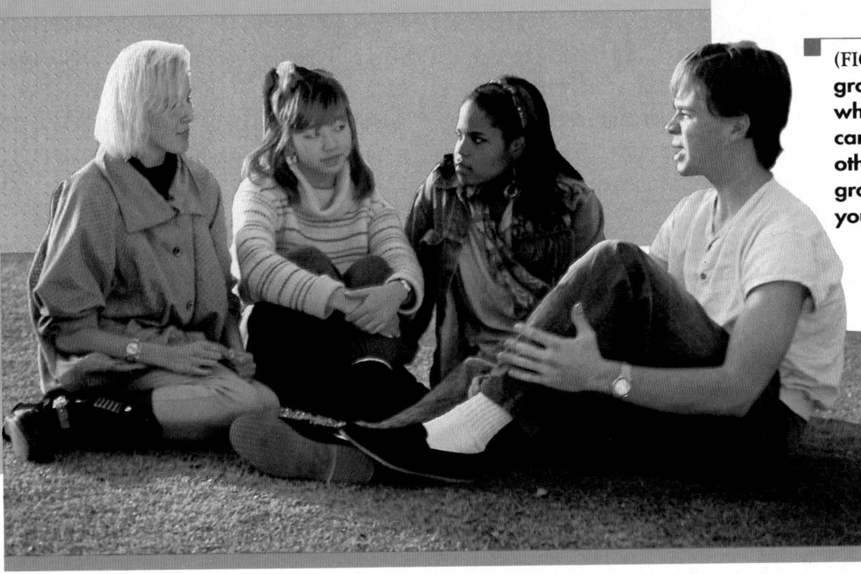

(FIGURE 8-5) **A support group is a group of people who trust each other and can talk openly with each other. Having a support group can help you build your self-esteem.**

She could use an "I" statement instead: "I sometimes have trouble making friends." She is then talking about *her* feelings only.

Another example of not using an "I" statement is when Lindsey said to her brother Scott, "You made me feel terrible when you told me that Anna is smarter than I am." Lindsey is transferring responsibility for her own feelings to Scott. She is saying that *Scott* is responsible for *her* feelings. To take responsibility for her own feelings, Lindsey could say, "When you said that Anna is smarter that I am, I felt hurt."

Although it is easier to speak in generalities, it is important to clearly state what we are feeling and saying.

Develop a Support Group

Few things can be as helpful in maintaining high self-esteem as having people with whom you can share your joys and sorrows—a **support group.** A support group is a group of people who trust each other and are able to talk openly with each other.

Your support group can consist of friends you trust or family members who care for you. A good support group will not exert any pressure on you. Instead, it will make you feel good about yourself.

Take a moment to write down the names of five of your friends who you would like in your support group. Make an effort to spend time with these people. Maybe your support group can get together at lunch or in the evening to discuss what is going on in your lives.

Self-disclosure—telling another person meaningful information about yourself—plays a central role in the development of positive self-esteem. That is because when you discuss your true feelings about yourself, it allows others to correct any distortions you express. By self-disclosing, you learn how you are perceived by others as they respond to you, and you can see yourself more accurately. You can also learn to better appreciate similarities and differences—the diversity among people—by sharing your feelings.

Self-disclosure usually happens gradually between people, as they learn to trust each other. Make sure you really trust the other person before you disclose anything extremely personal.

self-disclosure:

telling another person meaningful information about yourself.

support group:

a group of people who trust each other and are able to talk openly with each other.

Section 8.2

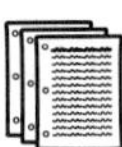

Section Review Worksheet 8.2

Assign Section Review Worksheet 8.2, which has students use the chapter to give advice in hypothetical cases.

Section Quiz 8.2

Have students take Section Quiz 8.2.

Reteaching Worksheet 8.2

Students who have difficulty with the material may complete Reteaching Worksheet 8.2, which has students complete a graphic showing steps to building self-esteem.

Journal 8D
Personal Skills

Have students write about one or more things they do well in the Student Journal. Encourage them to explain how they acquired this skill (natural ability, practice, competition) and how it makes them feel about themselves.

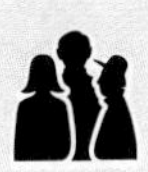

Cooperative Learning
How You Can Boost Your Self-Esteem

Have students work in small groups to sort out their reactions to the list in Figure 8-4. Have group members decide which 10 suggestions seem most useful and rank them. Then have all groups explain their choices.

Demonstration
Taking Responsibility

Invite the school guidance counselor to give examples of general complaints that avoid responsibility or misplace blame. He or she can show how such comments can be recast as "I" statements that clarify the problem and put the speaker in a position to do something about it.

Class Discussion
Identifying Support Groups

Ask students to name as many groups of people as they can that they or someone their age might associate with. Write the group names on the chalkboard. Ask: Among these groups, which ones are the most important? Which groups give people a sense of belonging? Which groups make a person feel good about himself or herself? Which groups can you trust?

Review Answers

1. To raise your self-esteem, assess your strengths and weaknesses, try not to judge yourself by unrealistic standards, decide that you are okay as you are, and change only the things you can change.

2. Answers may include using positive self-talk, being good at something, using "I" statements, developing a support group, resisting peer pressure, and acting with integrity.

3. Answers will vary depending on individual students' levels of self-esteem.

4. Answers will vary. Students may answer that people with high self-esteem feel good about themselves and have confidence in their abilities and judgment. Because of this they do not have to belittle others in order to feel superior. Also, people with high self-esteem appreciate their own worth and the worth of others. When a person appreciates the worth of others, he or she looks for positive qualities in the person instead of looking for and pointing out any negative qualities.

Resist Peer Pressure

Individuals who have low self-esteem usually do not have much confidence in their opinions or their decisions. Consequently, they are overly influenced by peers and by peer pressure.

Learning to trust yourself and your values builds confidence. The more you make your own decisions based on what you—not others—believe, the more confidence you will gain. This does not mean that you should ignore the advice or ideas of parents, friends, teachers, or others. It means that you should listen to your inner voice and make decisions based on what it is telling you.

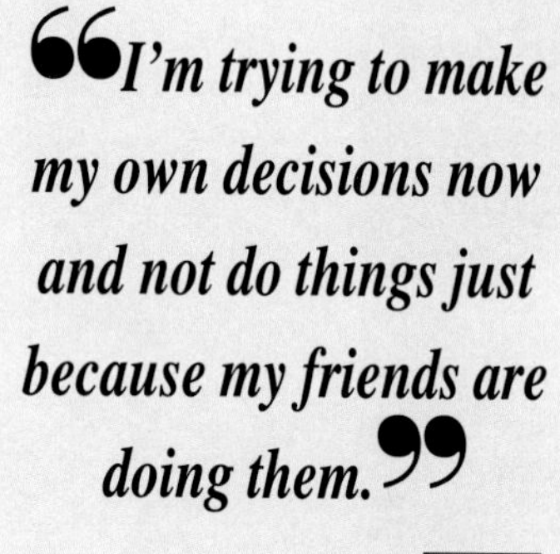

"I'm trying to make my own decisions now and not do things just because my friends are doing them."

Beatriz

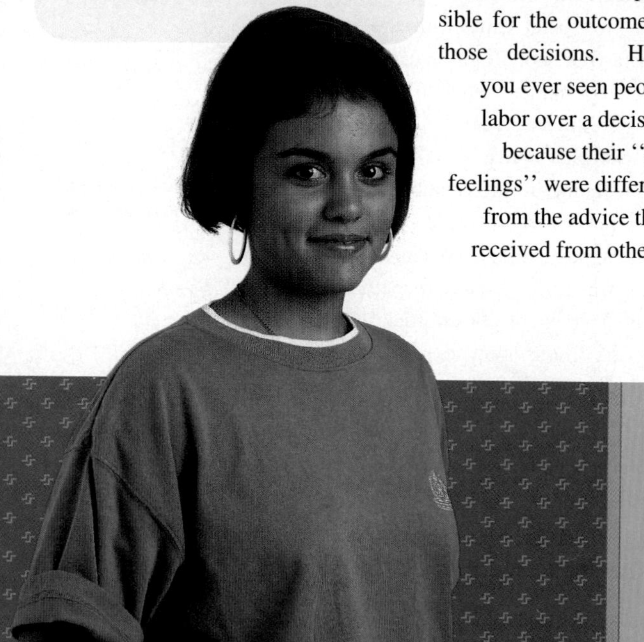

When you make your own decisions, you and you alone are responsible for the outcome of those decisions. Have you ever seen people labor over a decision because their "gut feelings" were different from the advice they received from others? You will notice that they tend to feel miserable afterward if they followed others' advice, only to find that their own path would have been the better one to take.

Act With Integrity

Once we appreciate our own worth we can begin to appreciate the worth of other people. People with healthy self-esteem do not act as if they are looking out for themselves. On the contrary, they treat other people with respect and compassion. They act in ways that will help other people maintain high self-esteem.

It's easy to take advantage of those with low self-esteem by manipulating them or bullying them into doing what we want. But it is our responsibility as people of integrity to refrain from doing so.

When you act with integrity and responsibility toward others, you will feel good about yourself, and that will improve your self-esteem even more.

Review

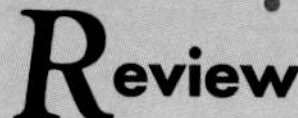

1. *Describe the most important way of raising your self-esteem.*
2. *Name at least three other ways to build your self-esteem.*
3. ***LIFE SKILLS: Building Self-Esteem*** *What steps will you take to improve your own self-esteem?*
4. ***Critical Thinking*** *Explain why people with high self-esteem do not have to put down other people in order to feel good about themselves.*

• • • TEACH continued

Extension

Building Your Skills

Some students may want to make a list of the things they do well and locate organizations in the community that would help them develop their special skills—community theaters, park district classes, community center facilities, privately owned businesses and shops.

ASSESS

Section Review

Have the students answer the Section Review questions.

Alternative Assessment

Retrain Yourself

Ask students to write a paragraph explaining why it is important to listen to the negative things you say to yourself and retrain yourself to say positive things to raise your self-esteem.

Closure

How Can You Improve?

Ask the class to define self-esteem and to give examples of ways people may build self-esteem.

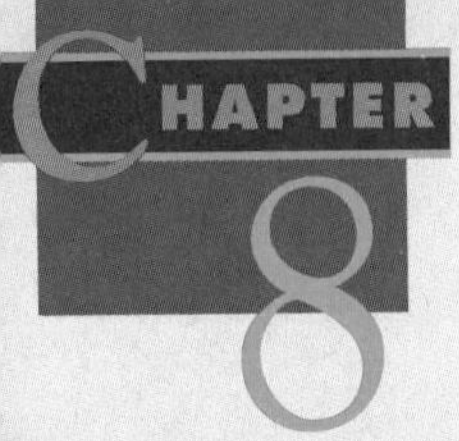

Highlights

Summary

- Self-esteem is the confidence and satisfaction you have in yourself. It is influenced by people and events of your early years.
- During early childhood, we make decisions about our own worth based on how we think others see us. As we grow older, we become better equipped to make these decisions ourselves.
- Media messages can lower one's self-esteem by presenting fashion models as unrealistic standards by which we judge ourselves. This can cause us to devalue ourselves because we look different.
- Accepting yourself is the most important part of raising your self-esteem.
- By cultivating your natural abilities, you will develop more confidence in yourself. Being good at one thing will make it easier for you to try out new skills and take positive risks.
- You can build self-esteem if you take responsibility for your feelings by using "I" statements. It is important to state clearly what you mean rather than to speak in generalities.
- Trusting and sharing with a support group can help a person maintain self-esteem.
- You can also raise your self-esteem by trying not to judge yourself by unrealistic standards, by deciding that you are okay as you are, and by using energy on changing only the things about yourself that you can change.
- Talking in a positive way to yourself about yourself, and believing it, can improve your confidence and self-esteem.

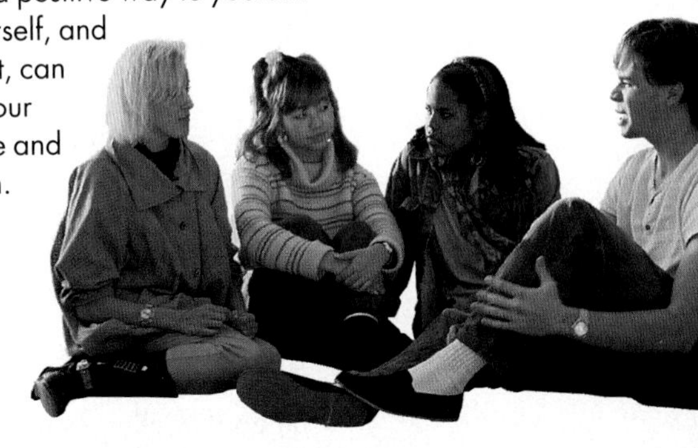

Vocabulary

self-esteem pride in and acceptance of yourself; your sense of personal worth.

body image the view a person has of his or her body.

positive self-talk talking in a positive way to yourself about yourself.

support group a group of people who trust each other and are able to talk openly with each other.

self-disclosure telling another person meaningful information about yourself.

Chapter 8 Highlights

Summary
Have students read the summary to reinforce the concepts learned in Chapter 8.

Vocabulary
Divide the class into small groups and give each group one of the following terms:

self-esteem
body image
positive self-talk
transferring responsibility
generalization
support group
self-disclosure
distortions

Have the groups develop definitions for their terms and create dramatic ways to illustrate the concepts.

Extension
Encourage students to make a "Who Am I?" file or book. In it they can keep a history of achievements, with photographs, summaries, etc. They may also devote a section to defining their positive qualities and things they enjoy doing. This can be expanded as they gain self-knowledge. Suggest that students complete their file or book with a list of positive changes they are making to improve the way they feel about themselves.

CHAPTER 8 ASSESSMENT

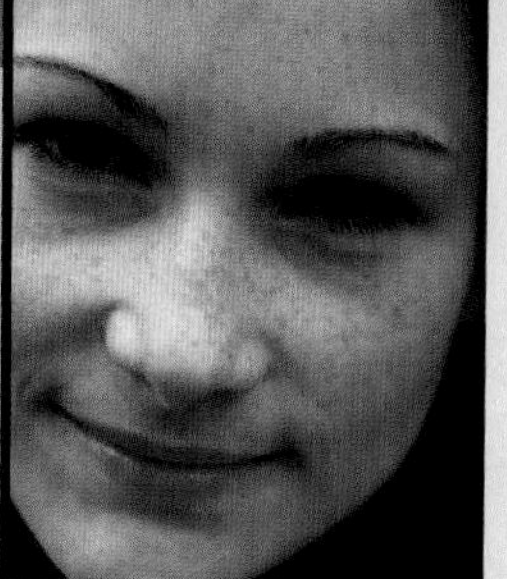

Chapter Review

CHAPTER REVIEW

Concept Review

1. self-esteem
2. body image
3. media
4. responsibility
5. strengths, weaknesses
6. positive self-talk
7. responsibility
8. support group
9. self-disclosure
10. peer pressure
11. integrity

Expressing Your Views

Sample responses:

1. If you do not have high self-esteem, you won't have confidence in yourself, you don't feel worthwhile, can't make good decisions, can't experience acceptance, or give and receive love. All of these factors negatively affect your relations with family and friends and how you do in school and at work. Low self-esteem has been linked to self-destructive behaviors, such as alcohol and other drug abuse, eating disorders, and suicide.

2. Sylvia needs to accept herself. She needs to use her energy to change the things she can and accept those things she cannot change. She needs to talk to herself in a positive way and take responsibility for her feelings by using "I" statements.

3. Jeremy needs to trust himself and his values. He needs to listen to his inner voice and make decisions based on what it is telling him.

Life Skills Check

Sample responses:

1. Answers will vary according to individual strengths and weaknesses.

2. I would tell Lee that he needs to act with integrity—to treat other people with respect and compassion.

Concept Review

1. The degree to which a person likes or feels good about oneself is ________.
2. Your ________ is how you see your appearance, fitness, and health.
3. Messages from the ________ often cause us to have a low self-esteem by telling us we must look a certain way to be attractive.
4. By deciding to take ________ for yourself and your own self-esteem, you can make changes in the way you view yourself.
5. You can learn to feel good about yourself by realistically accepting your ________ and ________.
6. ________ is talking in a positive way to yourself about yourself.
7. Communication improves when you take ________ for your feelings and words by being specific and using "I" statements.
8. Friends or family members with whom you can speak openly are a ________.
9. You can learn how you are perceived by others as they respond to you, and you can see yourself more accurately, through ________.
10. People with low self-esteem want to follow the crowd and often allow themselves to be influenced by ________.
11. When you act with ________ and treat other people with respect and compassion, you will feel good about yourself.

Expressing Your Views

1. Some psychologists think that an individual's self-esteem is the most important influence on mental well-being. Why do you think self-esteem is so important?
2. Sylvia hates school because she feels as though she has no friends. She feels shy around other students because she thinks they're all more attractive than she is. What can Sylvia do to boost her self-esteem?
3. Sunday night, Jeremy sneaked out of the house after midnight to ride around and drink beer with his friends. Jeremy didn't really want to go, but he was afraid his friends would think he wasn't "cool." After he got home, Jeremy realized he had been doing a lot of things lately that he didn't really want to do. He decided that from now on he would resist this kind of peer pressure. What could Jeremy do to change?

Life Skills Check

1. Assessing Your Health
You want to be able to accept yourself for what you are, but first you need to evaluate your self-esteem. As realistically as possible, make a personal inventory by listing as many strengths and weaknesses as you can about yourself. If your list of weaknesses is longer than your list of strengths, judge each weakness and decide whether you could view it in a more positive way. List ways you could improve your weaknesses and build on your strengths.

2. Building Self-Esteem
Lee appears to care only for his own feelings and becomes very defensive and upset if anyone criticizes his actions. You don't really consider yourself a close friend of his, but today he told you that he doesn't think anyone likes him much, and that he feels as if he doesn't have one true friend. How would you respond to this statement?

Projects

1. Work with a group to write a list of things individuals might hear as they are growing up that would build high self-esteem. Then write a list of things individuals hear that would prevent healthy self-esteem from developing. Compare your two lists and discuss the consequences that negative comments might have on the normal development of positive self-esteem.
2. Work with a group to create and produce a skit involving characters with healthy self-esteem and with poor self-esteem. Show how both personalities deal with problems. Then have the audience decide which qualities of healthy self-esteem are missing or are present.

Plan for Action

An individual's self-esteem has a great impact on his or her mental health. Create a plan to raise your own self-esteem.

Projects
Have students plan and carry out the projects for building self-esteem.

Plan for Action
Have students each imagine a character who has low self-esteem. The character may be unlike themselves. Each student should talk briefly about himself or herself, in character, stressing self-esteem issues. Other students then respond with ideas for improving the character's outlook: how can the character change appearance, attitudes, or behavior to improve self-esteem?

ASSESSMENT OPTIONS

Chapter Test
Have students take the Chapter 8 Test.

Alternative Assessment
Have students do the Alternative Assessment activity for Chapter 8.

Test Generator
The Test Generator (Macintosh® or IBM® format) contains an additional 50 assessment items for this chapter.

MANAGING STRESS

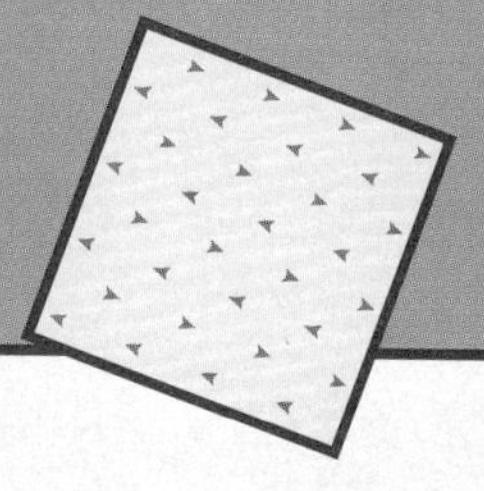

PLANNING GUIDE

TEXT SECTIONS	OBJECTIVES	TEXT FEATURES	OUTSIDE RESOURCES	NOTES
9.1 What Is Stress? pp. 191-196 1 period	• Define stress. • Describe the stress response. • Name at least four stress-related disorders.	• Section Review, p. 196	**TEACHER'S RESOURCE BINDER** • Lesson Plan 9.1 • Personal Health Inventory • Journal Entries 9A, 9B • Section Review Worksheet 9.1 • Section Quiz 9.1 • Reteaching Worksheet 9.1 **OTHER RESOURCES** • Making a Choice 9A • English/Spanish Audiocassette 3	
9.2 How to Manage Stress pp. 197-205 1 period	• Define stress intervention. • Explain why physical exercise is a good way to handle stress. ■ Use selective awareness to change your interpretation of a stressor. ■ Practice a relaxation technique that helps you to deal with stress.	• Check Up, p. 204 • LIFE SKILLS: Coping, p. 201 **ASSESSMENT** • Section Review, p. 205	**TEACHER'S RESOURCE BINDER** • Lesson Plan 9.2 • Journal Entries 9C, 9D • Life Skills 9A, 9B • Section Review Worksheet 9.2 • Section Quiz 9.2 • Reteaching Worksheet 9.2 **OTHER RESOURCES** • Making a Choice 9B • Transparencies 9A, 9B	
9.3 Managing Stress Is a Lifelong Process pp. 206-208 1 period	• Explain how a support group helps a person deal with stress. • Manage your time by setting goals and prioritizing. ■ Seek help if you or someone you know is overwhelmed by stress.	• LIFE SKILLS: Setting Goals, p. 207 **ASSESSMENT** • Section Review, p. 208	**TEACHER'S RESOURCE BINDER** • Lesson Plan 9.3 • Journal Entries 9E, 9F • Life Skills 9C, 9D • Section Review Worksheet 9.3 • Section Quiz 9.3 • Reteaching Worksheet 9.3	
End of Chapter pp. 209-211		**ASSESSMENT** • Chapter Review, pp. 210-211	**TEACHER'S RESOURCE BINDER** **OTHER RESOURCES** • Chapter Test • Alternative Assessment • Test Generator	

■ Denotes LIFE SKILLS objectives

• Items in blue are also part of the *Holt Health Activity Book.*

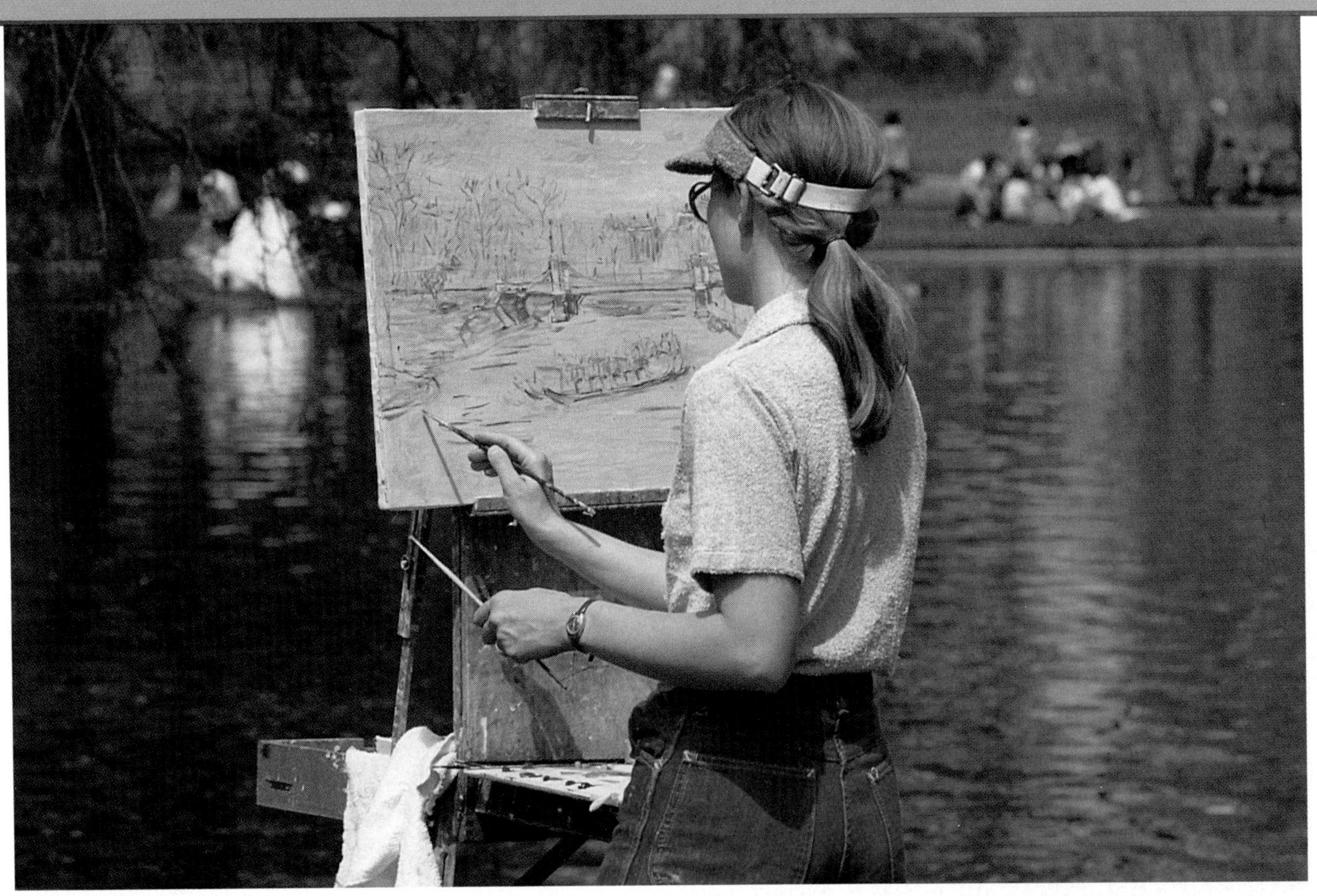

CONTENT BACKGROUND

Anxiety in Teenagers

A STUDY DONE BY THE RESEARCHERS AT the University of Minnesota Adolescent Health Program during the 1986-1987 school year found that a startling 20 to 25 percent of the 36,000 Minnesota teenagers surveyed reported high levels of stress, distress, or depression most or all of the time. The National Adolescent Student Health Survey (NASHS) found that of about 11,500 eighth and tenth graders surveyed, more than 45 percent reported that it was "very hard" or "hard" for them to cope with situations they considered stressful, both in school and at home. And although these findings indicate that many teenagers are stressed, very few seem willing to discuss these feelings with parents, teachers, or even other peers for fear of admitting to failure.

Some social scientists suggest that the best way to relieve the pressure these teenagers are under is to be supportive, reassuring, and understanding and to offer advice if asked. It is also important to remember that an adolescent's concerns and anxieties are *real,* but often teens think that authoritative figures such as parents and teachers don't take them seriously. Researchers at the University of Illinois recently conducted a study of 500 children aged nine to fifteen. They found that adolescents' seemingly strong emotional states vary widely on a daily basis and typically do not last for more than half an hour at a time. The researchers discovered that most of the teens surveyed are not "at war with themselves," and that the stress felt in various situations is natural and healthy.

What happens, though, when the stress becomes overwhelming? In addition to certain physical and emotional problems, some teens, like adults, turn to high-risk behaviors, the most

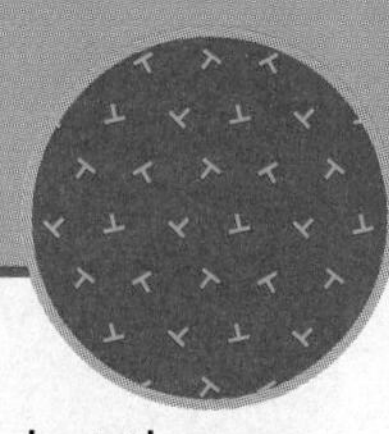

common of which is drug abuse. In fact, a 1989 Gallup Youth Survey found that 60 percent of the teenagers sampled named drug abuse as the most serious problem facing them. Research conducted at various institutions across the country indicates that while overall drug abuse is down among adolescents, the abuse of lethal drugs such as crack is on the rise, and alcohol consumption and smoking remain ominously high.

Unfortunately, stress—no matter what the age of the person—is unavoidable. However, as pointed out in the chapter, this does not mean that stress is unmanageable. Antistress strategies should be aimed at the causes of stress so that the stress can be eliminated. If this is not possible, stress should be temporarily reduced by treating its symptoms. In either case, high-risk behaviors should not be used to relieve anxiety.

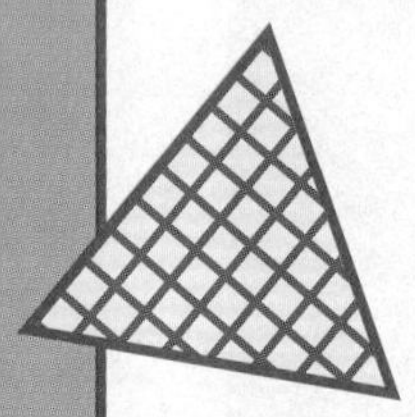

PLANNING FOR INSTRUCTION

KEY FACTS

- **Stress is a natural response that is experienced by all persons throughout their lives.**
- **Stress occurs when a new or unpleasant situation (stressor) causes a stress response.**
- **Stressors can be either positive (motivating) or negative (distressing).**
- **The stress response includes muscle tension, faster heart and breathing rates, release of adrenaline for quick energy, and digestive disturbances.**
- **Under stress, the body gears up for physical action (fight or flight). But if no physical action occurs, the stress is not released and illness can eventually result.**
- **About 60 to 80 percent of all physical and mental disorders are related to stress—either caused by it or made worse by it.**
- **Stress intervention techniques include elimination of the stressor, changing the interpretation of it (selective awareness), relaxation, and exercise.**
- **Many negative consequences of stress can be prevented by keeping physically healthy through regular exercise, balanced diet, adequate sleep, relaxation, and avoiding the use of tobacco, alcohol, and other drugs.**
- **A support group is your personal group of people whom you trust. Discussing problems with them can reduce stress.**
- **When a person is unable to cope with stress, help is available from professionals, including clergy, counselors, therapists, and hotline phone numbers for substance abuse and suicide.**

MYTHS AND MISCONCEPTIONS

MYTH: I am the only one who gets stressed-out about making mistakes or looking foolish.

Such self-doubts and fears affect all people at various times in their lives. Athletes, performers, and political candidates experience stress and self-doubt, too.

MYTH: All stress is bad.

Reasonable amounts of stress actually help us to be more alert, perform better, and accomplish more. A completely stress-free life would be boring and unproductive.

MYTH: I'm strong enough to get through life's worst problems without any help.

Anyone can become overwhelmed by extreme stress. When this happens, people should talk to a trusted adult or seek professional help.

VOCABULARY

Essential: The following vocabulary terms appear in bold-face type:

high blood pressure
stressor
stress response
stress
stress intervention
selective awareness
support group

Secondary: In addition, the following terms may require early attention:

meditation
progressive relaxation

FOR STUDENTS WITH SPECIAL NEEDS

LEP Students: Students may experience stress when they have difficulty expressing themselves in English. Such students may benefit from stress intervention if they interpret their situation positively. For example, if they know two languages, such knowledge enables them to read a wider variety of books, newspapers, and magazines; enables them to watch TV in either language; and enables them to enjoy the richness of two cultures. The ability to speak two languages can be an asset in finding a job as an adult.

Visual Learners: Have students collect newspaper and magazine photos of both stressed and happy faces. Ask them to write a description of how the stressed and happy faces differ.

Kinesthetic Learners: Students may find regular contact with a pet helpful in reducing stress. Have students report to the class on the stress-reducing effects of pets, using as references stress-management books and articles, which can be found through *Academic Abstracts* on CD or in *The Reader's Guide to Periodical Literature.*

ENRICHMENT

- Music can be stressful or relaxing, depending on its style and the listener's preference. Have students, working in pairs, experiment listening to two sequences of music, one they find stressful and another they find relaxing, and analyze how and why the sequences differ in their effect on people. Alternatively, try the same thing with stressful art and relaxing art.
- View 15 minutes of a dramatic movie or a TV soap opera. Have students analyze the stress situations and the stress responses in the characters' faces, voices, and actions. Ask them to suggest stress-intervention techniques that could be used in each situation.

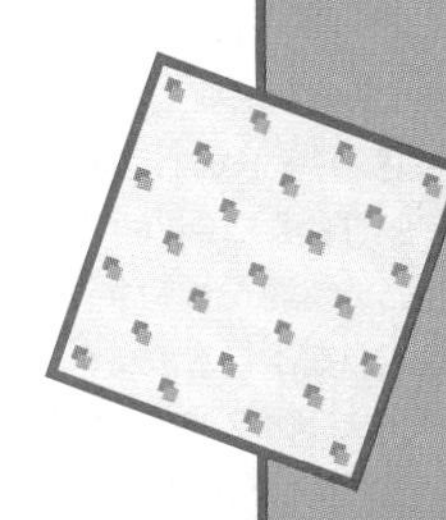

CHAPTER 9 CHAPTER OPENER

GETTING STARTED

Using the Chapter Photograph

Ask students to imagine they are feeling stressed-out after exams. Would the activity shown in the picture be a good way to relieve the stress? What other activities can you name that might help relieve stress? Why do such activities help relieve stress?

Explain to students that in this chapter they will learn how to recognize stress and some useful ways to deal with it.

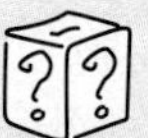

Question Box

Have students write out any questions they have about stress and put them in the Question Box. The Question Box provides them with an opportunity to ask questions anonymously. To ensure that students with questions are not embarrassed to be seen writing, have those who do not have questions write something else—such as something they already know about managing stress—on the paper instead.

Preview the questions and then answer them at appropriate points in the chapter. You may wish to allow students to write additional anonymous questions as they go through the chapter.

Personal Issues *ALERT*

Some of your students may have experienced—or may now be enduring—major stressors, such as a recent death in the family, divorce of parents, serious illness or accident, abuse, pregnancy, or suicidal thoughts. The practical advice in this chapter can especially benefit them. Always be alert to discomfort levels in students and provide opportunities for them to ask anonymous questions. Briefly remind the whole class about the counseling help that is available in your school and community.

CHAPTER 9

Managing Stress

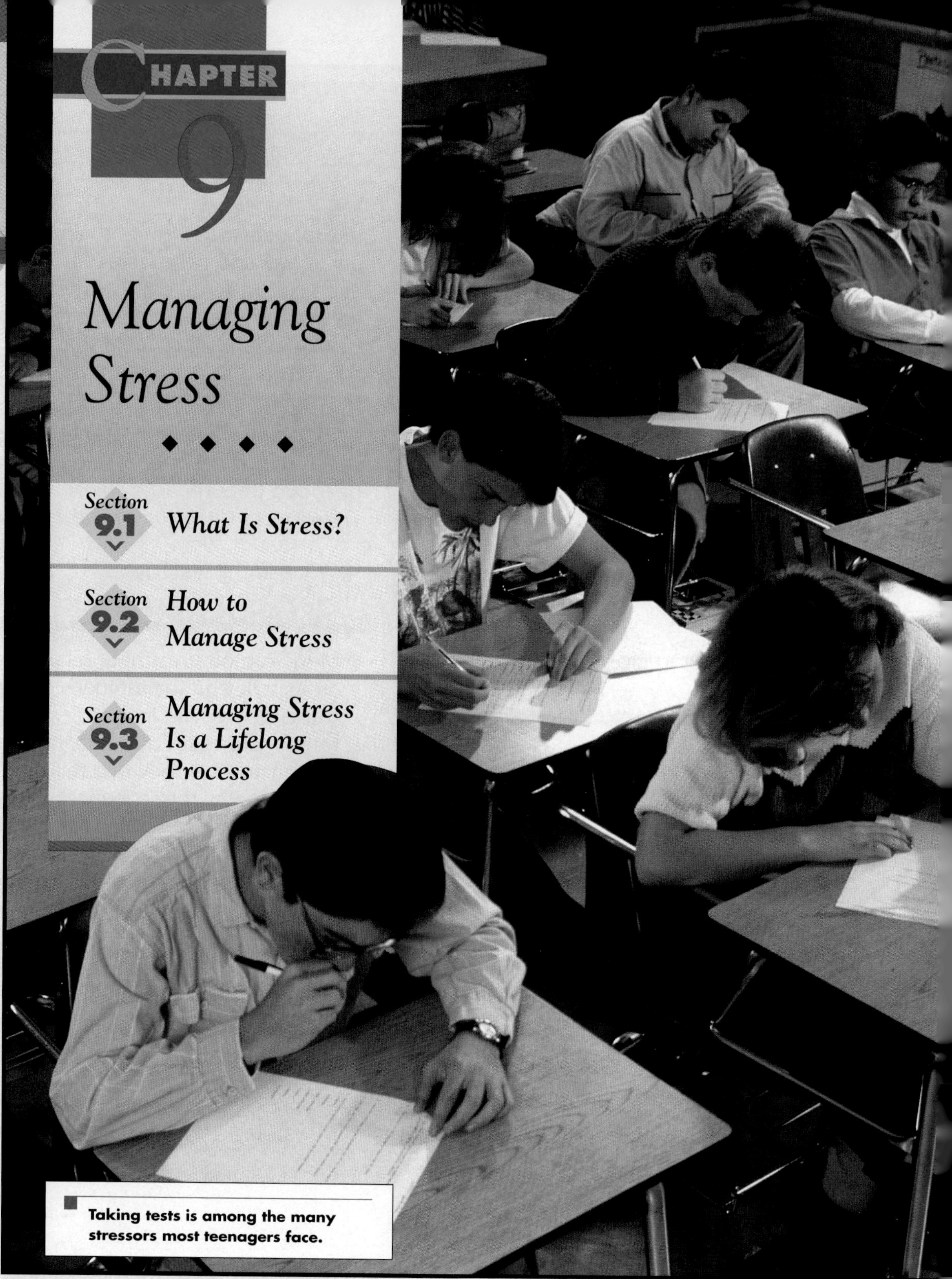

Taking tests is among the many stressors most teenagers face.

Raquel had no idea how she was going to do it. Getting up in front of her English class and giving a speech terrified her. What if she went totally blank and forgot everything she was going to say? Or what if she said something really stupid? What if everyone started laughing at her? What if . . . ? Just thinking about all the "what ifs" made Raquel's heart start to pound and her hands start to sweat.

She could pretend to be sick and stay home the day she was supposed to give her speech, but she knew she would have to give it anyway when she went back to school. There wasn't any way out of it, and it was making Raquel a nervous wreck. In fact, she was so stressed-out about it that she couldn't even concentrate on *writing* the speech.

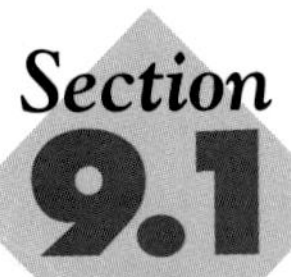

Section 9.1 What Is Stress?

Objectives

- *Define stress.*
- *Describe the stress response.*
- *Name at least four stress-related disorders.*

If you, like Raquel, have had physical reactions to a change in your life situation, you have experienced stress. It is perfectly natural to experience stress. All of us do. The key is learning how to manage stress so that it doesn't make you miserable or sick. In this chapter you'll find out about some techniques that can help you cope with the stress in your life.

Before you can cope with stress, you have to know how it develops. First, a situation arises that is new or potentially unpleasant. This situation is called a **stressor**. In Raquel's case, the stressor was the requirement that she give a speech to her English class. Raquel felt anxious, her heart raced, and her hands started sweating when she thought about the speech. What she was experiencing was a **stress response**—the mind and body's reaction to a stressor.

It is important to remember that stressors have only the *potential* to cause a stress response. For some people, giving a speech would not cause a stress response. It's only when a stressor *does* cause a stress response that stress results. Therefore, **stress** is defined as the combination of a stressor and a stress response.

Stressors

Stressors can occur in almost every area of life. You may feel stress at home if your parents or guardians are not getting along with each other or if they are getting a divorce. It can also be stressful if one of your

stress response: *the mind and body's reaction to a stressor.*

stress: *the combination of a stressor and a stress response.*

stressor: *any new or potentially unpleasant situation.*

Background

Five Stressor Categories

Psychologists identify five general stressor categories: biological (illness and problems one is born with); environmental (crowding, noise, poverty, disasters); thinking activities (exams, mental challenges); personal behavior (smoking, drinking alcohol, taking drugs, poor nutrition, poor sleep, little exercise); and life situations (death, relationships, personal events).

Section 9.1 Lesson Plan

MOTIVATE

Journal 9A
A Past Stressful Situation

This may be done as a warm-up activity. In the Student Journal in the Student Activity Book, have students write down at least one stressful situation they have experienced. Have them note the stress response they felt and what they did to relieve it.

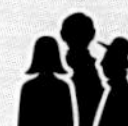

Cooperative Learning
Raquel's Situation

Have students form groups to discuss Raquel's situation. **What could Raquel do to relieve the stress?** *[Ask someone to help her prepare and practice the speech, breathe slowly and deeply, sit or lie down, and consciously relax.]* Students should also discuss how they have handled similar stressful situations.

TEACH

Class Discussion
Life Science Analogy

Stress affects all living things. Ask students to consider these analogies: **If you moved a flower from shady, damp woods into a sunny, dry yard, how would the move stress the plant?** *[Moving the plant changes its environment, including temperature and*

Background

Stress and the Immune System

The stress response prompts the adrenal glands to release two substances: (1) glucoticoid hormone, which provides quick energy and suppresses the immune system (to prevent allergic reactions that could hinder the body during fight or flight); and (2) adrenaline, which increases heart rate and blood pressure (to improve the body's performance). Thus the body is prepared for fight or flight. If the stress is prolonged, the immune suppression causes low resistance to allergens, bacteria, and viruses. Chronic stress can result in chronic illness.

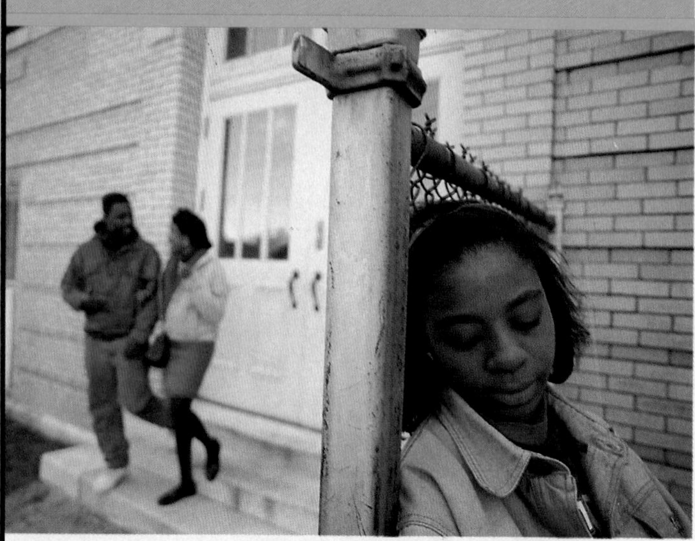

(FIGURE 9-1) **Stressors can come in many forms. If you are having trouble becoming part of a social group, you may experience stress as a result.**

parents remarries and you must move in with your new stepmother or stepfather. If you argue with your brother or sister, you might feel stress as a result.

At school, you may experience stress when you try out for a sport or the school play or when you are having trouble becoming part of a certain social group. You may feel stress if you don't have enough money to buy the right clothes for a school dance. Or you may experience stress if other students pick on you or make fun of you.

Many stressors involve our self-esteem. We fear that we will look foolish in front of other people whose opinions we care about. That is why Raquel experienced stress when she had to give a speech. She was worried about other people's opinions of her, which could affect her opinion of herself. If you have these kinds of self-doubts and fears, be comforted in knowing that you are not alone. People of all ages and all occupations want others to think well of them, and this is stressful for them, just as it is for you.

A stressor can be something as simple and common as trying to get paper clips untangled, hitting a red light when you're in a hurry, or getting a busy signal when you really need to talk with someone. If you let them, these kinds of "daily hassles" can add up and cause a tremendous amount of stress.

Even *positive* situations can be stressors. Getting married is a perfect example. It is a happy occasion, but because it involves a change in one's life situation, it can be just as stressful as a negative event. Making the all-star basketball team is another example of a positive life-changing event that can cause stress.

Having stressors is perfectly normal and healthy. Without them life would be boring, and *that* would be stressful. People need to have enough stressors to make life interesting, but not so many that they cause illness.

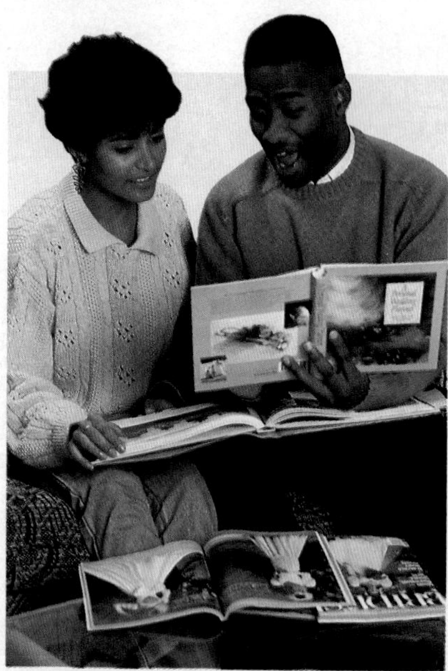

(FIGURE 9-2) **Even a positive event like getting married can be stressful, because it involves a change in one's life situation.**

• • • TEACH continued

wetness; the plant might wilt, stop growing, or even die.] **How is this like a family moving from one place to another?** *[Moving changes a family's environment, creating stress due to the change of social contacts, work, schools, climate, and so on.]* **If a pet is often hit or yelled at, what might its stress responses be?** *[It might become depressed, not eat well, hide, try to run away, or become aggressive and bite.]* **How is this like a person's response to similar stress?** *[Essentially the same]*

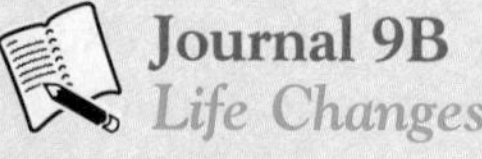

Journal 9B
Life Changes

Have students read the caption for Figure 9-2. Then, in the Student Journal, ask them to write about any situations listed in the figure that they have experienced in the past 12 months, and total their units.

Role-Playing
The Swim Party

Have students act out the following situation: The class is having a swimming party to celebrate the last day of school. But three students—Bill, Pam, and Jenny—are very uncomfortable with this. Bill can't swim and is afraid to admit it. Pam moved here only a month ago and doesn't know many students. Jenny feels very uncomfortable in a swimsuit. Assign students to

Life Changes of Teenagers

Life Event	Life-Change Units
Getting married	101
Being pregnant and unmarried	92
Experiencing the death of a parent	87
Acquiring a visible deformity	81
Going through a parent's divorce	77
Becoming an unmarried father	77
Becoming involved with drugs or alcohol	76
Having a parent go to jail for a year or more	75
Going through parents' separation	69
Experiencing the death of a brother or sister	68
Experiencing a change in acceptance by peers	67
Having an unmarried pregnant teenage sister	64
Discovering you are an adopted child	64
Having a parent remarry	63
Experiencing the death of a close friend	62
Having a visible congenital deformity	62
Having a serious illness requiring hospitalization	58
Moving to a new school district	56
Failing a grade in school	56
Not making an extracurricular activity	55
Experiencing the serious illness of a parent	55
Breaking up with a boyfriend or girlfriend	53
Having a parent go to jail for 30 or fewer days	53

Life Event	Life-Change Units
Beginning to date	51
Being suspended from school	50
Having a newborn brother or sister	50
Having more arguments with parents	47
Having an outstanding personal achievement	46
Seeing an increase in the number of arguments between parents	46
Having a parent lose his or her job	46
Experiencing a change in parents' financial status	45
Being accepted at the college of your choice	43
Being a senior in high school	47
Experiencing the serious illness of a brother or sister	41
Experiencing increased absence from home of mother or father owing to change in occupation	38
Experiencing the departure from home of a brother or sister	37
Experiencing the death of a grandparent	36
Having a third adult added to the family	34
Becoming a full-fledged member of a religion	31
Seeing a decrease in the number of arguments between parents	27
Having fewer arguments with parents	26
Having a mother who begins to work outside the home	26

(FIGURE 9-3) **Major changes in our lives can cause stress, even if they are positive events. To get an idea of how much your life has changed in the past year, add up the life-change units for the changes you experienced during the last 12 months. If your total score is less than 150, your life has changed little. If it is between 150 and 300, you have experienced moderate change. And if your score is over 300, your life has changed significantly.**

Background
Other Responses to Stress

Other responses related to stress include nervous behavior (nail-biting, finger-drumming), smoking, increased use of alcohol and medications, eating too little or too much, sleeping too little or too much, careless driving and being accident-prone, and being absent-minded.

Background
Stress and Illness

The connection between stress and illness is widely recognized. Dr. Hans Selye calls stress the "rate of wear and tear within the body." One study revealed that highly stressed air-traffic controllers had about five times the incidence of high blood pressure found in the general population. Allergists report that stress both initiates and worsens allergic attacks. Stress also appears to promote arthritis and some cancers. And the immune-system suppression that is part of the stress response allows attack by viruses and bacteria.

play the roles of the various students at the party. Afterward, have these students discuss the stressors and the stress responses they felt—including the stress of acting in these roles for this class.

Reinforcement
Physical and Nonphysical Threats

Students may wonder why our bodies respond identically to physical and nonphysical threats. Explain that humans evolved in a harsh environment, in constant physical threat from the natural elements and from animals and other humans. As a result, our stress response evolved as a survival mechanism. In today's environment, the old physical dangers to which our bodies are adapted are rare. Instead, our society provides nonphysical, emotional threats. Unfortunately, our environment has changed too fast for us to evolve new responses to nonphysical threats. Thus, when we feel threatened, our minds and bodies respond in the only way they know how—the physical stress response.

Class Discussion
Stress-Related Disorders

Invite students to talk about their own experiences with stress-related disorders and their observations of other people who have them. Ask if anyone in class has experienced getting a cold, tension headaches, TMJ syndrome, or other disorders at a stressful time. Refer to the list made on the chalkboard

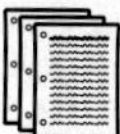

Personal Health Inventory

Have students complete the Personal Health Inventory for this chapter. The inventory asks students to rate the stressors in their life.

Making a Choice 9A

Stress in Your Life

Assign the Stress in Your Life card. The card requires students to discuss things they find stressful in their lives and to draw a cartoon showing the humorous side of a stressful situation.

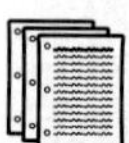

Section Review Worksheet 9.1

Assign Section Review Worksheet 9.1, which requires students to identify stressors, components of the stress response, and stress-related disorders.

The Stress Response

The stress response occurs because of the relationship between your brain and the rest of your body. Your brain recognizes a stressor and evaluates it. If your brain decides that the stressor is harmless, nothing happens to your body. But if the stressor is seen as a threat, your brain tells your body to produce certain chemicals called hormones that contribute to the stress response. During a stress response, the physical changes shown in Figure 9-4 occur.

Why does the brain tell the rest of the body to respond this way? It doesn't seem as though the stress response would help us at all. It certainly didn't help Raquel prepare for her speech. When could the stress response possibly be helpful to us?

Well, imagine that you are walking down the street and a huge dog suddenly leaps at you from behind a garbage truck, snarling, teeth bared, and ready to bite you. What do you do? Do you try to defend yourself against the dog, or do you run away as fast as you can? Whichever you do—fight the dog or run away—will require you to act immediately and with great physical effort.

The stress response makes it possible for you to protect yourself. Your body produces the hormone called adrenaline, which gives you the rush of extra energy you need. Your breathing speeds up, which helps get more oxygen throughout your body. Your heart beats faster, which increases the flow of blood to your muscles. And your muscles tense up, which prepares you to move quickly.

At the same time these changes are occurring, other changes are also taking place throughout your body. Because all

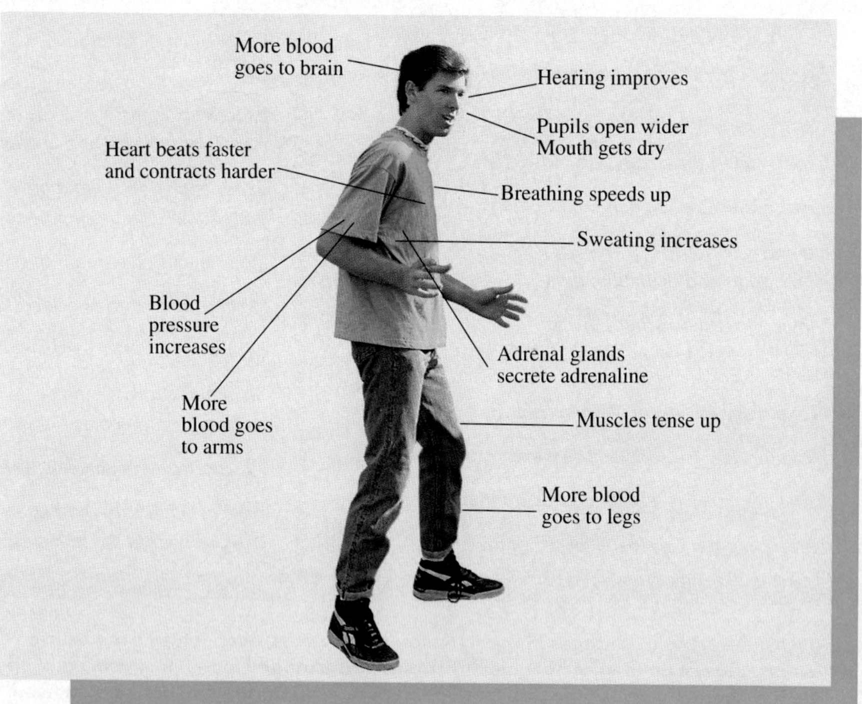

(FIGURE 9-4) **The physical changes of the stress response prepare the body to run away or stay and fight.**

• • • TEACH continued

earlier during class discussion and discuss which stressors might lead to stress-related disorders.

Extension

Clinic Visit

Suggest that students visit a mental health clinic to obtain pamphlets on dealing with stress. Display these in the classroom.

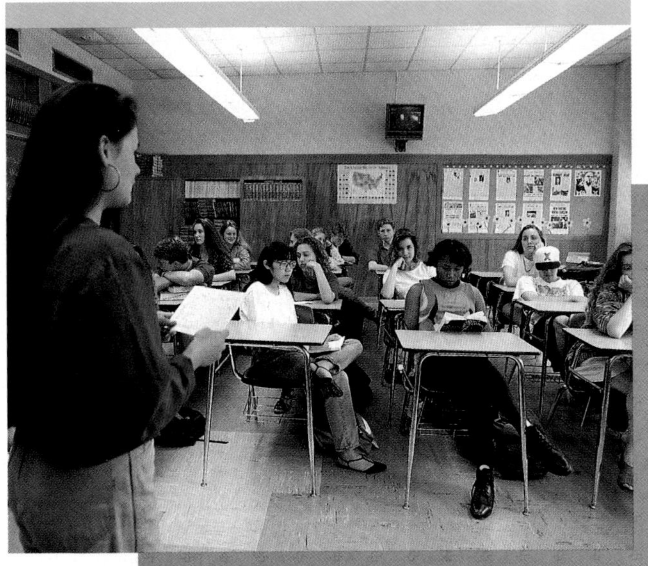

(FIGURE 9-5) **Giving a speech can cause exactly the same stress response as being attacked by an animal.**

your physical resources are mobilized to help you respond to danger, other body functions may take a back seat. The digestive system, for example, may begin to function strangely, causing diarrhea or constipation. Less saliva is produced, because it is a low priority to your body during times of physical danger. As a result, your mouth becomes dry.

The stress response is sometimes called the "fight-or-flight" response because it prepares you to either "fight" or "take flight." It prepares you to do something *physical.* So when you are physically threatened and need to respond physically, the stress response is helpful to you.

The problem is that your body responds the same way to a *nonphysical* threat as it does to a physical threat. In other words, giving a speech can cause exactly the same stress response as being attacked by an animal. But giving a speech, unlike defending yourself against an animal attack, does not require you to release stress in any physical way. The stress that is not released can make you physically ill.

Stress Can Make You Sick

It is estimated that from 60 to 80 percent of all physical and mental disorders are related to stress. Not all of these disorders, however, are *caused* by stress. Many of them are simply made worse by stress.

Allergies may be a good example of a stress-related disorder. Let's say that you are allergic to pollen. When there is a lot of pollen in the air, you have an allergic reaction. Your eyes sting, your nose runs, you sneeze, and you have trouble breathing. This is a completely physical reaction. It has nothing to do with stress.

But now imagine that you are under stress. Evidence indicates that when you are under stress, it may take a much smaller amount of pollen to cause the same allergic reaction.

Some of the other diseases and disorders that are suspected of being related to stress include the following:

The "fight-or-flight" response is discussed in greater detail in the Body Systems Handbook on pages 660-661.

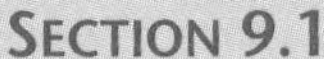

SECTION 9.1

Section Quiz 9.1

Have students take Section Quiz 9.1.

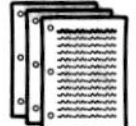

Reteaching Worksheet 9.1

Students who have difficulty with the material may complete Reteaching Worksheet 9.1. This worksheet requires students to identify stressors, symptoms of the stress response, and stress-related disorders in specific situations.

Review Answers

1. A combination of a stressor and a stress response

2. Feeling anxious, heart racing, hands sweating

3. Answers may include colds and flu, tension headaches, backache, coronary heart disease, high blood pressure, chronic fatigue, mental illness, and possibly cancer.

4. A stress-management program can help employees learn how to deal with and manage stress. As employees learn how to manage stress, they will experience less illness and, therefore, will be able to spend more days on the job and take fewer sick days.

high blood pressure: *a condition in which the blood pushes harder than normal against the inside of the blood vessels.*

- **Colds and Flu** Stress can weaken your immune system, the system of your body that defends against infection. As a result, a person under prolonged stress is more likely to become infected with cold and flu viruses. That person may also require more time than others to recover from these illnesses.

"I used to get a lot of headaches. Now that I'm doing relaxation exercises every day, they don't bother me as much."

— Sam

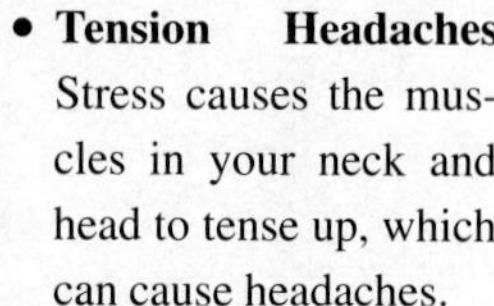

- **Tension Headaches** Stress causes the muscles in your neck and head to tense up, which can cause headaches.
- **Backache** Frequent tension in the muscles of the back can lead to backaches.
- **TMJ Syndrome** The joint that connects your upper jaw to your lower jaw is called the temporomandibular joint (TMJ). If stress causes a person to clench or grind the teeth, then pain in the joint, headaches, and dental problems can result.
- **Coronary Heart Disease** Prolonged stress can cause changes in your body that can lead to a heart attack. One of these changes is an increased amount of cholesterol in the bloodstream. Cholesterol is a fat-like substance that can clog the arteries that supply blood to the heart. If a blockage of blood to the heart occurs, a heart attack may result.
- **High Blood Pressure** Part of the stress response is an increase in blood pressure. **High blood pressure** can eventually cause the rupture of a blood vessel in the brain, resulting in the loss of speech, bodily movement, and even death.
- **Chronic Fatigue** Prolonged stress can cause a person to feel tired all the time. This type of fatigue is different from the feeling one gets after strenuous physical exercise. Chronic fatigue is a *long-term* loss of energy.
- **Mental Illness** Prolonged stress can wear down a person's psyche to the point that mental illness results. Damage to a person's mind can be just as devastating as damage to the body.

There is even some evidence that people under prolonged stress may be more likely than others to develop cancer.

Stress not only can make you ill, but also can lead to injuries. When you are under stress, you aren't able to concentrate very well, which could increase your chances of having an accident.

Review

1. *Define stress.*
2. *Describe the stress response.*
3. *Name at least four disorders that are caused by stress or made worse by stress.*
4. ***Critical Thinking*** *Many businesses offer stress-management programs to their employees. How could a stress-management program increase a company's profits?*

ASSESS

Section Review

Have students answer the Section Review questions.

Alternative Assessment

Present Level of Stress

Have students write a paragraph describing their current level of stress. Do they have any of the signs of a stress response; if so, can they say why? If they are feeling no stress, is this a typical condition for them, or do they expect it to change soon? Are they taking any specific steps to keep their stress level low?

Closure

Upcoming Stressful Situations

Ask students to list and describe one or more stressful situations they expect to face during the next 12 months. Stressful situations might include a prom, a playoff game, a driving test, moving, breaking up with a girlfriend or boyfriend, or a serious illness in the family. Have students save their list for the next section.

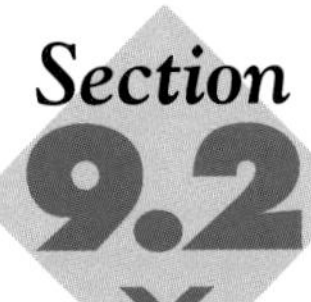

Section 9.2 How to Manage Stress

Objectives

- *Define stress intervention.*
- *Explain why physical exercise is a good way to handle stress.*
- *Use selective awareness to change your interpretation of a stressor.*
  LIFE SKILLS: Coping
- *Practice a relaxation technique that helps you to deal with stress.*
  LIFE SKILLS: Coping

In this section you'll learn how to manage stressors as they come up on a daily basis by using the stress model shown in below. Notice that the stress model consists of a series of steps, each step leading to the next. It is possible for you to take action to *stop* yourself from progressing from one step to the next.

The Stress Model

Step 1: A New or Potentially Unpleasant Situation (The Stressor) A situation triggers the stress.

Step 2: You Interpret the Situation as Threatening You interpret the situation as threatening, which leads to Step 3.

Step 3: Your Emotional Response You feel anxious, nervous, or insecure, which leads to the physical response in Step 4.

Step 4: Your Physical Response You experience the physical response, which leads to the negative consequences of Step 5.

Step 5: The Negative Consequences If nothing is done to relieve the stress, any number of consequences can result. School work may suffer, for example, as can a person's relationship with family and friends. A serious illness can also result from untreated long-term stress.

Signs of Stress

Physical Signs	Emotional and Mental Signs
Headaches	*Anxiety*
Dry mouth	*Frustration*
Teeth grinding	*Mood swings*
Shortness of breath	*Depression*
Pounding heart	*Irritability*
Indigestion	*Nightmares*
Diarrhea	*Nervous laugh*
Constipation	*Worrying*
Muscle aches	*Confusion*
Weight change	*Forgetfulness*
Fatigue	*Poor concentration*
Insomnia	*Loneliness*

(FIGURE 9-6) **This table shows some of the signs of stress. How many of these signs do you recognize in yourself? If you have more than a few, be sure to practice the stress interventions discussed in this chapter.**

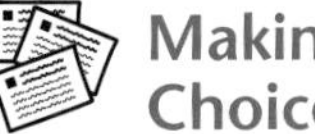

Making a Choice 9B

Stress Intervention Role-Play

Assign the Stress Intervention Role-Play card. The card requires students to describe a stressful situation, apply the stress model to the situation, identify stress interventions for the situation, and role-play the situation with and without the stress intervention. The class will discuss whether the stress interventions seemed successful.

Section 9.2 Lesson Plan

MOTIVATE

Journal 9C
Signs of Stress

This may be done as a warm-up activity. Ask students to study the signs of stress in Figure 9-6. In the Student Journal, have them write any of the signs that they experience when stressed. Tell them to annotate their list to show how often they experience each stress sign: D = daily, W = weekly, O = occasionally.

Class Discussion
A Personal Touch

Tell the students that studies rank your job as a teacher as very stressful. Then volunteer some examples of tasks or situations that a teacher deals with that are stressful. Indicate what the stressors are, such as overscheduling, difficult students, teaching concerns, and so on.

TEACH

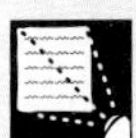

Teaching Transparency 9A
The Stress Road

Show this transparency (Figure 9-8) to introduce the stress model. The model presents the five stages of stress as towns along a highway. Keep the transparency displayed throughout this section for reference in teaching and for use by students.

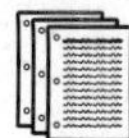

Life Skills Worksheet 9A

Creating a Relaxation Corner

Assign the Creating a Relaxation Corner Life Skills Worksheet, which encourages students to design a relaxation corner in their home, where they can go when they feel especially stressed out. (Use after relaxation techniques have been introduced.)

The following example will help you understand how the stress model works in a real-life situation.

Step 1. A New or Potentially Unpleasant Situation (The Stressor)	*Someone you are attracted to asks you to go to a movie with him or her.*
Step 2. You Interpret the Situation as Threatening	*You interpret this situation as threatening because you want to make a good impression and be able to go out with this person again. What if you say something dumb? What if this person doesn't think you are any fun?*
Step 3. Your Emotional Response	*During the movie, you start feeling nervous, doubtful, worried, and anxious.*
Step 4. Your Physical Response	*By the time the movie is over, you are sweating like crazy and your heart is racing in your chest.*
Step 5. The Negative Consequences	*You seem very nervous and you can't even talk about the movie later because you were too upset to pay much attention to it. The other person thinks you are strange and doesn't want to go out with you again.*

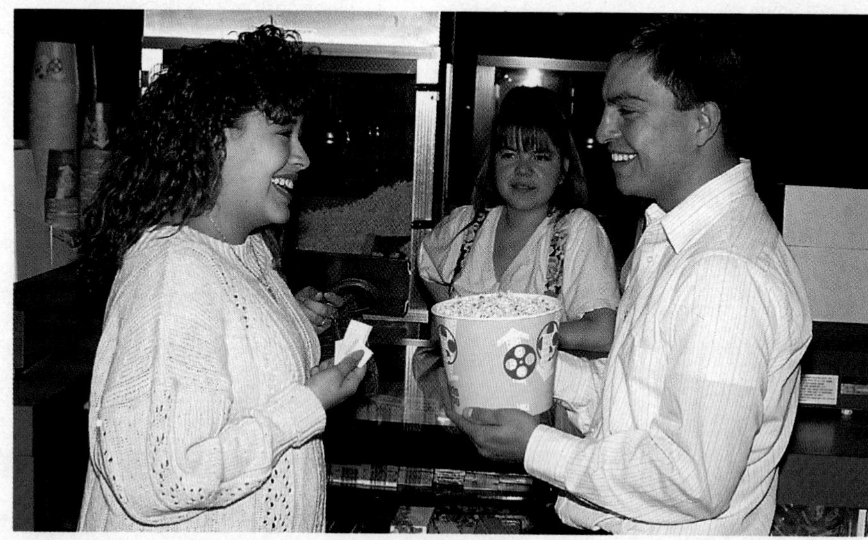

(FIGURE 9-7) **If you think positively, a situation such as a date is much more likely to turn out well. You can prevent a lot of stress by changing your interpretation of events.**

• • • TEACH continued

Game

The Stress Model

Have students form groups and play the Stress Model game to help them learn the five steps. Make sure the teaching transparency for the stress model is displayed for students' reference. Randomly choose a student to state Step 1 (a new or potentially unpleasant situation occurs), along with a stressor he or she makes up (example: failing an exam). Select another student to state Step 2 (interpret the situation), along with how he or she interprets the first student's stressor. (Is it a threat or not?) Continue with the remaining steps (3, emotional response—anxiety; 4, physical response—headache; 5, negative consequences—angry parents and possible punishment). Repeat the cycle until every student has had three turns.

Cooperative Learning

Stress Situations

Have students work in groups of four to write a stress situation, using the stress model. Tell them to write the five stress model steps down the left side of a sheet, and write what happens in each step on the right side. Have each group work with another group to critique and improve each other's situations.

This scenario can be much different. Imagine that you have the same life situation (being asked out), but this time you decide that you're going to *interpret* the situation positively. "I must be a really fun person," you think. "I must be desirable." Because you think of the situation this way, you won't feel nearly as nervous or insecure, and none of the negative things that happened in the first scenario will occur. You have stopped yourself from progressing from one step to the next.

Think of the stress model as a map of a road that goes through the towns of "A New or Potentially Unpleasant Situation," "You Interpret the Situation as Threatening," "Your Emotional Response," "Your Physical Response," and "The Negative Consequences." As with all roads, you can set up a roadblock anywhere along the way. Stress management is setting up roadblocks that prevent you from traveling to the next "town." The roadblocks you set up are stress interventions. A **stress intervention** is any action that prevents a stressor from resulting in negative consequences.

The following stress interventions, or roadblocks, are helpful in managing stress.

stress intervention: *any action that prevents a stressor from resulting in negative consequences.*

The Stress Model

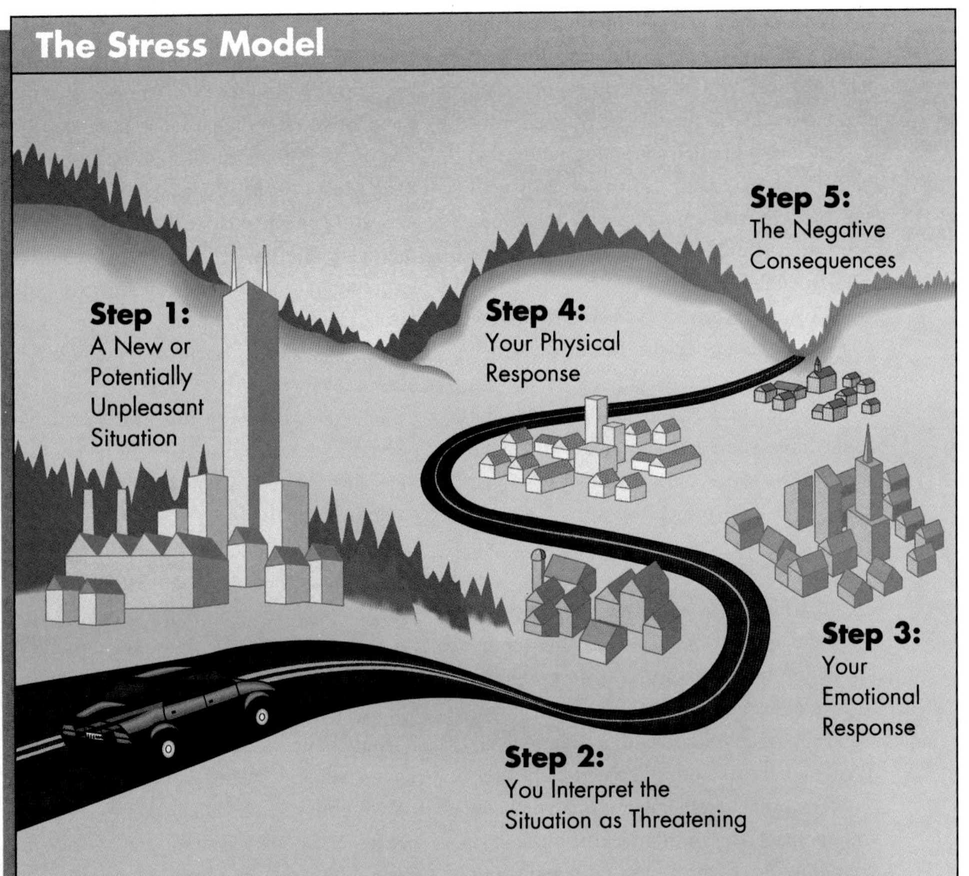

(FIGURE 9-8) **Think of the stress model as a map of a road that goes through different towns. As with all roads, you can set up a roadblock along the way.**

Section 9.2

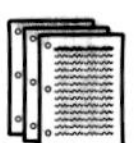

Section Review Worksheet 9.2

Assign Section Review Worksheet 9.2, which requires students to name the steps of the stress model, identify these steps in a specific situation, and suggest ways to intervene for each of the steps.

Section Quiz 9.2

Have students take Section Quiz 9.2.

Reteaching Worksheet 9.2

Students who have difficulty with the material may complete Reteaching Worksheet 9.2, which requires them to identify steps in the stress model and apply the stress model to a particular situation. It also asks students to choose among stress interventions for the situation.

Journal 9D
Dealing With Stressors

Ask students to create a three-column chart in the Student Journal. Explain that they are to list in the first column everyday situations that cause them stress. After they have read Eliminating Some Stressors, in the second column they should explain in a phrase or two how they can do it. After reading Changing Your Interpretation of a Stressor, have students write in the third column what positive aspect they can focus on through selective awareness.

Demonstration
Practicing Relaxation Techniques

Have students form small groups to practice some of the methods described in the text—meditation, progressive relaxation, body scanning, and imagery.

Class Discussion
Laughter Relieves Stress

Tell a joke in class or show cartoons from a book. Then discuss laughter as a method for reducing stress.

Class Discussion
Choosing an Intervention

Ask students to select some stressors from the chart they created in their Student Journal along with their intervention method. Have them write the

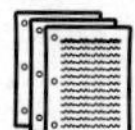

Life Skills Worksheet 9B

How Do You Communicate?

Assign the Communicating Effectively Life Skills Worksheet. The worksheet requires students to describe problems they have had communicating in the past week, to think about how miscommunication caused stress, to evaluate why there was a problem with communication, and to figure out concrete things they can do to communicate better.

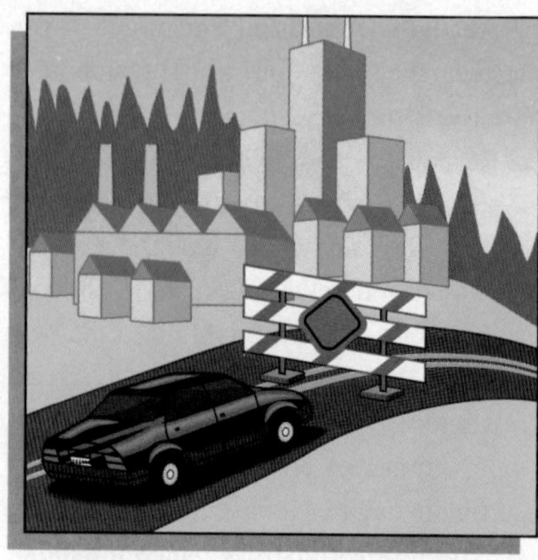

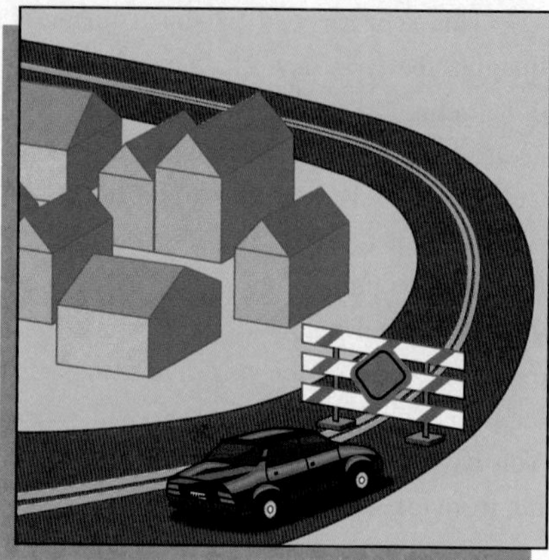

Eliminating Some Stressors

If you sat down and listed the situations that cause you stress, you would probably realize that you have a lot of stressors that occur regularly. These regular stressors are the easiest ones to anticipate and remove from your life. By getting rid of some of your stressors, you are setting up a roadblock—a stress intervention—in front of Step 1 of the stress model.

For instance, if it is very difficult for you to wake up in the morning, which causes you to be late to school or work, you could go to sleep earlier at night. Or you could have someone you live with make sure you wake up on time. Either way, you have stopped the progress of stress before it even starts by eliminating one of your stressors.

If someone at your school is mean to you, you could eliminate that stressor by just avoiding the person. If it isn't possible to avoid the person altogether, you could make sure that you are with a friend whenever you have to associate with that person.

The point to remember is that you have some control over the number of stressors in your life. One of the best ways of managing stress is to begin getting rid of some stressors in the first place. Which of *your* stressors can you eliminate?

selective awareness:

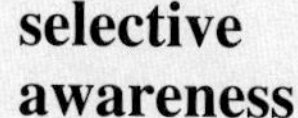

focusing on the aspects of a situation that help a person feel better (''thinking positively'').

Changing Your Interpretation of a Stressor

It would be impossible to get rid of all the stressors in your life. You can't control the fact that you didn't get the after-school job you wanted, for example, or that you will have a test in your Spanish class tomorrow.

But you *can* change the way you interpret a stressor. When you change your interpretation of a stressor, you are setting up a roadblock in front of Step 2 of the stress model. To do this, you can use what is called **selective awareness.** Selective awareness is choosing to focus on the aspects of a situation that help you feel better. Selective awareness can be thought of as ''thinking positively.''

If you don't get the job you want, you can think to yourself, ''At least I got some practice interviewing for a job, which will help me prepare for the next job interview.'' If you're nervous about a test, you can think: ''At least it will be over tomorrow, so I won't have to worry about it after that. Then I can do something fun.''

A college student named Tatyana gave her father a good lesson in selective awareness. She wrote him from college that she had fallen out of her dormitory window, cracked her skull, and had been taken to the hospital. While in the hospital, she wrote,

• • • TEACH continued

stressors on plain paper and place them anonymously in the Question Box. Draw the papers randomly from the box, and read the stressor. Then have the class suggest and discuss the best intervention for that stressor: elimination, selective awareness, relaxation, or exercise.

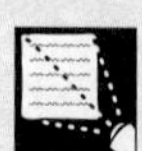

Teaching Transparency 9B

The Body Under Stress; The Body Relaxed

Use the transparency to help students identify physical symptoms they experience when going from a state of stress to a state of relaxation.

Extension

Stressful Occupations

Have students choose a profession or job they find interesting. Ask them to speculate about three stressors a person in this profession probably experiences daily. Then have them suggest a stress intervention strategy the person could use on the job.

she fell in love with a man who was on parole from prison for physically abusing his first wife. Tatyana told her father that she and this man were planning to run away to get married.

At the end of the letter, however, she told him that she hadn't really fallen out of a window, hadn't been taken to a hospital, and hadn't met anyone with whom she had fallen in love. "But," she wrote, "I *did* fail chemistry, and I wanted you to put that in its proper perspective." Tatyana's father was not very upset about her failing chemistry because he focused on the fact that something much worse could have happened. Now *that* is using selective awareness!

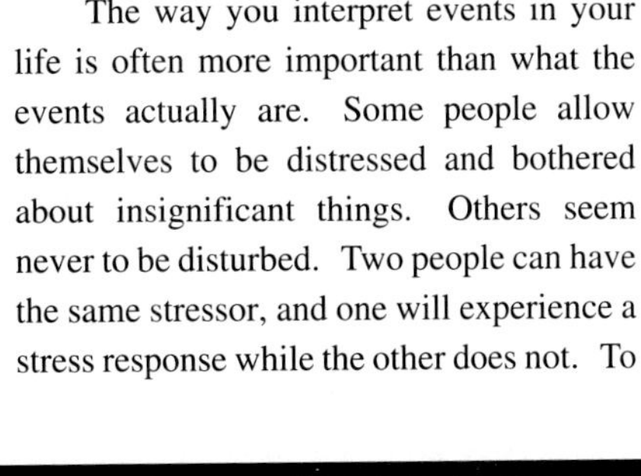

The way you interpret events in your life is often more important than what the events actually are. Some people allow themselves to be distressed and bothered about insignificant things. Others seem never to be disturbed. Two people can have the same stressor, and one will experience a stress response while the other does not. To

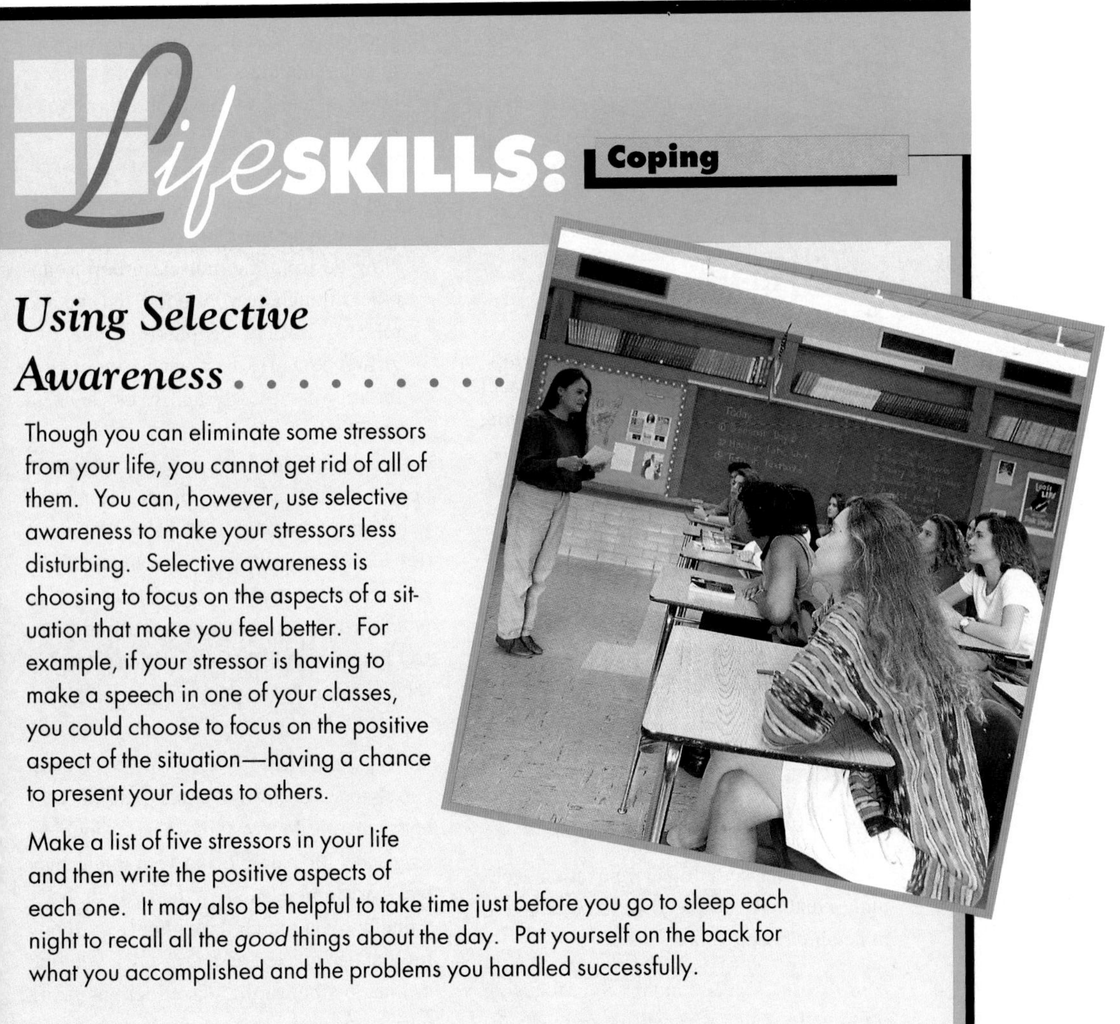

*Life*SKILLS: Coping

Using Selective Awareness

Though you can eliminate some stressors from your life, you cannot get rid of all of them. You can, however, use selective awareness to make your stressors less disturbing. Selective awareness is choosing to focus on the aspects of a situation that make you feel better. For example, if your stressor is having to make a speech in one of your classes, you could choose to focus on the positive aspect of the situation—having a chance to present your ideas to others.

Make a list of five stressors in your life and then write the positive aspects of each one. It may also be helpful to take time just before you go to sleep each night to recall all the *good* things about the day. Pat yourself on the back for what you accomplished and the problems you handled successfully.

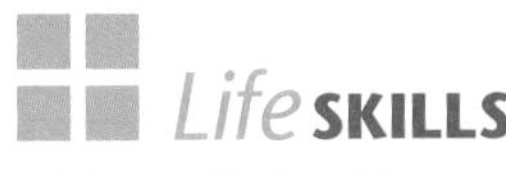

Life SKILLS

Using Selective Awareness

Ask volunteers to list five stressors and write some positive aspects of each.

Background

Progressive Relaxation

Progressive relaxation works systematically through the muscle groups: right arm/hand, left arm/hand, forehead, eyes, jaw, neck, shoulders/back, abdomen, right leg/foot, and left leg/foot. This takes time and practice to learn. An individual may want to use published guides to learn the method.

a great extent, each person determines how he or she reacts to situations and people.

The "Life Skills" activity on page 201 will help you to focus on the positive aspects of your stressors, rather than on the negative aspects.

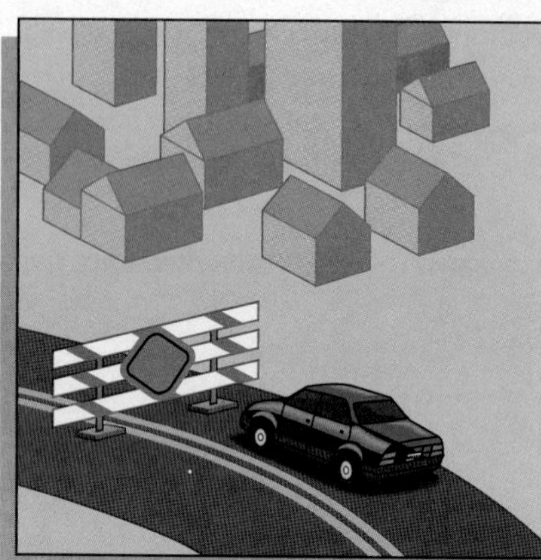

Using Relaxation Techniques

What if you're past the point of changing your interpretation of a situation? What if you are well on your way to becoming upset? One way to relieve your distress is to engage in some method of relaxation. When you do this, you are setting up a stress intervention in front of Step 3.

Different people relax in different ways. Some people like to listen to music. Others find that reading a book or watching television helps them relax. These activities have one thing in common: they take a person's mind off problems and hassles by focusing attention on the activity itself. Anything you do that "takes you away" for a while can be relaxing.

Here are some other relaxation techniques that have been shown to be effective in helping people relax.

Meditation Meditation involves focusing on something that is repetitive or unchanging. You can meditate by doing this simple, yet effective, exercise.

1. Sit down and close your eyes.
2. In your mind, repeat a word you find relaxing—maybe "calm," or "serene," or "one"—every time you breathe out.

After doing this for about 20 minutes you will probably feel relaxed and energetic.

Progressive Relaxation Some people prefer to be more active while relaxing. Progressive relaxation can meet this need. Here is how you do progressive relaxation.

1. First, tense the muscles in one part of your body. You might tense the muscles in your shoulders, for example. Notice how it feels to have those muscles *tensed*.
2. Then relax the same part of your body that you just tensed. Notice how it feels to have those muscles *relaxed*.
3. Now go from one muscle group to another throughout your body, tensing and relaxing. Many people find that this technique works best when you start at the top of the body and work down to your feet.

This is called progressive relaxation because you "progress" from one part of your body to another. Progressive relaxation is a good technique to use any time you feel tense. It is also a good technique to practice daily, so that when you find yourself in a stressful situation, you can quickly relax the muscles in your body.

Body Scanning Even when you feel tense, there is always some part of your body that feels relaxed. Your shoulders may ache, for example, but your thighs may feel warm and relaxed. When you do body scanning, you search throughout your body for that one relaxed part, and when you find it, imagine the warm, relaxed feeling being transferred to the rest of your body.

Autogenic Training You can relax by imagining that your arms and legs feel heavy, warm, and tingly. When they feel this way, it means that you have let go of muscle tension and dilated the blood vessels in your arms and legs. Once your body is relaxed, think of peaceful images—perhaps a relaxing day at the beach or walking under the stars.

Imagery Sitting quietly and thinking of certain images can help both your mind and body relax. Although you need to determine for yourself what images are relaxing to you, many people find the following images to be restful:

- the beach
- a park
- green pastures
- blue skies
- a starry night
- a meadow of flowers
- sunshine on your body
- a warm bath
- floating on water

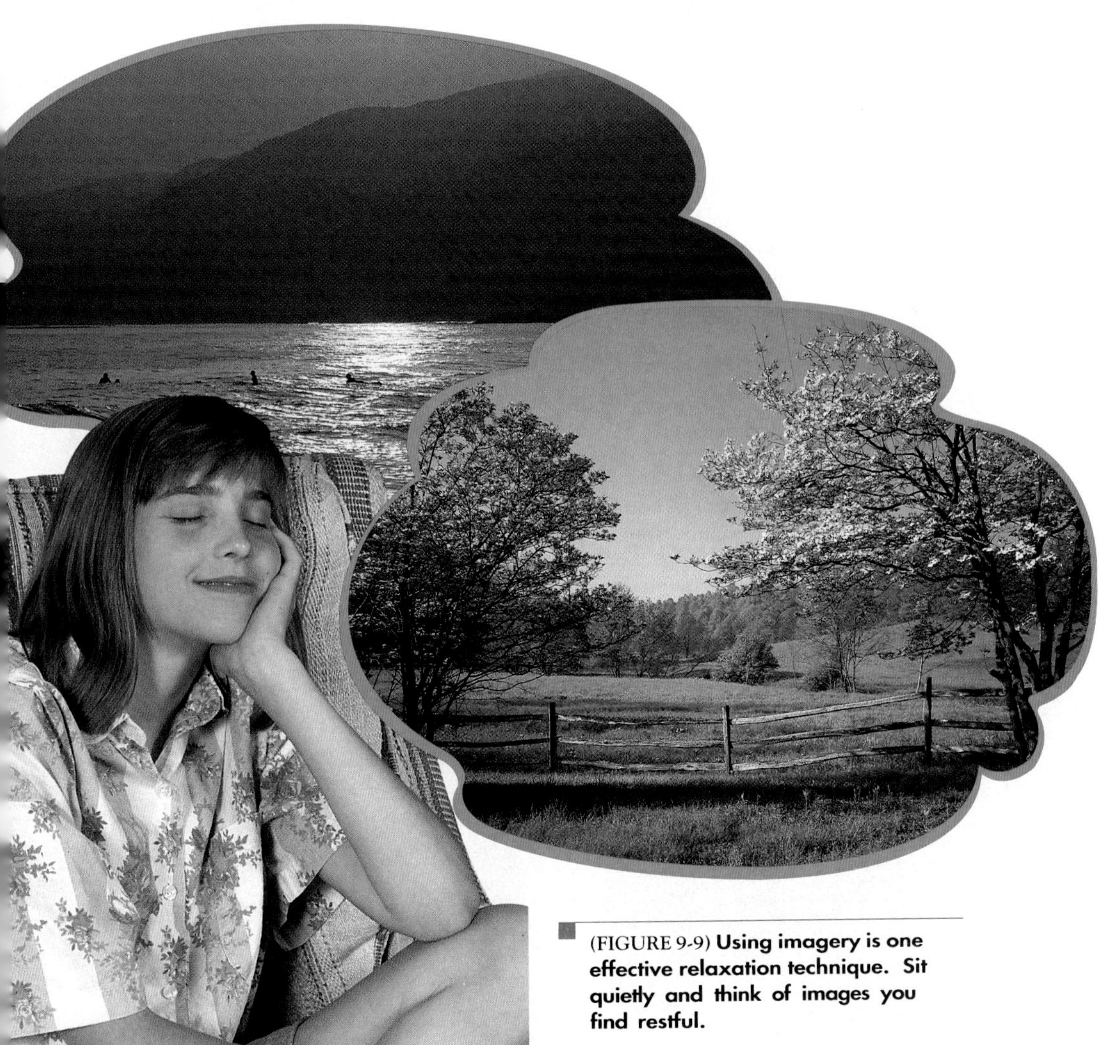

(FIGURE 9-9) **Using imagery is one effective relaxation technique. Sit quietly and think of images you find restful.**

SECTION 9.2

Background
Relaxation

Relaxation works best when done regularly. The key is to set aside the same time daily, in a comfortable and quiet place—no radio, TV, talking, or disturbing noises. It's also important to have the cooperation of those around you, to assure encouragement and uninterrupted time.

Check Up

Have students read the Check Up silently and answer the questions to themselves. Then ask for a show of hands on each question. Tell students to ask themselves the same questions at various times during the day. Ask them to assess whether they were tense all day or only at certain times.

Background

Using Physical Exercise

Occasional exercise does little good; general health and stress management need daily exercise. Warm-up exercises to stretch the body are very helpful. Good exercise activities include bicycling, swimming, aerobics, jogging, walking, racquetball, and tennis. A long-term benefit is that such exercise can be continued for a lifetime.

Check Up

How Tense Are You?

As you begin to read this, *freeze*. Don't move a bit. Now notice how your body is positioned.

1. Can you drop your shoulders? If you can, your shoulder muscles were unnecessarily tense.
2. Can you relax your forehead more? If you can, you were tensing the muscles in your forehead for no useful purpose.
3. Can you relax the muscles in your arms more? If you can, you were unnecessarily tensing them.
4. Check the muscles in your abdomen and legs. Are they contracted more than necessary?

Unnecessary muscle contraction is called bracing. Most of us don't even notice that we are bracing because it has become such a natural response to stressful lives. As a result of bracing, many people develop tension headaches, back trouble, or shoulder pain. You'll learn some relaxation techniques in Section 9.2 that will help you stop bracing.

Laughing Laughing is one of the easiest and most natural relaxation techniques known. You don't have to be taught how to laugh. Many people find that when they are under a lot of stress, it helps to watch a funny movie or television program or read a humorous book. Some studies have shown that laughing may even strengthen the immune system, and a stronger immune system is better able to fight off infections.

But laughing works as a relaxation technique only when you think something really is funny. Laughing because you feel nervous or embarrassed probably won't help you reduce stress.

Yelling or Crying Sometimes you just have to go off somewhere private and yell or cry. After a good yell or cry, a person can feel much more relaxed and able to deal with a stressor.

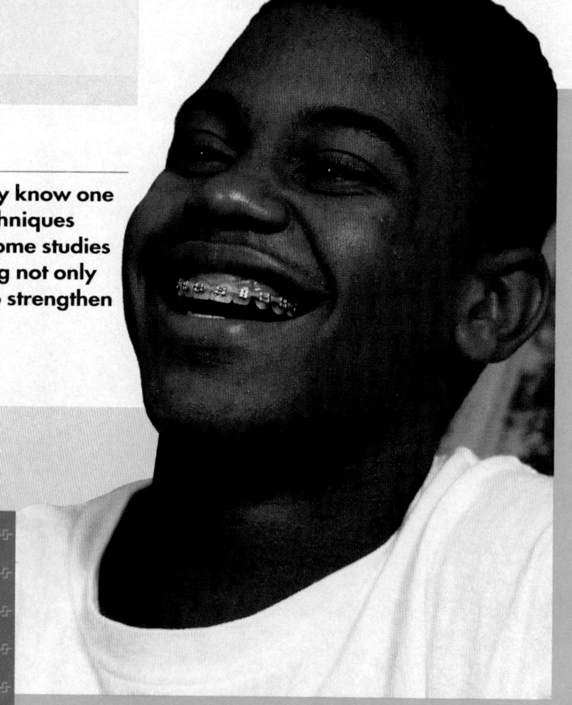

(FIGURE 9-10) **You already know one of the best relaxation techniques available—laughing. Some studies have shown that laughing not only relaxes you but may also strengthen your immune system.**

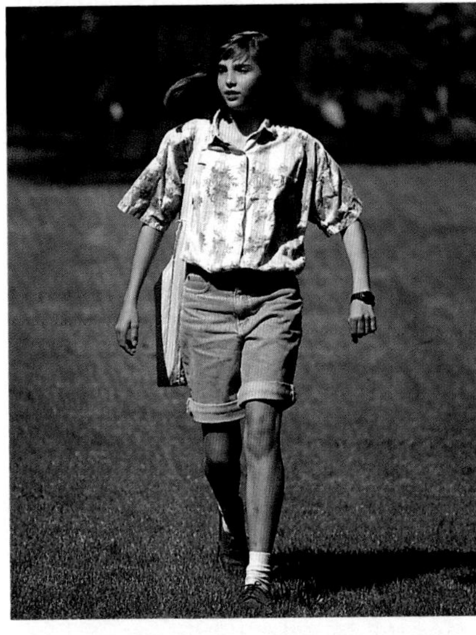

(FIGURE 9-11) **The stress response is harmful to you only if you don't do something physical. When you feel stressed, do a vigorous exercise such as walking at a brisk pace.**

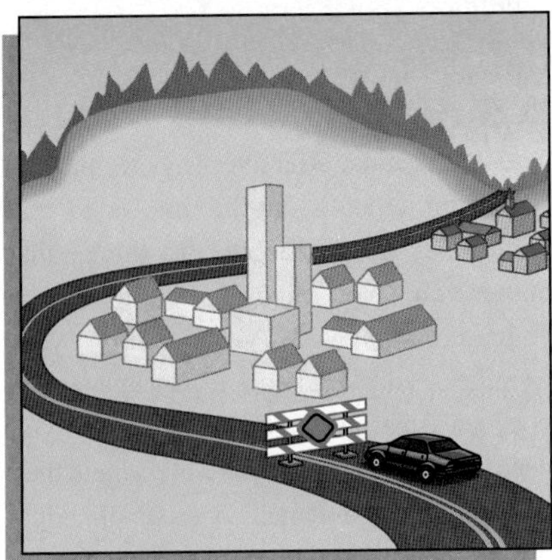

Using Physical Exercise

If you don't stop stress from progressing, you could end up with a variety of physical responses such as muscle tension, a racing heart, or high blood pressure. As you learned in Section 9.1, these changes are the result of the stress response, which prepares you to do something physical. The stress response is harmful to you only if you don't do something physical.

This is where exercise comes in. It sets up a stress intervention in front of Step 4 of the model by taking advantage of the body's readiness to do something physical.

Let's say you just had an argument with a friend. You are extremely angry. You can feel the muscle tension in your shoulders and you can feel your heart beating rapidly. If you take a jog around the neighborhood, or play basketball, or go for a swim, you *use* the tension in your muscles, and you *use* your increased heart rate to do something physical. You use the stress response to your advantage instead of allowing it to hurt you.

Review

1. *Define the term "stress intervention."*
2. ***LIFE SKILLS: Coping*** *Give one example of a stressor, and explain how a person could use selective awareness to change his or her interpretation of that stressor.*
3. *Why is physical exercise a good way to relieve stress?*
4. ***LIFE SKILLS: Coping*** *Practice a relaxation technique at least once, and describe how you felt afterward.*
5. ***Critical Thinking*** *Regular practice of a relaxation technique helps many people feel more energetic. Offer an explanation of this fact.*

Review Answers

1. Any action that prevents a stressor from resulting in negative consequences

2. Answers will vary. Accept any answer that shows an understanding and application of selective awareness.

3. Physical exercise enables the body to use the tension in the muscles, the increased heart rate, and some other physical changes that occur as part of the stress response in a positive, healthy way.

4. Answers will vary. Accept any answer that illustrates proper use of a relaxation technique.

5. Answers will vary. Relaxation techniques enable people to relax and become calm by taking their minds off problems as they focus their attention on a new activity. When a person feels calm or relaxed, he or she has more energy to devote to other activities rather than staying focused on the problem that caused the stress.

ASSESS

Section Review

Have students answer the Section Review questions.

Alternative Assessment

Which Roadblock?

Ask students to imagine being faced with four stressors at once: (1) it's final-exam week; (2) you had to give up your summer job because you must baby-sit your cousin across town for the summer; (3) the route to baby-sit is through a dangerous neighborhood; and (4) you lost your watch, which cost only $15, but you needed it badly to keep you on schedule. **How would you intervene for each stressor?** *[1—selective awareness; 2—selective awareness, relaxation, exercise; 3—elimination (find an alternate route, bicycle, or get a ride); 4—buy a new watch]*

Closure

Making It Work

Have students return to the list of stressful situations they compiled in the Closure feature of Section 9.1. Have them write beside each stressor an intervention they can use, and the specific thing they could do to make it work, such as how to eliminate the stressor, which specific positive thoughts to think, which relaxation method to use, or which exercise method to use.

Life SKILLS

Managing Your Time by Setting Goals and Prioritizing

Have students list their goals for tasks they want to complete today and prioritize them as described. Ask students to consider the following questions as they work on the list: Are there any activities or tasks I should say no to because I won't have enough time? Are there any goals that require me to get some help from others if I want to meet them? Who could I ask for help?

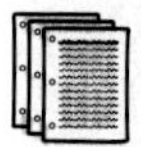

Life Skills Worksheet 9C

Evaluating Your Self-Esteem

Assign the Building Self-Esteem Life Skills Worksheet, which helps students build self-esteem by participating with a close friend in a guided discussion about self-doubts and strengths.

Section 9.3 Managing Stress Is a Lifelong Process

Objectives

- *Explain how a support group helps a person deal with stress.*
- *Manage your time by setting goals and prioritizing.*
  LIFE SKILLS: Setting Goals
- *Seek help if you or someone you know is overwhelmed by stress.*
  LIFE SKILLS: Using Community Resources

support group: *a group of people who trust each other and are able to talk to each other about their problems.*

You learned in Section 9.2 how to deal with stressors as they come up on a daily basis. You can also protect yourself from stress by continually practicing stress management throughout your lifetime.

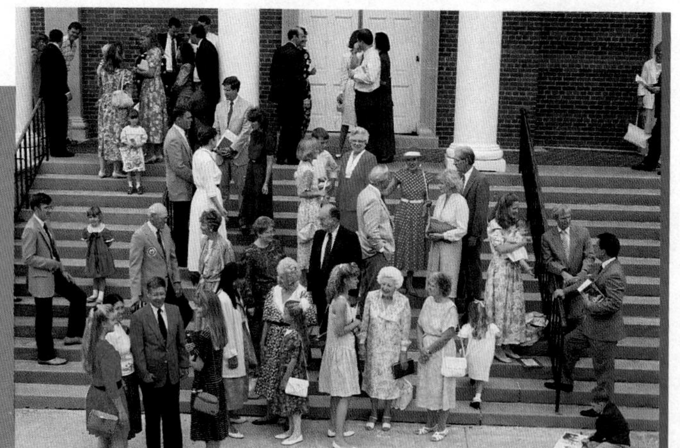

(FIGURE 9-12) **Many people find the support group they need in religious communities such as churches and synagogues. A support group is one of the most effective ways to manage stress throughout your lifetime.**

Physical Health

Many of the negative consequences of stress can be prevented by taking the following steps to keep yourself physically well:

- Exercise regularly.
- Eat a balanced diet.
- Get enough rest and sleep.
- Do one of the relaxation techniques discussed on pages 202-203 every day.
- Do not use tobacco, alcohol, or other drugs.

A Support Group

One of the most effective ways to manage stress throughout your lifetime is to talk with other people about the things that bother you. You might be able to discuss your stressors with your family, your friends, or your teachers. Find a few people you can trust and call on them when you need to talk, and be available when they need to talk to someone. A group of people like this is called a **support group.** Sometimes just talking about a stressor with a member of your support group can reduce the stress you're under.

A Spiritual Life

Many people find that having a spiritual life—a sense of connection with something greater than oneself—helps them get through times of great stress. Some people believe in a supreme being who provides

Section 9.3 Lesson Plan

MOTIVATE

Journal 9E
Stressful Life Stages

This may be done as a warm-up activity. Write the following life stages on the chalkboard: infancy, childhood, adolescence, adulthood, elderly. Ask students to write two stressors they think are important during each of the life stages. Tell them to write the life stage they believe is most stressful.

TEACH

Cooperative Learning
Devising a Health Program

Have students work in small groups, and have each group devise a physical health program. Ask them to plan a typical week, including exercise, meal patterns, sleep, and relaxation. Have the groups compare their plans.

Journal 9F
Support Groups

Have students construct a personal support group in the Student Journal, using the list on the chalkboard. Beside each category, have them write the names of individuals they trust to talk with about each type of problem.

Writing
Your Purpose in Life

Ask students to suppose their best friend has asked them two questions:

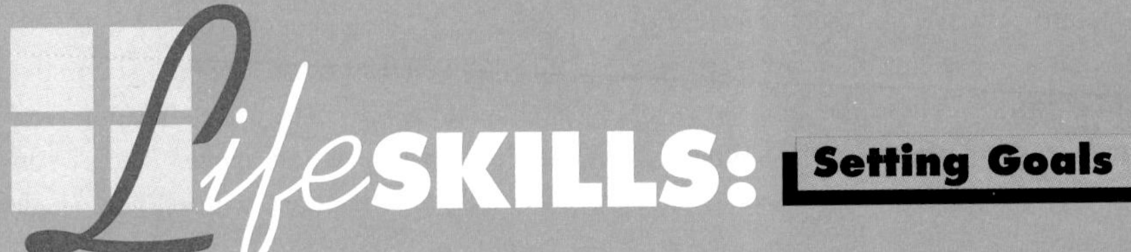

Managing Your Time by Setting Goals and Prioritizing

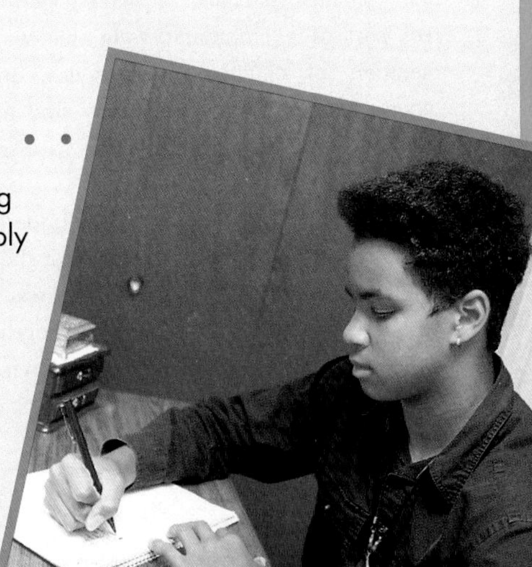

One common stressor for everyone is making enough time in the day. Sometimes we simply don't have enough time to do everything we want. The key to using time wisely is to set goals and prioritize them. The following steps will help you reduce the stress of "not enough time."

1. List your goals for today.
2. Prioritize your goals. Beside each goal, write either an "A," a "B," or a "C." The goals you label "A" are the ones you absolutely must get done that day. The ones labeled "B" are those you would *like* to get done. The goals labeled "C" are not very important and can wait until later.
3. During your day, do what is necessary to reach your "A" goals first, then your "B" goals. If you have some time left, you can attend to your "C" goals.

This strategy can be adapted for shorter or longer periods of time than a day. You can develop goals for a single morning, for example, or for a week, a month, and even a year.

The following suggestions may also help you manage your time:

- Learn to say no. Do not take on tasks that you have no time to complete.
- Work on one task at a time. Don't go back and forth between tasks. The time it takes to constantly reorient yourself is time wasted.
- Ask for help from others when you are pressured for time.

Life Skills Worksheet 9D

Finding Help When Stress is Overwhelming

Assign the Finding Help When Stress is Overwhelming Life Skills Worksheet, which encourages students to survey and evaluate one community resource that they could utilize in times of overwhelming stress.

Section Review Worksheet 9.3

Assign Section Review Worksheet 9.3, which requires students to fill in a chart identifying different ways to manage stress, whom they can turn to if stress becomes overwhelming, and when it is essential for a person to get help.

Section Quiz 9.3

Have students take Section Quiz 9.3.

Reteaching Worksheet 9.3

Students who have difficulty with the material may complete Reteaching Worksheet 9.3. This worksheet requires students to help reduce stress by prioritizing and scheduling activities.

"What do you believe about your purpose in life?" and "Does your belief help you deal with stress?" Have students write a letter to their friend, answering the questions. Explain that this will help them understand themselves better. Assure them that their thoughts are private and that no one will read their letters.

Class Discussion
Major Life Changes

Discuss the stressors of unplanned pregnancy, abuse, and suicide. Have students weigh the merits of people with such problems seeking help from various sources, such as clergy, a therapist, a doctor, a hospital, the police, and hot lines. Explore the impact upon family and friends of their seeking help.

Reinforcement
Seeking Help

Remind students that if stress ever overwhelms them, they should get help and not try to handle it alone. Emphasize that dangerous stressors, such as suicidal thoughts, pregnancy, sexual abuse, physical beatings, and psychological abuse are too much for one person to deal with alone. Remind students that even though there is the risk of hurting other family members in talking about one's problems, it is always better to seek help.

Extension
Using Support Groups

Have students test their individual support groups by selecting a problem

Review Answers

1. Talking with a trustworthy, helpful person about a stressor can reduce the stress a person is feeling. Also, the support person might be able to suggest ways to better cope with the stressor.

2. Answers will vary, depending on each individual student's goals.

3. You or the friend can talk with a trusting adult, or you or the friend can call the National Child Abuse Hot Line—1-800-422-4453.

4. Talk to an adult you can trust or look in the phone book under "Suicide" and call the local suicide-prevention hot line.

5. Tobacco is a stimulant; using tobacco can make a person feel even more stressed. Alcohol is a depressant; using alcohol can make the stress seem worse than it ordinarily would appear. Alcohol, along with other drugs, may make a person forget about a stressor for a very short time. Drugs do not, however, make the stressor go away, nor do they provide a long-term solution to dealing with the stressor.

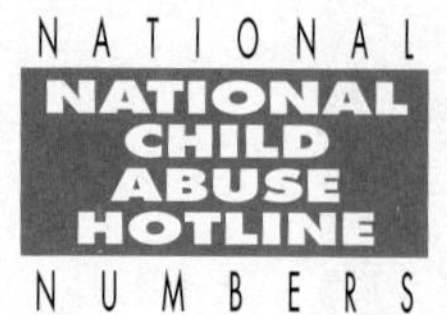

1-800-422-4453

comfort and guidance during hard times. And some people feel a strong connection with nature, which gives them a feeling of peace and a sense that they are part of a beautiful world. These are both ways of having a spiritual life. There are numerous other ways, perhaps as many ways as there are people.

Organized religions can help people deal with stress not only by offering spiritual guidance, but also by helping people feel part of a community. In this way, members of churches, synagogues, and other religious communities may find the support group they need to cope with the stressors in their lives.

Some people would not call themselves "spiritual," but they feel that their life has a purpose—to help relieve the suffering of others, for example, or simply to act with honesty and integrity. Believing that one's life has purpose and meaning can get a person through the worst of times.

Getting Professional Help

At times a person can feel overwhelmed by stress. This can happen to anyone, even those who practice stress management. If you ever feel unable to cope with the stress in your life, you can get help from a professional. You might know a minister, priest, or rabbi you can turn to. Or your school counselor might be someone you could talk with.

You could also talk to a therapist when you feel overwhelmed by stress. You'll learn in Chapter 7 about the different types of therapists and how to get in touch with them.

Some stressors cannot possibly be managed without the help of someone else. A person who is being physically, sexually, or emotionally abused should not be expected to deal with that stress all alone. If you are being abused, or if you know anyone who is being abused, you can talk with an adult you trust or call the hotline number shown at the left. The call is free, and you don't have to give your name. The person who answers the phone will tell you where to get help. Abuse is discussed in more detail in Chapter 20.

Sometimes stress can be so overwhelming that ending one's life seems like the only way out. If you or someone you know is thinking of suicide, get help immediately. Talk to an adult you trust or look in the phone book under "Suicide" and call your local suicide-prevention hotline. Chapter 11 of this book is devoted to discussing suicide prevention.

Review

1. *How does a support group help a person deal with stress?*
2. ***LIFE SKILLS: Setting Goals*** *Set your goals for the next week and divide them into tasks you must get done, tasks you would like to get done, and tasks that can wait until later.*
3. ***LIFE SKILLS: Using Community Resources*** *If you or someone you know were being abused, what could you do to get help?*
4. ***LIFE SKILLS: Using Community Resources*** *If you or someone you know were thinking of suicide, what could you do to get help?*
5. ***Critical Thinking*** *How could the use of tobacco, alcohol, or other drugs contribute to stress?*

• • • TEACH continued

from their Student Journal and actually talking to the person they indicated they could trust.

ASSESS

Section Review

Have students answer the Section Review questions.

Alternative Assessment

Suggesting Ways to Cope

Have students write a paragraph suggesting ways a student in the following situation could cope with the stress she faces: Ellen has an after-school job at a fast-food restaurant; she also helps her mother care for her younger brothers, who are 7 and 3 years old; she likes to participate in sports that often practice before school.

Closure

Testing the Relaxation Techniques

Ask students to choose one of the relaxation techniques described in the chapter and try it out the next time they feel a stress response coming on. Have students report back to the class on how successful the technique was for them.

Highlights

Summary

- A stressor is a new or potentially unpleasant situation.
- A stress response is a reaction of the mind or body to a stressor. Stress responses include release of adrenalin, faster heart rate, faster breathing rate, high blood pressure, tense muscles, and greater blood flow to the brain and legs.
- A stress response is helpful when a person is being physically threatened and needs to respond immediately.
- If not managed properly, stress can cause physical and mental disorders, or make such disorders worse.
- The stress model is a series of steps that describes how stress develops. If you know the stress model and the way it works, you can stop yourself from progressing from one step to the next.
- Using selective awareness, or focusing on the positive aspects of a stressor, is one way to cope with a stressful situation.
- Anything you do that takes you away from your worries for a while can help you relax and reduce stress. Relaxation techniques include listening to music, reading a book, meditating, progressive relaxation, body scanning, and imagery.
- Physical exercise can relieve muscle tension caused by stress.
- One of the most effective ways to manage stress throughout a lifetime is to develop a support system. A support system is a group of people you can talk to about your problems. Support systems usually include family members, friends, teachers, or clergy.
- When a person feels overwhelmed by stress, he or she can get professional help from counselors, therapists, and clergy.

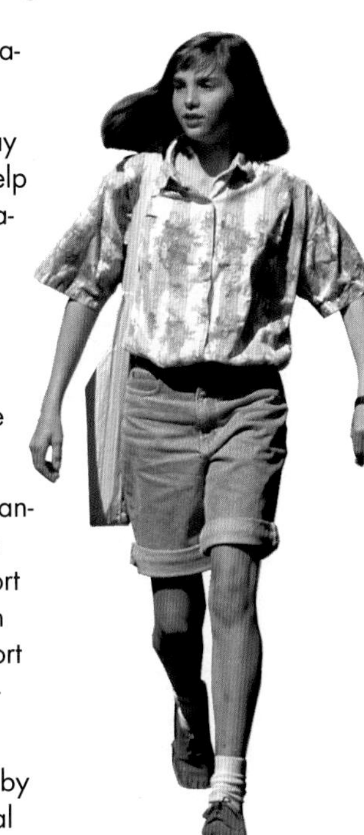

Vocabulary

stressor any new or potentially unpleasant situation.

stress response reaction of the mind and body to a stressor.

stress the combination of a stressor and a stress response.

selective awareness focusing on the aspects of a situation that help a person feel better ("thinking positively").

support group a group of people who trust each other and are able to talk to each other about their problems.

Chapter 9 Highlights Strategies

Summary

Have students read the summary to reinforce the concepts they have learned in Chapter 9.

Vocabulary

Have students review the definitions of *stressor, stress response, stress,* and *stress intervention,* then sketch a diagram showing their relation. Several diagrams are possible; the basic relation is:

Stressor + Stress Response = Stress

Stress Intervention

Extension

If students have a family member or friend who has a serious stress problem, suggest they share what they have learned in this chapter with that person. They might encourage the person to practice a relaxation technique or exercise along with them or go with them to a library or bookstore to find a helpful guide on stress intervention.

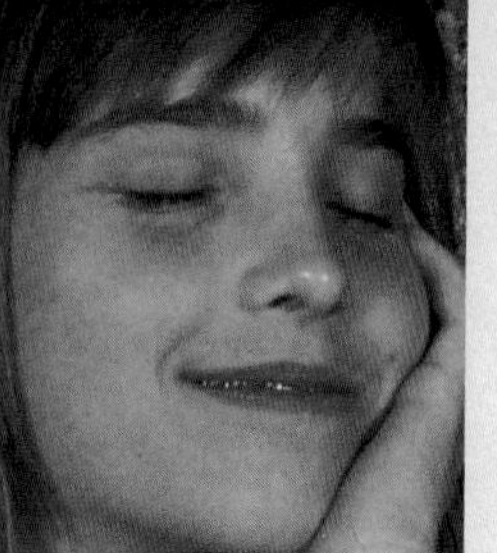

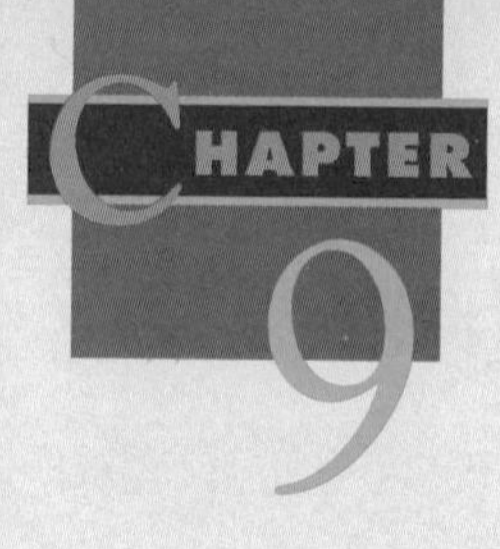

Chapter Review

Concept Review

1. How can stress be both bad and good for you?
2. What changes can occur in your body during a stress response?
3. Can positive situations be stressful? Explain.
4. Explain how stress can make you ill and lead to injuries.
5. Describe at least four other consequences of stress.
6. What are three ways to cope with stress?
7. At the end of a very stressful day, you find yourself unable to sleep. What can you do ?
8. Explain why progressive relaxation is a good way to manage stress.
9. What can you do to maintain your physical health during times of stress?
10. What is a support system? How can it help you?
11. What can a person do if he or she feels totally overpowered by stressful situations and has tried all the usual coping techniques?
12. Stress often results from taking on too many tasks. Name three ways to protect yourself from this kind of stress?

Expressing Your View

1. Exam time is always a stressful time for you. While you are studying, you seem to know the material well; but during the exam, your anxiety level is so high that you can't remember anything. What can you do to cope better with the stress, so that you can improve your grade on the next exam?
2. Name five jobs that you think are highly stressful. Name five jobs that you think are not stressful. Do you think everyone would classify these jobs as you did? Why, or why not?
3. Gary has been experiencing muscle tension and a rapid heartbeat. The problem seems to get worse every time he argues with his girlfriend. What advice would you give him?
4. Laughter usually has positive results in coping with stress. Describe a situation in which humor might be inappropriate or have a negative effect.

CHAPTER REVIEW

Concept Review

Sample responses:

1. People need enough stressors to make life interesting. Stress, however, can become bad for you when you can't control the stressors or relieve the stress. This type of stress can cause illness.

2. Your body releases adrenaline, which makes you breathe faster, your heart beat faster, your muscles tense, and your mouth feel dry.

3. Any event that involves a change in one's life situation, even a change that is positive, such as getting married, can be stressful.

4. Stress can make certain physical and mental disorders worse. Stress weakens the immune system and makes the body more susceptible to colds and flu. Because you can't concentrate very well when you are under stress, you can have an accident that may cause injuries.

5. Tension headaches, backache, TMJ syndrome, coronary artery disease, high blood pressure, chronic fatigue, mental illness

6. Eliminate some stressors, change your interpretation of a stressor (selective awareness), relaxation techniques, physical exercise

7. Use one of the various relaxation techniques.

8. It helps relax tense muscles that are often caused by stress.

9. Reduce or eliminate stressors and use various methods that are effective in controlling stress

10. A group of people you can trust and call upon if you need to talk. Sometimes just talking about a problem can reduce stress.

11. Get professional help.

12. Learn to say No, list your goal for the day, prioritize your goals, work on one task at a time, ask others for help

Expressing Your Views

Sample responses:

1. Try relaxation techniques before and during exams, talk with a counselor on how to take tests better

Life Skills Check

1. Coping
Your friend seems very impatient, competitive, and even hostile with her friends lately. You think that she has overburdened herself with activities and responsibilities. Describe some relaxation techniques that might ease her stress.

2. Coping
You just found out that your family will be moving to another city. You know there will be many benefits for your family, but all you can think about are the changes you will have to make. You feel worried and scared. Make a list of five positive aspects of moving that might make you feel better.

Projects

1. Work with a group to make a list of stressors in the everyday lives of people in a certain age category (children, teenagers, adults, or elderly people). Then interview two people in the age category your group chose, to find out what their greatest stressors are. Compare the results to your first list and discuss the results.
2. Write a short essay focusing on findings that show a definite relationship between physical disorders and stress.
3. Find out if you are managing your time wisely by making a pie graph that shows how much time you spend on your daily activities. For example, you might spend 5 percent on chores, 30 percent in school, 15 percent with friends, 10 percent on extracurricular activities, 5 percent on homework, and 35 percent sleeping. Analyze your graph and decide whether managing your time better will reduce your stress.

Plan for Action

List the greatest stressors in your life at this time and devise a plan to lower your stress level using the suggestions in this chapter.

Chapter 9 Assessment

2. Jobs that cause stress may require a lot of work in a short amount of time, may demand important decision making, or may make a person feel he or she has little control. Jobs that cause little stress may not have the pressure of time limits or may be enjoyable.
3. Try various methods in controlling stress, find out why he and his girlfriend argue, and try to resolve those problems. He must find ways to eliminate or reduce stressors.
4. When you feel nervous or embarrassed, or when you try to make a situation seem less serious because you do not know how to respond to the situation—such as laughing when you are with someone who is very ill, or laughing at a wake or funeral.

Life Skills Check

Sample responses:
1. Students may describe any of the relaxation techniques discussed in the chapter.
2. Answers will vary.

Projects

Have students plan and carry out the projects for managing stress.

Plan for Action

Have students work in pairs to role-play stressful situations such as interviewing for a summer job, performing in a school talent show, or taking a final exam. After developing a brief, stressful scene, have the person who is under stress describe any physical symptoms he or she feels; have the other person describe his or her response to the first person.

Assessment Options

Chapter Test

Have students take the Chapter 9 Test.

Alternative Assessment

Have students do the Alternative Assessment activity for Chapter 9.

Test Generator

The Test Generator (Macintosh® or IBM® format) contains an additional 50 assessment items for this chapter.

Coping With Loss

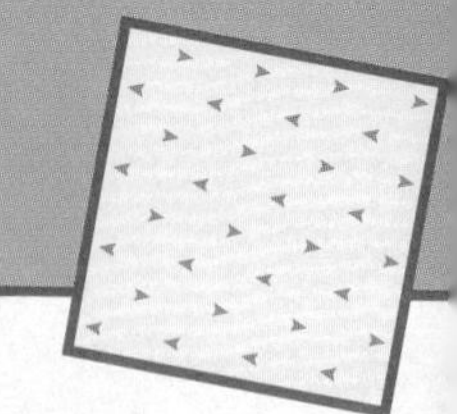

Planning Guide

TEXT SECTIONS	OBJECTIVES	TEXT FEATURES	OUTSIDE RESOURCES	NOTES
10.1 **Death and Dying** pp. 213-218 2 periods	• Describe the five stages terminally ill people generally pass through. • List three reasons why many people choose hospice care when they are terminally ill. • Describe the functions of a living will. ■ Learn how to be of help to someone who is dying.	• Check Up, p. 215 **ASSESSMENT** • Section Review, p. 217	**TEACHER'S RESOURCE BINDER** • Lesson Plan 10.1 • Personal Health Inventory • Journal Entries 10A, 10B • Life Skills Worksheet 10A • Section Review Worksheet 10.1 • Section Quiz 10.1 • Reteaching Worsheet 10.1 **OTHER RESOURCES** • Making a Choice 10A • Transparency 10A • English/Spanish Audiocassette 3 • Parent Discussion Guide	
10.2 **The Grieving Process** pp. 219-222 1 period	• List three reasons for having funerals or memorial services. ■ Learn how to deal with your own grief. ■ Learn how to give emotional support to someone who is grieving.	■ LIFE SKILLS: Communicating Effectively, p. 221 **ASSESSMENT** • Section Review, p. 222	**TEACHER'S RESOURCE BINDER** • Lesson Plan 10.2 • Journal Entry 10C • Life Skills Worksheet 10B, 10C, 10D • Ethics Worksheet • Section Review Worksheet 10.2 • Section Quiz 10.2 • Reteaching Worksheet 10.2 **OTHER RESOURCES** • Making a Choice 10B	
End of Chapter pp. 223-225		**ASSESSMENT** • Chapter Review, pp. 224-225	**TEACHER'S RESOURCE BINDER** • Chapter Test • Alternative Assessment **OTHER RESOURCES** • Test Generator	

■ Denotes LIFE SKILLS objectives

• Items in blue are also part of the *Holt Health Activity Book.*

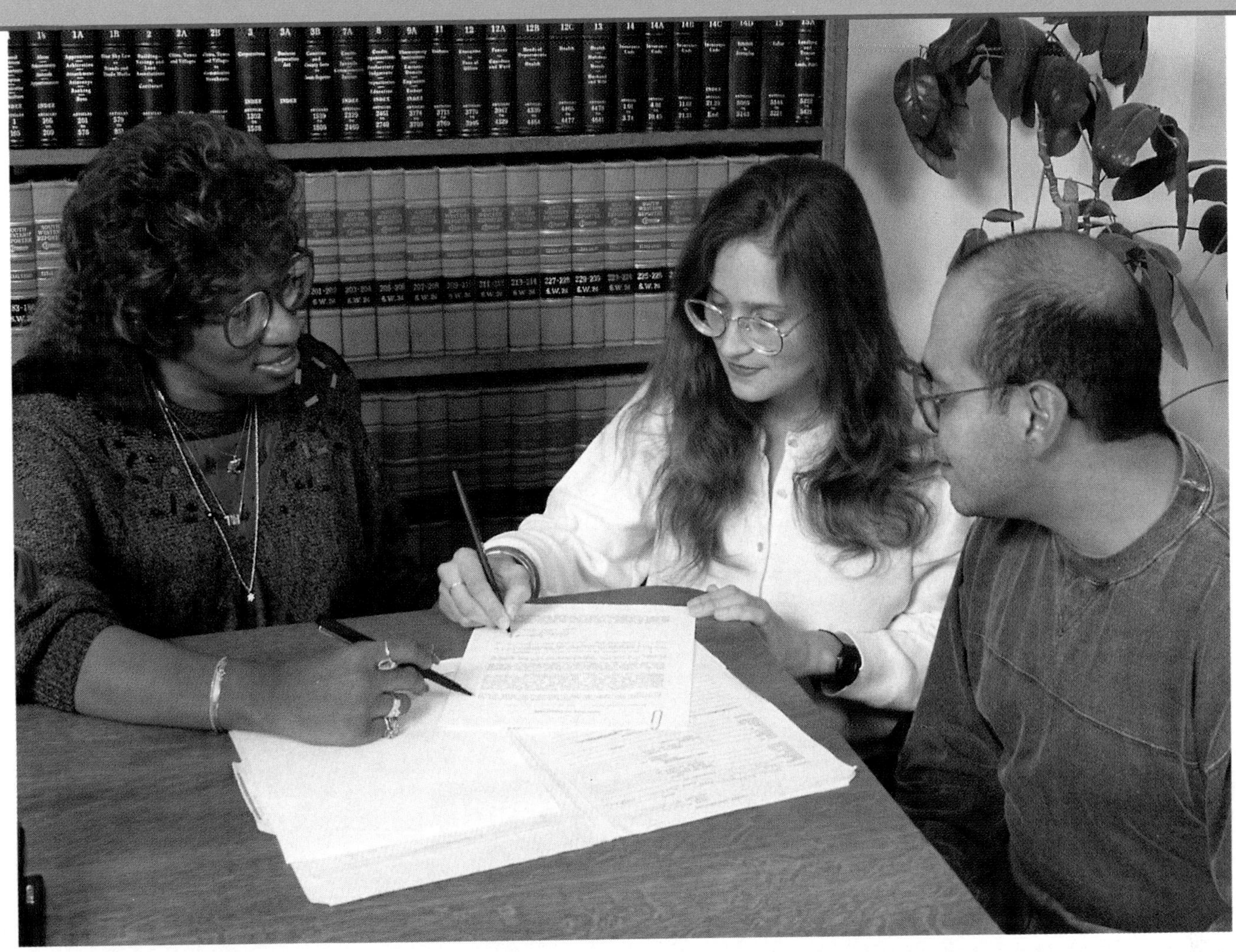

CONTENT BACKGROUND: The Living Will

EVER-CHANGING TECHNOLOGICAL MEDical advances, such as artificial hearts, sophisticated medications, and respirators and other life-support systems, have made the process of dying controversial. Whereas some people emphasize that these advances increase the length of a person's life, others believe they merely prolong the process of dying. Questions have been raised by physicians and their patients alike as to who decides whether a person should be allowed to die, when a person is actually dead, and what kinds of equipment can or should be used to maintain vital signs.

Two well-known cases—that of Karen Ann Quinlan, a comatose New Jersey woman kept alive via feeding tubes for 10 years, and that of Nancy Cruzan, a Missouri woman who remained unconscious for 4 years following an automobile accident—have impelled many people to sign living wills, which are documents that theoretically enable a person to determine which, if any, kinds of medical technology may be used to sustain life if he or she becomes terminally ill.

In order to generate a living will, a person must be mentally competent and at least 18 years of age at the time the document is drawn up. That person must sign the document in the presence of two witnesses. As long as the person generating the will is of sound mind, he or she can revoke it at any time.

According to recent polls, more than 80 percent of people living in the United States support the "right to die" and "death with dignity" philosophies. More than 40 of the 50 states recognize living wills. However, a living will is not a legally binding document. Interpretation of the verbiage in living wills often varies among physicians, between physicians and lawyers, and from state law to state law. As a result, a terminally ill person can be administered life-prolonging measures that he or she had never intended be used.

In the case of Nancy Cruzan, there was no living will document. As a result of the accident, she became unconscious and remained so for four years, at which point her family requested that the abdominal feeding tube that kept her alive be removed. The state of Missouri, however, ruled that the tube could not be removed. In a legal battle that reached the United States Supreme Court, Ms. Cruzan's family testified that she had never wanted to be kept alive in a vegetative state. The Supreme Court sided with the state in a decision handed down in July 1990, stating that states have the right to refuse removal of life-sustaining treatment from patients who have not made or cannot make their wishes known.

People who choose to sign living wills should state very specifically in writing *what* they will accept and refuse as treatment and *when* they want treatment begun and stopped. They should also make sure a notarized copy of the document is included in their medical file, and that at least one family member (along with a lawyer, and perhaps a clergy member), receive a copy as well.

PLANNING FOR INSTRUCTION

KEY FACTS

- **Recognizing the significance and permanence of death is tied to maturity. By adolescence, a person is capable of full awareness.**
- **The Harvard Medical School uses these criteria which must be met before an individual can be declared legally dead: unresponsiveness to painful stimuli, no breathing for over an hour, absence of reflexes, and failure of the brain to generate electrical impulse.**
- **Physician Elisabeth Kubler-Ross identified five stages most terminally ill patients pass through, with individual variations: denial, anger, bargaining, depression, acceptance.**
- **The dying person needs to find support, maintain control over some part of his or her life, and die with dignity.**
- **The dying person needs to communicate, to hear the truth, to have control over elements such as doctor choice and type of memorial service. One device that allows some control is a will.**
- **Hospice care gives to the dying person and his or her family as pain-free and calm an atmosphere as possible in which to prepare for death. Hospice care is given in the patient's home or in a homelike setting.**
- **Some people choose to sign a living will stating that they do not want life prolonged artificially if they have passed the point of possible recovery.**
- **Grief accompanies all loss; the most intense grief is involved in loss by death.**
- **Funerals and memorial services are held for the dead to symbolize an end to a life, to help survivors accept the finality of death and adjust to their loss, and to allow a show of support with a spiritual dimension.**

MYTHS AND MISCONCEPTIONS

MYTH: **You should not talk to a dying person about the impending death because it makes the person feel worse.**

Many people avoid a dying person or avoid talking about the illness because of their own discomfort. The terminally ill person often wants to be able to talk about what is happening; silence only compounds fears and depression.

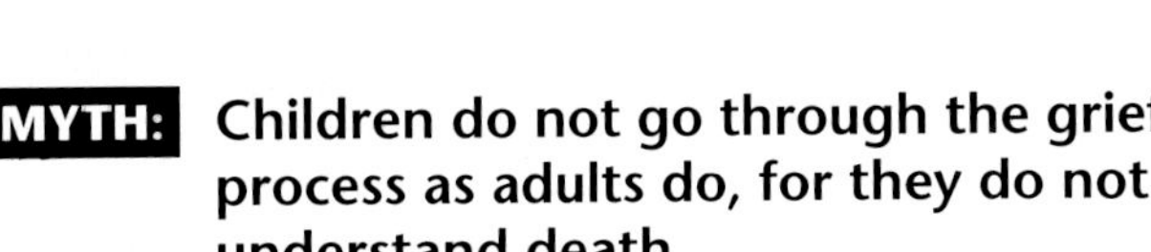

MYTH: Children do not go through the grief process as adults do, for they do not understand death.

Young children may not understand the permanence of death fully until perhaps age 10, and they may not fully understand until adolescence that everyone dies. But all children do go through a grief process.

MYTH: Children should not participate in the funeral or see the deceased person; it will only frighten and upset them.

Professionals often recommend that a youngster be able to see the person who has died; this is a visual, tactile confirmation beyond words. In addition, being with the family at the funeral home helps the child feel more secure and reduces irrational fears of abandonment.

MYTH: A person who does not show strong emotion outwardly when a loved one dies is not grieving.

Denial and shock may make a person feel numb. Adolescents particularly tend to experience denial, shock, and depression in ways that permit them to dampen emotions to a level that is manageable until they regain the strength to deal with their grief.

VOCABULARY

Essential: The following vocabulary terms appear in boldface type:

will	living will
hospices	cremation

Secondary: Be aware that the following terms may come up during class discussion:

coma	cardiopulmonary resuscitation (CPR)
funeral	life-support machines
memorial service	

FOR STUDENTS WITH SPECIAL NEEDS

Visual Learners: Have students gather, photograph, and draw images that to them best illustrate the key concepts of stages in dying, death with dignity, hospice care, and mourning for the dead. Have them arrange these images, along with the key words or phrases, in original collages.

LEP Students: Students can develop pantomimes that communicate emotions of the dying and bereaved and illustrate helpful responses by friends, family, and hospice workers. For each skit, the performers should write a simple explanation and read it to the audience after performing.

ENRICHMENT

- Give students library time to find books that contain poems or passages about death. After students read and select their favorite poems and excerpts, have them work in groups to collect the works into an illustrated volume of poems and quotes on the subject of death and how it affects the meaning of life. Some possible sources: Emily Dickinson, John Donne, Shakespeare, Elisabeth Kubler-Ross, Norman Cousins, Walt Whitman, John Keats, Dylan Thomas, Leo Tolstoy, Anton Chekhov.
- Encourage students to write a creative story about someone who is terminally ill. Describe how this person copes with the stages of dying. Include in the story the reactions of those around the dying person.

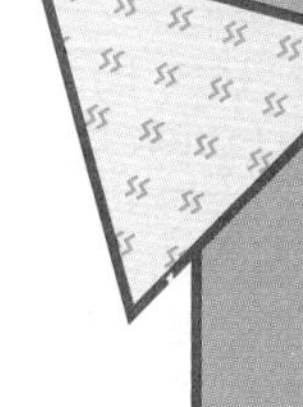

Chapter 10
Chapter Opener

Getting Started

Using the Chapter Photograph

Call students' attention to the photograph and ask, What is the situation here? What might the hospice worker be saying or doing for the terminally ill person? What might be some feelings the dying person is experiencing? Allow students several minutes to explore their own questions and thoughts about death before they write questions for the Question Box.

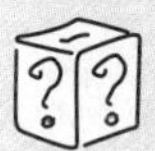

Question Box

The Question Box provides students with an opportunity to ask questions anonymously. To ensure that students with questions are not embarrassed to be seen writing, have students who do not have questions write something else—such as something they already know about hospice care, living wills, funerals, or coping with grief—on the paper instead.

Preview the questions and then answer them at appropriate points in the chapter. You may wish to allow students to write additional anonymous questions as they go through the chapter.

Chapter 10
Coping With Loss

Section 10.1 *Death and Dying*

Section 10.2 *The Grieving Process*

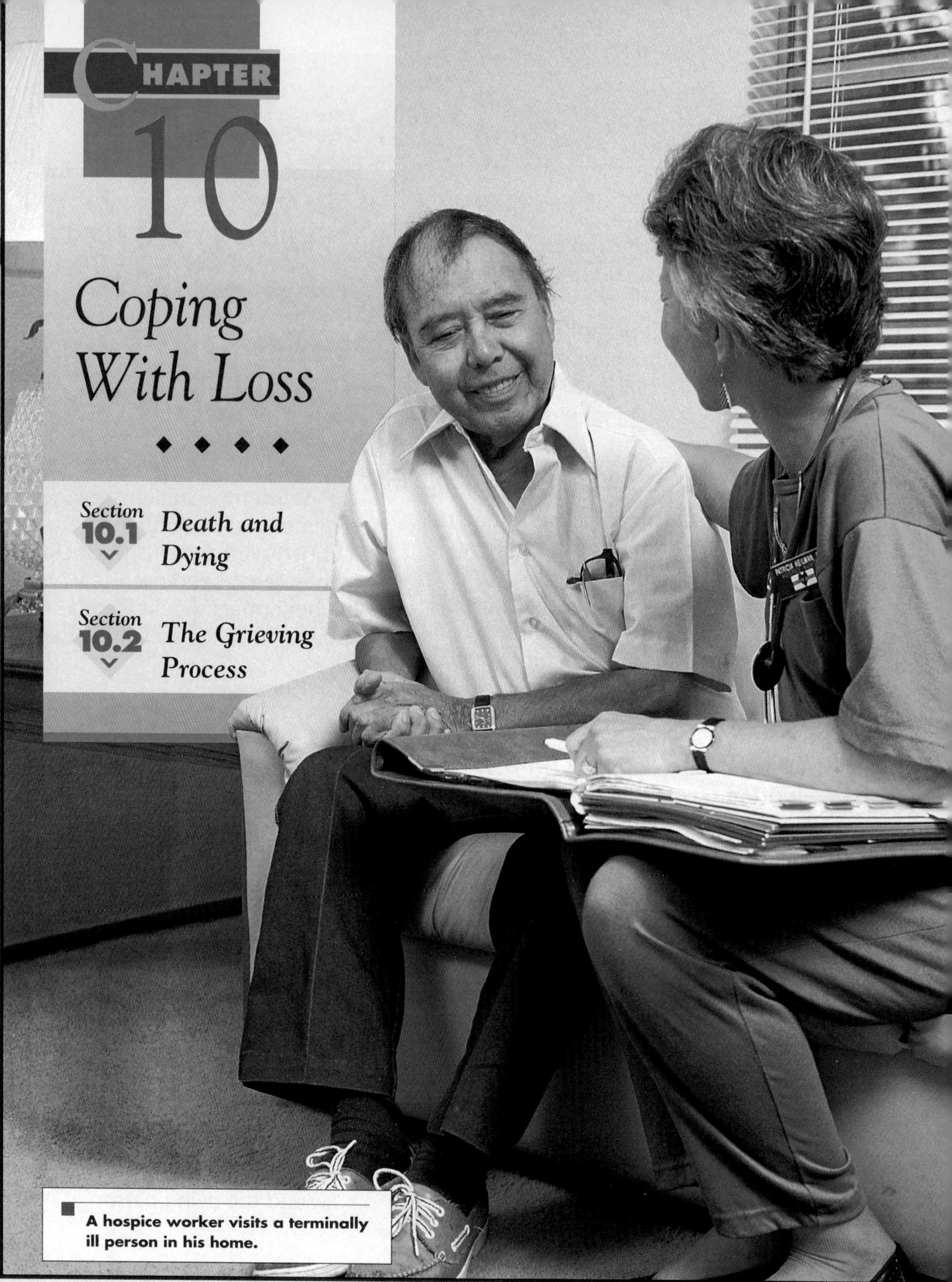

A hospice worker visits a terminally ill person in his home.

Personal Issues *ALERT*

Adolescents, who are just growing into a full realization of what death means, need to feel that they can discuss their feelings and questions openly. Some of your students will have suffered a loss and may be both relieved and eager to talk and learn that their feelings are normal. Sometimes the grief of children is misunderstood, or other family members are too upset to deal with the child's feelings, and feelings remain unresolved. However, the privacy of these students must be respected. Never use such students as "examples" or "experts." You may want to talk to them outside class to find out how they feel about sharing their emotions and experience.

Justin's brother, Chad, died last week. Chad had been in and out of the hospital for years with a serious illness; he died at home with his family close by. The funeral is over, and all the relatives have gone home. Now Justin has to go back to school. In a way this will be the hardest part, because he doesn't know how to act around his friends. What should he say? What will *they* say? He doesn't want to make anyone feel bad on his account. But he thinks it might help to talk with a friend about his brother.

Section 10.1 Death and Dying

Objectives

- *Describe the five stages terminally ill people generally pass through.*
- *List three reasons why many people choose hospice care when they are terminally ill.*
- *Describe the functions of a living will.*
- *Learn how to be of help to someone who is dying.*

LIFE SKILLS: Coping

If Justin were your friend, how would you help him? Would you feel embarrassed to say anything to him about his brother, afraid of saying the wrong thing? Most people would. Death is a topic that often makes us uncomfortable. But the more we know about it, the better we'll be able to help other people cope with death, and the better we'll be able to cope with our own losses.

Death is a natural part of life. Although we don't usually stop to think about it, death surrounds us all our lives. Even very young children are exposed to death—usually of pets or other animals. Children also learn about death through the media, especially from television. Those deaths seem remote and far away. By the time people become teenagers, however, most have known someone who has died. Often this is an older person, such as a grandparent, but sometimes it is a friend or brother or sister.

An understanding of death is greatly influenced by a person's age. For example, infants have no real concept of death. From age two to five, children recognize death but do not think it is permanent. Death is thought to be like sleep. From age five to nine, children come to view death as permanent, but not as something that could happen to them. Around age 10, children realize that death is inevitable and final. They know death happens but have trouble realizing it can happen to anyone at any time. Not until adolescence do most people have a full awareness of death.

SECTION 10.1

Background
Hospice

In medieval Europe, *hospice* meant "a refuge for weary travelers" and referred to the peace and refreshment provided by inns. Then religious orders began taking in the dying to provide nursing care and a final resting place for the end of their life, and the term shifted in meaning. The hospice concept as we know it originated with Dr. Cicely Saunders, who founded St. Christopher's Hospice in London in 1968.

Background
Living Will

Most people are not aware that a living will can be overridden by a family member. Once the patient is unable to respond, a loved one may have a change of heart and ask for resuscitation and/or life support. Medical staff then respond to the family member's wishes. For this reason, it is important for anyone making a living will to communicate his or her wishes in detail to family members.

Section 10.1 Lesson Plan

MOTIVATE

Journal 10A
Loss Experience

This may be done as a warm-up activity. Encourage students to write in the Student Journal in the Student Activity Book about some important loss they have experienced, such as a friend moving away, a parent leaving home due to divorce, or the death of a pet. Suggest that they describe their feelings about the loss and how those feelings have changed over time.

Class Discussion
Justin's Story

After students have read the story about Justin, ask: What would you say to Justin? Why? Encourage empathy for what Justin has gone through and what he must be feeling.

TEACH

Journal 10B
Feelings About Death

Give students time to recall the way they thought about death when they were small. Then have them write in the Student Journal in the Student Activity Book about how their thinking has changed as they have grown.

Check Up

Have students anonymously turn in their responses to the Check Up questions. Tally the results on the chalkboard and discuss reactions to the predominant feelings expressed. You might want to have them retake the Check Up at the end of the chapter to see if their attitudes have changed.

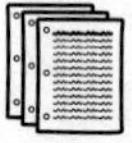

Personal Health Inventory

Have students complete the Personal Health Inventory for this chapter. The inventory helps them assess their own experiences and expectations with respect to death.

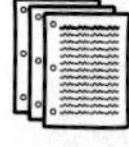

Life Skills Worksheet 10A

Helping Families Care for the Terminally Ill

Assign the Helping Families Care for the Terminally Ill Life Skills Worksheet, which has students list forms of assistance they can give families of the terminally ill.

When Does Death Occur?

According to the Harvard Medical School, all of the following criteria must be present for a person to be considered dead:

1. ***Unreceptiveness and unresponsiveness.*** *The patient is totally unresponsive to applied painful stimuli, such as poking with pins.*
2. ***Unresponsiveness in breathing.*** *For over an hour, the patient shows no spontaneous muscular contractions or breathing.*
3. ***Lack of reflexes.*** *The knee-jerk reflex is absent, or the pupil does not contract when light is pointed in the eye.*
4. ***Flat EEG.*** *For 20 minutes, the patient's brain does not generate an electrical impulse or brain wave.*

(FIGURE 10-1) **According to this definition, a person kept functioning by life-support systems is alive until the machines are shut off.**

When Does Death Occur?

In the past, people considered death to occur when the lungs and heart ceased to function. Scientific and technological advances, though, have made it more difficult to determine when death occurs.

Today, people whose heart and lungs have stopped are sometimes revived by cardiopulmonary resuscitation (CPR) or by a machine. Life-support machines can sometimes keep people "alive" if they cannot breathe or if their heart will not beat on its own. Machines can feed people if they cannot eat, and they can clean the blood if the body's organs cannot do it. Even when people are not emitting brain waves, they can still function artificially. When, then, is a person dead?

The Harvard Medical School has developed a definition of death that attempts to answer this question. According to this definition, the four criteria listed in Figure 10-1 must be met before an individual can be declared dead.

Stages in the Acceptance of Death

People who die suddenly do not have time to prepare for death. However, people who die from a terminal illness often have lots of time to think about death and to prepare for it.

Elisabeth Kubler-Ross, a noted physician, worked for years with patients dying from terminal illnesses. She identified five stages that most terminally ill patients go through when facing death. Understanding these stages can be valuable if you ever need to help a dying friend or relative.

Not all terminally ill people go through these stages in the same order. Some may skip a stage, revert to an earlier stage, or get stuck in one stage. People experience dying with the same individuality that they experience living.

Stage 1: Denial When told that death will soon come, a person's reflection is often shock and denial. Denial acts as a buffer and gives people a chance to think about the news. People may think, "It can't be true, not me." Or they may prefer to believe a cure will be found for their disease or that they will be the exception to the rule. At this point, it is helpful for patients to get a second opinion from a reputable physician to verify their condition. If you have a friend or relative in the denial stage, the best response is just to listen. Even if people who are dying talk about getting well soon,

• • • TEACH continued

Class Discussion

Life Cycle Concepts

Have students think about and verbalize their own concepts of the life cycle. Have volunteers suggest a diagram that illustrates this concept. Sketch the diagram on the chalkboard and erase the portion representing death. Ask, What happens to the concept of life cycle without death? Encourage students to express in their own words the perspective that death is a natural occurrence and part of living.

Case Study

Life-Support Systems

In 1975, a drug overdose at a party left Karen Ann Quinlan in a vegetative, comatose state, attached to a respirator. After some months, it became evident that she would not emerge from the coma, and without the respirator, would probably die. Although she had previously discussed with her family her wish to be allowed to die in such circumstances, the courts at first would not permit the family's doctors to remove life support. Some students may wish to research and report on the Quinlans' decade-long fight and what happened to Karen after life support was removed.

Demonstration

CPR

CPR is an important life-saving technique. Ask a health professional, such as a nurse or a representative from the local chapter of the Heart Association, to demonstrate the technique for the

it is better not to contradict them. That could force them to accept their death before they are ready.

Stage 2: Anger When people realize they are really going to die, they are likely to become angry. ''Why me?'' Anger is often directed at medical staff, family, or friends. People may feel they are being treated unfairly. After all, they may see someone who is mean and cruel but in perfect health. Why, then, should they have to die while this other person goes on enjoying life?

It is important to let them know they have a right to be angry, and that they can express their anger whenever they feel it. If the person gets angry at you, try to accept it without feeling hurt. Recognize that this is simply a stage that will pass. Providing an outlet for the anger can be helpful.

Stage 3: Bargaining Bargaining is a final attempt to avoid the inevitable. People who believe in God may promise to reform their lives in exchange for a miraculous recovery. Promises are made that will be fulfilled if death can be avoided.

Stage 4: Depression When bargaining fails and people realize their last hope is dimming, they are likely to feel depression. At this point, it might be helpful for you to encourage a dying person to discuss the depression. Sometimes dying people have practical problems that are worrying and depressing them. A friend or relative who is dying might want you to adopt a special pet. Sometimes dying people are depressed because they feel the loss of everything—friends, loved ones, home, and good health. Then it is most helpful just to be with them, often silently.

Stage 5: Acceptance Accepting your own death is hard to imagine, but most people who have terminal illnesses get to that point eventually. At this stage people have usually taken care of all personal matters. This includes wills, funeral arrangements, and bidding farewell to special people in their lives.

Check Up

How Do You Feel About Death?

On a separate sheet of paper, answer each of the following questions to determine how you feel about death. Use the following scale:

a = comfortable
b = somewhat comfortable
c = somewhat uncomfortable
d = uncomfortable

1. How comfortable are you talking about death and dying?
2. How comfortable would you feel if you had to visit and support someone you cared about who was terminally ill?
3. How comfortable would you feel if you had to provide support for a friend whose parent had died?
4. How comfortable would you feel about donating your kidneys for use upon your death?
5. How comfortable would you feel about signing a statement requesting that you not be kept alive if in a coma and on life-support mechanisms?
6. If you were legally responsible for someone being kept alive by life-support systems, and you knew the person would not want to remain in that state, how comfortable would you feel about ordering the withdrawal of the life-support equipment?

Death With Dignity

One of the most painful things about dying is that it can rob a person of dignity, especially in the impersonal atmosphere of a hospital, away from friends and family. Recognizing this, the helping professions

Making a Choice 10A

Wills

Assign the Wills card, which asks students to examine living wills and the emotions connected to inheritance.

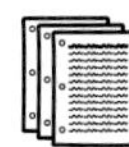

Section Review Worksheet 10.1

Assign Section Review Worksheet 10.1, which requires students to understand the stages in the acceptance of death, the advantages of hospices, and the functions of a living will.

Section Quiz 10.1

Have students take Section Quiz 10.1.

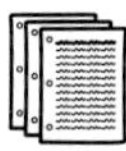

Reteaching Worksheet 10.1

Students who have difficulty with the material may complete Reteaching Worksheet 10.1, which requires them to sequence the stages in the acceptance of death and recognize the advantages of a hospice.

class. Follow the demonstration with a discussion of when CPR is appropriate.

Debate the Issue
Life-Support Systems

Divide the class into two teams to debate whether life-support mechanisms should be used to prolong the life of a person who will never regain consciousness or be able to function normally again.

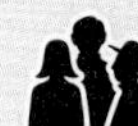

Cooperative Learning
Kubler-Ross Model

Divide the class into five groups and assign to each group one stage of the Kubler-Ross model to explore. Encourage each group to create a list of statements that would illustrate things a dying person might say at that particular stage. Then have them write possible responses they might give to help the person through the stage.

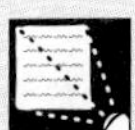

Teaching Transparency 10A
Acceptance of Death

Use this transparency to help students understand how they could help a dying person as he or she goes through the stages in the acceptance of death.

Reinforcement
Positive Ways to be Helpful

Help students list positive and practical things they could do for a friend or relative who is terminally ill.

Review Answers

1. Denial: When people are told that they will soon die, their reaction is usually one of disbelief. Anger: When people realize that they are really going to die, they are likely to become angry. Bargaining: People who believe in God may promise to reform their lives in exchange for a miraculous recovery. Depression: When people realize that bargaining will not work, their last hope has faded and they feel depressed. Acceptance: People have accepted their condition and that death will soon come.

2. Students may answer that hospices provide a homelike atmosphere; they can provide a program of medical care and counseling for the patient, as well as counseling for the family; hospices sometimes provide care in the patient's own home; hospices freely provide medication for pain; visitation with the patient is unrestricted; hospice services also include legal counseling, spiritual support, home nursing care, and nutritional counseling.

will: *a legal document describing what should be done with a person's possessions after the person's death.*

hospices: *places that offer housing, medical care, and counseling for terminally ill people, and counseling for the family.*

are exploring ways to allow dying people have more control over what happens to them, and to provide them with the support they need.

What Dying People Need Dying people, just like everyone else, want to communicate with others. They want to be able to express their feelings, and they need a caring group of family and friends to listen. Most also want the truth. When asked, at least 80 percent of people say they would like to be told if they had a terminal illness. Even if they are not told, most terminally ill patients already know or suspect they are going to die. They can tell by how people act and may even overhear parts of conversations about them.

Just like the rest of us, dying people want some control over things that affect them. To have that control, they need honest answers to their questions. Dishonesty not only prevents them from managing their remaining time, but it also damages their trust in others, which is so vital when everything else seems to be falling away.

What kinds of things do people who are dying want to control? They want to decide who their doctors will be, which treatments they will accept, and who will visit them. In addition, they often wish to control their own funeral or memorial service. Decisions such as whether there will be a burial or cremation, who will officiate at the service, and what will be included in the service can be made in anticipation of death. Also, they want to control what will be done with their possessions. Dying people are often comforted by knowing their possessions will be in the right hands after they die. This is best handled through a **will,** which is a legal document describing what should be done after death. It also may contain directions for the care of surviving family members or even pets.

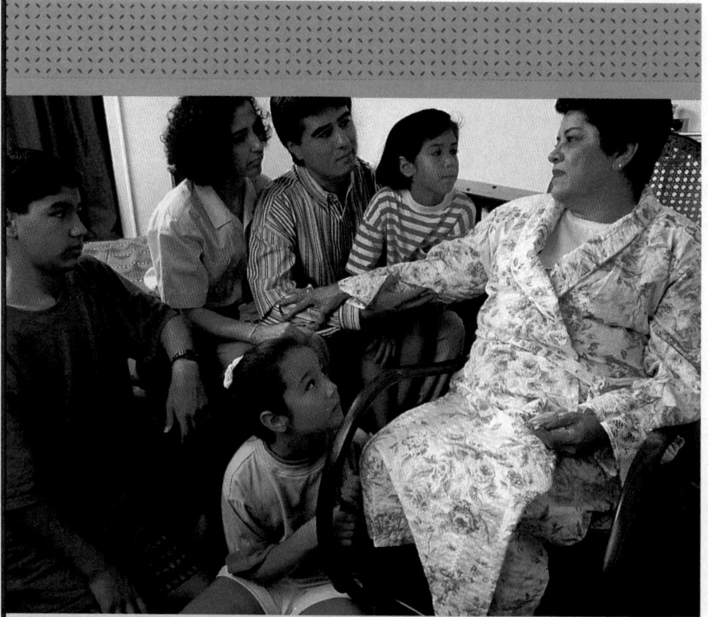

(FIGURE 10-2) **Dying people often want to express their feelings and need a warm group of family and friends to listen.**

Hospices Many people would rather die at home than in a hospital. **Hospices**—programs that care for terminally ill people—help fill this need. Hospices provide a homelike atmosphere even though the patient is away from home. Although they do not have a hospital's extensive equipment, they can provide a program of medical care and support for the patient, as well as support for the family. Sometimes hospices can provide care in the patient's own home through medical specialists who visit the patient.

The hospice approach has several unique features. For example, medications are freely administered for pain, reflecting the philosophy that the patient's remaining time should be as comfortable as possible. Families visit freely without restrictions on hours or age, and volunteers visit and talk with dying patients.

• • • TEACH continued

Here is a start:

- Stay in touch—and remember that holding a hand or hugging the person are important.
- Take a favorite food in a disposable container (phone first).
- Take the children out for a few hours or offer to stay with the dying person so that the family can go out, to give everyone a break.

Extension
Obituary

Make an optional assignment for students to write their own obituary, imagining that they have lived the full life they want for themselves. Tell students that the obituary should reflect their priorities, goals, and hopes for their life.

When hospice care is provided in the patient's own home, families learn to participate in the patient's care. They may administer medications or perform other tasks.

Family members receive counseling to work through their grief and to be better prepared to interact with the dying person. Other hospice services include legal counseling, home nursing care, and support for the grieving family after the patient dies.

People who choose to die in their own homes often prefer hospice care. For example, George Jeffrey, a 78-year-old man, began to feel ill and had extensive tests that showed he had advanced cancer. Mr. Jeffrey was a retired commercial artist who lived with his daughter and son-in-law and his grandchildren. He loved to play golf, spend time with his family, and watch sports on TV.

Mr. Jeffrey and his family chose to receive hospice care in the home. Mr. Jeffrey stayed in the family home and continued to use his favorite easy chair. He continued to watch sports on TV and visited a great deal with his family.

The family was told what to expect throughout the dying process. Nurses from the hospice program made regular visits to Mr. Jeffrey and his family. As the time of death approached, the nurse gently explained to the family what was happening.

When the moment of death was very near, the family's greatest concern was for Mr. Jeffrey. They wanted him to know how much they loved him. They wanted him to know they would be fine and that he could let go and pass from this life.

He died with great courage and dignity. Most of all, he died in an atmosphere of great love.

Living Wills Many ethical decisions surround the topic of death. Should life be preserved at all costs—even if the person is in a coma or in excruciating pain? Or should death simply be allowed to take its course without intervention?

The **living will** is one way to deal with this complex issue. A living will is a simple statement people can sign that instructs their doctors not to use medical equipment just to keep them breathing and their hearts beating when they have no chance for meaningful recovery. It tells the medical staff to let nature take its course. This takes the burden off their families and lets the medical staff know their wishes. An example of a living will is shown in Figure 10-3. Living wills should not be confused with regular wills. Living wills are concerned with life-support mechanisms, while regular wills deal with the distribution of material goods and instructions for the care of others.

living will

a document expressing a person's wish to be allowed to die in case of terminal illness or incurable injury rather than be kept alive by artificial means.

Review

1. *Describe the five stages terminally ill people generally pass through.*
2. *List three reasons why many people choose hospice care when they are terminally ill.*
3. *Describe the functions of a living will.*
4. ***LIFE SKILLS: Coping*** *You have a friend who is terminally ill and in the hospital. Your friend tells you the doctors are wrong and that he really isn't that sick. He wants to leave the hospital immediately and wants you to help him. What would you do?*
5. ***Critical Thinking*** *What types of patients might prefer hospital care to hospice care?*

Answers to Questions 1 and 2 are on p. 216.

3. A living will is a statement that people can sign instructing their doctors not to use medical equipment just to keep them breathing and their hearts beating when they have no chance for meaningful recovery.
4. Answers will vary. Students may answer that they would listen to their friend and suggest that he talk to his doctor about being released and then seek a second opinion. They should not contradict the patient's belief that he does not have a terminal illness.
5. Answers will vary. Patients who do not wish to die at home, who do not have family or friends to help them, or don't want to ask their family to help, might choose hospital care over hospice care.

ASSESS

Section Review

Have students answer the Section Review questions.

Alternative Assessment

Opinions on Hospice Care

Have students write a brief essay outlining their opinion about hospice care. They should explain what they think its value is, aspects they like or dislike, and needs they think hospice care does or does not meet.

Closure

Importance of Wills and Living Wills

With the class, develop a scenario in which a terminally ill patient talks about his or her concerns, makes a will, and arranges for a living will.

Living Will Declaration

FIGURE 10-3

To My Family, Doctors , and All Those Concerned with My Care

I, ______________________________, being of sound mind, make this statement as a directive to be followed if for any reason I become unable to participate in decisions regarding my medical care.

I direct life-sustaining procedures should be withheld if I have an illness, disease, or injury, or experience extreme mental deterioration, such that there is no reasonable expectation of recovering or regaining a meaningful life.

These life-sustaining procedures that may be withheld or withdrawn include, but are not limited to:

Surgery Antibiotics Cardiac Resuscitation Respiratory Support
Artificially Administered Feeding and Fluids

I further direct that treatment be limited to comfort measures only, even if they shorten my life.

You may delete any provison above by drawing a line through it and adding your initials.

Other personal instructions:

These directions express my legal right to refuse treatment, Therefore, I expect my family, doctors, and all those concerned with my care to regard themselves as legally and morally bound to act in accord with my wishes, and in so doing to be free from any liability for having followed my directions.

Signed ______________________________ *Date* _______________

Witness _______________________ *Witness* _______________________

Proxy Designaton Clause

If you wish, you may use this section to designate someone to make treatment decisions for you if you are unable to do so. Your Living Will Declaration will be in effect even if you have a designated proxy.

I authorize the following person to implement my Living Will Declaraton by accepting, refusing, and/or making decisons about my treatment and hospitalization:

Name ____

Address ____

If the person I have named above is unable to act on my behalf, I authorize the following person to do so:

Name ____

Address ____

I have discussed my wishes with these persons and trust their judgment on my behalf.

Signed ______________________________ *Date* _______________

Witness _______________________ *Witness* _______________________

Section
10.2 The Grieving Process

Objectives

- *List three reasons for having funerals or memorial services.*
- *Learn how to deal with your own grief.*
  LIFE SKILLS: Coping
- *Learn how to give emotional support to someone who is grieving.*
  LIFE SKILLS: Communicating Effectively

We experience grief when we suffer a great loss. People can grieve over losses other than death—the loss of a love relationship, for example, or even the loss of a treasured object. But grief is probably most intense when we lose someone through death.

The grief people feel when someone dies is influenced by several factors. For example, the feelings related to a sudden death are different from those resulting from death caused by a long illness. In one case, the death is an unexpected shock. In the other, you have time to prepare. Reactions to death also differ depending upon how close you were to the person who has died. However, regardless of who dies and how close you were to him or her, you will need to wrestle with the feeling of loss. Only the intensity of the loss will vary.

When people know a loved one is dying, they may go through the same stages of accepting death as the dying person. They may deny that death is imminent. They may become angry, sometimes at the patient, especially if they have been dependent on the dying person. They may spend a great deal of time praying and bargaining for the person to recover. They may get depressed. And, ultimately, they may come to accept the death and the need to survive in spite of it.

The loss of a parent through divorce is discussed in Chapter 19.

Dealing With Your Grief

Whether the death of someone close is anticipated or sudden, one thing is certain: expect the unexpected. No matter how much we plan and think about living without someone we love, we never really know how we will react to a death.

The loss of a love relationship is discussed in Chapter 17.

Ways to Deal with Your Grief

Speak to someone you can trust who will respect your feelings and keep your conversation confidential. This might be a close friend, teacher, coach, or school counselor. In some areas, there are support groups for the bereaved that your school counselor or a local hospital might know about.

It is important to get your feelings out. One way to do this would be to use phrases like: "I remember when ...." "I remember most about ...."

Talking about the future will stress the permanence of death and help with adjustment. For example, you can say: "We're really going to miss ...." "What I will miss the most is ...."

Be honest with yourself and others when discussing your feelings about death.

(FIGURE 10-4)

Background
Coping With Grief

Grief is different for young people than it is for adults. Because they do not react in the same ways as adults, children's and teens' grief may not be recognized. The intense emotions of grieving are so painful and frightening that a child may approach and avoid them over a long period. Denial provides a numbness that allows grieving youngsters to bring overpowering emotions to a manageable level until they have regained the psychological strength to deal with them. For many grieving teens, the second year after the death is harder than the first year, in part because the numbness is past and a flood of painful emotions must be dealt with.

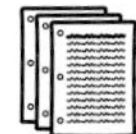
Life Skills Worksheet 10B

Support Groups for the Grieving

Assign the Support Groups for the Grieving Life Skills Worksheet, which asks students to locate resources available for grieving people, gather information about them, and compare them.

Section 10.2 Lesson Plan

MOTIVATE

Journal 10C
Justin's Feelings

This may be done as a warm-up activity. Have students review the story about Justin in the Chapter Opener and consider some of the feelings he is experiencing after losing his brother. Encourage them to use the Student Journal to describe one of Justin's possible emotions.

TEACH

Class Discussion
Grief Phases

Grief for someone dying or dead evolves in phases, in somewhat the same way the terminally ill experience stages in the progress of their illness. Have students talk about why the death of a loved one might cause feelings of denial, anger, and depression. *(The survivor is losing someone important, perhaps the emotional and economic center of his or her world.)*

Reinforcement
Grief Support Groups

Stress that releasing feelings of grief is an important part of the grieving process. Grief that is shared is less intensely suffered. Find out about grief support groups in your community and have students gather information to share with classmates.

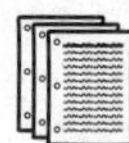

Life Skills Worksheet 10C

Writing a Condolence Letter

Assign the Writing a Condolence Letter Life Skills Worksheet, which asks students to write condolence letters under various circumstances.

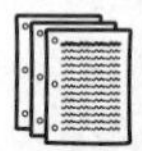

Life Skills Worksheet 10D

Helping Others Deal With Grief

Assign the Helping Others Deal With Grief Life Skills Worksheet, which asks students to prescribe appropriate supportive behavior for the grieving.

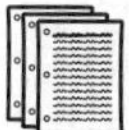

Ethics Worksheet

Assign the Ethics Worksheet for Unit 3.

Making a Choice 10B

Dealing With Guilt

Assign the Dealing With Guilt card, which asks students to examine strategies for dealing with guilt after a person's death and for avoiding such guilt by relating well to living people.

(FIGURE 10-5)

Ways to Help a Grieving Person

If you have a classmate who has lost someone through death, it is important to express your sympathy as a show of support. You might say: "I was sorry to hear about your brother's death. He was a great guy." But unless you're a close friend, don't ask for details.

Try to put the person in touch with others who are grieving. For example, teenagers who have lost a parent through death can be of great help to another teenager whose parent has just died.

Reassure the person that guilt, sadness, despair, and similar feelings are normal.

Listen, hold, and touch the grieving person. Let the person share the grief with you.

It is wise not to run away from feelings, because the hurt cannot be denied. It is best to let out the feelings, sharing them with people to whom you feel close. They can help by listening and by serving as a reminder that you are not alone.

During the grieving process, it may help to talk with a good friend about what you are experiencing. If you are a member of a church or synagogue, you may want to talk with your priest, minister, or rabbi. Organized support groups for people who have lost someone through death may also exist in your community. Another alternative is to talk to your school counselor or a therapist. Remember that seeking help is a sign of strength, not weakness. Figure 10-4 has some suggestions that can help you adjust to a death.

Helping Others Deal With Grief

If you know a person who is grieving, you can be of tremendous help. Try to imagine what would help if you were grieving. What would feel good to you would probably also feel good to someone else.

Communicate your concern. Express friendship. Let the person know you're there if needed. You can show you care by being comforting. Avoid saying things like "Don't cry, you'll get over it." Crying is a healthful way to release feelings of grief. Offer to help the grieving person adjust. You might be able to help with schoolwork or household chores.

As you try to help, let the person set the speed of the recovery. Everyone handles this type of situation differently. Allow the person to decide how you can help. For example, don't insist on giving advice if the person doesn't want it. Respect the grieving person's wishes and take your lead from him or her. And remember that a grieving person often needs support not only right after a death, but also a week, a month, or a year later.

If you are helping someone who is grieving, you might find the suggestions in Figure 10-5 helpful.

• • • TEACH continued

Role-Playing

Communicating Effectively

Partners can review "Helping Others Deal With Grief" for appropriate responses to a grieving friend. Some pairs may wish to repeat their impromptu dialogue for the class. Allow time for students to respond to such performances, pointing out what they think is most helpful and why.

Class Discussion

Funerals and Memorial Services

Use the following questions to help students explore the nature and importance of funerals and memorial services to the bereaved. **When might a family have a memorial service instead of a funeral for a loved one who has died?** *[When the body has been lost or cremated, or when the service has to be held long after the death.]* **Some adults feel that children should not attend the funeral of a loved one, but should be shielded from their grief. What would you say in response to an attitude like this?** *[The child misses a chance to realize that the death is real and final. The child is isolated from other family members at a vulnerable time and may feel terrified and abandoned. If the child feels that the dead person "went away" or "went to sleep" he or she may feel terrified that it will happen to another family member.]* Make the point to students, however, that no child should be forced to attend a funeral if he or she

Although negative emotions and readjustments accompany death, there are some positive outcomes. When families are close and communicate feelings openly, death can draw the survivors closer together and help them to grow from the experience.

Funerals and Memorial Services

When a person dies, the body is usually buried or cremated. When there is a burial, the body is placed in a casket and buried in a cemetery. In **cremation**, the body is reduced to ashes by intense heat. The ashes may be scattered or placed in an urn.

Within a few days of the death, there is almost always a funeral, which is a ceremony at which others pay respect to the person who died. Usually the body is in a casket, which is sometimes open, sometimes closed. A service is often performed that includes a speech praising the person who has died. This service may be held in a religious sanctuary or a funeral home

cremation
the complete reduction of the body to ashes by intense heat.

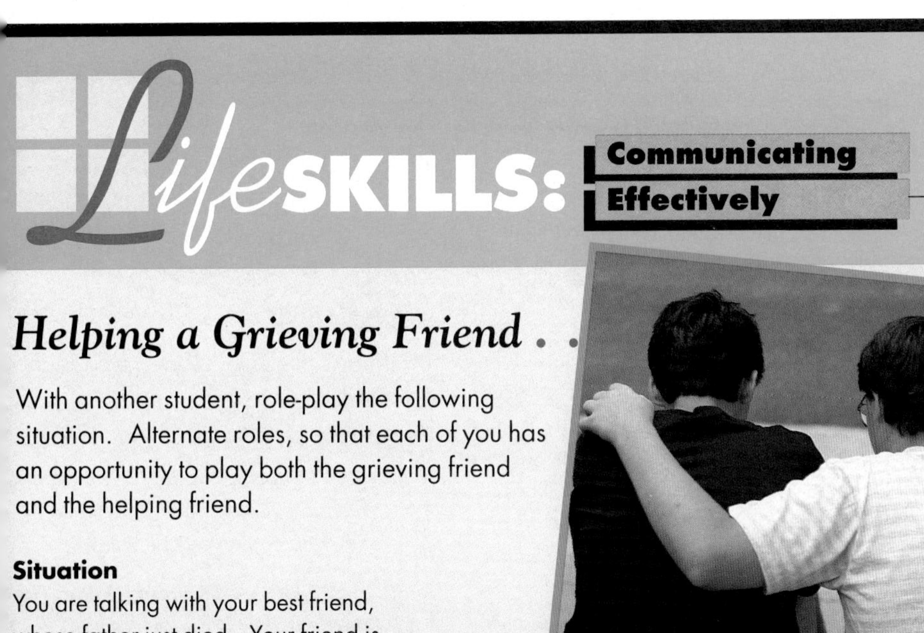

LifeSKILLS: Communicating Effectively

Helping a Grieving Friend . . .

With another student, role-play the following situation. Alternate roles, so that each of you has an opportunity to play both the grieving friend and the helping friend.

Situation

You are talking with your best friend, whose father just died. Your friend is really sad and needs to express his or her feelings. Using the guidelines in this chapter, talk with your friend and provide your support.

Here's one way you might start.

Friend: It doesn't seem real. I can't stop thinking Dad will come home after work, like he always did.

You: It's really tough, your dad dying. I know you miss him a lot.

is clearly terrified of going. The choice should be given.

Extension

Hospice Programs

Hospice programs work with grieving family members as well as with the dying. Encourage some students to visit a hospice center to learn more about ways to help someone work through his or her grief. Sources of information include trained hospice volunteers, the hospice library, and the hospice staff.

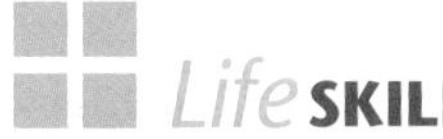

Life SKILLS

Helping a Grieving Friend

Pair students to complete the Life Skills activity. You may want to review the phases of grief with students and have them suggest statements a grieving person might make at any one of these junctures.

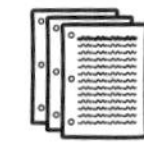

Section Review Worksheet 10.2

Assign Section Review Worksheet 10.2, which requires students to supply types and functions of services for the deceased and to classify appropriate and inappropriate ways of dealing with a grieving person.

Section Quiz 10.2

Have students take Section Quiz 10.2.

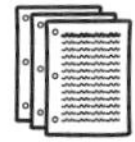

Reteaching Worksheet 10.2

Students who have difficulty with the material may complete Reteaching Worksheet 10.2, which has students supply ways to help a grieving person and to identify some benefits of funerals and memorial services.

Review Answers

1. Funerals and memorial services help people accept the finality of death and to adjust to their loss. These ceremonies are also a way for friends to show support to the grieving family. They also allow people to acknowledge the death spiritually.

2. Students might include the following in their answer: a good friend; family members; priest, minister, or rabbi; school counselor or therapist; teacher; coach; or an organized support group for people who have lost someone through death.

3. Students may answer that they would tell their friend that the grieving process takes a long time for many people to work through. Students may also relate their experiences with grief or the experiences of others.

4. Students may answer that just having someone there to listen to her would be of help. If this approach does not help Aunt Cindy work through the grief process, then she may need some professional help, such as a counselor, therapist, or support group.

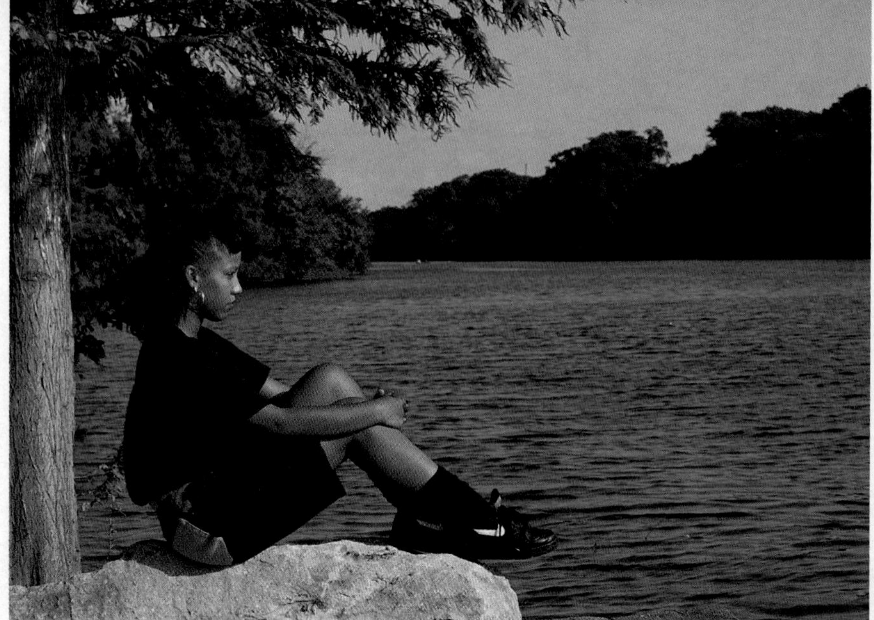

(FIGURE 10-6) **Grieving is a way to adjust to the idea that someone we love has died.**

chapel. When the body is to be buried, this indoor service is often followed by a short graveside service before burial.

Many times a memorial service is chosen instead of a funeral to pay respect to a person who has died. Memorial services differ from funerals in that the body is not present. Sometimes they take place after the body has been cremated or buried. Some memorial services are similar to funeral services, but others are more informal than traditional funerals.

Funerals and memorial services play an important role in helping people accept the finality of death and adjust to their loss. They can also allow people to observe the death spiritually.

In addition, these ceremonies provide a way for friends to show support to the grieving family. Seeing friends who knew and loved the person who has died can make the first few days of bereavement a little easier to bear.

Review

1. *Name three ways that funerals and memorial services help grieving people?*
2. ***LIFE SKILLS: Coping*** *If you were grieving over the death of a loved one, who could you talk with?*
3. ***LIFE SKILLS: Communicating Effectively*** *Your friend tells you that she just can't get over the death of her mother, who died two months ago. What would you say to reassure her that her feelings are normal?*
4. ***Critical Thinking*** *Your Aunt Cindy's husband died a month ago. She stays home all the time, crying frequently. What do you think would help her most?*

ASSESS

Section Review

Have students answer the Section Review questions.

Alternative Assessment

Ways to Help

Have students make a collage or poster representing ways to help a grieving friend. They can attach a written paragraph explaining the circumstances under which each type of help is appropriate or explain their work orally to the class.

Closure

Grief Process

Ask students to write a short story or a series of diary entries that chronicle the grief process as a teenager might experience it.

Highlights

Summary

- Most people do not have a full awareness of death until adolescence.
- A person can be declared legally dead if the following criteria are met: unreceptiveness and unresponsiveness, unresponsiveness in breathing, lack of reflexes, and a flat EEG.
- Most terminally ill patients go through specific stages: denial, anger, bargaining, depression, and acceptance.
- A will is a legal document that states what to do with possessions and may contain directions for the care of surviving family members or even pets.
- A hospice provides medical care in a homelike environment for a person who is dying. Hospice care might also include counseling for the patient and his or her family.
- A living will allows a person to make the decision to die instead of being kept alive by machines.
- Grieving people may go through the same stages as dying people in accepting death. It may help a grieving person to talk with someone about how he or she is feeling.
- A good way to help a grieving friend is to express your concern and let him or her know that you want to help.
- Funerals help people accept the finality of death, allow friends to show support, and let people observe death spiritually.

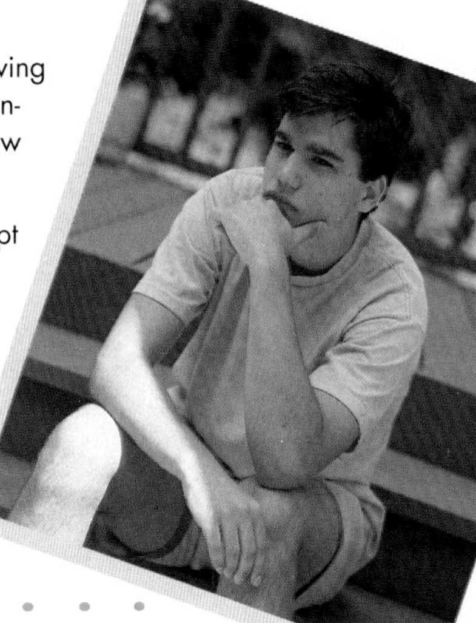

Vocabulary

will a legal document describing what should be done with a person's possessions after the person's death.

hospices places that offer housing, medical care, and counseling for terminally ill people, and counseling for the family.

living will a document expressing a person's wish to be allowed to die in case of terminal illness or incurable injury rather than be kept alive by artificial means.

cremation the complete reduction of the body to ashes by intense heat.

Chapter 10 Highlights Strategies

Summary

Have students read the summary to reinforce the concepts they have learned in Chapter 10.

Vocabulary

Have students use the four vocabulary terms and four other words or phrases from the chapter that were meaningful to them in a short essay that explains their attitudes toward dying and grief.

Extension

Have students work in groups to create a video, filmstrip, play, or series of artworks that teaches others about the ordeal of the dying and the bereaved and shows ways to help them through these trying periods.

CHAPTER 10 ASSESSMENT

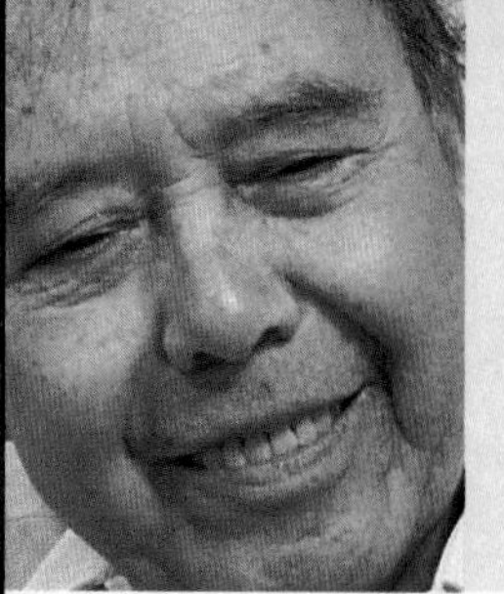

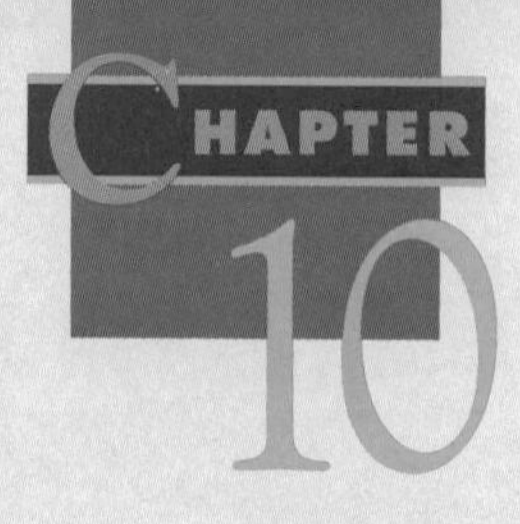

Chapter Review

Concept Review

1. Why might some people avoid a grieving person?
2. Describe a child's concept of death at various age levels.
3. List the four criteria for determining when death occurs.
4. Why is it helpful to know the five stages of accepting death identified by Elisabeth Kubler-Ross?
5. What are three needs of a dying person?
6. Why is it important to be honest with a dying person?
7. Describe some unique features of a hospice.
8. How is a regular will different from a living will?
9. How is the grief of a dying person similar to the grief of a survivor or other family member?
10. What factors influence the grief people feel?
11. What can you do during the grieving process to help adjust to a death? How can you help someone else deal with grief?
12. What is one positive outcome of death and grief?
13. How are burials different from cremations? How do funerals and memorial services differ?

Expressing Your Views

1. Your best friend just found out he has a terminal illness. He is convinced that a cure will be found soon and that he is not really going to die. It is hard for you to be around him because you are having trouble accepting the news too, but you want to help your friend if you can. How can you explain your friend's attitude? What would you do?
2. Your neighbor, who has two small children, is terminally ill. She has a full-time nurse at home so she doesn't need any kind of medical assistance. However, you want to help her in some way. What could you do?
3. Manuel has been grieving over his father's death for many months now. His friends don't understand his lingering depression. He is beginning to wonder if the grief he feels after all this time is normal and if it will ever go away. How could Manuel help himself?

CHAPTER REVIEW

Concept Review

Sample responses:

1. Most people are afraid they might say the wrong thing.

2. Infants have no real concept of death. Children ages 2 to 5 recognize death but do not think it is permanent. From ages 5 to 9, children see death as permanent, but not as something that could happen to them. At about age 10, children realize that death is inevitable, but have trouble realizing it can happen to anyone.

3. Unreceptiveness and unresponsiveness, unresponsiveness in breathing, lack of reflexes, flat EEG

4. It can help you understand and help a dying person.

5. They need to express their feelings; they need a group of family and friends to listen, and they need the truth.

6. So they can manage their remaining time, prepare for their death, and continue to trust supporting friends.

7. They provide medical care for the terminally ill in a home-like atmosphere or in the home. They provide counseling for the patient and family. Hospices administer medications to control pain and allow 24-hour family visitation. They also provide legal counseling, spiritual support, and nursing care.

8. A living will makes clear what lifesaving measures you will accept if you are suddenly hospitalized, while a regular will contains your instructions for the distribution of material goods and the care of others.

9. They both need to express their feelings, and both need a warm group of family and friends. Many survivors go through the same stages of grief as the dying person.

10. Sudden death and closeness to the person

11. Talk to someone about how I am feeling, talk about the future, and be honest with myself about my feelings. To help someone else deal with grief, I would let that person know that I care and that I'll be there if he or she needs me.

12. Death can draw the survivors closer and help them grow emotionally.

13. In a burial, the body is placed in a casket and buried. In a cremation, the body is reduced to ashes by intense heat. The ashes may be scattered or placed in an urn. A funeral is a service for the deceased in which the body (in a casket) is present; in memorial services, the body is not present.

Chapter 10 Assessment

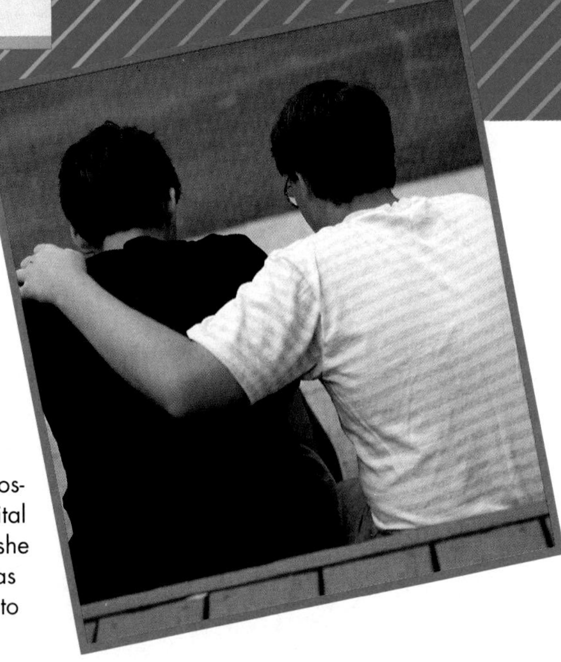

Life Skills Check

1. Coping
Beatrice is terribly depressed about her mother's death. She worries that her friends may get tired of hearing about it, but Beatrice does feel the need to share memories of her mother. Whom else could she talk to?

2. Communicating Effectively
Your aunt is terminally ill and has been in and out of hospitals for almost a year. She always dreads her hospital stays because she misses her children and pets when she is away from home. What would you suggest to her as an alternative to hospital care? What would you say to explain how the alternative care would be different?

Projects

1. Burial customs vary from culture to culture. Choose another country or culture and research its customs and attitudes toward death. Write a brief essay summarizing your findings and comparing that society's customs to those of our society.
2. Find a newspaper or magazine article about a family that had to make the decision whether to keep a loved one alive by life-support mechanisms, or an article about a situation where a family member carried out a patient's wishes through a living will. Bring the articles to class and discuss them in groups.
3. Interview a grief counselor or a psychologist about helping people deal with death. Then work with a group to prepare a pamphlet listing suggestions for individuals trying to cope with grief. Share copies of the pamphlet with other students in your school.

Plan for Action

Friends and family can support a dying person and each other. List three things you can do in the future to help a dying friend.

Expressing Your Views

Sample responses:
1. He is going through the denial stage. The best thing to do is to be with him and listen, but not dispute what he is saying.
2. I would be there to listen, to run errands, to watch the children, to prepare meals, and to help with chores.
3. Manuel can talk with someone he trusts about his feelings.

Life Skills Check

Sample responses:

1. A teacher, counselor, or religious leader

2. I would suggest hospice care. This would allow her to be at home with the support of visiting nurses and her family.

Projects

Have students share the results of the projects on death with other students in the school.

Plan for Action

Ask students to think about and then discuss what their immediate reaction would be if they learned tomorrow that they had a terminal illness. Then ask what their longer range concerns would be as they tried to plan for their own death and the consequences it would have for those around them.

Assessment Options

Chapter Test

Have students take the Chapter 10 test.

Alternative Assessment

Have students do the Alternative Assessment activity for Chapter 10.

Test Generator

The Test Generator (Macintosh® or IBM® format) contains an additional 50 assessment items for this chapter.

PREVENTING SUICIDE

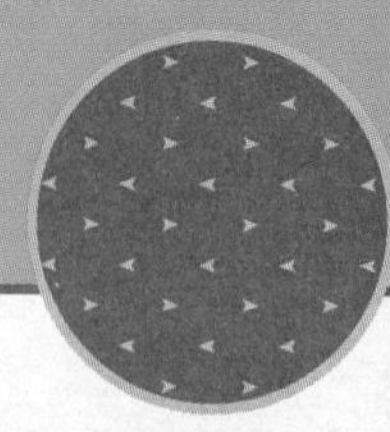

PLANNING GUIDE

TEXT SECTIONS	OBJECTIVES	TEXT FEATURES	OUTSIDE RESOURCES	NOTES
11.1 **Teenage Suicide: A Serious Problem** pp. 227-231 1 period	• Define suicide. • Understand how serious the problem of suicide is among teenagers. • Name three possible reasons for the increase in teen suicides. • Name at least three myths and facts about suicide.	**ASSESSMENT** • Section Review, p. 231	**TEACHER'S RESOURCE BINDER** • Lesson Plan 11.1 • Personal Health Inventory • Journal Entry 11A • Section Review Worksheet 11.1 • Section Quiz 11.1 • Reteaching Worksheet 11.1 **OTHER RESOURCES** • Transparencies 11A, 11B • Making a Choice 11A • English/Spanish Audiocassette 3	
11.2 **Giving and Getting Help** pp. 232-236 1 period	• List at least five warning signs of suicide. ■ Know strategies for dealing with someone who is suicidal. ■ Know how to use decision-making skills to help a friend in crisis. ■ Know what to do if you feel suicidal.	■ LIFE SKILLS: Solving Problems, p. 234 What Would You Do?, p. 235 **ASSESSMENT** • Section Review, p. 236	**TEACHER'S RESOURCE BINDER** • Lesson Plan 11.2 • Journal Entries 11B, 11C • Life Skills 11A • Section Review Worksheet 11.2 • Section Quiz 11.2 • Reteaching Worksheet 11.2 **OTHER RESOURCES** • Making a Choice 11B	
End of Chapter pp. 237-239		**ASSESSMENT** • Chapter Review, pp. 238-239	**TEACHER'S RESOURCE BINDER** **OTHER RESOURCES** • Chapter Test • Alternative Assessment • Personal Pledge • Test Generator	

■ Denotes LIFE SKILLS objectives

• Items in blue are also part of the *Holt Health Activity Book.*

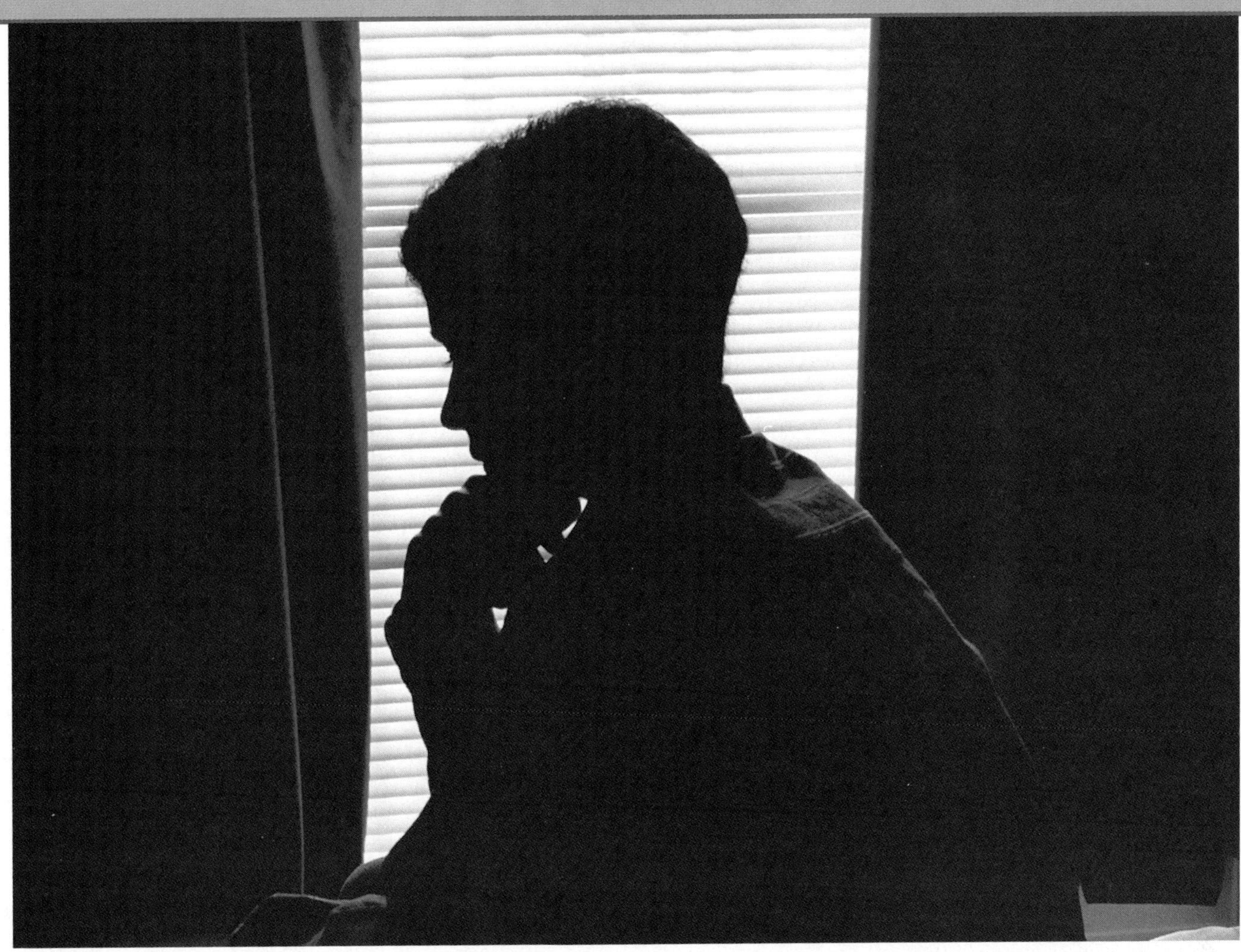

CONTENT BACKGROUND Teenage Suicide

SUICIDES AMONG YOUNG ADULTS AGES 15 to 19 have steadily increased since 1960. According to statistics compiled by the U. S. Department of Health and Human Services, 18 of every 100,000 Caucasian males in this age group committed suicide in 1987 as compared with 6 of 100,000 during 1960. Suicide rates among males of all other races increased from 4 per 100,000 in 1960 to 10 per 100,000 in 1987. About 2 of every 100,000 Caucasian adolescent females committed suicide in 1960. The rate in 1987 had risen to nearly 5 suicides per 100,000 females between the ages of 15 and 19. Females of all other races in the same age group who took their lives increased from 2 per 100,000 in 1960 to about 3 per 100,000 in 1987.

Suicide is the third leading cause of death—after accidental injuries and homicide—among Americans between the ages of 15 and 24. Although males in this age group are more likely to commit suicide than females, the 1987 National Adolescent Student Health Survey (NASHS) found that 42 percent of the 5,737 adolescent females polled said that they have "seriously thought" about ending their lives. Only 25 percent of the adolescent males surveyed answered similarly.

What makes these adolescents so depressed that suicide seems like the only option? Studies have revealed certain patterns. Nearly three-fourths of adolescents who attempt to end their lives are from broken homes. More than one-half of all teenage suicides or suicide attempts involve drugs—including alcohol—in some way. Eighty percent of all young adults who commit suicide have attempted suicide at some time in the recent past. About 12 percent of teenagers who

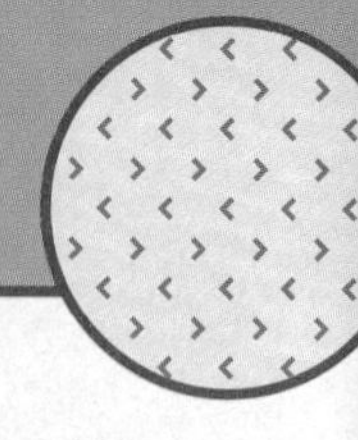

attempt suicide but fail will try again within 24 months and succeed at ending their lives.

Despite the alarming increase in the number of attempted suicides and actual suicides among teenagers in the United States over the past three to four decades, the NASHS found that fewer than half of the nearly 12,000 students surveyed were aware that a suicide-prevention hot line was available to them. Also, about 33 percent of those polled did not recognize the common signs displayed by a person who is likely to commit suicide. Over 36 percent didn't realize that people contemplating suicide often give away favorite possessions or change their appearance. And about one-third of the students, when asked whether people who talk about suicide actually go ahead with their decision, said they didn't know.

The topic of assisting a friend in a suicidal mindset provoked a range of responses among the students polled in the NASHS. Over 59 percent of the girls said they would find it "very hard" or "hard" to tell an adult about a friend contemplating suicide if they had promised they would not. Nearly 52 percent of the boys responded similarly. Relatively high percentages of students—about 32 percent of girls and about 30 percent of boys—responded that they would find it "very hard" or "hard" to tell the suicidal friend that he or she should get help from an adult. Also, about 37 to 41 percent of the students surveyed said it would be difficult for them to get help for the friend if the friend didn't want it.

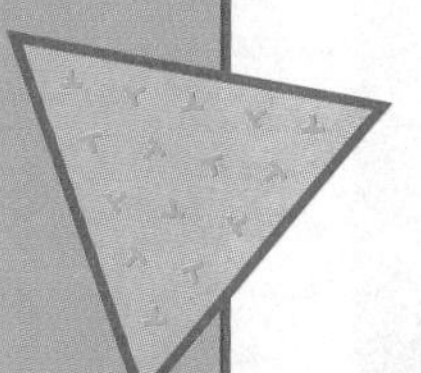

PLANNING FOR INSTRUCTION

KEY FACTS

- **Suicide is a serious problem for young people and the third leading cause of death for those ages 15 to 24.**
- **Some factors contributing to the increased suicide rate are family breakup and the ensuing sense of isolation it brings; increased mobility, which calls for continual readjustment; dysfunctional or abusive families; pressures to succeed; alcohol and drug use; and the romantic views of suicide presented in the media.**
- **For many, suicide seems like the only way out of extreme emotional pain.**
- **Most suicidal people reach out for help by talking about suicide and revealing deep emotional distress in a variety of ways.**
- **People who talk about suicide should always be taken seriously.**
- **While alcohol and drugs are not the cause of suicidal talk, they do interfere with a person's judgment and increase the likelihood of impulsive actions.**
- **The suicidal mindset is not a mental illness, an inherited tendency, or a permanent condition.**
- **If you feel suicidal, contact a trusted adult and ask for help.**
- **It is important to realize that there are various ways to solve difficult problems and that the pain will pass—but suicide is a permanent state.**

MYTHS AND MISCONCEPTIONS

MYTH: If you dare a suicidal person to attempt suicide, the person will not likely do it.

The dare may only strengthen the person's decision to commit suicide by convincing him or her that nobody really cares.

MYTH: Suicidal people always appear depressed and lonely.

Some suicidal people may suddenly become overly active and aggressive before attempting to commit suicide.

MYTH: Once a person attempts suicide and fails, he or she probably won't ever try it again.

Suicide victims have often tried several times to take their own lives.

MYTH: Secrecy is vital because information of a suicide attempt could ruin a person's future life.

If the suicide attempt is kept secret and professional help is not sought, there may be no future at all for the suicidal person.

VOCABULARY

Essential: The following vocabulary terms appear in boldface type:

suicide **suicidal mindset**

Secondary: Be aware that the following terms may come up during class discussion:

dysfunctional families sexual identity
depressed/depression therapist
self-esteem

FOR STUDENTS WITH SPECIAL NEEDS

Auditory Learners: Have students organize a mock radio panel presentation on teenage suicides. Topics that could be addressed include facts and myths about suicide, warning signs of suicide, and how to help suicidal people.

Kinetic and Visual Learners: Students will benefit from acting out situations in which one person gives warnings of suicide and another models helping behaviors (active listening, empathetic response, acknowledgment of the problem and its seriousness). A third person can act as a moderator who freezes the action to comment on what is being communicated and how it helps or harms the suicidal person.

ENRICHMENT

- Have students locate books and articles that discuss how the American family has changed in the twentieth century. Ask them to prepare a poster or write a song that illustrates how recent changes in society have strengthened or weakened the ability of family members to support one another.
- Clip newspaper or magazine advice columns that relate to some of the issues of the chapter (facing problems, building self-esteem, seeking support during a crisis) and allow students to study and discuss the articles. Then have interested students invent situations and write letters seeking help. Assign several students to study the letters and formulate replies that they think are helpful.
- Students might write a skit in which a suicide situation arises and is resolved by intervention. Encourage writers to use this as a forum to help dispel myths about suicide and educate themselves about how to help suicidal people.

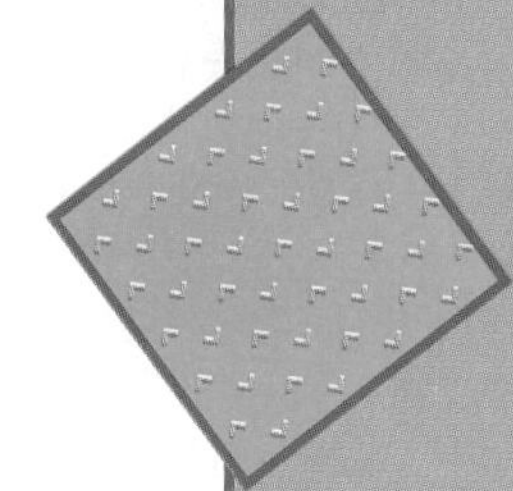

Chapter 11 Chapter Opener

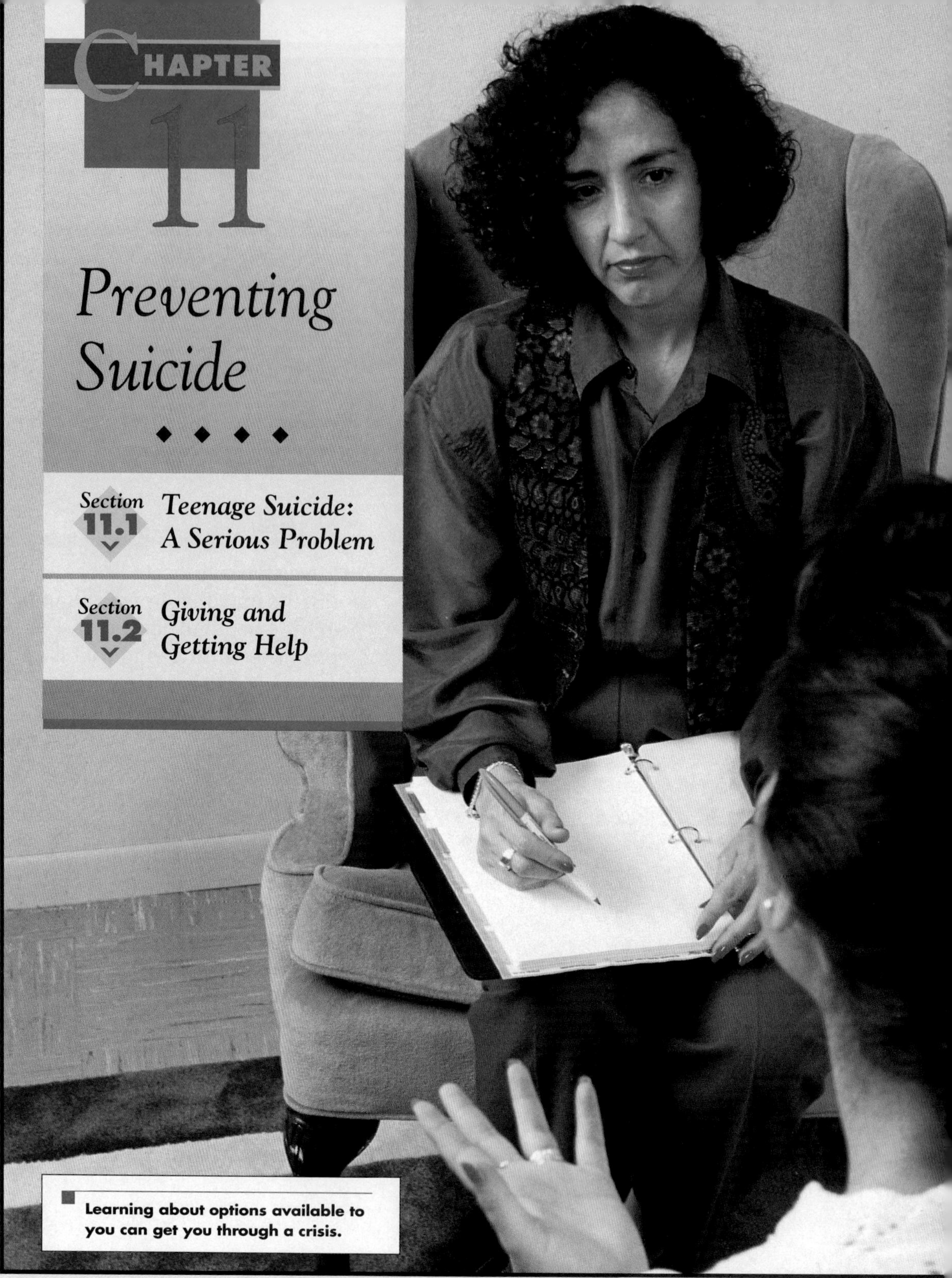

Getting Started

Using the Chapter Photograph

Have students look at the chapter photograph and think about Aaron's problems. What do you think Aaron decided to do about his problems? With whom did he discuss his feelings? Why do you think he made this decision? Students may also suggest thoughts that might be running through Aaron's mind and brainstorm other actions he might have taken.

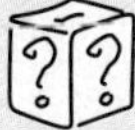

Question Box

Have students write out any questions they have about suicide and suicide prevention, and put them in the Question Box. The Question Box provides them with an opportunity to ask questions anonymously. To ensure that students with questions are not embarrassed to be seen writing, those who do not have questions should write something they already know about preventing suicide on the paper instead.

Personal Issues *ALERT*

Suicide is a difficult topic that can make both adults and students uncomfortable. In fact, references to suicide produce such anxiety in some people that suicide prevention can be hindered. Emphasize that understanding how people become suicidal, and how to help them, can save lives. Be aware that some students may be depressed or even suicidal, or may have family members who are. Such students may be encouraged by a respect for privacy, a calm and frank discussion, and an emphasis on the help that is available. By the same token, the students need reassurance that all people go through some periods of depression in their lives. Suicidal people differ in the degree and number of symptoms, and in their ability to cope.

Chapter 11

Preventing Suicide

Learning about options available to you can get you through a crisis.

After his father moved out, things got really bad for Aaron. After the divorce, Aaron lived with his mother, who was always on his case about something. He knew she was worried about money; his dad was always late with the child-support payment, and they could barely make ends meet.

Aaron couldn't concentrate on school anymore. He had flunked three tests in a row. If this kept up, he wouldn't be able to go to college. And even if he could get accepted by a college, there might not be enough money to pay for it. Aaron stayed awake at night, feeling desperate about his situation.

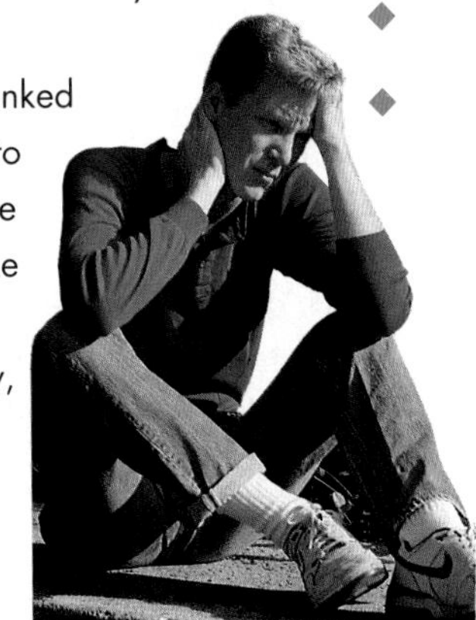

Then the worst thing of all happened. His girlfriend, Ashley, who had stuck by him through all his troubles, told Aaron she didn't want to see him anymore—she was going out with someone else now. His whole life seemed so hopeless that he wanted to go to sleep and never wake up.

Section 11.1 Teenage Suicide: A Serious Problem

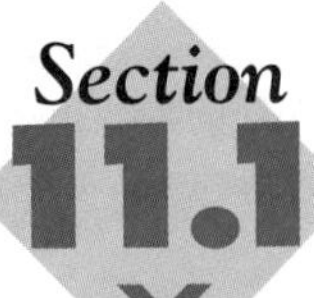

Objectives

- *Define suicide.*
- *Understand how serious the problem of suicide is among teenagers.*
- *Name three possible reasons for the increase in teen suicides.*
- *Name at least three myths and facts about suicide.*

Aaron reacted to the problems in his life by thinking about killing himself—committing **suicide.** He felt trapped. In his despair, he did not recognize that other options existed for him.

If you have ever been depressed like Aaron, you may have considered suicide. This is not unusual. Many people think about taking their own life when they feel extremely unhappy and hopeless. But if you have felt that suicide was the only way out of your troubles, you haven't learned about all the other options that exist.

In this chapter you will learn about the options available to you and your friends if life seems too painful to go on.

The Increase in Teen Suicides

Suicide is an increasingly serious problem among young people. The suicide rate among teenagers has quadrupled in the last 40 years. Suicide is the third leading cause

suicide: *the act of intentionally taking one's own life.*

Background
Statistics of Suicide

Suicide is the eighth leading cause of death in the United States. On average, about 28,000 people commit suicide each year in the United States. It is estimated that the number of people who attempt suicide is about 10 times this high. The group with the highest suicide rate in the nation is elderly white men who live alone.

Background
Suicide and Alcohol

Depression and suicide are strongly related to alcohol consumption on several levels. Alcoholics are often severely depressed. Consuming alcohol heightens or aggravates the symptoms of depression. For example, alcohol decreases appetite, can cause sleeplessness, and sharpens feelings of hopelessness. Only 1 percent of the general public commits suicide, but 6 percent to 29 percent of alcoholics commit suicide (1986).

Section 11.1 Lesson Plan

MOTIVATE

Journal 11A
Aaron's Situation

This may be done as a warm-up activity. Ask students to write in the Student Journal in the Student Activity Book a description of their feelings as they read about Aaron's situation. Suggest that they also describe how they would respond if he were their friend.

Writing
Aaron's Frame of Mind

Ask students to study the photograph of Aaron and write a descriptive paragraph or poem that reveals his frame of mind.

TEACH

Class Discussion
Suicide Awareness

Why do you think the suicide rate has increased so dramatically for young people? *[Students may list the reasons given in the book, but encourage them to list others as well. They may suggest that society moves much faster and is much more fragmented, making it hard to see "the big picture" and maintain emotional equilibrium, or they may cite a decline of values that support feelings of self-worth. A terminal illness or chronic pain may also be mentioned.]*

of death among people between the ages of 15 and 24. A recent study showed that about 1 in every 12 teenagers in the United States has attempted suicide.

Unfortunately, the reasons for the increase in teen suicide are not entirely clear. There are several factors that may contribute to the problem.

The rising divorce rate and breakup of families has created a situation in which many teenagers feel a sense of isolation and a lack of family support. Only a few decades ago, several generations of a family often lived in the same house. A young person usually had at least one close relative—a parent, a grandparent, an aunt, an uncle, or a cousin—to talk to. Today teenagers live in smaller families, with fewer adults around to offer emotional support.

Also, people today move from place to place more often than in earlier times. As a result of a parent's job loss or transfer to another city, children and teenagers often lose their old friends and must adjust to new schools. In times of trouble they may not be able to call on friends and relatives, who may be thousands of miles away.

Many teens live in troubled families, and feel that the love and care that they need is simply not there for them. Some teens may also experience physical, emotional, or sexual abuse.

Another factor may be the pressure to succeed in school and in future careers. Young people may feel like failures if they do not live up to their own or their parents' expectations.

The increased use of alcohol and drugs among teens also contributes to suicides. Although mind-altering substances may provide a temporary escape from emotional pain, they make things worse in the long run. Using alcohol and drugs damages a person's ability to solve everyday problems. And being drunk or high interferes with a person's judgment, and increases the chance that a person will act on a suicidal impulse.

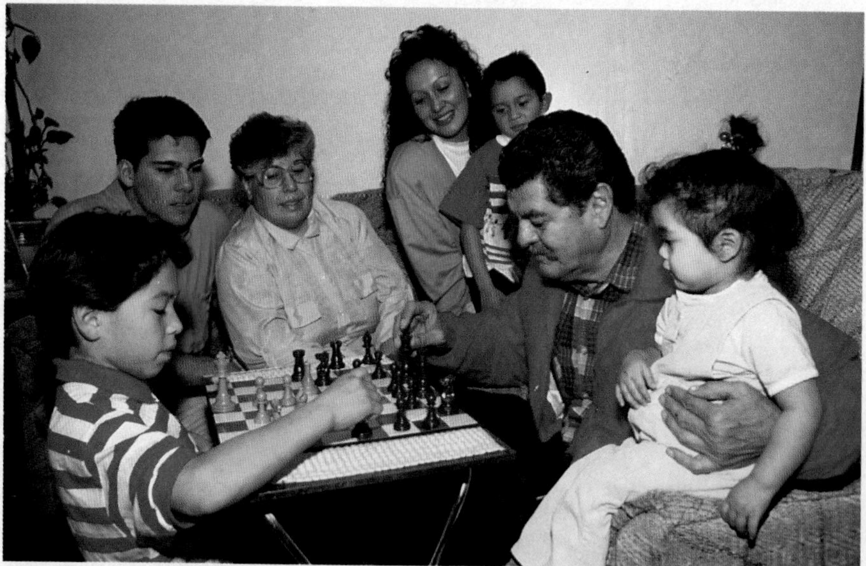

(FIGURE 11-1) **At one time, it was common for several generations of a family to live together. Teenagers in such families usually had at least one close relation to talk to.**

Background

Depression and Sunlight

Low levels of sunlight are linked to depression and depressive behavior. Experts say that people prone to depression should try to get two hours of sunlight each day.

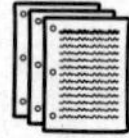

Personal Health Inventory

Have students complete the Personal Health Inventory for this chapter. The inventory helps them assess whether they show any warning signs of suicide.

Making a Choice 11A

Group Discussion

Assign the Group Discussion card. The card requires students to examine the meaning of, and feelings about, statements concerning suicide.

• • • TEACH continued

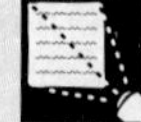

Teaching Transparency 11A

Suicide Rates

Use this transparency to complement the discussion of increased teen suicide rates in Section 11.1. It shows the actual and predicted suicide rates and population changes of 15- to 24-year-olds in the United States.

Class Discussion

Causes of Depression

What is the emotional condition that often accompanies suicidal thoughts? *[Depression]* You may wish to have students list specific examples of behaviors or incidents, such as the following, that could lead to or increase depression: feeling unloved, unresolved grief, very stressful experiences, low self-esteem.

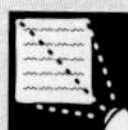

Teaching Transparency 11B

Myths and Facts

Show the transparency "Myths and Facts About Suicide" (Figure 11-3). Explain that in the past, anxiety and reluctance to talk about suicide have led to many wrong assumptions. Divide the class into pairs, assigning each pair one myth. Have them work out a brief dialogue in which one speaker believes the myth and the other must convince him or her of the facts.

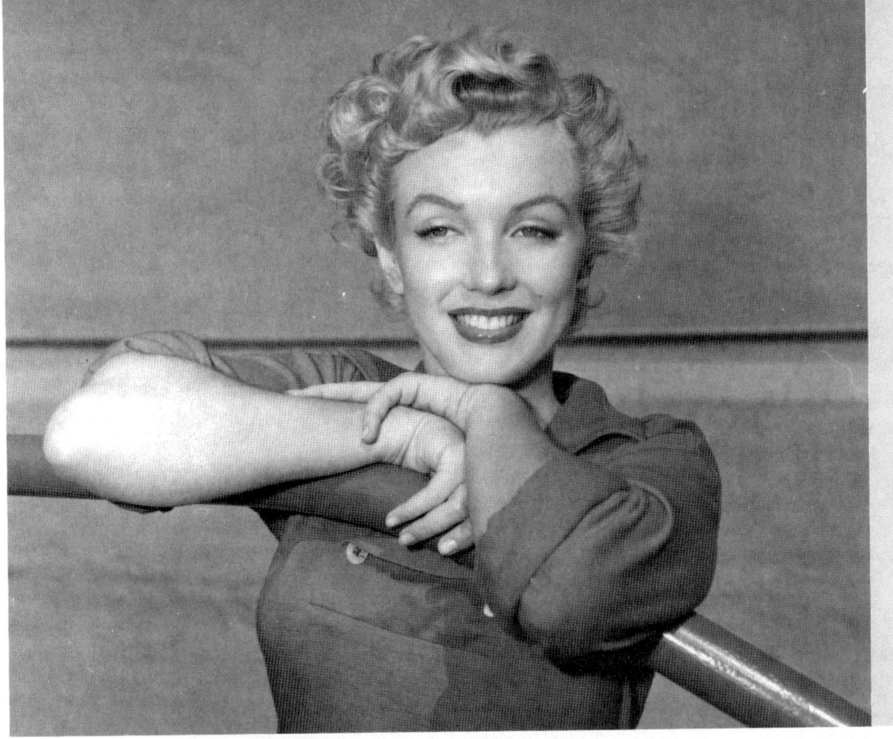

(FIGURE 11-2) **Marilyn Monroe committed suicide in 1962. Celebrities who commit suicide are sometimes made to seem like mythic figures.**

Finally, the popular media have romanticized suicide to a certain extent. When famous people kill themselves, they are sometimes made to seem like mythic figures. Suicide, such a message may seem to say, is glamorous and romantic. But once a celebrity is dead, he or she is not around to enjoy the romantic image. Suicide is not a glamorous act; it brings only death.

Why Would Someone Want to Die?

The reasons why young people try to kill themselves are many and complicated. Most people don't really want to die—they just want to end the emotional pain that they are suffering.

How can things get that bad? Life as a teenager can seem extremely stressful, especially if a person has low self-esteem. If someone who is already under great stress experiences a crisis, it may make life seem unbearable.

A crisis to one person would not necessarily seem like a crisis to another. To Aaron, losing his girlfriend was the last straw—he felt it pushed him over the edge. His girlfriend provided the only emotional support he had at that time. His father was gone, and his mother seemed preoccupied with keeping a roof over their heads.

When a person is depressed, events that at other times would be tolerable might seem impossible to bear. Moving to another town, not making a team or club, or the death of a pet could trigger a crisis in an already depressed person. Even an event that would seem trivial to others—having a bicycle stolen, for example—could be the last unbearable thing for an extremely depressed person.

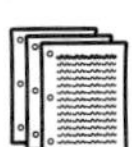

Section Review Worksheet 11.1

Assign Section Review Worksheet 11.1, which requires students to distinguish between myths and facts about suicide and to identify factors that could increase the risk of teen suicide.

Section Quiz 11.1

Have students take Section Quiz 11.1.

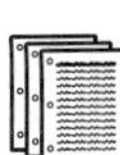

Reteaching Worksheet 11.1

Students who have difficulty with the material may complete Reteaching Worksheet 11.1, which requires them to identify myths and facts about suicide.

Class Discussion

Do They Really Want to Die?

In what sense is it true that a suicidal person doesn't want to die? *[The suicidal person wants the pain or problem to end, not life. He or she, however, is too immersed in depression and overwhelmed by feelings to see an end to the problem or options other than death.]*

Extension

What About the Terminally Ill?

Recent books about the right of terminally ill and painburdened patients to take their own lives include *Prescription Medicine: The Goodness of Planned Death* (Jack Kevorkian, 1991) and *Final Exit* (Derek Humphrey, 1992). Have students read one of these books and write a paper summarizing the author's main arguments, and stating their personal beliefs about suicide.

Myths and Facts About Suicide

Myth	Fact
Suicide usually occurs without warning.	*While some suicides may be impulsive, usually the person has thought about suicide for a long time.*
People who talk about killing themselves rarely commit suicide.	*Most people who commit suicide have talked about it before.*
If you ask a person if he or she is considering suicide, you will encourage that person to commit suicide.	*You will not cause a suicide simply by asking if someone is thinking about it. People who are not suicidal will not be affected by the question. People who are considering suicide will feel relieved that someone cares enough to ask and to listen to their problems.*
All suicidal people want to die.	*A suicide attempt is often a cry for help. The person may be asking for help to live.*
When a suicidal person suddenly seems calm and serene, there is no longer any danger of suicide.	*A suicidal person who suddenly acts calm and serene may have decided to commit suicide and therefore feels relief that a decision has been made.*
If someone makes a suicidal comment while drunk or high, it isn't very serious.	*People who are under the influence of alcohol or drugs may be at a greater risk of acting on suicidal thoughts because their judgment is impaired and they may be more impulsive.*
All people who commit suicide are mentally ill.	*Many people who feel suicidal are not mentally ill. They may be in a period of intense emotional crisis or in a deep depression.*
Once a person is suicidal, he or she will always be suicidal.	*Many people consider suicide for only a brief period in their lives. A person who attempts suicide and survives may never attempt it again if proper support and treatment is found.*
The tendency toward suicide is inherited and passed from parent to child.	*Suicide is a behavior and cannot be inherited. However, if a parent commits suicide, a child may see suicide as a way to solve problems.*

(FIGURE 11-3) **Because people avoid talking about suicide, many myths have arisen about the subject. Only by openly discussing suicide can people in trouble be recognized and helped.**

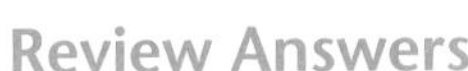

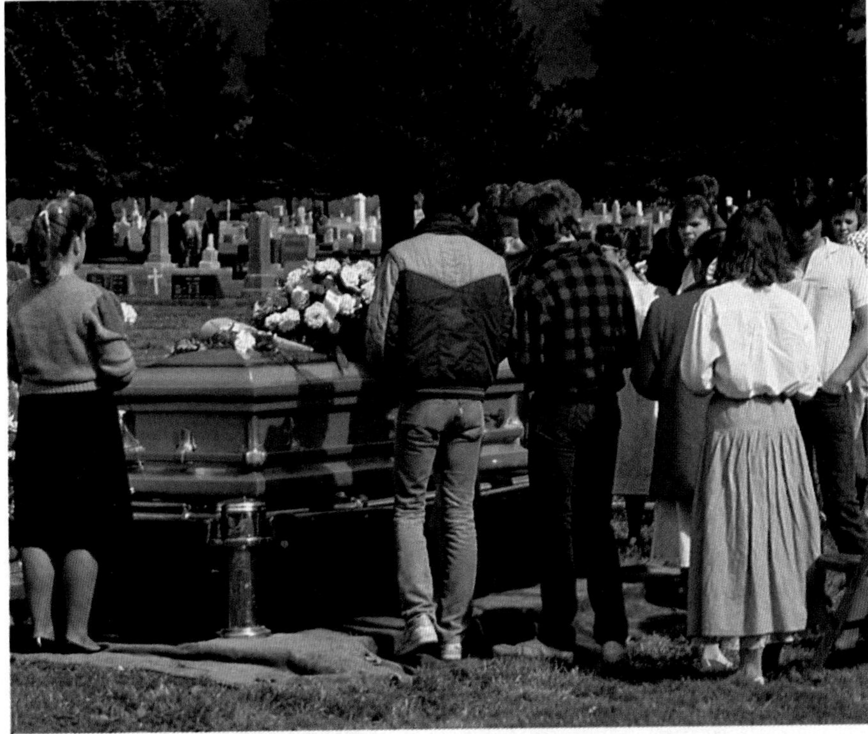

(FIGURE 11-4) **Suicide is a permanent response to what is usually a temporary problem.**

When people are in crisis situations, they may become confused and make poor decisions. They may develop ''tunnel vision,'' which is the inability to see all the options available. Aaron thought killing himself was the only way to solve his problems. When someone feels that suicide is the only solution to the problems of living, he or she is said to have a **suicidal mindset.**

But other solutions to problems always exist, even in the worst of situations. If Aaron had committed suicide, it would have been a permanent solution to a temporary problem. Aaron didn't really want to *die*. He just wanted to end his pain and suffering. The key to preventing suicide is getting help from people who can offer alternatives to ending one's life.

Review

1. *Define suicide.*
2. *Where does suicide rank among the causes of death of people aged 15 to 24?*
3. *Name three possible reasons for the increase in teen suicides.*
4. *Name three common myths about suicide and explain why each is not true.*
5. ***Critical Thinking*** *Describe some effects of alcohol and drug use that might increase the possibility that a person would attempt suicide.*

suicidal mindset:

the feeling that suicide is the only solution to the problems of living.

Review Answers

1. Suicide is the act of intentionally taking one's life.

2. Suicide is the third leading cause of death.

3. Answers will vary. Reasons may include divorce of parents; moving away from family and friends; dysfunctional families; pressure to succeed in school and in future careers; increased use of alcohol and drugs; glamorization of suicide by the media.

4. Answers will vary. Answers may include any of the myths and facts listed in Figure 11-3.

5. Alcohol and drugs may impair a suicidal person's judgment and make him or her act impulsively.

ASSESS

Section Review

Have students answer the Section Review questions.

Alternative Assessment

Alcohol and Drugs

Students can list several factors contributing to the suicide problem among young people and explain orally how alcohol and drug use increase the effects of these factors.

Closure

Teenage Suicide

Have students write a feature article on teenage suicide for a school newspaper, communicating facts about the seriousness of the problem, and dispelling common myths about suicide.

Background
Suicide and Sexual Identity

According to *The U.S. Department of Health and Human Services Task Force on Youth Suicide,* suicide is the leading cause of death among lesbian and gay youth. In fact, 30 percent of all youth suicides committed each year in the U.S. fall within this group. Schools can protect these young people from abuse of their peers and provide accurate information or referrals about homosexuality. Teens seeking information or answers concerning sexual identity issues can call The Out Youth Help Line, 1-800-969-6884.

Background
More Suicide Warning Signs

Indicators (in addition to those in the text) to be taken seriously are suicide notes, behavior that is much out of character (especially if it is self-destructive), drastic increase in use of alcohol and drugs, communication of a detailed plan for suicide, and talk about an available apparatus for killing oneself.

Section 11.2 Giving and Getting Help

Objectives

- *List at least five warning signs of suicide.*
- *Know strategies for dealing with someone who is suicidal.*
  LIFE SKILLS: Solving Problems
- *Know how to use decision-making skills to help a friend in crisis.*
  LIFE SKILLS: Making Responsible Decisions
- *Know what to do if you feel suicidal.*

It's hard to know how to help someone with such a serious and scary problem as suicide. You must do the best you can, but don't feel that the entire burden is on you. The worst thing a person can do is to feel responsible if a friend has committed suicide. If a person has killed him- or herself, no one is responsible but that person.

The first step is to try to determine if a friend feels suicidal. Statistics show that 80 percent of the people who attempt suicide have given warning signs. Study the table in Figure 11-7 so you will recognize possible warning signs of suicide.

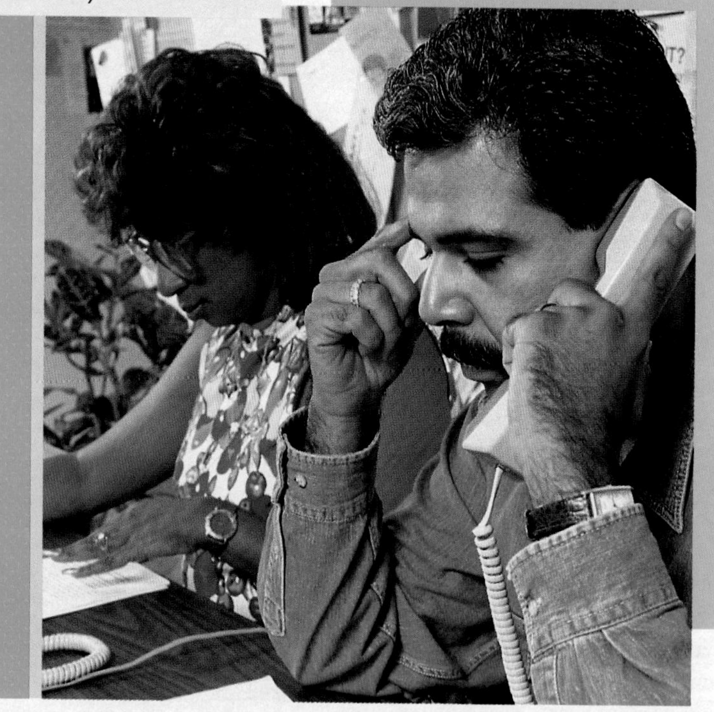

(FIGURE 11-5) **If you think a friend is suicidal, call a suicide hotline. The staffers there will assist your efforts to find help.**

Section 11.2 Lesson Plan

MOTIVATE

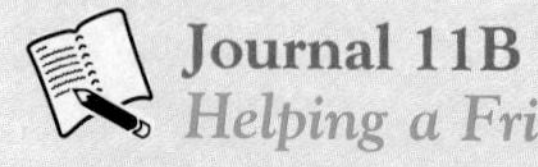

Journal 11B
Helping a Friend

This may be done as a warm-up activity. Stress that being able to turn to someone who cares can mean the difference between life and death for a suicidal person. Encourage students to write in the Student Journal several things they might do to help a friend who seems very depressed or makes suicidal threats.

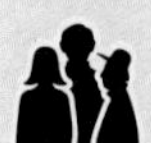

Cooperative Learning
Being a Good Listener

Many suicidal people can be helped in time if others listen to them and respond. Divide the class into small groups and develop a list of skills they think a person might need to be a good listener in such a situation. Student lists may have some of the following traits: good eye contact; comfortable relaxed posture, gestures, and slight leaning toward the speaker; reinforcing words and phrases that encourage communication and reflect what the speaker is feeling.

TEACH

Class Discussion
Suicide Warning Signs

Stress the importance of being sensitive to warning signs. **Why do many people fail to "hear" suicide warning signs or to take them seriously?** *[Some*

Intervention Strategies: What Should You Do?

Think back to Aaron at the beginning of this chapter. Assume that you are a friend of his and you've noticed that he has seemed really down lately. One night he says to you: "This may be the last time you will see me." Which of the following should you do?

1. Ask Aaron if he is thinking about committing suicide.
2. Avoid mentioning suicide but make an attempt to find out what is bothering Aaron.
3. Keep the talk light so as not to give Aaron any ideas about suicide.
4. Try to joke with Aaron about his problems and about suicide.

The first answer is the best one in this case. If Aaron isn't thinking about suicide, your mentioning it will not do any harm; you aren't going to make him suicidal by asking him if he is. But if Aaron is thinking about suicide, he urgently needs to discuss it. People who talk about suicide, or give any indication they are contemplating it, are often seeking help in the only way they know how.

Most suicidal people reach out to someone for help. In fact, many reach out repeatedly before they actually try to kill themselves.

If you have a friend who is suicidal, let your friend know you are listening and that you understand. Your friend may express feelings of being picked on, different, lonely, ugly, or stupid. Do not try to make your friend feel better by denying the feelings. Don't say, for example: "Oh, you're just imagining things. Snap out of it."

Be as understanding and patient as possible. To show you understand, you could say something like: "It must feel terrible to have all that pain and hurt feelings."

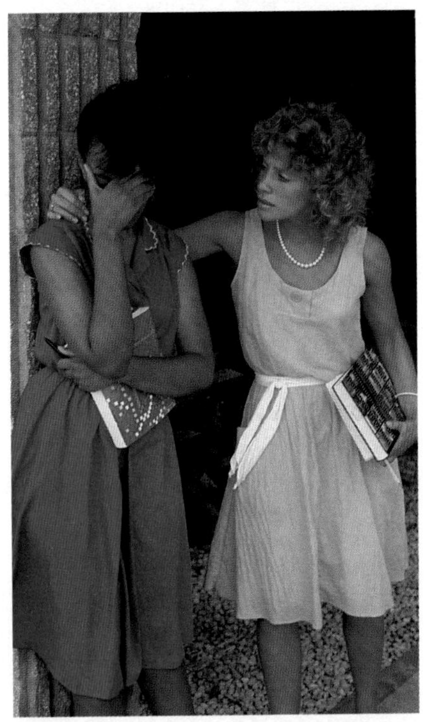

(FIGURE 11-6) **If a friend seems depressed and possibly suicidal, let him or her know that you're there, and that you care.**

Possible Warning Signs of Suicide

Prior suicide attempts
Direct statements about suicide
Indirect or subtle statements about suicide
Giving away prized possessions
Writing a will

(FIGURE 11-7) **Eighty percent of people who attempt or complete suicide give warning signs that are a cry for help.**

people don't want to hear something that raises their discomfort level so high, and they may set up psychological defenses to separate themselves from the communicator. Others feel concern but are immobilized by fear of involvement. Some dread what they think will be a prolonged involvement in an unpleasant situation; others think they will precipitate the suicide by acknowledging the threat of it.]

Reinforcement
Showing Concern

Point out that it never hurts to show concern for someone who is struggling with depression or an emotional crisis, even if he or she is not suicidal.

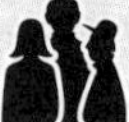

Cooperative Learning
Suicide Warning Signs

Divide the class into small groups and have each group develop descriptions of a person's behavior, statements, or situations that can be seen as warning signs of suicide. For example, "Joe loves sports cards and has a large collection. For weeks you have been begging him to sell you a prize card, but he has refused to part with it. Today he offers to give you his collection. You know he is upset about his poor grades this period, and he told you he hasn't been able to sleep much lately." You might have the students intersperse these descriptions with descriptions that do not include warning signals of suicide and read them to the class.

Life SKILLS

Helping a Suicidal Friend

Have students do the Life Skills activity, brainstorming the names of adults who can be called on to help a suicidal friend. Bring phone books to class and have students locate phone numbers for suicide hot lines, crisis intervention lines, suicide counselors, counseling services, human services clinics, and so on.

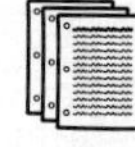

Life Skills Worksheet 11A

Peer Counseling Groups

Assign the Peer Counseling Groups Life Skills Worksheet, which requires students to investigate how peer counseling groups are organized to help in suicide prevention.

Making a Choice 11B

Helping a Friend in Trouble

Assign the Helping a Friend in Trouble card. The card asks students to discuss and role-play situations in which they could help a suicidal friend.

After discovering that your friend is suicidal, get help. Contact an adult who you feel is caring and in a position to help. This person could be a parent or other relative, teacher, school counselor, school nurse, religious leader, or neighbor. Such a person may be able to help your friend, and may also offer advice on other places to go for help.

You could also call your local suicide hotline. Look in the phone book under "Suicide" or "Crisis." The people staffing these phone lines will find help for you. You can also call the 911 emergency number or the police department.

Your friend might make you promise not to tell anybody. It may seem like a difficult decision to make—keeping a promise you made to a friend, or going for help. But by confiding in you, your friend is asking for help. To help your friend, you *must* break the promise and notify a trusted adult of the danger that exists.

Remember, though, that you are not responsible for your friend's life. Only he or she can make the decision to live.

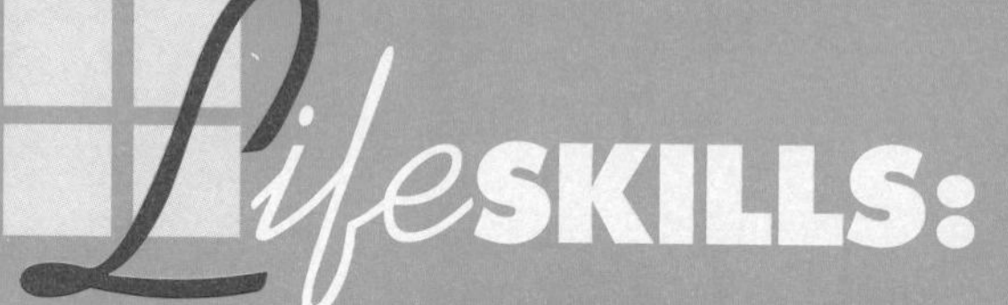

LifeSKILLS: Solving Problems

Helping a Suicidal Friend

A friend tells you that he is failing school and feels humiliated because his father is a teacher and has high expectations of him. He says he feels stupid and knows he'll never amount to anything. If that's the way his life is going to be, he says, he might as well kill himself. You listen and let him know you care about him and that you understand how bad he must feel. You offer to help him find assistance.

On a separate sheet of paper, write down the names of as many adults as you can think of who could help your friend.

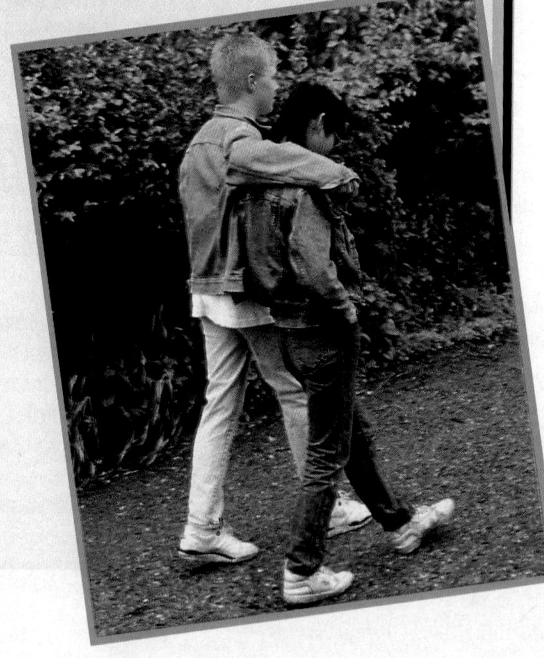

• • • TEACH continued

Journal 11C
Seeking Help

Encourage students to use the Student Journal to express their feelings about seeking help if they experience depression or consider suicide. They might express their fears about the risks they would be taking by talking to an adult and the difficulty of facing problems honestly. Ask that they list two things they learned in this chapter that would make them more willing to seek help.

Class Discussion
Getting the Best Help

Refer students to Figure 11-8 and ask: **Which of these adults would be most helpful to someone who is considering suicide?** Responses may vary, but ask students to express why they feel like they do.

Extension
Another Perspective

Ask students to select an adult they trust and can talk to easily. Have each student talk with the person about difficult situations and stresses he or she faced in teenage years and find out the person's perspective on those problems today. How did he or she cope as a teenager?

If You Feel Suicidal

If you ever feel that life is too painful to continue, you must ask for help. The reason you need help is that you are too confused and desperate to see all the alternatives to suicide.

Contact one of the adults listed in Figure 11-8, or any other adult you trust. You might be surprised to find out how much other people care for you and how willing they are to help you.

You may need professional counseling with a psychologist or therapist. At the very least, talk to a therapist to see if counseling is necessary. Therapists can offer options you hadn't thought of before. They can also help you learn new skills so that you can succeed in basic goals like making friends, coping with stress, or getting along with your family. Most important, they may remind you that no matter how bad things may seem, there are things you can do to help yourself feel better.

What Would You Do?

Making Responsible Decisions

You Made a Promise

Julia is your best friend. She has been acting depressed lately because her boyfriend broke up with her. Julia came to you and told you that she is thinking about killing herself. But she made you promise you would not tell anyone.

After you talk with her, you begin to wonder if you should tell anyone about Julia's problem. But you *did* promise not to and she *is* your best friend. What would you do?

Remember to use the decision-making steps:

1. **State the Problem.**
2. **List the Options.**
3. **Imagine the Benefits and Consequences.**
4. **Consider Your Values.**
5. **Weigh the Options and Decide.**
6. **Act.**
7. **Evaluate the Results.**

(FIGURE 11-8) **Help is available for those in crisis. Talk to a trusted adult if you (or a friend) are thinking of suicide.**

Some Adults Who Might Be Helpful in a Crisis

- Parent
- Grandparent, aunt, uncle, or other relative
- Teacher
- School counselor
- School nurse
- Therapist at a mental-health center
- Minister, priest, rabbi, or other religious leader
- Neighbor
- Person who staffs the local suicide hotline, the crisis hotline, or the 911 emergency number
- Person who answers the phone at the police department

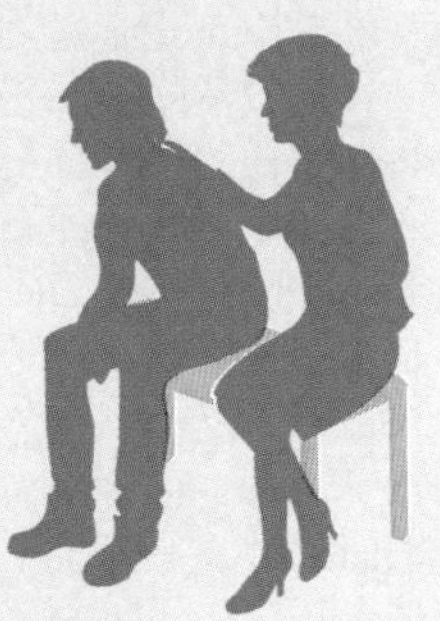

SECTION 11.2

What Would You Do?

You Made a Promise

Review the steps in the decision-making process briefly. Remind students, however, that in this case a decision must be made quickly. Therefore, it is important to decide before the fact how you will handle such a situation if it arises.

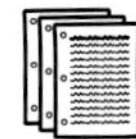

Section Review Worksheet 11.2

Assign Section Review Worksheet 11.2, which requires students to identify what to do if they or a friend feel suicidal.

Section Quiz 11.2

Have students take Section Quiz 11.2.

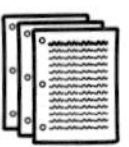

Reteaching Worksheet 11.2

Students who have difficulty with the material may complete Reteaching Worksheet 11.2, which requires them to identify warning signs of suicide and describe what a person could do to help someone who is suicidal.

Review Answers

1. Students may include any of the signs listed in Figure 11-7.

2. Students may ask the friend if he or she is thinking of suicide. They may let the friend know that they are listening and understanding. They may get help for the friend. Accept any answers that indicate students' understanding and ability to apply intervention strategies.

3. By confiding in the student, the friend is asking for help. To help the friend, the student must break the promise and notify a trusted adult of the situation.

4. Ask for help from a trusted adult or call the local suicide prevention crisis line.

5. Students may answer that a particular event, however trivial it may seem to someone else, may cause a person to feel suicidal if that person has been experiencing several stressful or depressing situations.

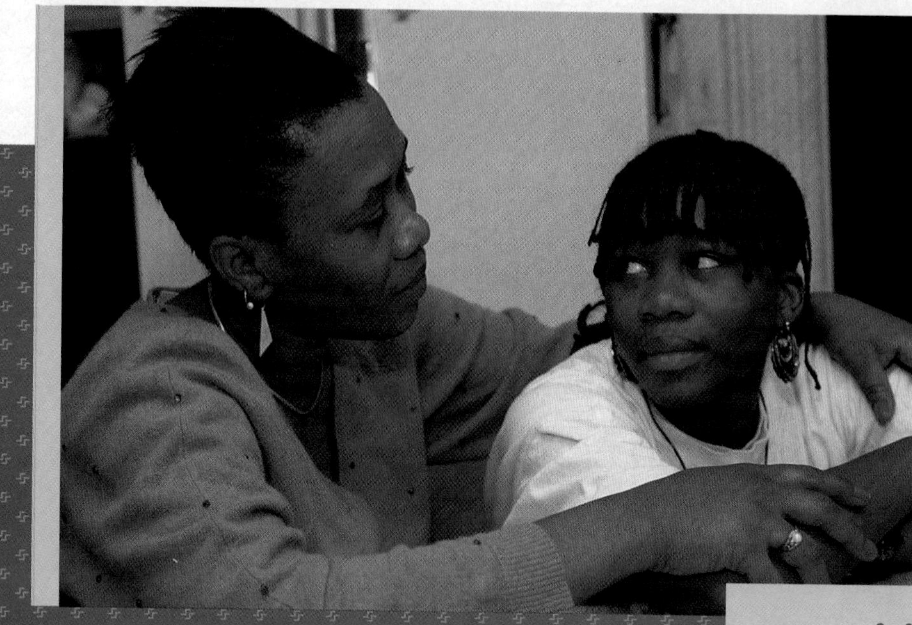

(FIGURE 11-9) **You might be surprised to find out how much other people care for you and how willing they are to help you.**

You need to be willing to take a risk—the risk of confronting and resolving your problems. If you are willing to talk openly and honestly about the things that are making you unhappy, you can create options for yourself that do not exist when you remain closed and depressed. Suicide is only one option out of thousands of options that life offers. If you choose it, then you won't have the chance to explore the others.

The teenage years are a difficult time for most people. Many adults who are now living happy lives once considered suicide or even attempted it when they were teenagers themselves.

The important thing to remember is that the pain *will* pass. Don't try to solve a temporary problem with the permanent solution of suicide. If you feel like hurting yourself, talk to a trusted adult now.

Review

1. *What are five signs that might indicate someone is suicidal?*
2. ***LIFE SKILLS: Solving Problems*** *Describe what you should do if your friend tells you he or she doesn't want to live.*
3. ***LIFE SKILLS: Making Responsible Decisions*** *Your friend made you promise that you would not tell anyone he was going to kill himself. Why should you break your promise?*
4. ***LIFE SKILLS: Coping*** *If you felt suicidal, how could you help yourself?*
5. ***Critical Thinking*** *Why do you think a particular situation will cause one person to feel suicidal, while another person in the same situation might not even be depressed?*

ASSESS

Section Review

Have students answer the Section Review questions.

Alternative Assessment

Ask students to write a letter to a counselor in which they express concern for a friend who exhibits some of the warning signs of suicide. Students may exchange letters and write a reply to the one they receive. Replies should show understanding of how to help a suicidal person.

Closure

Do's and Don'ts

Ask students to write a checklist of do's and don'ts for dealing with a person who may be suicidal. Suggest that they list four items in each column.

Highlights

Summary

- Suicide is one of the leading causes of death among people aged 15 to 24. The suicide rate among teenagers has quadrupled in the last 40 years.
- The following are possible reasons for the increase in teen suicides: (1) the rising divorce rate and breakup of families; (2) families moving from place to place more frequently; (3) absence of parental love and support in some families; (4) pressure to succeed in school and future careers; (5) increasing use of alcohol and drugs; and (6) romanticization of suicide by the media.
- Most people don't want to die but simply want to end the emotional pain they are suffering.
- Crises often seem more stressful if a person has low self-esteem. A crisis to one person may not be a crisis for someone else.
- Depression is a feeling that often accompanies suicide.
- When people are in crisis situations, they may become confused, make poor decisions, and be unable to see all the options available.
- Most people who attempt suicide display one or more warning signs. These signs or threats should always be taken seriously.
- Warning behaviors displayed by people thinking about suicide include mood swings, withdrawal, sadness, weight gain or loss, drop in grades, tiredness, inability to concentrate or make decisions, giving away prized possessions, and taking risks.
- If you think a friend is thinking about suicide, get help as soon as possible. Contact a caring adult or call your local suicide hotline number.
- If you are in pain and are thinking about suicide, know that counseling is available from mental-health professionals such as psychologists.
- A person who is willing to talk openly and honestly about problems has options that do not exist for a person who remains closed and depressed.

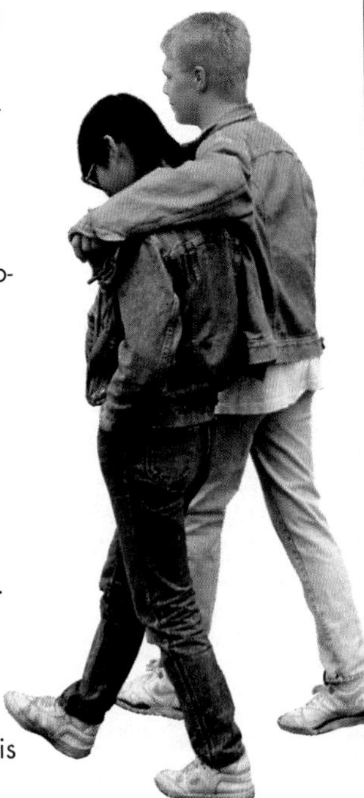

Vocabulary

suicide the act of intentionally taking one's own life.

suicidal mindset the feeling that suicide is the only solution to the problem of living.

Chapter 11 Highlights Strategies

Summary

Have students read the summary to reinforce the concepts they have learned in Chapter 11.

Vocabulary

Using the vocabulary words and at least five other key words or phrases from the chapter, students might create a concept map or drawing that shows the relationship of these words and phrases to one another and to the topic of teenage suicide. Suggest that students make their concept maps large enough to include illustrations that convey the concepts behind the words.

Extension

Have students contact local mental health organizations or the National Mental Health Institute by phone or letter and request information on giving and receiving help for depression and suicidal tendencies. Encourage them to organize this information into a display for the classroom.

Chapter 11 Assessment

Chapter Review

Concept Review

Sample responses:

1. Possible reasons include the rising divorce rate and breakup of families, families moving from place to place more frequently, some families not providing love and care to children, pressure to succeed, increasing use of alcohol and drugs, suicide being romanticized by the media.

2. Most people don't want to die but simply want to end the emotional pain they are suffering.

3. The teen may feel he or she is the cause of the divorce. The teen may also feel isolated and sense a lack of family support.

4. The depression may lead to a crisis situation in which the person becomes confused, makes poor decisions, or cannot see options available. Without seeing options, the person may view the situation as hopeless and for this reason attempt suicide.

5. They may decide to attempt suicide.

6. mood swings, withdrawal, sadness, weight gain or loss, drop in grades, tiredness, inability to concentrate or make decisions, giving away prized possessions, or taking risks.

7. Students may ask the friend if he or she is thinking of suicide. Students may let their friend know that they are listening and understand. Students may get help for their friend from parents, teachers, clergy, and school counselors.

8. By confiding in you, your friend is asking for help. To help your friend, you must break the promise and notify a trusted adult.

9. You will see options that you might not have seen before. Following through with these options may resolve the problems and you will not feel helpless and suicidal.

10. No. Once you receive help and resolve the problem(s) you will not feel as depressed; you will feel more in control and happier; you will learn new skills in dealing with various problems. A situation may never arise again in which you feel so hopeless, helpless, and depressed.

Expressing Your Views

Sample responses:

1. Talk with her about what may be bothering her and let her know that I am listen-

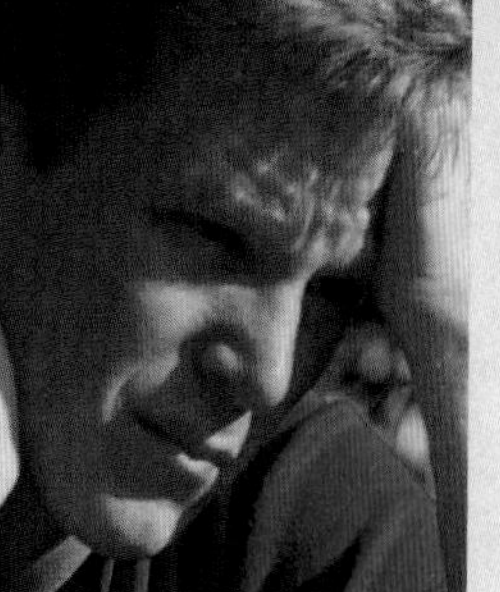

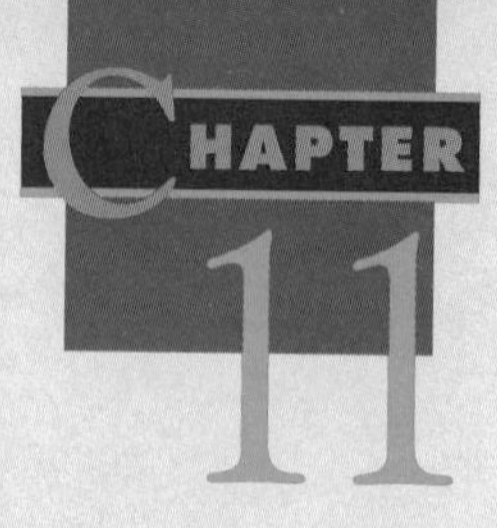

Chapter Review

Concept Review

1. Why is suicide a major problem among young people?
2. Is it true that all suicidal people want to die? Explain.
3. Explain why the breakup of families could contribute to the increase in teen suicides.
4. What makes the depression felt by a possible suicide victim different from the depression most people experience in everyday life?
5. What happens to people who are thinking of suicide when they find themselves in crisis situations?
6. Name six behavioral warning signs of suicide.
7. How can you help if a friend is in a suicidal situation? Who are some adults who could help?
8. If a friend who is suicidal confides in you about his or her intentions and swears you to secrecy, should you keep your promise? Explain.
9. If you feel suicidal, how can it be helpful to take the risk of confronting and resolving your problems?
10. If you consider suicide once, will you always be suicidal? Explain.

Expressing Your Views

1. A good friend of yours has lost a lot of weight pretty quickly. Her grades have been dropping and she seems withdrawn. All of this has happened since her boyfriend broke up with her. You are concerned about her. What should you do?
2. Will's parents have recently divorced, and soon he will have to move to another town. He has been very depressed and has started seeing a psychologist. His friends don't know the whole story, but they say that Will is getting counseling because he's not strong enough to handle his problems on his own. What would you say to Will's friends?
3. Randall seems antisocial because he is always alone. Twice in the past week he has started strange conversations with you that ended with a suicide threat. When you told a friend what had happened, the friend said not to worry, that Randall threatens suicide all the time just to get attention. What do you think? Should you be concerned?

CHAPTER 11 ASSESSMENT

Life Skills Check

1. Coping
Let's say that during the past year you became terribly depressed. Your spirits were so low that at one point you were thinking about suicide. Instead, you got professional counseling, and now you feel as though you are recovering. As part of your therapy, your counselor has asked you to write down a list of the things that make you happy. What would you include on your list?

2. Solving Problems
Suppose a friend calls you to come over to her house right away. When you arrive, she appears very upset and begins to talk about suicide and death. No one is at home except the two of you. What should you do?

Projects

1. Work with a group to design a suicide-prevention pamphlet, using the information in your textbook. Include myths and facts about suicide, some warning signs of suicide, a list of adults to contact in a crisis, and the free hotline number. Distribute copies of the pamphlet throughout your school or publish it in the school newspaper.
2. Work with a partner to make up a problem situation and then role-play, providing support and receiving support. Devise a positive way to act out how to cope with the situation.
3. Investigate the impact of the Vietnam experience on a soldier's suicidal tendencies. You might read a story or article written by a veteran or view a movie on this topic. You might also contact the Vietnam Veterans Outreach Program through a federal veteran's program and ask for statistics and information. Write a brief essay and share your findings with the class.

Plan for Action

Suicide is one of the leading causes of death among teenagers. Plan how you can prevent suicide in your life and in others' lives.

ing and I understand. Also, I would not attempt to make her feel better by denying any feelings she shares with me. If she is suicidal, I would get help.
2. That they do not fully understand the situation and that my best friend is stronger than most people, because my friend recognizes and admits feelings and is willing to risk confronting and resolving problems.
3. Randall may indeed be suicidal. I would be concerned and seek help for Randall by contacting a caring adult or calling the suicide hot line number.

Life Skills Check
Sample responses:
1. Answers will vary.
2. Be patient and understanding and let her know you are listening to what she is saying. Then get help as soon as possible by contacting a caring adult or calling the suicide hot line number.

Projects
Have students complete the projects on suicide.

Plan for Action
Ask the class to make a list of situations or incidents that are likely to make a teenager think of suicide. Then divide the class into groups and assign each group one of these situations. Have them come up with alternatives to suicide for the person who feels suicidal because of this life experience.

ASSESSMENT OPTIONS

Chapter Test
Have students take the Chapter 11 Test.

Alternative Assessment
Have students do the Alternative Assessment activity for Chapter 11.

Test Generator
The Test Generator (Macintosh® or IBM® format) contains an additional 50 assessment items for this chapter.

Issues in Health

ETHICAL ISSUES IN HEALTH

ISSUE: *Should terminally ill people have the right to determine how or when to die?*

Have students read the Ethical Issues in Health feature. Then ask them to name conditions under which a person—not necessarily themselves—might choose to die rather than continue living. These might include terminal illness, continuous pain, dependence upon machinery for breathing or other life-support functions, or paralysis. Emphasize that the list will be different for each person. Do the students feel that these conditions are easy or difficult to define? Would it depend on how the person felt at the time? How would you expect family members to respond to a death that was chosen?

Ethical Issues in Health

ISSUE: Should terminally ill people have the right to determine how or when to die?

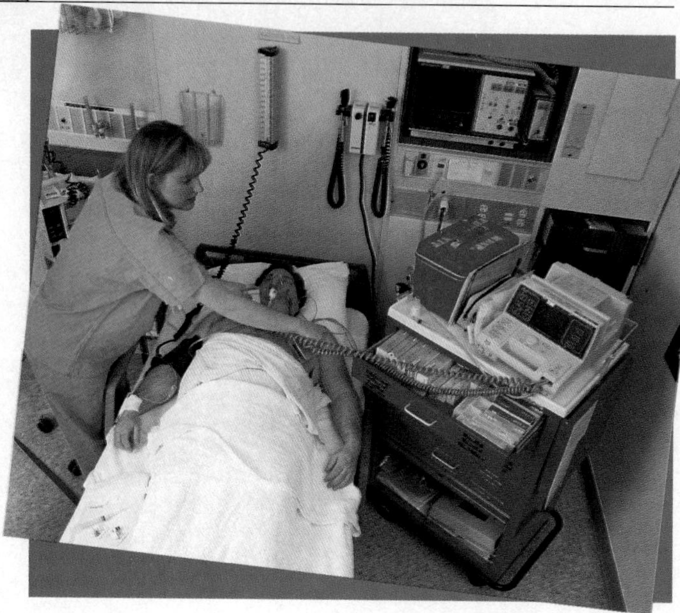

Death is the natural and inevitable end to life. Modern medical techniques, such as CPR and mechanical life support, have made it possible to avert death in situations where once a person certainly would have died. Modern technology is also capable of sustaining a person's life far beyond the point at which natural death would have occurred. Unfortunately, the technology to restore a healthy normal life to most of the people who survive with the aid of life-sustaining equipment does not exist. As a result, thousands of patients with no hope of recovery survive with mechanical support for weeks, months, and even years at great financial and emotional expense to their families and society.

Just as they did when they were healthy, people who are facing death need close relationships, honest communication, personal dignity, and control of their lives. Many people believe that the use of life-sustaining treatments, such as feeding through tubes and using equipment to maintain breathing and circulation, robs terminally ill patients of personal dignity and the right to control their lives. For this reason, many people believe that people with no hope of recovery should have the right to decide to die.

One way that people can retain control of their lives even when they are terminally ill is to establish a ''living will.'' Recognized by most states, a living will is a legal document that allows people to specify what measures they want taken if they should have a serious disease or injury that will ultimately and inevitably result in death. Such a document allows a person to choose between receiving life-sustaining treatment or refusing all life-sustaining treatment so that death can occur naturally. A living will is executed only when the patient becomes permanently unconscious.

Some people want to be able to decide how and when to die, should they become terminally ill. Those who support the legal right to control the conditions of their own deaths make up the ''right-to-die'' movement. Sometimes terminally ill people request assistance from friends and family in what is often called "assisted suicide" or "assisted death." When a physician helps terminally ill patients die at their request, it is called "euthanasia" or "physician aid in dying."

An increasing number of people faced with death, particularly those in the latter stages of AIDS, are asking their friends and physicians to assist them by injecting them with painkillers in large enough doses to cause death. In 1989, the suicide rate among people with AIDS in the United States was six times higher than the rate for other adults. The suicide rate among people with other terminal illnesses is unknown.

The issue of assisted death gained national media attention when Dr. Jack Kevorkian of Michigan was accused of murder for helping several people die with his controversial "suicide machine." Over the years, there have also been several highly publicized court trials of family members who caused the death of terminally ill loved ones suffering excruciating pain.

In the United States, a physician who causes the death of a terminally ill patient by injecting drugs or writing a prescription for the drugs can be charged with murder, even if it is at the request of the patient. A nonphysician who helps end a life upon request can also be charged with murder. However, very few people who have helped a terminally ill loved one die have been sentenced to jail. Laws legalizing assisted death have been introduced in several states, but as of 1992 the idea has been approved in only one state—California. In one country, the Netherlands, physicians who assist patients in dying are not prosecuted.

People in the "right-to-die" movement defend assisted death. They argue that the practice is ethical because dying people have the right to have some control over both their lives and their deaths, especially the length of time it takes to die. Those who oppose assisted death say that even those who are dying do not have the right to ask others to participate in an act that is illegal and morally wrong.

Situation for Discussion

Martha is a 35-year-old woman who has cancer. It began in an ovary and has now spread throughout many parts of her body. More than one physician has confirmed that Martha is terminally ill. She suffers excruciating pain and has asked her husband, a physician, to help her die by giving her a lethal dose of morphine.

a. If Martha's husband gives her enough morphine to cause her death, should he be tried for murder? Would he be morally right? Has he violated the oath to preserve life that all physicians take?

b. Is it ethical for Martha to ask her husband to help her die? Would it be more ethical for Martha to end her life without her husband's help than with his help?

c. What would you do if you were Martha? Martha's husband? Why?

UNIT 4

PROTECTING YOUR HEALTH IN A DRUG SOCIETY

CHAPTER OVERVIEWS

CHAPTER 12

THE USE, MISUSE, AND ABUSE OF DRUGS

Students learn that although drugs can be useful in the prevention, treatment, or cure of many illnesses, drugs cannot solve *all* their problems. The chapter suggests drug-free pain treatments, names the seven categories of drugs, and explains the differences among drug use, drug misuse, and drug abuse. A thorough discussion of over-the-counter and prescription drugs follows. Students learn about the effects of drugs on the body, including drug interactions, side effects, and allergies.

CHAPTER 13

ALCOHOL: A DANGEROUS DRUG

The chapter begins with a discussion of the short- and long-term effects of alcohol. Students learn some reasons why people drink and some reasons *not* to drink. Myths and facts about alcohol are presented, as are strategies for coping with pressure to drink. The chapter also covers the three phases of alcoholism, its probable causes, and its most important risks. Treatment options for alcoholics are discussed.

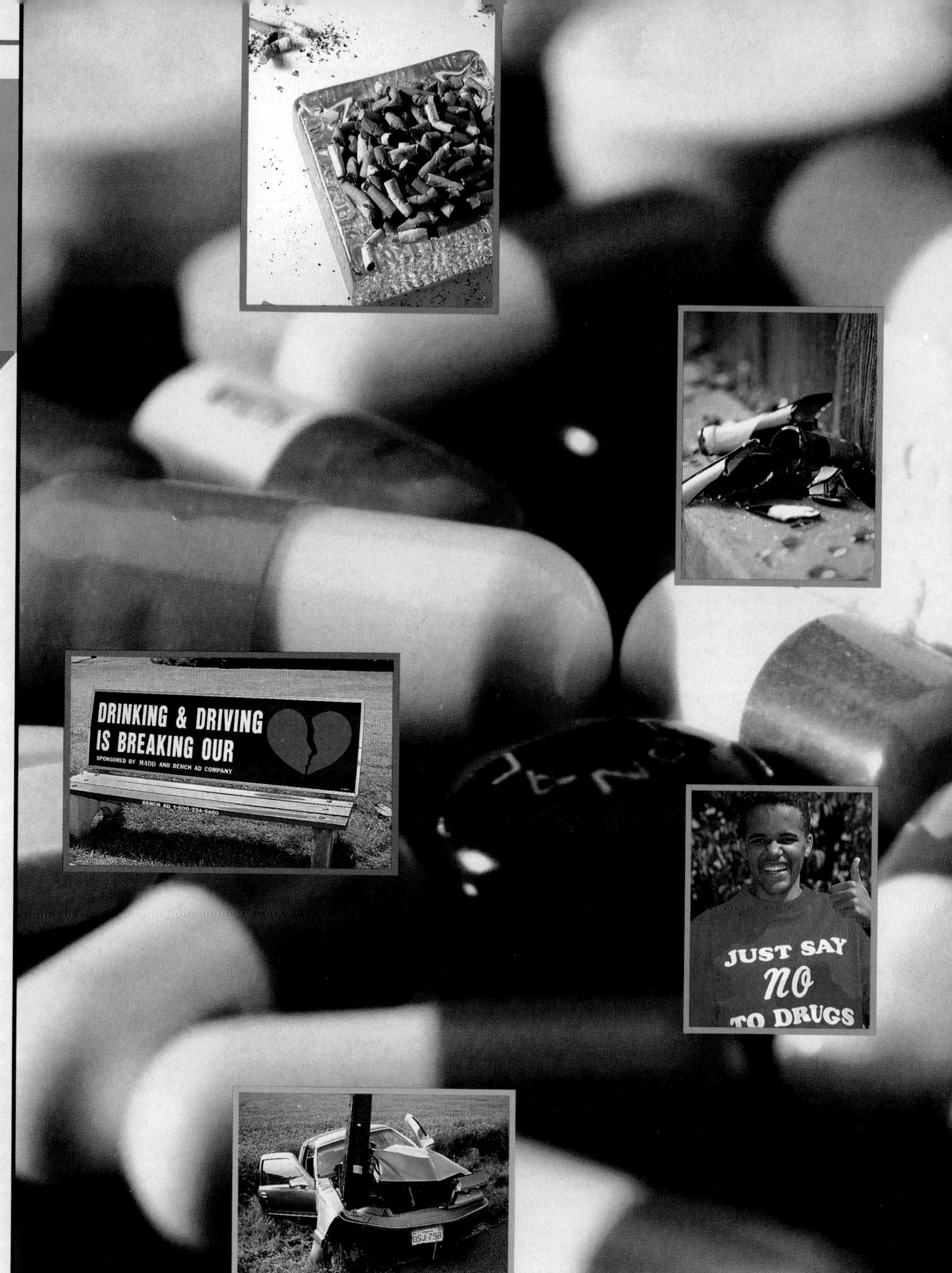

CHAPTER 14

TOBACCO: HAZARDOUS AND ADDICTIVE

Students learn about the chemicals in tobacco and study the effects of the three most poisonous chemicals in tobacco smoke. The prevalent smoking-related diseases, plus the risks of passive smoking and using pipes, cigars, and smokeless tobacco are discussed. An explanation of why people may begin smoking and reasons *not* to smoke are given. The chapter ends with suggested strategies for quitting smoking.

CHAPTER 15

OTHER DRUGS OF ABUSE

The dangers of drug abuse and ways it can damage society are discussed, followed by a thorough presentation of the psychoactive drugs of abuse, and their dangers and effects. Students learn that people should not try to overcome drug dependency on their own and that there is no such thing as a fully recovered addict. Options for recovering addicts and alternatives for those who consider abusing drugs are suggested.

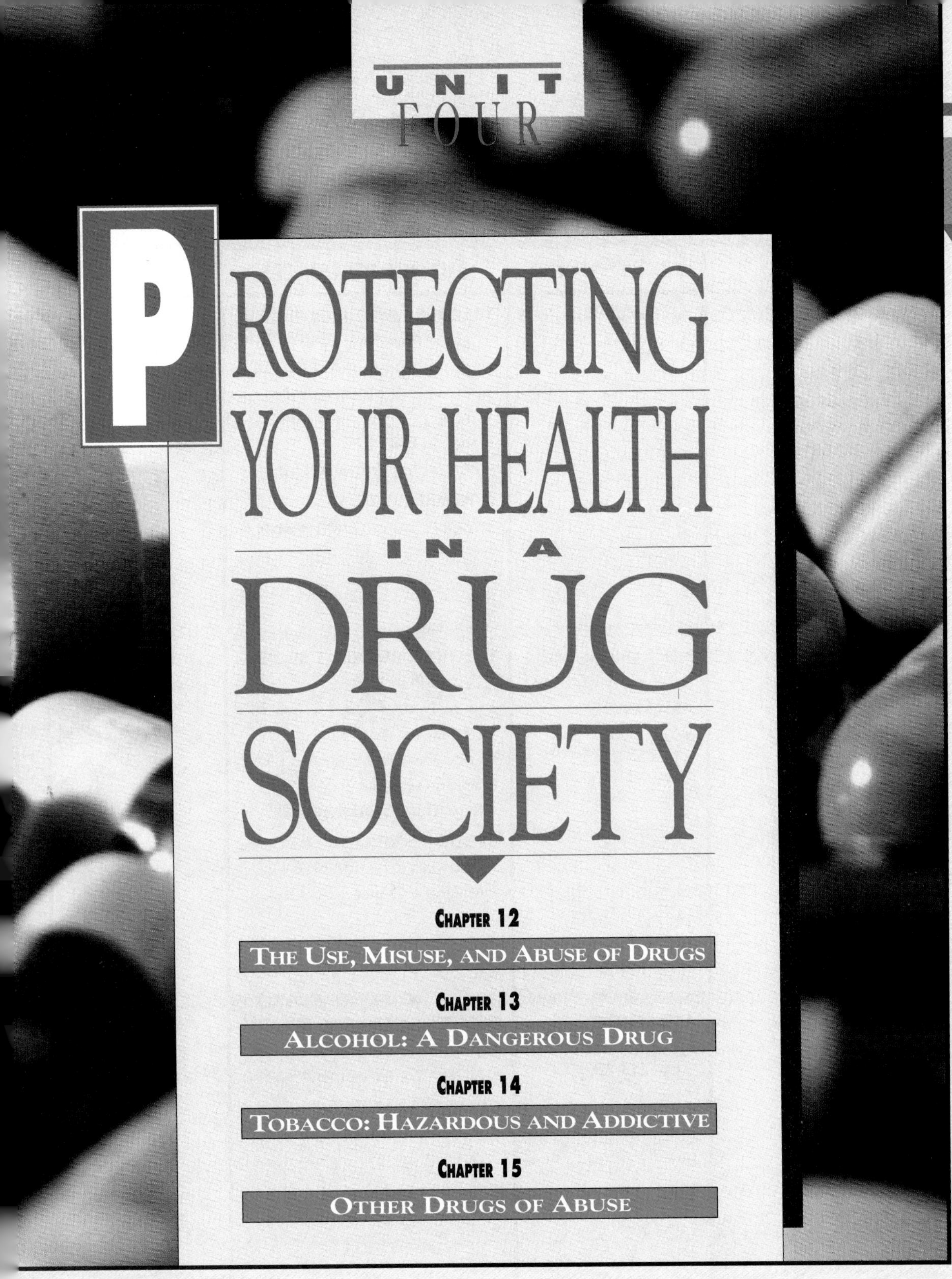

UNIT FOUR

PROTECTING YOUR HEALTH IN A DRUG SOCIETY

UNIT PREVIEW

This unit addresses the use of drugs—one of the most important health issues in our society. It provides students with the understanding of drug abuse they need to make responsible decisions. The reasons people use prescription drugs, over-the-counter drugs, alcohol, tobacco, and illegal drugs are explained and reasons *not* to use them given. Armed with the facts about the drugs, their dangers, and their effects, students are more likely to seek alternatives for dealing with their problems. The unit suggests these alternatives and offers suggestions for dealing with the pressure to use drugs. The five major health themes are emphasized throughout the unit, as indicated in the chart below.

THEMES TRACE

	WELLNESS	BUILDING SELF-ESTEEM	DECISION MAKING	DEVELOPING LIFE-MANAGEMENT SKILLS	ACCEPTANCE OF DIVERSITY AMONG PEOPLE
Chapter 12				pp. 252, 254	p. 246
Chapter 13		p. 272	p. 271	pp. 268, 272, 279–280	
Chapter 14	p. 294		pp. 292–294	p. 290	
Chapter 15		pp. 299–300	pp. 299–300	pp. 299, 311	

CHAPTER 12

THE USE, MISUSE, AND ABUSE OF DRUGS

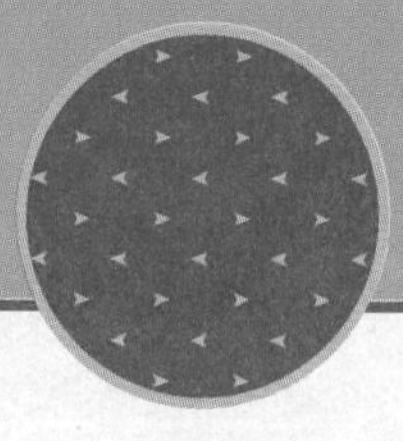

PLANNING GUIDE

TEXT SECTIONS	OBJECTIVES	TEXT FEATURES	OUTSIDE RESOURCES	NOTES
12.1 A Drug-Oriented Society pp. 245-249 1 period	• Name one problem with living in a drug-oriented society. • Name two ways to treat pain without using drugs. • Know the ways in which drug use, drug misuse, and drug abuse differ from each other.	**ASSESSMENT** • Section Review, p. 249	**TEACHER'S RESOURCE BINDER** • Lesson Plan 12.1 • Journal Entries 12A, 12B, 12C • Personal Health Inventory • Section Review Worksheet 12.1 • Section Quiz 12.1 • Reteaching Worksheet 12.1 **OTHER RESOURCES** • English/Spanish Audiocassette 4	
12.2 Over-the-Counter and Prescription Medicines pp. 250-256 1 period	• Describe three types of OTC medicines. • Know why prescription medications require a doctor's prescription. • Name three factors that may influence a medicine's effect. ■ Know how to read the label on a prescription medicine.	• LIFE SKILLS: Practicing Self-Care, p. 254 **ASSESSMENT** • Section Review, p. 256	**TEACHER'S RESOURCE BINDER** • Lesson Plan 12.2 • Journal Entries 12D, 12E, 12F, 12G • Life Skills 12A • Section Review Worksheet 12.2 • Section Quiz 12.2 • Reteaching Worksheet 12.2 **OTHER RESOURCES** • Transparencies 12A, 12B • Making a Choice 12A, 12B	
End of Chapter pp. 257-259		**ASSESSMENT** • Chapter Review, pp. 258-259	**TEACHER'S RESOURCE BINDER** • Chapter Test • Alternative Assessment **OTHER RESOURCES** • Test Generator	

■ Denotes LIFE SKILLS objectives

• Items in blue are also part of the *Holt Health Activity Book.*

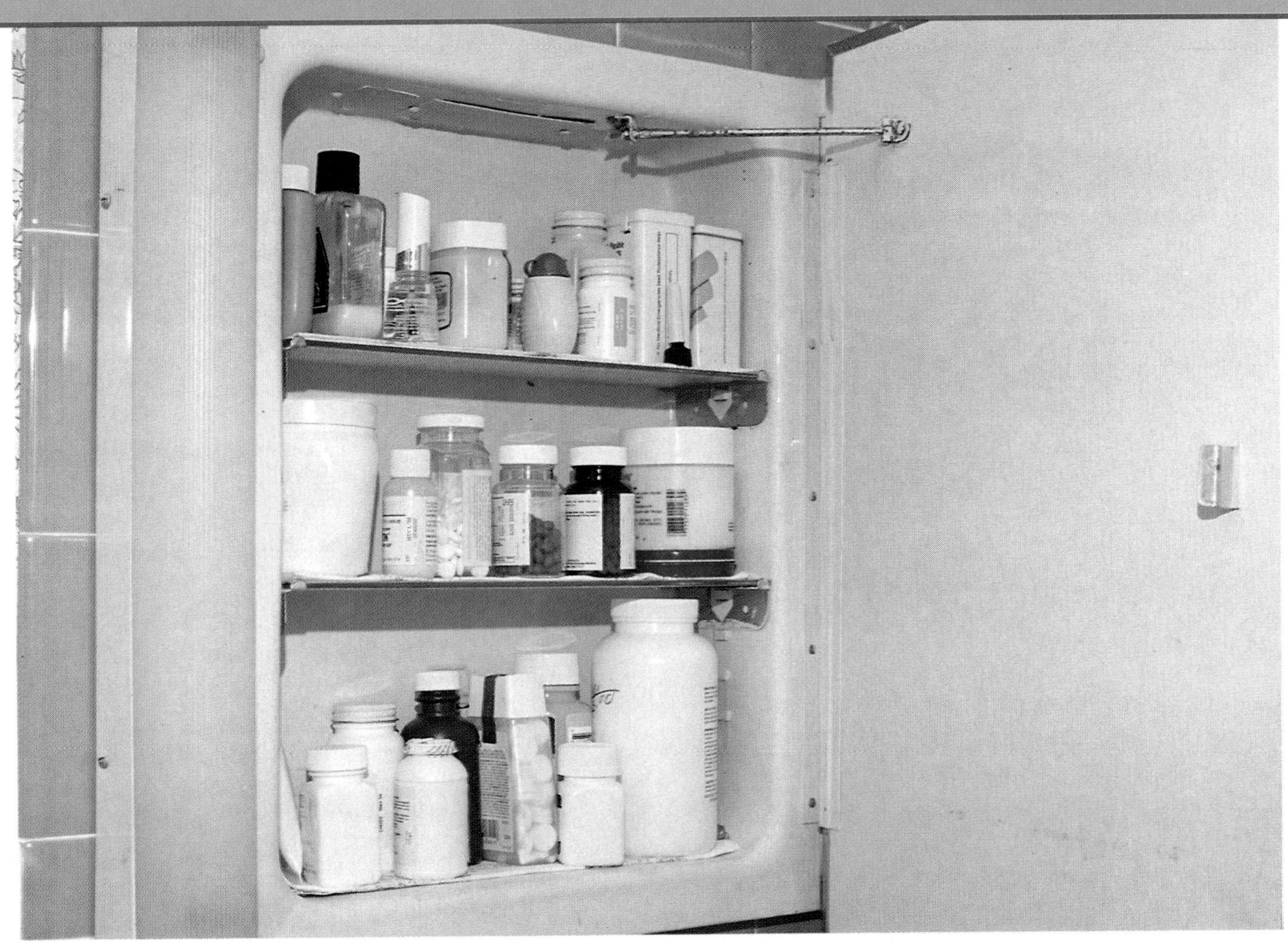

CONTENT BACKGROUND Dangers of Over-the-Counter Drugs

TREATING THE SYMPTOMS OF AILMENTS without looking for their root causes can lead to damaging consequences. The casual use of pills to stay awake and to lose weight is apparently an option for a certain number of teens. During the past month more than 4 percent of tenth graders have used nonprescription stay awake pills at least once. In the same group 1.3 percent of the males and 3.8 percent of the females have used nonprescription diet pills.

What motivates an individual to use chemicals of any type? There are three general motivators: (1) the need to escape pain or discomfort, (2) the need for a high, and (3) hereditary biochemical need activated by gateway drugs.

The most common motivator—encouraged by a tremendous volume of over-the-counter and prescription products—is the need or desire to escape pain or discomfort. The medications designed to meet this need are often used unnecessarily and unwisely.

Colds and allergies are common and make people uncomfortable. Therefore a large market exists for antihistamines and decongestants. Yet the wide availability and use of antihistamines, for instance, present a danger because the buyer may assume that any item sold at a grocery store must not be dangerous. On the contrary, antihistamines can be dangerous.

Triprolidine is an antihistamine used in many allergy medications. The effect of this ingredient on the motor coordination while driving is equivalent to a blood alcohol concentration of 0.05 percent—approximately the same effect as a couple of

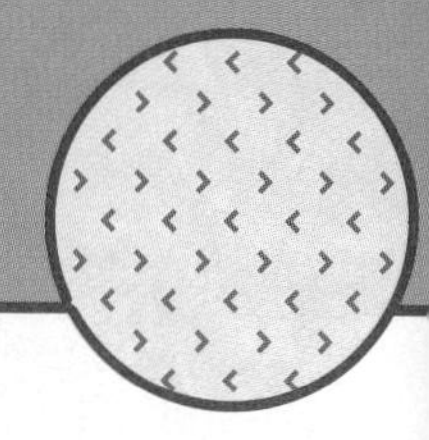

drinks. Diphenhydramine, another sedating ingredient in antihistamines, in a dose of 50 mg will slow driving simulator reaction time the same way a blood alcohol content of 0.1 percent will. Furthermore, driving impairment is evident even after the user no longer feels drowsy. According to a recent Gallup survey, "61% of those who take allergy medications that warn against driving say they ignore the warning and drive anyway." Compounding the problem of common antihistamine use is what happens when antihistamines and alcohol combine.

Given a choice, seeing a physician, purchasing a prescription medication, or buying a medication off the shelf, most individuals choose what seems to them the obvious solution: treat yourself.

As common as the cold is the headache that accompanies cold, flu, or stress. One solution to head pain is to take an over-the-counter analgesic. The most common are aspirin, acetaminophen, and ibuprofen. Some cold medications contain an analgesic, a decongestant, and an antihistamine. If a person takes an analgesic in combination with a cold medication, it is possible to get too much of the analgesic. An overdose of aspirin causes an acid-base imbalance in the body; acetaminophen overdose causes liver damage; and ibuprofen overdose causes gastric problems. Aspirin and the salicylate family in combination with certain viral conditions (notably chickenpox and flu) leads to Reye's syndrome, a life-threatening condition. Reye's syndrome presents itself at the tail end of the original illness. Its symptoms include severe tiredness, violent headache, disorientation, belligerence, and excessive vomiting. The bismuth subsalicylates in certain anti-diarrhea products can start Reye's syndrome in teens and children with flu or chickenpox symptoms.

Over-the-counter medications can also be dangerous to people with high blood pressure, glaucoma, diabetes, or kidney disease. Cough syrups can impair diabetic control because of their sugar and alcohol content. Decongestant nasal sprays, when used for more than a few days at a time, can create a withdrawal symptom that mimics the congestion the spray was designed to remedy. And some antacids should not be used in conjunction with tetracycline because the antibiotic cannot be absorbed properly.

Apparently innocent combinations of safe over-the-counter medications can lead to automobile accidents, liver damage, and even death. Clearly, use of chemicals is not the best way to handle the physical impairments encountered in daily life. Sometimes over-the-counter medication may be needed by a person who absolutely must function for a short time. After that it is best to let common, relatively minor complaints take their own course.

PLANNING FOR INSTRUCTION

KEY FACTS

- **Because we live in a drug-oriented society, people often think that drugs can solve all their problems.**
- **A drug is a substance that causes a physical or emotional change in a person.**
- **OTC drugs can be bought legally without a physician's prescription. Prescription drugs can only be purchased with a written order by a physician.**
- **Taking legal drugs properly in their correct amounts is drug use. Drug misuse is the improper use of drugs, such as taking the wrong amount, stopping its use too soon, or taking medicine prescribed for someone else. Drug abuse occurs when someone takes a legal drug for a nonmedical reason or an illegal drug for any reason at all.**
- **Medicines do at least one of four things: fight bacteria and other disease-causing organisms, protect the body from disease, influence the circulatory system, and affect the nervous system.**
- **The three most common kinds of OTCs are analgesics, which relieve pain; sedatives, which help a person sleep; and stimulants, which make a user more alert.**

- **Drugs can cover up a symptom without curing a disease.**
- **The right dosage of a drug varies according to the person's age, height, weight, and gender.**

MYTHS AND MISCONCEPTIONS

MYTH: Even though two drugs were prescribed by different physicians, it's okay to take them at the same time.

It can often be dangerous to take two drugs at the same time. If a physician did not know that a patient was taking a drug prescribed by another physician, he or she might prescribe a drug that could interact with the first drug and cause serious effects.

MYTH: You don't have to read all the literature that accompanies a prescription.

The literature that accompanies some drugs provides very important information about the effects of the drug.

MYTH: If you have the same symptoms as someone else, it's all right to finish his or her prescription medicine.

It is never safe to take another person's prescription drug, because the prescription was tailored to the other person's needs.

VOCABULARY

Essential: The following terms appear in boldface type.

drug	**psychoactive effect**
effect	**analgesic**
prescription	**sedative**
drug use	**stimulant**
addiction	**dose**
medicine	**side effect**
drug misuse	**drug allergy**
drug abuse	

Secondary: Be aware that the following terms may come up during class discussion.

antacid	drug interaction
antibiotic	inhalants
antihistamine	strep throat
appetite suppressant	throat culture
barbiturates	tranquilizer

FOR STUDENTS WITH SPECIAL NEEDS

Less-Advanced Students: Have students create a mobile, poster, or other visual display in which the chapter's vocabulary is highlighted. They could write each of the terms on one side of a card or a cutout shaped like a pill or bottle, and the definition on the other side.

LEP Students: Have students for whom English is a second language look to see if prescription and over-the-counter medications in their home have directions in their native language. If not, have students ask pharmacists near their home if directions in their native language are available for most drugs. Have them prepare a list of precautions they have learned about in class that may help their family.

ENRICHMENT

- Have students write a report on the warnings that should accompany medications. They may want to interview family members, adults, and other teenagers about the drugs they take as medicine. Have them ask family members whether they have been warned that certain foods should not be in the stomach when their medication is taken. They may also want to ask if their relatives were warned of the danger of taking two different medications at one time. If students do research before writing their report, one reference book is *Drugs and the Human Body: With Implications for Society—3rd ed.,* by Ken Liska.
- Have students debate whether it is fair that antibiotics are issued only by prescription in the United States, while they may be purchased over the counter in certain other countries.

CHAPTER 12

CHAPTER OPENER

GETTING STARTED

Using the Chapter Photograph

Ask students when they might take any of the OTC preparations in the photograph. Discuss whether or not they think people can overdo using these drugs. Ask them if they know of other ways to get rid of a headache without taking medication. Mention that the chapter will discuss the use, misuse, and abuse of drugs. Ask students how they might explain the differences in the meanings of these three terms.

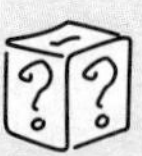

Question Box

Have students write out any questions they have about the use, misuse, and abuse of drugs and put them in the Question Box. The Question Box provides students with an opportunity to ask questions anonymously. To ensure that students with questions are not embarrassed to be seen writing, have students who do not have questions write something else—such as something they already know about drugs—on the paper instead.

Preview the questions and then answer them at appropriate points in the chapter. You may wish to allow students to write additional anonymous questions as they go through the chapter.

Personal Issues *ALERT*

The discussion of drug use may make students uncomfortable for several reasons. Students who have to take prescribed medicine may feel that others will think they are doing something wrong. Be sure to mention that drugs save the lives of many people. Other students may have someone close to them who abuses drugs or alcohol. Care must be taken to avoid any references that may bother these students.

CHAPTER 12

The Use, Misuse, and Abuse of Drugs

◆ ◆ ◆ ◆

Section 12.1 *A Drug-Oriented Society*

Section 12.2 *Over-the-Counter and Prescription Drugs*

Our society depends on drugs to cure every ache and pain.

Everything had gone wrong for Marisa today. The math test was a complete disaster. She had left her health assignment at home. Worst of all, she had a big fight with her best friend. By the time Marisa got home she was crying, and she had a terrible headache.

Without thinking about it, she went to her mother's medicine chest to find a pain reliever for her headache. As she swallowed the pills, Marisa looked at her puffy face in the bathroom mirror. She wished she could take a drug that would make her forget about her bad day.

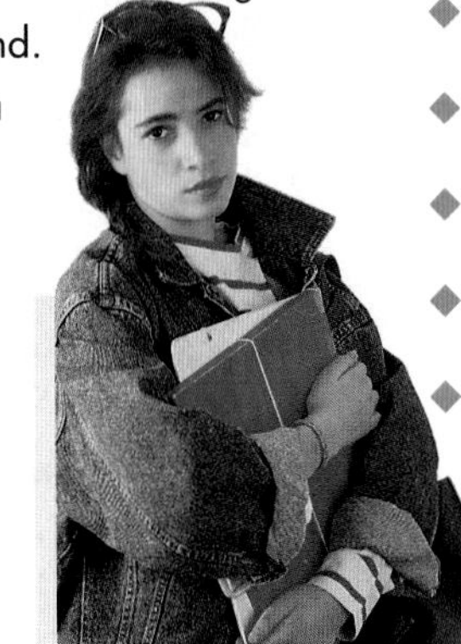

Section 12.1 A Drug-Oriented Society

Objectives

- *Name one problem with living in a drug-oriented society.*
- *Name two ways to treat pain without using drugs.*
- *Know the ways in which drug use, drug misuse, and drug abuse differ from each other.*

We live in a drug-oriented society. The commercials we see on television make this clear. Have a headache? Take a painkiller. Is your stomach acting up? No problem—get some antacids. Feeling tired? Grab a cup of coffee. Want to relax? Have a beer. One reason our society has become so dependent on drugs is that we are constantly hearing about how great they are.

Every year, pharmaceutical companies spend about $25 billion on advertising. The alcohol industry spends an additional $18 billion to $20 billion. As a result, it is hard to find a magazine or a television program that doesn't feature at least one drug advertisement. In addition, many sports events are sponsored by beer manufacturers.

The message we receive from all the advertising is clear: If we take a drug, we'll feel better.

What is so bad about this message? After all, some drugs can save lives. Before the development of effective medicines, there was little relief for severe pain, and even minor infections could become deadly. Today, drugs can prevent, treat, or cure most illnesses. The problem is that many people think drugs can solve *all* their problems.

Healthier Options

Marisa's headache resulted from her stressful day at school. When she got home, she could have done some physical exercise that would have relaxed her, or she could have performed one of the relaxation exercises

Background
Variable Drug Effects

Some substances act like drugs in some people yet have no effect whatsoever on other people. Monosodium glutamate (MSG) is a flavor enhancer used in many foods. Most people have no problems after eating foods with MSG. However, others experience heart palpitations and nausea. Nutmeg, a common kitchen spice, causes distortions of time and space in some people; however, most people do not experience these effects.

Section 12.1 Lesson Plan

MOTIVATE

Journal 12A
Headaches and Stress

This may be done as a warm-up activity. Encourage students to write down their reactions to Marisa's response to the events of the day. Have them include how they would probably respond to the same kinds of problems.

Cooperative Learning
Marisa's Response

Have students form small groups to discuss why Marisa's first response was to take a pill to relieve her headache. Have them consider what influences people to take a pill or a capsule whenever they have the slightest pain.

TEACH

Class Discussion
A Pill for Every Problem

Discuss with students the emphasis in society on taking drugs for almost every possible ailment. **What do you think "a drug-oriented society" means?** *[A society in which taking a drug is the solution for every problem, including slight pains, stress, and just being tired]* **Why was Marisa wrong to**

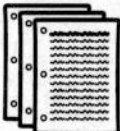

Personal Health Inventory

Have students complete the Personal Health Inventory for this chapter. The inventory helps them assess their own behavior with respect to misusing drugs.

described in Chapter 9. Chances are, either of these would have made her head feel better.

Next time you have a headache or stomachache, ask yourself if the pain you are feeling has something to do with stress. If it does, see if physical exercise or a relaxation exercise makes you feel better, or just try talking to someone about your anxiety. You may find that the pain goes away without the use of a drug.

If you're feeling depressed or anxious about something, know that drinking alcohol or taking a drug will not solve your problem. The effects of these drugs last for a short period of time, and when they wear off, you might feel worse than you did before. Instead, you might try to find someone you can talk to. A parent, a friend, or a teacher may be able to offer some support.

drug: *a substance that causes a physical or emotional change in a person.*

What Is a Drug?

A **drug** is any substance that causes a physical or emotional change in a person. All drugs can be placed into one of the following seven categories: herbal drugs, over-the-counter drugs, prescription drugs, tobacco products, alcohol, illegal drugs, and unrecognized drugs.

Cultural DIVERSITY

Medicines From the Rain Forest

People in so-called developing cultures are helping in the development of powerful new medicines. These cultures, which have existed for thousands of years in the tropical rain forests of the world, have already contributed a tremendous amount to the contents of our medicine cabinets. Tropical rain forests, shown in green on the map, are areas along the equator that have great amounts of rainfall and a huge number of different living things.

Quinine is an excellent example of a medicine that came to us from the rain forest. Made from the bark of the *Cinchona* tree in the Andean tropical forest of South America, quinine was long used as a medicine by the native people. Only later did people in more "advanced" societies discover that quinine cured malaria, an often fatal disease transmitted by mosquitoes.

Rain forest cultures introduced us to another important drug called curare. In the South American rain forest, native people extracted curare from woody vines and dipped their arrows into it to paralyze the animals they shot. In our society, curare serves not as a poison but as a muscle relaxant that is used during surgery.

Finally, fully 70 percent of the plants known to be useful in the treatment of cancer come from rain forests. We know about most of these cancer-fighting plants from the native people who live where the plants grow.

• • • TEACH continued

think that problems can be solved by taking a pill? *[Pills may just be an escape that keep her from facing her real problem.]* **What are the dangers in taking a pill whenever you want to feel better?** *[A person who takes a pill for every problem does not develop strength and problem-solving techniques to face the bigger trials that may present themselves later on.]* **What are some actions you can take when you are upset by the way things are in your life?** *[Students may discuss ideas mentioned in the book, or they may add their own suggestions.]*

Journal 12B
Ways to Cope

Have students write in the Student Journal in the Student Activity Book any of the ideas given in the class discussion that they think may help them personally to overcome anger, stress, or sadness. Ask them to include examples of the occasions when the ideas may work for them.

Role-Playing
Positive Alternatives to Drugs

Have students role-play a situation in which a teenager is upset after not making the team or after having an argument at home or with a friend. One student takes a pill to relieve the bad feeling. Another student uses a more positive approach.

Herbal Drugs Herbal drugs, such as herbal teas, can be classified as drugs because they have an **effect**, though mild, on the body. Because they are so mild, herbal drugs are not controlled by law.

Over-the-Counter Drugs Over-the-counter (OTC) drugs can be legally bought without a doctor's prescription. Two examples of OTC preparations are aspirin and cough medicines.

Prescription Drugs Prescription drugs are drugs that require a doctor's prescription to buy. A **prescription** is a doctor's written order to a pharmacist that a patient be allowed to purchase a drug. A prescription includes the drug's name, directions for use, and amount of the drug to be used. Prescription drugs are usually more powerful than over-the-counter drugs.

Tobacco Products Tobacco products contain the drug nicotine. Examples of tobacco products are cigarettes, cigars, snuff, and chewing tobacco.

Alcohol Beer, wine, and distilled liquors all contain the drug alcohol.

Illegal Drugs Illegal drugs are substances that cannot be legally sold, purchased,

effect:

the influence a drug has on the body, the mind, or both.

prescription:

a doctor's written order for a specific medicine.

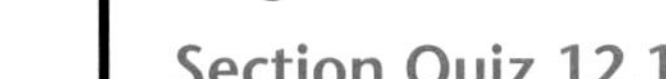

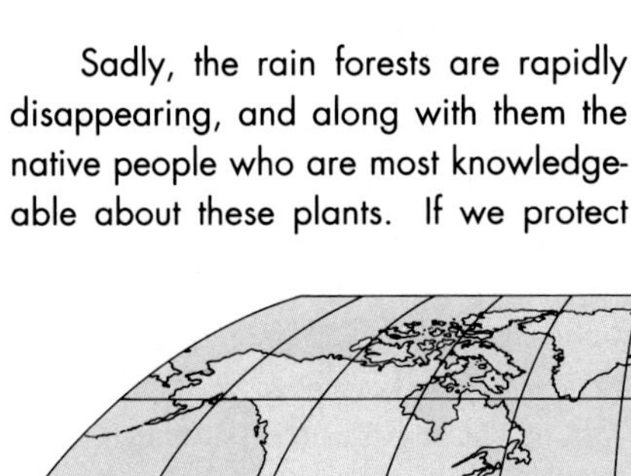

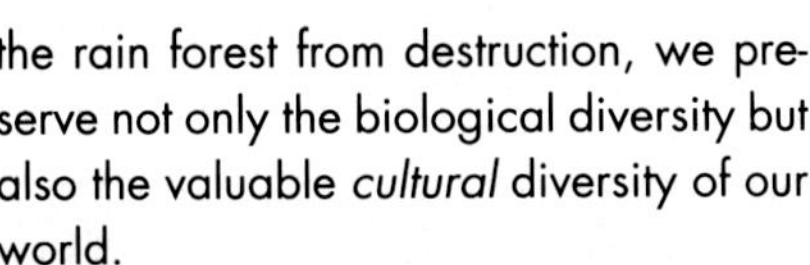

Sadly, the rain forests are rapidly disappearing, and along with them the native people who are most knowledgeable about these plants. If we protect the rain forest from destruction, we preserve not only the biological diversity but also the valuable *cultural* diversity of our world.

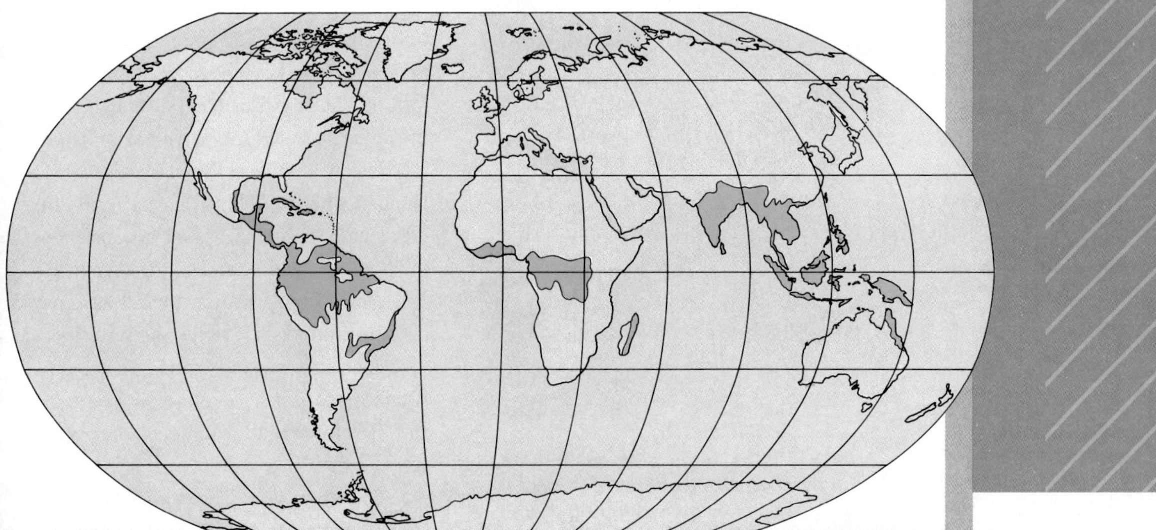

Section 12.1

Section Review Worksheet 12.1

Assign Section Review Worksheet 12.1, which requires students to suggest means other than taking drugs for solving problems and to identify characteristics of drug use, drug misuse, and drug abuse.

Section Quiz 12.1

Have students take Section Quiz 12.1.

Reteaching Worksheet 12.1

Students who have difficulty with the material may complete Reteaching Worksheet 12.1, which requires them to recognize characteristics of drug use, misuse, and abuse.

Reinforcement

Caution in Using Drugs

After students read about the seven categories of drugs, mention that all drugs, even those prescribed by a physician, should be used only according to the directions. Discuss why even OTC drugs have to be used with discretion.

Role-Playing

Drug Use, Misuse, and Abuse

Have students make up skits that show examples of drug use, drug misuse, and drug abuse. The class should judge which category is being presented by the skit. Caution them to make a distinction between misuse and abuse, so that both categories are not included in the same skit.

Game

Drug Use, Misuse, and Abuse

Have cards prepared with examples of drug use, misuse, and abuse or ask students to prepare cards. Have a student read a card and identify the example given as use, misuse, or abuse of a drug. You may also ask them to explain why the example does not belong to one of the other categories.

Background
Caffeine

Besides being present in coffee, caffeine is a drug that is present in many medications, such as tablets for cold symptoms and migraine headaches. All cola drinks, except those that are decaffeinated, also have caffeine. Even a slice of chocolate cake has a very small amount of this drug. Caffeine is a powerful stimulant of the central nervous system. In very high doses, caffeine stimulates the brain so much that it can cause convulsions and even death.

drug misuse: *improper use of a drug.*

drug use: *taking a medicine properly and in its correct dosage.*

drug abuse: *intentional improper use of a drug.*

psychoactive effect: *an effect on a person's mood or behavior.*

addiction: *a condition in which the body relies on a given drug to help it function.*

or used. Powder cocaine, marijuana, crack cocaine, and heroin are all examples of illegal drugs.

Unrecognized Drugs Unrecognized drugs are found in products that are not usually classified as drugs. One example of an unrecognized drug is caffeine. Caffeine is an ingredient in coffee and colas.

Inhalants are another kind of unrecognized drug. Certain substances, when inhaled, cause a lightheaded feeling. Examples of inhalants are gasoline, spray paint, and correction fluid for paper. As you will learn in Chapter 15, inhalants are extremely dangerous.

Drug Use, Misuse, and Abuse

Taking drugs properly and in their correct amounts is called **drug use.** Let's say you wake up one morning with a sore throat and a high fever. You go to the doctor, who takes a throat culture and tells you that you have strep throat. The doctor gives you a prescription for antibiotics, which fight the bacteria that cause strep throat. When you take the antibiotics as the doctor directs, you are practicing proper drug use.

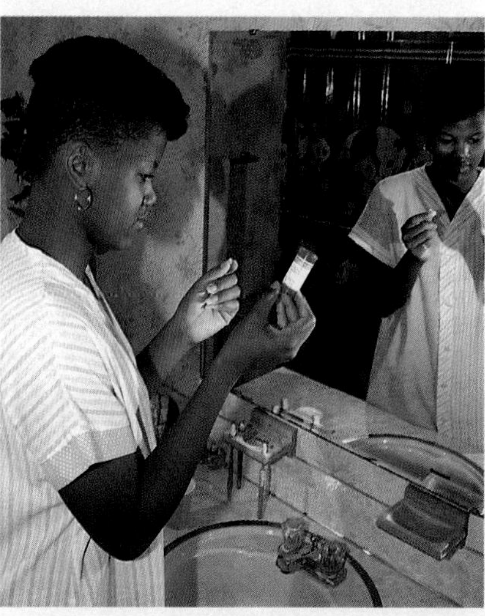

(FIGURE 12-1) **Some illnesses require medications for treatment. Using drugs correctly means taking them exactly as directed and in their proper doses.**

Drug misuse is the improper use of a drug. One way of misusing drugs is to take the wrong amount of a prescribed drug. If your doctor told you to take two tablets of a certain medicine each day, but you take *four,* you are misusing the drug. Taking too much of a medicine can lead to an overdose, which can be dangerous and even fatal.

Another way to misuse a drug is to stop taking it too soon. If the doctor told you to take two tablets a day until you finished the entire bottle, but you quit as soon as you felt better, you would be misusing the drug.

Taking medicine prescribed for someone else is another example of drug misuse. If you have a sore throat and take the medicine that is prescribed for your sister's sore throat, you are misusing a drug. Taking medicine prescribed for someone else can be very dangerous.

Drug abuse occurs when a person takes a legal drug for a nonmedical reason, or an illegal drug for any reason at all. A person who takes cough medicine to get high is abusing drugs, even though cough medicine is legal. A person who smokes marijuana is abusing drugs because marijuana is illegal. Other instances of drug abuse include smoking crack cocaine, sniffing powder cocaine, and taking heroin.

Many drugs that are abused have psychoactive effects. A **psychoactive effect** is an effect on a person's mood or behavior. Alcohol, caffeine, nicotine, tranquilizers, and heroin are all examples of psychoactive drugs.

The abuse of a drug can lead to **addiction.** When a person becomes addicted to a drug, it means that he or she has developed a

• • • TEACH continued

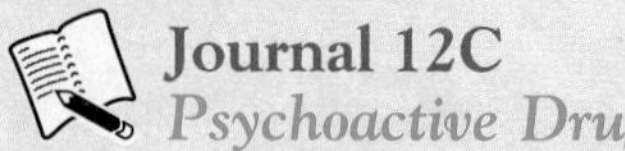

Journal 12C
Psychoactive Drugs

Have students write in the Student Journal their concerns about psychoactive drugs. Ask them to write their goals in life and how taking drugs could prevent them from reaching those goals.

Extension
Placebos

Interested students may wish to find out the effects of placebos on diseases. Have them find out why placebos can have a positive effect on disease.

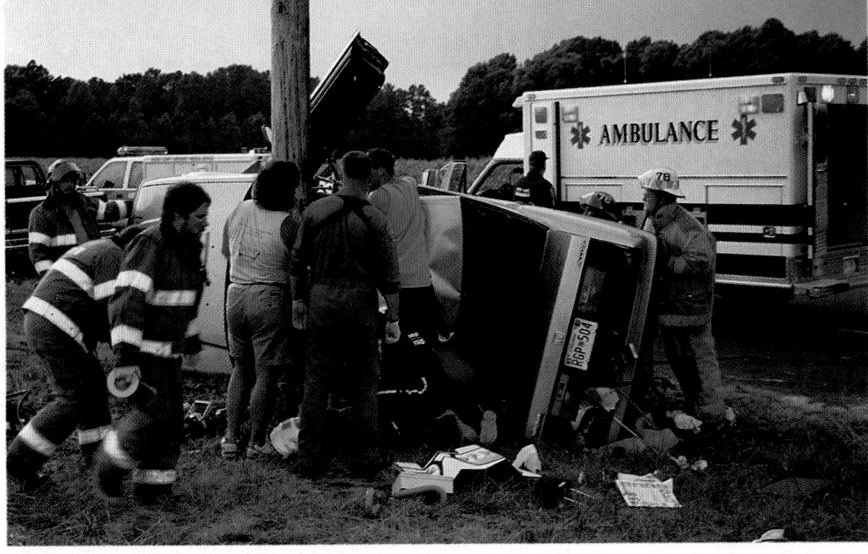

(FIGURE 12-2) **Abusing alcohol or other psychoactive drugs can be deadly.**

physical need for the drug and suffers withdrawal symptoms if unable to take the drug. Some common withdrawal symptoms are nausea, cramps, trembling, and nervousness. Drug abuse and addiction are discussed in more detail in Chapters 13, 14, and 15.

Psychoactive Drug Use and Risk Behaviors

One of the dangers of using psychoactive drugs is that they impair a person's ability to make good decisions. Someone who normally behaves responsibly might not be able to make the right decisions when under the influence of a psychoactive drug.

Joshua, for example, has decided to delay sexual intercourse until marriage. Usually he has little trouble sticking to his decision. But what if he gets drunk or high? Chances are, his decision will be harder to remember and harder to carry out. Not only would Joshua violate his own values if he had sexual intercourse, but he would also increase his risk of causing an unwanted pregnancy or getting a disease that is transmitted sexually. This can be especially dangerous today, when the risk of getting AIDS can make the wrong decision a life-threatening one.

In addition, studies have shown that the use of psychoactive drugs is strongly associated with an increased risk of serious injury and violence. What this can mean is that you have a much greater chance of getting hurt in an accident or getting into a fight if you are drunk or high.

Review

1. *What is one problem with living in a drug-oriented society?*
2. *What are two ways to treat pain without the use of drugs?*
3. *Define drug use, drug misuse, and drug abuse. How do they differ?*
4. ***Critical Thinking*** *Why might a person who has abused a drug be more likely to get AIDS than a person who has not?*

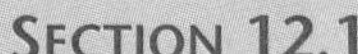
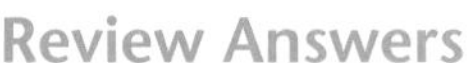

SECTION 12.1

Review Answers

1. Answers may include: people get the message that if they take a drug they will feel better, and some people think that drugs can solve any and all problems.

2. Answers will vary but may include physical exercise and relaxation exercises. If your pain is caused by stress, try talking to someone you can trust about your anxiety.

3. Drug use is taking drugs properly and in their correct amount. Drug misuse is the improper use of drugs, which may be unintentional. Drug abuse is using a legal drug for a nonmedical reason or an illegal drug for any reason at all and is almost always intentional.

4. When a person abuses a drug, the drug may impair that person's ability to make reasonable decisions. That person may be more likely to engage in sexual intercourse without any protection and thus expose himself or herself to HIV, which causes AIDS.

ASSESS

Section Review

Have students answer the Section Review questions.

Alternative Assessment

Drug Use, Misuse, or Abuse?

Have students explain in their own words how drug use, misuse, and abuse are different. They could make a chart to display the differences.

Closure

Perspective on Drug Use

Have students explain the effects of drugs on the quality of life, both positive and negative.

Background
Food and Medications

Certain foods can make a medication act more slowly, more quickly, or not at all. For example, the calcium in milk, cheese, and yogurt can interfere with absorption of the antibiotic tetracycline. Taking a drug with soda pop or fruit or vegetable juice may cause the drug to dissolve too quickly. Liver and green leafy vegetables keep drugs taken to prevent blood clotting from working. A chemical called tyramine found in aged cheese, sour cream, liver, bananas, and soy sauce can react with medication for high blood pressure and actually drive up the blood pressure. Because of reactions such as these, it is important to read the literature accompanying all drugs.

Section 12.2 Over-the-Counter and Prescription Drugs

Objectives

- *Describe three types of OTC medicines.*
- *Know why prescription medications require a doctor's prescription.*
- *Name three factors that may influence a medicine's effect.*
- *Know how to read the label on a prescription medicine.*
  LIFE SKILLS: Practicing Self-Care

stimulant: *a drug that speeds up body functioning.*

medicine: *a substance used to treat an illness or ailment.*

analgesic: *a medicine that relieves pain.*

sedative: *a drug that slows down body functioning and causes sleepiness.*

Over-the-counter and prescription drugs are two kinds of **medicines**. Most medicines do at least one of four things: they battle bacteria and other organisms that cause disease; they protect the body from disease; they influence the circulatory system; or they affect the nervous system. For more information on the different types of medicines, see Figure 12-3.

Over-the-Counter (OTC) Drugs

OTC drugs are medicines that you can buy without a doctor's prescription. Three of the most common types of OTC drugs are analgesics, sedatives, and stimulants.

Analgesics are used to relieve pain. Three types of analgesics are aspirin, acetaminophen, and ibuprofen.

Sedatives are drugs that slow down body functioning and make you sleepy. OTC preparations that have sedatives in them include mild sleeping pills and allergy medications that contain antihistamines.

Stimulants are the opposite of sedatives; they make you more alert. The type of stimulant that is most commonly used in OTC medicines is caffeine. OTC preparations that contain caffeine include some headache remedies, cold remedies, and appetite suppressants.

Most people think that OTC preparations are completely safe. Unfortunately, no drug is free of risk. Aspirin can lead to stomach irritation and bleeding, and it also may be associated with a serious disease called Reye's syndrome. A number of people who have taken aspirin for chickenpox or flu have suffered this illness, which is why doctors now recommend that you use acetaminophen to treat any symptoms of these infections. Salicylates, the ingredients in aspirin that are believed to be linked to Reye's syndrome, are also contained in some other OTC medications. Teenagers suffering from flu and chickenpox should take special care to read all OTC labels carefully and to avoid all preparations that contain salicylates.

In addition, some OTC medicines can be misused or abused. Antihistamines can cause drowsiness and dizziness, which is why a person who has taken them should not try to drive. Over-the-counter appetite suppressants, which contain caffeine and a stimulant drug called phenylpropanolamine (PPA), can cause high blood pressure and increased heart rate.

One final warning about OTC preparations: Remember that sometimes pain is a helpful symptom of infection. By covering up a symptom with an OTC preparation instead of treating its cause, you may be making your infection worse than it already is.

Section 12.2 Lesson Plan

MOTIVATE

Journal 12D
Uses of Medications

This may be done as a warm-up activity. Encourage students to list in the Student Journal the OTC drugs and prescription drugs they are familiar with. Tell them to write what each drug is used for.

TEACH

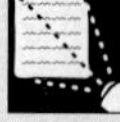

Teaching Transparency 12A
Drug Types and Effects

Use the table "Some Common Drug Types and Their Effects" (Figure 12-3) to help students classify drugs according to four types of action they cause.

Cooperative Learning
Drug Action Symposium

Divide the class into four groups, according to the four types of actions caused by drugs, as shown in Figure 12-3. Each group will discuss and study the drugs that deliver one type of action shown on the chart: (1) protects body from disease, (2) battles organisms that cause disease, (3) influences the circulatory system, (4) influences the nervous system. Have each group work together to understand the action of each type of drug, its effects, and

Some Common Drug Types and Their Effects

Type of Drug	Type of Action	Effect	How Available
Vaccines	*Protect body from disease*	*Cause body to set up agents to fight a specific disease before exposure*	*Doctor's office or clinic*
Antisera	*Protect body from disease*	*Stronger than vaccines; cause body to set up agents to fight a specific disease after exposure*	*Doctor's office or clinic*
Penicillin (antibiotic)	*Battles organisms that cause disease*	*Kills bacteria*	*Prescription*
Tetracycline (antibiotic)	*Battles organisms that cause disease*	*Slows down growth and reproduction of bacteria*	*Prescription*
Digitalis	*Influences circulatory system*	*Increases force of heart contractions, corrects irregular heartbeat*	*Prescription*
Diuretics	*Influence circulatory system*	*Relieve body of excess water and salt*	*OTC or Prescription*
Vasodilators	*Influence circulatory system*	*Enlarge veins and arteries to increase flow of blood*	*Prescription*
Antiarrhythmics	*Influence circulatory system*	*Work to correct irregular heartbeat*	*Prescription*
Hypertensives	*Influence circulatory system*	*Work to prevent high blood pressure*	*Prescription*
Analgesics (aspirin, acetami-nophen, ibuprofen)	*Influence nervous system*	*Relieve pain, lower fever, reduce joint swelling (note: aspirin and ibuprofen have this last effect: acetaminophen does not)*	*OTC or, in some cases, prescription*
Stimulants	*Influence nervous system*	*Prevent sleep, heighten awareness*	*OTC or, in some cases, prescription*
Barbiturates	*Influence nervous system*	*Relieve anxiety, insomnia, prevent certain types of seizures*	*Prescription*
Tranquilizers	*Influence nervous system*	*Relieve anxiety, insomnia; milder than barbiturates*	*Prescription*

(FIGURE 12-3) **Medicines can battle diseases and sometimes prevent them completely. Most OTC preparations, however, treat symptoms and do not fight infections.**

how it is available. Have them do this for each drug listed on the chart. Have groups report on their category.

Class Discussion
Drug Types and Effects

Refer to the table "Some Common Drug Types and Their Effects" and ask **How do vaccines differ from antisera?** *[Vaccines cause the body to create antibodies before exposure. Antisera cause the body to set up agents after exposure. Antisera are stronger than vaccines.]* **How do penicillin and tetracycline differ in their effects?** *[Penicillin kills bacteria; tetracycline slows down growth and reproduction of bacteria.]* **How do analgesics influence the nervous system?** *[They relieve pain, lower fever, reduce swelling.]*

Journal 12E
Nonprescription Medications

Have students write in the Student Journal which of the following OTC medicines they may have taken at some time: an analgesic, a sedative, and a stimulant. Have them include the reason for taking each medication.

Class Discussion
"Analgesics: Their Effects and Hazards"

After students have looked at the table "Analgesics: Their Effects and Hazards," ask **Which analgesic would you use if aspirin irritates your stomach?** *[Acetaminophen]* **Why should children**

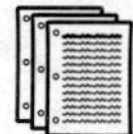

Life Skills Worksheet 12A

Being a Wise Consumer

Assign the Being a Wise Consumer Life Skills Worksheet, which requires students to compare the packaging and cost of a brand-name OTC drug and its generic version.

Making a Choice 12A

Using Drugs Safely

Assign the Using Drugs Safely card. The card requires students to generate and discuss reasons for following safety guidelines when using medicines

Making a Choice 12B

Reasons for Drug Use

Assign the Reasons for Drug Use card. The card asks students to look for explanations for the extensive use of drugs in our society.

Analgesics: Their Effects and Hazards

Analgesic	Effects	Potential Hazards
Aspirin	*Relieves pain, reduces fever, reduces swelling*	*Causes stomach irritation and bleeding, associated with Reye's syndrome in children and adolescents, can cause overdose.*
Acetaminophen	*Relieves pain, reduces fever*	*Risk of overdose, may cause liver damage in high doses.*
Ibuprofen	*Relieves pain, reduces fever, reduces swelling*	*Can cause stomach irritation and bleeding.*

(FIGURE 12-4) **Although analgesics are easily available, they are not without risk. If you must use these preparations, make sure that you take them according to their instructions and in their proper dose.**

Read the labels of all OTC preparations before you buy them. The labels should provide complete information about the correct amount to take and possible undesirable effects.

Prescription Drugs

Prescription drugs are usually more powerful than the medicines you can buy over the counter. For this reason, they cannot be purchased without a doctor's prescription.

dose: *the exact amount of a drug.*

A prescription always has a required **dose**—the correct amount of a drug to be taken at one time or at stated intervals. If you are using a prescribed medication, make sure you take the right dose each time. Be sure that you finish the entire dose, even if the signs and symptoms of your disease have completely disappeared. It is particularly important that you continue taking antibiotics for an infection as long as the doctor instructs. Even though you may start to feel better after a few days, the bacteria that caused the infection may not be completely eliminated. If you stop taking the antibiotics too soon, the remaining bacteria can cause the infection to return.

Finally, prescription drugs can be abused. Some drugs that are prescribed, such as barbiturates and tranquilizers, have very strong psychoactive effects. They can also be addictive, which is why it is very important to take drugs like these only if they are prescribed for you.

It is extremely important that you follow the instructions on the label of any prescription medication. Remember that they are prescribed for a particular person with a particular condition. The only person who should be taking the medicine is the person whose name appears on the label. Even if you and your friend think you have the same

• • • TEACH continued

and adolescents avoid using aspirin for chickenpox or flu? *[Some children and adolescents who have taken aspirin for these diseases developed Reye's syndrome.]* **What caution must be taken when using acetaminophen?** *[It may cause liver damage in high dosages.]*

Journal 12F

Taking Antibiotics

Have students write in the Student Journal the name of an antibiotic they have taken. Ask them to write down any special directions that they had to follow, such as taking the medication on an empty stomach or a certain number of hours before or after a meal. Have them explain why they think these precautions must be taken.

Class Discussion

Prescribed Medication

Ask: **Why do you think you need a prescription to purchase many of the drugs on the market?** *[Prescribed drugs are more potent than OTC drugs, and a physician needs to consider a patient's overall condition to determine whether a certain drug would have a harmful effect on him or her.]*

illness, don't take his or her prescription medication. It could be that you don't have the same illness or that you are allergic to the medication offered to you.

Effects of Drugs on the Body

When a drug enters the body, it is absorbed into the bloodstream. Once there, the drug travels to the parts of the body it will affect.

One factor that influences the effect of a drug is the dose that has been taken. The amount of drug that is right for a person will vary according to that person's age, height, weight, and gender, among other factors. In general, the heavier a person is, the higher a dose he or she will require. All medicines have recommended doses.

In addition, the way a drug is administered, or taken, has a very important impact on its effect. Medicines are usually either swallowed or injected. Injected medicines go directly to the bloodstream, which is why they have faster effects than medicines that are swallowed.

Guidelines for Appropriate Use of Medicines

Things You Should Remember About Use of Medicines
Don't mix medications without checking with a physician or pharmacist. When more than one drug is taken the results are often unpredictable.
Don't take a prescription medication unless it was prescribed for you. If you ever have an allergic reaction to a drug or food, make sure you tell a physician before using the same or another medication.
Don't use over-the-counter drugs for long periods of time. You may be delaying diagnosis of a serious problem.
Don't ever conclude that if a little bit of a drug makes you feel good, that more will make you feel better. Never take more of a medication than you are directed to.
Don't use a medicine prescribed for someone else, even if you seem to have the same problem.
If you get a prescription from a physician for a medicine, always ask how long you should continue to take the medicine.
Keep all drugs away from children.

(FIGURE 12-5) **Keep in mind these basic safety rules for the proper use of medications. Medicines are anything but helpful when they are misused.**

SECTION 12.2

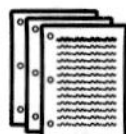

Section Review Worksheet 12.2

Assign Section Review Worksheet 12.2 which requires students to decide whether statements concerning OTC drugs, prescription drugs, and the effects of drugs are true or false and to correct any false statements.

Section Quiz 12.2

Have students take Section Quiz 12.2.

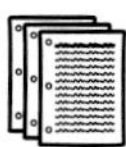

Reteaching Worksheet 12.2

Students who have difficulty with the material may complete Reteaching Worksheet 12.2, which requires students to complete a diagram and questions concerning the characteristics of OTC drugs.

Case Study
Misuse of a Medication

A patient was regularly using decongestant nose drops for a sinus condition, every half-hour. He became addicted to the medication and began to suffer from terrifying hallucinations at night. When he stopped using the nasal decongestant, the hallucinations stopped. He did, however, have to be treated for withdrawal symptoms. Emphasize that although medications are helpful, they can also harm someone unless they are used responsibly.

Debate the Issue
The Approval Process

Have students debate the question: Should the Food and Drug Administration approval process be speeded up for new drugs that might help AIDS patients?

Class Discussion
Drug Absorption

Ask: **Why do some prescriptions state that the patient should take a medication on an empty stomach?** *[If the medication enters the bloodstream through the stomach lining, food in the stomach can slow down the absorption process.]* **Why do injected medicines work faster?** *[Injected medicines go directly to the bloodstream.]*

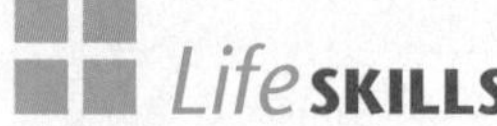

How to Read a Prescription Label

Have students review the Life Skills activity. Discuss what they can learn by reading a prescription label. Tell students to make up a prescription label for penicillin (ordered for themselves) with all the appropriate information.

When a medicine is taken orally—by mouth—it is often absorbed into the bloodstream through the stomach lining. This process can take a long time, especially if there is food in the stomach that can slow down the absorption process. The food can also protect the stomach lining from irritation, which is why doctors recommend that certain medicines should always be taken with a meal.

Drug Interactions Sometimes the effect of a medicine can be made either greater or smaller if there is already another drug in your system. This influence, called drug

LifeSKILLS: Practicing Self-Care

How to Read a Prescription Label . . .

All prescription drugs should have clearly marked labels. If you have a medication prescribed for you, make sure you read the label carefully before beginning your treatment. The prescription number is often at the very top of the label, and your name should be underneath. If your name is not on the label, do not take the medicine. One of the most dangerous things you can do is take a prescription drug that has been prescribed for someone else.

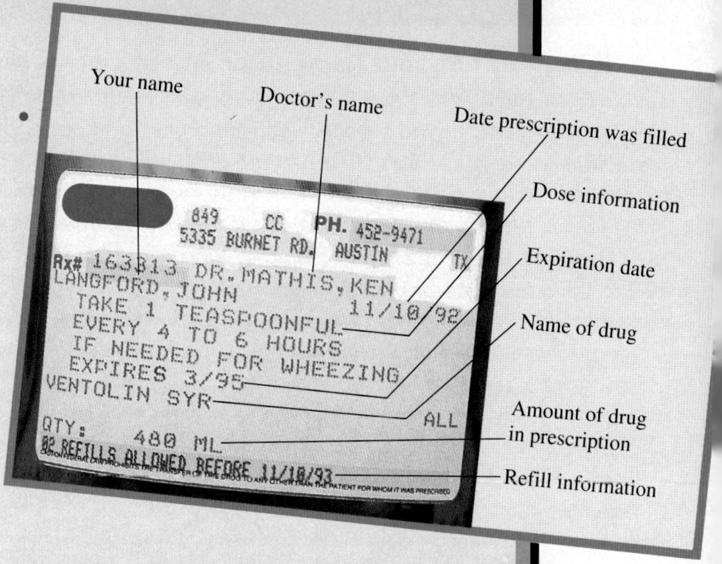

Your name
Doctor's name
Date prescription was filled
Dose information
Expiration date
Name of drug
Amount of drug in prescription
Refill information

849 CC PH. 452-9471
5335 BURNET RD. AUSTIN TX
Rx# 163313 DR. MATHIS, KEN
LANGFORD, JOHN 11/10/92
TAKE 1 TEASPOONFUL
EVERY 4 TO 6 HOURS
IF NEEDED FOR WHEEZING
EXPIRES 3/95
VENTOLIN SYR ALL
QTY: 480 ML
02 REFILLS ALLOWED BEFORE 11/10/93

Next to your name, your doctor's name should be listed, along with the date the prescription was filled. Underneath your name are directions explaining how often you should take the drug and how much you should take each time. This is followed by the drug's expiration date—the final date the drug can be safely used—and the name of the drug.

The bottom of the label should list the amount of the drug contained in the entire prescription dose, and should also provide instructions on how many times (if at all) the prescription can be refilled.

Not all labels will follow this exact order, but they all should contain this same information.

• • • TEACH continued

Reinforcement
Drug Administration

Have students recall the ways drugs enter the body by drawing the outline of a body and labeling the places where drugs enter the body.

Journal 12G
Drug Allergies

Ask students to write in the Student Journal if they are allergic to any drug and the symptoms of the allergy.

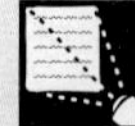

Teaching Transparency 12B
Information on Drug Labels

Use this transparency to make students aware of the important information contained on the labels of prescription and OTC drugs.

Extension
Information from Pharmacists

Suggest that students visit a pharmacy to find out what kinds of information a pharmacist gives with prescription drugs, beyond the literature provided by the pharmaceutical companies.

How drugs enter the body

1. Asthma medications, which are inhaled, directly affect the respiratory system.

2. Some medicines are placed under the tongue. These are absorbed into the bloodstream very quickly.

3. The medicines stored in transdermal patches are absorbed into the bloodstream through the skin.

4. Medicines that treat skin ailments such as cuts or burns can be applied topically, or directly onto the skin.

5. When medicines are swallowed, they are often absorbed into the bloodstream through the stomach.

6. Drugs can be injected either through a muscle or through a vein. Medicines that enter the body in this way have very strong effects, because they travel immediately to the bloodstream.

7. Some drugs that are swallowed enter the bloodstream through blood vessels that supply the intestine.

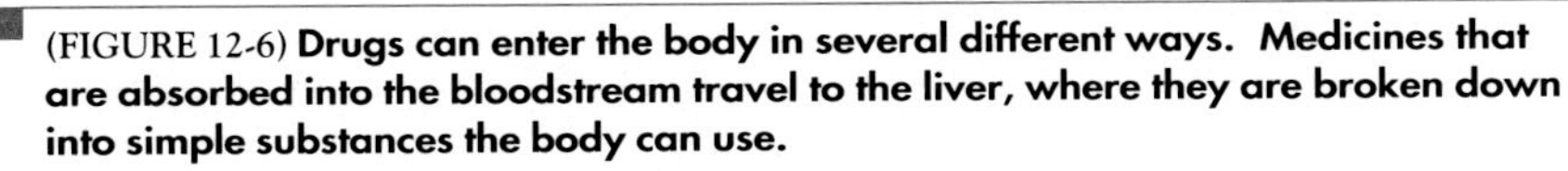

(FIGURE 12-6) **Drugs can enter the body in several different ways. Medicines that are absorbed into the bloodstream travel to the liver, where they are broken down into simple substances the body can use.**

Background

Dangerous Interactions

Emphasize that harmful reactions may occur when drugs interact. When a tranquilizer is taken with another brain depressant such as an antihistamine, analgesic, or alcohol, oversedation can occur. For example, the drug triazolam, sometimes taken for jet lag, can cause amnesia if combined with alcohol. Also, nicotine reduces the potency of some prescription medications. The drugs affected by nicotine range from painkillers such as Darvon, to tranquilizers such as Valium, to sleeping pills. Smokers need different doses and/or a different frequency of administration of these kinds of drugs.

Review Answers

1. Analgesics, sedatives, and stimulants

2. Prescription medicines have a required dosage and are usually more powerful than OTC medicines. Some prescription medicines can be abused because they have psychoactive effects and are addictive.

3. Dose, the way the drug is administered, and drug interactions

4. Answers may include your name; the name of the medicine prescribed; directions on how to take the medicine; the name of your physician; the date the medicine expires; how many times the prescription can be refilled; and the pharmacy's name, address, and phone number.

5. Answers may include the following: a person may be allergic to the drug; there may be a drug reaction if the person is already taking another drug; the drug may not be appropriate for the other person's illness or condition.

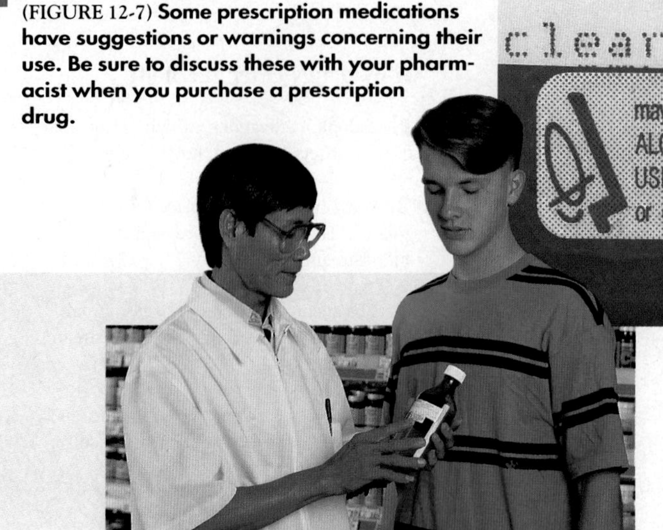

(FIGURE 12-7) **Some prescription medications have suggestions or warnings concerning their use. Be sure to discuss these with your pharmacist when you purchase a prescription drug.**

interaction, is very difficult to predict. A drug interaction can be dangerous. For example, combining a prescribed barbiturate with alcohol has been known to cause coma or death.

Avoiding a harmful drug interaction is another good reason to read all label information on any OTC or prescription medication you buy. If you have specific questions about how certain medicines interact, ask your doctor.

side effect: *an effect that accompanies the expected effect of a drug.*

drug allergy: *an unwanted effect that accompanies the desired effect of a drug.*

Side Effects and Allergies If you've ever taken a cold medicine that contains an antihistamine, you may have found that in addition to feeling your nasal passages clear, you felt a bit drowsy. The drowsiness you felt is called a **side effect**, because it is an effect that comes in addition to the drug's desired effect. Other common side effects of medicines include nausea, dizziness, and headaches.

A medicine can also have unpleasant effects when the person taking it has a **drug allergy**. Drug allergies occur when your body mistakes the medicine you have taken for a disease-causing agent, and tries to reject it.

Symptoms of drug allergies include a rash, a runny nose, and a quickened heart and breathing rate. If you think you may be allergic to a medicine, make sure you talk with your doctor before you take that medicine again. Allergies get worse each time they occur. If their early effects are ignored, they can eventually be fatal.

Review

1. *Name three types of OTC medicines.*
2. *Name two reasons why prescription medicines require a doctor's prescription.*
3. *What are three factors that can influence the effect of a medicine?*
4. **LIFE SKILLS: Practicing Self-Care** *What are three important things to look for on a prescription label?*
5. **Critical Thinking** *Using your knowledge of drug effects and how they are influenced, explain why it can be dangerous to use a prescription drug that has been prescribed for someone else.*

ASSESS

Section Review

Have students answer the Section Review questions.

Alternative Assessment

Medication Do's and Don'ts

Have students draw up a list of safeguards to be followed when taking either an OTC or prescription drug.

Closure

Have students briefly summarize the main points of the section. Ask them to explain how the information they learned will affect their future behavior.

Highlights

Summary

- We live in a drug oriented society.
- Physical exercise or a relaxation exercise can often relieve pain without drugs.
- Drugs can be classified as herbal drugs, over-the-counter drugs, prescription drugs, tobacco products, alcohol, illegal drugs, and unrecognized drugs.
- You can misuse a prescribed drug by taking the wrong dosage, by stopping it too soon, or by taking medicine prescribed for someone else.
- Drug abuse occurs when a person deliberately takes a legal drug for a nonmedical reason or an illegal drug for any reason.
- Psychoactive drugs such as alcohol, caffeine, nicotine, tranquilizers, and heroin impair a person's ability to make good decisions. The use of these drugs has been found to be associated with an increased risk of serious injury and violence.
- Three of the most common types of over-the-counter drugs are analgesics, sedatives, and stimulants. They should be taken according to the label directions.
- Drugs can sometimes cause side effects or allergies. Nausea, drowsiness, dizziness, and headaches are common side effects. Symptoms of drug allergies include a rash, a runny nose, and a quickened heart rate.

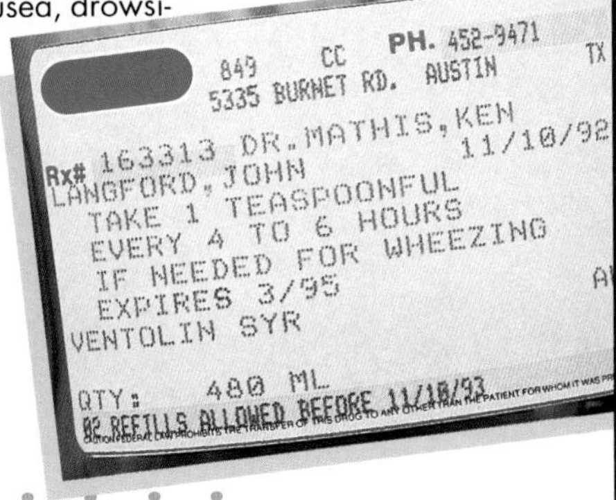

Vocabulary

drug a substance that causes a physical or emotional change in a person.

prescription a doctor's written order for a specific medicine.

drug use taking a medicine exactly as directed.

drug misuse unintentional improper use of a drug.

drug abuse intentional improper use of a drug.

psychoactive effect an effect on a person's mood or behavior.

addiction a condition in which the body relies on a given drug to function.

analgesic a medicine that relieves pain.

sedative a drug that slows down body functioning and causes sleepiness.

stimulant a drug that speeds up body functioning.

Chapter 12 Highlights Strategies

Summary

Have students read the summary to reinforce the concepts they learned in Chapter 12.

Vocabulary

Have students work in groups to make up skits in which they use the vocabulary terms and their definitions.

Extension

Have students examine magazines to find advertisements for OTC drugs. Ask them to make a chart that shows the different kinds of drugs advertised and the ages of the people to whom the ads were directed. Tell students to tally their results and prepare a report on their findings.

CHAPTER 12 ASSESSMENT

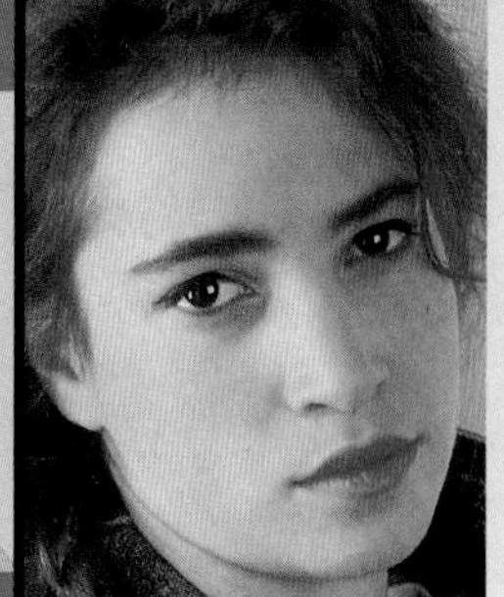

Chapter Review

Concept Review

1. Give examples of drug use, drug misuse, and drug abuse.
2. Advertisements suggest that drugs make you feel better. How can this be a negative message?
3. Explain two differences between over-the-counter drugs and prescription drugs.
4. What are some ways you can misuse a drug?
5. What are some drugs that have psychoactive effects? What are the risks of abusing these drugs?
6. What does it mean when a person becomes addicted to a drug? How might a person know if he or she is physically dependent on a drug?
7. Antibiotics and vasodilators are two types of medicines. Name two things that medicines can do to your body.
8. What are some dangers of taking (a) aspirin? (b) appetite suppressants?
9. Why should a person who is taking antihistamines not drive a car?
10. Why is it important to finish a prescribed medication?
11. How are medicines usually administered? How does the method used have an impact on its effect?
12. What can happen if you take a drug when another drug is already in your system?
13. Define drug allergies and name two symptoms of them. What happens if they are ignored?

Expressing Your Views

1. Mario hurt his knee during hockey practice. That night he took some of his friend's prescription medicine for pain. Should Mario have taken this? Why or why not?
2. Your friend has had a fever and runny nose for several days. She has been taking ibuprofen along with an over-the-counter cold remedy to ease her suffering. How is this risky behavior? What would you advise her to do?
3. It seems as if you have had a stuffy nose forever. You have been using a nasal spray for about a month. You realize it is not healthy to take drugs for a long time, but every time you stop using the spray, you can barely breathe through your nose. What do you think has happened?

CHAPTER REVIEW

Concept Review

1. Drug use: taking prescription drugs according to the directions on the label. Drug misuse: because you missed a scheduled dose of a prescription drug, you take twice the amount this time to "catch up." Drug abuse: taking cocaine.

2. You can solve any and all problems by taking drugs.

3. Prescription drugs require a prescription; over-the-counter drugs do not. Prescription drugs are often more powerful, have psychoactive effects, and can be addictive.

4. Taking the wrong amount, not taking all the prescribed medication, and taking medicine prescribed for someone else

5. Alcohol, caffeine, nicotine, tranquilizers, and heroin. The risks are addiction and possible change in mood or behavior.

6. The person has developed a physical need for the drug and will suffer withdrawal symptoms if he or she does not take it. A person will know he or she is addicted because he or she will suffer withdrawal symptoms if he or she tries to stop taking the drug.

7. They battle bacteria and other organisms that cause disease; they protect the body from disease; they influence the circulatory system; they affect the nervous system.

8. Aspirin can lead to stomach irritation and bleeding and may be associated with Reye's syndrome. Appetite suppressants can cause high blood pressure and increased heart rate.

9. They can cause drowsiness and dizziness.

10. If antibiotics are stopped too early, the bacteria may not be eliminated and the infection could return.

11. Swallowed or injected. Injected medicines go directly into the bloodstream and therefore usually act more quickly than those that are swallowed.

12. You can have a drug interaction.

13. A drug allergy occurs when the body mistakes the medicine for a disease-causing agent and tries to reject it. Symptoms include a rash, a runny nose, and quickened heart and breathing rates. The results can be fatal.

Life Skills Check . . . . . .

1. Practicing Self-Care
You have had a sore throat and fever for several days. You haven't been eating well because it is painful to swallow. The doctor prescribed a medicine for strep throat, but shortly after you take the directed dosage your stomach starts to hurt. What could be the matter?

2. Practicing Self-Care
Your mother had been having trouble sleeping for a long time. Then her doctor prescribed a sleeping medication, or barbiturate, for her. She's been taking the medication for a week, and has been sleeping better. Last night when you went out to dinner with her, she had a glass of wine. Did she take a risk by drinking alcohol? Explain.

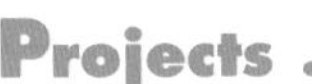

Projects . . . .

1. Select an advertisement for an over-the-counter drug. Analyze the claims and benefits and determine the accuracy of the ad. How does the ad try to sell the drug? Is the drug really needed? Rewrite the ad, giving suggestions for relieving the problem without use of the drug.
2. Invite a pharmacist to the classroom or visit a local pharmacy. Ask the pharmacist about over-the-counter drugs, prescription drugs, warnings, and directions for use.
3. Three common types of over-the-counter drugs are sedatives, analgesics, and stimulants. Go to the store and compare name brands, lists of ingredients, directions, and prices. Record your findings on a chart, and display it in the classroom.

Plan for Action . . . .

You have a choice regarding how much you rely on drugs to relieve symptoms of illness. Devise a plan to restrict your reliance on drugs.

Chapter 12 Assessment

Expressing Your Views

1. No; taking medicine for someone else is a form of drug misuse and can be very dangerous.
2. She may be covering up her symptoms and making the infection worse. She should stop taking both medications and consult her doctor.
3. Your body probably has built up a tolerance for the spray. This is a form of addiction.

Life Skills Check

1. You may be misusing the medicine. Read the prescription label to see if you should be taking the medicine with food.
2. Yes. Never mix alcohol with any medications because of drug interaction.

Projects

Have students plan and carry out the projects on drugs.

Plan for Action

Have students discuss their personal plans to avoid misusing and abusing drugs. They should use all they have learned in the chapter to come to decisions about their own behavior with regard to using drugs for medication, using them only when necessary, and always according to directions.

Assessment Options

Chapter Test

Have students take the Chapter 12 Test.

Alternative Assessment

Have students do the Alternative Assessment activity for Chapter 12.

Test Generator

The Test Generator (Macintosh® or IBM® format) contains an additional 50 assessment items for this chapter.

CHAPTER 13

ALCOHOL: A DANGEROUS DRUG

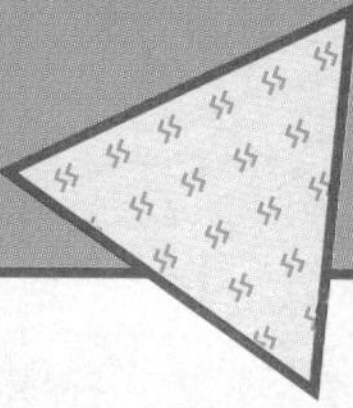

PLANNING GUIDE

TEXT SECTIONS	OBJECTIVES	TEXT FEATURES	OUTSIDE RESOURCES	NOTES
13.1 **Effects of Alcohol on the Body** pp. 261-266 1 period	• Discuss the effects of intoxication. • Name two diseases caused by long-term alcohol abuse.	**ASSESSMENT** • Section Review, p. 266	**TEACHER'S RESOURCE BINDER** • Lesson Plan 13.1 • Personal Health Inventory • Journal Entry 13A • Section Review Worksheet 13.1 • Section Quiz 13.1 • Reteaching Worksheet 13.1 **OTHER RESOURCES** • Transparencies 13A, 13B • Parent Discussion Guide • English/Spanish Audiocassette 4	
13.2 **Teenagers and Alcohol** pp. 267-273 2 periods	• Name two reasons why some people drink. • Name four reasons not to drink. • Discuss myths and facts about alcohol. ■ Name at least three ways you could refuse alcohol if a friend offers it to you. • Use the decision-making steps to decide whether to take a ride with someone who has been drinking.	• What Would You Do?, p. 271 ■ LIFE SKILLS: Resisting Pressure, p. 272 **ASSESSMENT** • Section Review, p. 273	**TEACHER'S RESOURCE BINDER** • Lesson Plan 13.2 • Journal Entry 13B • Life Skills 13A, 13B, 13C • Section Review Worksheet 13.2 • Section Quiz 13.2 • Reteaching Worksheet 13.2 **OTHER RESOURCES** • Transparencies 13C, 13D • Making a Choice 13A	
13.3 **Alcohol Abuse and Alcoholism** pp. 274-277 1 period	• Know the three phases of alcoholism. • Name the most important risks of alcohol abuse. • Know the ways in which a family can be damaged by a family member's alcoholism.	**ASSESSMENT** • Section Review, p. 277	**TEACHER'S RESOURCE BINDER** • Lesson Plan 13.3 • Journal Entries 13C, 13D • Section Review Worksheet 13.3 • Section Quiz 13.3 • Reteaching Worksheet 13.3 **OTHER RESOURCES** • Making a Choice 13B	
13.4 **Hope for Recovery** pp. 278-280 1 period	• Discuss the treatment options for alcohol abuse. ■ Learn how to get help if you or someone you know abuses alcohol.	**ASSESSMENT** • Section Review, p. 280	**TEACHER'S RESOURCE BINDER** • Lesson Plan 13.4 • Journal Entry 13E • Life Skills 13D • Section Review Worksheet 13.4 • Section Quiz 13.4 • Reteaching Worksheet 13.4	
End of Chapter pp. 281-283		**ASSESSMENT** • Chapter Review, pp. 282-283	**TEACHER'S RESOURCE BINDER** • Chapter Test • Alternative Assessment • Personal Pledge **OTHER RESOURCES** • Test Generator	

■ Denotes LIFE SKILLS objectives

• Items in blue are also part of the *Holt Health Activity Book.*

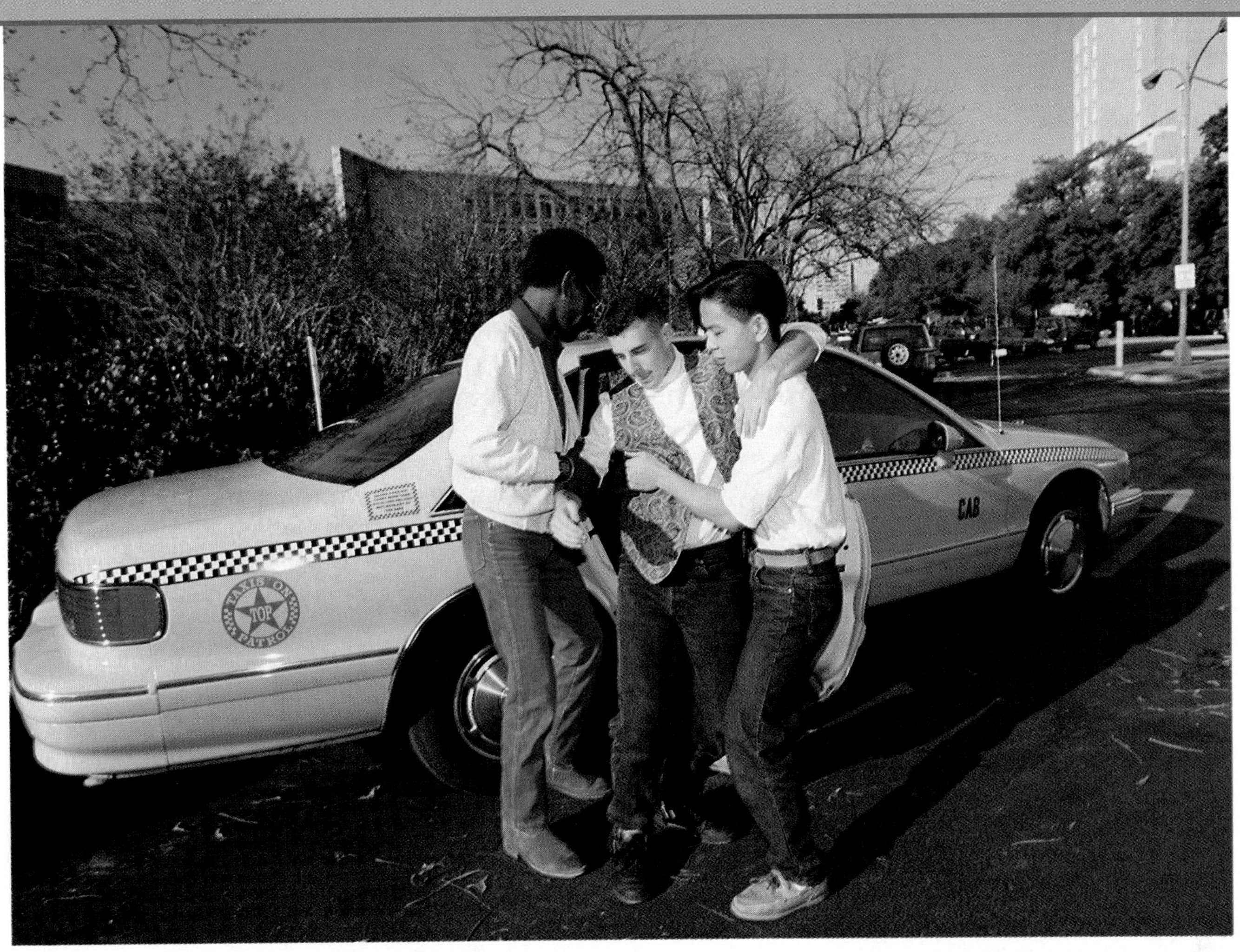

CONTENT BACKGROUND

Alcohol Use and Abuse Among Teens

IN 1991 THE *JOURNAL OF THE AMERICAN Medical Association* reported the results of a survey conducted on alcohol use by ninth- through twelfth-grade students in the United States. Of 11,631 students included in the survey, 10,235 had consumed alcohol at some time in their lives. The National Adolescent Student Health Survey (NASHS), conducted in the fall of the 1987-1988 school year, revealed similar results on teenage alcohol use and abuse. Of 11,419 eighth- and tenth-grade students polled, 83 percent reported having consumed alcohol on at least one occasion. Nearly 4,800 of these adolescents said they had drunk alcohol in the month before the survey, and 3,654 said that they had consumed five or more alcoholic beverages on a single occasion two weeks before the survey.

There are an estimated 17 million alcoholics in the United States. Of these, 4.25 million are teenagers. Even though some experts on substance abuse consider alcohol use one of the leading health problems in teenagers, fewer than half (43 percent) of those students polled in the NASHS perceived that consuming five or more drinks once or twice on the weekend presented a great health risk.

Unfortunately, this misperception of alcohol not being a dangerous drug continues or worsens as teens enter college. For example, several studies at colleges and universities in Massachusetts have revealed that twice as many students attending Boston College were admitted to local hospitals in 1990 as a result of accidents related to drinking than in the previous school year. The

University of Massachusetts at Amherst reports that 80 percent of the cases treated at the student health facility on any weekend are results of alcohol abuse. The Harvard School of Public Health conducted a survey of freshmen attending 14 different colleges in Massachusetts. It found that of over 1,500 respondents who drink at least once a week, 82 percent of the females and 92 percent of the males reported that they drink at least five alcoholic beverages each time.

It often takes years for alcoholism to develop in an adult. In teens, however, this disease can develop in as little as one year of steady drinking. Alcohol abuse is associated with malnutrition, toxic hepatitis, cirrhosis, certain kinds of cancers, pancreatitis, hypertension, and cardiovascular diseases. Alcohol abuse is also a contributing factor in 30 percent of all suicides, 85 percent of incidents of domestic violence, over 50 percent of all automobile deaths, 65 percent of all accidental drownings, and 60 percent of all cases of reported child abuse.

What can be done to diminish or even eliminate this "epidemic"? Until recently, education on any kind of substance abuse was often limited to high school students. Some alarming statistics regarding alcohol and its widespread use among young Americans, however, have caused educators to begin such courses at much earlier ages.

In addition to education on substance abuse in the elementary and middle schools, legislation has been enacted in many states to raise the legal drinking age from 18 to 21. Also, some states have redefined, or are considering redefining, intoxication by lowering the legal limit of the blood alcohol level (BAL) from 0.1 to 0.08. The states that have modified their definition of intoxication, California for example, have reported an increase in arrests of people who are drunk and driving and a dramatic decrease in traffic fatalities.

Although it would be impossible to eliminate alcohol use and abuse from our society completely, most social scientists believe that educational efforts at a relatively young age might, at the very least, encourage young people to postpone their choice to drink on a regular basis. Groups such as Students Against Driving Drunk (S.A.D.D.) and Mothers Against Drunk Driving (M.A.D.D.), along with tough drunken driving laws, are needed to increase public awareness of the hazards of drunken driving and to curb the abuse of this drug among today's youth.

PLANNING FOR INSTRUCTION

KEY FACTS

- **In the United States, anyone under the legal drinking age who drinks alcohol is breaking the law and can be arrested, fined, and can acquire a criminal record.**
- **When an alcoholic drink is consumed, the alcohol travels quickly through the bloodstream to all cells in the body, including the brain.**
- **Blood alcohol level (BAL) is the percentage of alcohol in a person's blood. It is affected by gender, weight, the drinking rate, and whether there is food in the stomach.**
- **The short-term effects of alcohol abuse include reduced inhibitions and coordination, behavior changes, poor judgment, loss of control, slowed reflexes, alcohol breath, flushed face, and frequent urination. The long-term effects of alcohol abuse are serious and include liver disease, heart disease, brain damage and memory loss, and an increase in the rate of getting certain cancers.**
- **Teens often drink alcohol to relax, to be sociable, to numb emotional pain, to feel independent, to rebel, for excitement, and because they believe the advertising that portrays drinking as desirable.**
- **The American Medical Association calls alcoholism a disease that develops in three phases—abuse, dependence, and addiction.**

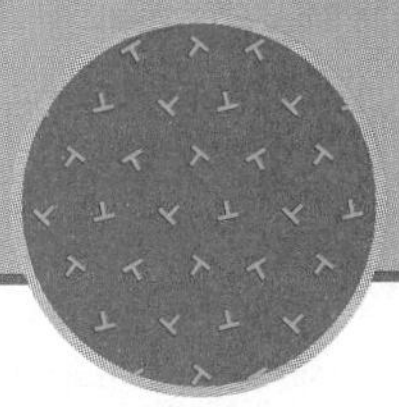

- Alcoholism's causes are uncertain but are believed to be a combination of psychological, environmental, and physical factors.
- Alcoholics Anonymous (AA) is the most widely used self-help organization for alcoholics. Al-Anon and Alateen are companion organizations for codependent families and teens.

MYTHS AND MISCONCEPTIONS

MYTH: Alcohol stimulates you, makes you livelier, and helps you do things better.

Just the opposite is true, because alcohol is a depressant that slows down the nervous system. The "loosening up" commonly experienced when drinking is really a relaxation of inhibitions, which encourages people to behave in ways they normally are afraid to.

MYTH: I can drive just as well after a few beers—in fact, I can drive even better.

This is completely disproved by tests showing that even low levels of alcohol slow reactions. People feel they can drive because drinking creates a false feeling of confidence.

MYTH: Brandy will warm you up when you are at a football game, snowmobiling, skiing, or hunting.

Actually, drinking alcohol cools the body. Alcohol causes blood vessels near the skin to dilate so that more blood flows there, causing the sensation of warmth described in this myth.

VOCABULARY

Essential: The following vocabulary terms appear in boldface type:

blood alcohol level (BAL)
intoxicated
hangover
hepatitis
cirrhosis
alcoholism
withdrawal
fetal alcohol syndrome (FAS)

Secondary: Be aware that the following terms may come up during class discussion:

inhibitions
esophagus, pharynx, larynx
binge
sexually transmitted diseases (STD)
predisposition
codependent

FOR STUDENTS WITH SPECIAL NEEDS

At-Risk Students: Have students think of a personal experience in which alcohol played a role: witnessing an argument between people who had been drinking, seeing a person drunk, seeing a photograph of a car crash, listening to parents at a party, or trying alcohol themselves. Have them write brief descriptive stories or poems in which they express how they felt during the experience.

Less-Advanced Students: Have students bring to class newspaper and magazine articles about alcohol-related traffic accidents, or have them take notes on such accidents during newscasts. Ask them to highlight the blood alcohol level (BAL) when indicated, and place these articles on the classroom bulletin board.

ENRICHMENT

- Have students interview adults in their community to discover their opinions about alcohol use. What effect does drinking have on a person's life? on life in the community? Is responsible drinking possible? desirable? Should people be allowed to drink at 18? Should young people be given alcohol at home to learn how to handle it? Students should agree on a list of questions, conduct the survey, then create a bar graph poster showing the results.
- Several noted recovering alcoholics, such as former President Gerald Ford's wife, Betty, have written books about their experiences. Have students select such a book and report on how the person became an alcoholic and how he or she began recovery.
- Have students research and report on attitudes toward alcohol in other countries. Have them compare and contrast these attitudes to those in the United States.

Chapter 13
Chapter Opener

GETTING STARTED

Using the Chapter Photograph

What is happening in this photograph? *[The policeman is checking the driver's level of intoxication.]* **What might have happened if the driver were driving drunk and had not been stopped by the officer?** *[The driver could have been involved in or involved someone else in a serious accident.]* **What would you do if your friend, who was drunk, wanted to drive home from a party?** *[Try to talk the person out of driving; take the car keys]* Explain to students that in this chapter they will learn about alcohol abuse and why it is so dangerous. If the young person in the photograph continued to drive drunk, he would be breaking a law.

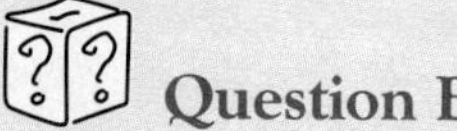

Question Box

Have students write out any questions they have about alcohol and alcohol abuse and put them in the Question Box. The Question Box provides students with an opportunity to ask questions anonymously. To ensure that students with questions are not embarrassed to be seen writing, have those who do not have questions write something else—such as something they already know about alcohol and its abuse—on the paper instead.

Preview the questions and then answer them at appropriate points in the chapter. You may wish to allow students to write additional anonymous questions as they go through the chapter.

Personal Issues *ALERT*

Alcohol abuse is so prevalent that many of your students probably have been touched by it in some way. They may know someone who was injured in a drunken-driving accident, they may have a girlfriend or boyfriend who drinks, they might know an alcoholic, or they might even be alcoholics themselves. An alcoholic student or one with an alcoholic family member may have trouble dealing with the material in this chapter. Such a student may fear exposure of the problem and may not want to discuss it.

If you sense that anyone in class has this problem, remind the entire class of counseling assistance available in your school and local area.

Chapter 13

Alcohol: A Dangerous Drug

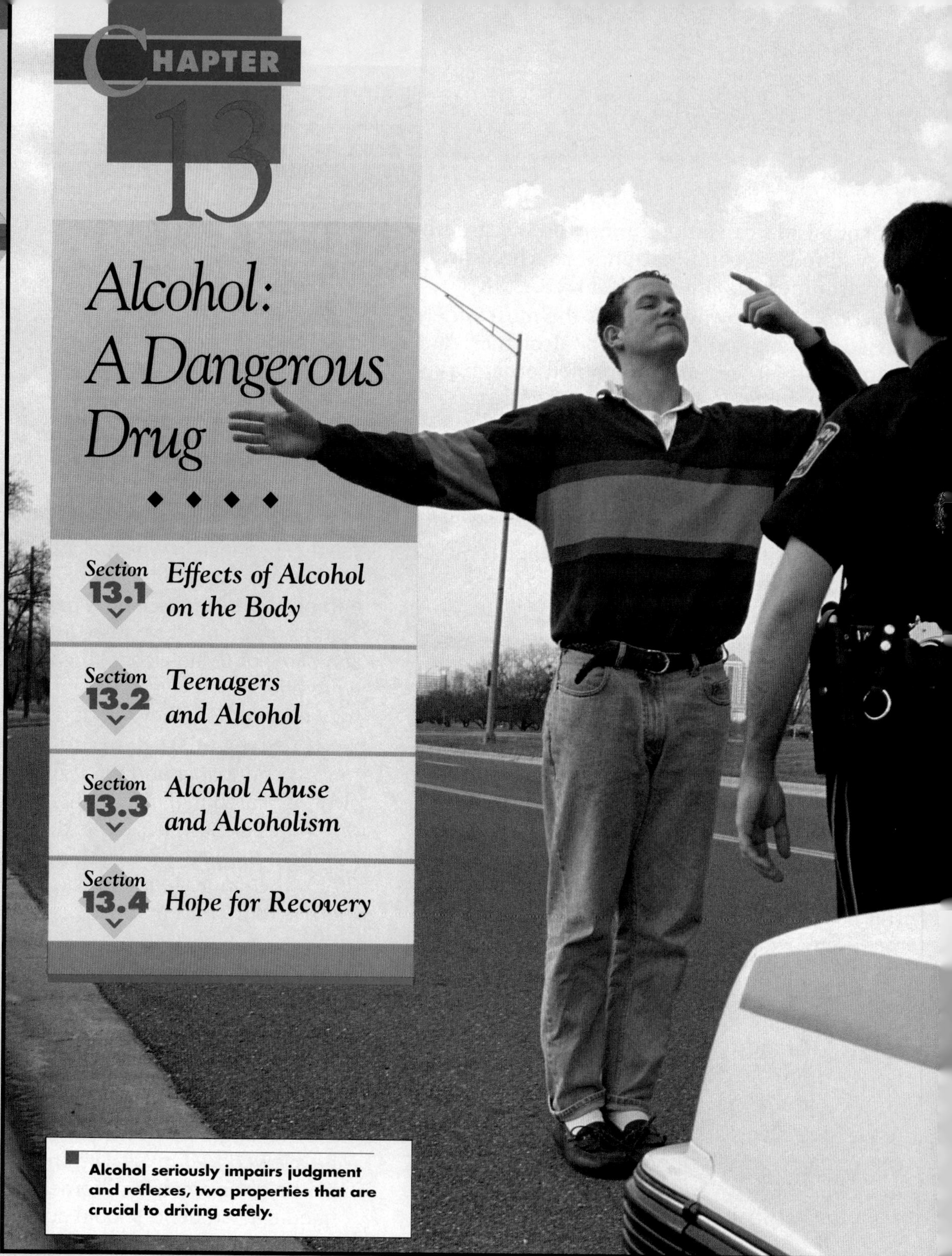

Alcohol seriously impairs judgment and reflexes, two properties that are crucial to driving safely.

Navorn was excited. School was out for the summer, and she had a great summer job lined up. Now she was celebrating at an end-of-school-year party, but it was getting late. Navorn saw Billy heading out the back door, and she was about to ask him for a ride home. Then she noticed that he seemed pretty drunk. So she asked a friend who hadn't been drinking for a ride.

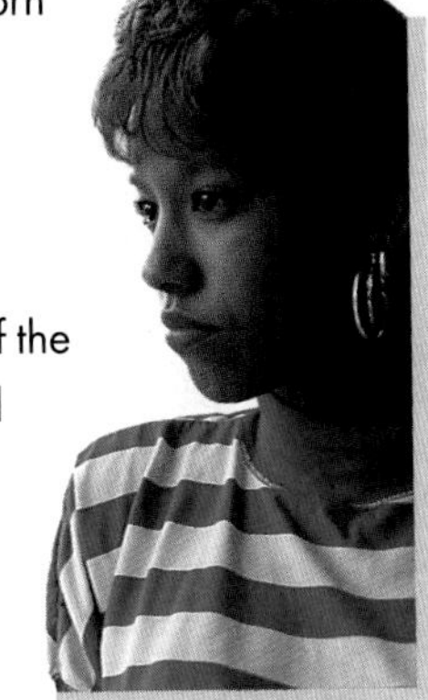

The next day she heard the news. Billy had lost control of the car on his way home. It crashed into a ditch and hit several trees. Billy didn't make it. If Navorn had taken a ride with Billy, she might have been killed too.

Section 13.1 Effects of Alcohol on the Body

Objectives

- *Discuss the effects of intoxication.*
- *Name two diseases caused by long-term alcohol abuse.*

Alcohol may be the most misunderstood drug. It is widely advertised and is often consumed at parties and restaurants. But alcohol is also a very dangerous drug that kills thousands of people every year and addicts millions more. It tears families apart and is involved in more than half the violent crimes committed in the United States. And, for Americans under 21, it is an illegal drug.

One reason alcohol is illegal for teenagers has to do with what happened to Billy. Drunken-driving crashes kill between 3,000 and 4,000 teenagers every year. These numbers were even higher a few years ago, when some states allowed people as young as 18 to drink. Highway safety experts think the raised legal drinking age is responsible for saving many thousands of lives.

More and more people are deciding not to drink alcohol. They have made this decision not only because they worry about drunken-driving, but also because they don't like what alcohol does to their bodies. Like any drug, alcohol changes the way your body functions. These changes are unhealthy, and can be very dangerous.

When Alcohol Enters the Body

Your friend Leo loves beer. He says it's a better thirst quencher than any other drink, which is why he likes to have one with his lunch. He tells you he knows there's going to be a lot of beer at Sandra's party and that it should be a pretty great time.

The party is in full gear when Leo arrives. It doesn't take him long to find out where the beer is. From that moment on, Leo's evening is ruined.

Background

Types of Alcohol

There are many different types of alcohol. Consumers commonly encounter three types: ethanol, ethylene glycol, and isopropyl alcohol. Ethanol is used in alcoholic beverages, varnish, medications such as cough syrup, and gasohol (mixed with gasoline). For drinking, ethanol is produced by fermenting grapes or other fruits to make wines, sugar cane to make rum, and various grains to make beer, whiskey, vodka, and so on. Ethylene glycol is used as automobile antifreeze, and isopropyl alcohol is used in cosmetics and as rubbing alcohol. Ethylene glycol and isopropyl alcohol both are poisonous.

Section 13.1 Lesson Plan

MOTIVATE

Journal 13A
Alcohol: Good or Bad?

This may be done as a warm-up activity. Have students turn to the Student Journal in the Student Activity Book. Ask them to write their responses to these questions: How do you think drinking alcohol might be good for you? How might it be bad for you?

Class Discussion
Alcohol at a Party

Have students discuss Navorn's decision not to ride with Billy because he was drunk. **What could she have done to stop him from driving?** *[Persuaded him not to drive, found someone to take him home, sent him home in a taxi cab, had everyone physically block him from leaving, hidden his car keys, talked him into sleeping the night there, called his family, and so on]* Have you or anyone you know ever been in a situation similar to Navorn's? Describe the situation and the outcome.

TEACH

Cooperative Learning
Questionnaire

Have students work in four groups to develop questions in four subject areas: drinking and teens, drinking in families, social attitudes toward drinking, and legal aspects of alcohol use. Have

Background
Alcohol Content

Alcoholic beverages vary widely in their alcohol content. Fermented drinks include beer, containing 2 to 6 percent alcohol, and wine, containing 7 to 24 percent. Distilling increases alcohol content to make whiskey, gin, rum, vodka, and other hard liquors, with an alcohol content of 12 to 55 percent. "Proof" is twice the alcohol percentage, so a whiskey that is 50 percent alcohol is 100 proof. Except for beer, all types of alcoholic beverages must be labeled to show the percentage of alcohol. The Federal Food and Drug Administration prohibits beer labels from stating the alcohol content to discourage promotion and purchase of beer on the basis of its intoxication potential. Beers commonly are 5 percent alcohol, although some states limit it to 3.2 percent.

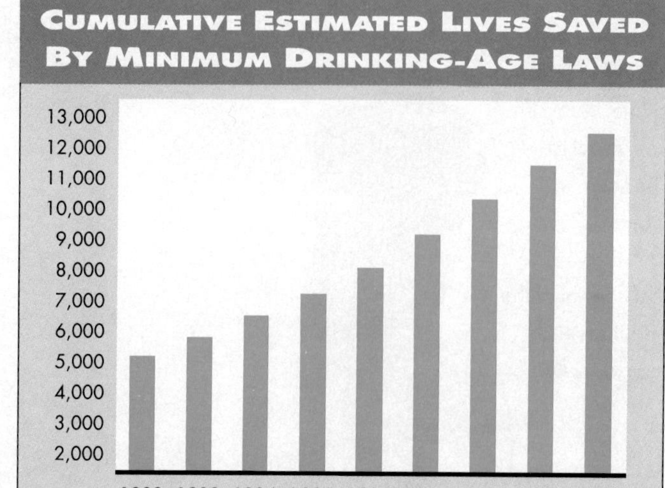

(FIGURE 13-2) **Experts believe that minimum-drinking-age laws have saved more than 11,000 lives.**

blood alcohol level (BAL): *a way to measure the level of alcohol in a person's body.*

Each gulp of beer Leo swallows makes its way first into his stomach and then into his small intestine. From his stomach and small intestine, the alcohol is absorbed into his bloodstream. Once the alcohol has been absorbed, it travels in the bloodstream to all Leo's cells and tissues, including his brain. Within *minutes,* Leo is feeling the effects of the beer.

Eventually the alcohol reaches Leo's liver, which breaks it down into carbon dioxide and water. The more Leo drinks, the harder his liver will have to work to help rid his body of alcohol. In fact, it will take Leo's liver more than an hour to break down the alcohol in each bottle of beer he drinks.

intoxicated: *being affected by alcohol. Effects of intoxication can range from mild lightheadedness to severe and complete loss of judgment and reflexes.*

Blood Alcohol Level One drink is enough to interfere with a person's judgment and reflexes. And the more a person drinks, the more alcohol interferes with judgment and reflexes.

The percentage of alcohol in a person's bloodstream is called the **blood alcohol level (BAL).** A person's BAL can be influenced by gender, body weight, the amount of food in the stomach, and the rate of drinking.

If after a few beers Leo has a BAL of 0.1, it means that .1 percent, or 1/1000, of his blood is pure alcohol. That is enough for Leo to be declared legally **intoxicated**, or drunk, in most states. It is also enough to impair his judgment and vision, which will make him a very dangerous driver. If he keeps drinking, Leo's BAL will keep getting higher.

Short-Term Effects of Alcohol After a few beers, Leo starts feeling relaxed. He's had a rough day at school, but now he can't remember why.

His face feels flushed and very warm, because the alcohol he has drunk has dilated, or widened, the blood vessels near his skin. He also has to urinate constantly, as his body tries to get rid of the alcohol in his system.

On his way to the bathroom Leo knocks over an empty chair. He is too drunk to notice what he did, and when he

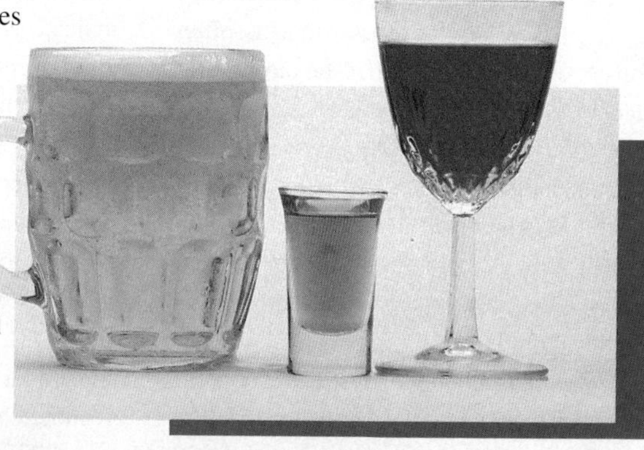

(FIGURE 13-3) **A 12-ounce bottle of beer, an 8-ounce glass of wine, and a 1.5-ounce glass of whiskey all have about the same alcohol content.**

• • • TEACH continued

them combine their questions into a survey they can administer to a sample of other students in the school or complete themselves. Have students present their results in a written report or a set of pie graphs.

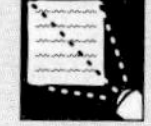

Teaching Transparency 13A
Alcohol in the Body

Display the transparency showing how alcohol is distributed through the body (Figure 13-4). Have a volunteer trace and describe the pathway that alcohol takes to reach the brain and other organs. Ask students to explain how the body disposes of the alcohol.

Demonstration
BAL

Pose the following question and then demonstrate how you arrive at the answer using math. **How much alcohol is in one serving of liquor?** *[The alcohol percentage in a bottle of liquor is typically 40 percent. Convert 40 percent to a decimal (.4, or four-tenths, of the liquor is pure alcohol). Then multiply 1.5 (ounces of liquor in one drink) times .4. The answer is .6 (ounce of alcohol in one drink.)]* **If the liver breaks down about 0.4 ounce of alcohol in 1 hour, how long will it take to get rid of all the alcohol from the drink?** *[Divide .6 ounce by .4 ounce per hour. The answer is 1.5 hours.]*

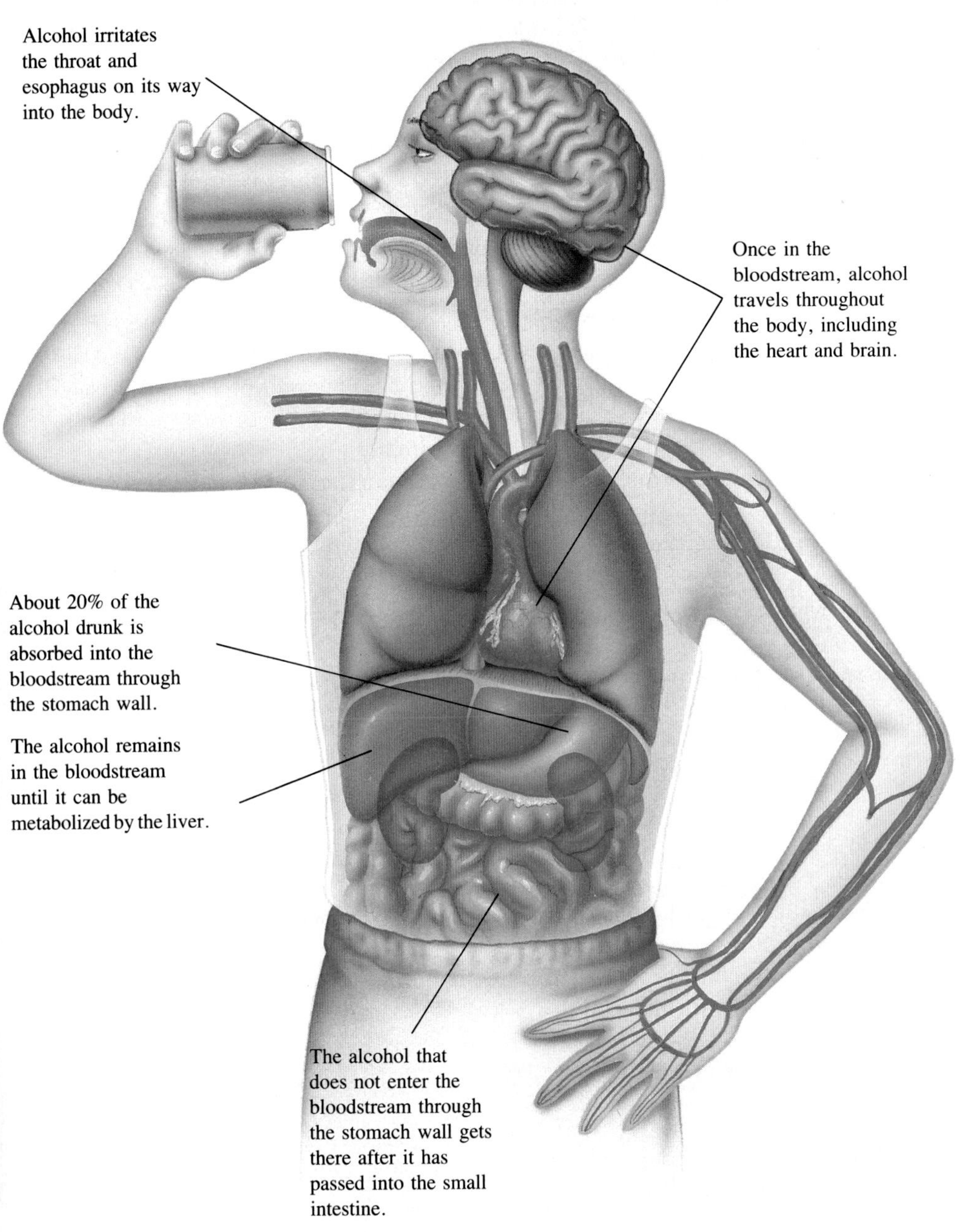

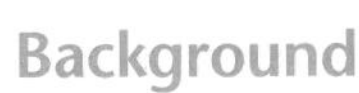

Alcohol irritates the throat and esophagus on its way into the body.

Once in the bloodstream, alcohol travels throughout the body, including the heart and brain.

About 20% of the alcohol drunk is absorbed into the bloodstream through the stomach wall.

The alcohol remains in the bloodstream until it can be metabolized by the liver.

The alcohol that does not enter the bloodstream through the stomach wall gets there after it has passed into the small intestine.

(FIGURE 13-4) **The alcohol in one 12-ounce bottle of beer reaches the bloodstream very quickly. It then remains in the bloodstream until it is metabolized—a process that takes more than an hour for each bottle of beer.**

Background
Effects Differ by Sex

If a man and a woman weigh the same, the woman probably will be affected by the same amount of alcohol sooner than the man. This is due to differences in their body fat (women have more fatty tissue) and rate of metabolism.

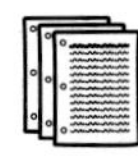

Personal Health Inventory

Have students complete the Personal Health Inventory for this chapter. The inventory helps students assess whether they abuse, are dependent on, or are addicted to alcohol.

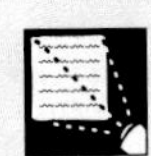

Teaching Transparency 13B
Blood Alcohol Level and Its Effects

Show the transparency titled *Blood Alcohol Level and Its Effects* (Figure 13-6). Point out that the BAL is for a 140-pound person, and ask: **If you weigh less than 140 pounds, would the same amount of alcohol affect you more, or less?** *[More, because the same dose of alcohol would spread through a smaller quantity of blood, raising the BAL.]* **Which affects you more—a drink before dinner, or during a meal?** *[A drink on an empty stomach affects you more, because the alcohol is very quickly absorbed by it. Eating food along with or before taking a drink spreads the absorption of alcohol over a longer time and causes a lower BAL.]*

Class Discussion
Myths and Facts About Alcohol

Discuss the "Myths and Facts About Alcohol" (Figure 13-5). **We know that beer, wine, and hard liquors are equally intoxicating. But beer and wine coolers often pose a greater hazard for teenagers than hard liquor. Why?** *[They are cheaper, more widely available, and their lower alcohol content misleads some into believing that a person can't get as drunk on them.]*

Debate the Issue
Setting the Legal Drinking Age

Divide the class into two teams and have the teams debate whether teenagers should be allowed to drink

Background
Costs of Alcohol Use

Americans drink over 5 billion gallons of beer each year (24 gallons per person), nearly 600 million gallons of wine, and over 400 million gallons of distilled liquors. In 1990 alcohol killed over 65,000 Americans and cost us over $100 billion.

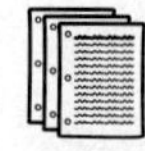

Section Review Worksheet 13.1

Assign Section Review Worksheet 13.1, which requires students to evaluate possible long-term and short-term effects of alcohol.

Section Quiz 13.1

Have students take Section Quiz 13.1.

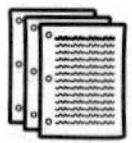

Reteaching Worksheet 13.1

Students who have difficulty with the material may complete Reteaching Worksheet 13.1, which requires them to list effects of alcohol on the body.

Myths and Facts About Alcohol

Myth	Fact
You can't get as drunk from beer, wine, or wine coolers as you can from "hard" liquor like vodka and scotch.	*A bottle of beer, a glass of wine, and a wine cooler all have around the same amount of alcohol as a shot of a distilled spirit like vodka or scotch. Therefore, they are just as intoxicating.*
A person who looks and acts sober is sober.	*Not everyone shows the effects of alcohol in the same way. Even people who seem completely sober are dangerous drivers if they have been drinking alcohol.*
Alcohol can't be as dangerous as illicit drugs because it is easily available to people over the age of 21.	*Even though alcohol is a legal drug for Americans over 21, when it is abused it is just as dangerous as many illicit drugs.*

(FIGURE 13-5) **Myths about alcohol not only are untrue, but also can be dangerous to believe—particularly if a person is drinking and driving.**

hangover:
uncomfortable physical effects brought on by alcohol use. Symptoms of a hangover include headache, nausea, upset stomach, and dizziness.

returns from the bathroom he trips over it. Laughing loudly, he struggles to get up from the floor. Leo may find this funny, but his lack of coordination and inhibition has resulted from a serious event; the alcohol in his bloodstream has entered his brain, changing the way it functions.

Leo sees Roberto leaving the party with a girl Leo used to date. The sight enrages him, and he grabs Roberto and shoves him against the wall. Roberto just shakes his head, rolls his eyes, and walks away.

Leo finds some more beer and sits in the kitchen, drinking by himself.

The next thing he knows, Leo is waking up on a kitchen floor—a kitchen floor he doesn't recognize. ''Oh yeah,'' he realizes, ''I guess I passed out in Sandra's kitchen.'' He has a dull headache, a sick stomach, and he feels very dizzy. Leo has a **hangover.** ''Just my luck,'' he says out loud.

Actually, Leo *was* pretty lucky. He could have seriously hurt Roberto or himself if Roberto hadn't ignored him. If Leo had tried to drive home, he could have easily had a wreck.

Leo's hangover lasts until late in the afternoon. (Nothing but time makes a hangover go away.) As a result, he plays poorly at basketball practice. ''Okay, so I got drunk last night,'' Leo tells you when you ask him if he's all right. ''What are you—my mother?''

Leo feels bad about what happened at the party but refuses to believe that it had anything to do with alcohol. That means he'll probably drink again soon.

• • • TEACH continued

at age 18. Remind students that both the pro and con teams should be able to refute one another's arguments with solid evidence.

Blood Alcohol Level and Its Effects

Number of Drinks in a 1-hour Period (140-pound person)	Approximate Blood Alcohol Level	Effects on Body
1	.025	*Feeling of relaxation, warmth, and well-being; slight impairment of judgment*
2	.05	*Inhibitions are lessened; judgment impaired, behavior can become impulsive*
3	.075	*Reflexes and coordination impaired; speech and hearing slightly affected*
4	.1	*Legally drunk in most states; vision, hearing, judgment, reflexes, coordination impaired*
6	.161	*Intoxication; coordination seriously affected; vision blurred, speech and hearing severely impaired*
8	.215	*Intoxication extreme; no control over thoughts and perceptions; walking and even standing become difficult*
12	.321	*Intoxication severe and dangerous; nervous system may become affected, coma and death can result*

(FIGURE 13-6) **This table shows the estimated blood alcohol level and its effects on a 140-pound person. A person's blood alcohol level will vary according to a number of factors, such as weight and gender.**

Review Answers

1. A person who is intoxicated may become angry, behave impulsively and without inhibitions, and lose his or her reflexes. Coordination will become impaired, making the person clumsy. With increased levels of intoxication, the person can have difficulty walking and standing.

2. Answers will vary. Students may answer hepatitis, cirrhosis, heart disease, and cancer.

3. Answers will vary. Students should point out the short-term effects and consequences of intoxication as well as some possible long-term consequences. Students may also suggest alternative ways to enjoy oneself at a party, other than drinking alcohol.

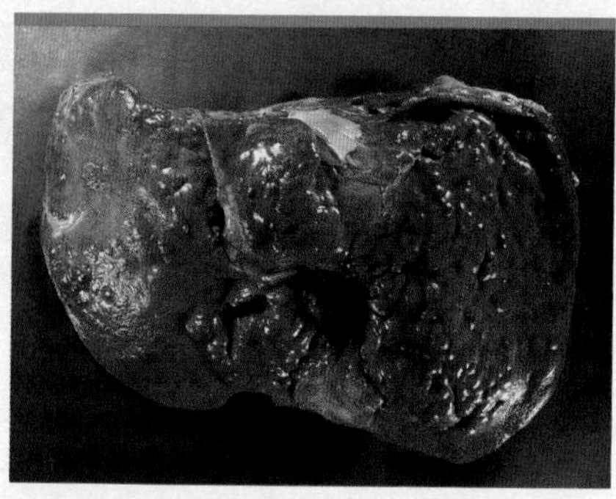

(FIGURE 13-7) **A normal liver (left), and a liver with cirrhosis (right). Cirrhosis is an incurable, untreatable disease caused by alcoholism.**

Long-Term Effects

Over a period of time, the alcohol Leo drinks can seriously damage his body.

First, alcohol can harm his liver. As you now know, the liver works hard to break down the alcohol in his body into carbon dioxide and water. The liver does this job well, but pays a price each time. Studies show that even small doses of alcohol leave fat deposits on liver cells. The livers of alcoholics are often damaged beyond repair.

hepatitis: *an inflammation of the liver that can be caused by long-term alcohol abuse. Symptoms of hepatitis include high fever, weakness, and a yellowing of the skin.*

cirrhosis: *a condition in which liver cells are replaced by useless scar tissue. Cirrhosis can be caused by long-term alcohol abuse.*

One liver disease that can result from alcohol abuse is **hepatitis** (hep-uh-TY-tis). Hepatitis is an inflammation or infection of the liver that can cause fever, a yellowing of the skin, weakness, and sometimes death. More information about hepatitis can be found in Chapter 21.

Another liver disease caused by alcohol abuse is **cirrhosis** (sur-OH-sis), which occurs when liver cells are permanently replaced with useless scar tissue. People with cirrhosis often suffer serious digestive problems, because their livers are no longer able to metabolize food properly. Research shows that people with cirrhosis who continue to drink have only about a 50 percent chance of living more than five years.

Alcohol can also damage the heart. It causes fat deposits to develop on heart muscle, which can interfere with the heart's ability to pump blood through the body. For this reason, alcoholics have a greater chance of developing heart disease than those who don't drink or do so moderately.

Alcohol kills brain cells. Unlike those in other parts of the body, the cells in the brain cannot be replaced. Loss of brain cells can lead to irreversible memory damage.

Finally, long-term alcohol abuse can also increase one's chances of suffering cancers of the liver, esophagus, pharynx, and larynx.

Review

1. *Explain how a person's behavior changes when he or she is intoxicated.*
2. *Name two diseases caused by long-term alcohol abuse.*
3. ***Critical Thinking*** *What could you say to Leo to persuade him to change his drinking habits?*

ASSESS

Section Review

Have students answer the Section Review questions.

Alternative Assessment

Lifelong Drinking Habits

Tell students about a girl who started drinking several cans of beer a day in high school and has continued this habit into adult life. She is now 45 years old, has a job and family, and still drinks several cans of beer a day. Have students describe what alcohol-related problems she might face in the future.

Extension

Alcohol Laws

Have students contact your state's alcoholic beverage control agency to learn about the alcohol laws in your state. Ask students to prepare a report or poster summarizing their findings.

Closure

Feelings About Drinking and Driving

Have students assess their feelings about drinking. Then have them summarize orally their feelings about drinking and driving.

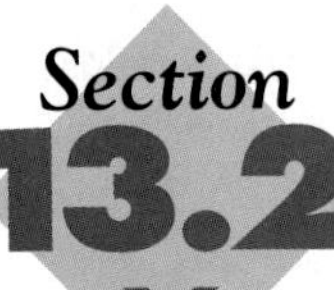

Section 13.2 Teenagers and Alcohol

Objectives

- Name two reasons why some people drink.
- Name four reasons not to drink.
- Discuss myths and facts about alcohol.
- Name at least three ways you could refuse alcohol if a friend offers it to you.
  LIFE SKILLS: Resisting Pressure
- Use the decision-making steps to decide whether to take a ride with someone who has been drinking.
  LIFE SKILLS: Making Responsible Decisions

If you watch a sporting event on television, or read a magazine, or drive a few miles on the highway, you are certain to see an advertisement for alcohol. Have a drink, the advertisements seem to say, and you can be like the people pictured—cool, glamorous, and sophisticated. Many people believe the ads and drink to fit the image they see.

Some people think they have to drink to be relaxed, to be social. But as Leo experienced, drinking alcohol can make a person angry and aggressive. In this way, it can make a person *less* social.

Other people may drink to ease emotional pain. You saw how Leo forgot what was disturbing him after he had a few beers. Many teenagers who are having problems at home or at school may be looking for something to help them forget their worries. It's completely understandable to feel this way. But alcohol tends to add to a person's problems, rather than solve them.

Some teenagers drink because it makes them feel independent. Others do so to rebel, or for excitement.

But whatever the reason, if you drink alcohol, you are putting your life on the line.

Drunken Driving

Alcohol severely damages judgment, reflexes, and vision. These effects happen to a person even if he or she doesn't *feel* drunk. In other words a person with a high blood alcohol level may not necessarily be slurring words, reeling, and staggering, but still is in no shape to be behind a wheel.

Blood Alcohol Level and Its Effects on Driving Ability

BAL	Decrease in Driving Ability
.04—.06	12%
.07—.09	23%
.10—.12	30%

(FIGURE 13-8) **As this table shows, a person does not have to be legally drunk (a BAL of .10) to be a dangerous driver. A blood alcohol level of .04 or above can severely impair judgment, coordination, and vision, which are all important to safe driving.**

Background

Teenage Drinking

A person must be 21 or older to purchase alcoholic beverages in most states. Despite these laws, alcohol is the drug most used, and abused, by teenagers. Virtually every high school student tries alcohol; two-thirds use it to some degree, and 5 percent use it daily. One estimate is that about 150 out of every 1,000 high school students may have an alcohol problem.

Section 13.2 Lesson Plan

MOTIVATE

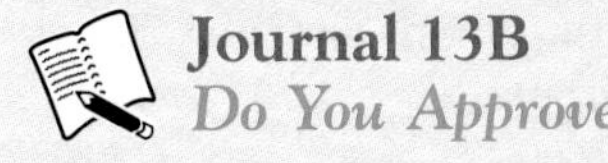

Journal 13B
Do You Approve?

This may be done as a warm-up activity. In the Student Journal in the Student Activity Book, have students answer the following questions: Is our state law that prohibits drinking alcohol until a certain age a fair law? Why? If you have friends who drink, do you approve, disapprove, or not care?

TEACH

Class Discussion
Selling Beer

Have students recall beer ads they have seen and heard. On the chalkboard, write the heading GIMMICKS THAT SELL BEER and list the gimmicks as students provide them (for example, cool and refreshing, sports, sex, beautiful scenery, fun activities, social enjoyment, friendship, reward for a job well done).

Have students address the categories one by one to explain, first, how the connection with desirable rewards is made and, second, why the connection is false. For instance, beer is associated with sports by being sold in sports bars; drinking doesn't promote physical health, and real people who drink a lot don't look like the models in the ads.

Social Standards

Teaching students to say no to alcohol is complicated by our culture's double standard for drinking. Students see adults advocating sobriety yet drinking too much on holidays and laughing at alcoholic community leaders. It may also seem paradoxical to teens that they are generally considered adult enough to drive, vote, marry, and serve in the armed forces, yet are not considered adults when it comes to alcohol. Thus, teaching students to say no to alcohol requires the support of their parents or guardians as well as the teacher's efforts.

A person doesn't have to be legally drunk in order to be dangerous on the highway. As little as one alcoholic beverage can cause enough impairment to cause a car crash. Figure 13-8 shows how different blood alcohol levels can affect a person's driving ability.

There are things you can do to minimize your risk of getting involved in a drunken-driving incident. First, don't drink. Of all reasons to turn down alcohol, this may well be the most important.

Second, don't accept a ride with anyone who has been drinking, even if he or she swears that you have nothing to worry about. Instead, call a sober person to pick you up. Maybe you can persuade the person you're with to come with you. You may want to show a parent or guardian a copy of the contract prepared by Students Against Driving Drunk (S.A.D.D.). This agreement guarantees that parents or guardians who are called for a ride home will pick up their teenagers—no questions asked. A copy of the contract is shown in Figure 13-10.

Binge Drinking

Remember that alcohol has very serious effects on the body. What you should also know is that alcohol is a poison. If a person drinks enough of it at one time, it can cause immediate death.

Although the amount of alcohol necessary to kill a person varies, a blood alcohol level of about .4 percent is usually enough to put a person in a coma and on the verge of death. For a 140-pound person, that's about 15 to 17 drinks in a one-hour period.

Binge drinking—drinking large amounts of alcohol quickly—can easily cause death by alcohol poisoning. Binge drinking is a very serious problem among teenagers and young adults who take part in drinking games.

Drunk Driving: Facts and Numbers

Two out of every five Americans will be involved in an alcohol-related traffic accident in their lifetime.

About 540,000 people are injured every year in alcohol-related crashes. About 43,000 of these people are seriously injured.

Traffic crashes are the greatest single cause of death for Americans between the ages of 5 and 34. Alcohol is involved in at least half of these crashes.

About 25,000 people die each year in drunken-driving accidents. This translates to 500 deaths each week, 71 every day, 1 every 20 minutes.

Between 7 P.M. and 3 A.M. on weekends, in some parts of the country, 10 percent of all drivers are legally impaired or drunk.

(FIGURE 13-9) **Studies show that drivers between the ages of 16 and 24 are three times as likely to die in a drunken-driving crash as older drivers.**

• • • TEACH continued

Role-Playing

Drunk Driving

Have students role-play the aftermath of drunken-driving accident:

Leo and Debbie leave a party after consuming beer and wine coolers. As he drives her home, Leo smashes into a utility pole. Debbie hurtles through the windshield and dies from a head injury. Leo has severe head and chest injuries requiring extensive surgery. Neither was wearing a seat belt.

Assign the following roles: police officer, newspaper reporter, parents and sister of Leo, single mother of Debbie, and child who witnessed the accident.

Reinforcement

Blood Alcohol Level

Direct students' attention to Figure 13-8, "Blood Alcohol Level and Its Effects." Explain the significance of the numbers by providing these examples:

- A "23 percent decrease in driving ability" means that a driver is about one-fourth slower in hitting the brakes when a child steps out in front of the car or when another driver pulls out in front.
- It means you lose about one-fourth of your alertness.
- It means you lose about one-fourth of your visual sharpness, which is especially dangerous at night. It's like dimming the headlights.

CONTRACT FOR LIFE

A Contract for Life Between Parent and Teenager

The SADD Drinking-Driver Contract

Teenager I agree to call you for your advice and/or transportation at any hour, from any place, if I am ever in a situation where I have been drinking or a friend or date who is driving me has been drinking.

Signature

Parent I agree to come and get you at any hour, any place, no questions asked and no argument at that time, or I will pay for a taxi to bring you home safely. I expect we would discuss this issue at a later time.

I agree to seek safe, sober transportation home if I am ever in a situation where I have had too much to drink or a friend who is driving me has had too much to drink.

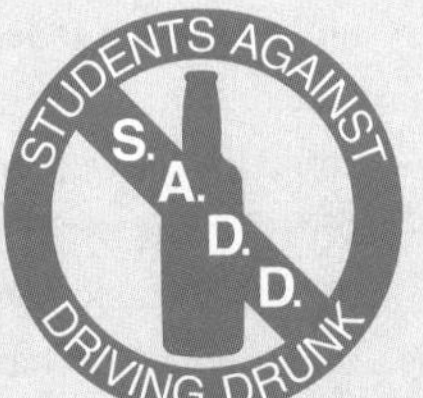

Signature

Date

S.A.D.D. does not condone drinking by those below the legal drinking age. S.A.D.D. encourages all young people to obey the laws of their state, including laws related to the legal drinking age.

Distributed by S.A.D.D., "Students Against Driving Drunk"

(FIGURE 13-10) **S.A.D.D. published this contract between parents and teenagers for the sake of reducing the amount of drunken-driving incidents. This organization does not approve, however, of alcohol use among teenagers.**

Making a Choice 13A

Alcohol-Free Activities

Assign the Alcohol-Free Activities card. The card requires students to list activities that cannot or should not be done by people who have been drinking.

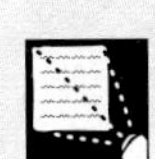

Teaching Transparency 13C
Drunk Driving: Facts and Numbers

Show the transparency *Drunken Driving: Facts and Numbers* and demonstrate how many in the class will be involved in alcohol-related traffic accidents in their lifetimes by having 40 percent of the class stand up. Then illustrate the 540,000 injured in alcohol-related crashes each year by comparing this number to city populations they may be familiar with. **If one person dies in an alcohol-related accident every 20 minutes, how many will die during this class period? How many will die today?** *[Two or three during class; (25,000 a year ÷ 365 days = 68 today)]*

Demonstration
Who Is Legally Drunk?

Prepare one index card for each student. Write LEGALLY DRUNK on 10 percent of the cards, and SOBER DRIVER on the remaining cards. Distribute the cards at random, face down, and ask the students which of them have a card that says "legally drunk" without turning the cards over. (This demonstrates that you can't tell which driver out of every 10 is drunk.) Have students turn over their cards to discover who is legally drunk. Explain that a driver should drive defensively and assume that all other drivers may be drunk.

Class Discussion
Contract for Life

Give students a moment to read S.A.D.D.'s "Contract for Life" and then dis-

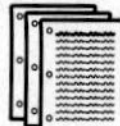

Life Skills Worksheet 13A

Assign the Hidden Persuasion Life Skills Worksheet, which has students spot hidden attempts at persuasion to drink alcohol.

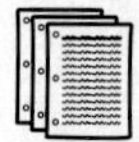

Life Skills Worksheet 13B

Resisting Peer Pressure

Assign the Resisting Peer Pressure Life Skills Worksheet. It requires students to examine strategies for resisting pressure to drink, taking into consideration their peer group, their own personal style, and their objectives.

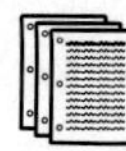

Life Skills Worksheet 13C

Building Self-Esteem

Assign the Building Self-Esteem Life Skills Worksheet, which requires students to explore strategies for raising self-esteem and to detect causes for low self-esteem.

Blood Alcohol Level's Effect on Death Risk

BAL	Chance of Dying
.02—.04	1.5 times as likely
.05—.09	11 times as likely
.10—.14	48 times as likely
.15+	380 times as likely

(FIGURE 13-11) **Drinking alcohol in any amount can put a person's life in danger.**

Breaking the Law

People under 21 break a law every time they have any alcohol (except under special circumstances, such as religious purposes). Like all crimes, getting caught drinking alcohol under the age of 21 can lead to arrest, a fine, and even a criminal record. Many teenagers have decided that they'd rather not risk their futures by drinking alcohol now. In addition, driving while under the influence of alcohol is illegal for people of all ages. A person does not have to be in an accident in order to be caught driving drunk—the driver of any car exceeding the speed limit or noticeably weaving through traffic is subject to inspection and a possible blood alcohol level test.

Losing Control

One of the best reasons not to drink is that alcohol can make a person lose control. Drinking to the point of intoxication can remove inhibitions completely. As a result, drunk people may find themselves doing things they regret.

For example, Krystal and Claudio are the school's most popular couple. Wherever they go is *the* place to be. Whatever they do, everyone wants to do too. It's a secret, but one thing they *haven't* done is have sexual intercourse.

Claudio lives with his grandmother, who happens to be out of town for the weekend. He takes advantage of this opportunity, and throws the year's wildest party. By the end of the night, everyone is very drunk, including Claudio and Krystal. The house is severely damaged: the stereo is broken beyond repair, and part of the carpet has been badly burned.

Claudio doesn't know any of this yet, because Krystal has suddenly decided she's ready to have sex with him. The two of them have stumbled to his bedroom.

Hours later, Claudio wakes up, horrified and ashamed. He hadn't wanted it to be like that. How could he have been so stupid? He knows they both made a mistake and that it's too late to go back now. What if Krystal gets pregnant? What about sexually transmitted diseases? Claudio knows that if they hadn't been drunk, they wouldn't have lost control.

Teenagers who drink are much more likely to get pregnant and also to suffer sex-

• • • TEACH continued

cuss what it says. Ask: Would you and your parent or guardian be willing to sign this contract, and stick by it? Do you think either you or the other signer might ever violate the contract? Why? If your parent or guardian is unwilling to sign the contract, is there another adult whom you deeply trust that you could get to sign the contract? Ask the following question, if needed: If you are not willing to sign this contract, suppose you have a friend killed in a drunken-driving accident tonight. Would you reconsider signing the contract?

Debate the Issue
Prohibition

Divide the class into two teams to debate the pros and cons of passing a law prohibiting the use of alcohol. Suggest that before students begin the debate they find out about the positive and negative effects of Prohibition in the 1920s in the United States, which outlawed all alcoholic beverages containing more than 0.5 percent alcohol.

Writing
Learning to Drink at Home

Tell students to picture a family gathering at which teenagers 13 to 18 are allowed to drink beer and wine. The parents feel that it's better the kids learn to hold their liquor at home than drink with their friends away from home. Have students write a paragraph explaining why the parents' rea-

ually transmitted diseases, such as AIDS, than those who don't. In fact, teenagers who use alcohol make up one of the fastest growing groups of people with AIDS in the United States.

Standards Set by Parents or Guardians

Many teenagers decide not to drink because they want to abide by the standards set by their parents or guardians. Chances are that a lot of students in your class have decided not to drink for this reason.

An Alcohol-Free Life

People who choose not to drink do so because they like being sober. They find that being drunk interferes with a lot of activities they enjoy—like taking part in sports, or going to the movies, or socializing with friends, or reading. Being sober allows them to get the most out of the things that make them happy.

What Would You Do ?

Making Responsible Decisions

He Doesn't *Seem* Drunk

You're at a party, and it's getting late. Your friend Cliff, who drove you to the party, tells you he's sober enough to take you home. He doesn't seem drunk at all, but you know he's had at least four or five drinks. What would you do?

Remember to use the decision-making steps:

1. **State the Problem.**
2. **List the Options.**
3. **Imagine the Benefits and Consequences.**
4. **Consider Your Values.**
5. **Weigh the Options and Decide.**
6. **Act.**
7. **Evaluate the Results.**

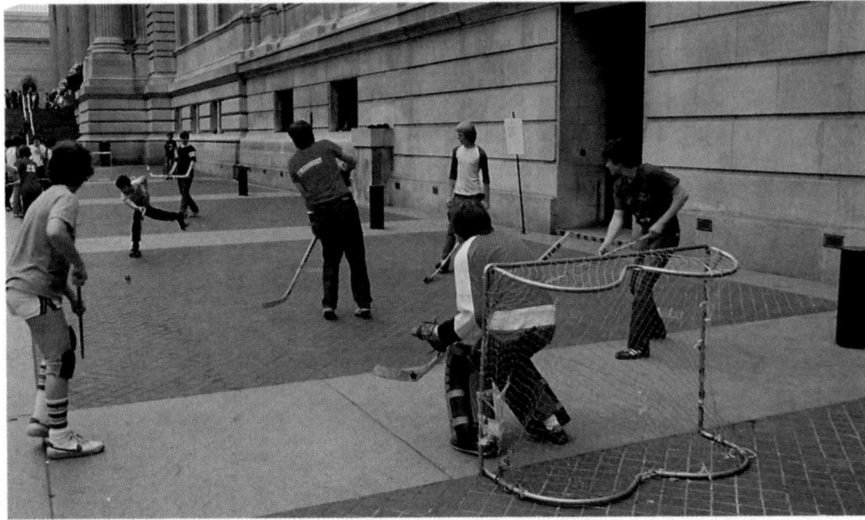

(FIGURE 13-12) **Life's healthiest and happiest activities never include drinking alcohol.**

What Would You Do ?

He Doesn't *Seem* Drunk

Have students read the description of the situation. Ask students how they would handle it. What would they say to Cliff, who does not appear drunk and may not acknowledge that he shouldn't drive? How would they find alternative transportation for themselves and for him? They should use the seven decision-making steps to help them make a reasonable choice.

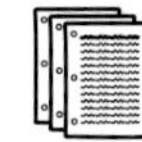

Section Review Worksheet 13.2

Assign Section Review Worksheet 13.2, which requires students to examine consequences of drinking.

Section Quiz 13.2

Have students take Section Quiz 13.2.

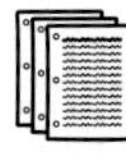

Reteaching Worksheet 13.2

Students who have difficulty with the material may complete Reteaching Worksheet 13.2, which requires them to list the reasons people drink or do not drink.

soning is wrong and what the dangers are of allowing teens to drink.

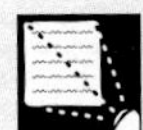

Teaching Transparency 13D
Reasons Not to Drink

Use the Reasons Not to Drink transparency to summarize information on the risks of alcohol use.

Cooperative Learning
Anti-drinking Advertisements

Have students form small groups to write anti-drinking ads that would appeal to teenagers. Tell them to be as creative as they wish and that the ads can be humorous.

Extension
Anti-drinking Organizations

If there is a chapter of S.A.D.D., M.A.D.D., or R.I.D. (Remove Intoxicated Drivers) in your school or community, have a representative meet with the class to explain their mission in stopping drunken driving.

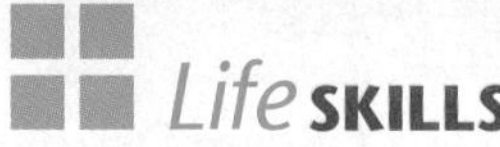

Life SKILLS

To Turn Down Alcohol

Have students individually use the seven decision-making steps in deciding whether to ride home with Cliff. Evaluate their decisions in a class discussion.

Review Answers

1. Answers may include: to appear cool, glamorous, or sophisticated; to feel relaxed; to be sociable; to ease emotional pain; to feel independent; to rebel; for excitement.

2. Answers may include: drinking and driving causes accidents; binge drinking can cause a person to go into a coma, or even death; purchasing alcohol in most states is illegal for anyone under the age of 21; drinking causes a person to lose control; drinking may lead to an unwanted pregnancy or to sexually transmitted diseases, including AIDS; drinking may go against parents' or guardians' standards.

Saying No Thanks

You may find yourself in the position of having to turn down a drink at a party. There are a lot of ways to do this, but in general, the less you make of it, the easier it's going to be. If someone asks you if you want a drink, try just saying "no thanks." Remember that you don't owe anyone any explanations.

For many teenagers, saying no to alcohol is a matter of self-esteem. In general, the higher a person's sense of confidence and responsibility are, the better he or she may be at resisting pressure.

See the Life Skills activity below for some situations that test your ability to turn down alcohol.

LifeSKILLS: Resisting Pressure

To Turn Down Alcohol

It's never easy to decide not to do something a lot of other people are doing. Still, resisting pressure to drink alcohol is one of the healthiest decisions you can ever make. If you do have to turn down alcohol, it may help to have some idea of what you want to do or say. On a separate sheet of paper, write down what you would do or say in each situation.

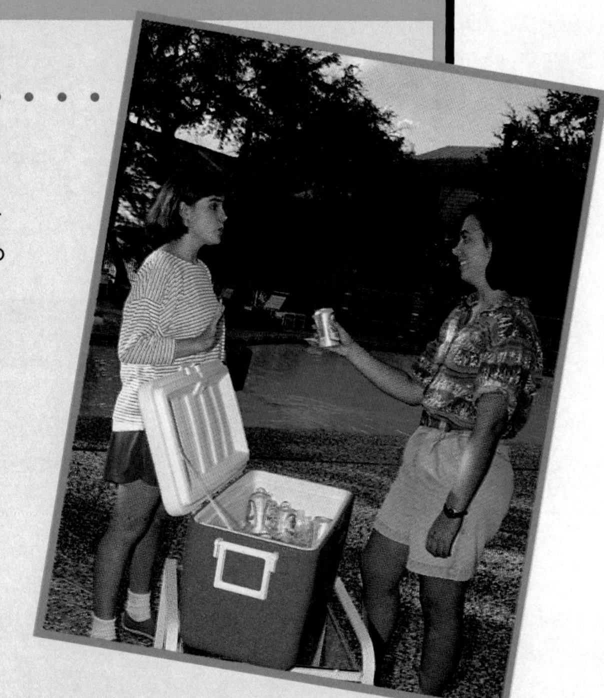

1. You're at a party, and a friend is about to get herself a beer. She asks if you want one.
2. You're with a group of friends who are passing around a bottle of liquor. The bottle comes to you, and you realize everyone is watching.
3. Four friends are sitting at a table playing a drinking game. They ask you to join them.
4. You're attracted to someone who likes to drink. The first time you're out together, he or she asks if you want to share a bottle of wine with dinner.

You don't have to make a big deal about the fact that you have chosen not to drink. But be firm about your decision. It is, after all, the right one.

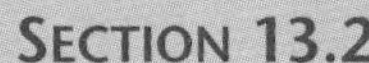

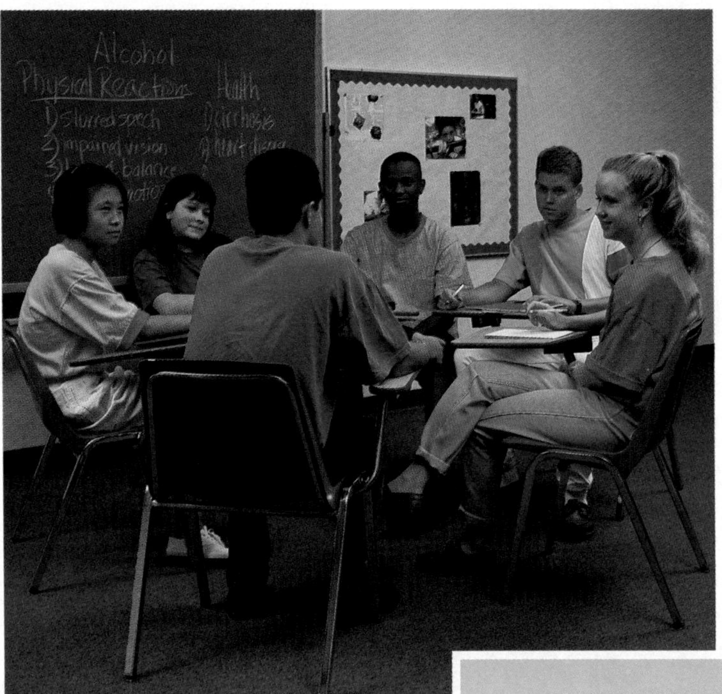

(FIGURE 13-13) **Talking about peer pressure and other issues with fellow students often helps teenagers resist the urge to use alcohol.**

Getting Involved

One of the most rewarding things you can do with your spare time is to volunteer for an anti-alcohol cause. This could mean planning an alcohol-free dance or other activities that bring people together without alcohol. You might want to think about organizing a discussion group for students in your school to talk about peer pressure or other things that tempt them to try alcohol.

In addition, look into joining your school or community chapter of S.A.D.D. or Remove Intoxicated Drivers (R.I.D.). Encourage your friends to volunteer with you. If you have trouble persuading them, remind them that drunken-driving crashes kill one teenager every three hours. Any organization that is working to bring that number down is worth the time and effort you put into it.

Review

1. *Name two reasons why some people drink.*
2. *What are four good reasons not to drink?*
3. *What are two myths a lot of teenagers hear about alcohol?*
4. ***LIFE SKILLS: Resisting Pressure*** *Name three ways you could refuse alcohol if a friend offers it to you.*
5. ***LIFE SKILLS: Making Responsible Decisions*** *Name two possible short-term negative consequences of accepting a ride with someone who has been drinking.*
6. ***Critical Thinking*** *Why are people who are intoxicated more likely to get into automobile crashes than people who are sober? Be specific.*

Section 13.2

Answers to Questions 1 and 2 are on p. 272.

3. Answers may include: you can't get as drunk from beer, wine, or wine coolers as you can from hard liquor; a person who looks and acts sober is sober; having a cup of coffee or a cold shower can make a person less drunk.

4. Answers will vary. Students may answer, "No thanks" or "I don't want to break the law" or "I don't like the taste of alcohol."

5. Answers will vary. Students may answer, being involved in a drunken-driving accident and being injured.

6. Alcohol impairs coordination, vision, judgment, and reaction time, all of which decrease a person's ability to control a car.

ASSESS

Section Review

Have students answer the Section Review questions.

Alternative Assessment

Point out that many adults drink heavily on holidays, especially at Christmastime and on New Year's Eve. **Why do so many people drink heavily on these holidays? What are some good reasons not to drink on these holidays?** *[Holiday traffic is heavier and therefore creates more opportunities for accidents; winter weather may make driving hazardous; hangovers reduce the enjoyment of the season.]*

Closure

Using Common Sense

Have students suggest responses to friends who say the following:

- My mom drinks, even at work, and nobody knows it. Why shouldn't I drink?
- People say alcohol is just another drug, but it's not—it's legal.

Background
Causes of Alcoholism

Alcoholics were once believed to be morally weak people who could stop drinking if they only tried harder. But in the 1950s the American Medical Association (AMA) defined alcoholism as a disease instead of a character flaw. According to the AMA's *Encyclopedia of Medicine,* alcohol addiction is caused by interaction of personality, environment, and the addictive nature of the drug. This medical association identifies several factors that can contribute to addiction: drinking heavily for a long time, availability and affordability of alcohol, social acceptance, stress from loneliness or loss, hormonal factors in women, and insecure personalities.

Section 13.3 Alcohol Abuse and Alcoholism

Objectives

- *Know the three phases of alcoholism.*
- *Name the most important risks of alcohol abuse.*
- *Know how alcohol can affect an unborn child.*
- *Know the ways in which a family can be damaged by a family member's alcoholism.*

alcoholism: *the state of being psychologically and physically addicted to alcohol.*

According to the American Medical Association, alcoholism is a disease just like cancer or heart disease. Most people who have this disease pass through three phases: abuse, dependence, and addiction.

Abuse

When a person who drinks alcohol cannot do so in moderation or at appropriate times, he or she is abusing alcohol. There are more people who abuse alcohol than you may realize. Every person who drives drunk, for example, is abusing alcohol. People who become violent or angry when they are drunk, or do things they wouldn't do when they are sober, are abusing alcohol.

Leo, Claudio, and Krystal are examples of teenagers who are abusing alcohol. In reality, all teenagers who drink alcohol are abusing it, because they are doing something illegal.

People who abuse alcohol regularly can suffer in many ways. They often do poorly in school or at their jobs. And they are likely to engage in risky behaviors, such as having unprotected sex.

Signs of Alcohol Abuse

Odor on the breath	*Frequent absences*
Intoxication	*Unexplained bruises or accidents*
Difficulty focusing, glazed eyes	*Irritability*
Uncharacteristically passive or aggressive behavior	*Loss of memory (blackouts)*
Decline in personal appearance or hygiene	*Changes in peer-group associations and friendships*
Decline in school or work performance	*Damaged relationships with family members or close friends*

(FIGURE 13-14) **Every teenager who drinks alcohol is an alcohol abuser.**

Section 13.3 Lesson Plan

MOTIVATE

Journal 13C
Do You Like the Way It Tastes?

This may be done as a warm-up activity. In the Student Journal, have students tell whether they like the taste of alcoholic beverages and explain their answer.

TEACH

Class Discussion
Signs of Alcohol Abuse

Write the following on the chalkboard:

Drinking → Abuse → Dependence → Addiction → Recovery

Explain that not all drinking leads to abuse, but when it does, this is the path it often follows. **What are signs of abuse?** *[Examples: drunken driving, poor schoolwork, behavioral changes]* Write them on the chalkboard under *abuse.* **What are signs of psychological dependence?** *[Need alcohol to function; constant desire for it; no withdrawal symptoms if drinking stops]* **What are signs of addiction?** *[Alcohol first priority; neglect everything else; withdrawal symptoms if drinking stops]*

Debate the Issue
Who Is Responsible?

Divide the class to debate the following topic: Alcoholics should not be held responsible for any crime they commit; they can't help being drunk,

Risk Factors for Alcoholism

Risk Factors You Cannot Control	Risk Factors You Can Control
Genes	*Drinking before the age of 21*
Environment	*Associating with people who drink*
	Bending to peer pressure
	Drinking beyond moderation
	Drinking at inappropriate times
	Drinking alone

(FIGURE 13-15) **Most risk factors for alcoholism can be avoided. For this reason, alcoholism is a preventable disease.**

Dependence

People in the dependence phase of alcoholism feel they need the drug to function properly. They have a very strong and constant desire for alcohol. At this point this desire is a psychological one only, which means that they are not yet physically addicted to alcohol. Even so, alcohol is beginning to dominate their lives.

Addiction

Eventually the dependence on alcohol becomes physical as well as psychological. Those who are physically dependent on alcohol suffer unpleasant withdrawal symptoms if they don't have a regular fix. Studies show that teenagers can become physically dependent, or addicted, much more quickly than adults. Teenagers who abuse alcohol can become addicted to it in as little as one to two years. It takes most adults about 5 to 20 years of alcohol abuse to become addicted.

Once a person becomes both psychologically and physically dependent on alcohol, he or she is an alcoholic.

Being addicted to alcohol means putting the drug before everything else. Alcoholics often neglect their jobs, their responsibilities, even their families, because their one focus—the one thing they think about—is on getting more alcohol. Sometimes they will substitute alcohol for food, which can lead to serious health problems such as malnutrition.

They may also be in a constant state of denial. People who are completely addicted to alcohol may resent any suggestion that they may have a drinking problem. They often claim that they can quit any time they want. In reality, such people usually need assistance in order to stop drinking.

Causes of Alcoholism It's not completely clear why some people can drink alcohol without becoming addicted, while others become alcoholics.

SECTION 13.3

Background

Genetic Predisposition to Alcoholism

Genetic predisposition is believed to be one factor in becoming an alcoholic. About half of the Asian people—Japanese, Chinese, Koreans, and others—however, have a genetic predisposition *not* to become alcoholics. In people with this genetic makeup, drinking causes nausea, sweating, and other unpleasant symptoms. This may be a factor in Japan's low rate of alcoholism, which is about half that in the United States. Some Native Americans also have this genetic makeup.

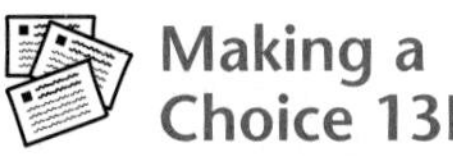

Making a Choice 13B

Who Is Vulnerable

Assign the Who Is Vulnerable card. The card asks students to discuss traits and experiences that may predispose young people to drink alcohol.

because of a genetic predisposition. Allow each side to state its case and make counterarguments. Explain that doctors and psychologists have argued for years whether alcoholics are people who drink too much and thus become addicted, or whether they are genetically predisposed to drinking. There is no single cause of alcoholism, but a combination of factors.

Journal 13D
Risk Factors

Go over the six risk factors that everyone can control (Figure 13-15). Reach a consensus on what each category means—for example, "drinking beyond moderation" might mean anything beyond one or two drinks; "drinking at inappropriate times" might mean drinking when one gets up in the morning. Then have students turn to the Student Journal and evaluate themselves on the risk factors they can control. Suggest that students put each of the risk factors in a vertical list and before each, write *Never, Rarely, Sometimes,* or *Often.*

Reinforcement
Fetal Alcohol Syndrome

Refer students to Figure 13-17. **Explain that this child is deformed because its mother drank while she was pregnant. What's the best way to prevent FAS?** *[Don't drink.]* Explain

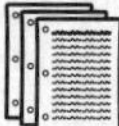

Section Review Worksheet 13.3

Assign Section Review Worksheet 13.3, which requires students to identify elements and consequences of alcohol abuse and alcoholism.

Section Quiz 13.3

Have students take Section Quiz 13.3.

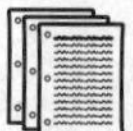

Reteaching Worksheet 13.3

Students who have difficulty with the material may complete Reteaching Worksheet 13.3, which requires them to classify statements according to alcohol abuse, alcohol dependence, and alcohol addiction.

fetal alcohol syndrome (FAS):

a set of birth defects that can occur when a pregnant woman drinks alcohol. These defects include low birth weight, mental retardation, facial deformities, and behavioral problems.

Some evidence shows that children of alcoholics are more likely than others to become alcoholics as adults. And some evidence indicates that the likelihood of becoming an alcoholic may be inherited through genes.

But it is difficult to separate the possible effects of genetic traits from environmental factors. Children who grow up in alcoholic families are less likely than others to get their emotional needs met. So when they get older, they may use alcohol to numb their emotional pain.

Alcoholism probably results from a combination of psychological, environmental, and physical factors.

(FIGURE 13-16) **Living with an alcoholic family member can be confusing and lonely. But with proper treatment, the families of alcoholics can fully recover—regardless of whether the alcoholic they are living with does.**

Fetal Alcohol Syndrome

When a pregnant woman drinks alcohol, every bit of the drug in her system passes into the bloodstream of her unborn child. Babies who are exposed to alcohol in this way are at risk of suffering from a set of defects known as **fetal alcohol syndrome (FAS).** These defects include low birth weight, mental retardation, facial deformities, and behavioral problems.

No one is exactly sure how much alcohol must reach the unborn child in order for FAS to occur, so many doctors advise women not to drink alcohol at all while they're pregnant. Women who are not addicted to alcohol have no trouble following this suggestion. Alcoholic women, however, may have difficulty staying away from alcohol for nine months.

Alcohol and the Family

Dennis's two sons love to be with him when he is sober. That's when he is warm and affectionate—that's when they know that he loves them. It's when he's drunk that everything becomes unpredictable. While drunk, he has beat them more times than they want to remember.

This behavior is not unusual—it is estimated that between 50 and 80 percent of all family violence involves alcohol.

But the damage alcoholism has caused Dennis's family goes beyond physical violence. The two sons don't talk about it, but they know that they must avoid their father when he is drunk. They also must make excuses for him when he is too intoxicated to go to work. They spend their time wondering what Dennis will be like at the end of the day. Will he have gone to work? Will he threaten them? Or will he be kind and loving, and make promises they know he won't keep? Dennis's addiction has taken over his entire family.

• • • TEACH continued

that FAS children generally require special medical care costing many thousands of dollars. Who do you think should pay for this special medical cost—the parents, a national health-care program, the government? Would it be fair to levy a special tax on alcohol or the alcoholic beverage manufacturer? Why or why not? Stress that the entire FAS problem could be prevented by not drinking.

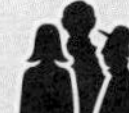

Cooperative Learning

Alcohol and the Family

Divide the class into groups of four or five students to discuss what Dennis's family should do to help him and themselves. Ask them to recommend specific steps for Dennis, such as throwing away the liquor, or going for counseling; for the family, such as taking him to court or leaving him. Then have the groups compare notes and reach a consensus on the best approach for Dennis and his family.

Extension

History of Alcohol

Have students use encyclopedias to discover the history of alcohol use in the United States from colonial times to the present, including the temperance movement and Prohibition during 1918–1933.

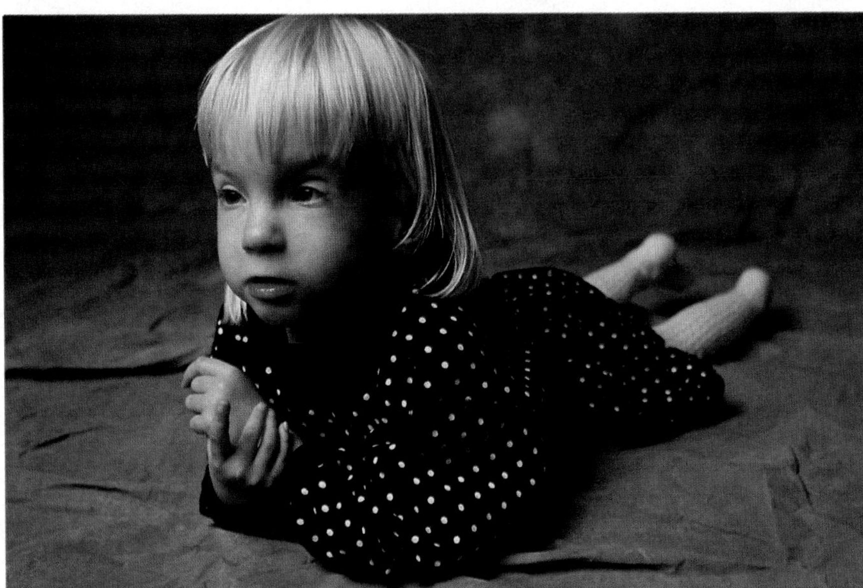

(FIGURE 13-17) **Fetal alcohol syndrome is a set of birth defects that can affect the babies of women who drink alcohol while pregnant.**

Being controlled by a family member or a loved one's addiction is sometimes called being codependent. Teenagers who have an alcoholic parent often don't know what to expect when they come home from school. Some have learned that if they don't take responsibility for something, no one in the family will. They may find themselves doing responsible jobs at home, such as making sure the utility bill is paid, that teenagers from nonalcoholic families usually don't have to worry about. And even though they are doing so much for the family, these teenagers often feel as though they are somehow to blame for everything. They may think that they're constantly in the way.

The important thing for them to know is that their parent's drinking is *not* their fault, and that they can get help.

In the next section you'll learn about treatment for alcoholism and about the help available for family members of alcoholics.

Review

1. *What are the three phases of alcoholism?*
2. *What are three dangers of alcohol abuse?*
3. *Explain how a pregnant woman's drinking can affect her unborn child.*
4. *How can a parent's alcoholism affect the children?*
5. ***Critical Thinking*** *What do you think are some psychological and sociological factors that can cause a person to become an alcoholic?*

Review Answers

1. Abuse, dependence, addiction
2. Answers will vary but may include drunk driving, violent behavior, breaking the law, doing poorly in school or on the job, engaging in risky behaviors, neglecting or abusing family and friends, and having health problems.
3. It may result in fetal alcohol syndrome, which includes defects such as low birth weight, mental retardation, facial deformities, and behavioral problems.
4. Answers will vary. Accept answers that indicate a variety of abusive behaviors by parents with this disease, such as physical abuse, mental abuse, and emotional abuse.
5. Answers will vary. Psychological factors might include desire to numb emotional pain and to feel relaxed; sociological factors might include to be one of the group, or to bend to peer pressure because everyone else is drinking.

ASSESS

Section Review

Have students answer the Section Review questions.

Alternative Assessment

Drinking Behavior

Ask students to recall Leo, who liked beer with lunch. Have them write a paragraph explaining which stage of alcoholism Leo is in, how they can tell, and what other signs of alcohol abuse Leo exhibits.

Closure

Still a Problem

Discuss the following question: **Given all the problems with alcohol abuse and alcoholism, why do people in our society continue to drink?** *[Alcohol relaxes people, relieves physical and emotional discomfort, and makes people high; it is legal, unlike other drugs; it is widely available; it is heavily advertised; it is culturally sanctioned.]*

Background
Repeated Treatment

More than half of the alcoholics who undergo treatment are able to abstain from alcohol. But it is not unusual for an alcoholic to resume drinking, especially in response to a trauma such as the loss of a loved one or a job. Thus, alcoholics sometimes must go through withdrawal and treatment more than once.

Background
Alcoholics Anonymous

Alcoholics Anonymous (AA) was founded in Akron, Ohio, by two alcoholics, salesman Bill W. and surgeon Dr. Bob (AA does not use last names; hence the organization's name). A desire to stop drinking is the only prerequisite to becoming a member. No membership or attendance records are kept and no fee is charged—the meetings run on donations. AA is completely independent of government and religious and other organizations. AA has over 1 million members in the United States and over 2 million worldwide.

Section 13.4 Hope for Recovery

Objectives

- *Discuss the treatment options for alcohol abuse.*
- *Learn how to get help if you or someone you know abuses alcohol.*
  LIFE SKILLS: Using Community Resources

withdrawal: *the process of discontinuing a drug to which the body has become addicted.*

In order to quit drinking, an alcoholic must first admit that he or she is powerless over alcohol. Then the process of recovery can begin. Sometimes a person who is addicted to alcohol can reach this conclusion by himself or herself. Other times it may take intervention by friends and family to get an alcoholic to this point. But no matter how it happens, a person who has admitted this has completed the first step of the recovery process.

Withdrawal

When an alcoholic quits drinking, he or she goes through **withdrawal.** Withdrawal is the process of discontinuing a drug to which the body has become addicted. During withdrawal, a person may suffer extreme

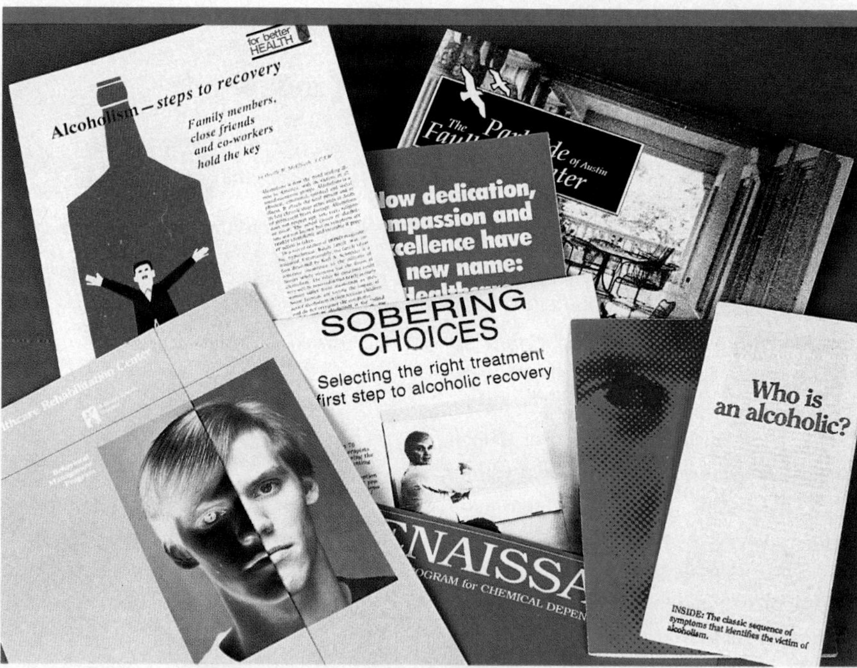

(FIGURE 13-18) **All alcoholics who want to overcome their addiction must first admit that they are powerless over alcohol.**

Section 13.4 Lesson Plan

MOTIVATE

Journal 13E
Attitudes Toward Drinking Now

This may be done as a warm-up activity. In the Student Journal, ask students to write about whether their attitudes toward drinking and alcohol abuse have changed based on what they learned in this chapter and, if it has changed, how it changed.

TEACH

Class Discussion
Getting Into Treatment

Write the following sequence on the chalkboard:

Admit → Quit → Withdrawal → Recovery

Have students explain how they are interrelated and then supply withdrawal symptoms and features of recovery programs as you write them. **Why must alcoholics first admit that they are powerless over alcohol?** *[Unless they admit they are powerless over alcohol, they can't be helped to get well.]* **Does quitting drinking mean slowing down, or stopping entirely?** *[Stop entirely]* **Why should withdrawal be medically supervised?** *[The seizures during withdrawal can be dangerous, and various prescription drugs are used to aid withdrawal.]* **During recovery, why do families undergo counseling as well as the alcoholic?**

nervousness, headaches, tremors, or seizures. Ordinarily these symptoms would go away once the alcoholic has some alcohol. But there is no such relief for a person who has decided to quit drinking. The withdrawal phase of recovery usually lasts no more than a few days. Those going through it, however, may want to be under constant medical supervision.

Inpatient and Outpatient Programs

Alcoholics who have gone through withdrawal are no longer physically addicted to alcohol. Now the harder part comes, because they have to stop being emotionally addicted as well. People who have at one time depended on alcohol to help them cope with problems may want a drink whenever times are hard. And because they are alcoholics, having just one drink is likely to make them physically and emotionally addicted once again. That's why patients in treatment programs are not allowed any alcohol at all.

Some recovering alcoholics decide to join hospital inpatient programs, which means that they live at the hospital while receiving treatment. Others choose to move home after completing withdrawal, and to participate in hospital outpatient programs. After going through withdrawal, patients in both programs receive counseling in order to understand why they became addicted to alcohol, and to help them cope with life without it. This may come in the form of individual sessions, or in group therapy, which gives the patient the opportunity to talk to other people going through the same thing. Many hospitals also offer therapy sessions and education classes for families of alcoholics, who are also in a recovery process—living with an alcoholic can be as damaging as being one.

Alcoholics Anonymous

There are many self-help programs for alcoholics. By far the most widely used of these is Alcoholics Anonymous (AA). Many hospital treatment programs require their patients to attend AA meetings. In addition, AA has helped a large number of alcoholics stop drinking without any other form of treatment.

The AA method for recovery involves 12 steps. The first and perhaps most important of these is for the alcoholic to recognize that he or she is powerless over alcohol.

Through regular meetings and shared experience, AA members bring themselves and each other closer to their goal of a life that is free of alcohol, and full of emotional, physical, and spiritual well-being. Such a goal, AA members know, can only be reached one day at a time. For this reason, many recovering alcoholics attend AA meetings every day, and learn to celebrate every day, week, month, and year they conquer without alcohol.

To find out about AA meetings in your area, look in the phone book under "Alcoholics Anonymous."

Al-Anon and Alateen

Having a parent, a sibling, or a spouse who is an alcoholic can make a person feel alone and lost. Al-Anon and Alateen were formed to bring people who are feeling this way together.

Al-Anon is designed to help family members talk about the problems of living with an alcoholic. Alateen was specifically designed to help teenagers cope with the same situation.

Meetings at Al-Anon and Alateen are very much like those of AA. People who feel like talking about their experiences can do so. Those who would rather just listen don't have to say anything. Knowing that

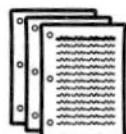

Life Skills Worksheet 13D

Using Community Resources

Assign the Using Community Resources Life Skills Worksheet, which requires students to locate all the resources available for breaking addiction and staying off alcohol, gather information about them, and compare them with one another.

Section Review Worksheet 13.4

Assign Section Review Worksheet 13.4, which requires students to identify steps to recovery and resources for recovery.

Section Quiz 13.4

Have students take Section Quiz 13.4.

[Because living with an alcoholic can be as damaging as being one.]

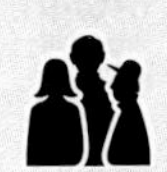

Cooperative Learning
Finding Out About Available Services

Divide the class into five groups to research alcohol treatment, therapy, and support available in your area. Each group should prepare a report showing their contacts, addresses, and phone numbers, and present to the class a summary of the services.

Case Study
Classroom Visit

Contact the local AA chapter and ask for an alcoholic to visit the class to be interviewed for this case study. Ask students to prepare questions before the visit and review them with the class. Have each student write a summary of the interview.

Reinforcement
Abstinence

A recovering alcoholic's abstinence must be permanent. Reinforce this fact by asking these questions: **How soon after recovery is it safe for an alcoholic to enjoy one small glass of wine at a special occasion?** *[Never. He or she must never drink again.]* **If a recovering alcoholic has a bad cold, should he or she take a spoonful of a cold remedy that contains alcohol?** *[No. He or she must never have any form of alcohol.]*

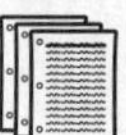

Reteaching Worksheet 13.4

Students who have difficulty with the material may complete Reteaching Worksheet 13.4, which requires them to recall the steps and the rationale of the recovery process.

Review Answers

1. A person can join an inpatient program, an outpatient program, or a self-help program.

2. Look in the phone book under "Alcoholics Anonymous" for a number to call, or call the Al-Anon Family Group Headquarters hotline: 1-800-344-2666.

3. Call the Al-Anon Family Group Headquarters hotline: 1-800-344-2666.

4. Students might answer that living with an alcoholic can be damaging because it can make other family members feel alone and lost. Often the other family members feel as though they are to blame for everything and that they are constantly in the way.

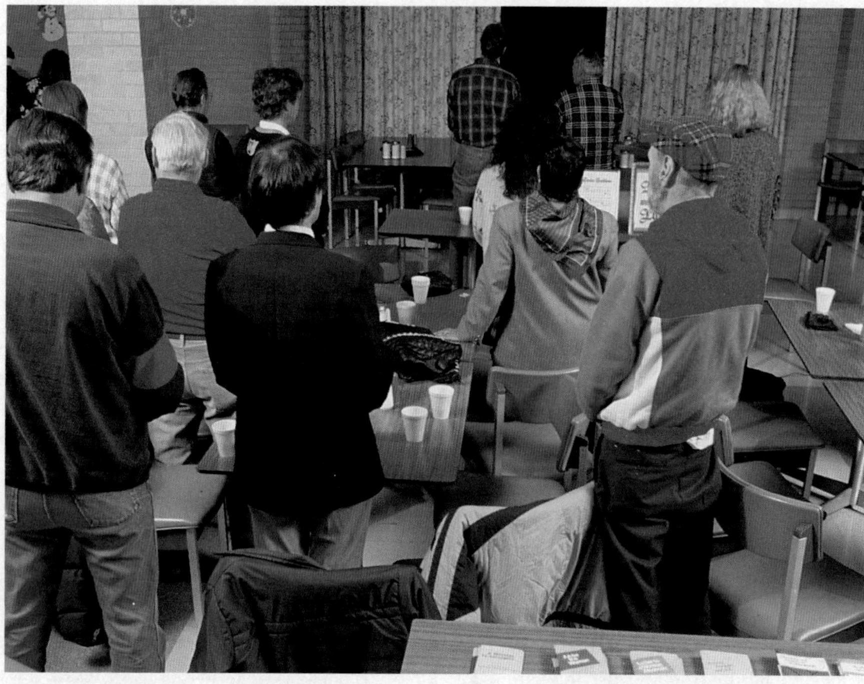

(FIGURE 13-19) **Alcoholics Anonymous is the most widely used and the most successful of the self-help programs. It has helped many alcoholics stop drinking without hospital treatment.**

NATIONAL
AL-ANON FAMILY GROUP HEADQUARTERS HOTLINE
NUMBERS

1-800-344-2666

other people are going through the same thing can make some very difficult situations less painful.

One of the most important goals of groups like Al-Anon and Alateen is to help people realize that they can get help whether or not the alcoholic they are living with gets treatment. Even if the alcoholic keeps drinking, the family members can improve their own lives.

To find out about Al-Anon and Alateen meetings in your area, look in the phone book under "Alcoholics Anonymous." The person who answers the phone can tell you about meetings in your town. Or you can call the Al-Anon Family Group Headquarters free hotline number shown at the left. They keep a list of Al-Anon and Alateen groups throughout the country.

Review

1. *Describe three ways a person can begin recovery from alcoholism.*
2. ***LIFE SKILLS: Using Community Resources*** *How could you find out about meetings of Alcoholics Anonymous in your area?*
3. ***LIFE SKILLS: Using Community Resources*** *How could you find out about meetings of Alateen in your area?*
4. ***Critical Thinking*** *Do you agree with the statement: "Living with an alcoholic can be as damaging as being one?" Why or why not?*

• • • TEACH continued

Extension
Drug Therapy

Many recovering alcoholics take the drug disulfiram (it makes them quite sick if they drink). Have students research this drug to discover what it does, how it works, and why it is so helpful to a recovering alcoholic.

ASSESS

Section Review

Have students answer the Section Review questions.

Alternative Assessment
Going It Alone

An alcoholic has decided that she is stronger than alcohol, will quit drinking by locking herself in a room, and will begin an alcohol-free life without anyone's help. Have students write an explanation of why she probably will fail.

Closure
Self-Esteem

Ask students to explain the relationship between self-esteem and the ability to resist alcohol. What is that relationship? Can low self-esteem be improved? Can damaged self-esteem be rebuilt?

Highlights

Summary

- One drink can impair a person's judgment, reflexes, and vision enough to cause an automobile accident.
- Drinking alcohol can cause hangovers, damage the liver and heart, kill brain cells, and increase a person's chances of getting cancers of the liver, esophagus, pharynx, and larynx.
- Minimize your risk of getting involved in a drunken-driving incident by not drinking, and by not accepting a ride with anyone who has been drinking.
- Alcohol can be deadly if a person drinks enough of it at one time.
- Teenagers who drink are much more likely to get pregnant and to contract sexually transmitted diseases, such as AIDS, than those who don't.
- Alcoholics and the people who are close to them can be helped by groups and programs such as Alcoholics Anonymous, Al-Anon, and Alateen.

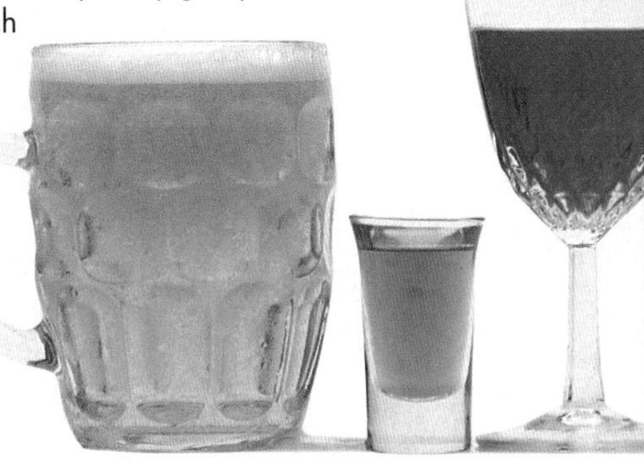

Vocabulary

blood alcohol level (BAL) a way to measure the level of alcohol in a person's body.

intoxicated being affected by alcohol. Effects of intoxication can range from mild lightheadedness to severe and complete loss of judgment and reflexes.

hangover uncomfortable physical effects brought on by alcohol use. Symptoms of a hangover include headache, nausea, upset stomach, and dizziness.

hepatitis (hep-uh-TY-tis) an inflammation of the liver that can be caused by long-term abuse. Symptoms of hepatitis include high fever, weakness, and a yellowing of the skin.

cirrhosis (sur-OH-sis) a condition in which liver cells are replaced by useless scar tissue. Cirrhosis can be caused by long-term alcohol abuse.

alcoholism the state of being psychologically and physically addicted to alcohol.

fetal alcohol syndrome (FAS) a set of birth defects that can occur when a pregnant woman drinks alcohol. These defects include low birth weight, mental retardation, facial deformities, and behavioral problems.

withdrawal the process of discontinuing the use of a drug to which the body has become addicted.

Chapter 13 Highlights Strategies

Summary

Have students read the summary to reinforce the concepts they have learned in Chapter 13.

Vocabulary

Discuss the definitions of blood alcohol level (BAL), fetal alcohol syndrome (FAS), alcoholism, co-dependent, withdrawal, and recovering alcoholic. Ask if there are any terms students are uncertain about.

Extension

Hold an anti-drinking poster competition, and display the posters in places where they will be seen by everyone in the school. The posters might address common myths about alcohol and might advocate never drinking and driving.

Chapter 13 Assessment

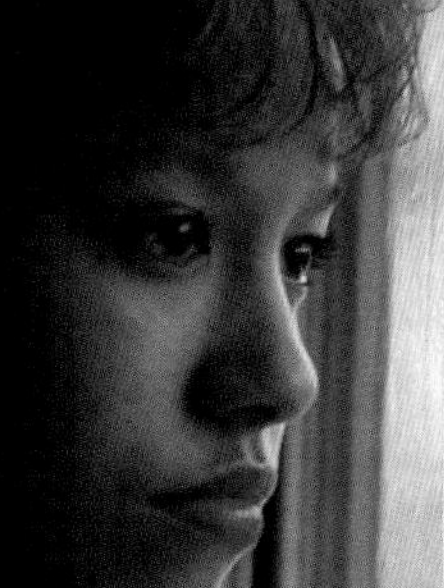

Chapter Review

Concept Review

1. How does alcohol affect the mind and body?
2. What is one way that drinking alcohol can make an individual less social?
3. How does alcohol affect a person's driving? What are two consequences of driving drunk?
4. What is S.A.D.D.? What is the purpose of their "Contract for Life"?
5. How is saying "no" a matter of self-esteem?
6. What are some signs that a person has a drinking problem?
7. How is the dependence stage of alcoholism different from the addiction stage?
8. Why can some people drink alcohol without becoming addicted, while others become alcoholics?
9. What does being codependent mean?
10. What is the first step in recovering from alcoholism?
11. What help is available for a problem drinker?

Expressing Your Views

1. You're about to leave a party with a friend, but then you realize that both of you have had too much to drink. What should you do?
2. People who drink at parties often try to get everyone else there to drink as well. Why do you think people who drink try to pressure others to drink?
3. Mothers Against Drunk Driving (M.A.D.D.) is an organization that promotes stricter penalties for people who drive drunk. Contact this organization to find out what your state's acceptable blood alcohol level is and what the local and state penalties are for drunken driving. Do you think these penalties are fair and adequate? Why or why not?

Chapter Review

Concept Review

Sample responses:

1. Alcohol interferes with a person's judgment, reflexes, coordination, vision, speech, and hearing. A person may at first feel relaxed and uninhibited; he or she may be impulsive. With very high blood alcohol levels, a person could go into a coma and die.

2. Drinking alcohol lessens a person's inhibitions and judgment. This can lead to obnoxious behavior, such as laughing loudly and being rude. It can also cause a person to become angry and aggressive.

3. Drinking alcohol severely impairs a person's judgment, reflexes, and vision, making the person incapable of controlling a car or reacting quickly enough to avoid an accident. Being arrested for drunk driving and being involved in an accident are two consequences of driving drunk.

4. Students Against Driving Drunk; to reduce the number of drunk-driving incidents.

5. In general, a person with high self-esteem also has a higher sense of confidence and responsibility, making it easier to say no to drinking.

6. The person may do poorly in school or at work and engage in risky behavior. Also, he or she has a strong desire for alcohol and may make up excuses to drink.

7. People in the dependence stage have a strong desire for alcohol. This desire is psychological only. In the addiction stage, the dependence on alcohol is both psychological and physical.

8. There is some evidence indicating a predisposition to alcoholism may be inherited through genes.

9. Being controlled by a family member's or loved one's addiction to alcohol.

10. The alcoholic must first admit that he or she is powerless over alcohol.

11. Inpatient and outpatient programs, as well as self-help programs, such as Alcoholics Anonymous

Expressing Your Views

Sample responses:

1. Do not drive and do not let my friend drive; instead get a ride home from someone who has not been drinking or call my parents for a ride home

2. Most people don't want to drink alone.

3. Answers will vary depending on state laws.

Chapter 13 Assessment

Life Skills Check

1. **Using Community Resources**
   Charlie's mother is an alcoholic. Sometimes she's asleep on the living room couch when Charlie comes home from school. Other times she's awake, but impatient with Charlie and quick to get angry over small things. Charlie knows she needs help, and would also like to talk to someone about how his mother's drinking affects him. What can Charlie do to get help?

2. **Resisting Pressure**
   Movies, television, and advertisements often seem to encourage audiences to drink by making alcohol consumption seem appealing and sophisticated. What can you do to resist this pressure to drink?

3. **Communicating Effectively**
   You think your friend may have a drinking problem because she always smells like alcohol, and because she often seems drunk. What could you say to persuade her to contact a group that could help her with her problem?

Projects

1. Make a poster advertising Al-Anon and Alateen meetings. Display these posters throughout the school. Include suggestions and illustrations to help the problem drinker. You might also write to these organizations for any additional information to display.

2. Create a bulletin board to show alcohol's effect on various parts of the body such as the brain, kidneys, liver, stomach, and heart. Include illustrations and labels, along with diseases brought about by alcohol abuse.

Plan for Action

About half of all fatal driving accidents are related to alcohol use. Devise a plan to ensure that you will always drive sober.

Life Skills Check

Sample responses:

1. He can contact Al-Anon or Alateen.

2. Know the dangers of drinking and know that the right decision is not to drink

3. I could tell her that I know something is wrong and there are people, including myself, who are willing to stand by her and help her. I would suggest she call Alcoholics Anonymous to find out where in the community help is available to her. I would also encourage her to attend a meeting and offer to go with her for support.

Projects

Have students plan and carry out the projects within the school.

Plan for Action

Ask students to recall the photograph at the start of the chapter. Do they know more now about what might happen if they were persuaded to drink alcohol? Do they have better ideas for resisting such pressure? Ask students to suggest arguments they'd make if pressured to drink with friends.

Assessment Options

Chapter Test

Have students take the Chapter 13 Test.

Alternative Assessment

Have students do the Alternative Assessment activity for Chapter 13.

Test Generator

The Test Generator (Macintosh® or IBM® format) contains an additional 50 assessment items for this chapter.

CHAPTER 14

TOBACCO: HAZARDOUS AND ADDICTIVE

PLANNING GUIDE

TEXT SECTIONS	OBJECTIVES	TEXT FEATURES	OUTSIDE RESOURCES	NOTES
14.1 **The Effects of Tobacco on the Body** pp. 285-291 1 period	• Name three major chemicals in tobacco. • Name two kinds of diseases smoking can cause. • Name one disease smokeless tobacco can cause. • Know the difference between mainstream and sidestream smoke. ■ Know how to request that a person not smoke in your presence.	■ LIFE SKILLS: Communicating Effectively, p. 290 **ASSESSMENT** • Section Review, p. 291	**TEACHER'S RESOURCE BINDER** • Lesson Plan 14.1 • Personal Health Inventory • Journal Entry 14A • Life Skills 14A • Media Worksheet • Section Review Worksheet 14.1 • Section Quiz 14.1 • Reteaching Worksheet 14.1 **OTHER RESOURCES** • Transparencies 14A, 14B • English/Spanish Audiocassette 4	
14.2 **A Tobacco-Free Life** pp. 292-294 1 period	• Know two reasons why people start using tobacco. • Know three reasons not to use tobacco. • Know two strategies you can use to quit smoking.	**ASSESSMENT** • Section Review, p. 294	**TEACHER'S RESOURCE BINDER** • Lesson Plan 14.2 • Journal Entries 14B, 14C • Life Skills 14B • Section Review Worksheet 14.2 • Section Quiz 14.2 • Reteaching Worksheet 14.2 **OTHER RESOURCES** • Making a Choice 14A, 14B	
End of Chapter pp. 295-297		**ASSESSMENT** • Chapter Review, pp. 296-297	**TEACHER'S RESOURCE BINDER** • Chapter Test • Alternative Assessment • Personal Pledge **OTHER RESOURCES** • Test Generator	

■ Denotes LIFE SKILLS objectives

• Items in blue are also part of the *Holt Health Activity Book.*

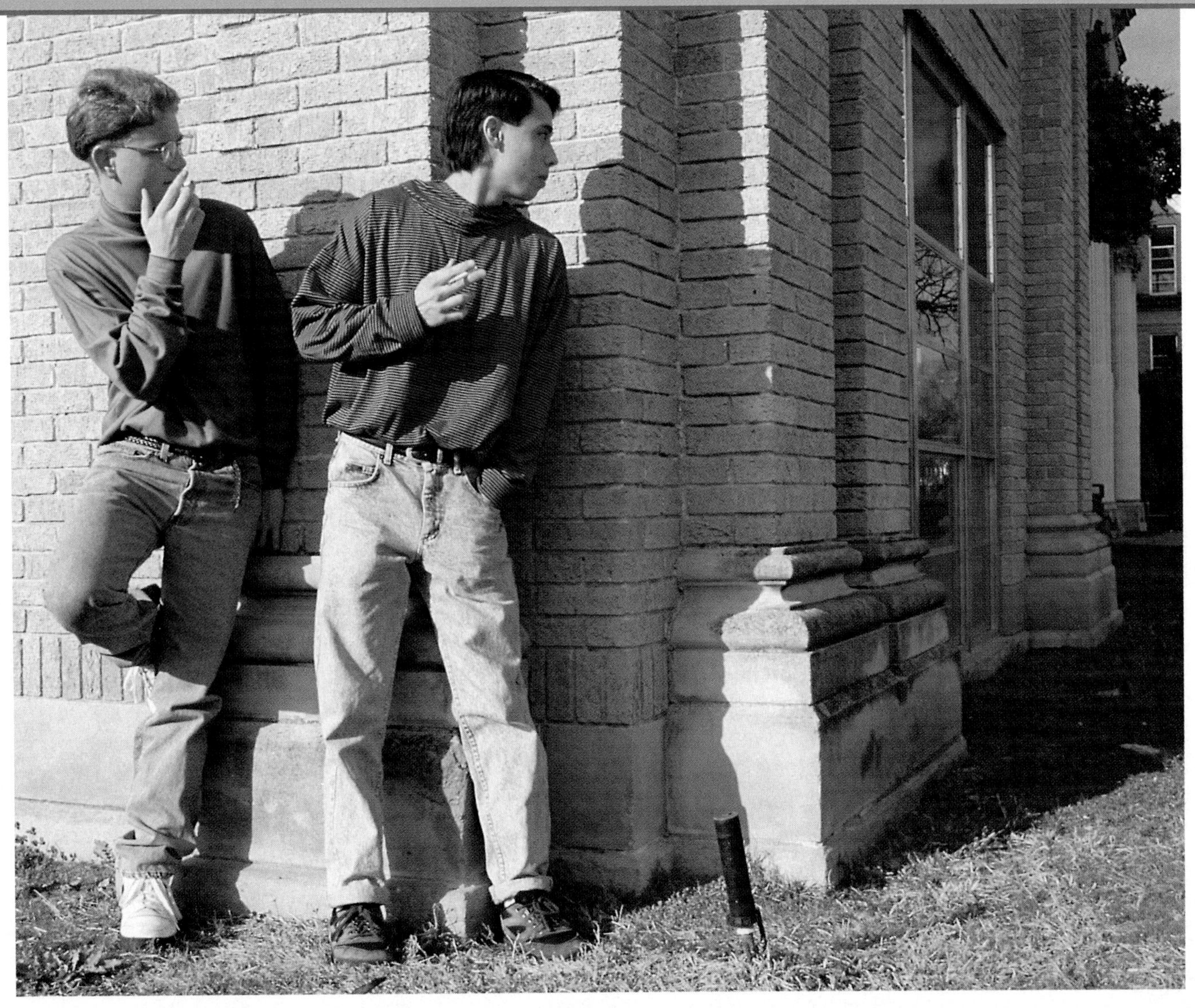

Content Background Cigarettes and Teens

The number of cigarettes smoked in 1990–worldwide–was 5.37 trillion, an increase of 170 billion over the 1989 figure. And it is estimated that about 20 percent, or 250 million, of the people who live in developed nations will die from smoking-related diseases an average of 23 years sooner than people who do not smoke.

Around the globe, adolescents make up a large proportion of the people who smoke. Most of these young people begin the cigarette habit before reaching the age of 16. In the United States alone, over 3,000 adolescents start smoking every day.

Cigarette advertising is one of the main reasons young adults start smoking. Cigarettes are the single most frequently advertised product on billboards. In the print media, cigarette advertisements are second only to advertisements for automobiles in most frequently advertised product. Cigarette advertisements generally depict smokers as successful, glamorous people who engage in healthful activities such as sports despite their unhealthful choice to smoke. Health-care professionals blame these advertisements for enticing American children under the age of 18 to spend millions of dollars annually on cigarettes.

According to the Centers for Disease Control and Prevention (CDC) in Atlanta, Georgia, adolescent smokers aged 12 to 18 overwhelmingly prefer the most heavily advertised brands.

Another major factor contributing to the increase in the number of young smokers is the lax enforcement of laws prohibiting sales of cigarettes to minors. Some experts argue that reducing young people's access to tobacco will curb cigarette smoking by minors, but others disagree, believing that tobacco access laws—like their alcoholic beverage counterparts—encourage young people's use of cigarettes.

A program carried out in a Chicago suburb during 1988 and 1989 seems to support the hypothesis that limiting access reduces adolescents' experimentation with, and addiction to, cigarettes. Letters detailing the Illinois law regulating the sale of cigarettes were sent to merchants. Antismoking legislation and education programs were enacted. Sales of cigarettes to 12- and 13-year-olds fell from about 70 percent of attempts to less than 5 percent after one and a half years of active enforcement accompanied by stiff penalties.

Fewer youth were trying cigarettes in the first place. Two months before legislation was enacted, nearly 50 percent of the junior high students had smoked cigarettes at least once. Two years after the program had gotten underway, however, fewer than 25 percent of students at the same age had experimented with cigarettes.

Suggestions for preventing teenage smoking include the following:

- **support and enactment of legislation that prohibits distribution of free samples**
- **enforcement of current legislation**
- **stiff fines or loss of licenses for those who make illegal sales**
- **ban of cigarette vending machines.**

Antismoking groups also encourage parents and guardians to emphasize to adolescents the negative effects of smoking:

- **cancers and other diseases**
- **the stench associated with tobacco smoking**
- **stained teeth and fingernails**
- **the cost–over $600 per year for one pack of cigarettes per day.**

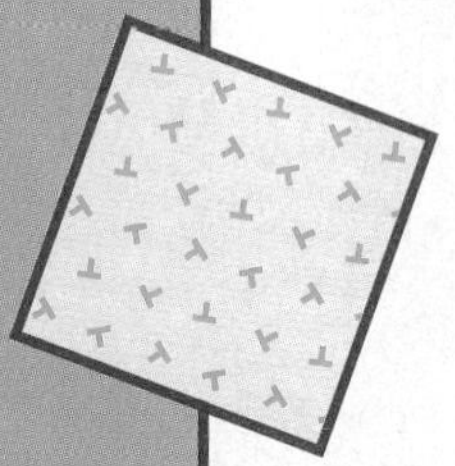

PLANNING FOR INSTRUCTION

KEY FACTS

- **Tobacco contains about 400 poisonous chemicals. The most poisonous are nicotine, tar, and carbon monoxide.**
- **Smoking is the most avoidable cause of death in the United States, yet smoking kills 434,000 Americans every year.**
- **Smoking causes over 80 percent of the lung cancers in the United States. It is the number-one cause of cancer deaths in women and the number-two cause in men.**
- **Smoking causes many kinds of cancer; respiratory diseases such as chronic bronchitis and emphysema; and cardiovascular disease.**
- **Sidestream smoke kills about 50,000 nonsmokers a year.**
- **Smokeless tobacco causes cancers of the mouth and throat.**
- **People start using tobacco because of peer influence, parental example, and advertising.**
- **Reasons *not* to use tobacco include respiratory illnesses and cancer; shortness of breath; loss of taste and smell; bad-smelling breath, hair, and clothing**
- **To quit smoking, set a quitting date, decide whether to quit "cold turkey" or to taper off, prepare your environment, seek help, and find a safer way to handle stress.**

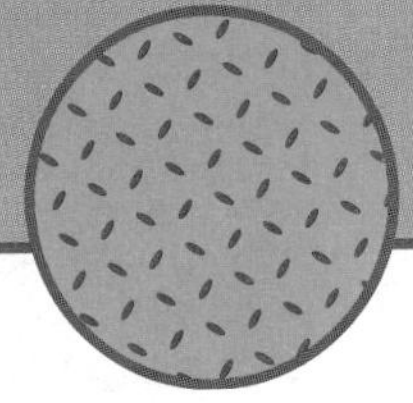

MYTHS AND MISCONCEPTIONS

MYTH: Smoking makes you feel better.
Nicotine is a stimulant drug that can give smokers a temporary lift. Smoking also calms some people. But these effects require increasing doses, leading to addiction. In the long run, smoking makes people feel worse.

MYTH: Low tar, low nicotine cigarettes are safe to smoke.
No cigarettes are safe. Smokers of low tar, low nicotine cigarettes tend to inhale more deeply and to smoke more cigarettes so that they receive similar levels of toxic substances.

MYTH: Smokeless tobacco is safe.
It is not safe to use snuff or to chew tobacco. They create the same addiction to nicotine that smoking does. In addition they damage teeth, gums, and cheeks and can cause cancers and heart disease.

VOCABULARY

Essential: The following vocabulary terms appear in boldfaced type.

nicotine
psychoactive substance
addictive
tar
carbon monoxide
cancer
chronic bronchitis
emphysema
chewing tobacco
mainstream smoke
sidestream smoke
passive smoker

Secondary: Be aware that the following terms may come up during class discussion.

cilia
nicotine poisoning
prostate cancer
cardiovascular disease
atherosclerosis
stroke
snuff
nicotine patch

FOR STUDENTS WITH SPECIAL NEEDS

Visual Learners: Have students prepare a display of anti-smoking posters, available from organizations such as the American Cancer Society, and cigarette ads from magazines. Use the display as the basis for a class discussion of the feelings that tobacco companies try to evoke in people to get them to smoke a particular brand, such as the need to belong, the desire to be popular, and the desire to be successful.

At-Risk Students: Have students conduct a survey of adults or teenagers they know who have successfully quit smoking cigarettes. They should prepare a list of questions, which might cover reasons for smoking in the first place, reasons for quitting, and methods used to quit. Have them present their findings to the class in an oral report, skit, or set of graphs.

ENRICHMENT

- Have students research the use of tobacco in Native-American cultures, the early tobacco trade, its economic importance to America, and its impact on American slavery.
- Have students find out how much is spent on tobacco advertising, how many people see the ads, how they affect sales, and what efforts are being made to make advertising less appealing to teens.

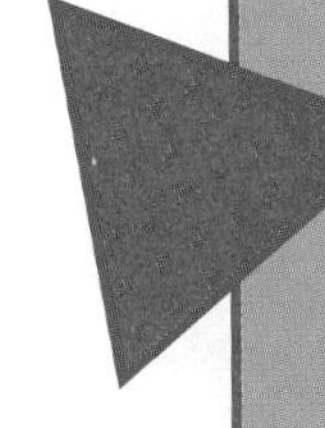

CHAPTER 14
CHAPTER OPENER

GETTING STARTED

Using the Chapter Photograph

Ask students to read the cigarette warning labels. Ask why they think people continue to use tobacco despite the warnings. Have them review the similar government warning on alcoholic beverage containers and discuss why people continue to drink despite the warning.

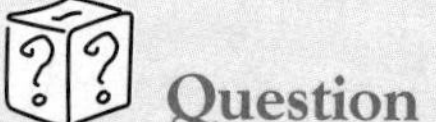

Question Box

Have students write out any questions they have about smoking or other tobacco use and put them in the Question Box. The Question Box provides students with an opportunity to ask questions anonymously. To ensure that students with questions are not embarrassed to be seen writing, have students who do not have questions write something else—such as something they already know about tobacco—on the paper instead.

Preview the questions and then answer them at appropriate points in the chapter. You may wish to allow students to write additional anonymous questions as they go through the chapter.

CHAPTER 14

Tobacco: Hazardous and Addictive

◆ ◆ ◆ ◆

Section 14.1 *The Effects of Tobacco on the Body*

Section 14.2 *A Tobacco-Free Life*

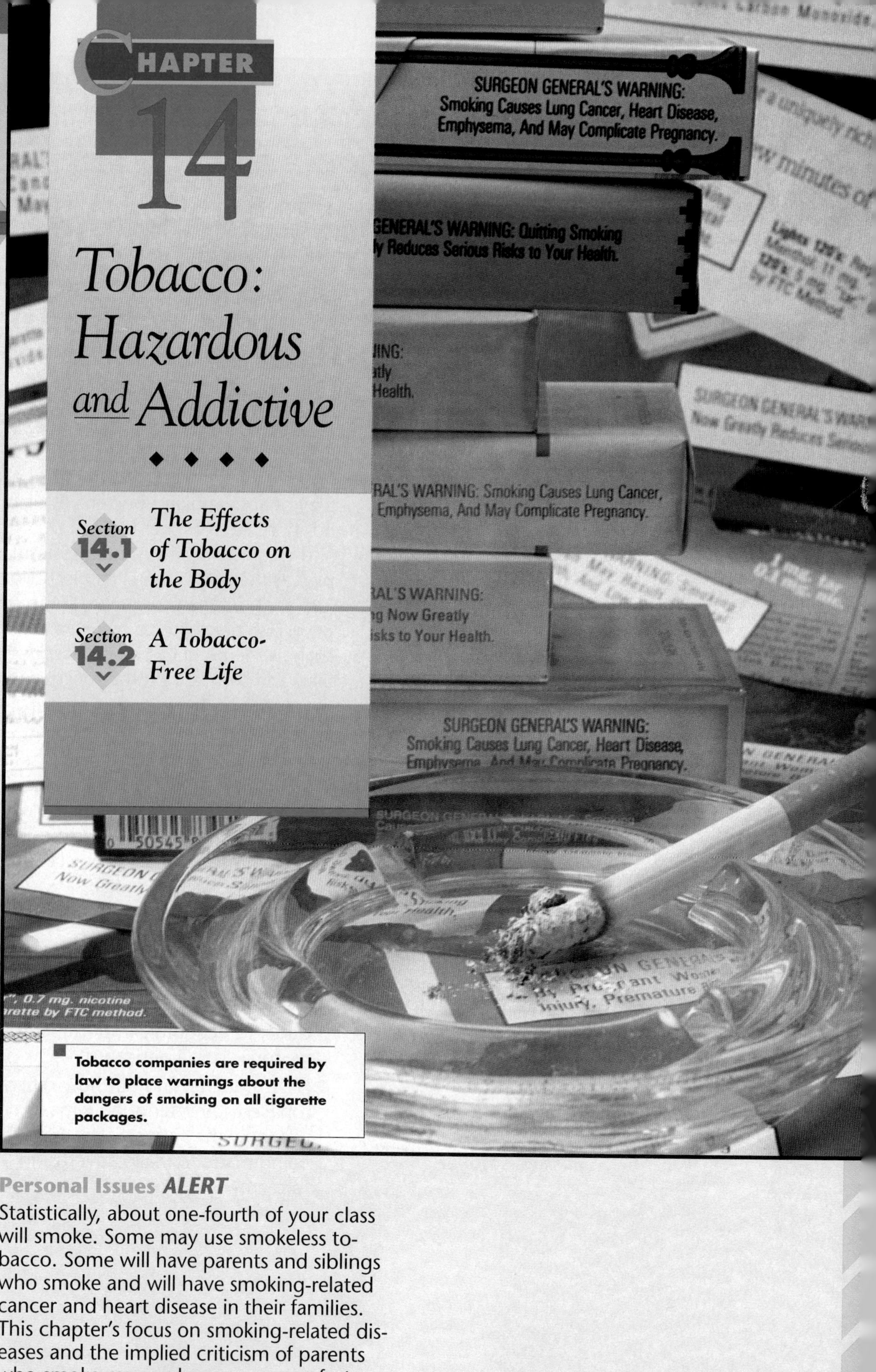

Tobacco companies are required by law to place warnings about the dangers of smoking on all cigarette packages.

Personal Issues *ALERT*

Statistically, about one-fourth of your class will smoke. Some may use smokeless tobacco. Some will have parents and siblings who smoke and will have smoking-related cancer and heart disease in their families. This chapter's focus on smoking-related diseases and the implied criticism of parents who smoke may make some uncomfortable. But help students recognize that if peer pressure encourages one to smoke, then discomfort from facing the facts can encourage one to quit.

Ethan has been smoking a pack of cigarettes every day for the past year. He didn't get hooked right away. In fact, the first few times he smoked, he got really sick. But soon he got used to it, and then he began to enjoy smoking. Now he finds it hard to get through each hour without smoking a cigarette. His girlfriend, Mara, hates his habit. She finds it really unattractive—his hair and clothes always reek of cigarette smoke. More important, she's worried about his health. He's always short of breath, and sometimes he coughs for minutes on end until his throat is raw. Mara knows he has to quit. The problem is, how can she persuade Ethan to give up cigarettes?

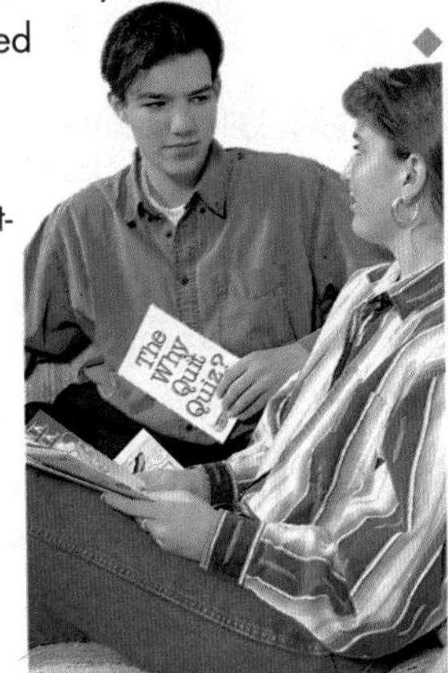

Section 14.1 The Effects of Tobacco on the Body

Objectives

- *Name three major chemicals in tobacco.*
- *Name two kinds of diseases smoking can cause.*
- *Name one disease smokeless tobacco can cause.*
- *Know the difference between mainstream and sidestream smoke.*
- *Know how to request that a person not smoke in your presence.*
  LIFE SKILLS: Communicating Effectively

Mara hopes that if she can scare Ethan enough about the risks of smoking, he'll find the courage and willpower to quit. She found some books and pamphlets on smoking and disease, and she is teaching Ethan some interesting facts. For example:

- Illnesses caused by smoking kill 434,000 Americans every year. That number is higher than the amount of Americans killed by the AIDS virus since its discovery.
- Cigarette smoking is considered the most avoidable cause of death in the United States.
- The death rate from heart disease is 70 percent higher for smokers than for nonsmokers, and over 90 percent of lung cancer cases are caused by smoking.
- Tobacco smoke also creates a health hazard for all those around the smoker who rely on the same air supply. Each year an estimated 50,000 nonsmokers die from exposure to tobacco smoke released into the air by smokers.

The Chemicals of Tobacco

Tobacco contains more than 4,000 chemicals. More than 401 of these chemicals are poisonous. When Ethan smokes a cigarette

Background
Smoking: America's Gift to the World

The Maya peoples of Mexico and Central America originated tobacco smoking, probably for religious rituals. Columbus and other early explorers introduced tobacco in Europe. As people grew addicted to nicotine, tobacco became a valuable crop. Modern cigarettes became popular after 1915, with annual consumption exceeding 600 billion around 1980. Since the peak year of 1963, U.S. per capita cigarette consumption has declined from over 4,300 per year to about 3,000 per year.

Section 14.1 Lesson Plan

MOTIVATE

Journal 14A
Feelings About Smoking

This may be done as a warm-up activity. In the Student Journal in the Student Activity Book, have students express their feelings about smoking. If they are smokers, ask them to tell how they feel when smoking. If they don't smoke, have them tell how they feel about the smoke of others.

TEACH

Class Discussion
Does Ethan Have the Right to Smoke?

Have students name some problems Ethan's smoking might cause. These might include his health, the cost of his addiction, the risk of serious diseases, the hazard to Mara when she breathes his smoke, and her negative feelings. Does Ethan have the right to smoke, even when it affects someone he loves? Does Mara have the right to convince him to stop smoking? Solicit ideas on how Mara might convince Ethan to give up smoking.

Game
Name Your Poison!

Have students write five questions on index cards about the three most poi-

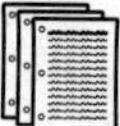

Personal Health Inventory

Have students complete the Personal Health Inventory for this chapter. The inventory helps them assess their own behavior with respect to the hazardous and addictive nature of tobacco.

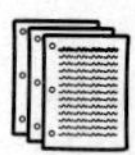

Life Skills Worksheet 14A

Communicating Effectively

Assign the Communicating Effectively Life Skills worksheet. This worksheet helps students consider different ways to communicate with smokers who may or may not be violating the rights of nonsmokers in particular situations.

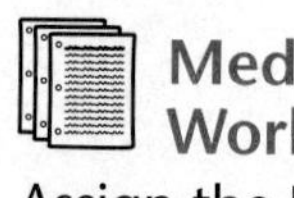

Media Worksheet

Assign the Media Worksheet for Unit 4.

What's Really In Cigarettes?

(FIGURE 14-1) **It would be hard to find a list of ingredients that are more hazardous than those in tobacco.**

addictive: *causing a physical dependence; a person who is addicted to a drug requires that substance in order to function normally.*

tar: *solid material in tobacco smoke that condenses into a thick liquid.*

nicotine: *an addictive chemical found in tobacco.*

psychoactive substance: *a substance that causes a change in a person's mood and behavior.*

he inhales every one of those chemicals, and every one of those poisons. Mara did some math and figured out that since Ethan is smoking one pack of cigarettes a day, he inhales these chemicals 70,000 times a year. Three of the most poisonous chemicals in tobacco smoke are tar, nicotine, and carbon monoxide.

Nicotine Nicotine is the psychoactive chemical in tobacco. A **psychoactive substance** causes a change in a person's mood and behavior. Nicotine is also the reason Ethan is hooked on smoking—it is a very **addictive** drug. A person who is addicted to a drug has trouble functioning without it. Because Ethan is addicted to nicotine, if he were to quit smoking his body would go through a physical withdrawal. The withdrawal symptoms of nicotine include irritability, headache, restlessness, and anxiety. These symptoms are unpleasant, but temporary. Sooner or later Ethan's body would stop reacting in this way. Ethan is also psychologically dependent on nicotine. This means that he has a constant craving for it. A psychological addiction can be as difficult to overcome as a physical one.

Tar Tobacco smoke contains tiny pieces of solid matter called **tar**. When these tiny particles enter the lungs, they condense and form a sticky coating on the bronchial tubes. The bronchial tubes are lined with tiny hairs called cilia, which beat back and sweep away agents that cause disease. When the

• • • TEACH continued

sonous chemicals in tobacco. (Examples: Which poison in tobacco is a psychoactive substance? *[Nicotine]* Which poison makes smokers short of breath? *[Carbon monoxide]*) Divide the class into two teams and give half the cards to each team. Have teams take turns asking each other the questions. Then have them trade cards and repeat.

Reinforcement
The More You Smoke, the Worse You Get

Emphasize that the effects of smoking are cumulative. The earlier you start, the more years you smoke, the more cigarettes you smoke, the more you inhale, and the more of each cigarette you smoke—the worse the effects. Compare smoking to slow poisoning with cyanide: daily small doses accumulate until a person dies. Point out that people who abruptly stop smoking get much better and live longer.

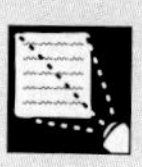

Teaching Transparency 14A
How Smoking Affects Your Body

Show the transparency of Figure 14-2. Point to each organ as you explain how smoking affects it. Ask students to define terms, such as cancer, cilia, and emphysema, as they arise.

cilia are damaged, they can't do their job. Ethan's cigarette habit puts a quart of tobacco tar into his lungs and cilia each year. If Ethan doesn't quit smoking soon, his cilia will be so damaged that they will not be able to protect him from getting a serious respiratory disease.

Carbon Monoxide As the cigarette burns, it releases an extremely dangerous gas called **carbon monoxide**. Carbon monoxide interferes with the blood's ability to carry oxygen. This is why Ethan is always so short of breath—he's not receiving as much oxygen as he should be.

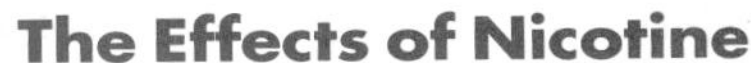

The Effects of Nicotine

Every time Ethan takes a puff of a cigarette, the nicotine he inhales travels to his bloodstream and then to his brain. This entire process takes only seven seconds, so Ethan will start feeling the effects of the nicotine immediately. This means that Ethan's heart will beat more quickly, his blood pressure will increase, and he will begin to feel more alert and energetic. These effects last for only about 30 minutes, which is why Ethan usually craves another cigarette about half an hour after he has finished his last one.

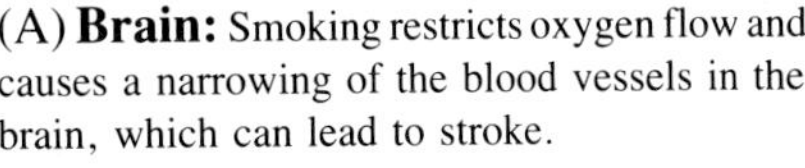

carbon monoxide:

a poisonous gas released by burning tobacco.

(A) **Brain:** Smoking restricts oxygen flow and causes a narrowing of the blood vessels in the brain, which can lead to stroke.

(B) **Lungs:** Cigarette smoke introduces cancer-causing agents directly to the lung tissue. It also impairs the cilia's ability to clear these and other harmful foreign substances from the lungs, increasing the risk of lung cancer and emphysema.

(C) **Heart:** Nicotine increases heart rate and blood pressure, and constricts the blood vessels, which can lead to a heart attack.

(D) **Stomach:** Cigarette smoke can lead to ulcers.

(E) **Intestines:** Cigarette smoke can also cause ulcers in the small intestine.

(F) **Bladder:** Smoking can cause cancer of the bladder.

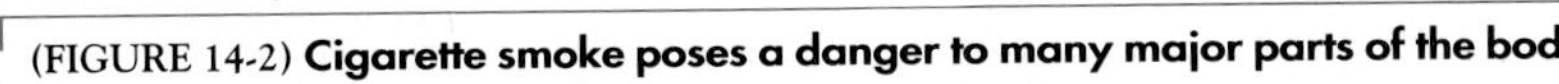

(FIGURE 14-2) **Cigarette smoke poses a danger to many major parts of the body.**

Background

The Price of Smoking

Cigarette manufacturing is one of the most profitable businesses in the United States. Unlike the cost of cigarette manufacturing, the price of smoking is very high. Yearly medical costs are $22 billion, lost time from work and school due to smoking-related illness amounts to $43 billion, and damage from fires started by cigarettes has a price tag of $400 million.

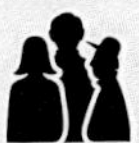

Cooperative Learning

Questioning Smokers

Form small groups. Have each group share observations about smokers: Do they know someone who smokes? When and how much do the people smoke? Are the smokers considerate of nonsmokers nearby? Do they have any symptoms of smoking (cough, hoarse voice)? Does their smoking affect nearby nonsmokers in any way?

Class Discussion

Is Smokeless Tobacco Safer?

Write the following headings on the chalkboard: CIGARETTE, CIGAR, PIPE, and SMOKELESS. Ask students to name the diseases that are caused by each as you write them on the chalkboard. (Cigarettes: lung cancer, chronic bronchitis, emphysema, atherosclerosis, heart attack, stroke; cigars: stomach cancer, cancer of the larynx; pipes: cancers of the tongue, lips, stomach, larynx; smokeless: cancers of the mouth, throat, tongue, cheeks, gums) Point out that lung cancer and respiratory disease are not caused by smokeless tobacco because this tobacco is not burned and thus doesn't produce tar and carbon monoxide. **Is smokeless tobacco safer to use than cigarettes?** *[No. Smokeless tobacco doesn't cause lung cancer or respiratory disease, but it causes other cancers and heart disease.]*

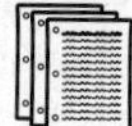

Section Review Worksheet 14.1

Assign Section Review Worksheet 14.1, which requires students to complete charts on the health problems caused by tobacco products and the effects of chemicals in cigarette smoke.

Section Quiz 14.1

Have students take Section Quiz 14.1.

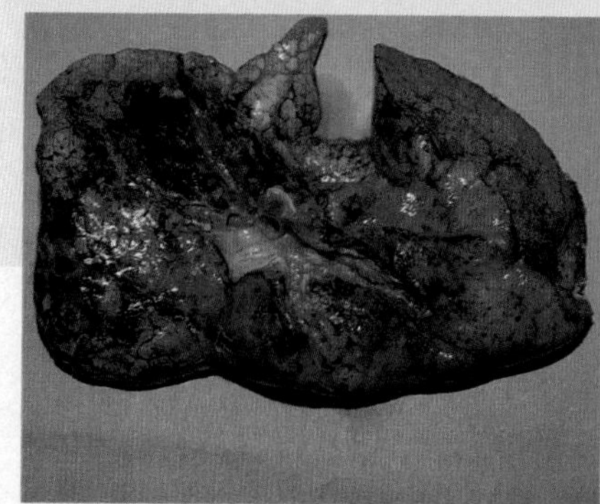

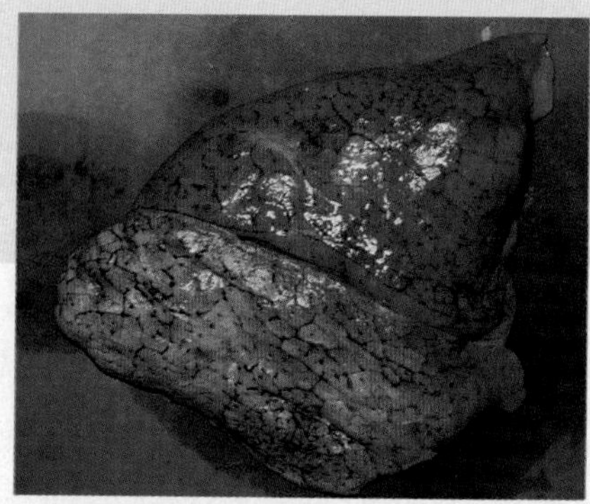

(FIGURE 14-3) **A cancerous lung (left) and a healthy lung (right). The white areas on the otherwise blackened lung show the development of lung cancer.**

cancer:

a disease caused by the formation and growth of deadly cells that attack and replace healthy cells.

Mara discovered why Ethan felt sick the first few times he smoked. When a person's body isn't used to nicotine, a condition called nicotine poisoning can result. Symptoms of nicotine poisoning include lightheadedness, rapid pulse, cold clammy skin, nausea, and sometimes vomiting and diarrhea. "I can't believe you kept smoking when it made you so sick," she told him.

Smoking and Disease

People who smoke put themselves in danger of developing a smoking-related disease. And mothers who smoke risk harming not only themselves but also their newborn and unborn children. For a list of these risks, see Figure 14-4. The risk of getting a smoking-related disease is highest among people who have smoked for a long time, who started smoking at a young age, and who smoke heavily. Mara figures that since Ethan started smoking as a teenager, he'll be at a very high risk of suffering a smoking-related disease if he doesn't quit soon.

Cancer Tobacco is a major cause of several types of cancers. **Cancer** is a dangerous disease caused by the formation and growth of malignant, or deadly, cells that attack and replace healthy cells. This can happen anywhere in the body. One major type of cancer caused by smoking is lung cancer. Lung cancer is the most common cause of cancer deaths among both American men and women and the second most common type of cancer among American men and women.

The bronchial tree, which is the hollow tubing that connects breathing passages from the mouth and nose to the lungs, produces a combination of saliva and mucus called sputum. Over a period of time the chemicals in cigarette smoke may cause changes in the cell genes of the sputum. These changes can lead to lung cancer.

There is no effective treatment for lung cancer. Every year, 120,000 Americans die from this disease. According to studies, cigarette smoking causes 80 percent of all cases of lung cancer in the United States.

Other cancers caused by smoking include cancers of the larynx, esophagus, bladder, kidney, and pancreas.

• • • TEACH continued

Demonstration

Model of Lungs

To show students how smoking affects your lungs, you can make a model of lungs. Poke a small hole in a clear plastic bottle near the top. Fill the bottle with cotton balls. Insert a cigarette into the bottle top and press clay around it to seal. Exhale by squeezing the air out of the bottle, leaving the small hole uncovered. Next, inhale by covering the small hole with your finger and let the bottle reinflate to its original shape.

Writing

Mainstream vs. Sidestream Smoke

Reinforce the distinction between mainstream smoke and sidestream smoke. Then have students write answers to these questions as you read them: **Is it right for one person to light a cigarette and fill the air with sidestream smoke, without asking the others? Why or why not? What should the smoker do instead?** *[Quit smoking or find a place to smoke.]* **Is smoking a dangerous form of air pollution? Why?** *[Yes. Sidestream smoke promotes several diseases.]* Then discuss whether people should tolerate air pollution from a cigarette any more than they would tolerate air pollution from a garbage incinerator.

Respiratory Diseases Ethan has a persistent cough because his smoking habit has caused mucus to accumulate in his respiratory tract. Over a period of time this condition can cause a respiratory disease such as chronic bronchitis or emphysema.

Chronic bronchitis is an inflammation of the bronchial tubes in the lungs and the production of excessive mucus. This results in a chronic cough and breathing difficulties. Smokers with chronic bronchitis often wake up in the morning coughing and spitting up mucus. Chronic bronchitis can eventually lead to emphysema.

Emphysema is a disease in which tiny air sacs in the lungs are ruptured, or torn. Under normal circumstances, these air sacs absorb oxygen coming into the body and help push carbon dioxide out of the body. When torn, they lose the ability to do this. This is why a person with emphysema is always short of breath. People with advanced emphysema constantly struggle for air. Sometimes they can't breathe without the help of a special oxygen tent.

Emphysema may last for years and is often fatal. Eighty percent of emphysema cases are related to smoking.

Cardiovascular Disease As you learned earlier in this section, nicotine increases heart rate and blood pressure, and carbon monoxide makes the circulatory system work very hard to deliver oxygen to the body's cells. Over a period of time, both of these chemicals put a great deal of strain on the body's blood vessels and cause cardiovascular disease, or disease of the heart and blood vessels. More than 120,000 smokers in the United States die every year from cardiovascular diseases.

Smoking can lead to atherosclerosis, which is the buildup of fat on the blood vessel walls. This can increase the chance that a blood vessel will become blocked or break near the heart, resulting in a heart attack. Another type of cardiovascular disease, a stroke, can occur if a blood vessel breaks or becomes blocked near the brain.

Pipes, Cigars, and Smokeless Tobacco

"Maybe," Ethan said, "I could get my fix of nicotine from something else, like a cigar, a pipe, or even chewing tobacco." Mara and Ethan did some research and found that people tend to inhale the smoke from cigarettes more deeply than they do the smoke from cigars or pipes. For this reason, cigarettes are the most dangerous of

chronic bronchitis:

an inflammation of the bronchial tubes in the lungs and the production of excessive mucus.

emphysema:

a disease in which the tiny air sacs of the lungs lose their elasticity.

Reasons Mothers Shouldn't Smoke

The baby could weigh less than he or she should and have serious health problems.

The baby could be born too early.

The baby could grow more slowly after he or she is born.

The baby could have learning problems and have trouble in school.

A miscarriage could occur.

The baby has a higher chance of dying from "Sudden Infant Death Syndrome" (SIDS).

There is more of a chance that the child will smoke as an adult.

Nicotine in cigarettes is a poison. The baby of a woman who smokes will drink this poison in her breast milk.

(FIGURE 14-4) **Pregnant women and mothers who smoke risk harming not only themselves but also their unborn and newborn children.**

SECTION 14.1

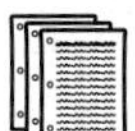

Reteaching Worksheet 14.1

Students who have difficulty with the material may complete Reteaching Worksheet 14.1.

Debate the Issue

Should All Smoking Be Banned?

Pose these questions:

- Should people be allowed to smoke anywhere? What about around babies or young children? around their pets? around elderly people? sick people? people with allergies? people with asthma?
- Should patients, visitors, and hospital personnel be allowed to smoke in hospital rooms? in bed? when gassing up their cars? during droughts in pine forests and grasslands?
- Is it fair to forbid adults to smoke? After all, adults are not forbidden to drink alcohol.

Then divide the class into two teams to debate the question: Should all smoking be banned?

Role-Playing

Would You Please Not Smoke Here?

Have students role-play the situations at right:

- In a group of friends, one person asks permission to smoke.
- In a group of strangers in a waiting room, one person asks the others for permission to smoke.
- In a group of friends, one lights up without asking.
- In a group of strangers in a waiting room, one person lights up without asking permission.
- In a restaurant, three people at a table light up in a nonsmoking sec-

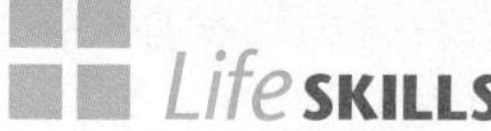

Life SKILLS

A Cigarette With Dinner?

Have students consider the situation described in the text and then have them propose solutions.

chewing tobacco: *a form of smokeless tobacco that is placed between a person's cheek and gum.*

the three. But even so, cigars and pipes have their own hazards. Pipe smokers have been known to suffer cancers of the tongue and lip, and certain types of cancers, such as cancer of the stomach and larynx, are more common among people who smoke cigars and pipes than among those who smoke cigarettes.

Smokeless Tobacco Smokeless tobacco comes in two forms. **Chewing tobacco** is placed between a person's cheek and gum. When this tobacco is chewed, it releases juices that contain nicotine and other chemicals. These juices mix with the saliva and are absorbed into the bloodstream.

The second kind of smokeless tobacco, snuff, is ground tobacco that is inhaled through the nose or placed between the cheek and gum. The nicotine and other chemicals are then absorbed into the blood-stream through the mucous membranes of

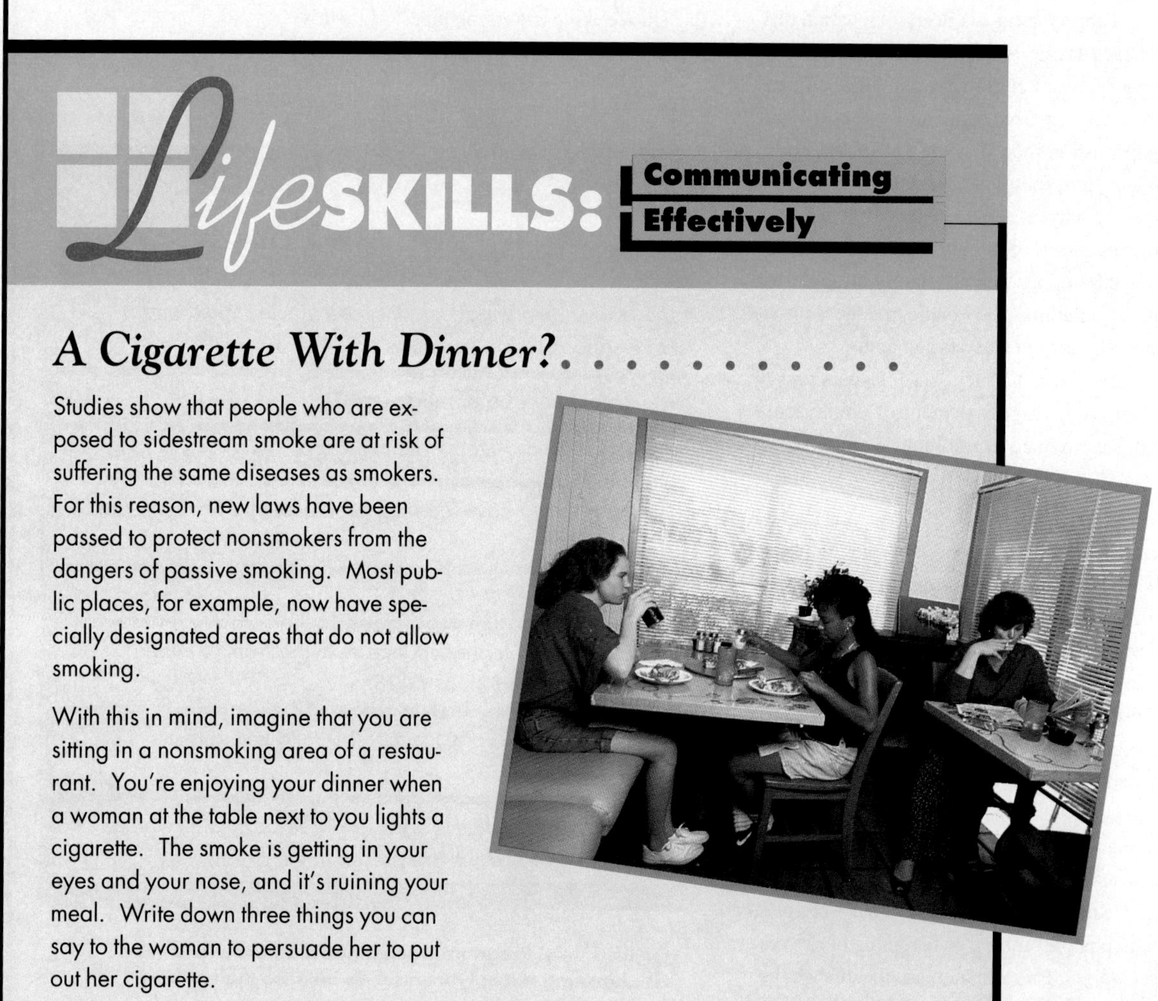

LifeSKILLS: Communicating Effectively

A Cigarette With Dinner?

Studies show that people who are exposed to sidestream smoke are at risk of suffering the same diseases as smokers. For this reason, new laws have been passed to protect nonsmokers from the dangers of passive smoking. Most public places, for example, now have specially designated areas that do not allow smoking.

With this in mind, imagine that you are sitting in a nonsmoking area of a restaurant. You're enjoying your dinner when a woman at the table next to you lights a cigarette. The smoke is getting in your eyes and your nose, and it's ruining your meal. Write down three things you can say to the woman to persuade her to put out her cigarette.

• • • TEACH continued

tion, refuse to douse their cigarettes, and claim that nonsmoking areas violate their civil rights.

After acting out each scenario, discuss how to handle each situation.

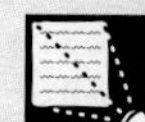

Teaching Transparency 14B
Smoking Is Glamorous

Use the Smoking Is Glamorous transparency to highlight the messages cigarette ads try to convey. Have students analyze the ad and name actual ads that contain the same message.

Extension
Ask the Experts

Have students use materials obtained from the American Cancer Society, American Lung Association, American Heart Association, and public health agencies to create an antismoking bulletin board. Encourage them to share the literature they obtained with friends who smoke.

the nose or mouth. Once in the bloodstream, the nicotine travels to the brain.

Both snuff and chewing tobacco can cause cancer of the mouth and throat, and chewing tobacco can also lead to cancer of the tongue, cheek, and gums.

The Risks of "Passive" Smoking

Mara saved her biggest weapon for last. If Ethan couldn't be persuaded to quit smoking to save his own health, maybe he would do so for hers. "It's dangerous for me to be around you when you smoke," Mara told him. "It could make me sick—it could even kill me."

Mara had learned that a burning cigarette releases two types of smoke:

- **Mainstream smoke** passes through the tobacco and filter when the smoker inhales.
- **Sidestream smoke** rises from the cigarette during the time the smoker is not inhaling.

Almost 75 percent of the smoke that comes from a burning cigarette is sidestream smoke. Sidestream smoke enters the environment and affects anybody who happens to be around. A person who inhales the sidestream smoke of a cigarette is a **passive smoker**. Sidestream smoke contains twice as much tar and nicotine, and three times as much carbon monoxide, as mainstream smoke. After 30 minutes in a smoke-filled room, a passive smoker has inhaled almost as much carbon monoxide as someone who has just smoked a cigarette.

Passive smokers are at an increased risk of suffering both lung cancer and heart disease. Sidestream smoke can also aggravate a person's allergies and cause respiratory infections. When Mara told Ethan these facts, he agreed to quit smoking.

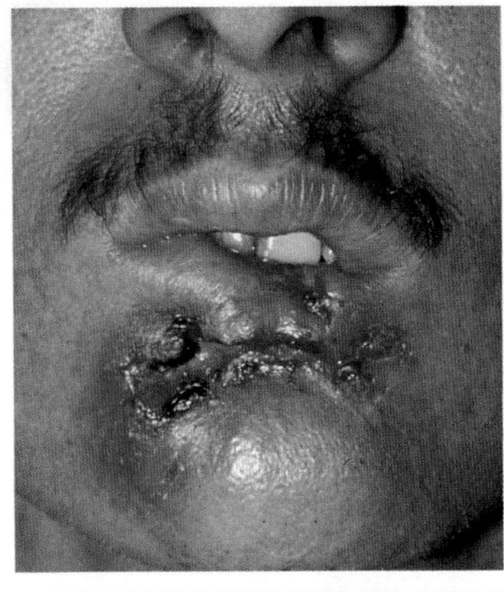

(FIGURE 14-5) **Chewing tobacco can lead to serious facial deformities as well as certain types of cancer.**

Review

1. *What are three major chemicals in tobacco?*
2. *What are two major types of diseases caused by smoking?*
3. *What is one disease caused by smokeless tobacco?*
4. *Define mainstream and sidestream smoke. How do they differ?*
5. ***LIFE SKILLS: Communicating Effectively*** *What can you say if a person sitting next to you in a nonsmoking area lights a cigarette?*
6. ***Critical Thinking*** *If cigarettes did not contain tar, would they be safe to smoke?*

mainstream smoke: *smoke that is inhaled directly into the mouth through a cigarette, pipe, or cigar.*

sidestream smoke: *smoke that enters the environment from burning tobacco.*

passive smoker: *A nonsmoker who is exposed to the sidestream smoke of a cigarette, cigar, or pipe.*

Section 14.1

Review Answers

1. Tar, nicotine, carbon monoxide
2. Cancer, respiratory diseases, cardiovascular disease
3. Cancer of the mouth and throat
4. Mainstream smoke passes through the tobacco and filter when the smoker inhales; sidestream smoke rises from the cigarette during the time the smoker is not inhaling. Two differences between mainstream and sidestream smoke are that mainstream smoke is filtered, whereas sidestream smoke is not; and mainstream smoke is inhaled by the smoker, whereas sidestream smoke is inhaled by the smoker and by all those around the smoker.
5. Students may answer that they could point out to the smoker that this is a nonsmoking section and that they would appreciate it if the person could refrain from smoking while sitting in this section.
6. No; tobacco contains thousands of other chemicals that are harmful to one's health.

ASSESS

Section Review

Have students answer the Section Review questions.

Alternative Assessment

Why Is Tobacco Hazardous and Addictive?

Have students write a paragraph explaining why tobacco is both hazardous and addictive.

Closure

Setting an Example

Tell students to look ahead to a time when they may have children of their own. Ask them: **What is the best way to teach your children not to use tobacco?** *[Set a good example by not using it yourself.]*

Background
Why Are There No Cigarette Ads on TV?

Cigarette companies were the largest advertisers on TV and radio until Congress banned their ads in 1971. Now they are leaders in magazine and newspaper ads, billboards, bus ads, and point-of-sale ads. In magazines, cigarette ads often appear on the back cover, a high-visibility placement. Cigarette makers get around the ban on TV ads by financing sporting events on TV.

Background
Antismoking Information

The following organizations in the Blue Pages or White Pages of telephone directories have information on smoking.

- American Cancer Society (Antismoking pamphlets, videos, posters, and comics.)
- American Lung Association (pamphlets, and some offices have school packets)
- American Heart Association (pamphlets)
- Government health service (pamphlets)

Section 14.2 A Tobacco-Free Life

Objectives

- *Know two reasons why people start using tobacco.*
- *Know three reasons not to use tobacco.*
- *Know two strategies you can use to quit smoking.*

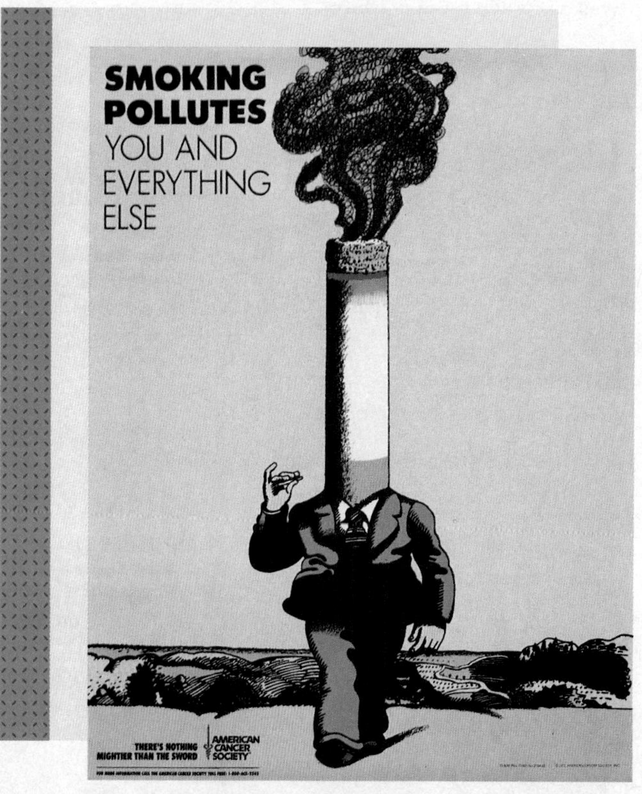

(FIGURE 14-6) **An advertisement from the American Cancer Society. Antismoking organizations are working to destroy the myth that smoking makes people glamorous and attractive.**

Every package of cigarettes and smokeless tobacco carries a warning from the Surgeon General on the dangers of tobacco use. These dangers are well known and well documented. Probably because these risks are so well understood, fewer people today use tobacco than ever before. But even so, more than 72 million Americans ignore these warnings and use tobacco products.

People use tobacco for different reasons. Peer influence and a parent's example may give someone the impression that it's O.K. to use tobacco. For example, Ethan's father has always smoked, and many of his friends smoke as well. If neither his dad nor his friends were smokers, Ethan might never have started smoking.

Another factor that may influence a person's decision to smoke is advertising. Models in cigarette and smokeless tobacco advertisements usually look glamorous and attractive. They can make tobacco use seem very appealing. Some organizations are working to destroy this idea by publishing posters showing the less attractive features of the habit.

Reasons Not to Use Tobacco

Just as peer pressure can tempt you to use tobacco, the influence of friends can help you make the decision *not* to use it. Many teenagers are aware of tobacco's dangers.

Having parents who don't use tobacco can also help a person make the same decision. Most parents realize how harmful tobacco is. They wouldn't want to see their sons or daughters jeopardize their lives by using a dangerous product.

Section 14.2 Lesson Plan

MOTIVATE

Journal 14B

Why Do Some People Smoke, But Not Others?

This may be done as a warm-up activity. Ask students to think about three smokers they know and write in the Student Journal in the Student Activity Book why they think each one smokes. Then, have them think about three nonsmokers they know and give reasons why they think each of them doesn't smoke.

TEACH

Class Discussion

Why Do Teens Smoke?

Ask students why teens smoke and write their reasons on the chalkboard. In discussing peer pressure, ask volunteers to describe situations where they have felt pressured to smoke. Have students think about their friends who smoke or don't smoke, and whether these people's parents do or do not have the cigarette habit. In discussing advertising, have students cite some of the messages that advertisers use to promote smoking among teenagers. **Of the three major reasons, which do you think has the strongest effect on teens?** *[Parental pressure]*

Four Good Reasons to Avoid Tobacco

1. *It's dangerous: Using tobacco causes cancer and can lead to high blood pressure, cardiovascular disease, and various lung disorders.*
2. *It's expensive: Smoking a pack of cigarettes a day costs more than $700 a year. Chewing a container of tobacco every two days costs about $500 a year.*
3. *It leaves an unpleasant odor: The smell of tobacco lingers on your breath, in your hair, and on your clothes.*
4. *It's unattractive: Tobacco can leave dark stains on your fingers and on your teeth. In addition, many teenagers find the sight of a person smoking or chewing tobacco unappealing.*

(FIGURE 14-7)

As Figure 14-7 indicates, using tobacco is an expensive, smelly, and unattractive habit. But the most important reasons not to use tobacco products are that they can damage your health and shorten your life. As you learned earlier in this chapter, the diseases caused by smoking and chewing tobacco are serious and often fatal.

Quitting Smoking

If you avoid smoking altogether, you'll never have to worry about its health risks. But if you are a regular smoker, know that if you quit your habit for good, you can dramatically reduce your chances of getting a serious disease. If Ethan can stay away from cigarettes for five years, his chances of getting lung cancer will decrease by 50 percent. And in 15 years, his chances of suffering *any* smoking-related illness will be almost as low as a person who has never smoked. But even a few days after he stops smoking, Ethan will begin to feel less winded and healthier.

Some smokers are worried that they will gain weight if they stop smoking. In fact, most people don't gain weight. What they do gain is a sense of confidence about themselves. It's a great feeling to overcome a habit that once controlled you.

Even though it is difficult to quit, you can do it. Lots of people do. Here are some strategies that may help you:

Set a Quitting Date Select a date to quit before you actually do so. If possible, choose a time when your level of stress is relatively low. For example, it may be easier to quit smoking when you are on vacation than when you are studying for final exams.

Decide Your Approach Different approaches work for different people. Many people prefer the ''cold turkey'' approach. They decide that, after the quitting date they have selected, they will never smoke again. Others prefer to gradually cut down the number of cigarettes they smoke, until they quit completely.

Prepare Your Environment If you decide to quit cold turkey, throw away all smoking materials and ashtrays in your

Life Skills Worksheet 14B

Resisting Pressure

Assign the Resisting Pressure Life Skills worksheet. This worksheet helps students define their own reasons for not smoking and select the best way to resist the pressure to smoke in particular situations.

Making a Choice 14A

Bulletin Boards About Smoking

Assign the Bulletin Boards About Smoking card. This card requires students to make bulletin boards dealing with reasons to quit smoking and alternatives to smoking.

Making a Choice 14B

Tobacco-Free Life Skit

Assign the Tobacco-Free Life Skit card. This card requires students to write a skit that could be presented to younger students to convince them never to start smoking.

Demonstration

Reasons to Avoid Tobacco

High up on the chalkboard, write in large letters: *WE HAVE SPECIAL REASONS NOT TO USE TOBACCO!* Then tell students:

- If you are an athlete or exercise regularly, please stand under the sign.
- If you play a brass or wind instrument in the band, please come up.
- If you, or anyone in your family, has allergies, asthma, problems breathing, chronic colds, or coughs, please come up.
- If anyone in your family has ever had cancer, heart disease, or lung disease, please come up.
- If you have a younger brother or sister, please come up.
- If you think that someday you may become a parent, please come up.
- If you want to live a full, healthy life and lower your risk of cancer, lung disease, or heart disease, please come up.

Join the group yourself, and close by pointing out that everyone has special reasons for not using tobacco.

Journal 14C

Confidential Tobacco Survey

Have students interview at least 10 tobacco users they know and ask them if they would like to stop and if so why. Ask them to record the information in the Student Journal.

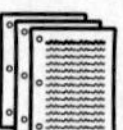

Section Review Worksheet 14.2

Assign Section Review Worksheet 14.2, which requires students to answer questions about why people start using tobacco products, why they should not use them, and how to quit smoking.

Section Quiz 14.2

Have students take Section Quiz 14.2.

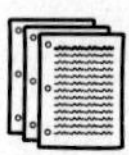

Reteaching Worksheet 14.2

Students who have difficulty with the material may complete Reteaching Worksheet 14.2.

Review Answers

1. Peer influence, parent's example, advertising
2. Damage to one's health, shortening of one's life, and tobacco is an expensive, smelly, unattractive habit.
3. Set a quitting date, decide your approach, prepare your environment, get help if you need it, and find other ways to cope with stress.
4. Students may answer that it would be harder to quit because the person trying to quit would be around cigarettes all of the time.

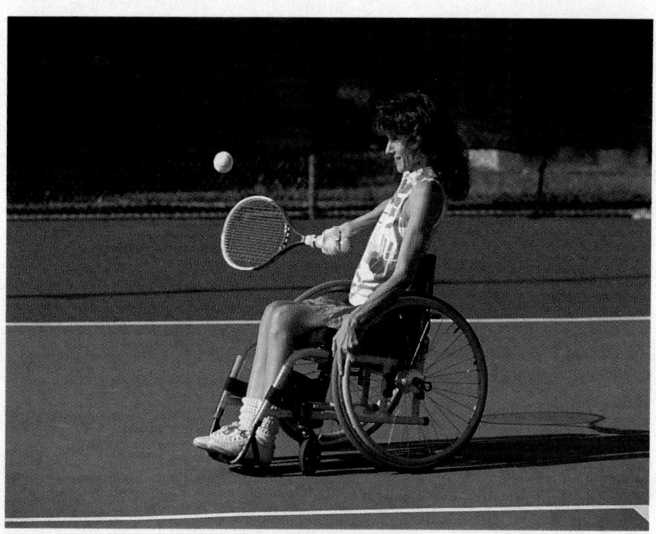

(FIGURE 14-8) **Quitting smoking enables a person to participate in and enjoy healthy, strenuous exercise.**

house and car. If you decide to cut down, keep only one day's supply of cigarettes on hand at a time. If you have decided to smoke eight cigarettes the first day, for example, throw away the rest of the pack or have a friend keep it for you. That way, you won't be tempted to smoke more than you have allowed yourself.

Get Help if You Need It Most people who try to quit smoking need a lot of help and support. Make sure your friends and family know that you are planning to quit, and that you may need to turn to them when times get hard. You may also find it easier to quit with other people than on your own. Most towns and communities offer workshops especially designed to help people stop smoking. Check your yellow pages for a program near you.

Some people find that nicotine gum or nicotine patches (squares soaked in nicotine and placed on the skin) help them stop smoking without suffering nicotine withdrawal symptoms. Nicotine gum and patches are available only by prescription.

Find Other Ways to Cope With Stress Most people who smoke want a cigarette most when they are under stress. There are healthier ways to handle anxiety. Getting regular exercise, for example, can be very relaxing. Try taking a long walk once a day. As your health and your wind improve, you'll be able to exercise for longer periods of time. In addition, the stress-management exercises described in Chapter 9 can help you cope with stress much more effectively than smoking.

After You Quit

Once you have stopped smoking for good, you'll start feeling better, both physically and psychologically. That feeling of being constantly short of breath will go away, and you'll even discover that the food you eat smells and tastes better. Although you may not have realized it, smoking dulls your senses of taste and smell.

In addition, you will enjoy the great sense of achievement that accomplishing a major goal can give you. By quitting smoking, you will have conquered a major addiction and taken a large step toward a long, healthy life.

Review

1. *What are two reasons why people start using tobacco?*
2. *What are three good reasons not to use tobacco?*
3. *What are two things you can do to help yourself quit smoking?*
4. ***Critical Thinking*** *Why might it be harder for a person to quit if his or her friends and parents smoke?*

• • • TEACH continued

Extension

Do Quit-Smoking Devices Help?

Have students visit a pharmacy and ask the pharmacist questions about nicotine gum and skin patches. How effective are they? Why are they available only by prescription? What do they cost? Does the pharmacist know of a local quit-smoking program?

ASSESS

Section Review

Have students answer the Section Review questions.

Alternative Assessment

What Would You Tell a Child About Tobacco?

Ask students to think of a child who looks up to them, such as a little sister or brother or a neighbor's child. What advice would they give this child about using tobacco?

Closure

Why Do We Allow Tobacco Use At All?

Discuss these questions: Given all the negative aspects of tobacco, why do people continue to use it? Why do we allow the sale of tobacco?

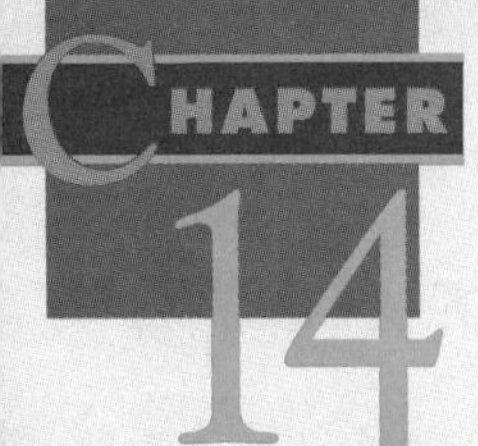

Highlights

Summary

- Tobacco smoke contains more than 4,000 chemicals; three of the most poisonous are tar, nicotine, and carbon monoxide.
- Nicotine, the psychoactive chemical in tobacco, leads to both psychological and physical dependence.
- Tar can damage the lining of the bronchial tubes, leaving a person vulnerable to several respiratory diseases.
- Carbon monoxide is a poisonous gas that interferes with the blood's ability to carry oxygen.
- Some diseases caused by smoking include cancer, chronic bronchitis, emphysema, and cardiovascular disease.
- Smoking pipes and cigars can lead to cancers of the lip, tongue, stomach, and larynx.
- Smokeless tobacco can cause cancers of the mouth, throat, tongue, cheek, and gum.
- Passive smokers are at an increased risk of suffering both lung cancer and heart disease.
- Factors that may cause a person to start using tobacco include peer pressure and a parent's example. The same influences, however, can also help a person make the decision not to using tobacco.
- Once you decide to quit smoking, choose a plan and accept support from friends and family. Substituting other activities will help you cope with your day-to-day stresses.

Vocabulary

nicotine an addictive chemical found in tobacco.

tar solid material in tobacco smoke that condenses into a thick liquid.

carbon monoxide a poisonous gas released by burning tobacco.

chewing tobacco a form of smokeless tobacco that is placed between a person's cheek and gum.

mainstream smoke smoke that is inhaled directly into the mouth through a cigarette, pipe, or cigar.

sidestream smoke smoke that enters the environment from burning tobacco.

passive smoker a nonsmoker who is exposed to the sidestream smoke of a cigarette, cigar, or pipe.

Chapter 14 Highlights Strategies

Summary

Have students read the summary to reinforce the concepts they learned in Chapter 14.

Vocabulary

Have students look at the vocabulary list and ask about any terms they do not understand.

Extension

Have students investigate the smoking regulations in their town or city. Is smoking permitted in public buildings? Is smoking regulated in restaurants, theaters, and shopping centers? How long have any regulations been in effect?

CHAPTER 14 ASSESSMENT

CHAPTER REVIEW

Concept Review

1. c.
2. d.
3. d.
4. a.
5. a.
6. b.
7. d.

Expressing Your Views

Sample responses:

1. Smoking is deadly. Smoking is addictive, and the more you smoke the more likely you are to become addicted to tobacco and the more likely you are to get colds, bronchitis, heart disease, lung cancer, and other cancers.

2. I would approach management with the facts on passive smoking and ask if I could have a space to work in that was free of tobacco smoke.

3. Athletes may chew tobacco because of their own peer group behavior or because they started to chew tobacco at an early age and are now addicted to it. Some athletes may feel pressure to perform and use the tobacco thinking it will relieve some of the stress. Since young children look up to athletes, these children may be influenced to try chewing tobacco simply because they want to be like their hero.

4. Answers will vary with students' opinions. Most students, however, should answer that more regulations should be placed on the advertising of tobacco because of the influence advertising has on people to begin or to continue to use tobacco products.

Life Skills Check

Sample responses:

1. I would tell my aunt that cigarette smoke bothers me and ask her to ask her friend to refrain from smoking while in the car.

2. I would tell her that smoking is doing more harm than good. She should stop smoking and find healthy ways to deal with the stress. She could get regular exercise or try relaxation exercises. I would encourage her in her decision to stop smoking.

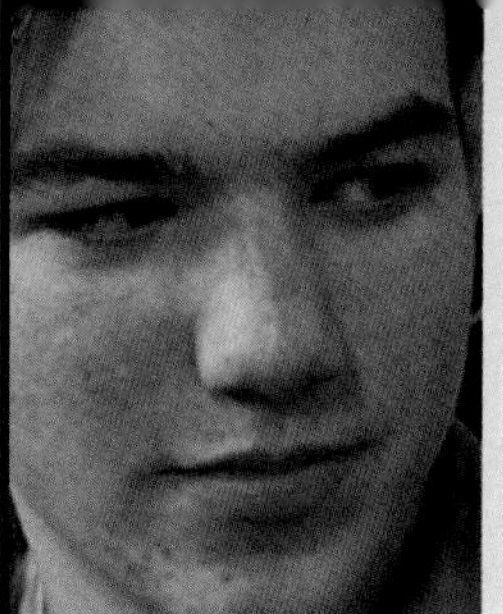

Chapter Review

Concept Review

1. What substance causes the largest number of avoidable deaths in the U.S.?
a. alcohol
b. nicotine
c. tobacco
d. carbon monoxide

2. Which of the following happens to most people the first few times they smoke?
a. nausea
b. clammy skin
c. rapid pulse
d. all of these

3. Which is a harmful effect of tobacco use?
a. respiratory disease
b. heart disease
c. cancer
d. all of these

4. Emphysema is
a. a deadly respiratory disease.
b. a cardiovascular disease.
c. nicotine poisoning.
d. a form of cancer.

5. Which of the following statements is true about smoking?
a. Passive smoking carries health risks.
b. Smokeless tobacco is a safe form of tobacco.
c. Pipe or cigar smokers are not at risk for developing cancer.
d. all of these

6. Which of the following statements about tobacco users is NOT true?
a. Even a light smoking habit can leave a person winded.
b. Tobacco users often have low blood pressure.
c. Tobacco users become physically dependent.
d. Smokers want a cigarette most when under stress.

7. Which of the following may influence people to use tobacco?
a. peers
b. parents
c. advertising
d. all of these

Expressing Your Views

1. Yesterday you caught your 13-year-old brother smoking a cigarette. What would you say to him to discourage him from smoking?

2. What would you do if you worked in an area where smoking was allowed? What are some ways to protect nonsmokers from environmental tobacco smoke?

3. You often see certain athletes using chewing tobacco. Why do you think they do this? Do you think the sight of them chewing tobacco will influence young people?

4. Do you think more or fewer regulations should be placed on the advertising of tobacco products? Explain.

CHAPTER 14 ASSESSMENT

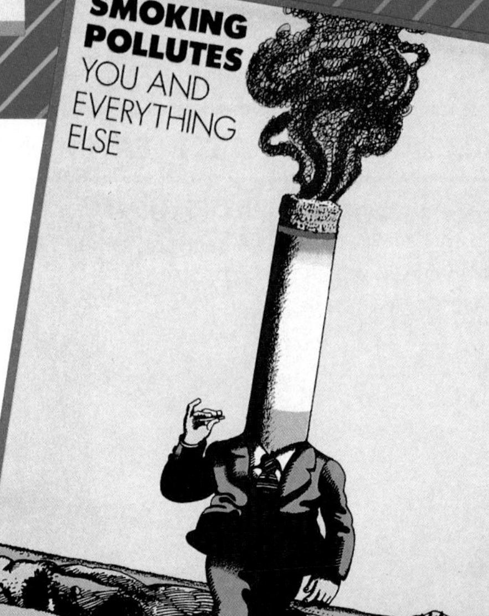

Life Skills Check

1. **Communicating Effectively**
   You are going on a long road trip with your aunt that the two of you have been planning for weeks. At the last minute she tells you that a friend of hers, who is a smoker, will be riding for at least half of the trip with the two of you. Cigarette smoke bothers you, especially when it's in a closed area like a car. What would you do?

2. **Communicating Effectively**
   Your friend wants to quit smoking, but she says she's under tremendous stress at school, at her after-school job, and at home. She's afraid the anxiety will be overwhelming. What would you say to her?

Projects

1. Write to your local chapter of the American Lung Association, American Heart Association, or American Cancer Society for information on the effects of using tobacco and about ways to quit using it. Share this information with the class.
2. Find a magazine advertisement for smokeless tobacco and display it on one side of a poster board. Beside it, draw an ad showing health hazards linked to smokeless tobacco. Display your poster in the classroom or around your school.
3. Research the current cost of a pack of cigarettes and figure out how much money a smoker would spend in a year if he or she smoked a pack a day. Then talk to smokers and ask them to list things they would buy, other than cigarettes, with this amount of money.

Plan for Action

Using tobacco is a very dangerous habit. If you use tobacco, list five reasons to quit. If you do not use tobacco, list five reasons not to start.

Projects

Have students plan and carry out the projects for anti-smoking education.

Plan for Action

Have students work in small groups to devise a plan to convince a friend or relative to quit smoking. Have them share ideas of how to counter the smoker's expected objections.

Personal Pledge

Have students read and sign the personal pledge for Chapter 14.

ASSESSMENT OPTIONS

Chapter Test

Have students take the Chapter 14 Test.

Alternative Assessment

Have students do the Alternative Assessment activity for Chapter 14.

Test Generator

The Test Generator (Macintosh® or IBM® format) contains an additional 50 assessment items for this chapter.

CHAPTER 15

OTHER DRUGS OF ABUSE

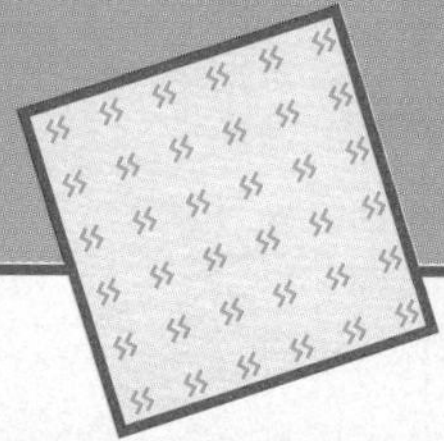

PLANNING GUIDE

TEXT SECTIONS	OBJECTIVES	TEXT FEATURES	OUTSIDE RESOURCES	NOTES
15.1 **Drug Abuse and Addiction** pp. 299-301 2 periods	• Name two important dangers of drug abuse. • Name two ways in which drug abusers can damage society. ■ Know how a person can become addicted to a drug.	**ASSESSMENT** • Section Review, p. 301	**TEACHER'S RESOURCE BINDER** • Lesson Plan 15.1 • Personal Health Inventory • Journal Entry 15A • Section Review Worksheet 15.1 • Section Quiz 15.1 • Reteaching Worksheet 15.1 **OTHER RESOURCES** • Making a Choice 15A • English/Spanish Audiocassette 4 • Parent Discussion Guide	
15.2 **The Effects of Drugs of Abuse** pp. 302-312 4 periods	• Know the effects of one category of psychoactive drugs. • Name two dangers of crack cocaine. ■ Know how to avoid inhalant fumes. ■ Discuss what you would say to a friend who is thinking of taking anabolic steroids.	■ LIFE SKILLS: Communicating Effectively, p. 311 **ASSESSMENT** • Section Review, p. 312	**TEACHER'S RESOURCE BINDER** • Lesson Plan 15.2 • Journal Entries 15B, 15C, 15D, 15E • Life Skills 15A • Section Review Worksheet 15.2 • Section Quiz 15.2 • Reteaching Worksheet 15.2 **OTHER RESOURCES** • Transparency 15A	
15.3 **Treatment for Dependency** pp. 313-316 1 period	• Name two things everyone should know about treatment for drug dependency. • Know three options for recovering drug abusers. • Know a healthy option to abusing drugs.	**ASSESSMENT** • Section Review, p. 316	**TEACHER'S RESOURCE BINDER** • Lesson Plan 15.3 • Journal Entries 15F, 15G • Life Skills 15B • Section Review Worksheet 15.3 • Section Quiz 15.3 • Reteaching Worksheet 15.3 **OTHER RESOURCES** • Making a Choice 15B • Transparency 15B	
End of Chapter pp. 317-319		**ASSESSMENT** • Chapter Review, pp. 318-319	**TEACHER'S RESOURCE BINDER** • Chapter Test • Alternative Assessment • Personal Pledge **OTHER RESOURCES** • Test Generator	

■ Denotes LIFE SKILLS objectives

• Items in blue are also part of the *Holt Health Activity Book.*

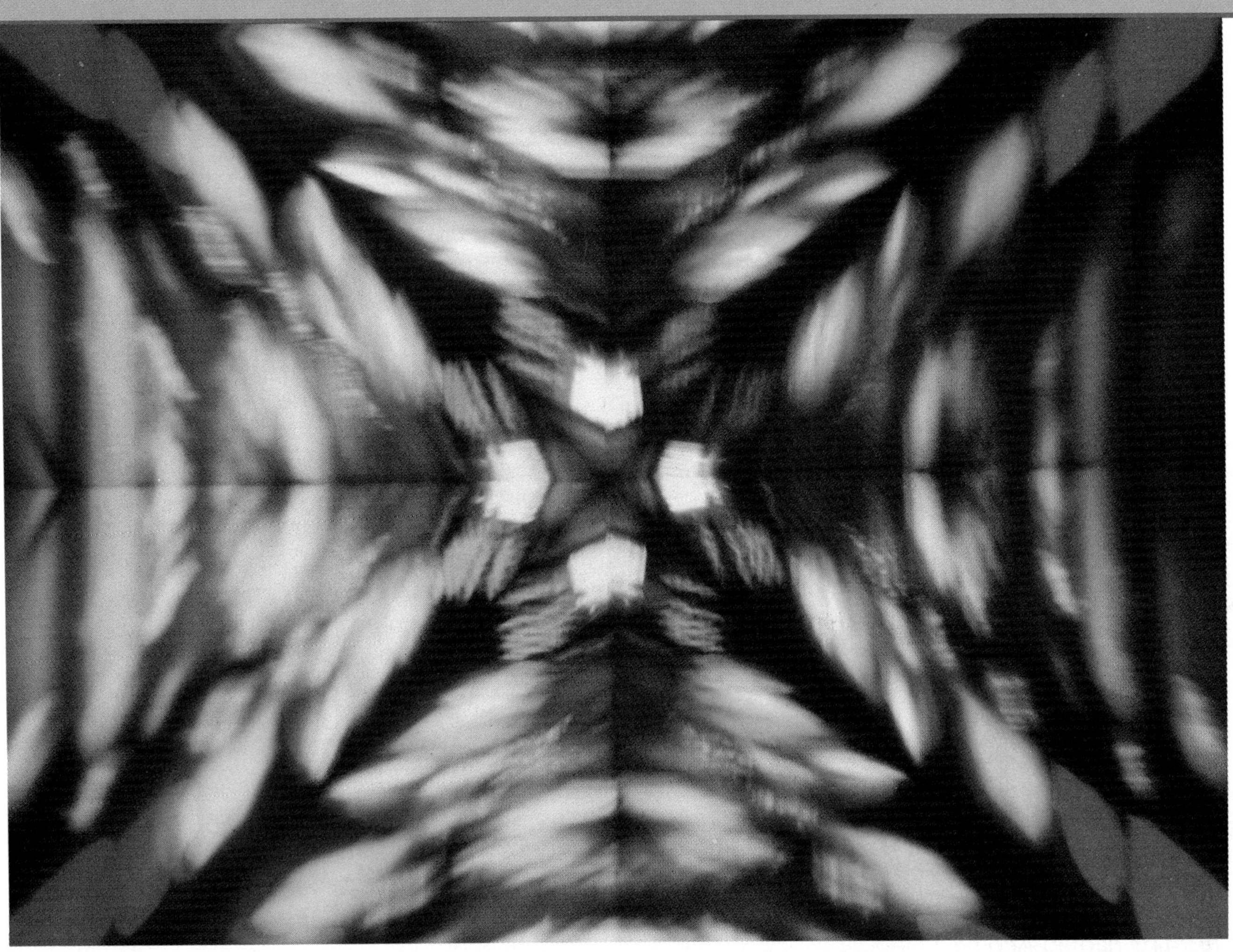

Content Background

Abuse of Hallucinogenic Drugs Among Teenagers

In early 1992, Dr. Louis Sullivan, then secretary of the United States Department of Health and Human Services, announced that according to a 1991 survey of nearly 15,500 high school graduating seniors, abuse of illegal drugs by these adolescents was at its lowest level since the survey was begun in 1975. Dr. Sullivan further stated that educational programs were the primary reason for a 4 percent decrease in the abuse of several illegal drugs. The survey reported a 1.6 percent decrease in the abuse of cocaine, a 4 percent fall in the abuse of marijuana, and a nearly 0.5 percent decline in heroin abuse.

However, surveys conducted by other medical and health organizations point to an increase in drug abuse among adolescents. According to studies published in *The Journal of the American Medical Association,* the abuse of psychoactive substances by adolescents has dramatically increased over the past two decades. The journal reported that abuse of such substances on a daily basis is twice as common in high-school-aged males as in their female counterparts. Furthermore, the increased abuse of psychoactive drugs is seemingly related to an increase in teenage suicide and suicidal behavior, which includes suicide attempts as well as thinking about and planning suicide. For example, from 1950 to 1980, the suicide rate among 15- to 19-year-old Caucasian males increased more than 300 percent. The suicide rate for this same period among females increased only 67 percent.

A nationwide study, known as the National Adolescent Student Health Survey (NASHS), conducted in 1987 found that some younger students are also taking psychedelic drugs. Of the 11,419 eighth- and tenth-graders sampled, 4.7 percent (537) had tried psychedelic drugs such as acid (LSD), angel dust, mescaline, peyote, and psilocybin in their lifetimes. While these percentages are small, they do suggest that some younger adolescents are trying psychedelic drugs at least once or twice. These findings emphasize the critical need for drug education to begin at younger ages.

While relatively few of those students polled in the NASHS reported that they had abused psychedelic drugs, the abuse of the hallucinogenic drug lysergic acid diethylamide, or LSD (commonly known as acid), is on the rise among slightly older American adolescents. Results of surveys taken in 1990 and 1991 by the University of Michigan and the National Institute on Drug Abuse revealed that more high-school-aged seniors had taken LSD than cocaine in the year before each survey. In fact, of the 26,000 high school seniors polled in 1991 nationwide, 2,418 Caucasian males and 1,300 of their female counterparts had abused hallucinogens—almost always LSD—during the previous year. In a poll of alternative high schools in Seattle, Washington, 90 percent of the students surveyed reported having tried hallucinogenic substances during the 1991 academic year alone. These statistics indicate the magnitude of our nation's drug problem.

Statistics gathered by the United States Drug Enforcement Administration (DEA) and the Parents' Resource Institute for Drug Education (PRIDE) suggest that some of the reasons for the increased abuse of LSD among American teenagers include its availability and relatively low cost. Also, many teens hold the misconception that because LSD is not physically addictive, it's a "safe" drug. Furthermore, many teens who abuse the drug also fail to realize that some of the consequences of taking acid, even once, include severe short-term memory loss, paranoia, repeated visual hallucinations, persistent panic attacks, nightmares, and even psychosis.

As with any kind of substance abuse, the information and training provided in our school system is essential in combating the problem. Drug education classes are being taught across the country to younger and younger students. Attention is also being focused on high-risk children—those with poor learning skills; runaways; those who have been abused and neglected by their families; children with drug-abusing parents; and those exposed to high crime rates, violence, and drug availability. For these and all children it is important to begin the anti-drug use educational process an early age.

PLANNING FOR INSTRUCTION

KEY FACTS

- **Although peer pressure to use drugs can be intense, self-esteem and knowledge about drugs can help a teenager to resist.**
- **Stimulants are drugs that cause alertness. Caffeine and cocaine are natural stimulants; amphetamines are synthetic stimulants.**
- **Hallucinogens such as LSD, PCP, and ecstasy distort the senses, making it difficult to distinguish what is real from what is not.**
- **Narcotics such as morphine, codeine, and heroin are drugs derived from the opium poppy plant; they relieve pain but are very addictive.**
- **Sedative-hypnotics are drugs that depress the body system and cause sleepiness. Barbiturates are prescribed sedatives that relieve severe anxiety and insomnia. Benzodiazepines are prescription tranquilizers that relieve minor anxiety and insomnia.**
- **Anabolic steroids (drugs used by people to develop muscles and body strength) cause liver and heart damage, in addition to high blood pressure.**
- **Drugs taken during pregnancy may pass into the fetus's bloodstream, causing the child to be born with deformities, retardation, slow reflexes, and learning disabilities.**

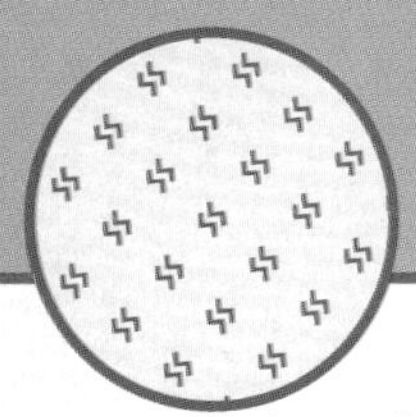

- **One should not try to overcome drug addiction without professional help.**

MYTHS AND MISCONCEPTIONS

MYTH: You can't do any harm just trying drugs once or twice.

People have died taking crack for the first time. After trying drugs once or twice, some people try them repeatedly until they are addicted.

MYTH: Cocaine causes no major health problems.

An overdose of cocaine can cause death. Some people are hypersensitive to cocaine and die from exposure to small amounts. The sudden rise in blood pressure from cocaine can cause a stroke, resulting in paralysis or death. Some people have epileptic seizures from cocaine.

MYTH: Marijuana is a safe drug.

Marijuana is detrimental to driving ability and often results in accidents. Smoking marijuana may have greater ill effects on the lungs than smoking tobacco since the marijuana is smoked unfiltered.

VOCABULARY

Essential: The following terms appear in boldface type.

psychoactive drug	**flashback**
addicted	**depressant**
physical dependence	**designer drugs**
withdrawal	**inhalants**
psychological dependence	**narcotic**
stimulant	**overdose**
hallucinogen	**sedative-hypnotics**
hallucination	**anabolic steroid**

Secondary: Be aware that the following terms may come up during class discussion.

euphoria	methadone
amphetamine	student-assistance program
barbiturates	

FOR STUDENTS WITH SPECIAL NEEDS

Visual Learners: For students who learn best visually, you may wish to show the video series *Straight Talk About Drugs.* This series contains three videos: *Tranquilizers and Sedatives; Stimulants and Narcotics;* and *Psychedelics, PCP, and Dangerous Combinations.* The series provides information about the effects of drugs, addiction, the dangers of combining drugs, and rehabilitation programs. The videos may be available at your library or can be obtained at Guidance Associates, Communications Park, Box 3000, Mount Kisco, NY 10549. Call 1-800-431-1242.

At-Risk Students: Have students create a newspaper for circulation among younger students that carries an antidrug message. They could do this by collecting articles from newspapers and magazines or by writing their own feature stories, news stories, cartoons, and editorials.

ENRICHMENT

- Arrange for a speaker—a nurse, doctor, counselor, or rehabilitated drug abuser who wishes to warn others away from the drug scene—to address the class and to answer questions. Have students prepare by submitting anonymous questions they would like answered by the speaker. After the talk, have students discuss their reactions and any topics raised by the talk.
- Have students write a story related to teenagers and the drug-abuse problem. For example, they may write about the peer pressure a teenager faces, or about someone who is tempted to take drugs in order to become "one of the crowd."

CHAPTER 15 CHAPTER OPENER

GETTING STARTED

Using the Chapter Photograph
Ask students how the teenager in the picture is helping to convey an anti-drug message and why her effort is important.

Question Box
Have students anonymously write out any questions they have about drugs and drug abuse and put them in the Question Box. To ensure that students with questions are not embarrassed to be seen writing, have students who do not have questions write a fact they already know about drugs on the paper instead.

Preview the questions and then answer them at appropriate points in the chapter. You may wish to allow students to write additional questions as they go through the chapter.

Personal Issues *ALERT*
The discussion of drugs and drug abuse may make students uncomfortable. Students may know someone with a drug problem or someone in their family may be dependent on drugs. In addition, a student may be struggling because of peer pressure to try drugs. Lesbian and gay youths are three times as likely to abuse drugs or alcohol as heterosexual youths. Prepare the class to be respectful of privacy, tolerant of others' problems, and sensitive during class discussions or activities.

CHAPTER 15 Other Drugs of Abuse

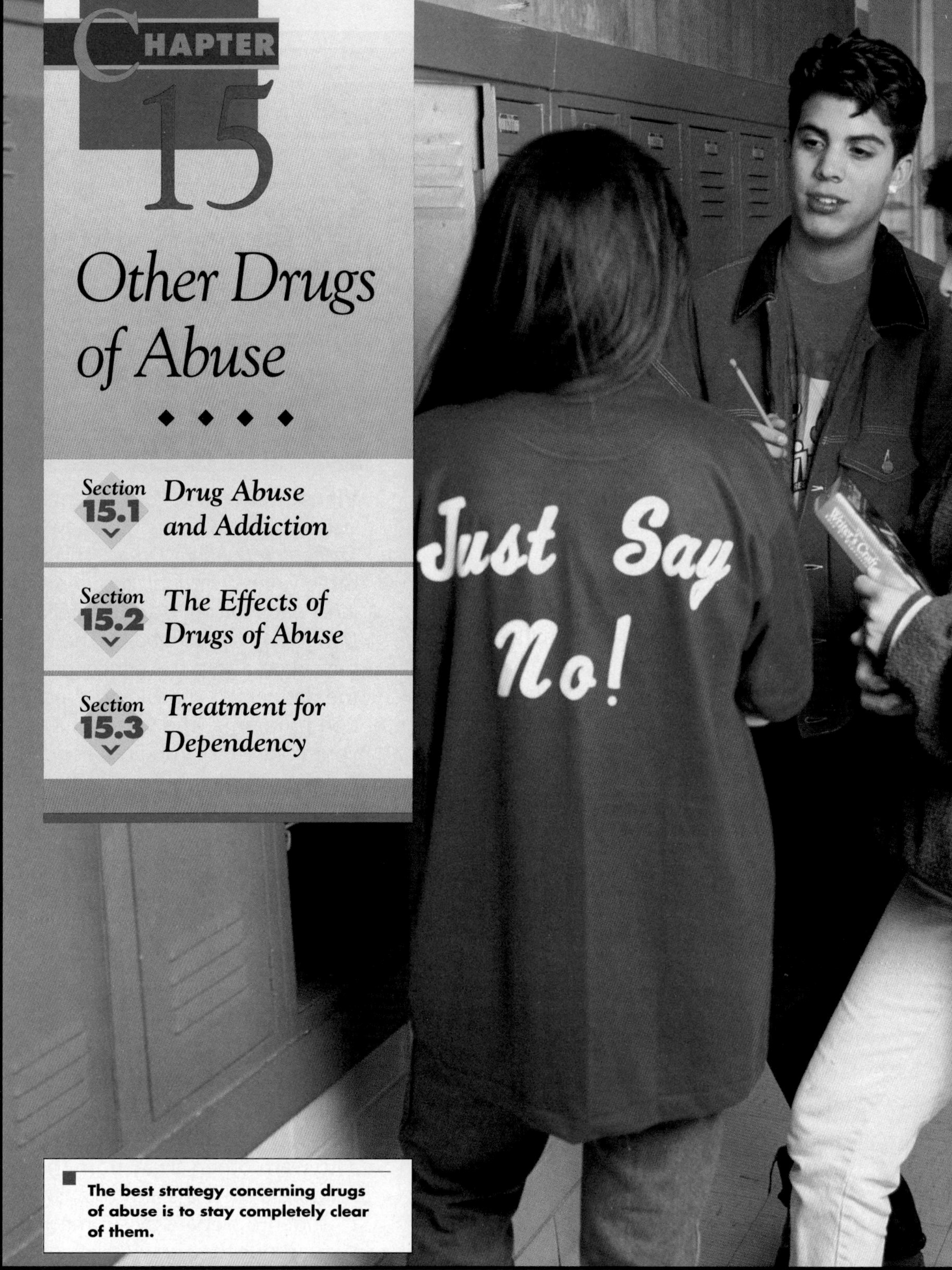

The best strategy concerning drugs of abuse is to stay completely clear of them.

Max always looked forward to the weekends. Every Saturday night he would get together with the same four friends, and they would always find something fun to do. Sometimes they'd grab a hamburger and see a movie. Other times they'd just go to someone's house and watch a ballgame. Then one night one of Max's friends wanted everyone to smoke marijuana. Max really didn't want to try it, but he did, and didn't like it. Now his friends are talking about getting ahold of some crack. This Saturday night they're supposed to get together and smoke it. This time Max knows he won't be joining his friends—but he doesn't know what to tell them.

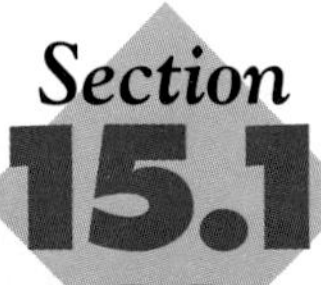

Section 15.1 Drug Abuse and Addiction

Objectives

- *Name two important dangers of drug abuse.*
- *Name two ways in which drug abusers can damage society.*
- *Know how a person can become addicted to a drug.*
  LIFE SKILLS: Resisting Pressure

It turned out that Max's friend Troy didn't want to try crack either. They told the others their decision and spent Saturday night at Troy's house watching basketball on television. They also talked about the pressure they felt to do drugs with their friends.

If you've ever been under peer pressure to do something you didn't want to do, you probably know how difficult it can be. You may have felt as though you had to choose between your friends and your own values. This is especially true when it comes to **psychoactive drugs** of abuse. A psychoactive drug is a drug that affects a person's mood and behavior. Making the decision to abuse them can be deadly.

psychoactive drug:
a drug that affects a person's mood and behavior.

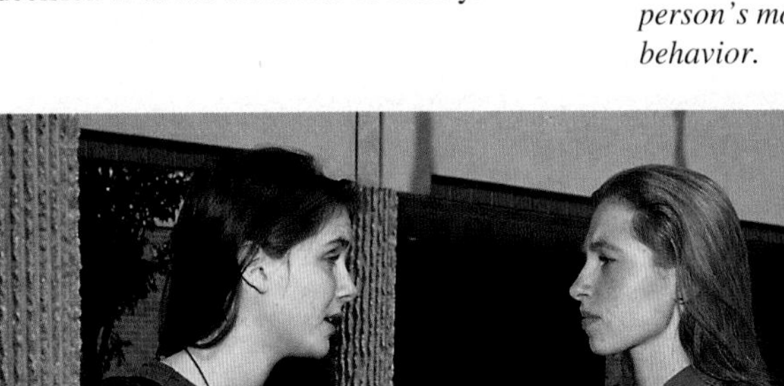

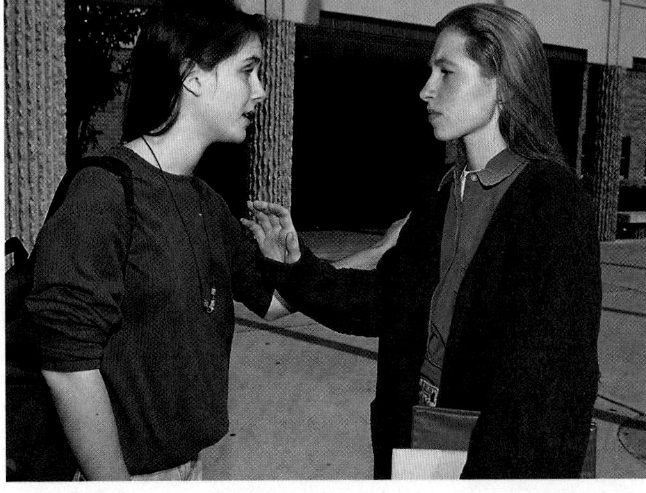

(FIGURE 15-1) **Knowing how to resist peer pressure is an important skill to have—especially when it comes to drug abuse.**

SECTION 15.1

Background
Drug Testing
In general, employers may use random drug testing if there is reasonable suspicion of ongoing drug use. Employers often couple testing with education and rehabilitation programs. Even in jobs that do not directly affect public safety, testing is becoming more common. It may include pre-employment screening, random testing, or testing following a specific incident that has raised suspicion.

Background
Addiction
Addiction is the direct result of physical changes induced by a drug. When a drug creates an overabundance of neurotransmitter molecules, for instance, certain nerve cells in the brain respond by creating fewer receptors. Then, if the drug supply is suspended, the nerve pathway is no longer able to function normally. Renewed supplies of the drug are necessary to keep the pathway functioning normally. The nerves will eventually readjust if the drug is withdrawn slowly.

Section 15.1 Lesson Plan

MOTIVATE

Journal 15A
Pressure to Use Drugs
This may be done as a warm-up activity. Encourage students to record in the Student Journal in the Student Activity Book their concerns about being pressured by friends to try drugs. They may also write their feelings about Max and his decision.

TEACH

Class Discussion
Dealing With Peer Pressure
To help students understand the problems caused by psychoactive drugs, ask: **Why are psychoactive drugs of abuse so dangerous to use?** *[These drugs affect your mood and behavior.]* To help students deal with peer pressure, ask the following questions: **How can peer pressure be a factor in taking a drug of abuse?** *[It's hard to turn down a friend's pressure on you to do something, even though you don't want to.]* **What can you do to avoid falling into the drug trap?** *[Be aware of your own values and don't let anyone make you feel less worthwhile because you don't give in to their demands. You may need to find other friends.]*

Role-Playing
Not Caving In to Peer Pressure
Have students role play a situation in which one member of a group stands

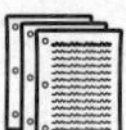

Personal Health Inventory

Have students complete the Personal Health Inventory for this chapter. The inventory helps them assess their behavior with respect to drug abuse.

Making a Choice 15A

Pressure to Take Drugs

Assign the Pressure to Take Drugs card. The card asks students to discuss alternatives to drug use and how drug abusers affect people around them.

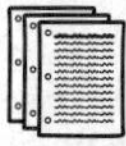

Section Review Worksheet 15.1

Assign Section Review Worksheet 15.1, which requires students to complete statements and a chart about drug abuse and addiction.

Section Quiz 15.1

Have students take Section Quiz 15.1.

REMINDER

To *use* a drug means to take a medicine exactly as directed. To *misuse* a drug is to take a medication improperly. To *abuse* a drug is to take a legal drug for a nonmedical reason, or an illegal drug for any reason at all.

Luckily for Max, he had the self-esteem and the knowledge necessary to make the right choice. He was also lucky that he had Troy to talk to about his decision. It's important to have a high opinion of yourself in order to cope effectively with peer pressure. When it comes to drug abuse, it's also important to know as much as you can about the risks you would face if you *didn't* make a good decision. Abusing drugs is highly dangerous for two reasons:

1. It can make a person lose control of the ability to make responsible decisions. Many who abuse drugs act irresponsibly, and sometimes violently.
2. It can cause a person to become **dependent**. A person who is dependent on a drug is controlled by a psychological or physical desire for it.

addicted:

the state of being physically dependent on a drug.

Drug Abuse

On Monday, Max and Troy found out that their friends had stolen a car after smoking crack on Saturday night. They had been caught by the police and were waiting to find out what would happen to them. Max and Troy think their friends would not have stolen the car if they hadn't been under the influence of crack.

People who abuse drugs place themselves, their families, and their society in danger. According to studies, more than 35 percent of all crimes in the United States are committed by people who are under the influence of illicit drugs. That number continues to grow, as drugs like crack have become widespread in many American cities and towns.

Drug abuse also plays a major role in many cases of child abuse and other instances of family violence. Finally, people who drive while under the influence of drugs are just as dangerous to society as those who drive drunk.

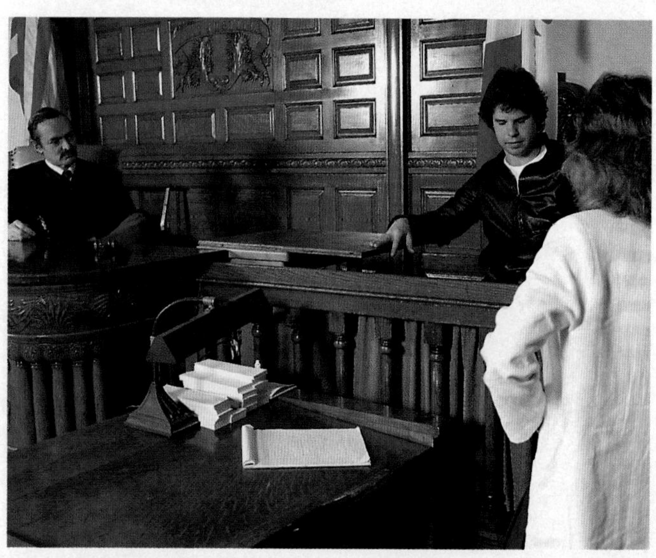

(FIGURE 15-2) **Drug abuse contributes to more than 35 percent of the crimes committed in the United States.**

The Addiction Process

When a person is **addicted** to a drug, it means that his or her body has grown so used to the presence of the drug that it can't function without it. A lot of people think that drug addiction is something that could never happen to them. They believe that no matter how many times they take a certain drug, they will always have the power to stop when they want to. It's important to know that this isn't so. Addiction is a physical process. No matter how strong and invulnerable people may feel, the truth is that if they abuse addictive drugs, they will become physically dependent.

Just as you couldn't do without getting any sleep for a week, people who are addicted to drugs find it very difficult to function without the substance their bodies have come to demand.

Tolerance The body of a person who regularly uses or abuses a drug will eventually

• • • TEACH continued

up to friends who are pressuring him or her to use drugs. The challenge will lie in the way the resisting member uses facts to refute the peers who are exerting pressure.

Role-Playing
It Can't Happen to Me!

Have students role-play a situation in which one friend is trying to convince the other that just trying crack once won't do any harm. The other person should use what he or she has learned so far about the effects of crack on the body. This person should make it clear that no matter how strong drug users think themselves to be, they can become physically dependent.

Class Discussion
How Drugs Affect the Body

After students learn about tolerance of a drug, ask: **What does forming a tolerance to a drug mean?** *[This means that higher and higher doses of the drug are needed to produce the same effect.]* **What are some physical withdrawal symptoms?** *[nausea, vomiting, sleeplessness, and seizures]*

Extension
Is This Fair or Foul?

Some communities are trying to help police locate drug dealers. Newspapers print forms that a reader can clip out and send to the police. A reader who knows of drug dealing in the neighborhood can write names and locations on the form. This method helps keep the

form a resistance, or **tolerance**, to that substance. This means that higher and higher doses of the drug will be required in order to produce the same effects. If Max's friends were to abuse crack regularly, for example, they would soon discover the need to take more and more of the drug in order to get the same ''high'' they felt the first time they smoked it.

Crack cocaine is not the only type of drug whose use leads to tolerance. Many people who take prescription medications that relieve pain or anxiety also find that after a while they must increase the amount of drug they take in order to get the same relief that one or two pills used to give them. Tolerance is the first step in the addiction process.

Dependence Many psychoactive drugs will cause a person to become dependent. A drug dependency can be physical, psychological, or both. **Physical dependence**, or addiction, occurs when a person's body comes to expect the presence of a drug. If it doesn't receive the drug it expects, the body will go through a physical **withdrawal**. Common withdrawal symptoms include nausea, vomiting, and sleeplessness. People who have developed a very high tolerance for a drug may suffer more serious and dangerous withdrawal symptoms, such as seizures. In general, the more addictive and powerful a drug is, the more serious its withdrawal symptoms will be.

A drug doesn't have to lead to tolerance and addiction in order to cause dependence. Many psychoactive drugs can lead to **psychological dependence**. People who are psychologically dependent on a drug are controlled by a constant craving for that substance. Some people with this type of dependency associate certain drugs with a feeling of happiness that they can't seem to find anywhere else.

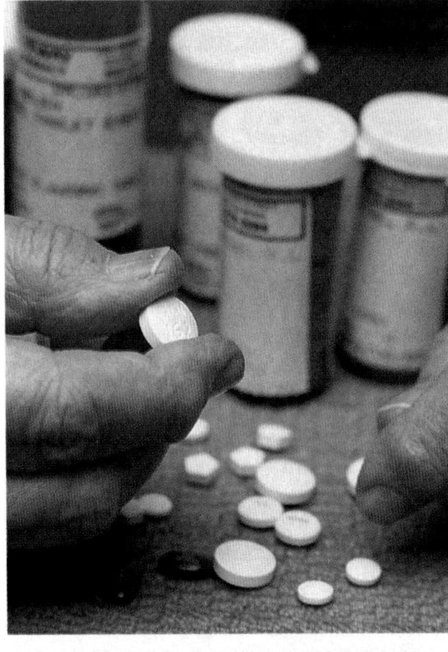

(FIGURE 15-3) **Illegal drugs are not the only substances that can cause addiction. Some prescription medications can lead to tolerance and psychological and physical dependence.**

Review

1. *What are two important dangers of drug abuse?*
2. *What are two ways in which drug abusers can damage society?*
3. *What are two major steps of the addiction process?*
4. ***LIFE SKILLS: Resisting Pressure*** *How would you have told Max's friends that you didn't want to smoke crack?*
5. ***Critical Thinking*** *Explain how a person who abuses a drug that is not physically addictive can still become dependent on that drug.*

REMINDER

Alcohol and nicotine are also addictive, psychoactive drugs of abuse.

physical dependence: *a condition in which the body becomes so used to the presence of a drug that it needs it in order to function.*

withdrawal: *the body's reaction when it doesn't receive a drug it depends upon.*

psychological dependence: *a constant desire to take a psychoactive drug.*

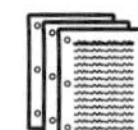

Reteaching Worksheet 15.1

Students who have difficulty with the material may complete Reteaching Worksheet 15.1, which asks them to determine the letters needed by completing statements to make a hidden message.

Review Answers

1. Answers may include irresponsibility, violence, and dependency.
2. Answers may include an increase in crime, child abuse, family violence, and accidents.
3. The two steps are tolerance and dependence.
4. Answers will vary. Students may answer that they would say they do not use drugs.
5. Psychoactive drugs can cause a psychological dependence in which the person associates a certain drug with a feeling of happiness that he or she cannot seem to find anywhere else.

reader who supplied the names anonymous. Some people fear that the names of innocent people could be supplied to police. Ask students to write their opinions of this practice.

ASSESS

Section Review

Have students answer the Section Review questions.

Alternative Assessment

Drugs Among Teenagers

Ask students at what age they think drug education should begin. Have them discuss how what they have learned about drugs will help them to avoid the pitfalls of drug abuse.

Closure

The Effects of Drugs

Discuss with students whether they think learning about the effects of drugs on the body will deter teenagers from taking drugs.

Section 15.2 The Effects of Drugs of Abuse

Objectives

- Know the effects of one category of psychoactive drugs.
- Name two dangers of crack cocaine.
- Know how to avoid inhalant fumes.
- Discuss what you would say to a friend who is thinking of taking anabolic steroids.
  LIFE SKILLS: Communicating Effectively

stimulant: *a drug that causes alertness and speeds up the activity of the body.*

Psychoactive drugs of abuse fall into several categories according to the effects they have on the body. Of course, different drugs have different effects. A person who has taken cocaine will act very differently, for example, from a person who has taken marijuana. Still, it is important to know that every drug works by influencing a specific part of the body. This means that even if you have convinced yourself that a psychoactive drug you take will not affect you, it will. Once you have taken a psychoactive drug, you have limited control over the effects it has on you. For some information on the effects of specific psychoactive drugs, see Figure 15-9 on pages 308-309.

People who take drugs of abuse often lose control of themselves in certain situations and suffer impaired judgment. Things that require concentration, such as driving a car or making an important decision, can become difficult and often impossible when a person is under the influence of a psychoactive drug.

Stimulants

As you learned in Chapter 12, **stimulants** are drugs that cause alertness. Caffeine is the mildest of the stimulants, which is why it is legal to buy and to use. Other stimulants, such as cocaine and amphetamines, have much stronger effects and can be very dangerous.

Caffeine Caffeine is a naturally occurring stimulant. Aside from over-the-counter medications, caffeine can be found in some colas, in tea, and in coffee. A person who drinks a beverage containing caffeine will feel its effects within about 30 minutes. This is because caffeine is absorbed very quickly into the bloodstream through the gastrointestinal tract, and then travels to every part of the body, including the brain.

There is some evidence that caffeine stimulates the mind and body because it interferes with a chemical the brain produces called adenosine. Adenosine may normally influence certain effects in the brain that make a person weary and tired. Caffeine blocks adenosine from achieving these effects, which means that a person who has taken caffeine will be much more alert and much less tired than someone who has not. In high doses, caffeine can make a person irritable, nervous, and unable to sleep.

There is some evidence that caffeine can lead to tolerance and physical dependence. Regular coffee drinkers who give up their habit have been known to suffer such withdrawal symptoms as headache, irritability, drowsiness, and anxiety.

Cocaine and Crack Like caffeine, cocaine is a stimulant derived from an organic,

Section 15.2 Lesson Plan

MOTIVATE

Journal 15B
Saying No to Drugs

This may be done as a warm-up activity. Have students write in the Student Journal in the Student Activity Book their reasons for not taking drugs.

TEACH

Class Discussion
Losing Control With Drugs

What is one way in which drugs differ? *[Different drugs affect specific parts of and have different effects on the body.]* **Why is driving a car when using psychoactive drugs so dangerous?** *[These drugs make you lose your ability to concentrate, which is necessary when driving a car.]* **Why wouldn't you trust someone taking psychoactive drugs with a responsible job?** *[Someone taking these drugs would probably have difficulty making important decisions.]*

Class Discussion
Categories of Drugs of Abuse

What are stimulants? *[Stimulants are drugs that cause alertness.]* **How does caffeine work to stimulate the mind and body?** *[It interferes with a chemical the brain produces called adenosine. Ordinarily, adenosine makes a person feel tired. Caffeine blocks adenosine from doing this and the person feels alert and*

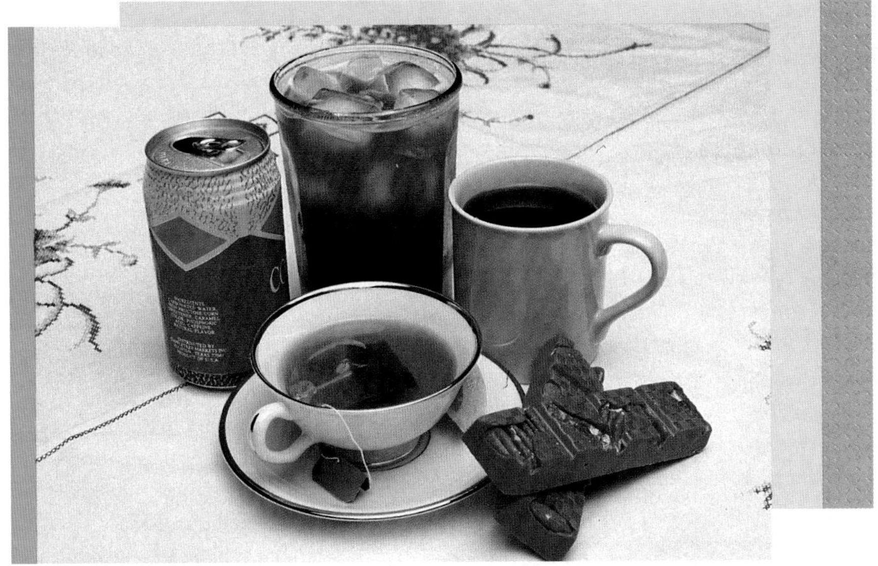

(FIGURE 15-4) **Caffeine is a major ingredient in coffee, tea, chocolate, and certain soft drinks.**

or naturally grown, plant. But it is much more dangerous and addictive. Cocaine is inhaled through the nose, injected, or smoked. When it is inhaled, it enters the bloodstream through the lining of the mucous membrane of the nose, and then travels to the brain. When cocaine is injected or smoked, it reaches the bloodstream more quickly than when it is inhaled.

Someone who has just inhaled cocaine may feel a sense of euphoria, or pleasure. This feeling usually begins within moments after the cocaine has been taken and will last for about 15 minutes.

One important thing to know about this sense of pleasure is that it is often followed by irritability, anxiety, and exhaustion. These feelings will actually last for a longer time than the pleasurable emotions the drug first caused. Cocaine users find that in order to get the sense of pleasure back, they need to take the drug again.

An especially addictive form of cocaine is crack. Because crack (also called rock) is smoked, it gets to the brain very quickly. This means that a person who uses it will feel its physical effects immediately.

There are many reasons why cocaine and crack are so dangerous. For one thing, they are extremely addictive. You read that a person who inhales cocaine wants to take more of the drug as soon as the effects wear off. This is true to an even greater extent for crack, since crack's effects are so strong and so immediate. Breaking an addiction to cocaine or crack is very difficult. A person going through cocaine withdrawal may experience an intense and constant craving for the drug and a severe loss of energy, as well as severe depression and anxiety.

In addition, crack and cocaine both cause severe psychological dependence. Many crack and cocaine abusers find that they are happy only when they are high. Ending a psychological dependence can be as difficult as breaking a physical one.

But even without their addictive qualities, crack and cocaine are highly dangerous

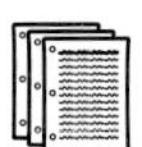

Life Skills Worksheet 15A

Making Responsible Decisions

Assign the Life Skills Worksheet 15A, which has students examine the decision-making process involved in drug use.

less tired than he or she would without caffeine.] **What happens when people take high doses of caffeine?** *[They become irritable, nervous, and cannot sleep.]*

Role-Playing
Effects of High Doses of Caffeine

Have students role-play a situation in which one member has drunk several cups of coffee to keep awake, in order to study for a test. The person with all the caffeine is excitable and cannot sleep. After not sleeping all night, the student is exhausted and unable to think when taking the test.

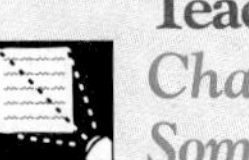

Teaching Transparency 15A
Characteristics of Some Drugs of Abuse

Show the transparency of the chart "Characteristics of Some Drugs of Abuse" (Figure 15-9). Ask several volunteers to interpret the information contained in the chart. **What does the chart tell you about whether a person can become psychologically or physically dependent on caffeine?** *[Moderately]* **Which drugs may cause death with long-term use?** *[LSD, PCP, inhalants, heroin, barbiturates, benzodiazepines]* **Which drugs are highly addictive?** *[cocaine, amphetamines, heroin, barbiturates, benzodiazepines]*

Journal 15C
Personal Risk

Have students use the Student Journal to write their feelings about the personal risks of drug abuse.

Background
The Debate About Amphetamines
Amphetamines were first used to treat asthma, obesity, and to improve athletic performance. By 1947, the medical community became aware that amphetamines were being abused. Abusers began taking up to 30 tablets a day in order to lose weight. Soon these people experienced a mental and physical deterioration. The benefits of these drugs for weight loss are short term. They cause nervousness and excitation of the central nervous system. Since the drugs suppress hunger, the dieter never learns how to deal with hunger.

Facts on Crack

Crack is a form of cocaine that has been chemically altered so that it can be smoked. Because the process changes the cocaine into a chemical "base," crack belongs to a category of cocaine known as freebase.

Crack looks like small lumps or shavings of soap, but has the texture of porcelain. In some parts of the country crack is called "rock" or "readyrock."

The immediate effects of smoking crack are dilated pupils and a narrowing of blood vessels. Crack also causes increases in blood pressure, heart rate, breathing rate, and body temperature.

Crack can constrict the heart's blood vessels, making it work harder and faster to move blood through the body. In some people, this stress may trigger chest pain or heart attack, even for first-time users.

Crack can cause brain seizures, which are a disturbance of the brain's electrical signals. Some users have suffered strokes after using crack—the increase in blood pressure that the blood causes may rupture blood vessels.

Repeated use of crack without experiencing problems does not guarantee freedom from seizures in the future. The next dose—used in the same amount in the same way—can produce a fatal seizure.

Violent, erratic, or paranoid behavior can accompany the use of crack. Hallucinations are also common. Other psychological effects may include profound personality changes.

Crack is particularly alarming because it causes an intense stimulation of the reward center of the brain by allowing the brain chemical dopamine to remain active longer than normal. This causes changes in brain activity and triggers an intense craving for more of the drug, thus creating a powerful psychological dependence on the drug.

(FIGURE 15-5) **Smoking crack even once can be fatal.**

drugs. Cocaine constricts the body's blood vessels, making it harder for blood to circulate. This can put a strain on the heart, and it can even cause a heart attack. For this reason, trying crack or cocaine even once can be fatal.

Amphetamines In contrast to caffeine and cocaine, amphetamines—another type of stimulant—are not derived from natural substances. They are synthetic drugs, which means they are produced or manufactured in laboratories.

Amphetamines are prescription drugs that do have some medical use. Some doctors prescribe amphetamines to treat certain childhood behavioral disorders.

When amphetamines are abused, they can cause tolerance, psychological dependence, and addiction. A person who abuses amphetamines will feel an extreme sense of alertness and an initial feeling of pleasure. Like the effects of cocaine, these pleasurable feelings don't last for a very long time, and they are replaced by a sense of depression and anxiety.

One particularly dangerous form of amphetamine is called ice. Like crack, ice can be smoked. Remember that when a drug is smoked, it will reach the brain much more quickly than when it is taken orally or injected. Ice is very addictive. Its effects include dilated pupils, short attention span, and extreme talkativeness. Ice stays in the system for a very long time. Unlike those of crack, the effects of ice can be felt for several hours.

Hallucinogens

Hallucinogens such as LSD and PCP are very powerful psychoactive substances because they distort the senses. When the senses are affected in this way, it's not always easy to tell what's real from what is not. This is why people on hallucinogens

• • • TEACH continued

Class Discussion
"Facts on Crack"

To help students understand and assimilate the information in the chart "Facts on Crack," ask the following questions: **Why does crack use often trigger heart attacks?** *[Crack causes the blood vessels to constrict, making the heart overwork as it tries to move blood through the body.]* **Why does crack cause strokes in some people who use it?** *[The increased blood pressure caused by the drug may rupture blood vessels, which causes a stroke.]* **Why is crack so addictive?** *[It causes an intense stimulation of the reward center of the brain. This triggers an intense craving for more of the drug.]*

Cooperative Learning
Campaigning Against Crack

Have students work in cooperative groups to produce slogans that will point out the dangers of crack. Have them refer to the chart "Facts on Crack" and the information in the text. Ask them to make posters that will display their slogans.

Debate the Issue
Should Amphetamines Be Used for Weight Control?

Hold a class debate on the topic: Should amphetamines be used for controlling the appetite? Have students do some research on the addictiveness of amphetamines, as well as on their effects on weight control. Al-

often forget where they are and may have difficulty keeping track of time. In some cases, hallucinogens have caused people to believe they have special powers. Three powerful hallucinogens are LSD, PCP, and a designer drug called ecstasy.

LSD Lysergic acid diethylamide, or LSD, is made from a type of fungus that grows on rye and other grains. The effects of LSD are not always easy to predict. Sometimes the drug will stimulate the body like cocaine. Other times it acts as a **depressant**, which is a drug that slows down body functions such as heart rate and blood pressure.

A person who has taken LSD will begin to feel its effects within about 30 to 90 minutes. At first the user may feel a rise in body temperature and a loss of appetite. Eventually, the effects reach the senses. At this point the user may begin to see and hear things that are not there. This type of effect is known as a **hallucination**. At the same time, he or she may be experiencing huge emotional swings. People on LSD often feel incredibly happy one moment, and on the verge of tears the next.

Some LSD experiences are extremely frightening. Users can become panicked, confused, and extremely anxious. Some people have become so upset and scared while on the drug that they have killed themselves.

Sometimes a person who has had a bad LSD experience will suddenly start feeling the drug's effects again, long after the experience is over. This is called a **flashback**. People can experience flashbacks without warning, sometimes months after they have taken their last dose of LSD. Flashbacks can be as frightening and dangerous as the bad experiences that prompted them.

PCP Another dangerous hallucinogen is PCP. Also known as ''angel dust,'' PCP is usually sprinkled on tobacco or marijuana cigarettes and smoked. PCP has been known to cause severe mental disturbances. People on PCP often act violently toward others or toward themselves.

The mental disturbances caused by PCP may disappear after a few hours. Sometimes, though, they last for a much longer time. People who take PCP may feel the drug's effects for several weeks.

Designer Drugs Some very powerful psychoactive drugs can be created by making slight changes in the chemistry of drugs that already exist. These are called **designer drugs**. One type of designer drug is MDMA, also called ecstasy.

Ecstasy is an illegal drug that is very close in its chemical makeup to amphetamines. Like amphetamines, it causes psychological and physical dependence. People who have used ecstasy say it makes them feel relaxed and happy. It can also cause confusion, depression, sleep problems, and severe anxiety. The physical effects of ecstasy include blurred vision, nausea, faintness, and chills and sweating.

Because ecstasy is a fairly new drug of abuse, not much is known about its long-term dangers and effects. Some studies with laboratory animals, however, show that using this drug over a long period of time causes brain damage in laboratory animals.

Marijuana and Hashish

Marijuana and hashish are organic drugs that come from the Indian hemp plant. It is not certain whether marijuana and hashish are physically addictive, but people have been known to become psychologically dependent on both drugs.

The psychoactive ingredient in both marijuana and hashish is a chemical called delta-9-tetrahydrocannabinol, or THC. Both drugs are usually smoked, although they can be eaten as well.

depressant: *a drug that slows body functioning.*

designer drugs: *synthetic drugs that are similar in chemistry to certain illegal drugs.*

hallucination: *imaginary sights and sounds, often induced by the use of a hallucinogen.*

flashback: *an unexpected return to an unpleasant LSD experience, often months after the original experience ended.*

hallucinogen: *a drug that distorts a person's senses.*

low presentations, counterarguments, and questions from the audience.

Class Discussion
Hallucinogens

After the students have read about hallucinogens, ask: **What happens during a hallucination?** *[During a hallucination, a drug user begins to see and hear things that are not there.]* **What causes some users of LSD to kill themselves?** *[They become so frightened and confused by the experience that they think the only way out is to kill themselves.]* **What is a flashback?** *[Long after the experience is over, an LSD user can suddenly start feeling the drug's effects again, with all the terrifying moments relived.]*

Journal 15D
Coping With Stress

Ask students to use the Student Journal to write about how they cope with stress. Have them be specific about positive actions they take to help them when stress is a problem.

Role-Playing
Positive Measures Against Stress

Ask students to role-play a situation where one member of the group is under terrible pressure at home and is considering taking drugs. Have the others in the group provide other ways to solve the pressure problem instead of escaping to drugs.

Marijuana and hashish have very relaxing effects. In fact, people who use these drugs can become so relaxed that they may find it difficult to finish sentences, to speak, or even to remember their own thoughts. They may also suffer a loss of coordination. For these reasons, driving a car or operating other machinery is very dangerous for people who are high on marijuana or hashish.

The effects of both drugs make many people anxious and may even cause a state of panic. It can be very frightening not to have control over your own thoughts and coordination.

inhalants: *chemicals that produce strong psychoactive effects when they are inhaled.*

Inhalants

Inhalants are chemicals that produce strong psychoactive effects when they are inhaled. Certain glues and paint thinners contain inhalant fumes. Another type of inhalant is nitrous oxide, or "laughing gas," which some dentists use as a form of analgesic.

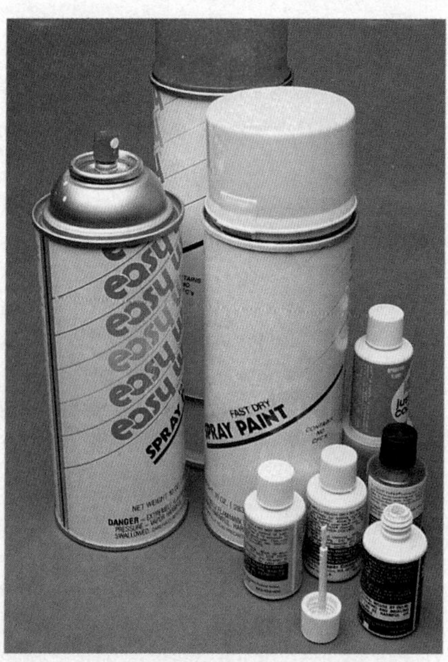

(FIGURE 15-6) **Some paint thinners and glues contain inhalant fumes.**

Inhalants enter the bloodstream and travel to the brain immediately after they are inhaled. A person abusing inhalants will experience an initial feeling of lightheadedness and giddiness. These effects last for a very brief period of time, and are often replaced by dizziness, nausea, and headache. Like marijuana, inhalants can interfere with a person's coordination, thoughts, and perceptions.

The best way to prevent inhalant abuse is to know what kinds of products contain dangerous fumes. It's best to avoid these products completely, but if you have to use them, make sure you read the label and follow the instructions.

If you feel yourself getting lightheaded while using one of these products, go outside until the feeling goes away. Make sure that you close all containers after you have finished with them. Inhalants are very powerful drugs of abuse. You wouldn't want to leave yourself or anyone else exposed to their dangers.

narcotic: *a drug with pain-relieving and psychoactive properties that is made from the opium plant.*

Heroin and Other Narcotics

Narcotics, which are drugs that have been derived, or made, from the opium poppy plant, are something of a double-edged sword. Some narcotics serve useful medical purposes, because they relieve pain so effectively. Morphine and codeine are two narcotic preparations used in hospitals for patients in severe pain.

On the other hand, narcotics are among the most physically addictive drugs of abuse. All narcotic medications should be taken only under the strict orders and observations of a doctor.

Not all narcotics have medical uses. One type of narcotic, heroin, is a very powerful, very addictive drug that is illegal to buy, sell, and use.

• • • TEACH continued

Reinforcement

Dangers of Heroin

Why are heroin addicts at risk of contracting AIDS? *[Heroin addicts usually inject heroin into their veins. Since they may share a needle with an HIV infected person, they are at risk of introducing the HIV virus into their bloodstream.]* **What happens when abusers overdose on heroin?** *[Their breathing slows down so much that they lose consciousness, go into a coma, and often die.]*

Role-Playing

A Right Way and a Wrong Way to Use a Prescribed Drug

Have students dramatize a right way and a wrong way to use a prescribed drug such as a sleeping pill or a tranquilizer. Students should demonstrate that the user should use the pills exactly as prescribed. Usually, the prescription is for a temporary condition and is not refilled. They should also include in their dramatizations that the patient should tell the physician if he or she is taking any other drugs at the time. The drug should not be taken with alcohol.

Class Discussion

Anabolic Steroids

Tell students that anabolic means "to build up." Ask students why the steroids used by athletes are called anabolic steroids. Have students discuss why steroid use is dangerous to their health. Students may recall that ath-

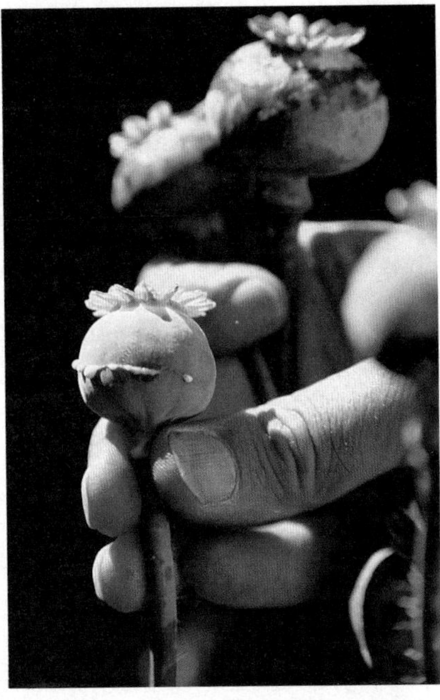

(FIGURE 15-7) **Heroin and other narcotics are all made from the opium poppy plant.**

Like all narcotics, heroin causes tolerance to the drug. People who are addicted to heroin have to keep increasing their doses in order to get the same effects. For this reason they run the constant risk of overdose. Large doses of heroin can severely depress the respiratory system. This can lead to a loss of consciousness, coma, and even death.

Heroin is most often bought and sold on the street, which means that it has some additional dangers. For one thing, drug dealers selling heroin often "cut" or mix the drug with other substances. People who buy heroin never know if the drug they are taking is pure.

In addition, people who use heroin usually inject the drug into their veins. Heroin users who share dirty or contaminated needles run the risk of infecting themselves with hepatitis or AIDS. One of the fastest-growing groups of AIDS sufferers in the United States is intravenous drug abusers.

overdose:

a serious, sometimes fatal, reaction to a large dose of a drug.

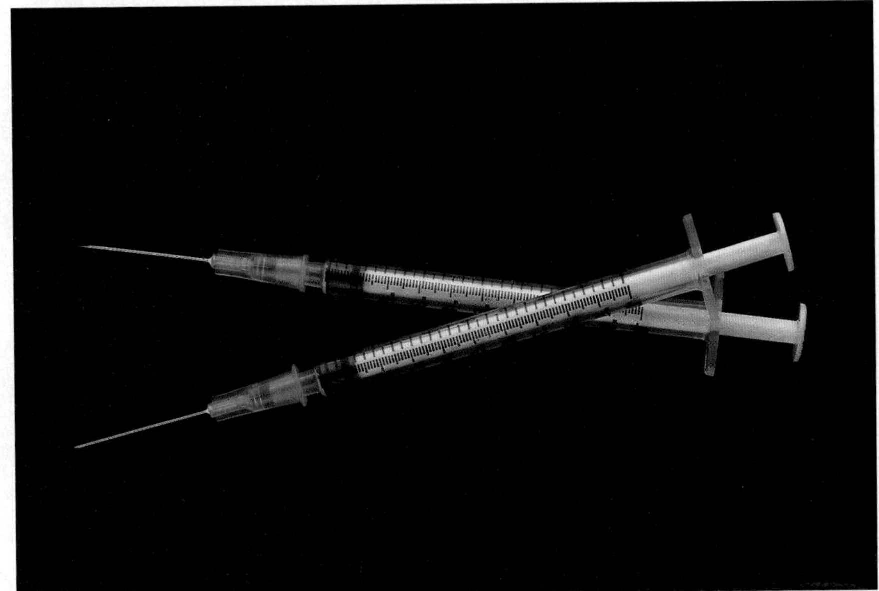

(FIGURE 15-8) **Intravenous drug users who share contaminated needles are at a high risk of contracting HIV.**

letes have been sent home from the Olympics and have been deprived of gold medals for using steroids. Ask students to use Figure 15-11 to help them decide how the judges of an athletic event might be able to tell before testing that an athlete is using steroids.

Journal 15E
Would You Take Steroids?

Encourage students to think about and write in the Student Journal their feelings about the use of steroids to improve athletic ability.

Cooperative Learning
Risks of Using Steroids

Have students work in cooperative groups to discuss the problem athletes face of taking or not taking steroids. Ask them If they knew steroids would help them win an important athletic contest, would they be tempted to take them? Have students list the opinions of the group and then share and debate these with the class.

Class Discussion
Drugs and Pregnancy

Why is taking drugs during pregnancy such a dangerous act? *[A fetus is very sensitive to any chemicals, some of which may cause facial and body deformities, retardation in growth and learning, brain damage, slowed reflexes, and severe learning disabilities. In addition, the fetus may be born with the same addiction as its mother.]* **What is the effect of marijuana use during**

Characteristics of Some Drugs of Abuse

Drug	Short-Term Effects	Long-Term Effects
Caffeine	*Increased alertness, decreased appetite, elevated heartbeat*	*Irritability, insomnia, anxiety*
Cocaine	*Increased alertness, euphoria, excitement, decreased appetite, elevated heartbeat*	*Restlessness, anxiety, insomnia, possible nasal damage when sniffed*
Amphetamines	*Increased alertness, euphoria, excitement, decreased appetite, elevated heartbeat*	*Restlessness, anxiety, insomnia*
LSD	*Illusions and hallucinations, poor perception of time and distance*	*Increased delusions and panic, psychosis, flashbacks, death*
PCP	*Illusions and hallucinations, poor perception of time and distance*	*Increased delusions and panic, psychosis, flashbacks, death*
Marijuana and Hashish	*Relaxation, breakdown of inhibitions*	*Possible psychosis, impaired breathing when smoked*
Inhalants	*Relaxation, euphoria, impaired coordination*	*Hallucinations, brain damage, death*
Heroin	*Relaxation, relief of pain and anxiety, euphoria*	*Weight loss, stupor, sickness, death*
Barbiturates	*Relaxation, euphoria, drowsiness, impaired coordination, sleep*	*Brain and/or liver damage, confusion, irritability, sickness, death*
Benzodiazepines (minor tranquilizers)	*Relaxation, euphoria, drowsiness, impaired coordination, sleep*	*Brain and/or liver damage, confusion, irritability, sickness, death*

(FIGURE 15-9) **Some drugs of abuse are more addictive and more powerful than others. All of these substances, however, have their dangers.**

• • • TEACH continued

pregnancy? *[Increased risk of low birth weight, delay in physiological development, and abnormalities of the nervous system]* **What effect do cocaine and heroin use have on the fetus?** *[The baby may be born with the same addiction.]*

Extension

Advice of the Athletic Director

Have students interview their athletic director or coach about the use of steroids to improve athletic ability. Have them share what they learned with the class.

Effects of Overdose	Psychological Dependence	Physical Dependence
Restlessness, irritability, insomnia	*Moderate*	*Moderate*
Restlessness, irritability, insomnia, psychosis, death	*High*	*High*
Restlessness, irritability, insomnia, psychosis, death	*High*	*High*
Anxiety, hallucinations, psychosis, stupor, panic, death	*Low*	*None*
Anxiety, hallucinations, psychosis, stupor, panic, death	*High*	*Low*
Stupor, paranoia, possible psychosis	*Moderate*	*Moderate*
Stupor, death	*Unknown*	*Unknown*
Stupor, death	*High*	*High*
Slurred speech, stupor, death	*High*	*High*
Slurred speech, stupor, death	*High*	*Moderate*

Section Review Worksheet 15.2

Assign Section Review Worksheet 15.2, which requires students to correct false statements about the effects of drug abuse.

Section Quiz 15.2

Have students take Section Quiz 15.2.

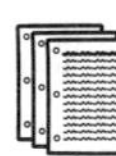

Reteaching Worksheet 15.2

Students who have difficulty with the material may complete Reteaching Worksheet 15.2, which requires them to complete a concept map about the effects of drug abuse.

Background
Use of Tranquilizers

Tranquilizers are meant for those who have a severe or incapacitating anxiety, panic, or tension. They are not designed to treat someone suffering from the ordinary tension of everyday life. The latter kind of tension is normal and can help motivate a person to attain worthwhile goals. Users of tranquilizers such as Valium develop withdrawal symptoms after taking large doses for a few days, moderate doses for a few months, or small doses for a few years. Combining alcohol with Halcion to aid sleep can cause amnesia.

sedative hypnotics:

drugs that depress the body system and cause sleepiness.

Sedative-Hypnotics

Sedative-hypnotics are drugs that depress the body system and cause sleepiness. Some common names for sedative-hypnotics are tranquilizers, sleeping pills, and sedatives.

The two major kinds of sedative-hypnotics are barbiturates and benzodiazepines. Barbiturates are prescribed preparations that relieve anxiety and insomnia. They are also very addictive, abused drugs that are illegally bought and sold. Secobarbital and pentobarbital (sold under the brand names Seconal and Nembutal) are two common types of barbiturates.

Benzodiazepines (which are sometimes called minor tranquilizers) are prescription medications prescribed to relieve minor anxiety and insomnia. Some common benzodiazepines are diazepam (sold under the brand name of Valium), chlordiazepoxide (Librium), and chlorazepate (Tranxene).

Although benzodiazepines are not as powerful as barbiturates, they are still addictive drugs of abuse. Like barbiturates, the benzodiazepines are often sold illegally to drug abusers.

Drugs and Pregnancy Facts

The infants of women who use marijuana when they are pregnant are at increased risk of suffering low birth weight, delay in physiological development, and nervous system abnormalities.

Women who use cocaine when they are pregnant are at increased risk of suffering hemorrhage (heavy bleeding), premature delivery, and miscarriage.

Heroin use during pregnancy increases the likelihood of stillbirth and infant death.

The babies born to women who are addicted to narcotics such as heroin will suffer withdrawal symptoms within 72 hours of birth. These symptoms, which may last for 6 to 8 weeks, include restlessness, tremors, disturbed sleep, sweating, vomiting, stuffy nose, diarrhea, high-pitched crying, and seizures.

(FIGURE 15-10) **Women who abuse drugs while they are pregnant endanger the lives and well-being of their unborn babies.**

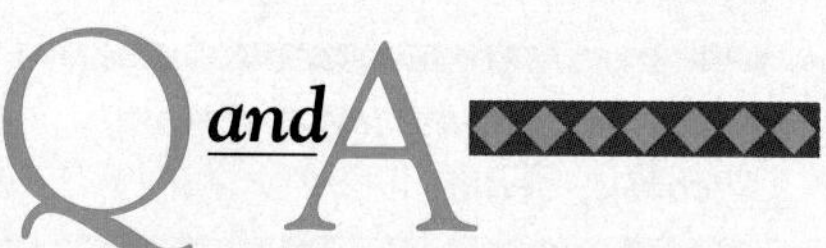

Q. Can sniffing cocaine kill a person?

A. There have been several instances in which a person has died from sniffing cocaine.

Q. Is marijuana as dangerous as alcohol?

A. Yes. Both alcohol and marijuana impair a person's judgment, lessen coordination, and diminish reflexes. A person who has had alcohol or marijuana should never try to drive. Both substances can also cause long-term damage to the body. Finally, both alcohol and marijuana are illegal substances for teenagers in the United States.

Drugs and Pregnancy

Many drugs a woman takes when she is pregnant pass into the bloodstream of her unborn child. For this reason, women who are pregnant should always check with their doctor before using any medications. This is particularly true during the first several weeks of pregnancy, when the fetus is especially sensitive to any chemicals that may cause damage.

What if a drug abuser were to get pregnant? Drugs of abuse can pose very serious dangers to the growth and development of an unborn child. Babies born to women who abused drugs when they were pregnant have suffered such damage as facial and body deformities, retardation in growth and learning, brain damage, slowed reflexes, and severe learning disabilities. In addition, there is evidence that babies born to women who are addicted to drugs such as heroin and crack are born with the same addictions as their mothers.

LifeSKILLS: Communicating Effectively

Should She Use Steroids?

Jessie hits the swimming pool every morning at 6:00. By the time you wake up every day, she's already been swimming for an hour. No wonder she's captain of the girl's varsity swim team, and that she swims the anchor leg on the freestyle and medley relay teams. Still, Jessie says, practice isn't enough to get her a college scholarship.

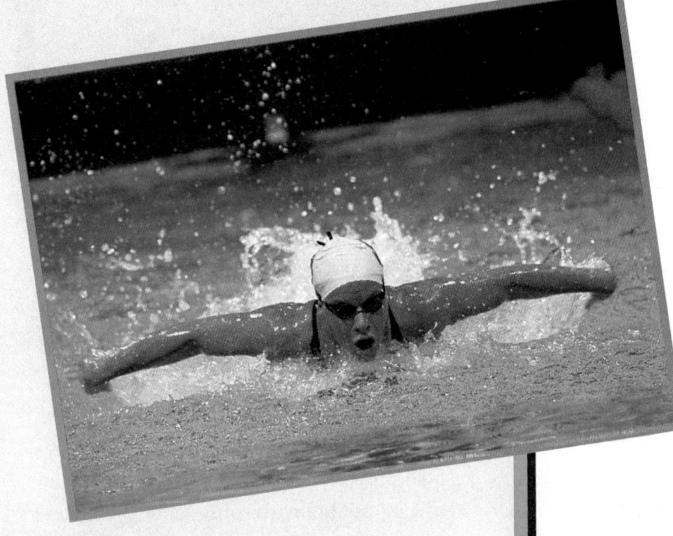

Unfortunately, Jessie's greatest goal is to swim for a big university team. You find it hard to believe that Jessie isn't good enough to qualify, but she insists that there are hundreds of other girls who are bigger, stronger, and faster. That's why she's thinking about using steroids. She says she knows some people who have used them. "You should see their muscles," Jessie says "They blow me away every time I swim with them." "Come on, Jessie," you say. "Not every good swimmer uses steroids."

"Yeah, but I'll have to if I want to get a scholarship."

You know Jessie's serious, and that you'll have to talk her out of using steroids. What are some good arguments you can use?

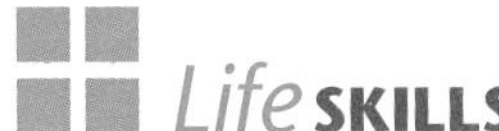

Life SKILLS

Should She Use Steroids?

Have students do the Life Skills exercise in the text, answering the questions on paper.

Review Answers

1. Answers will vary. Be sure students' explanations include behavior, physiological changes, sensations, and health consequences.
2. Answers may include addiction, violent behavior, increased risk of heart attack, and death.
3. Answers may include: read the label and follow the instruction; use only in an open, well-ventilated area; and close all containers after you have finished.
4. Answers will vary. Students should include in their answers that steroids have dangerous side effects that far outnumber any benefits.
5. Yes. If a person does not follow the directions on the prescription label or those given by the doctor exactly, the person may misuse the drug and take too much of it or take the drug too often. This misuse can lead to abuse and addiction.

Profile of a Steroid Abuser

Social	*Recent changes in friends* *Obsession with health, exercise, weight lifting*
Physical	*Rapid weight gain and muscle development* *Increased body hair* *Deepening of voice* *Acne* *Hair loss* *Breast enlargement (males)* *Difficulty urinating* *Elevated blood pressure* *Stomach upset* *Jaundice* *Swelling of extremities*
Mental Changes	*Increased aggression* *Hyperactivity, irritability* *Auditory hallucinations* *Paranoid delusions* *Manic episodes* *Depression and anxiety* *Panic disorders* *Suicidal thoughts*

(FIGURE 15-11) **People who abuse steroids show certain social, physical, and mental symptoms.**

Anabolic Steroids

anabolic steroid: *an artificially made, complex substance that can temporarily increase muscle size.*

One of the most widespread problems in both professional and amateur sports is the use of **anabolic steroids** among athletes. Made to resemble the male hormone testosterone, anabolic steroids were originally developed and used to treat people suffering from a blood condition called anemia, as well as certain bone and joint disorders.

Because they can help a person gain weight and develop muscles, anabolic steroids have become very popular drugs of abuse. Athletes have used them to help them run or swim faster, or to make them stronger. But the dangers of abusing anabolic steroids far outnumber what some people may think of as benefits.

For example, anabolic steroids can cause liver and heart damage, as well as very high blood pressure. Anabolic steroid abusers have been known to act aggressively and even violently. For more characteristics of anabolic steroid abuse, see Figure 15-11.

Athletes who use anabolic steroids may think they are at an advantage in competition. Anabolic steroids can be easily detected, however, and any athlete caught with anabolic steroids in his or her system is automatically disqualified from most competitions.

Review

1. *Explain the effects of one category of psychoactive drugs.*
2. *Name two dangers of crack cocaine.*
3. *What is a good precaution to take if you have to use a product with inhalant fumes?*
4. ***LIFE SKILLS: Communicating Effectively*** *If your friend wanted to take anabolic steroids to get stronger, what would you say to him or her?*
5. ***Critical Thinking*** *Is it possible for a person using drugs for medical purposes to become addicted? Explain your answer.*

ASSESS

Section Review

Have students answer the Section Review questions.

Alternative Assessment

A Drug-Free World

Ask students to speculate what it would be like if there were no drugs of abuse in the world.

Closure

What Stands Out Most

Ask students what made the most vivid impression on them as they learned about the effects of various drugs of abuse.

Section 15.3 Treatment for Dependency

Objectives

- *Name two things everyone should know about treatment for drug dependency.*
- *Know three options for recovering drug abusers.*
- *Know a healthy alternative to abusing drugs.*

Fighting a dependency to any drug is not easy. Most people who are addicted to drugs are psychologically dependent on them as well. The goal of all drug-treatment programs is to help a person battle not only the drug dependency itself but also the reasons why the drug abuse started in the first place. Fortunately, there are many options for people in this situation.

There are two things everyone who decides to seek treatment for a drug dependency should know. First, no one should try to overcome a drug dependency on his or her own. *Everyone* needs help when it comes to addiction or dependence. Another thing to realize about drug dependency is that there is no such thing as a *recovered* drug addict. Even if a person has not abused drugs for years, the chance that the person will relapse by abusing a drug again, and will become dependent again, is always there. Every recovering drug addict learns to take life without drugs one day at a time.

Methadone Maintenance Programs

People who are addicted to heroin have an especially difficult time overcoming their dependence. Their bodies have become so used to the presence of heroin that the withdrawal process can be very painful.

Some heroin addicts choose methadone maintenance to help them go through the withdrawal process. Like heroin, methadone is a narcotic. But its effects are not

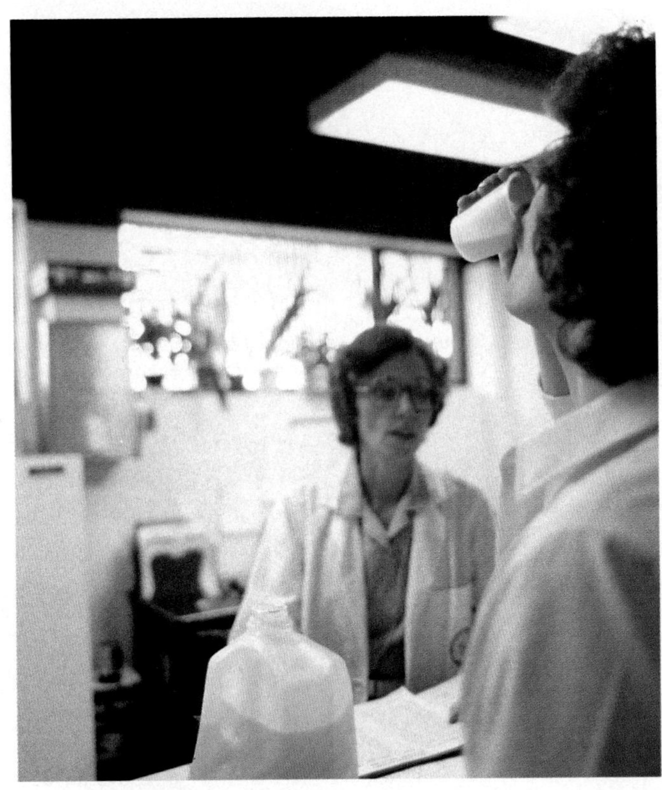

(FIGURE 15-12) **Methadone, a narcotic without the powerful effects of heroin, may help a person endure the painful process of heroin withdrawal.**

Background
Methadone in Treatment of Heroin Addicts

Methadone is used in the treatment of heroin addicts. It suppresses withdrawal symptoms for 24 to 32 hours. It is legal and is effective when taken orally, avoiding dirty needles and the possibility of spreading AIDS. However, many addicts continue to take heroin along with methadone. The long-term percentage of cures is low. Methadone itself is addictive. Some patients sell the methadone that is supposed to carry them through the weekend. A drug called LAAM—chemically related to methadone—suppresses heroin withdrawal symptoms for 48 to 72 hours. Since a supply of LAAM need not be given for the weekend, there is less possibility of its being sold on the street.

Section 15.3 Lesson Plan

MOTIVATE

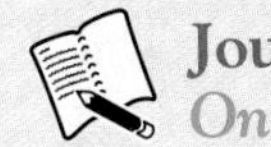

Journal 15F
On Seeking Help

This may be done as a warm-up activity. Have students write in the Student Journal what they would do if they were using drugs and wanted to stop. To whom would they turn for help? What would be their reasons for quitting drugs?

Class Discussion
Fighting Dependency

Why is it important for a person who has become addicted to a drug to find out why he or she became addicted in the first place? *[If the person is not able to solve the problem that caused the addiction, the person may fall back into drug use again.]* **What are two things someone must remember when seeking treatment for dependency on drugs?** *[Everyone needs help when it comes to drug addiction; there is no such thing as a recovered drug addict.]* **Why does a person addicted to heroin have such a difficult time during treatment?** *[The withdrawal process is very painful because the body has become dependent upon the drug.]*

Cooperative Learning
Helping a Friend on Drugs

Have students work in cooperative groups to discuss how they would handle the problem of a friend who

Background

Causes of Addiction

Researchers claim that there does not seem to be an addiction-prone personality. However, people differ in their ability to withstand stress and peer pressure, which may be a factor in drug addiction. Rehabilitation must help addicts to be aware of these differences and help them overcome them.

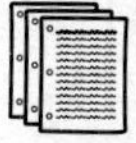

Life Skills Worksheet 15B

Where to Get Help

Assign the Life Skills Worksheet 15B, which requires students to find out about help for drug abusers in their community.

Making a Choice 15B

A Family Disease?

Assign the A Family Disease? card. The card asks students to discuss the meaning of the term "family disease" when applied to drug addiction.

nearly as powerful or as appealing. People who go through methadone maintenance are able to provide their bodies with the narcotic they crave. The dosages of methadone are gradually decreased until the withdrawal process has been completed.

Withdrawing from a physical addiction is only the first step in the recovery process. The next hurdle all drug addicts must clear is the psychological dependency they have formed.

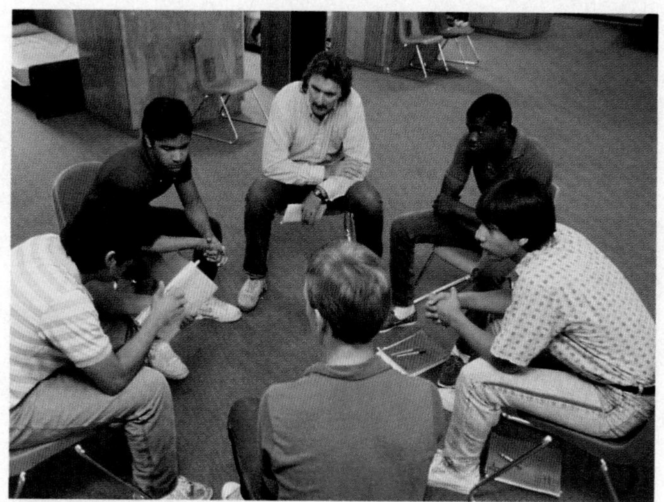

(FIGURE 15-13) **Group therapy sessions play an important role in all inpatient and outpatient drug-treatment programs.**

Inpatient and Outpatient Programs

Programs in hospitals and special treatment centers provide help for addicts going through withdrawal. Some recovering drug abusers need to live at the center while they receive treatment. Others will choose to stay at home and participate on an outpatient basis.

Although some programs provide methadone maintenance for recovering addicts, many treatment facilities help their patients go through withdrawal without the use of chemicals.

Inpatient and outpatient programs rely very heavily on education, one-on-one counseling, and group therapy to help recovering patients overcome their psychological dependencies. This is a very important part of the treatment process. In sessions, addicts talk to each other or to a counselor about the reasons why they started abusing drugs, and why they want to stop relying on them now.

Self-Help Programs

There are also programs available for drug abusers who want to quit without the help of professional counselors. Self-help programs like Narcotics Anonymous work in the same way as Alcoholics Anonymous. The first step those who join NA must take is to admit that they are powerless over their dependence on drugs. From there, recovering abusers help one another stay drug free by attending regular meetings and through listening to and supporting each other one day at a time.

Options for Teenagers

Many teenagers who abuse drugs want to quit but aren't sure how to go about doing it. Most hospital and treatment-center programs have special divisions for teenagers with drug problems. Even so, some teenagers may find it intimidating to go to a stranger and admit that they have a problem with drugs.

For this reason, many schools now have student assistance programs available for students. Student assistance programs are set up to offer students information and sometimes to refer them to places that can help them overcome a drug dependency. Schools that don't provide student assistance programs usually have guidance counselors to perform the same functions. In addition, many towns and communities

needs help in dealing with drug dependency. Have them discuss whether they would tell a counselor or would go directly to the friend.

Class Discussion

Teenagers Trying to Quit Drugs

What could teenagers do who are trying to quit drugs? *[Schools have school assistance programs or guidance counselors to refer them to places that can help them overcome a drug dependency. The Yellow Pages in the phone book lists state and local councils on drug abuse.]* **When might you seek help from an intervention counselor?** *[If you have a friend who isn't seeking help for drug dependency, you might want help in knowing how to confront the friend with his or her need for help.]*

Role-Playing

Peer Pressure

Have students role-play situations in which drugs are being used and nonusers are being urged to participate. One scene could take place at a gym and involve steroids, another could involve a school playground and marijuana, a third scene could involve a cafeteria and tranquilizers.

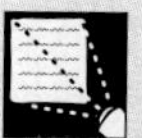

Teaching Transparency 15B

The Cost of Illegal Drugs

Use this transparency to show the extent of the illegal drug problem in the United States. The tables show the estimated amounts of money spent on illegal drugs by all Americans, by high school students, and by college students.

have state or local councils on drug abuse that can provide referral services for teenagers seeking treatment. State and local councils on drug abuse should be listed in your yellow pages.

A guidance counselor or student assistance program can also refer students to intervention counselors. If you know someone who is dependent on drugs and who isn't seeking the help he or she needs, you may want to think about using a formal group intervention strategy. Intervention means confronting a drug addict with his or her dependency and strongly encouraging him or her to seek treatment. If you decide that you want to use intervention, make sure you talk to an expert first.

If you have a drug abuse problem, there is nothing to be ashamed or embarrassed about. The important thing is to

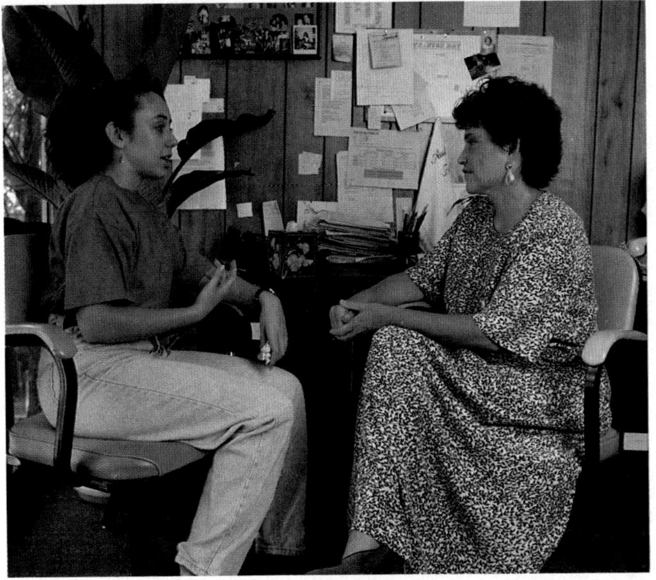

(FIGURE 15-15) **School guidance counselors can help teenagers with drug dependencies get proper treatment.**

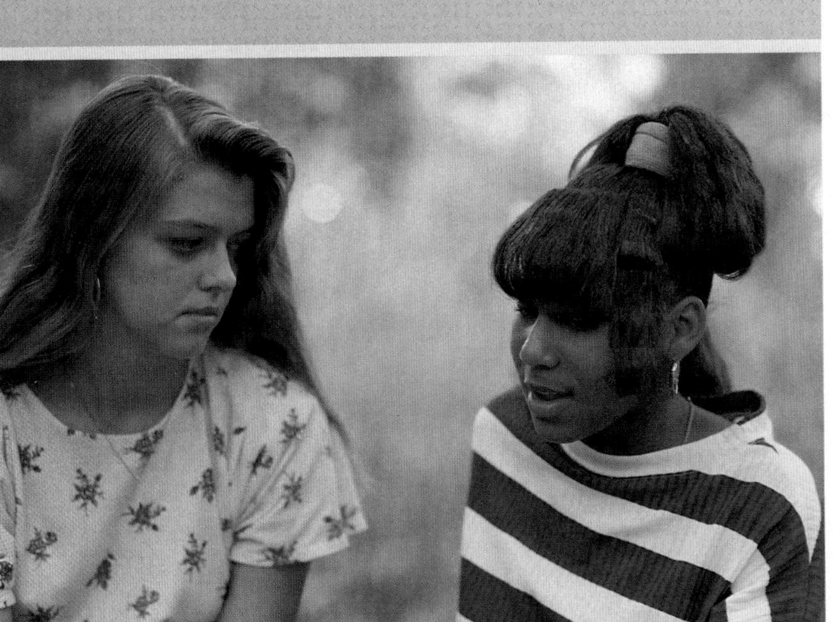

(FIGURE 15-14) **Sometimes having a friend to talk to can make hard times less painful.**

NATIONAL
NATIONAL PARENTS' RESOURCE INSTITUTE FOR DRUG EDUCATION (PRIDE)
NUMBERS
1-800-241-7946

NATIONAL
NATIONAL COCAINE HOTLINE
NUMBERS
1-800-262-2463

SECTION 15.3

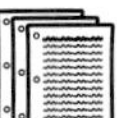

Section Review Worksheet 15.3

Assign Section Review Worksheet 15.3, which has students complete statements about treatment for drug dependency.

Section Quiz 15.3

Have students take Section Quiz 15.3.

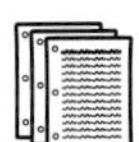

Reteaching Worksheet 15.3

Students who have difficulty with the material may complete Reteaching Worksheet 15.3, which has them complete a maze dealing with recovery from drug addiction and dependency.

Journal 15G
Options to Drugs

Have students write in the Student Journal the alternatives to taking drugs as a solution for everyday problems. Ask them which alternative they would choose and why.

Extension
Crisis Intervention

Have students visit a community clinic, family counseling center, or other agency that deals with people in crisis over drugs. Have them write questions ahead of time and prepare a brief report afterward about the kinds of problems drug users face and how they are being helped.

Review Answers

1. No one should try to overcome a drug dependency on his or her own; there is no such thing as a recovered drug addict.

2. Methadone maintenance programs for heroin abusers, in- and outpatient programs, self-help programs

3. Talking to someone you feel you can confide in about problems

4. A person who has abused drugs in the past most likely will have the tendency to abuse drugs again in certain circumstances. Therefore, a recovering drug abuser must learn to take life without drugs one day at a time.

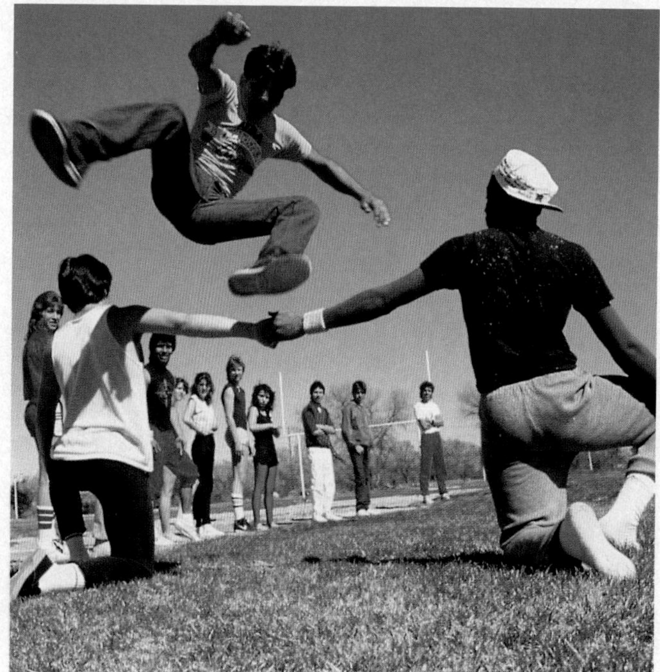

(FIGURE 15-16) **Life's too short to be wasted on drugs.**

NATIONAL
NATIONAL DRUG INFORMATION AND REFERRAL LINE
NATIONAL INSTITUTE ON DRUG ABUSE
NUMBERS
1-800-662-4357

admit you do have a problem and get help. One thing you *shouldn't* try to do is recover by yourself. Remember, no one can overcome a drug dependency on his or her own—everyone needs help. Talk to someone in the student assistance program at your school, or call one of the hotline numbers listed in the margin. Once you have admitted you have a drug problem and you have made the decision to seek help, you have taken a major step toward recovery.

Finally, if you have thought about abusing drugs, know that there are other options. Life can be very difficult. Many teenagers face struggles in their day-to-day lives—such as poverty, family problems, or depression—that can make it very hard to get through each day. Teenagers in these situations sometimes may feel a sense of hopelessness about themselves and the world around them. Why not take a drug, they may think, if it makes things easier for a while?

If you have felt this way, you're not alone. But taking drugs is the *worst* thing you can do. Their effects don't last forever, and when they end, you are left with the same feelings you had before—only worse. People who abuse drugs or alcohol often act impulsively and even dangerously. A person who is drunk or high, for instance, is more likely to commit suicide than a person who isn't.

There are people you can talk to about the things that are troubling you. If you don't think you can confide in a parent or close friend, you may want to speak to a coach, a teacher, or a religious leader. If they can't help you, they may be able to refer you to someone who can. The important thing to remember is that pain does pass and life can get better. Drugs may seem like a temporary solution, but in the long run they don't solve problems—they only add to them.

Review

1. *What are two things everyone should know about treatment for drug dependency?*
2. *Name three options for recovering drug abusers.*
3. *What's a healthier way to deal with problems than abusing drugs?*
4. ***Critical Thinking*** *Explain the reasoning behind the following statement: "There is no such thing as a recovered drug abuser."*

ASSESS

Section Review

Have students answer the Section Review questions.

Alternative Assessment

Why Take the Risk?

Ask students to explain what makes drugs of abuse so attractive that people will take risks to obtain and use them. What kinds of personality traits and experiences make people most vulnerable to using drugs?

Closure

Letter of Advice

Ask students to write a brief letter to Josephine, a young woman who is thinking about taking drugs to help her face her problems. Tell them to make it clear that adding drugs to her problems will only make them worse.

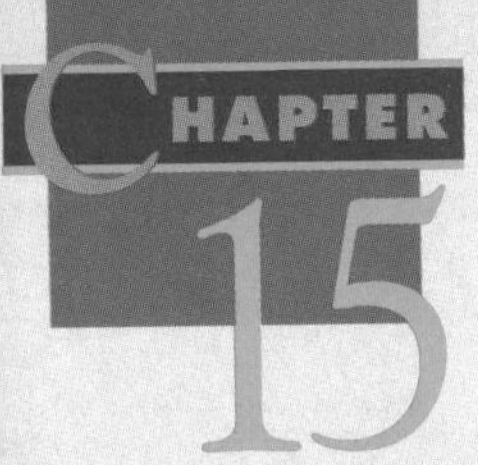

Highlights

Summary

- One reason why drug abuse is dangerous is that it can cause a person to act irresponsibly.
- Continued drug abuse can lead to psychological or physical dependence, or both.
- Caffeine, cocaine and crack, and amphetamines are all examples of stimulants.
- Hallucinogens such as LSD and PCP are very dangerous psychoactive substances, because they distort the senses.
- Marijuana can impair a person's judgment and coordination.
- Certain types of glues contain inhalant fumes that produce strong psychoactive effects when inhaled.
- Narcotics are highly addictive drugs. Some narcotics such as morphine and codeine have some medicinal value. The narcotic heroin, however, has no medical purpose and is illegal to buy, sell, and use.
- Steroid abuse can lead to very high blood pressure and can severely damage the heart and liver.
- No one should ever try to overcome a drug addiction on his or her own.
- There is no such thing as a recovered drug abuser. Even if a person has not abused a drug in years, there is always a chance that person will abuse, and become dependent on, drugs again.
- Methadone maintenance programs, inpatient and outpatient programs, and self-help programs are three options for recovering drug abusers.

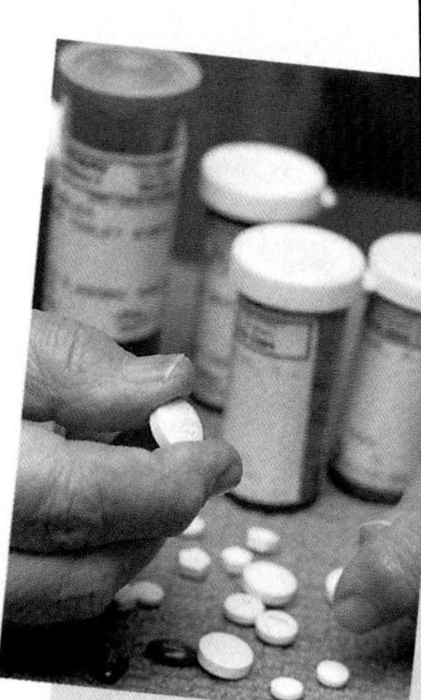

Vocabulary

psychoactive drug a drug that affects a person's mood and behavior.

stimulant a drug that causes alertness and speeds up the activity of the body.

hallucinogen a drug that distorts a person's senses.

narcotic a drug with pain-relieving and psychoactive properties that is made from the opium poppy plant.

sedative-hypnotics drugs that depress the body system and cause sleepiness.

anabolic steroid an artificially made, complex substance that can sometimes increase muscle size.

Chapter 15 Highlights Strategies

Summary

Have students read the summary to reinforce the concepts they learned in Chapter 15.

Vocabulary

Have students write a paragraph about drugs of abuse using the vocabulary words correctly.

Extension

Have students make anti-drug abuse posters to be displayed in the community. The posters may contain myths about what drugs do for you, ways to stay drugfree, or what to do if you need help in getting off drugs.

CHAPTER 15 ASSESSMENT

CHAPTER REVIEW

Concept Review

1. mood, behavior
2. physical
3. tolerance
4. physical, psychological
5. cocaine
6. crack, cocaine
7. synthetic
8. hallucinogenic
9. flashback
10. marijuana, hashish
11. narcotic
12. liver, heart
13. recovered

Expressing Your Views

Sample responses:

1. Sharon is building up a tolerance to the medication. I would tell her to inform her doctor so that he or she can change the medication before she becomes addicted to it.

2. Barry could be addicted to amphetamines. I would encourage him to talk to someone in the student assistance program or to his counselor about the situation. I would support Barry if he decided to overcome his addiction and encourage him as he goes through a drug-abuse program.

Life Skills Check

Sample responses:

1. I would tell him not to use cocaine or crack under any circumstances. He does not have to explain to anyone why he doesn't want to try them. All he has to do is say No. Cocaine and crack are addictive drugs; people on cocaine and crack often behave violently; cocaine and crack can be fatal, even the first time they are used.

2. I would use the decision-making steps. Some reasons for not using drugs are that they are dangerous and addictive; I could lose control of my behavior; my parents do not approve; and using drugs goes against my own values.

Projects

Have students plan and carry out the projects on drug abuse.

Personal Pledge

Have students read and sign the Personal Pledge for Chapter 15.

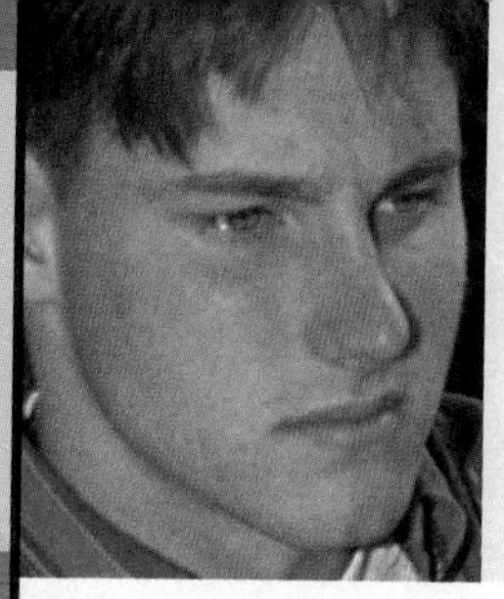

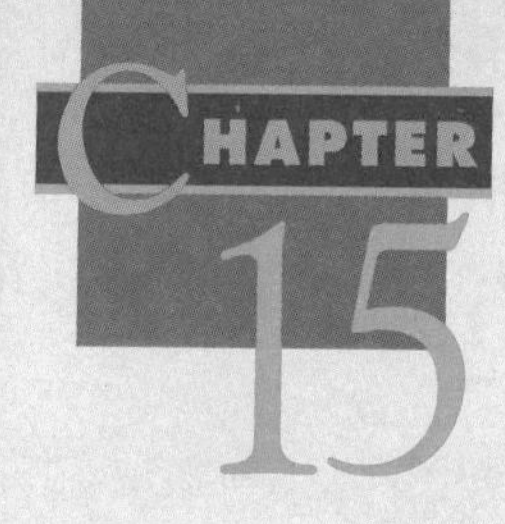

Chapter Review

Concept Review

1. A psychoactive drug is a drug that affects a person's ________ and ________.
2. Addiction is a ________ process.
3. ________ is the first step in the addiction process.
4. ________ dependence occurs when a person's body comes to expect the presence of a drug. ________ dependence is a strong desire to repeat the use of a drug for emotional reasons.
5. When ________ is inhaled, it enters the bloodstream, then travels to the brain.
6. Statistics show that half of all prisoners in the U.S. are ________ or ________ users.
7. ________ drugs such as amphetamines are drugs produced or manufactured in laboratories.
8. People on ________ drugs often forget where they are, may have difficulty keeping track of time, and may believe they have special powers.
9. A ________ is an unexpected return to an unpleasant LSD experience, often months after the original experience ended.
10. ________ and ________ are two organic drugs that come from the Indian hemp plant.
11. Morphine, codeine, and heroin are examples of ________ drugs.
12. Steroids can cause ________ and ________ damage as well as high blood pressure.
13. There is no such thing as a ________ drug addict, because even if a person has been off of drugs for years, that person could become dependent again.

Expressing Your Views

1. Your friend Sharon, who has been taking a prescription medication for several weeks, confides to you that she is having to take increasingly greater amounts of the drug in order to get the same pain relief she once got with the recommended dosage. Why is this happening to her? What would you tell her?
2. Your friend Barry takes amphetamines whenever he has to study for a test. "They keep me going," he's told you. But he's been absent from school a lot, and whenever you see him he's moody and anxious. What could be wrong with Barry? How can you help him get the treatment he needs?

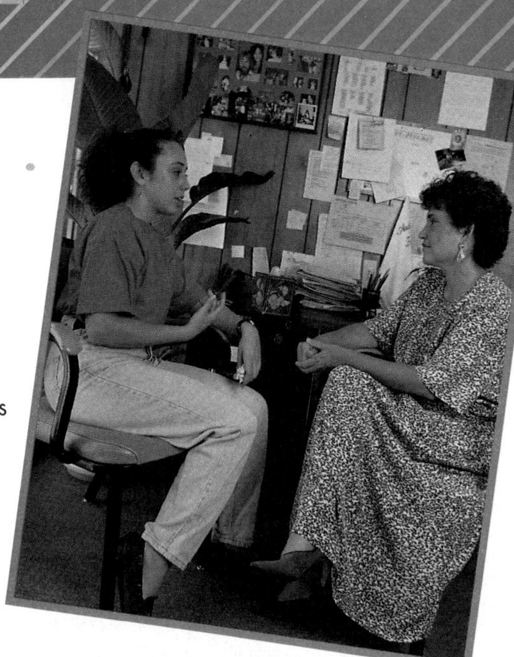

Life Skills Check

1. **Communicating Effectively**
Your younger brother is planning to attend a party. You found out that several of the people there will be using cocaine and crack. What advice should you give him?

2. **Resisting Pressure**
While on a camping trip, two of your friends try to persuade you to try PCP. They assure you that the drug's effects will be gone by the time you return home the next day. You feel uneasy about using drugs, but you are also worried about what your friends will think if you refuse—saying no isn't easy. What should you do? What are some good reasons to say no?

Projects

1. Work with a partner to create a poster that describes information about different types of drugs. The following information could be included: street names, how the drug is taken, the physical and mental effects of the drug, and any other descriptive information. Display your poster in the classroom.

2. Work with a small group. Imagine that all of you in the group are parents. What kind of policies would you set to discourage your children from abusing drugs? What could you do to encourage your children to follow healthy practices?

3. Certain athletes and other well-known personalities have had highly publicized bouts with drug abuse. Research the experience of one such celebrity. Why do you think this person may have turned to drugs? What other options do you think he or she may have had? Present the results of your research to the class.

Plan for Action

Life isn't easy for anyone, but people who abuse drugs when times are hard make things even worse for themselves. What are two things a person can do to cope with problems in a healthy way?

Plan for Action

Have students discuss the nature of addiction to drugs. **What is the difference between addiction to cocaine and a liking for certain foods?** *[In addiction, the body is physiologically changed so that it requires the drug to function normally; a preference does not have physical consequences when denied.]* **Is it possible to become addicted to a substance you try just once or twice?** *[Yes, crack is an example.]* **Are there circumstances when addiction to a drug is acceptable?** *[Yes; for instance, when morphine is used in high doses to treat terminally ill patients.]*

ASSESSMENT OPTIONS

Chapter Test
Have students take the Chapter 15 Test.

Alternative Assessment
Have students do the Alternative Assessment activity for Chapter 15.

Test Generator
The Test Generator (Macintosh® or IBM® format) contains an additional 50 assessment items for this chapter.

Issues in Health

EVALUATING MEDIA MESSAGES

How Bad Can It Be if Athletes Do It?

Have students read the Evaluating Media Messages feature. Ask students how they would respond to Joel's habit of chewing tobacco. Would it offend them? Would they want to try it themselves? Can they think of another reason Joel may be so insistent? *(Tobacco is addictive and Joel may be habituated to it.)* What problems might Joel have in giving it up? *(Overcoming addiction; giving up a habit he associates with people he admires or with people he sees a lot)*

Have interested students find out the number of young people who use smokeless tobacco. Have them choose a particular age range for their research. What percentage use smokeless tobacco? What percentage of young people in the same age range smoke cigarettes? Have students create pie graphs indicating the proportion of young people who have both habits.

Evaluating Media Messages

How Bad Can It Be If Athletes Do It?

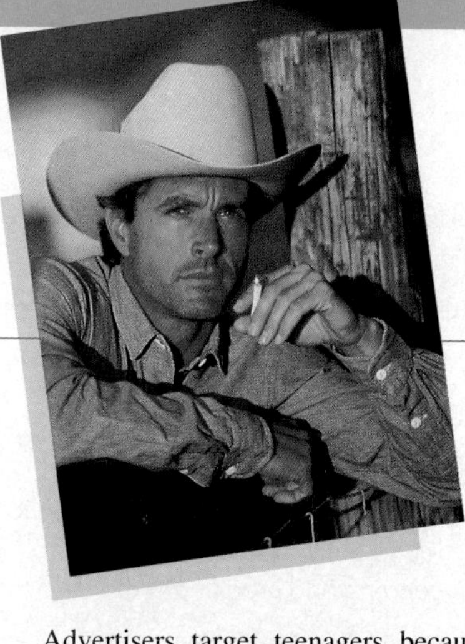

Joel and Lucinda were walking home from school when Joel pulled out a pouch of chewing tobacco and put some in his mouth. Lucinda was horrified. "What are you doing with that stuff, Joel?" she cried.

"Oh, come on, Lucinda," Joel said. "It's not like I'm smoking cigarettes—I mean I'm not bothering anyone, and it's not going to give me cancer."

"You're wrong," Lucinda replied. "My uncle used to do it, and he got cancer of the mouth."

"So what?" Joel replied. "Your uncle's probably an old man who would've gotten cancer anyway."

"No, actually he was in his twenties when he got sick."

"Well, look at all the pro athletes who chew tobacco and dip snuff. Those guys are in great shape, so it must be okay."

"Joel, my uncle played college baseball. He was in great shape too," Lucinda informed him.

Joel is one of a growing number of teenage boys who use smokeless tobacco (chewing tobacco and snuff). While smoking has declined among teenagers in the United States, the use of smokeless tobacco has risen. In fact, the number of 17- to 19-year-old males using smokeless tobacco increased by a multiple of 8 during the 1980s. Researchers believe this increase resulted from the skillful marketing efforts directed at teens by tobacco companies.

Advertisers target teenagers because they are aware that teenagers can be very easy to influence. For instance, it is well known that many teens experience low self-esteem and a sense of being powerless. So advertisers portray people in tobacco ads as just the opposite—mature, self-confident, and independent. Such images make using tobacco very attractive to people who are looking for ways to appear more mature, to feel more confident, or to assert their individuality. Teens can fight back, but they must carefully evaluate the media messages in tobacco ads to combat their effect.

When evaluating a media message, it is helpful to refer to a simple model of communication. The SMCR model below breaks communication into four parts.

1. The *Source* of the communication creates a message that can be verbal, nonverbal, visual, or musical.
2. The *Message* is what the source wants to say.
3. The *Channel* is the means by which the message is transmitted. In mass media this could be television, magazines, newspapers, radio, etc.
4. The *Receiver* interprets the message on the basis of his or her individual experiences and values.

Joel's comments to Lucinda indicate how he has been affected by media messages about smokeless tobacco. For example, one message that frequently appears in smokeless tobacco ads is that the product is good because it does not produce smoke, which bothers many people. Joel, the receiver, obviously agrees with the reasoning in this message; but Lucinda objects. "Sure, there's no smoke," she explains, "but when you use that stuff, you still do things that upset a lot of people—like spitting, drooling, and leaving smelly, wet tobacco in soft-drink cans." Joel may not have thought about how other people see these behaviors, because smokeless-tobacco ads don't mention them. Once he has considered Lucinda's remarks, he might evaluate messages about smokeless tobacco differently.

Joel's belief that chewing tobacco can't be very dangerous because athletes do it is an example of association, a very effective marketing tool. It is also an example of how powerful nonverbal communication can be. In using association, the source (an advertiser) makes a connection between something receivers like and the product the source wants to sell. If the channel is television or some other type of visual media, just the picture of a healthy athlete using smokeless tobacco can convey the false impression that the habit is not dangerous. Linking healthy athletes to unhealthy substances such as tobacco is actually a mixed message. When analyzed, mixed messages can be recognized as containing conflicting information.

Tobacco companies employ association not only by using athletes in their ads but also by giving free samples of smokeless tobacco to athletes—particularly major-league baseball players. The free samples are tremendously effective because millions of fans see their heroes using the products during televised games. To try to eliminate the association of athletes with smokeless tobacco, the National Cancer Institute and the National Institute for Dental Research have recently begun working with major-league baseball teams to help players quit using smokeless tobacco.

Media images make tobacco use attractive to people who want to feel more mature and confident.

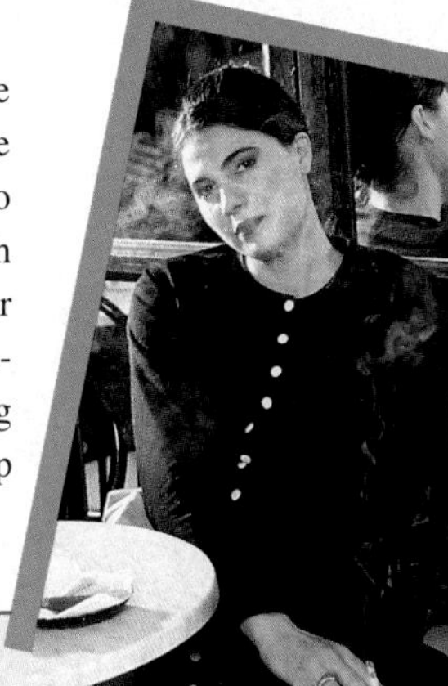

Critical Thinking

1. Find several tobacco or alcohol ads and analyze them using the SMCR Model.
2. Identify one product—tobacco, alcohol, antacid, cold medicine, pain reliever, diet pill—that you have bought or wanted to buy because of a media message. Evaluate the message by asking yourself the following questions:
   - Who is the source?
   - What is their message?
   - How will they benefit if I do as they wish?
   - How will I benefit if I do as they wish?
   - What are my values?
   - What is best for me?
3. What can you do do to convince a friend who has started using smokeless tobacco to stop?

UNIT 5

Family Life, Sexuality, and Social Health

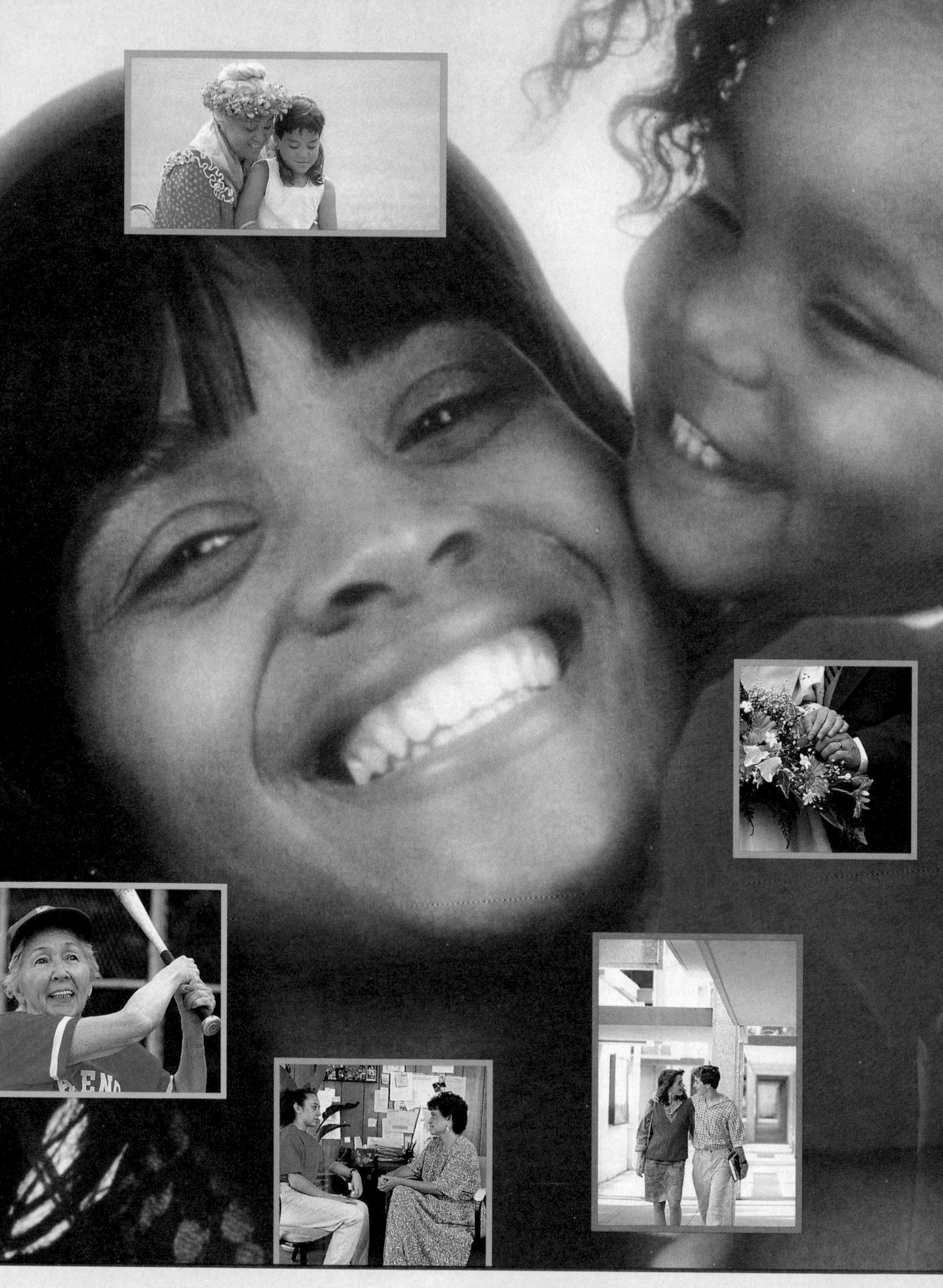

CHAPTER OVERVIEWS

CHAPTER 16

REPRODUCTION AND THE EARLY YEARS OF LIFE

This chapter describes the male and female reproductive systems and explains their functions in detail. Disorders of the reproductive systems are described, and proper care of the reproductive organs is discussed. Students learn about the development of human beings from fertilization of the egg through childhood.

CHAPTER 17

ADOLESCENCE: RELATIONSHIPS AND RESPONSIBILITIES

Students learn about the physical, emotional, and mental changes that occur during adolescence. To help them be more successful in interpersonal relations, such as friendships, family life, and dating, the students also learn effective communication techniques. The chapter discusses sexuality and the possible consequences of sexual intimacy. Finally, students learn skills for responsible sexual behavior.

CHAPTER 18

ADULTHOOD, MARRIAGE, AND PARENTHOOD

This chapter covers the stages of adulthood, the process of aging, and the needs of the elderly. It also explains the reasons why people get married, the ingredients that go into a successful marriage, and the difficulties teenagers may face in marrying early. It ends with a discussion of parental responsibilities.

CHAPTER 19

FAMILIES

Students learn the functions of a family, the different types of families, how families have changed, and the characteristics of a healthy family. Students also receive information on coping with divorce and living in a dysfunctional family.

CHAPTER 20

PREVENTING ABUSE AND VIOLENCE

This chapter describes the forms of child, spouse, and elder abuse, and names sources of help for abusive families. It also defines sexual assault and acquaintance rape and suggests ways to avoid them. Students learn about risk factors related to homicides, the reasons why some teenagers join gangs, and some ways to avoid violence.

UNIT FIVE

FAMILY LIFE, SEXUALITY, AND SOCIAL HEALTH

UNIT PREVIEW

The life stages of human beings from conception to old age are covered in this unit. The in-depth treatment of reproduction, adolescence, and sexuality provides students a sound basis for making responsible decisions about sexual behaviors. Students learn that the decisions they make at each stage of their life affects their short- and long-term wellness. The unit gives information to help students deal with family problems such as divorce and abuse. They also learn how to reduce their risks of being victims or perpetrators of sexual assault and other violent conflict. The five major health themes are emphasized throughout the unit, as indicated in the chart below.

THEMES TRACE

	WELLNESS	BUILDING SELF-ESTEEM	DECISION MAKING	DEVELOPING LIFE-MANAGEMENT SKILLS	ACCEPTANCE OF DIVERSITY AMONG PEOPLE
Chapter 16		pp. 347–348		pp. 330, 337	
Chapter 17		pp. 372–373	pp. 356, 370, 373–374, 376, 379	pp. 357–363, 368–369, 375, 377–380	pp. 355, 366–367, 370
Chapter 18	pp. 389, 392		pp. 385–386	pp. 388, 393–394	p. 391
Chapter 19		pp. 413–414	p. 412	pp. 409–410, 413–414	pp. 404–407
Chapter 20			p. 422	pp. 423, 428, 430–431	

Reproduction and the Early Years of Life

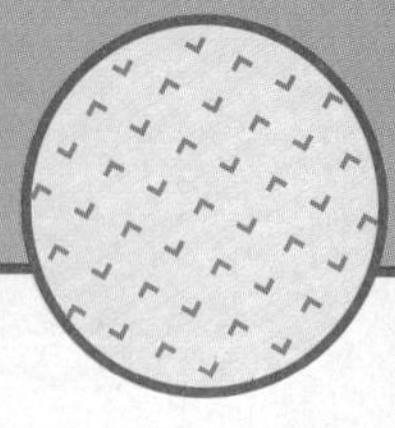

Planning Guide

TEXT SECTIONS	OBJECTIVES	TEXT FEATURES	OUTSIDE RESOURCES	NOTES
16.1 The Male Reproductive System pp. 325-330 1 period	• Name the major organs of the male reproductive system. • Explain the two functions of the testes. • Trace the path of the sperm from the testes to the outside of the body. • Describe how the sperm meets the egg and fertilizes it. ■ Describe how to do a testicular self-examination.	**ASSESSMENT** • Section Review, p. 330	**TEACHER'S RESOURCE BINDER** • Lesson Plan 16.1 • Personal Health Inventory • Journal Entry 16A • Section Review Worksheet 16.1 • Section Quiz 16.1 • Reteaching Worksheet 16.1 **OUTSIDE RESOURCES** • Transparency 16A	
16.2 The Female Reproductive System pp. 331-338 2 periods	• Name the organs of the female reproductive system. • Trace the path of the egg from the ovary to the uterus. • Explain how the uterus changes during the menstrual cycle. ■ Describe how to do a breast self-examination.	**ASSESSMENT** • Section Review, p. 338	**TEACHER'S RESOURCE BINDER** • Lesson Plan 16.2 • Journal Entry 16B • Life Skills 16A • Section Review Worksheet 16.2 • Section Quiz 16.2 • Reteaching Worksheet 16.2 **OUTSIDE RESOURCES** • Transparencies 16B, 16C	
16.3 Pregnancy, Birth, and Childhood Development pp. 339-348 2 periods	• List the substances that can pass from the mother to the placenta. • Describe the events that occur during birth. ■ Use self-talk about childhood experiences to increase your self-esteem.	■ LIFE SKILLS: Building Self-Esteem, p. 347 **ASSESSMENT** • Section Review, p. 348	**TEACHER'S RESOURCE BINDER** • Lesson Plan 16.3 • Journal Entries 16C, 16D • Life Skills 16B • Section Review Worksheet 16.3 • Section Quiz 16.3 • Reteaching Worksheet 16.3 **OUTSIDE RESOURCES** • Transparencies 16D, 16E • Making a Choice 16A, 16B	
End of Chapter pp. 349-351		**ASSESSMENT** • Chapter Review, pp. 350-351	**TEACHER'S RESOURCE BINDER** • Chapter Test • Alternative Assessment • Personal Pledge **OUTSIDE RESOURCES** • Test Generator	

■ Denotes LIFE SKILLS objectives

• Items in blue are also part of the *Holt Health Activity Book*.

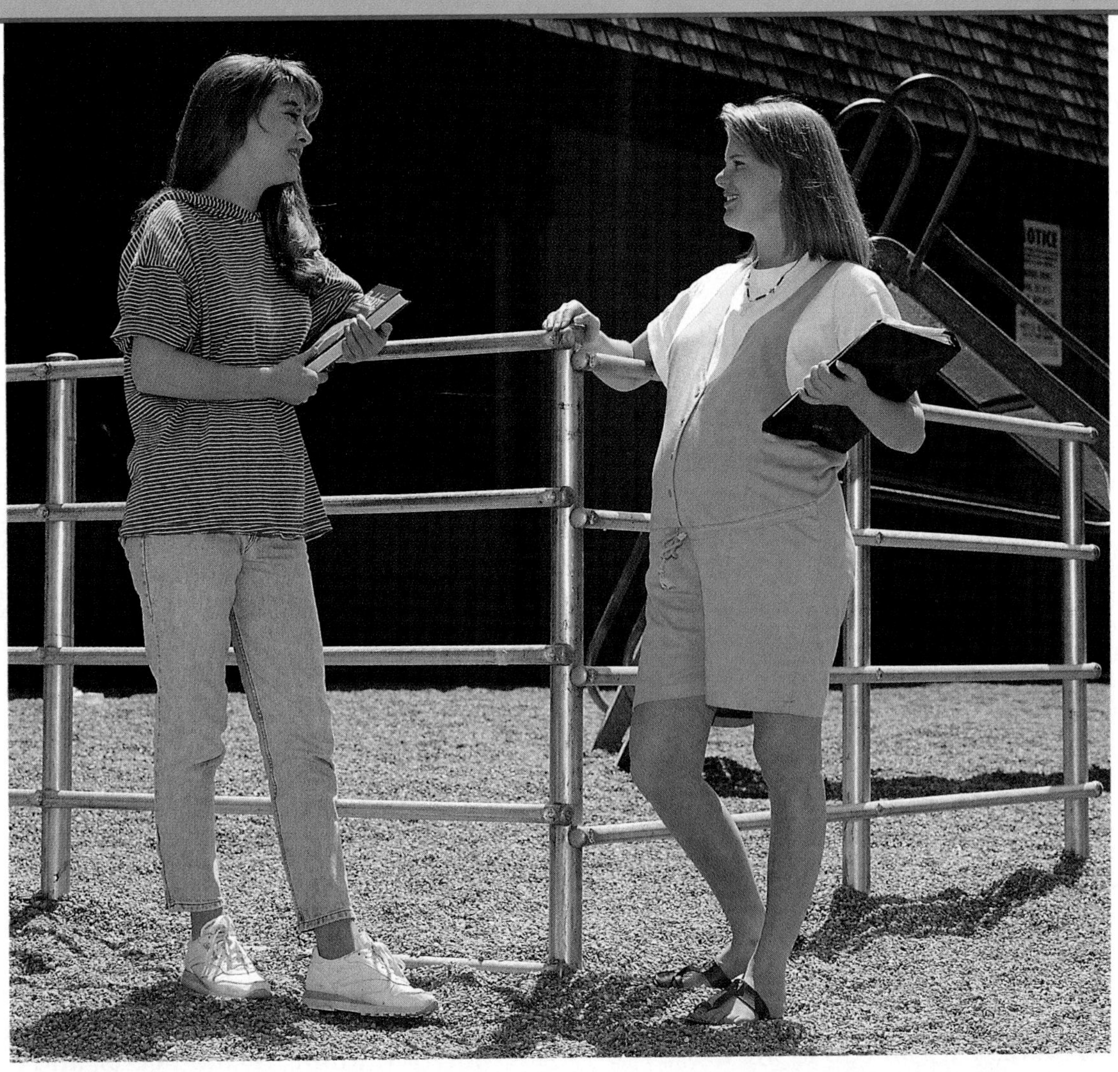

CONTENT BACKGROUND

Sexual Activity Among Adolescents

ACCORDING TO SURVEYS, ADOLESCENTS in this country are becoming sexually active at a much younger age and at a much faster rate than their predecessors in the sixties, seventies, and eighties. The Urban Institute and the National Survey of Family Growth have found that 27 percent of female adolescents aged 15, and 33 percent of males of the same age say that they regularly have sex. By the age of 16, 34 percent of girls and 50 percent of boys are sexually active. At 17, just over half (52 percent) of the females and 66 percent of the males surveyed "go all the way." By the age of 18, nearly three-fourths of all teenagers have sexual intercourse on a regular basis.

Because most teenagers are regularly having sexual intercourse by the 11th grade and only about half of these sexually active teens are using contraceptives, the teenage birthrate in the United States is the highest among all Western countries. Each year in this country, half a million teenage girls give birth. Of these teenage mothers, about 50 percent never finish high school and usually rely on welfare as their only means of support. Studies have also shown that if girls between the ages of 15 and 16 have one child, they are very likely to have at least one more child before they reach the age of 20.

Experts feel that the most effective means of preventing teenage pregnancies (five out of every six such pregnancies are unintentional and about 40 percent of teen pregnancies end in abortion) is a combination of strong parental guidance and support, extensive courses in sex education at a relatively early age, and accessible health care. Regarding sex education, although a 1989 study of over 4,000 teachers revealed that 86 percent of them recommended abstinence as the best alternative to prevent teenage pregnancy, less than half told their students where they could obtain contraceptives.

Recent studies have shown that school-based health clinics located in the high school or in nearby buildings seem to be quite effective in preventing teen pregnancies. Teens who have access to such clinics are more likely than not to use contraceptives. The first such clinic in the United States was in St. Paul, Minnesota, and the teenage birthrate in that area dropped 50 percent between 1976 and 1984. In fact, Minnesota still has the lowest teen pregnancy rate in the country—only 7.5 percent of the babies born in the state are to mothers under the age of 20. Mississippi, where such clinics are not as numerous, has the highest national percentage (20.8) of infants born to teenage mothers.

It is difficult for young adults to make decisions about these high-risk behaviors. Today's young people should receive explicit and extensive courses in sex education that begin in the middle schools and junior highs. The education must be supplemented with available counseling on such matters as well as any necessary treatment or preventive measures that can be taken.

PLANNING FOR INSTRUCTION

KEY FACTS

- **A sperm unites with an egg in the process of fertilization, and an embryo immediately begins to develop.**
- **Testes, suspended in the scrotum, make sperm and produce the hormone testosterone, which causes male sex characteristics to develop.**
- **Men should be alert for possible disorders of the reproductive system, such as twisting of the testes, undescended testes, inguinal hernia, infertility, and prostate enlargement or cancer.**
- **The female reproductive system produces eggs and provides a place for fertilization to occur. It also provides shelter and nourishment for the fetus until birth.**
- **Interior parts of the female reproductive system include the vagina, the cervix, the uterus, the Fallopian tubes, and the ovaries.**
- **The ovaries produce eggs and sex hormones. Each ovary contains thousands of eggs, but only one is released each month.**
- **Women may suffer from disorders of the reproductive system such as menstrual cramps, premenstrual syndrome, vaginitis, toxic shock syndrome, ovarian cysts, and cancer.**
- **The fertilized egg, a single cell, begins to divide and is then called an embryo.**
- **The cervix holds in place the developing baby and the fluids surrounding it. When the baby is fully developed, the uterus begins to contract and the cervix opens so that the baby can emerge.**
- **Growth and development continue after birth through the stages of infancy, childhood, and adolescence.**

MYTHS AND MISCONCEPTIONS

MYTH: During menstruation, a woman should not swim or exercise strenuously because she is in a weakened state.

Menstruation is a normal body function and does not require restriction of any accustomed activity. Actually, exercise may help relieve cramps.

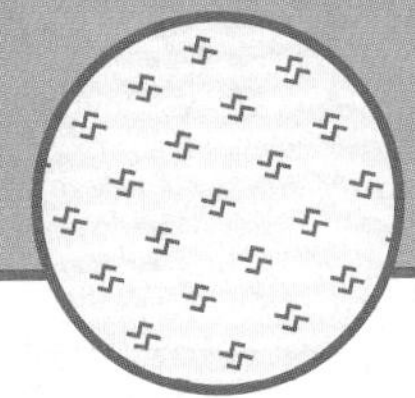

MYTH: **Douching after sexual intercourse is an effective means of birth control.**

After intercourse, sperm are already in the vagina and uterus. Douching may actually force sperm farther along toward the egg.

MYTH: **Penis size is directly related to sexual performance.**

The size of a man's penis has nothing to do with his ability to perform sexually, to satisfy a woman, or to make a woman pregnant.

MYTH: **Miscarriage may occur if the mother works, exercises, or experiences a fright or fall.**

Most aspects of daily life do not contribute to miscarriages. Factors that *do* contribute to miscarriage are abnormalities of the fetus, problems with the shape or function of the woman's uterus or cervix, genital infections, a chronic disease in the mother (such as diabetes), or the mother's use of alcohol and tobacco.

VOCABULARY

Essential: The following vocabulary terms appear in boldface type:

sperm	**ovaries**
egg	**ovulation**
fertilization	**uterus**
testes	**Pap test**
penis	**embryo**
vagina	**fetus**
cervix	

Secondary: Be aware that the following terms may come up during class discussion:

scrotum	circumcision
testosterone	infertility
erection	clitoris
ejaculation	sex hormones
orgasm	menstrual cycle
menstrual cramps	contractions
placenta	labor
umbilical cord	

FOR STUDENTS WITH SPECIAL NEEDS

Visual Learners: Students will benefit from a display of images that trace the development of a human from conception through birth and the first 10 years of life. Have students locate pictures or make drawings that represent conception, pregnancy, childbirth, infancy, and the stages of childhood. These can be placed on a time line fixed to a bulletin board, wall, or chalkboard.

Auditory Learners: Have students write the parts of the male and female reproductive systems on index cards. On the other side of each card, students should write the location and function of the part. These cards may be used as flash cards by students working in pairs or groups.

ENRICHMENT

- Have students write imaginative narrative accounts from the point of view of the developing embryo and fetus. Suggest that they imagine the environment in the uterus and the changes occurring in the developing individual. They might use a diary format to chronicle events in each trimester of development, childbirth, and the first moments of life outside the mother's body.
- Have students research the subject of circumcision, looking for information to answer the following questions: What percentage of boys are circumcised? At what age is the operation usually performed? What benefits are said to result? Are there any dangers or disadvantages of circumcision? Students may wish to hold a debate on the merits of circumcision following their research.

CHAPTER 16
CHAPTER OPENER

GETTING STARTED

Using the Chapter Photograph

Have students look at the photograph. **How has Tonya's body changed?** *[She has gained weight and her abdomen has expanded due to the growth of the baby inside her. Her breasts are getting larger in preparation for breast feeding. Hormones are being produced to maintain the pregnancy.]* **How might Tonya's and Sabrena's attitudes toward pregnancy and raising children differ?** *[Students might respond that Tonya is older and more mature than Sabrena and, thus, is probably less anxious and uncertain about having a child.]*

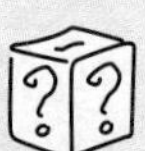

Question Box

Have students write out any questions they have about the reproductive organs, conception, pregnancy, birth, and early childhood, and put them in the Question Box. The Question Box provides them with an opportunity to ask questions anonymously. To ensure that students with questions are not embarrassed to be seen writing, have those who do not have questions write something else—such as something they already know about the reproductive system—on the paper instead.

Personal Issues *ALERT*

Many teenagers feel that their bodies should develop within a time frame and physical norms approved of by their peers. Stress that rate of maturation and individual development vary greatly among perfectly normal individuals. Also be aware that many students may be uncomfortable discussing sexual intercourse, conception, pregnancy, childbirth, and parenting issues. Some students may be dealing with these realities themselves. Others may be reluctant to participate in open discussion of these topics for ethnic or religious reasons. Be ready to answer student questions matter-of-factly and respect student privacy; insist on the use of correct terms; and be ready to accept differing values.

CHAPTER 16

Reproduction and the Early Years of Life

A couple embrace their newborn baby.

Sabrena's older sister, Tonya, is pregnant. Tonya and her husband have been married for four years, and they have been looking forward to having a baby. Sabrena is extremely excited and can't wait to see her new niece or nephew. She has started thinking about what it would be like to have a baby. Sabrena isn't even sure she wants to have children. The idea of being responsible for a child's safety and well-being is pretty frightening. She's glad she doesn't have to make a decision about having children for a long time. Right now, she thinks, she will just enjoy her sister's baby.

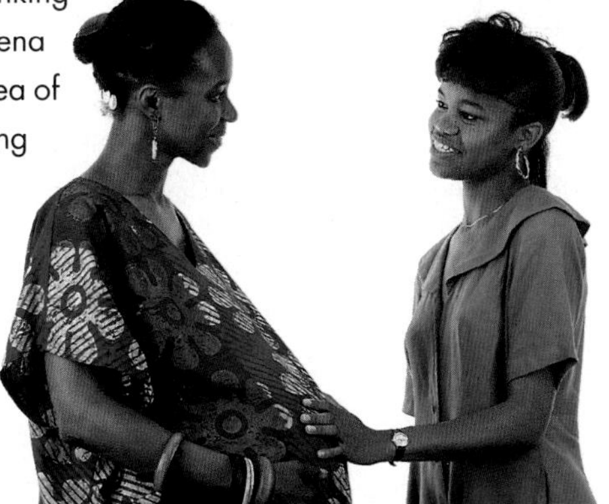

Section 16.1 The Male Reproductive System

Objectives

- *Name the major organs of the male reproductive system.*
- *Explain the two functions of the testes.*
- *Trace the path of the sperm from the testes to the outside of the body.*
- *Describe how the sperm meets the egg and fertilizes it.*
- *Describe how to do a testicular self-examination.*
  LIFE SKILLS: Practicing Self-Care

Every person who has ever lived is the result of a process that began when a cell from a man, called a **sperm,** joined with a cell from a woman, called an **egg** or ovum. The male and female reproductive systems work together to bring the sperm and the egg together. This union of sperm and egg is called **fertilization.** Each sperm and each egg contains one-half of the instructions needed for the development of a new, unique human being.

The process of producing a new individual is called *reproduction.* In humans, the term reproduction means simply "having children."

One job of the male reproductive system is to produce sperm and transport them into the body of a woman. Look at Figure 16-1, which shows the parts of the male reproductive system. The parts that you can see from the outside are the penis and the scrotum. The scrotum is the loose sac under the penis. Inside the scrotum are two testes, which produce the sperm. Connecting the testes and the penis are the two vas deferens, which are tubes through which the sperm travel. Along the way are glands that produce fluids that nourish and protect the sperm.

fertilization: *the union of a sperm and an egg.*

sperm: *male reproductive cell; contains one-half of the instructions needed for the development of a new human being.*

egg: *female reproductive cell, also called an ovum; contains one-half of the instructions needed for the development of a new human being.*

Background
Vasectomy

Vasectomy is a means of male sterilization in which the vas deferens tubes are cut and tied in two places. The operation usually is performed in a doctor's office and takes about 15 minutes. Vasectomy is not immediately effective because sperm may remain in the tubes above the places where they were cut and tied. The man should use birth control until a final sperm count is made at the doctor's office (about three months after surgery). After a vasectomy, a man can still have an erection and ejaculate (sperm make up only 5 percent of the semen).

Section 16.1 Lesson Plan

MOTIVATE

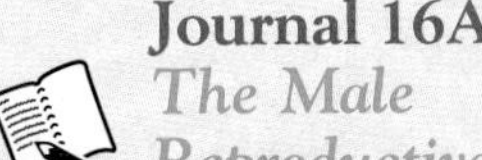

Journal 16A
The Male Reproductive System

This may be done as a warm-up activity. Have students turn to the Student Journal in the Student Activity Book and write all the facts they know about the male reproductive system. Then have them list statements they have heard but do not know to be true. After they read the first section, have them refer to their journal to confirm the correctness of their facts and try to prove or disprove unproven statements.

Class Discussion
The Human Reproductive System

Discuss how the human reproductive system differs from other body systems. Point out that unlike other body systems, the reproductive system differs tremendously between the sexes. Have students name primary differences in the male and female reproductive systems of which they are aware.

TEACH

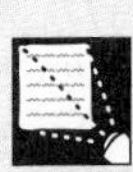

Teaching Transparency 16A
The Male Reproductive System

Show the transparency of the male reproductive system (Figure 16-1). Have students describe the functions of vari-

testes: *male reproductive structures that make sperm and produce the male hormone testosterone.*

The Testes

The **testes**, which are also called testicles, are two egg-shaped structures that hang inside the scrotum.

The testes have two functions. The first function of the testes is to make the sperm. The testes hang away from the body so that the temperature inside them is slightly cooler than the rest of the body. The temperature in the testes is very important to the sperm-making process. If the temperature is too high, the testes will make defective sperm that cannot fertilize an egg. The testes produce about 50,000 sperm every *minute*.

The second function of the testes is to produce the male sex hormone testosterone. Testosterone is necessary for the production of sperm and also for the development of male sex characteristics.

At puberty, the amount of testosterone in the male body increases, which causes boys' bodies to change. Coarse, curly hair called pubic hair begins to grow on the lower part of the abdomen around the penis. Similar coarse hair grows under the armpits. Teenage boys also begin to grow a beard on the lower part of the face. Some men—but not all men—grow hair on the chest. Testosterone is also responsible for a man's well-defined muscles, heavier bones, and deeper voice.

The Vas Deferens and the Urethra

The sperm must be able to travel to the outside of the body in order for reproduction to occur. Follow along the red line in Figure

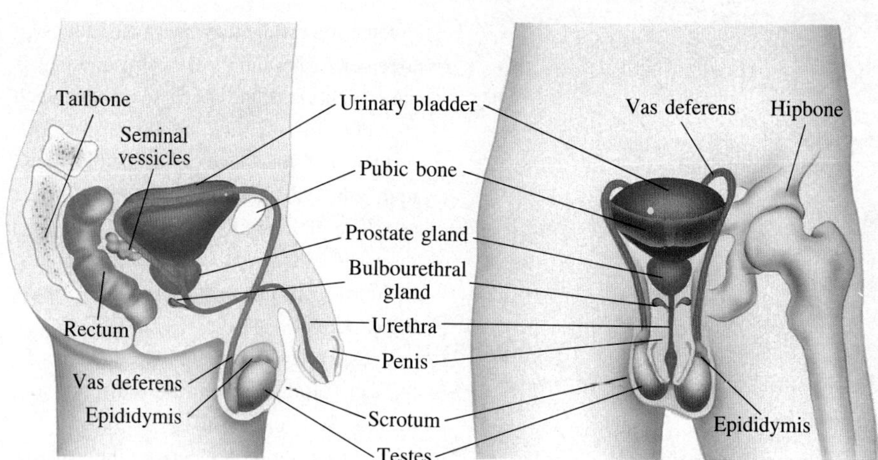

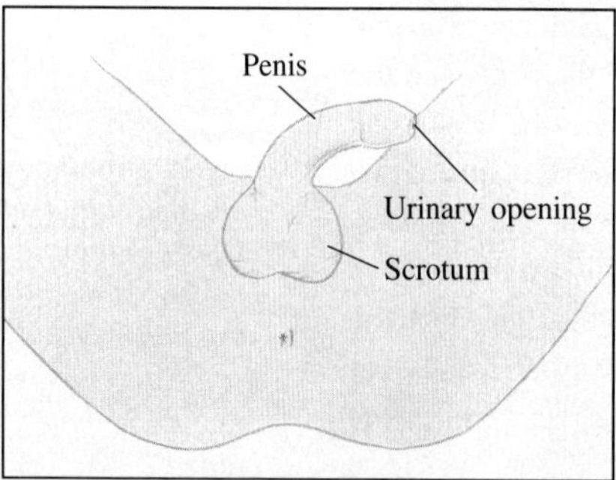

(FIGURE 16-1) **The function of the male reproductive system is to make sperm that fertilize the egg of the woman. Sperm are made in the testes and exit the body through the penis. The small diagram at the left shows the parts of the male reproductive system that can be seen from the outside.**

• • • TEACH continued

ous parts, tell how sperm are produced and protected, and trace the path sperm take out of the body.

Demonstration
Sperm and Egg Size

Tell students that an egg cell is about 0.005 in. in diameter, or about the size of a sharp pencil point. A sperm cell is so small it cannot be seen without a microscope. Help students visualize the size of sperm by measuring off a 1-in. length on the chalkboard. Explain that it would take 480 sperm placed end to end (including the tails) to stretch this distance.

Demonstration
Sperm Travel

To help students comprehend the difficulty of the sperm's journey to the egg, have them refer to a metric ruler. Explain that sperm swim at a rate of about 1 to 4 mm per minute. Have students compute how far sperm would move in an hour and measure this distance on the ruler. *(The sperm would move 60 to 240 mm.)*

Reinforcement
Circumcision

Reassure students that circumcision is neither bad nor good, but is simply a choice some parents make. The presence or absence of the foreskin does not affect health or sexual performance.

16-2 to see the route the sperm take to leave the body.

After sperm are made in a testis, they travel to a structure called an epididymis, which is a tightly coiled mass of tubules located at the top of each testis. The sperm become fully mature while they are in the epididymis. After about two to ten days, the sperm leave the epididymis and travel through a tube called the vas deferens. Men have two of these tubes.

The vas deferens tubes lead to the urethra, which is the tube that runs through the center of the penis. The sperm leave the body through the urethra. The urethra is also the tube through which urine leaves the body during urination.

As the sperm travel through the vas deferens and the urethra, they pass by glands that add fluids to the sperm. These fluids nourish and protect the sperm, as well as enable the sperm to move on their own. The addition of these fluids to the sperm creates the fluid called semen.

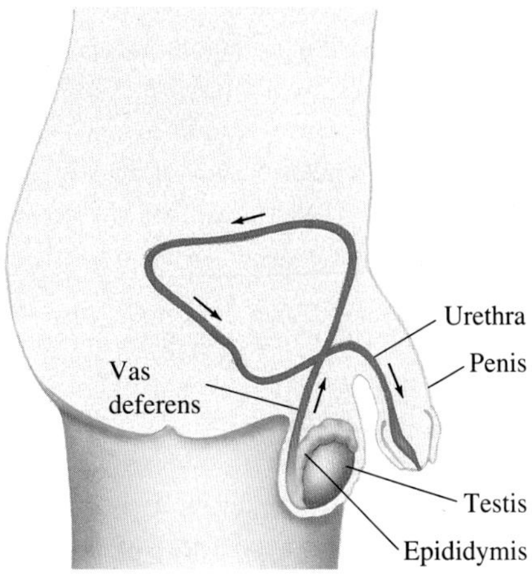

(FIGURE 16-2) **The red line shows the path of the sperm. The sperm are made in the testis, mature in the epididymis, and then travel through the vas deferens and the urethra to reach the outside of the body.**

The Penis

The **penis** is the body part that makes it possible for the sperm to reach the inside of a woman's body. When a man becomes sexually excited, the arteries leading to his penis open wider, allowing more blood to flow into the penis. At the same time, some of the veins in the penis close or narrow so that less blood flows out.

The accumulated blood causes the penis to become larger, longer, firmer, and to point upward instead of hanging downward. When a man's penis is in this state, he is said to have an erection. An erection makes it possible for the penis to be inserted into the vagina of the woman.

Ejaculation The process by which semen leaves the man's body is called ejaculation. During ejaculation, muscles around the urethra and base of the penis contract. The contraction is what moves the sperm out of the body. When a man ejaculates, he is said to have an orgasm.

Ejaculation can occur even while a man is sleeping. Especially among teenagers, the levels of testosterone may rise and fall somewhat unpredictably. These hormone fluctuations can cause frequent erections and then ejaculation during sleep. Ejaculation during sleep is called a nocturnal emission or a "wet dream." Nocturnal emissions are very common in adolescent and adult males and are perfectly normal.

penis:

male reproductive structure that deposits sperm inside the female body.

Sperm's Journey

During sexual intercourse, the sperm are deposited inside the woman's body, only a few inches away from the egg. But from a sperm's point of view this is a long and difficult journey.

SECTION 16.1

Background

Orgasm and Ejaculation

The Cowper's glands, seminal vesicles, and prostate gland all secrete fluids to protect and nourish the sperm. The Cowper's glands secrete fluid just before orgasm. This fluid may contain hundreds of thousands of sperm. Therefore, withdrawal is not a reliable method of birth control. Ejaculation is a reflex action controlled by the autonomic nervous system. But, because it can be influenced by impulses from the higher brain centers, ejaculation may be delayed or prevented.

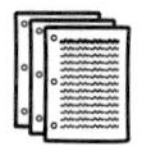

Personal Health Inventory

Have students complete the Personal Health Inventory for this chapter. The inventory helps them assess their care of the reproductive system.

Reinforcement

Care and Prevention

Stress the importance of cleaning and protecting the genitals. Males should wear a protector while participating in athletic events and strenuous exercise. Point out that fitted clothing is OK, but clothing that is too tight can cause pain in the groin.

Extension

Update on Disorders

Have students visit the library to find articles on one of the disorders of the male reproductive system discussed in the section. Several students might visit the local chapter of the American Cancer Society to get information about testicular and prostate cancer. Ask them to prepare a panel discussion giving the class a health update on any additional information, new findings or treatments, and suggestions for prevention of these disorders.

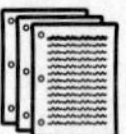

Section Review Worksheet 16.1

Assign the Section Review Worksheet for Section 16.1, which asks students to complete sentences describing structures and functions of the male reproductive system.

How are sperm able to make the trip? First, each sperm has a tail that whips back and forth, which propels the sperm forward. Second, sperm are streamlined and very small, much smaller than most cells in the human body. Their streamlined shape and small size make it easier for them to swim quickly.

The semen in one ejaculation contains 40 million to 300 million sperm. Why are so many sperm released, if only one will join with an egg?

First, the vast majority of sperm will never make it to an egg. They will become trapped in mucus or die on the way to the egg.

Second, even though only one sperm can actually fuse with an egg, the presence of many sperm is necessary for this to happen. The egg is protected by a layer of many smaller cells. Sperm contain enzymes that loosen this layer of cells. Only after *many* sperm have released their enzymes can *one* sperm make it all the way inside the egg. After one sperm has made it inside, a protective shield forms, which prevents other sperm from fusing with the egg.

Circumcised or Uncircumcised?

Some men are circumcised and some men aren't. Circumcision is an operation in which a fold of skin—called the foreskin—is cut from around the tip of the penis. Circumcision is usually done when a baby boy is two to eight days old. Parents may choose whether or not to have their male infants circumcised.

Figure 16-4 shows the difference between a male who has been circumcised and one who hasn't. Though they look different, circumcised and uncircumcised penises function in exactly the same way.

Males who have not been circumcised should pull the foreskin back when they wash. Cleaning under the foreskin prevents the buildup of a secretion that can cause irritation and odor in uncircumcised males.

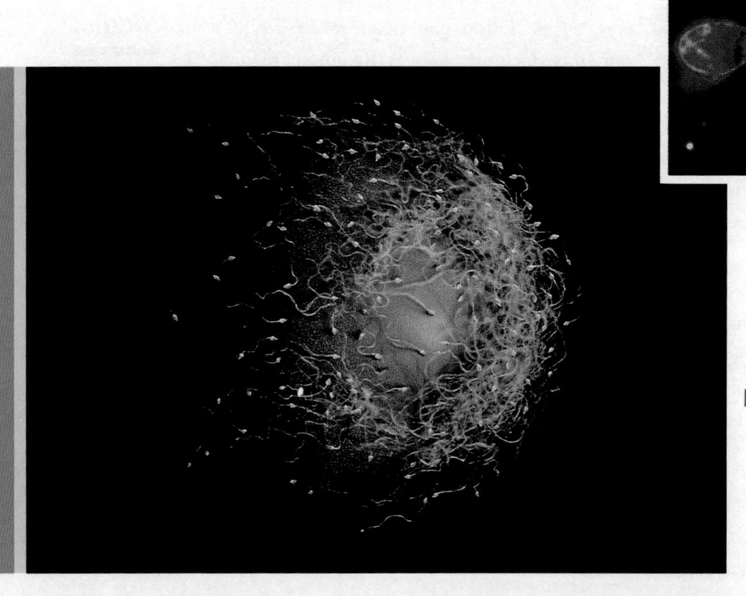

(FIGURE 16-3) **(Top) Sperm use their long tails to swim toward an egg. (Left) After one sperm has made it inside the egg, a protective shield prevents the other sperm from entering.**

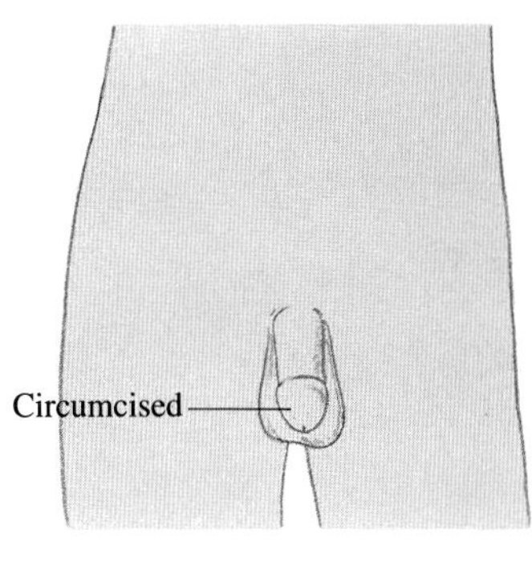

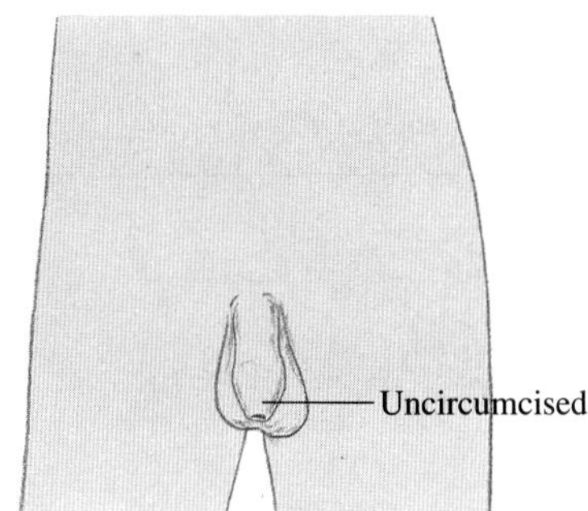

(FIGURE 16-4) **Parents decide whether to have their newborn boys circumcised. Though they look different, circumcised and uncircumcised penises function in the same way.**

Disorders of the Male Reproductive System

Even men who take good care of their reproductive systems can have something go wrong. But if a man knows as much as possible about male disorders, he will be better prepared to seek the correct treatment.

Testicular Torsion Testicular torsion means "twisted testis." However, that's not exactly accurate. It is the spermatic cord, which suspends each testis in the scrotum and contains many blood vessels, that can become twisted during strenuous exercise or even during sleep. The condition is very rare, but it is an emergency. Men who experience pain in the groin should seek medical treatment *immediately*, since testicular torsion can destroy the testes.

Undescended Testes When some males are born, one or both of their testes remain inside the body rather than hanging loose in the scrotum. This condition is called undescended testes. If the testes do not descend into the scrotum by the age of two, medical treatment is necessary. Undescended testes are more likely than others to develop cancer. And they interfere with developing healthy sperm, which can lead to infertility. Any male who thinks he may have this condition should seek medical treatment.

Inguinal Hernia Sometimes part of an intestine protrudes into the scrotum through a weakness in the abdominal wall. This condition is called an inguinal hernia. Inguinal hernias can be painful and usually require surgery to correct.

Infertility The condition of being unable to reproduce is called infertility. Both men and women can be infertile. Infertility in a man means that he has too few sperm or that his sperm are unable to fertilize an egg. Male infertility can be caused by any number of factors, such as exposure to harmful chemicals or X-rays, the development of testicular mumps as an adult, and other infections. Medical treatments are available for many kinds of male infertility.

Enlarged Prostate Gland As men get older, the prostate gland frequently gets bigger, which obstructs the outlet of the urinary bladder. The result is difficulty with urination. An enlarged prostate gland can be dangerous, and also uncomfortable.

Prostate and Testicular Cancers Older men are also more likely to get cancer of the prostate gland, which requires surgical treatment. Prostate cancer is the most common cancer in American men (and the second most common cause of cancer deaths in American men).

Background

Cancers

Testicular cancer accounts for 12 percent of all cancer deaths in males 15 to 34 years of age. Presence of an undescended or partially descended testicle places a man at much greater risk of developing testicular cancer.

Prostate cancer by itself kills a relatively small number of men. However, if it is not detected early, and cancer cells spread beyond the prostate, there is an 80 percent chance that death will result within 10 years. Presently, surgical removal of the prostate gland is the principal method of ridding the body of this cancer.

Section Quiz 16.1

Have students take Section Quiz 16.1.

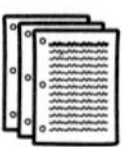

Reteaching Worksheet 16.1

Students who have difficulty with the material may complete Reteaching Worksheet 16.1, which requires them to identify structures, functions, and disorders of the male reproductive system.

Review Answers

1. Testes
2. Testes
3. Passage of semen during ejaculation and passage of urine during urination
4. A tail that whips back and forth, its small size, and its streamlined shape
5. Stand in front of a mirror and look for any swelling on the scrotum. Roll each testicle gently between the thumbs and fingers while feeling for any lumps, enlargements, tenderness, or change in texture. Report any abnormalities to a physician.
6. When the vas deferens are cut and tied off, mature sperm from the epididymis cannot travel to the urethra and to the outside of the body.

How to do a testicular self-examination:

1. Do the examination each month. The best time is after a warm bath or shower, when the scrotum is relaxed.

2. Stand in front of a mirror and look for any swelling on the scrotum.

3. Examine each testicle by rolling it gently between your thumbs and fingers, as shown in the diagram at the right. Feel for any lumps, enlargements, tenderness, or change in texture.

4. If you notice any abnormalities, report them to your doctor.

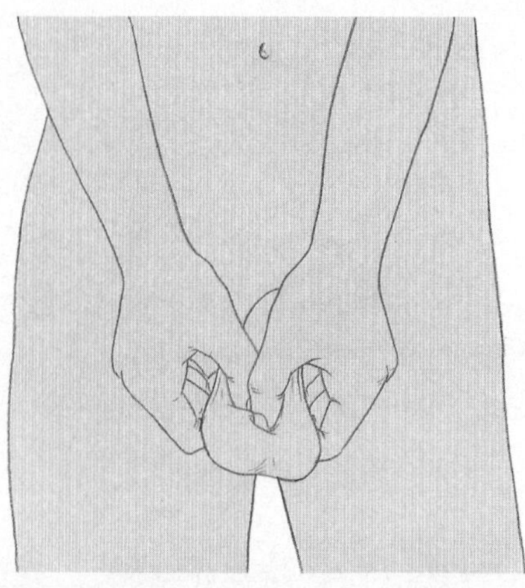

(FIGURE 16-5) **If testicular cancer is treated early, there is an excellent chance of recovery. Males should perform a monthly examination of their testes to detect any abnormalities as soon as possible.**

Testicular cancer is cancer of the testes. It usually occurs in males between the ages of 15 and 35. The good news about testicular cancer is that if it is noticed and treated early, there is an excellent chance of cure. To make sure that this kind of cancer is detected early, men should do a monthly examination of their testes. See Figure 16-5 for instructions in performing a testicular self-examination.

Care of the Male Reproductive System

Males need to follow a few simple steps to take care of their reproductive organs:

1. Wash the penis and scrotum daily, and check for any sores or bumps.
2. Don't wear extremely tight clothing. Tight clothing over the external reproductive organs can cause pain.
3. Do the testicular self-examination shown in Figure 16-5 once a month to detect lumps or other abnormalities.

Review

1. *Which male structure makes sperm?*
2. *Where is the male hormone testosterone produced?*
3. *What two functions does the male urethra serve?*
4. *What characteristics of sperm make it possible for them to swim quickly?*
5. ***LIFE SKILLS: Practicing Self-Care*** *Briefly describe how to do a testicular self-examination.*
6. ***Critical Thinking*** *A vasectomy is an operation in which the vas deferens are cut and tied off. Explain why a vasectomy is a very effective method of preventing pregnancy.*

ASSESS

Section Review

Have students answer the Section Review questions.

Alternative Assessment

Male Reproductive System

Ask students to create an outline that documents the production of sperm, their journey, and the fertilization of an egg. The principal parts of the male reproductive system should be identified in the outline.

Closure

Paragraph Description

Have students describe the functions of the male reproductive system and explain how they are carried out.

Section

16.2 The Female Reproductive System

Objectives

- *Name the organs of the female reproductive system.*
- *Trace the path of the egg from the ovary to the uterus.*
- *Explain how the uterus changes during the menstrual cycle.*
- *Describe how to do a breast self-examination.*
  LIFE SKILLS: Practicing Self-Care

The job of the female reproductive system is to produce an egg and to provide a place where the egg and the sperm can join. After the egg and sperm join, the fertilized egg begins its development into a new individual. The female reproductive system provides the new individual with shelter and nourishment for the nine months before birth. And after birth, the breasts of women are able to provide nourishment in the form of milk. Because of this, breasts are considered to be part of the female reproductive system.

The parts of the female reproductive system, except for the breasts, are shown in Figure 16-6.

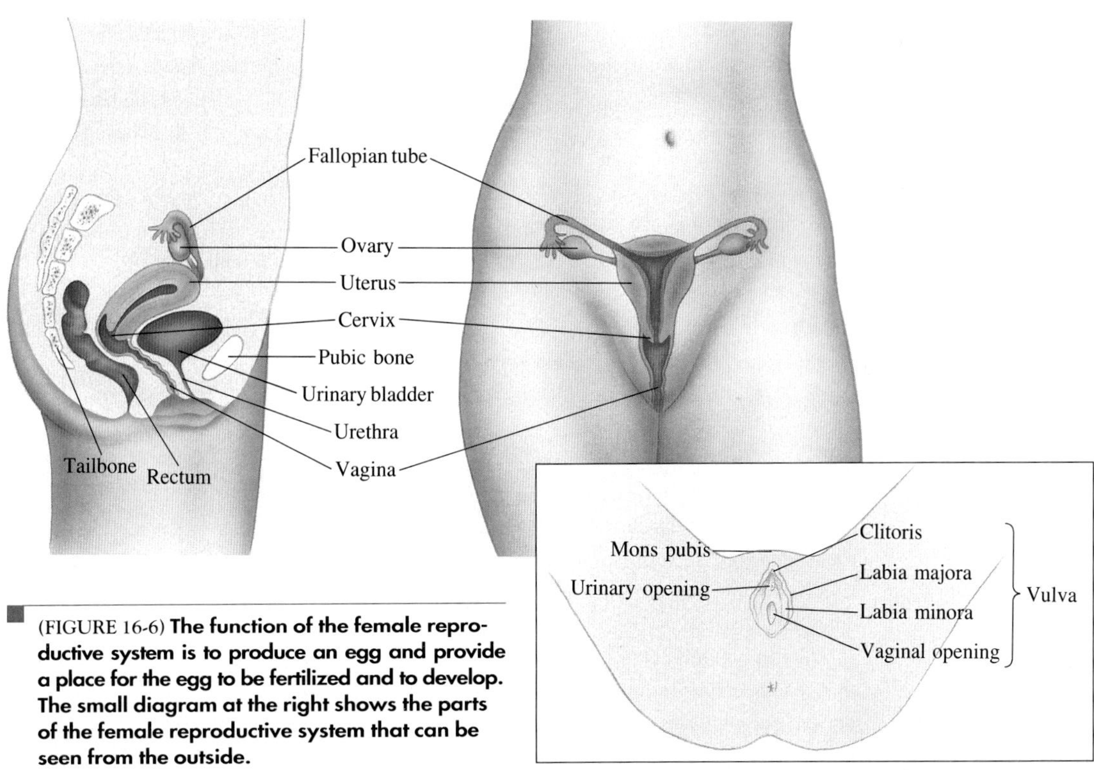

(FIGURE 16-6) **The function of the female reproductive system is to produce an egg and provide a place for the egg to be fertilized and to develop. The small diagram at the right shows the parts of the female reproductive system that can be seen from the outside.**

Background

The Egg

In most women, only about 400 eggs actually mature over a lifetime. Each egg matures within a follicle, or a sac made of cells, which bursts open when the egg is ready for release. At this time, the follicle is about the size of a pea. The empty follicle is then known as the corpus luteum. The egg does not travel on its own. Rather, fringes and tiny hairs in the Fallopian tube draw the egg in and sweep it along. The walls of the tube also contract to help move the egg.

Section 16.2 Lesson Plan

MOTIVATE

Journal 16B
The Female Reproductive System

This may be done as a warm-up activity. Have students use the Student Journal to state the facts they know about the female reproductive system and to list statements they have heard but do not know to be correct. As they read the section, students can verify their facts and unproven statements.

Cooperative Learning
Changes at Puberty

In small groups, have students list changes in the female body that occur during puberty. *(Broadening of the hips, development of breasts, beginning of menstruation.)* Compile a class list that can be added to as students read this section.

TEACH

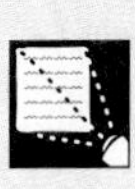

Teaching Transparency 16B
The Female Reproductive System

Show the transparency of The Female Reproductive System. Have them point out specific parts of the female reproductive system, describe their functions, and trace the path of the egg from the ovary to the uterus.

Background
Hymen and Tampon Use

The hymen is a thin skin over the vaginal opening. Not all women have one, and the hymen may vary in thickness. A girl's hymen may have a hole in it large enough to admit a tampon. (A broken hymen does not necessarily mean a girl has had sexual intercourse; nor does an intact one mean she has not.) However, some girls have difficulty inserting tampons. This may be due to a somewhat thick hymen or to muscle tension. Some doctors recommend that young girls use sanitary pads instead of tampons until they have been menstruating for two years, in part because of the possibility of toxic shock syndrome.

ovaries: *female reproductive structures that produce eggs and female sex hormones.*

ovulation: *the release of an egg from an ovary.*

vagina: *female reproductive structure that receives the sperm.*

cervix: *the base of the uterus, which bulges down into the vagina; has a small opening through which sperm can enter the uterus.*

The Vulva

All the parts of the female reproductive system that can be seen from the outside are together called the vulva.

The bone in the center of the lower part of the body is called the pubic bone. Women have extra fat in front of the pubic bone that forms padding that men don't have. The mound formed by the extra padding is called the mons pubis.

The other parts of the vulva are located between the upper part of the thighs. The two larger folds of skin are called the labia majora. At puberty, pubic hair begins to grow on the mons pubis and the labia majora. Inside the labia majora are two smaller folds of skin called the labia minora.

In between the labia minora is the clitoris. Like the penis, the clitoris is the source of greatest sexual excitement and has the capacity to become erect. It is covered by a hood of skin that is connected to the labia minora.

Below the clitoris is the opening of the urethra. Unlike the urethra of the man, the woman's urethra does not have a role in reproduction. The only purpose of the woman's urethra is to provide a way for urine to pass out of the body. Below the urethra is the opening of the vagina.

The Vagina and Cervix

The **vagina** is a muscular tube that receives the sperm. At one end of the vagina is the opening to the outside of the body. At the other end of the vagina is a part of the uterus called the **cervix**, which bulges down into the vagina. In the center of the cervix is a small opening through which sperm can enter the uterus.

During birth, the baby must pass through the cervix and the vagina. For this reason, the vagina is sometimes called the birth canal.

The Ovaries

The two **ovaries** are located in the lower part of the abdomen, one on each side. Like the testes, the ovaries have two major functions. The first function of the ovaries is to produce the eggs. Ovaries usually produce only one mature egg at a time.

The second major function of the ovaries is to produce sex hormones. At puberty, the female sex hormones cause a girl to develop breasts, wider hips, pubic and underarm hair, and a rounded body shape. After puberty, these hormones continue to control the monthly release of an egg and the menstrual cycle.

Before a female baby is born, her ovaries begin the development of several hundred thousand eggs. However, the process stops before the eggs are completely mature. All of the eggs in the ovaries remain in this "half-mature" state until puberty. After puberty, hormones cause one of the eggs to complete the process of maturing about once a month. The release of an egg from an ovary is called **ovulation.** After ovulation, the egg is ready to be fertilized by a sperm from the man.

Follow the path of the egg as it travels to meet the sperm in Figure 16-7. The arrow shows the path of the egg.

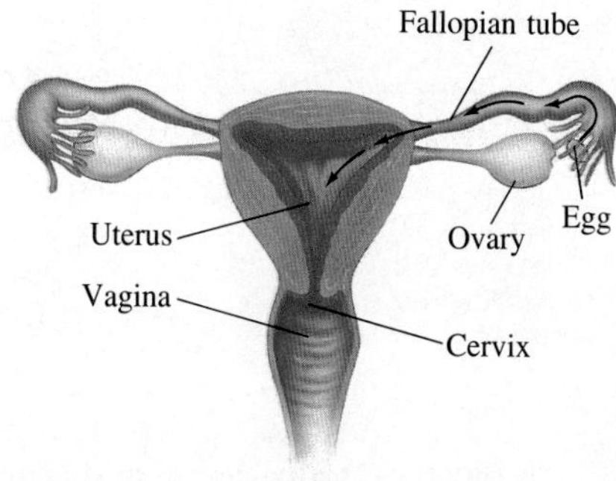

(FIGURE 16-7) **About once a month an egg is released from a woman's ovary, and travels through the Fallopian tube into the uterus.**

• • • TEACH continued

Class Discussion
Design of the Female Reproductive System

Discuss with students how the parts of the female reproductive system are well-designed to carry out their functions. For example, the vagina is muscular and able to stretch. The cervix remains small but it enlarges during labor to allow birth to occur. The uterus has thick walls, richly supplied with blood, and is also very stretchable. Be sure the students understand that the egg moves along the Fallopian tube to the uterus, whether or not it is fertilized. Ask: **Why is this movement preferable to the egg remaining in the ovary until fertilized?** *[Possible reasons could include short life span of sperm, brief period of time during which the mature egg can be fertilized, and the need for the embryo to implant quickly in the uterus.]*

Reinforcement
Menstrual Cycles

Reassure female students that there is a wide range of patterning that is considered normal for menstrual cycles. In addition, while the cycle is becoming established during puberty, it often varies a great deal. Also, outside factors such as illness or stress can delay the onset of a period.

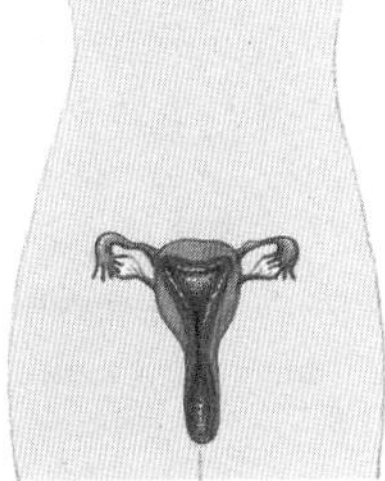

1. Day 0-Day 5: The uterine lining begins to thicken.

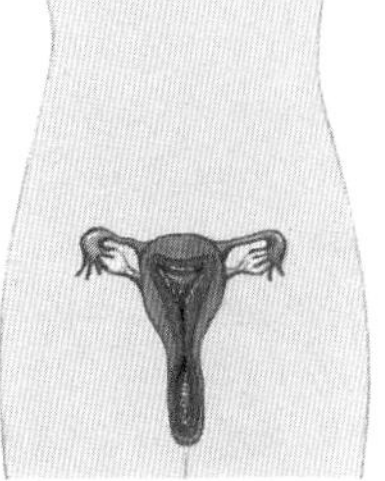

2. Day 5-Day 14: The uterine lining continues to thicken until ovulation occurs, around day 14.

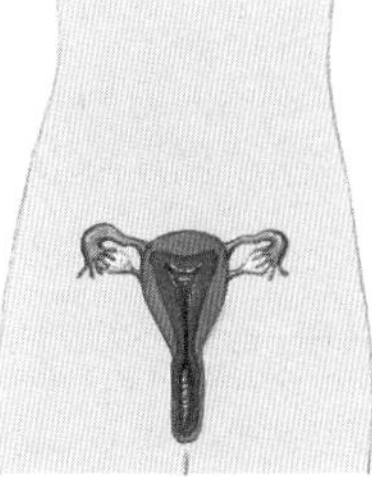

3. Day 15-Day 28: The thickened uterine lining awaits a fertilized egg. If the egg is not fertilized, the egg begins to break down.

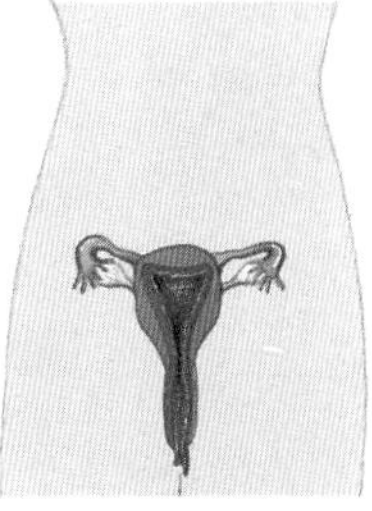

4. Menstruation: The lining is being shed and is flowing from the woman's body. The cycle begins again.

(FIGURE 16-8) **This diagram shows what happens inside the uterus if the egg is not fertilized. During the menstrual cycle, the uterine lining gets thicker and thicker. If the egg is fertilized, the lining will be maintained, and the uterus will expand to many times its usual size. If the egg is *not* fertilized, however, the lining is shed and flows from the body during the menstrual period.**

The Fallopian Tubes

Even though an ovary releases an egg, the egg and sperm do not join in the ovary. They join together in one of the Fallopian tubes. When an egg has matured, fluid sweeps it from the ovary into one of the Fallopian tubes. These tubes provide a way for an egg to travel from the ovary to the uterus.

If the egg meets the sperm as it travels through the upper third of the Fallopian tube, it can be fertilized. If the egg is not fertilized within 12 to 24 hours after it is released from the ovary, the egg begins to break down and can no longer be fertilized. In either case, the egg continues to float toward the uterus. The egg reaches the uterus about four or five days after it was released from the ovary. If it has been fertilized, it will grow and eventually become a baby. If the egg has not been fertilized, it will simply dissolve in the uterus.

The Uterus

The **uterus** is a hollow, muscular organ about the size of a fist. It is sometimes called the womb. The main job of the uterus is to provide a place for a baby to grow before birth. During pregnancy, the uterus is able to expand to many times its usual size.

uterus:

the hollow muscular organ that provides a place for the baby to grow before birth; also called the womb.

The Menstrual Cycle

The uterus undergoes cyclical changes (approximately on a monthly basis), which prepare it to receive and nourish a fertilized egg. These changes in the uterus are called the menstrual cycle.

During the menstrual cycle, the inner lining of the uterus thickens, and many tiny blood vessels grow into this thickened lining. The changes in the uterine lining are caused by a hormone called progesterone.

Class Discussion
Multiple Births

Initiate a discussion of multiple births by asking students the following questions: **If a woman's ovaries contain many eggs and a man releases millions of sperm during an ejaculation, why is only one egg usually fertilized?** *[Eggs mature in the ovaries at different times, and usually only one mature egg is released during each menstrual cycle.]* **What might happen if two eggs were released from the ovaries at the same time?** *[Two different sperm might fertilize them. Fraternal twins would result. These twins, unlike identical twins, would not look exactly alike.]* **What would happen if one egg were fertilized and later divided into two separate balls of cells?** *[Identical twins would result.]*

Demonstration
Larger Than Life

Ask for five volunteers, each of whom will sketch one structure of the female reproductive system (ovaries, Fallopian tubes, uterus, cervix, vagina). Designate a triangular area of the classroom as the female reproductive system and have students place their sketches within the triangle to show the proper position of each structure. Then name a phase of the menstrual cycle (such as ovulation) and have each volunteer describe any changes that his or her structure is undergoing at that time.

SECTION 16.2

Background
Monthly Cycles

The word *menstruation* is derived from the Latin word *menses,* meaning "month." The hormones that initiate puberty in females and control the menstrual cycle are estrogen and progesterone. Low levels of estrogen and progesterone trigger menstruation. A high level of estrogen triggers ovulation, and a high level of progesterone causes the uterine lining to thicken.

Once these changes have occured, one of two things happens, depending on whether the egg has been fertilized by a sperm.

If the egg *has* been fertilized, hormones are released that tell the uterus to maintain its thickened lining. The woman is pregnant.

Most of the time, though, the egg has not been fertilized and the woman is not pregnant. The thickened uterine lining breaks down, and the woman menstruates.

Except during pregnancy, most women release an egg approximately every month from puberty until about age 50. Even if a woman has many children, only a small percentage of her eggs will be fertilized and result in pregnancy.

Menstrual Fluid If the egg has not been fertilized and the woman is not pregnant, the blood vessels of the lining begin to close up and then to break. The cells of the lining begin to come loose from the inside of the uterus. Blood from the broken blood vessels helps to wash these cells out of the uterus. This mixture of blood and cells is called menstrual fluid. The amount of menstrual fluid varies from woman to woman. Some women may have a light menstrual flow—only about a tablespoon of menstrual fluid each cycle. Others have a heavy flow —eight or more tablespoons each cycle.

The Menstrual Period The menstrual fluid passes through the opening of the cervix and through the vagina to the outside of the body. The time during which the menstrual fluid is flowing to the outside of the body is called the menstrual period. Most women have menstrual periods that last from three to seven days.

After the menstrual period is completed, the uterus prepares a new thickened lining. This lining will be ready for the next egg that is released from the ovary and travels down the Fallopian tube to the uterus.

The average menstrual cycle lasts about 28 days. This is the time from the first day of a menstrual period until the first day of the next menstrual period. However, the length of the menstrual cycle varies. One woman might have a 25-day cycle while her best friend has a 35-day cycle. Yet another woman might have a cycle that is a different length each month. This is called an irregular cycle. Irregular cycles are especially common during the first few years after a girl begins to menstruate. In addition, a woman who usually has a regular cycle may occasionally have a period earlier or later than usual.

The age at which a girl has her first menstrual period also varies from individual to individual. Most girls begin to menstruate between the ages of 12 and 14. However, it is not unusual for a girl to have her first period as young as age 9 or 10. Other girls do not have a period until they are 17 or 18. Beginning menstruation at 10 or 13 or 18, having a regular 28-day cycle or one that's shorter or longer—all of these individual differences are perfectly normal.

Disorders of the Female Reproductive System

The following conditions are the most common or the most serious of the disorders that affect women.

Menstrual Cramps Menstrual cramps are a very common problem for females, especially teenagers. These are cramps felt in the lower abdominal area that are caused by the uterus contracting to expel its lining. Those who have cramps usually have them the first day or two of their menstrual periods, but sometimes the cramps last longer.

Warm baths and exercise can sometimes relieve cramps. However, medication is usually required for severe cramps. The nonprescription medications that are

• • • TEACH continued

Demonstration
Breast Self-Examination

Emphasize to female students the importance of a monthly self-examination of the breasts. If possible, ask a representative of the American Cancer Society to visit the class and demonstrate the technique of self-examination, using a model.

Reinforcement
Pap Test

Stress the importance of a yearly Pap test for sexually active women (or any woman over age 20). The procedure involves gently scraping cells from the cervix, transferring some of these cells to a slide, and examining them for abnormalities.

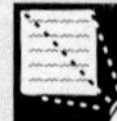

Teaching Transparency 16C
Fertility Testing

Use this transparency to review the parts of the male and female reproductive system described in the text. Refer to the graph of basal body temperature when discussing fertility testing procedures.

Extension
Feminine Products

Ask students to research and report on feminine hygiene products. Some students might study recent articles and

most effective in relieving cramps contain ibuprofen. If ibuprofen does not relieve cramps, a doctor should be consulted. He or she may prescribe medication that alleviates menstrual cramps. Cramps will usually decrease in severity as a woman gets older.

PMS (Premenstrual Syndrome) Some women experience a combination of problems before their menstrual periods called PMS (premenstrual syndrome). PMS seems to be most common among women in their thirties. The physical symptoms are swelling and tenderness of the breasts, a bloated feeling, constipation, headaches, and fatigue. The emotional signs of PMS are depression, crying, anxiety, and anger. A female with PMS may have all of these signs and symptoms or may have only a few. PMS usually occurs for one to three days before menstruation, but some women may have PMS for two weeks before each menstrual period.

Researchers do not yet know why some females have PMS and others do not. Nor do they know exactly *what* causes PMS, though hormonal fluctuations may be responsible.

Doctors recommend that those with PMS reduce their intake of salt and sugar and completely avoid caffeine (in coffee and colas) and nicotine (in tobacco). They also recommend regular physical exercise and relaxation exercises, such as those described in Chapter 9. If a woman follows these recommendations for several months and still has PMS, she should seek medical treatment. A doctor may also prescribe medication to relieve the signs and symptoms of PMS.

Vaginitis An infection of the vagina is called vaginitis. Most women will have vaginitis sometime during their lives. The signs and symptoms may include itching or soreness of the vulva, an unpleasant odor, a thick fluid from the vagina, and sometimes a burning sensation during urination. Vaginitis can be caused by a fungus, bacteria, or protozoa, and each kind of vaginitis requires a different kind of treatment. If a woman has any of the symptoms of vaginitis, she should seek medical treatment to get the correct medication.

It is important to know that *most* fluids from the vagina are perfectly normal. If the fluid is clear or whitish and nonirritating, it is probably normal. Many factors besides an infection can create vaginal fluids—sexual excitement and hormonal changes, are two examples. All women have these kinds of secretions. It is only when the fluid is irritating that a woman should become concerned about a possible infection.

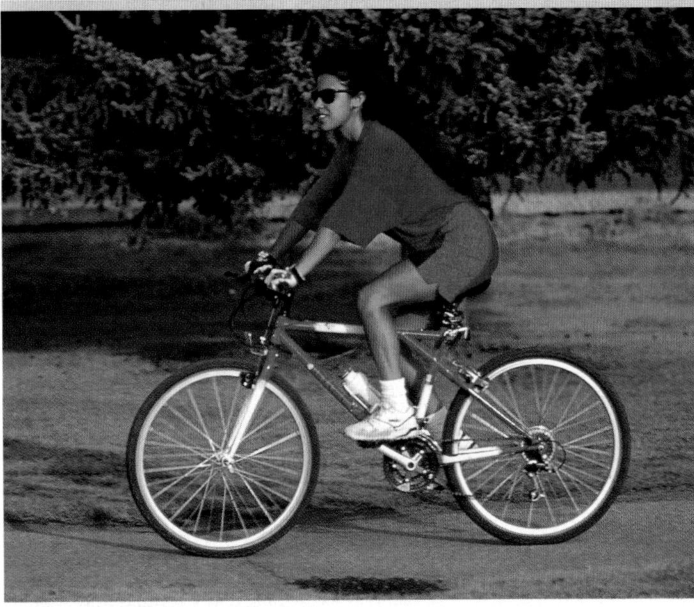

(FIGURE 16-9) **Getting plenty of exercise can help alleviate the pain and tension that sometimes accompany a woman's menstrual period.**

Life Skills Worksheet 16A

Mammography

Assign the Mammography Life Skills Worksheet, which asks students to investigate local mammography testing programs.

brochures for facts regarding which products are useful and which are unnecessary or potentially harmful. Others might analyze the advertising of feminine products to expose fallacies and illogical appeals used to promote unnecessary products.

Background
Disorders

Ovarian cysts often grow where a follicle has enlarged but failed to break open and release an egg. Many cysts are fluid-filled; some are solid. Most are harmless and go away by themselves; however, those that grow large can cause pain, abdominal swelling, or even abnormal menstruation and require surgery for removal.

Endometriosis is a disorder affecting some 5 million women in the United States. In the past, conventional surgery has been the only option to alleviate this condition. Now, thanks to laser laparoscopy, there is a quicker, safer option. A laparoscope (a thin, lighted telescope) is inserted through a small incision in the abdomen and used to view the reproductive organs and guide the laser. The laser is inserted through a second small incision and used to destroy unwanted tissues.

Toxic Shock Syndrome Toxic shock syndrome is an infection that is very rare but also very dangerous. Toxic shock syndrome is caused by bacteria and is often associated with the use of highly absorbent tampons.

The signs and symptoms of toxic shock syndrome are high fever, nausea, diarrhea, dizziness, and a sunburn-like rash. The rash is often on the palms of the hands and the bottoms of the feet. A woman who has these signs and symptoms should remove the tampon and then go to a hospital emergency room immediately, because toxic shock syndrome can cause death.

Ovarian Cysts An ovarian cyst is a growth on an ovary. A woman with an ovarian cyst may experience pain or may have no signs or symptoms at all. Large cysts must be surgically removed, but small cysts sometimes disappear without any treatment.

Cancers Cancer can occur in any part of the female reproductive system. Doctors recommend that women have a yearly pelvic examination to detect cancers early. The earlier cancer is caught, the more successful the treatment. During the examination, the doctor will do what is called a **Pap test,** in which cells from the cervix are removed and tested for cancer. This test is painless and saves many lives every year.

Pap test: *a medical procedure in which cells from the cervix are removed and tested for cancer.*

Women should also get in the habit of checking their breasts for lumps and other abnormalities each month. Figure 16-10 demonstrates how to do a breast self-examination. Most lumps found this way are not cancerous, but any lump should be checked out by a doctor to make sure.

Sexually transmitted diseases (STDs) can cause infertility. The relationship between STDs and infertility is discussed in Chapter 22.

Doctors recommend regular mammograms (an X-ray of the breast), beginning when a woman is about 35 years old. If cancer of the breast is caught and treated early, there is an excellent chance of recovery. For this reason, regular breast self-examinations can be lifesaving.

Infertility Women, like men, can be infertile—unable to have children. The most common cause of female infertility is failure to ovulate—to release an egg. Another common cause is scar tissue in the Fallopian tubes, which prevents the sperm from reaching the egg. The scar tissue may have been the result of an infection or previous surgery. Endometriosis may also result in infertility. Endometriosis is a condition in which tissue from the endometrial lining of the uterus grows somewhere else in the abdomen. Many cases of infertility can be treated medically.

Care of the Female Reproductive System

The female reproductive system may seem more complicated than the male system, but actually it doesn't require much more care. Females should take the following simple steps to keep everything working smoothly.

1. Wash the external reproductive organs daily with a mild, nonirritating soap. Feel for any unusual bumps or sores.
2. Don't use feminine ''hygiene'' sprays. They can cause irritation. If daily washing doesn't keep a woman clean and fresh-smelling, she should seek medical help. An unpleasant odor may be a sign of an infection. Remember, though, that vaginal secretions have a unique scent that is perfectly normal. As a girl gets older, she gets better at telling the difference between the usual healthy scent and the odor that means infection.
3. Don't use douches unless they are medicinal douches recommended to you by your doctor. Like sprays, douches are usually unnecessary, and they can cause irritation.

How to do a breast self-examination:

Do the breast self-exam once a month. Two or three days after your menstrual period ends is the best time, because your breasts are less likely to be tender or swollen.

1. Stand in front of a mirror and look carefully at your breasts. Look for anything unusual, such as discharge from the nipples, puckering, dimpling, or scaling of the skin.

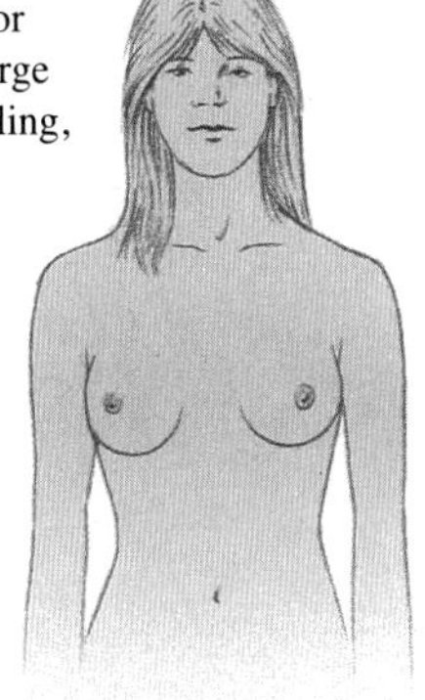

2. Clasp your hands behind your head and press your hands forward. Do you notice any change in the shape of your breasts since the last time you did a breast self-exam?

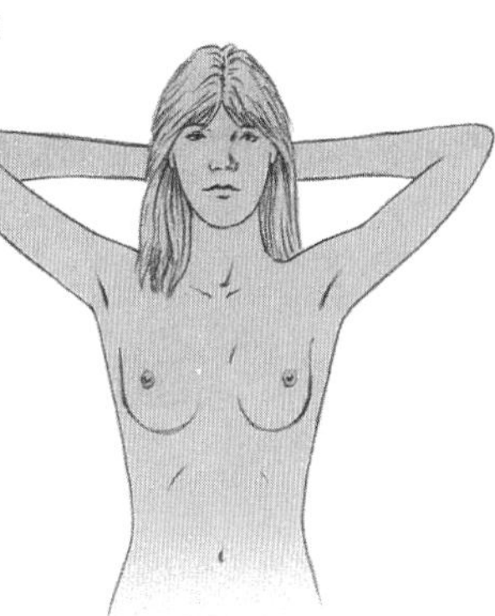

3. Press your hands firmly on your hips and bow slightly forward and pull your shoulders and elbows forward. Do you notice any change in shape of your breasts since the last time you did a breast self-exam?

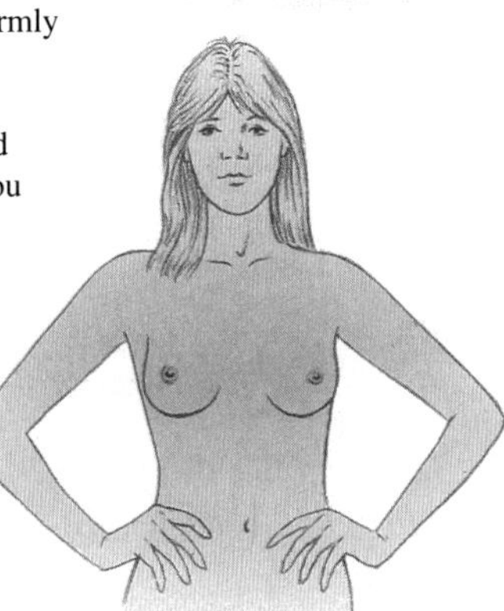

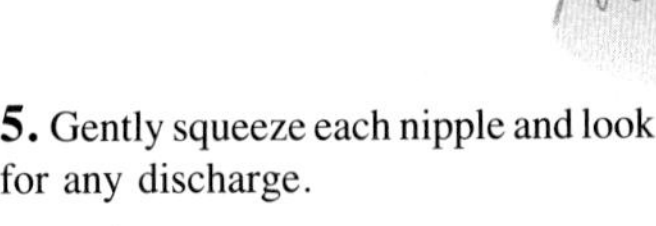

4. Raise your left arm. Use your fingers to examine your left breast. Beginning at the outer edge of your breast, press the flat part of your fingers in small circles, moving the circles slowly around the breast. Make sure to include the area between the breast and the armpit and also the armpit itself. Do you feel any unusual lump under the skin? Now repeat this step on your right breast with your right arm raised.

5. Gently squeeze each nipple and look for any discharge.

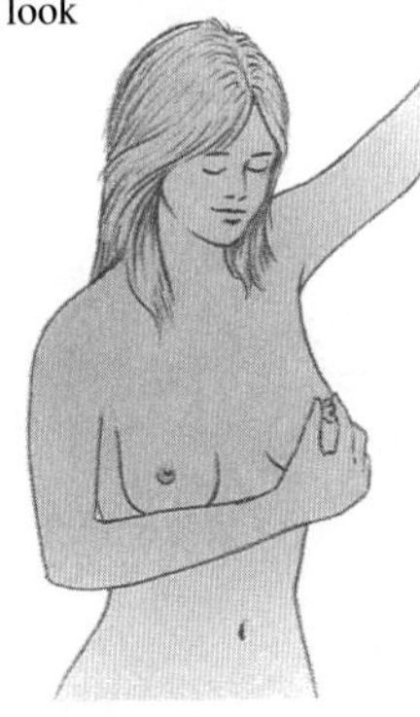

6. Lie down and put a pillow or folded towel under your left shoulder. Raise your left arm. Examine your left breast in the same way you did in Step 4. Repeat on your right breast.

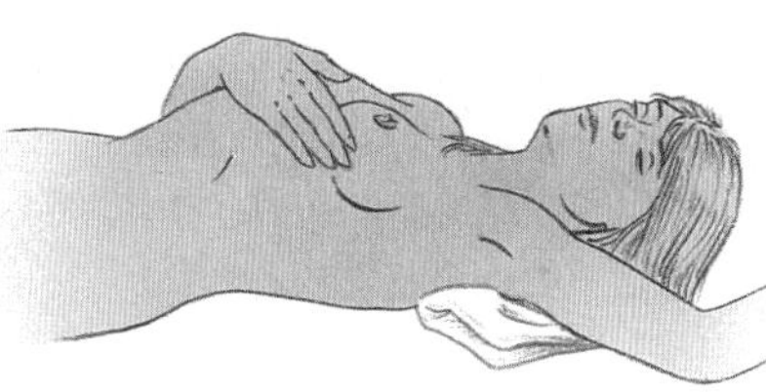

(FIGURE 16-10) **Breast self-examination should be done once a month to become familiar with the usual appearance and feel of your breasts. Most lumps are not cancerous, but any lump should be checked out by a doctor to make sure.**

SECTION 16.2

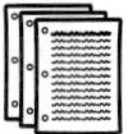

Section Review Worksheet 16.2

Assign Section Review Worksheet 16.2, which requires students to complete a network and a chart showing the functions and disorders of the female reproductive system.

Section Quiz 16.2

Have students take Section Quiz 16.2.

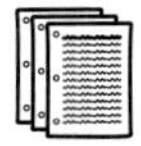

Reteaching Worksheet 16.2

Students who have difficulty with the material may complete Reteaching Worksheet 16.2, which requires them to complete sentences describing structures, functions, and disorders of the female reproductive system.

Review Answers

1. Ovary
2. Fallopian tube
3. It breaks down and is shed.
4. Stand before a mirror and look at each breast for anything unusual. Repeat, clasping hands behind your head and pressing hands forward, and pressing hands on hips and bowing forward. Raise each arm in turn and use the fingers of the other hand to feel the breast and armpit for any lumps. Gently squeeze each nipple and look for any discharge. Lying down, repeat the examination of each breast.
5. When the Fallopian tubes are cut and tied off, sperm cannot travel through the tubes to meet and fertilize an egg.

4. During menstruation, change sanitary pads or tampons often—at least every three hours. In addition, do not use highly absorbent tampons.
5. Visit a gynecologist, family physician, or pediatrician once a year to make sure that the reproductive system is healthy. A gynecologist is a physician who specializes in caring for the female reproductive system. Young women should start getting yearly gynecological exams at the age of 18, or earlier if they are sexually active.
6. Do a monthly breast self-examination to find lumps or other abnormalities. Figure 16-10 shows how to do the breast exam. The best time to do the self-examination is a few days after a menstrual period, when the breasts are less likely to be tender.

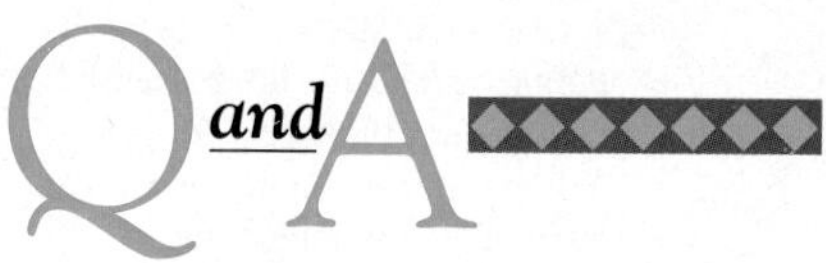

Q: I'm almost 14 years old and I still haven't started having menstrual periods. Could there be something wrong with me?

A: It is not abnormal for a girl to be 14 or 15 years old before she begins to menstruate. A girl who has reached the age of 16 and has not menstruated should probably see a doctor to make sure she doesn't have a medical problem.

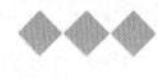

Q: Someone told me that a woman can't get pregnant the first time she has sexual intercourse. Is this true?

A: No. A woman is just as likely to get pregnant the first time as at later times.

Q: Can a woman get pregnant even if she doesn't have an orgasm during sexual intercourse?

A: Yes, pregnancy can occur whether or not a woman has an orgasm.

Review

1. *Which female structure produces the eggs?*
2. *In which structure do the egg and the sperm join?*
3. *What happens to the thickened uterine lining if fertilization does not occur?*
4. ***LIFE SKILLS: Practicing Self-Care*** *Briefly describe how to do a breast self-examination.*
5. ***Critical Thinking*** *A tubal ligation is an operation in which the Fallopian tubes are cut or tied off. Explain why tubal ligation is a very effective method of preventing pregnancy.*

ASSESS

Section Review

Have students answer the Section Review questions.

Alternative Assessment

Newspaper Health Column

Have students write an imaginary newspaper health column answering letters from teens with questions about the female reproductive system. Encourage them to use the information they learned in this section to answer the letters.

Closure

Female Life Cycle

Have volunteers use the chalkboard to summarize and illustrate what happens to an egg from the time a female is born until she conceives an offspring.

Section 16.3 Pregnancy, Birth, and Childhood Development

Objectives

- List the substances that can pass from the mother to the placenta.
- Describe the events that occur during birth.
- Use self-talk about childhood experiences to increase your self-esteem.
  LIFE SKILLS: Building Self-Esteem

For most new parents, the birth of a child is both exciting and a little scary. Raising a child can bring a great deal of happiness and a sense of accomplishing something that is truly worthwhile. When parents see themselves in the shape of a nose or a funny way of laughing, they know that something of themselves will live on after they are gone.

But having a child is also a tremendous responsibility. Parenthood means sacrifices and sleepless nights, losing freedom and gaining worries. The decision of whether to have children is important and shouldn't be taken lightly. This decision will be discussed in Chapter 18. In the rest of this chapter, you'll learn what happens after the sperm and the egg join.

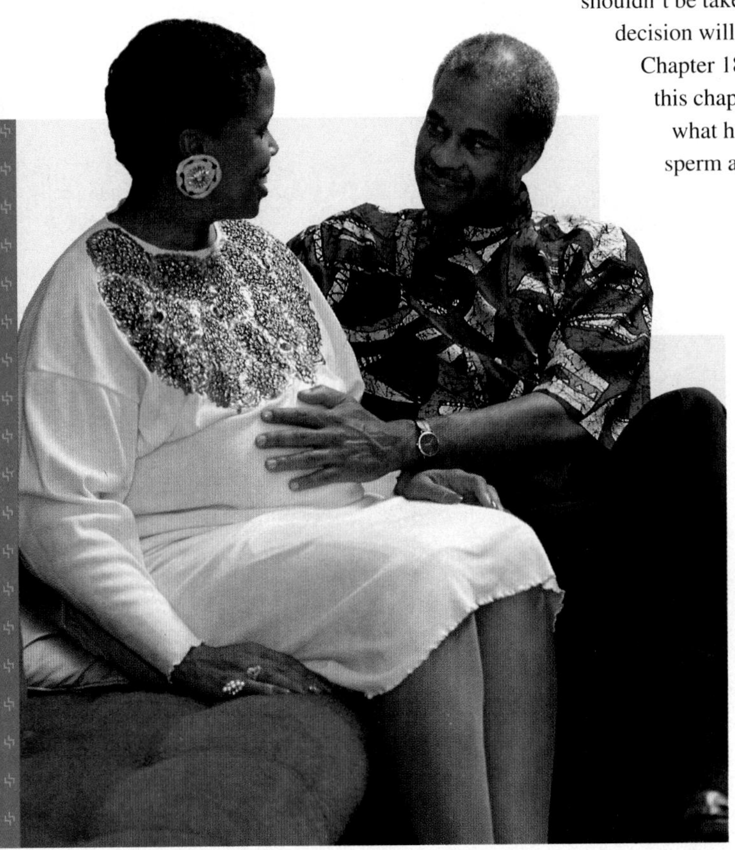

(FIGURE 16-11) **Parenthood can be one of the most fulfilling experiences in life, but it is also a tremendous responsibility.**

Section 16.3 Lesson Plan

MOTIVATE

Journal 16C
Feelings About Becoming Parents

This may be done as a warm-up activity. Refer students to the photograph shown in Figure 16-11. Ask: How do you think the man and woman feel about becoming parents? Have students write in the Student Journal what they think it would be like to become a parent.

Writing
Stages of Life So Far

Have students write a descriptive paragraph, poem, or short story about stages they feel they have passed through since birth. For each stage, they might describe the physical and psychological gains that were made.

TEACH

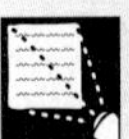

Teaching Transparency 16D
Fertilization

Show the diagram outlining the fertilization of the egg and the path of the fertilized egg to the uterus (Figure 16-12). Have students describe the changes the embryo undergoes during this journey and explain what happens to it when it reaches the uterus.

Background
Ectopic Pregnancy

If a fertilized egg implants itself anywhere other than the uterus, an ectopic pregnancy results. Ninety-five percent of ectopic pregnancies occur in a Fallopian tube. Most such pregnancies end early because this tube is not a hospitable environment for the embryo's development. As the embryo grows, the tube is stretched and hemorrhage often occurs. If the embryo becomes large enough the tube will burst, creating a dangerous situation that requires immediate medical attention. Ectopic pregnancy is the seventh leading cause of maternal death, primarily because the condition is hard to diagnose. Ectopic pregnancy now occurs in 1 out of every 100 pregnancies, and the number is increasing.

embryo:
a fertilized egg after it has divided into two cells.

Implantation

Before fertilization, the sperm and the egg are two separate cells, each containing *one-half* of the information needed for the development of a new person. After fertilization, there is only one cell, but it contains *all* of the material needed for the development of a new person.

After the sperm fertilizes the egg in the Fallopian tube, the fertilized egg continues to travel toward the uterus. Figure 16-12 shows the path of the egg.

About 30 hours after fertilization, the egg divides into two cells and is now called an **embryo.** The embryo divides into four cells, the four cells into eight cells, and so on. By the time the embryo reaches the uterus, about four days after fertilization, it is made of a hundred or more cells.

As the embryo comes to rest on the soft, thick lining of the uterus, it begins to burrow into the lining. By the 10th day after fertilization, the embryo contains thousands of cells and is completely buried in the uterine wall. This process is called implantation.

From Mother to Baby

As the embryo implants itself in the wall of the uterus, it is beginning to use up all of the nutrients that were stored in the egg before fertilization. If the embryo is to survive, it must have a way to obtain everything it needs from the mother as it grows. The placenta is the structure that allows the embryo to get what it needs from the mother. The placenta is an organ shaped like a disc that rests against the inner wall of the uterus. It is connected to the embryo by a structure called the umbilical cord.

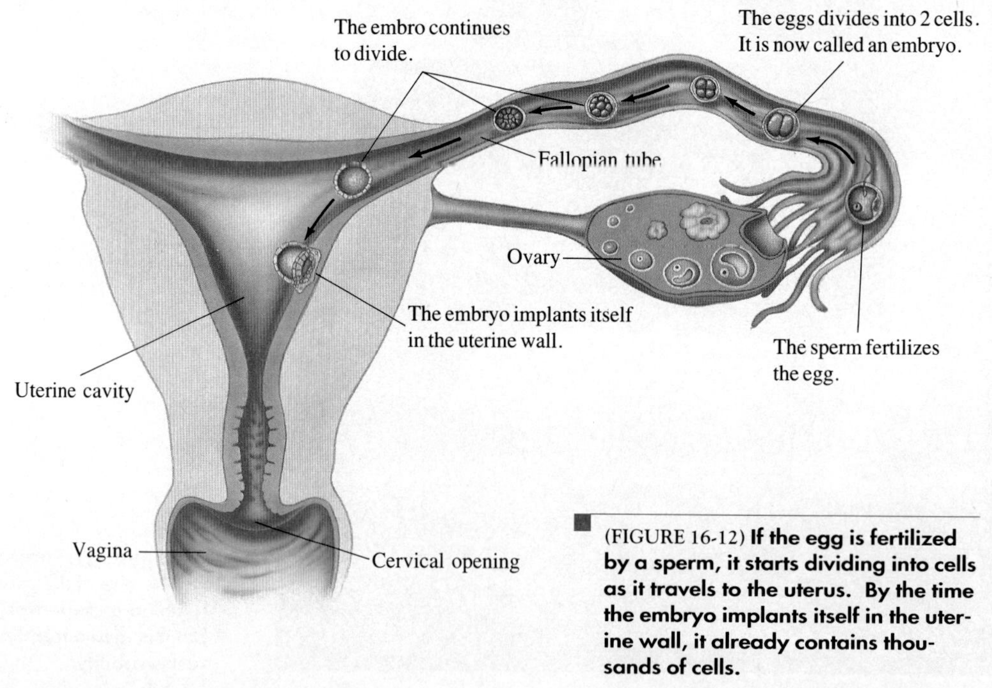

(FIGURE 16-12) **If the egg is fertilized by a sperm, it starts dividing into cells as it travels to the uterus. By the time the embryo implants itself in the uterine wall, it already contains thousands of cells.**

• • • TEACH continued

Demonstration
Crossing the Placental Barrier

Divide an area of the chalkboard into two parts. One part will represent the mother's blood, the other the developing baby's blood. Provide students with a list of substances that are exchanged in the placenta. These include oxygen, carbon dioxide, and wastes. Ask students to draw arrows on the chalkboard, showing the movement of these substances between the mother and baby.

Reinforcement
Prenatal Care

Poor prenatal care is one major cause of the low birth weight and high mortality rate for infants born to teenage mothers. Have students suggest a list of do's and don'ts for a pregnant woman. Write these on the chalkboard as students explain why each is important. *(The developing baby requires good food and plenty of fluid intake by the mother. Toxins and other harmful substances taken in by the mother go directly to the blood of the embryo or fetus, where they can retard development or cause defects or congenital diseases. For these reasons, it is important that women who are pregnant eat well, drink plenty of healthful fluids, avoid alcohol, tobacco, and most drugs, and get the proper amount of exercise and rest.)*

(FIGURE 16-13) **Oxygen and nutrients travel from the mother to the fetus through the umbilical cord.**

The mother's blood does not flow into the baby. Instead, pools of blood are formed that bathe the outside of the embryo's blood vessels. Even though the mother's blood and the embryo's blood come very close to each other, they do not mix in the placenta.

Oxygen and nutrients from the mother's blood diffuse across the walls of the embryo's blood vessels in the placenta. The oxygen and nutrients then travel through the blood vessels in the umbilical cord to the baby.

Viruses and drugs can also pass from the mother's blood to the baby's blood. Some viruses and drugs can cause the baby to develop abnormally. For this reason, pregnant women should take good care of their health and avoid exposure to diseases. In addition, a pregnant woman should never take any drug without checking with her doctor first. This includes alcohol and drugs that can be bought without a prescription, such as aspirin and cold remedies.

Changes During Pregnancy

Once the embryo has implanted itself in the uterus, it grows rapidly. A heart and brain begin to form. Eyes appear and the face takes shape. Small buds on the sides of the body become arms and legs. Internal organs like the lungs, stomach, and liver are developing. The embryo floats in a warm, fluid-filled sac called the amniotic sac.

Eight weeks after fertilization occurs the embryo is only 30 mm long (a little over 1 in. long). However, all the major organ systems of its body are formed and growing. From the ninth week until birth, it is called a **fetus.**

fetus:

a developing individual from the ninth week of pregnancy until birth.

Background
Calculating Date of Birth

The human period of gestation is 280 days, or about 9 months. To calculate the approximate date of a baby's birth, first determine when the pregnant woman's last period began. Then count back three months from the first day of this period and add seven days plus one year.

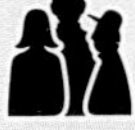

Cooperative Learning
Stages of Development

Divide the class into small groups and assign each group a stage of embryo or fetal development to explore in depth. You might assign the stages shown in Figure 16-14. Allow out-of-class or library time for students to locate information in books, magazines, and pamphlets. For each stage, have them tell what happens to the developing baby and how it can be affected by the mother's actions.

Role-Playing
Issues in Pregnancy

Allow students to show their understanding of pregnancy, fetal development, and childbirth by role-playing several situations that call for a counselor, parent, friend, or doctor to help a woman make decisions. The following are some possible scenarios:

A young woman thinks she might be pregnant and asks a parent or friend what she should do.

A pregnant woman who smokes (or drinks, or takes drugs) sees her doctor for a checkup.

A young woman is six weeks pregnant and doesn't know what to expect. She talks to a counselor.

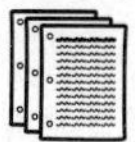

Life Skills Worksheet 16B

Home Pregnancy Tests

Assign the Home Pregnancy Tests Life Skills Worksheet, which requires students to examine and compare different brands of pregnancy testing kits.

Making a Choice 16A

Knowledge About Reproduction

Assign the Knowledge About Reproduction card. The card requires students to discuss their attitudes toward learning about the reproductive systems.

Making a Choice 16B

Thoughts About Having Children

Assign the Thoughts About Having Children card. The card asks students to examine their plans and feelings about having a family.

(FIGURE 16-14)

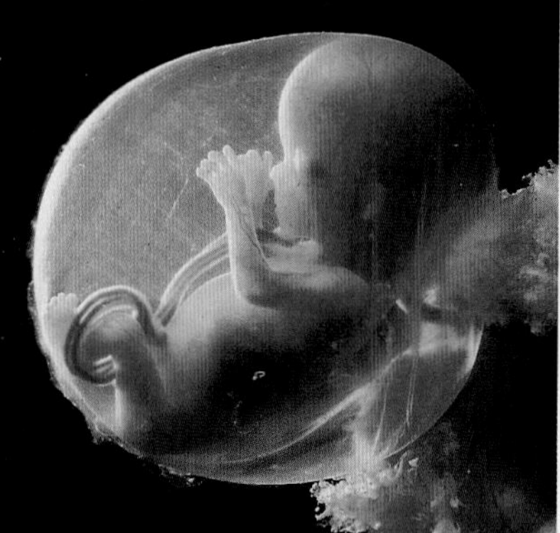

16 weeks

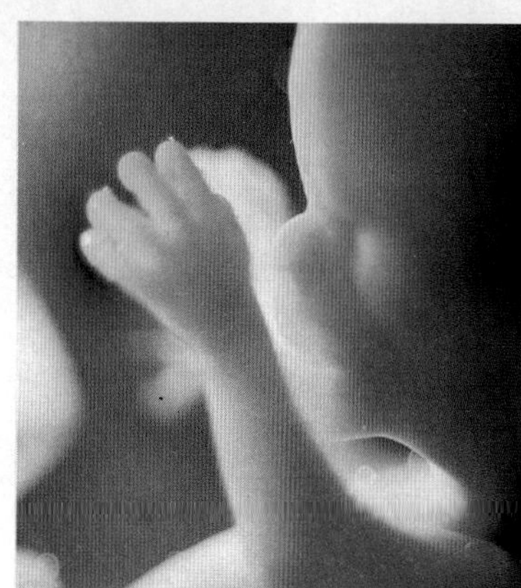

12 weeks

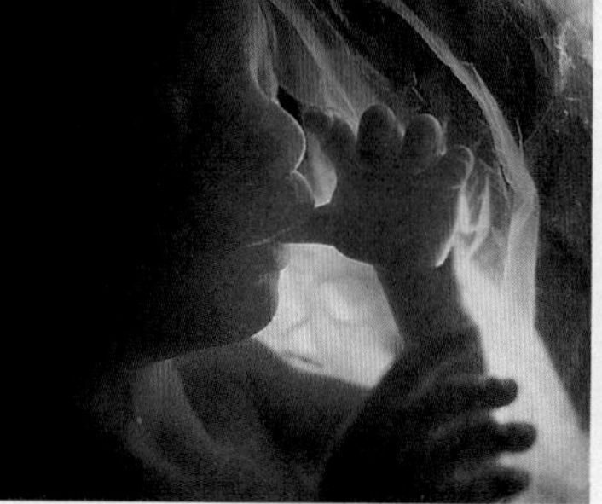

18 weeks

Development Inside the Uterus

By the End of 12 Weeks
- Brain enlarging
- Arms and legs forming
- Bones forming
- Heart and blood system fully functioning
- Digestive system forming
- About 4 inches long

By the End of 16 Weeks
- Mother can feel fetal movements
- About 5 inches long

By the End of 18 Weeks
- Skin begins to grow
- Hair can be detected on upper lip and on eyebrows
- About 6 inches long

By the End of 24 Weeks
- Mouth can open, close, and swallow
- Eyes can open and close
- About 9 inches long

Full Term
- Features, organs fully formed
- About 15 inches long

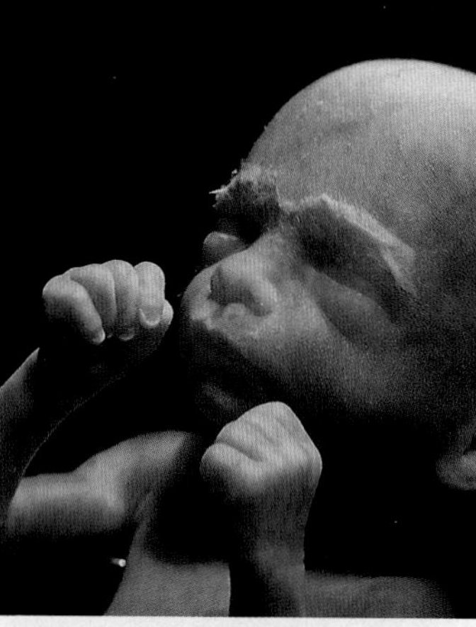

24 weeks

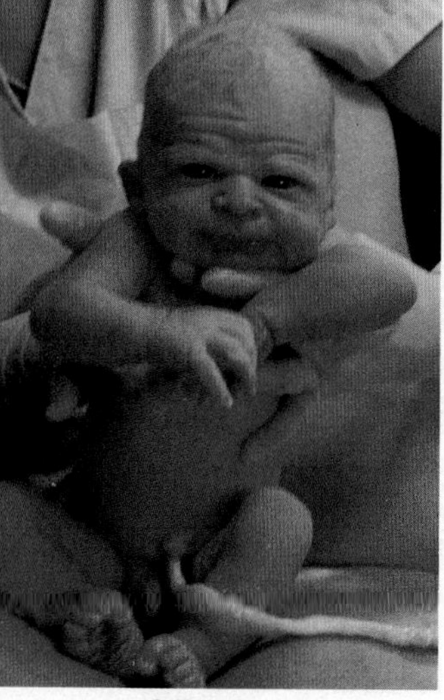

full term

Pregnancy Tests

When a female misses a menstrual period, it is a sign that she *might* be pregnant. However, a number of other reasons, like stress and illness, might also explain a missed period. A missed period is not a very reliable indicator of pregnancy.

An accurate pregnancy test detects a hormone called HCG (human chorionic gonadotropin). Three weeks after fertilization, a pregnant female will probably have enough HCG in her blood and urine for a positive test result. Doctors and health clinics can administer these tests.

Pregnancy "test kits" can be obtained at drug stores. These kits also test for the presence of HCG. However, they must be administered correctly to be accurate. If a negative result is obtained, the test should be done again. If the result is positive, the woman should visit a doctor or clinic to do another test to confirm the result.

• • • TEACH continued

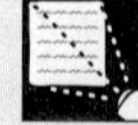

Teaching Transparency 16E
Stages of Childbirth

Show the transparency of the stages of childbirth (Figure 16-15). Have students explain the changes and events that are illustrated in each picture. The transparency may also prove useful for reference in answering questions students may have about childbirth, such as: What if the baby is not in the right position? How is a baby removed by Caesarean section?

Demonstration
Growth of the Fetus

To dramatize the rapid growth of a fetus, supply students with the following information and have them work in groups to use materials that will demonstrate the change in length and weight of a developing baby at different stages of pregnancy. Students will need to be supplied with rulers, scales, and modeling materials such as clay or wood.

End of	Size of Fetus
Month 1	.25 in. (0.6 cm)
Month 3	3 in. (7.6 cm); 1 oz. (28.3 g)
Month 5	12 in. (30.5 cm); 1 lb. (453.6 g)
Month 7	14–15 in. (35.6–38.1 cm); 2–2.5 lb. (907.2–1,134 g)
Month 9	18–20 in. (45.7–50.8 cm); 7–9 lb. (3,175.2–4,082.4 g)

Childbirth

The stages of the birth of a child are shown in Figure 16-15. By the time the baby is ready to be born, it has usually moved so that its head is down against the cervix. The cervix is a ring of very strong muscles at the lower part of the uterus. These muscles are able to hold a developing baby and surrounding fluids inside the uterus without relaxing until the baby is ready to be born.

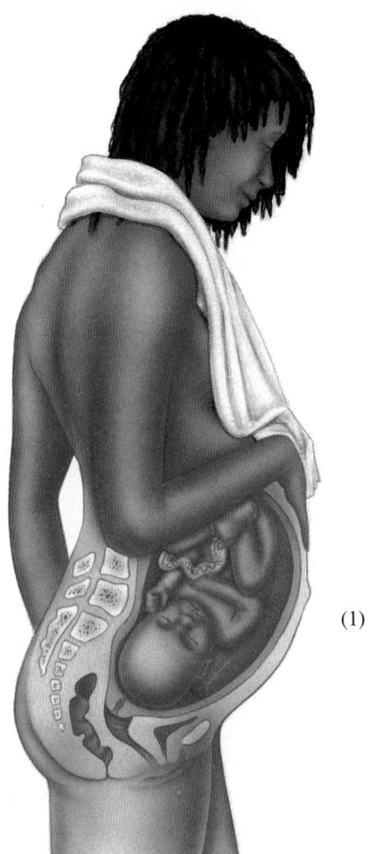
(1)

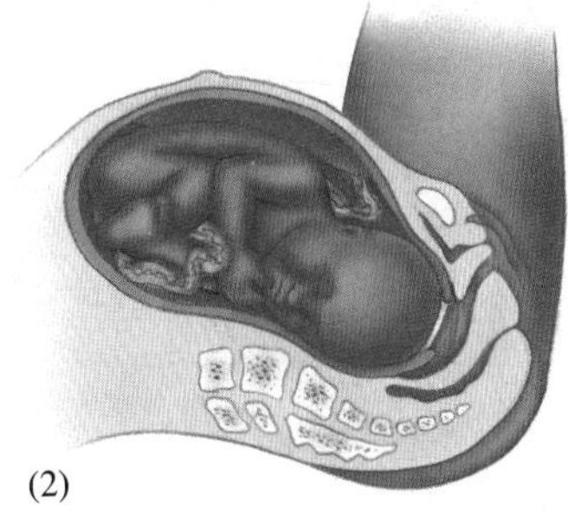
(2)

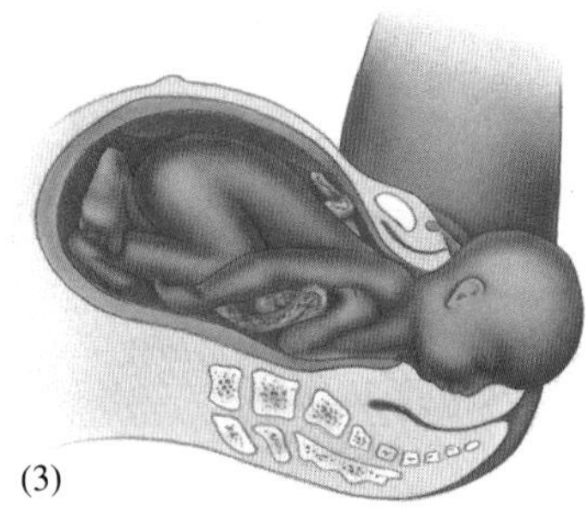
(3)

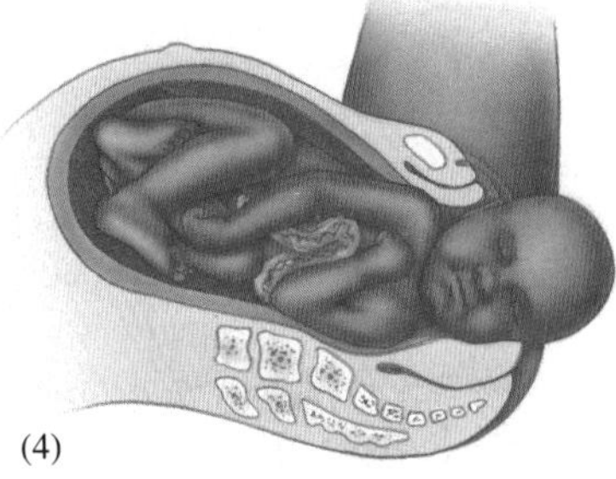
(4)

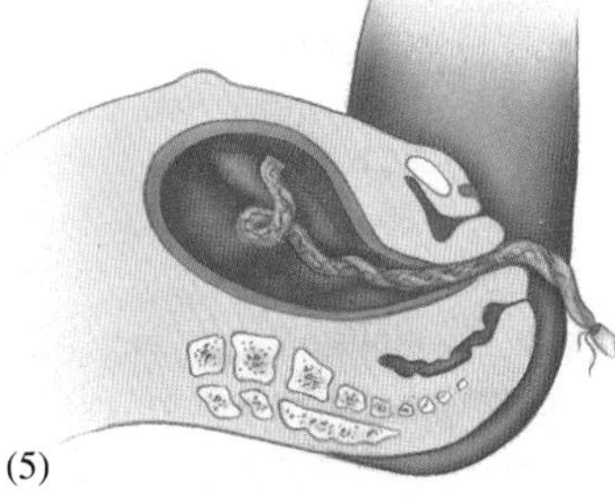
(5)

(FIGURE 16-15)

The birth of a child These drawings show various stages of childbirth. (1) A month or two before birth, the fetus drops to a lower position. (2) In the first stage of delivery (dilation), strong uterine contractions cause the cervix to dilate. (3) By the end of this stage, the cervix has completely dilated, the membranes surrounding the baby have ruptured, and the head has begun to extend into the birth canal. (4) During the second stage (expulsion), the head emerges fully and the shoulders rotate. (5) By the third stage (placental), the baby has been born. The uterus expels the placenta and the umbilical cord.

SECTION 16.3

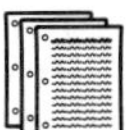

Section Review Worksheet 16.3

Assign Section Review Worksheet 16.3, which requires students to identify stages during pregnancy, childbirth, and childhood development.

Section Quiz 16.3

Have students take Section Quiz 16.3.

Debate the Issue

Surrogate Motherhood

You may wish to give students background on surrogate motherhood and have the class debate whether it should be legal. Students may also locate information in articles, using the *Reader's Guide to Periodical Literature.* Allow time for arguments, counterarguments, and rebuttals.

Extension

Memoirs

Students might be interested in writing a book of memoirs from their childhood, including milestones of physical growth and growing independence. Memories of infancy could be provided by questioning parents, guardians, or siblings, watching videotapes their parents made, or referring to a baby book or medical records.

Background
Baby's Head Shape
The bones in the head of a newborn are very pliable and soft. This allows them to shift position during delivery, letting the baby's head pass through the birth canal. For this reason, a baby's head may look misshapen at birth. Within a few days, it returns to normal shape.

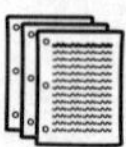

Reteaching Worksheet 16.3
Students who have difficulty with the material may complete Reteaching Worksheet 16.3, which requires them to sequence stages in development before and after birth.

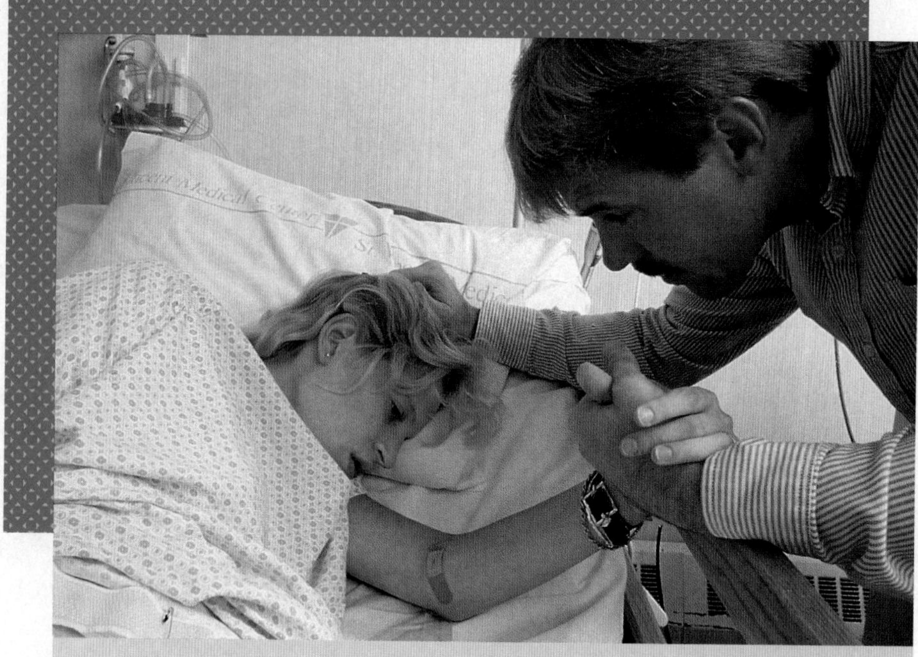

(FIGURE 16-16) **It is now common for the father of the baby to take part in childbirth by providing comfort and encouragement to the woman in labor.**

Birth defects are discussed in Chapter 24.

Near the end of the pregnancy, muscles in the walls of the uterus begin to contract. Weak, irregular contractions may occur for several weeks before birth. When it is time for the baby to be born, the contractions become much stronger and last longer. They also start to come at regular intervals, closer and closer together. The final stage of pregnancy, when contractions are strong enough to push the baby out of the mother's body, is called labor. Labor usually takes between five and twenty hours.

The contractions press the baby's head against the cervix and force it to open wide enough for the baby to pass through. The baby then passes through the vagina and out into the world. Within a few seconds the baby takes its first breath. The baby no longer needs the placenta, so the umbilical cord is cut.

The placenta then separates from the wall of the uterus. About half an hour after the baby is born, the placenta and the umbilical cord are pushed out of the uterus. The process of childbirth is complete.

More and more, hospitals are allowing fathers, friends of the mother, and even brothers and sisters of the newborn to be present at the birth. And some women choose to deliver their children at home with the help of a midwife—a nurse trained in childbirth—or a doctor. Some women receive pain-relieving medicine during labor and delivery. Others prefer to go without medication. In addition, many women take childbirth classes that help them and their birthing partners prepare for the process ahead.

Though most pregnancies and births go smoothly and normally, complications sometimes occur. Figure 16-17 describes some complications of pregnancy and birth.

Complications of Pregnancy and Birth

Complication	Description
Ectopic pregnancy	*The embryo becomes implanted in the Fallopian tube or somewhere else in the abdomen besides the uterus. The embryo dies and sometimes must be removed by surgery.*
Miscarriage	*The embryo or fetus is expelled from the uterus prematurely. Miscarriages may be caused by a genetic defect, illness in the mother, drugs the mother has taken, or other factors. Miscarriages usually occur during the first three months of pregnancy.*
Toxemia	*The pregnant woman has high blood pressure, swelling, and protein in the urine. Toxemia must be treated in the hospital. Untreated toxemia can result in convulsions, coma, and the death of both mother and fetus. It is most common among teenagers, older women, and women who already had health problems.*
Rh incompatibility	*A woman's blood produces a substance that attacks a substance in the fetus's blood. This may occur if the woman is Rh negative and the fetus is Rh positive. The problem can be avoided by injections that prevent a woman's blood from making the Rh substance.*
Premature birth	*A baby is born before it is fully developed. A baby is considered to be premature if it is born before the 37th week of pregnancy. Premature babies are placed in incubators, which are special containers that protect the baby while it continues to develop.*
Cesarean section	*If delivery through the birth canal is considered to be dangerous for any reason, an operation called a cesarean section is performed. An incision is made through the abdomen and uterus, and the baby is taken from the mother's body.*
Multiple births	*Two or more infants are born together. Two infants are called twins, three are called triplets, and four are called quadruplets. The birth of five infants—quintuplets—is extremely rare.*
Stillbirth	*A fully developed fetus is born dead.*

(FIGURE 16-17) **Most pregnancies and births go smoothly and normally, but complications sometimes occur.**

Background
Cocaine Babies

Babies born to cocaine-addicted mothers are an increasing medical and educational problem. One New York health professional estimated in 1990 that 11 percent of urban mothers giving birth are addicted to drugs. From 1987 to 1988, the number of "cocaine babies" born in Illinois rose 79 percent. Nationwide, there are hundreds of thousands of such babies. These babies are born with drugs in their systems; a great number of them die very quickly; many more are permanently damaged, physically and mentally. Those who are not permanently damaged still spend weeks withdrawing from the drugs; they are cranky and jittery, flail their fists, and do not eat well. Cocaine babies who have permanent damage will present problems and costs to society for years, as the burden of their care and special educational needs becomes more evident.

Background

Postpartum Period

The time following childbirth is called the postpartum period. During these few weeks, hormonal changes in the mother cause the breasts to secrete a substance (colostrum) that helps bolster the baby's immunity. The hormone prolactin stimulates the production of milk by the mammary glands. The mother may experience some symptoms of depression, known as "postpartum blues," which are both psychological and hormonal in origin. This period may cause the new mother to feel somewhat overwhelmed. It typically lasts only a short time, however.

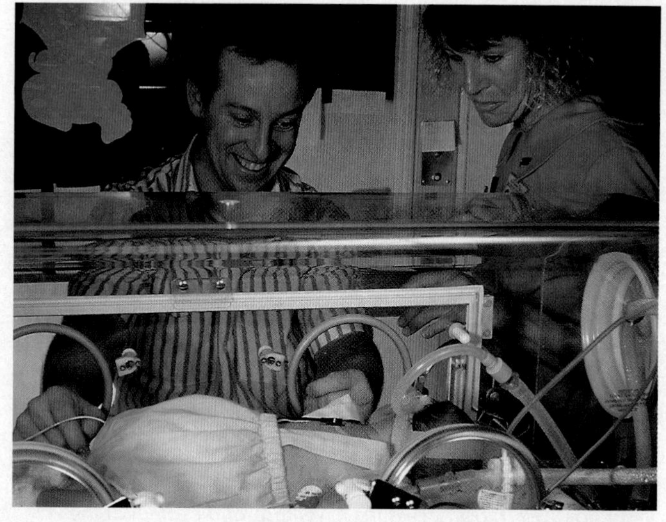

(FIGURE 16-18) **Babies who are born before they are fully developed are called premature babies. This premature infant weighed only 1 pound, 14 ounces at birth. Even babies this small respond to a parent's care.**

Infancy Through Childhood

Imagine what it was like living in the womb. You didn't have to eat or breathe, and you didn't have to adjust to different temperatures and different environments. Suddenly, all of that changed. After you were born, food had to be taken into the mouth, and air into the lungs. And you had to let it be known that you needed something (for example, you were cold and needed to be covered with a blanket).

After you were born, you continued to grow and develop. You grew taller and stronger throughout infancy and childhood, and you are probably *still* growing. In addition, you developed in other ways. About a month after you were born, you started to smile when you saw a human face. By six months, you could recognize the familiar people who cared for you, and you probably cried when a stranger tried to hold you. A few months later, you could sit up by yourself and play with simple toys.

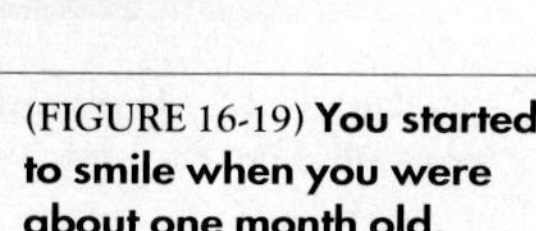

(FIGURE 16-19) **You started to smile when you were about one month old.**

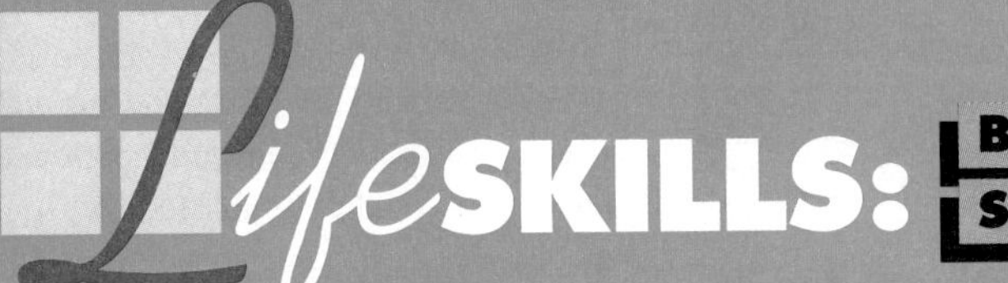

Using Self-Talk About Childhood Experiences. . . .

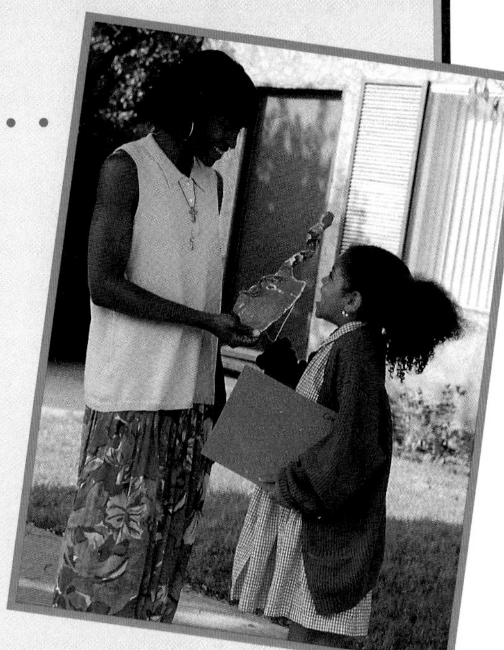

Your childhood experiences were probably the most important influences on your self-esteem. Some of the experiences made you feel great about yourself. Others, unfortunately, were painful and made you feel terrible. The following activity will help you understand *why* you feel the way you do about yourself, and it may help you increase your self-esteem.

1. Make a list of five childhood experiences that made you feel good about yourself.
2. Make a list of five childhood experiences that made you feel bad about yourself.
3. Go down your first list and say positive things to yourself about each item. For example, if one of your positive childhood experiences was winning an award for a piece of art you did, you can say to yourself, "I'm proud that I can draw so well."
4. Now go down your second list; only this time say something to yourself to counteract the *bad* feelings. If you learned to read later than many children, for example, you can say to yourself, "Well, at least I learned to read, which is something a lot of people never learn to do."

This kind of talking to yourself is called self-talk. Self-talk is a very effective way of making the most of positive experiences and minimizing the effect of negative ones.

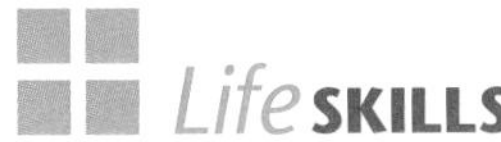

Using Self-Talk About Childhood Experiences

Have students complete the Life Skills activity in the text, writing the two lists and working through self-talk responses to each item listed.

Review Answers

1. Oxygen and nutrients
2. Weak, irregular contractions are first noticed. The contractions then become stronger and last longer, and come at closer, regular intervals. The contractions finally become strong enough to push the baby out of the mother's body. The cervix dilates, or widens, to a diameter of about 10 cm.
3. Answers will vary depending on individual students' childhood experiences. Students' self-talk responses should be positive and minimize the effect of the negative experience.
4. The AIDS virus may cross the placenta and in this way be transmitted to the fetus.

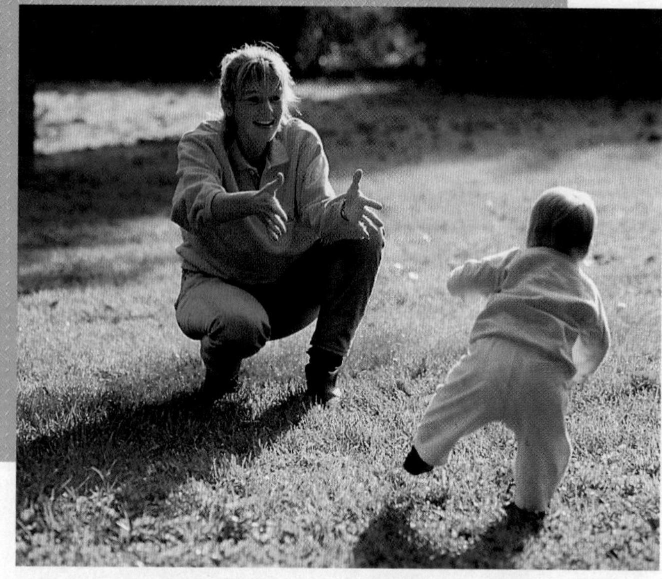

(FIGURE 16-20) **Most babies begin to walk when they are about one year old.**

When you were about one year old, you were determined to learn to walk. No one has to teach a baby how to pull itself up onto its own two feet and take its first steps. In fact, it would be difficult to stop a baby from learning to walk!

As a toddler, you were also teaching yourself how to talk. The sounds you had been hearing all your life began to have meaning and you struggled to imitate them. You may have learned that "ba-ba" could cause an adult to give you a bottle of milk or that your mother was delighted when you waved and said "bye-bye."

During your childhood years, you learned how to be more independent. You learned to go to the cabinet for food when you were hungry, rather than sitting in your room and crying until you were fed. You were allowed to go to a friend's house by yourself. You learned how to cross the street safely. You went to school.

School occupied a major part of your day, and you learned a great deal there. Of course you learned a lot of facts, but you also learned how to get along with people different from you and your family.

These years prepared you for adolescence. Without your childhood experiences you wouldn't be able to make friends, you wouldn't be able to study and learn well, and you wouldn't feel confident that you could make effective decisions.

If you do the Life Skills activity on page 347, it may help you to understand the early influences on your life. What happens to us during childhood deeply affects our self-esteem.

You also grew *physically* in preparation for adolescence. Your height and weight increased quite a bit and your coordination improved. These and other physical changes would be even more dramatic as you approached puberty. In the next chapter you'll learn about the changes that occur during adolescence.

Review

1. *What substances pass from the mother to the fetus through the placenta?*
2. *Describe how uterine contractions and the cervix change during labor.*
3. ***LIFE SKILLS: Building Self-Esteem*** *Think of one negative event of your childhood and use self-talk to minimize its effect on your self-esteem.*
4. ***Critical Thinking*** *AIDS is caused by a virus. Explain how the AIDS virus may be transmitted from a pregnant woman to her developing child.*

ASSESS

Section Review

Have students answer the Section Review questions.

Alternative Assessment

Stages of Pregnancy and Childbirth

Separate the class into groups and have each group be responsible for explaining a stage of pregnancy or childbirth. Allow a variety of methods of presentation, but require that they explain what happens to both the mother and the child during the stage for which they are responsible.

Closure

Beliefs About Parenthood

After students have read and discussed this section, have them write in the Student Journal a statement of their beliefs about parenthood and their future plans for having a family.

Highlights

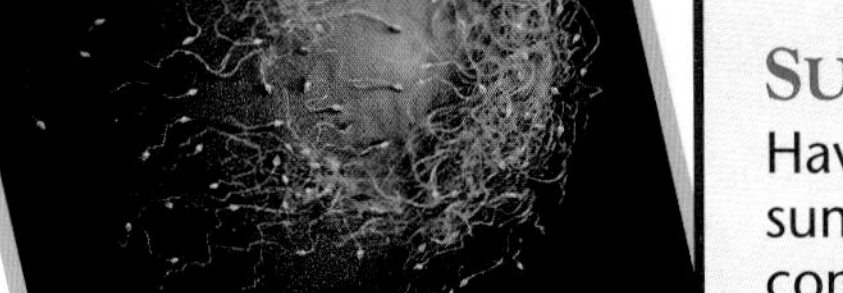

Summary

- The union of sperm and egg is called fertilization.
- The testes, vas deferens, urethra, and penis are the major organs of the male reproductive system.
- The testes make sperm and produce the male hormone testosterone. The amount of testosterone increases at puberty, causing boys' bodies to change.
- Even though only one sperm can fuse with the egg, the presence of many sperm is necessary for this to happen.
- In the female, the vagina, the ovaries, the Fallopian tubes, and the uterus make up the internal reproductive system.
- The ovaries produce eggs and sex hormones. After puberty, these hormones control the monthly release of an egg .
- The egg and sperm join in one of the Fallopian tubes.
- The uterus provides a place for a baby to grow before birth.
- Monthly breast self-examinations and yearly visits to a gynecologist for a Pap test can help keep a female's reproductive system healthy.
- The embryo implants itself on the wall of the uterus and gets oxygen and the nutrients it needs from its mother through the placenta and umbilical cord.

Vocabulary

sperm male reproductive cell; contains one-half of the instructions needed for the development of a new human being.

egg female reproductive cell, also called an ovum; contains one-half of the instructions needed for the development of a new human being.

fertilization the union of a sperm and an egg.

testes male reproductive structures that make sperm and produce the male hormone testosterone.

ovaries female reproductive structures that produce eggs and female sex hormones.

uterus the hollow muscular organ that provides a place for the baby to grow before birth; also called the womb.

embryo a fertilized egg after it has divided into two cells.

fetus a developing individual from the ninth week of pregnancy until birth.

Chapter 16 Highlights Strategies

Summary

Have students read the summary to reinforce the concepts they have learned in Chapter 16.

Vocabulary

Ask students to select 20 to 30 of the words they consider most important in the chapter and make a crossword puzzle or other word game using the words. The best of these efforts could be duplicated for a timed class competition.

Extension

Arrange for students to visit a prenatal clinic, obstetrician's office, or public health department to see firsthand how and where pregnant women are given care, or to hear good prenatal care described. If possible, allow students to see the equipment used, and to ask questions about the expected pattern of development and problems that could arise.

Chapter 16 Assessment

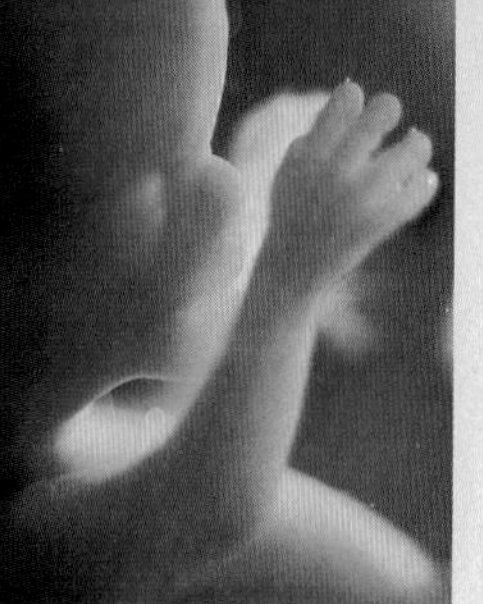

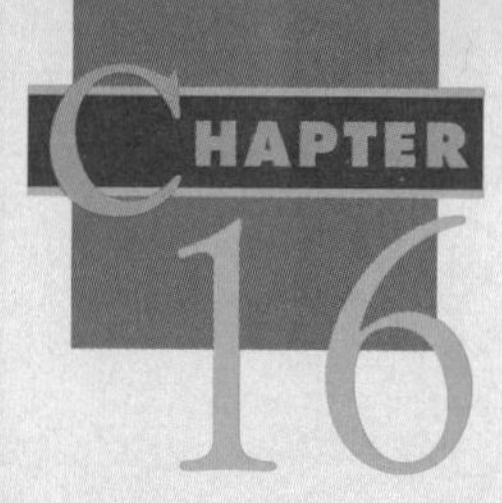

Chapter Review

Concept Review

1. Sperm is made in the
   a. urethra. c. penis.
   b. testes. d. testosterone.

2. When a sperm joins with an egg, it is called
   a. ovulation. c. ejaculation.
   b. premenstrual syndrome. d. fertilization.

3. A disorder of the male reproductive system is
   a. circumcision. c. undescended testes.
   b. toxic shock syndrome. d. epididymis.

4. The female reproductive system includes
   a. the ovaries. c. the uterus.
   b. the Fallopian tubes. d. all of these.

5. Egg cells and female sex hormones are produced in the
   a. ovaries. c. vagina.
   b. cervix. d. vulva.

6. When the uterus sheds its lining, it is called
   a. premenstrual syndrome. c. vaginitis.
   b. ovulation. d. menstruation.

7. Which of the following behaviors provides good protection for young women against breast cancer?
   a. monthly self-examinations
   b. loose-fitting clothing
   c. yearly mammograms
   d. body cleanliness

8. From the mother, the fetus can receive
   a. viruses. c. nutrients.
   b. oxygen. d. all of these.

Expressing Your Views

1. A married couple has been trying to start a family but so far has been unsuccessful. What might be some reasons for this? What could be suggested to this couple as a solution to their problem?

2. Millions of sperm are released in one ejaculation. Why do you think so many are released if only one is needed to fertilize an egg?

3. You're 16, and you have had only one menstrual period, five months ago. Should you be concerned? What should you do?

4. Every month when it is time for your menstrual period you feel tired and depressed. Are these feelings unusual? What can you do to relieve them?

Chapter Review

Concept Review

1. b **5.** a
2. d **6.** d
3. c **7.** a
4. d **8.** d

Expressing Your Views

Sample responses:

1. The woman may not be releasing an egg or there may be scar tissue in the Fallopian tube that keeps sperm from reaching the egg. The woman may have endometriosis. The man may have a low sperm count or abnormal sperm. The couple should see their doctor to determine the cause of their infertility. Many cases of infertility can be treated medically.

2. A large number of sperm are released to ensure that some will reach the egg. Many sperm die during their journey through the female reproductive tract. The head of the sperm contains an enzyme that breaks down the outer layer of the egg. Many sperm are needed to break down this layer so that one sperm can enter the egg.

3. No. Early menstrual cycles can be irregular. To ease my concern, I can see my doctor and discuss any questions I have with him or her.

4. No. Take a warm bath and/or exercise; a nonprescription pain reliever that contains ibuprofen will also help relieve menstrual cramps.

Life Skills Check

1. See his doctor immediately, as the swelling and soreness could be a sign of a serious problem.

2. Answers will vary depending upon the characteristic of their personalities students wish to change.

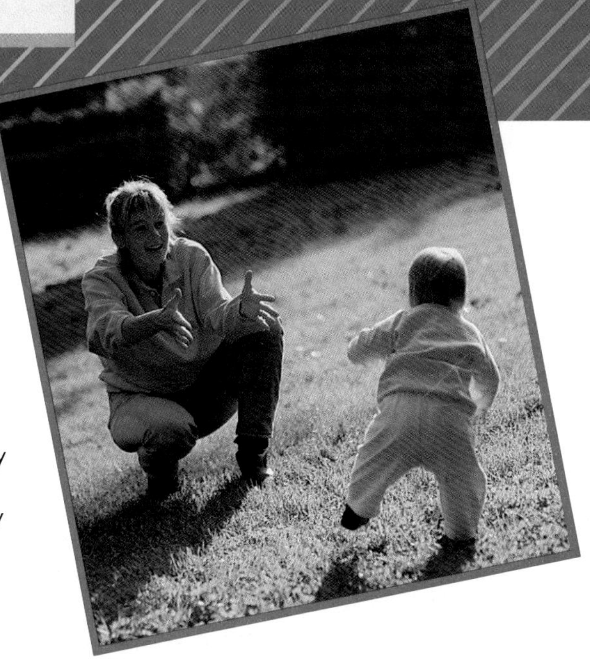

Life Skills Check

1. **Practicing Self-Care**
   A friend has confided in you that he has been having soreness and swelling in his testes. He is hesitant to visit a doctor. What advice would you give him?
2. **Building Self-Esteem**
   Most people have sides to their personality that they would like to change in order to feel better about themselves. Think of one aspect of your personality you think you would like to change. How could you change this trait or at least develop it to be more positive?

Projects

1. Invite a representative from the American Cancer Society to discuss breast and testicular self-examinations with the class. Ask him or her to bring, if possible, models of the testicles and breasts in order to instruct the class, as well as any pamphlets describing the procedure. Prepare at least one question to ask the representative.
2. Suppose you had to teach a course on male and female reproduction. Work with a group to develop an outline you would use to cover the information you have learned in this chapter. Groups could then present the outlines in an oral report.

Plan for Action

Males and females need to follow only a few basic steps to take care of their reproductive organs. Plan a daily, monthly, and yearly routine to ensure a healthy reproductive system and to prevent disorders from occurring.

Projects

Have students complete the projects for reproduction and the reproductive system.

Plan for Action

Have students work in groups to compile a list of five actions they think are most important for the health of a mother and fetus, and five behaviors or qualities they think are most important in caring for infants and children. Have the whole class compare lists and compile final checklists of Healthy Moms and Babies, and Raising Healthy Families.

ASSESSMENT OPTIONS

Chapter Test

Have students take the Chapter 16 Test.

Alternative Assessment

Have students do the Alternative Assessment activity for Chapter 16.

Test Generator

The Test Generator (Macintosh® or IBM® format) contains an additional 50 assessment items for this chapter.

ADOLESCENCE: RELATIONSHIPS AND RESPONSIBILITIES

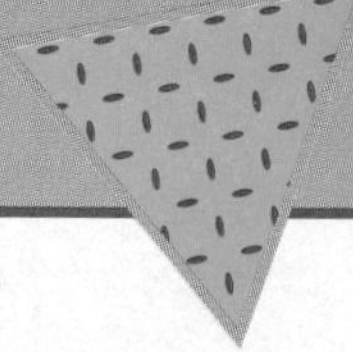

PLANNING GUIDE

TEXT SECTIONS	OBJECTIVES	TEXT FEATURES	OUTSIDE RESOURCES	NOTES
17.1 Changes During Adolescence pp. 353-356 1 period	• Describe how puberty affects the male body. • Describe how puberty affects the female body. • Describe the nonphysical changes that occur during adolescence.	**ASSESSMENT** • Section Review, p. 356	**TEACHER'S RESOURCE BINDER** • Lesson Plan 17.1 • Personal Health Inventory • Journal Entries 17A, 17B • Life Skills 17A • Section Review Worksheet 17.1 • Section Quiz 17.1 • Reteaching Worksheet 17.1 **OTHER RESOURCES** • Transparency 17A • Parent Discussion Guide • English/Spanish Audiocassette 5	
17.2 Communicating Effectively pp. 357-363 1 period	■ Learn how to use "I" messages instead of "you" messages. ■ Learn active-listening skills. ■ Learn a method of verbally resisting pressure. ■ Learn a method of resolving conflict.	■ LIFE SKILLS: Communicating Effectively, p. 358 **ASSESSMENT** • Section Review, p. 363	**TEACHER'S RESOURCE BINDER** • Lesson Plan 17.2 • Journal Entry 17C • Life Skills 17B • Section Review Worksheet 17.2 • Section Quiz 17.2 • Reteaching Worksheet 17.2	
17.3 Relationships With Peers pp. 364-369 1 period	• Describe how to make and keep a friend. • Name three functions that dating serves. ■ Name three actions that will help you cope with a breakup.	**ASSESSMENT** • Section Review, p. 369	**TEACHER'S RESOURCE BINDER** • Lesson Plan 17.3 • Journal Entry 17D • Section Review Worksheet 17.3 • Section Quiz 17.3 • Reteaching Worksheet 17.3	
17.4 Sexuality and Responsibility pp. 370-376 1 period	• Describe the difference between sexual and emotional intimacy. • Name three possible consequences of teenage pregnancy. • Know the benefits of sexual abstinence. ■ Consider how a pregnancy now would affect your life goals.	■ LIFE SKILLS: Setting Goals, p. 375 **ASSESSMENT** • Section Review, p. 376	**TEACHER'S RESOURCE BINDER** • Lesson Plan 17.4 • Journal Entry 17E • Section Review Worksheet 17.4 • Section Quiz 17.4 • Reteaching Worksheet 17.4 **OTHER RESOURCES** • Making a Choice 17A	
17.5 Skills for Responsible Sexual Behavior pp. 377-380	■ Learn how to deal with internal pressures to become sexually intimate. ■ Learn how to resist pressure to become sexually intimate. ■ Apply the decision-making model to decisions about your own sexual behavior.	• What Would You Do?, p. 379 **ASSESSMENT** • Section Review, p. 380	**TEACHER'S RESOURCE BINDER** • Lesson Plan 17.5 • Life Skills 17C • Section Review Worksheet 17.5 • Section Quiz 17.5 • Reteaching Worksheet 17.5 **OTHER RESOURCES** • Transparency 17B • Making a Choice 17B	

■ Denotes LIFE SKILLS objectives

• Items in blue are also part of the *Holt Health Activity Book.*

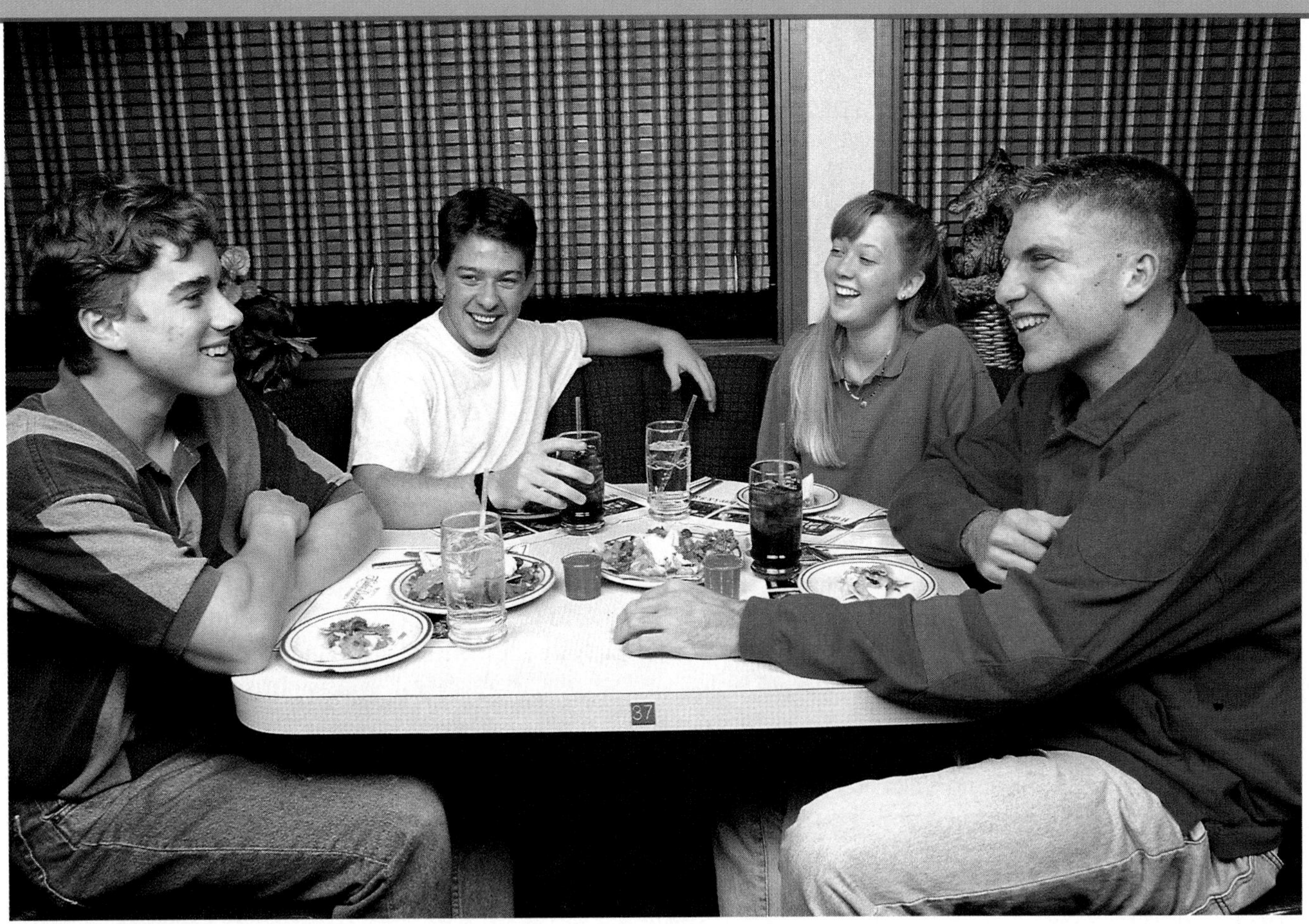

CONTENT BACKGROUND Teenage Homosexuality

According to widely accepted estimates, between 4 percent and 10 percent of adults in the United States are homosexual. Among high school students, as many as one in ten may be discovering he or she is gay or lesbian. This can be a difficult discovery to make, and the statistics bear this out. Of teens who commit suicide, for instance, 30 percent are gay or lesbian. These teens are two to three times more likely to attempt suicide. Homosexual teens are frightened by the homophobic threats of older teens and often feel uncertain of their own worth as well as safety. As a result, they are vulnerable to depression, academic difficulties, drug use, and becoming runaways.

The future may not look better to teenage homosexuals. In the larger society, gays are not welcome in the military, and few homosexual politicians, business people, teachers, and other professionals are open about their orientation. The fear of "outing," or having one's homosexual orientation publicized against one's wishes, testifies to the power of discrimination. Gay couples are not recognized by law, which complicates matters of insurance, sick leave, parenting, and inheritance.

Homosexuality was at one time classified by the American Psychiatric Association as a disorder. This classification was dropped in 1974, owing in part to pioneering research by Dr. Evelyn Hooker at U.C.L.A. The American Psychological Association has an active committee that seeks to extend gay and lesbian rights. A growing number of authorities see homosexuals as having no more psychological disturbances than heterosexuals. They attribute any increased disturbances in the homosexual population to the social stigma and oppression they face.

Homosexual teens typically receive no sex education or information appropriate to their orien-

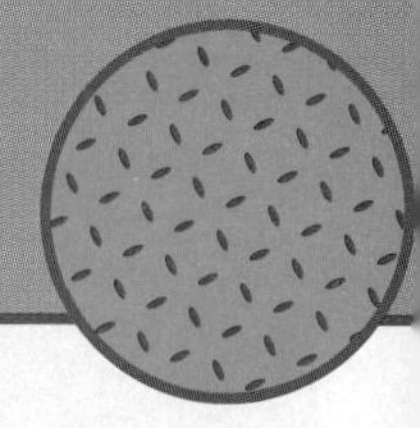

tation. This is largely because many people believe that assisting or educating gay and lesbian students is condoning behavior that they view as immoral or unnatural.

Some major organizations, such as the National Education Association, the American Academy of Pediatrics, and the Child Welfare League of America, advocate efforts to help gay and lesbian youth. The Fairfax County schools in Virginia, the Project 10 program in Los Angeles, and the New York City and San Francisco school systems have moved ahead despite community opposition. Fairfax County has developed a curriculum on homosexuality; Los Angeles has a dropout prevention program and in-school discussion groups. San Francisco schools each have at least one identified gay or lesbian teacher or counselor for students to talk to. Alternative high schools in both New York and San Francisco have special programs set up for gay students, giving them counseling and individualized instruction.

Some opponents of homosexual education in schools fear that open discussion encourages otherwise heterosexual students to become homosexual or bisexual. Research suggests otherwise. Homosexuality appears to have a genetic component. One study found, for instance, that 52 percent of identical twins of homosexual men were homosexual as well; only 22 percent of fraternal twins and 11 percent of adopted brothers of gay men were also gay. Studies by Dr. Gunther Dorner and his associates suggest a neuroendocrine predisposition to homosexuality in men. Such research may suggest that homosexuality is not necessarily a learned behavior. It is clearly important to educate all students about homosexuality.

Additional information can be obtained from the following: The Campaign to End Homophobia, in Cambridge, Massachusetts; the Equity Institute, in Amherst, Massachusetts; and the National Lesbian and Gay Task Force, in Washington, D.C.; and by calling the National Lesbian and Gay Hotline (1-800-221-7044) or by calling the Out Youth Austin Hotline (1-800-969-6884).

PLANNING FOR INSTRUCTION

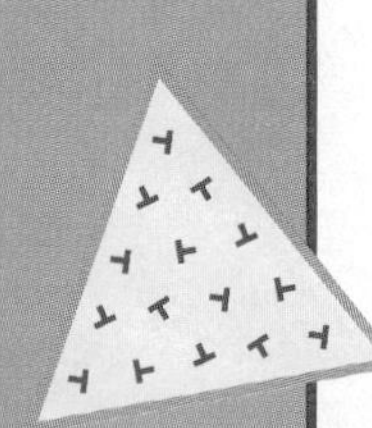

KEY FACTS

- **Adolescence is a time of change in bodies, emotions, mental abilities, and social life, lasting from two to four years, beginning as early as age eight.**
- **Puberty is the period of physical development during which males and females become able to produce children. Hormonal changes cause various physical changes, including sperm production in boys, ovulation and menstruation in girls, and growth and increased sex drive in both.**
- **The four levels of communication are information giving, directing or arguing, exploring, and self-disclosing.**
- **Nonverbal communication includes eye contact, facial expression, and body positions. If your nonverbal messages disagree with your words, you send a mixed message.**
- **Sexuality is everything that makes one a sexual person. Most people are heterosexuals (attracted to the opposite sex); some are homosexuals (attracted to the same sex).**
- **Emotional intimacy is sharing thoughts and feelings, respecting, and trusting. Sexual intimacy is genital touching and intercourse.**
- **Teen pregnancy jeopardizes emotional, social, and intellectual growth; endangers the health of mother and baby; disrupts academic and career plans; and creates stress.**
- **Sexual abstinence is a positive, responsible decision, waiting until one is older and ready to build lasting relationships. It requires skill in self-control, resisting pressure from others and learning other ways to show love.**

MYTHS AND MISCONCEPTIONS

MYTH: Adolescence is a miserable time for both the adolescent and the family.

The physical, mental, and emotional changes during adolescence, are not in themselves negative. They prepare the young person for adulthood.

MYTH: Teens don't listen to their parents.

Teens appear not to listen to their parents only because the values the parents are trying to instill have already been absorbed.

MYTH: Teens who become pregnant are just being careless.

Carelessness is one factor. Pressure to have sex is another. But for some teens becoming pregnant is intentional.

VOCABULARY

Essential: The following vocabulary terms appear in boldface type:

puberty
hormones
nocturnal emissions
nonverbal communication
mixed message
active listening
relationship
empathy
heterosexuals
homosexuals
sexual intimacy
emotional intimacy
sexual abstinence

Secondary: Be aware that the following terms may come up during class discussion:

endocrine glands
pituitary gland
larynx
estrogen
progesterone
menstruation
ovulation
toxemia

FOR STUDENTS WITH SPECIAL NEEDS

LEP Students: Students might benefit from the active-listening technique in Section 17.2. Give students extra practice in this method by helping them prepare cards with the chapter's vocabulary words and definitions. Have them take turns reading aloud and actively listening to the words and definitions.

At-Risk Students: Emphasize to students the social, educational, and financial penalties of teen pregnancy. Then ask them to write short, fictional stories about a teenage girl who becomes pregnant and how the pregnancy affects her life plans.

ENRICHMENT

- Have students use library resources to research the work of Erik Homburger Erikson, a psychoanalyst best known for his study of the adolescent *identity crisis.* Ask them to prepare a report on his life and contributions and present a summary to the class.
- Arrange for a practicing youth psychologist to visit the class and answer students' questions about adolescence, communication, and responsible sexual behavior.

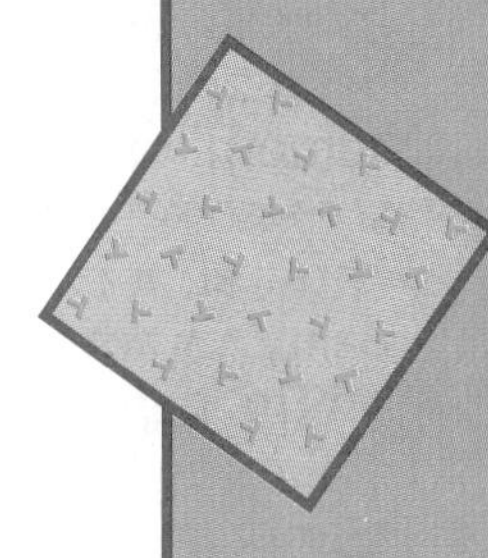

Chapter 17
Chapter Opener

GETTING STARTED

Using the Chapter Photograph

Ask students to speculate about who the girl in the photo is talking to—her mother, her teacher, her boyfriend, or another girl. Ask them what their social lives would be like if there were no telephones. Explain that this chapter will focus on changes that occur during the teen years and on managing relationships with others.

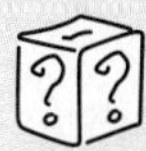

Question Box

Have students write out any questions they have about puberty, sexuality, and relationships and put them in the Question Box. The Question Box provides students with an opportunity to ask questions anonymously. To ensure that students with questions are not embarrassed to be seen writing, have students who do not have questions write something else—such as something they already know about puberty, sexuality, or adolescence—on the paper instead.

Preview the questions and then answer them at appropriate points in the chapter. You may wish to allow students to write additional anonymous questions as they go through the chapter.

Chapter 17

Adolescence: Relationships and Responsiblities

◆ ◆ ◆ ◆

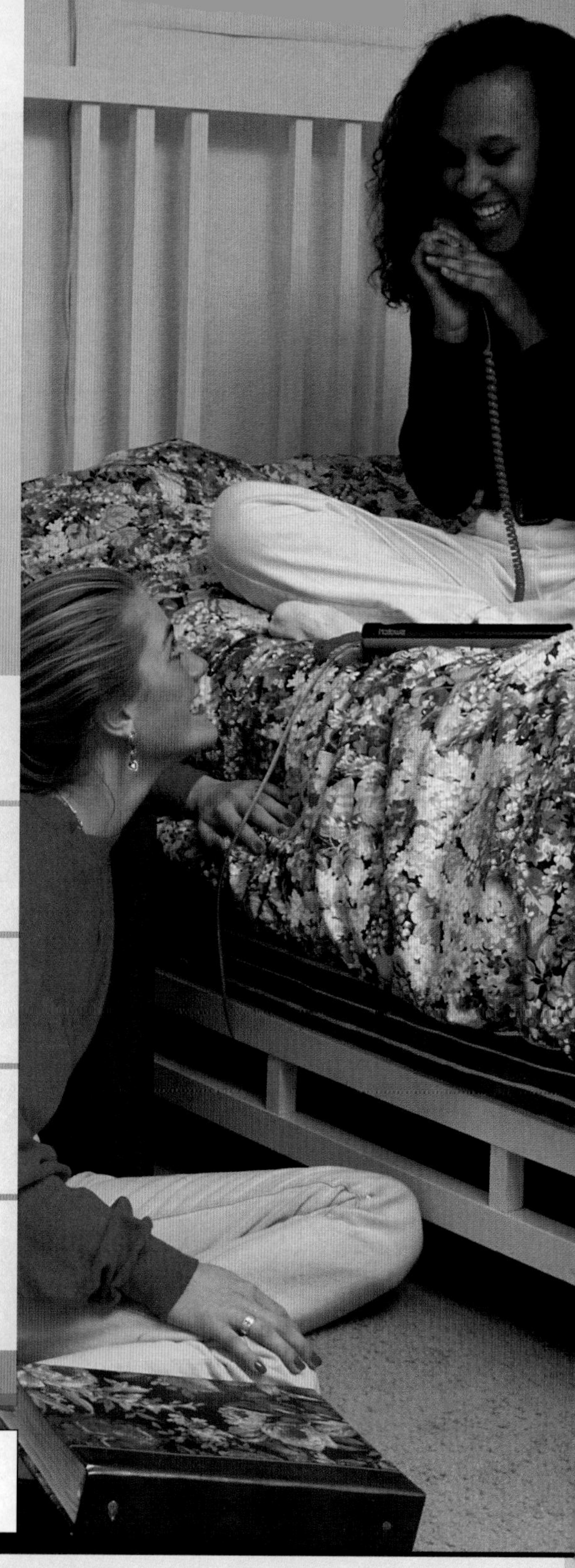

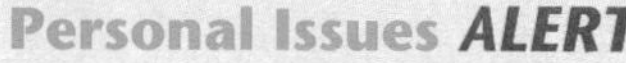

Social interactions become very important during the adolescent years.

Personal Issues *ALERT*

Discussion of the sensitive physical and emotional changes of adolescence may embarrass some students because they are going through these changes themselves. Also, some may be involved in intimate relationships and be sensitive about discussing such matters. Some may have questions that they feel are too personal—or even too simple—to bring up before the class, so provide opportunities for them to ask anonymous questions via the Question Box. As always, respect their privacy.

"She must think I'm such a jerk," Martin mutters unhappily to himself as he hurls his books into his locker. Every time he gets up the nerve to say hello to Caitlyn, he immediately clams up if she says "Hi" back. Martin has it bad for Caitlyn. But even though he's attracted to her, he's also afraid of her, afraid that she will reject him. Martin thinks he isn't good-looking, and he feels awkward and gawky. "How could Caitlyn possibly want to go out with me?" he thinks to himself. To make matters worse, Martin's body seems to betray him at every turn, with sweaty palms and embarrassing sexual arousal. Although many people Martin's age go through the same thing, he is convinced that he is the only one with these problems.

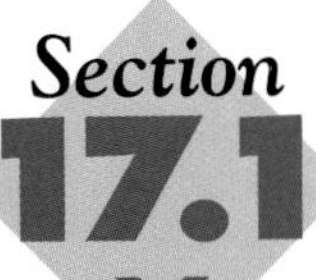

Section 17.1 Changes During Adolescence

Objectives

- *Describe how puberty affects the male body.*
- *Describe how puberty affects the female body.*
- *Describe the nonphysical changes that occur during adolescence.*

Martin doesn't realize it, but virtually everyone suffers similar discomforts during adolescence. If he could read Caitlyn's mind, he would probably find that she, too, has many of the same feelings.

Adolescence is a time of change—changing body, changing emotions, changing mental abilities, and changing social life. All these changes can cause feelings of awkwardness. It helps to know as much as possible about what is going on, and it also helps to realize that the changes are perfectly normal.

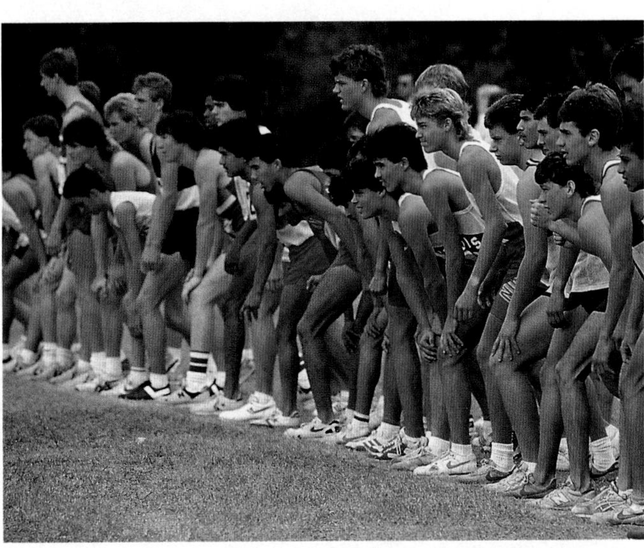

(FIGURE 17-1) **People go through puberty at different rates. Don't worry if you are maturing faster or slower than your friends.**

SECTION 17.1

Background

Body Odor

In early adolescence, activity in the sweat glands increases. Body odor is caused not by perspiration itself—which is odorless—but by bacteria acting upon it. Washing the skin with soap slows the growth of bacteria, helping to eliminate odor. Antiperspirants and deodorants can cut down the amount of perspiration and hide odor, but they do not prevent it. Careful daily washing is the best way to control body odor.

Background

The Teen Years: Developing Your Self

Adolescence is the time of developing self and independence. Moodiness and rebelliousness peak during ages 13 to 16. The root of this behavior is a lack of self-confidence, evident in the over-concern for appearance and peer acceptance. Relationships with parents and authority figures such as teachers often become strained, and continuing communication is essential. In normal teen development, self-confidence, independence, and maturity increase in the later teen years.

Section 17.1 Lesson Plan

MOTIVATE

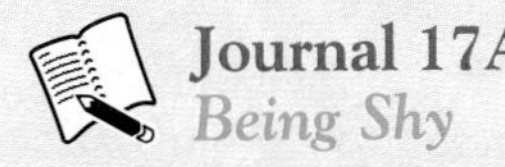

Journal 17A

Being Shy

This may be done as a warm-up activity. Ask students to think about Martin's situation, and ask if they ever have felt shy with a person they like. Ask what Martin should do—remain silent and hope Caitlyn will talk to him, or work up his courage and ask her out? Then, in the Student Journal in the Student Activity Book, have students relate a situation in which they felt shy and describe steps they could have taken to overcome their shyness.

TEACH

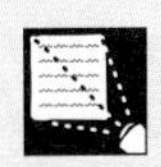

Teaching Transparency 17A

Physical Changes During Adolescence

Show the transparency of changes that occur during puberty (Figure 17-2). Divide the class into small groups. Tell each group to make a chart titled PUBERTY, with three headings: BOYS, GIRLS, and BOTH. Have them read the text and study the transparency, naming items for a student recorder in each group to list in the proper columns on the chart, and raising questions for the recorder to note. Discuss the charts and respond to any questions listed by the recorders.

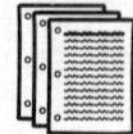

Personal Health Inventory

Have students complete the Personal Health Inventory for this chapter. The inventory helps them assess their own progress in adolescence, including physical, intellectual, emotional, and social growth.

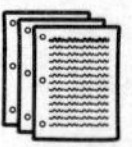

Life Skills Worksheet 17A

Taking Care of Yourself

Assign the Taking Care of Yourself Life Skills Worksheet, which gives students information about caring for their reproductive system and asks them to list things they need to buy, habits they need to change, and information they need to find to practice self-care.

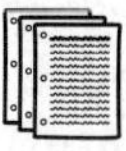

Section Review Worksheet 17.1

Assign Section Review Worksheet 17.1, which requires students to categorize changes of puberty as changes in males, changes in females, or nonphysical changes.

Section Quiz 17.1

Have students take Section Quiz 17.1.

puberty:

the period of physical development during which people become able to produce children.

hormones:

chemical substances, produced by the endocrine glands, which serve as messengers within the body.

REMINDER

The endocrine glands are discussed in greater detail in the Body Systems Handbook on pages 660–661.

Physical Changes

The most dramatic changes during the adolescent years are the physical ones. You grow taller and larger, and enter the time of life called **puberty.** Puberty is the period of physical development during which people become able to produce children. Both males and females go through puberty. The age at which people begin puberty varies widely, from as young as 8 to as old as 16. It usually takes from two to four years for all of the changes of puberty to be completed.

Puberty is triggered by the release of specific **hormones**. Hormones are chemical substances, produced by the endocrine glands, which serve as messengers within the body.

The pituitary gland, located in the brain, releases hormones that send the message to other endocrine glands that it is time for them to begin releasing the hormones that cause puberty.

In males, the pituitary gland releases hormones that cause the testes to manufacture increased amounts of the hormone testosterone. Testosterone causes many of the changes of puberty. A boy notices that his testes and penis begin to grow larger and that pubic hair appears around his genitals. He gets taller and stronger. Later, hair

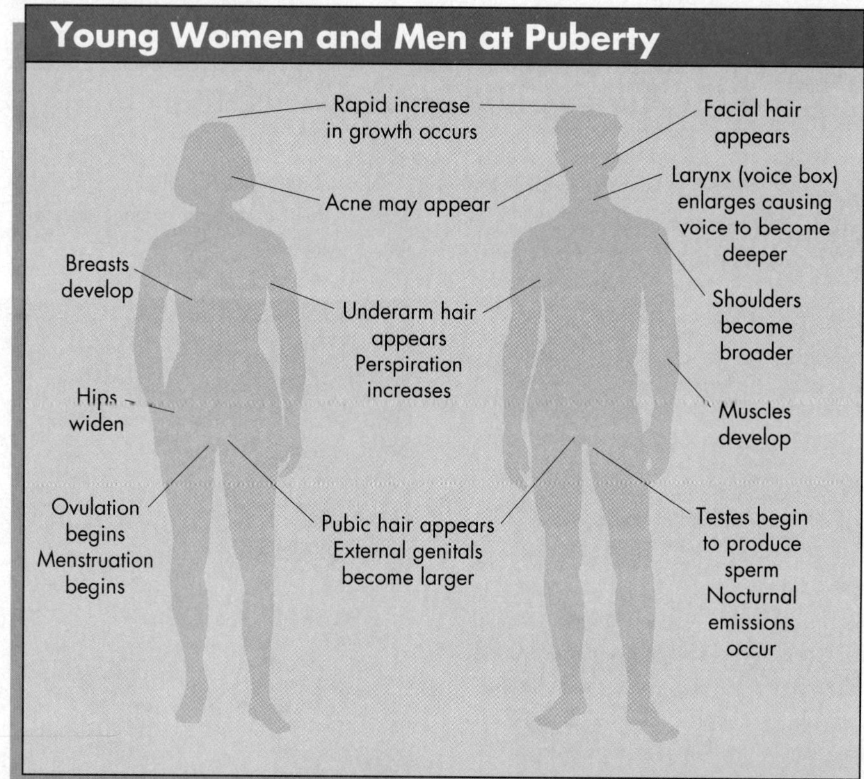

(FIGURE 17-2) **Puberty is the time of life in which people become able to produce children. Among other changes, males begin to produce sperm, and females begin to ovulate.**

• • • TEACH continued

Writing

Nonphysical Changes During Adolescence

Ask students to write a brief paragraph that (1) compares their emotions now to their emotions when they were 10 years old, (2) compares the kinds of problems their minds can solve now to those they could solve when they were 10, or (3) relates things they now can do independently that required an adult's help when they were 10. Ask volunteers to read examples and use these for class discussion on the nonphysical changes of adolescence.

Journal 17B

Concerns About Adolescence

Have students write in the Student Journal in the Student Activity Book any concerns they may have about the changes they are undergoing as teenagers. Their concerns might include physical changes, emotional changes, or feelings toward others.

Extension

Gathering Information

Ask students to visit a public health facility or family doctor to obtain pamphlets on understanding the changes and problems that occur during adolescence and have them display these in the classroom.

grows under his arms and on his face. Testosterone also causes the larynx (voice box) to enlarge, resulting in the lower and deeper male voice. Before the voice stabilizes, however, it may break unpredictably for a while.

These types of changes may be welcome, but another aspect of puberty usually isn't. The increase in testosterone levels causes the oil glands to increase their production of oil. When these glands become clogged, acne can result.

An important part of male puberty is the beginning of sperm production by the testes, when boys start to experience **nocturnal emissions** (''wet dreams''). Nocturnal emissions are ejaculations of semen that occur during sleep. They are perfectly normal and no cause for alarm. Once sperm production has begun, a male is capable of causing pregnancy in a female.

In females, the pituitary gland releases hormones that cause the ovaries to produce the hormones estrogen and progesterone, the major female sex hormones. The female sex hormones cause female changes at puberty. The uterus, Fallopian tubes, vagina, and clitoris grow in size. The breasts also start to grow, and pubic hair appears around the genitals. A girl grows taller, and her hips widen.

During puberty, a girl begins to ovulate and to have menstrual periods. The first menstrual period usually occurs between the ages of 12 and 14, but it is not unusual for a girl to have her first period as young as 9 or as old as 17. Once a female has begun ovulation and menstruation, she is capable of becoming pregnant. As a result of hormonal changes during puberty, both males and females experience an increased sex drive and may find that they feel sexually aroused around some people.

Teenagers tend to develop at the same rate as their parents did. That does not mean, however, that all teenagers develop at the same rate. If you are developing at a faster or slower rate than other people your age, don't worry. You are almost certainly developing normally. If you are concerned, speak to a health professional or other trusted adult.

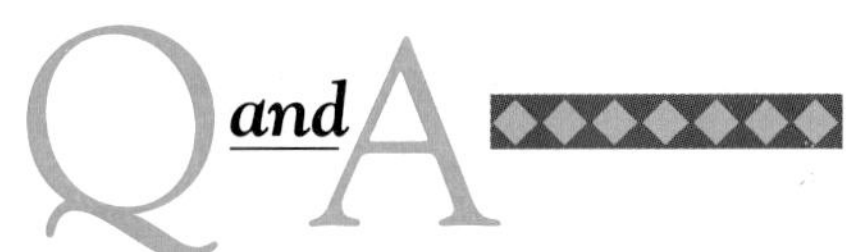

Q: Is it possible for a girl to get pregnant before she has had her first menstrual period?

A: Actually it is possible, but only if she has had her first ovulation. Ovulation occurs two weeks before menstruation. A girl does not always feel ovulation and may not know when she is ovulating. So if she has sexual intercourse, she could become pregnant after her first ovulation but before her first menstrual period.

Q: I'm 14 years old, and I think I'm getting breasts. But I'm a guy! What's the matter with me? Should I see a doctor?

A: Don't worry. Swelling around and beneath the nipples is quite common among boys going through puberty. It will eventually go away. The swelling is caused by hormonal changes. Sometimes the area can be painful and tender to the touch. Only about 2 percent of boys with this swelling have anything medically wrong with them. But if you continue to be concerned, visit a health professional to have it checked out.

REMINDER

Ovulation is the release of an egg from an ovary.

nocturnal emissions:

ejaculations of semen that occur during sleep.

SECTION 17.1

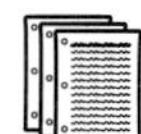

Reteaching Worksheet 17.1

Students who have difficulty with the material may complete Reteaching Worksheet 17.1, which requires them to fill in a flow chart that outlines the causes of puberty and the physical changes males and females undergo during this period.

Review Answers

1. The boy's body grows larger; increased oil production may cause acne; facial hair appears; larynx enlarges, which causes a deeper voice; shoulders become broader; muscles develop; penis and testes increase in size; pubic and underarm hair appears; sperm production begins; nocturnal emissions occur; perspiration increases.

2. The girl's body grows in size; increased oil production may cause acne; breasts develop; hips widen; sexual organs increase in size; ovulation and menstruation begin; pubic and underarm hair appears; perspiration increases.

Answers to Questions 1 and 2 are on p. 355.

3. Emotions may be more intense or a person may react to various familiar situations with different emotions; a person may recognize and better control his or her emotions; mental growth involves thinking more logically and abstractly; social growth involves moving from being dependent on people to being more independent; there is an increasing awareness of the feelings of others.

4. People experiencing puberty may constantly wonder whether body changes taking place in them are normal. If an adolescent is developing faster or slower than others, he or she may feel self-conscious, awkward, and unattractive. These feelings can negatively affect a person's self-concept and he or she may tend to withdraw.

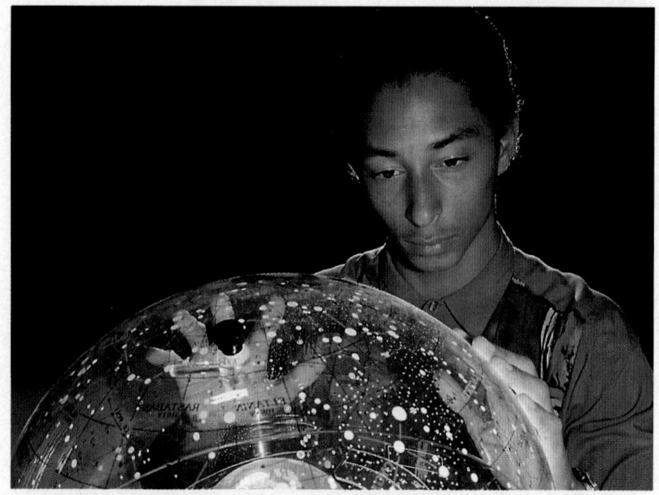

(FIGURE 17-3) **Your mental abilities improve during adolescence, allowing you to think and reason in a logical, abstract manner.**

Other Changes

At the same time that your body is developing, your emotions, mental abilities, and social abilities are also changing.

As you mature, you experience emotions for different reasons than before, or perhaps you feel them more intensely. Things that didn't bother you when you were younger might cause you distress now. And at the same time, you might be totally unaffected now by things that used to make you angry.

With maturity, you can better recognize and control emotions. If you can control your emotions, you can prevent them from having a negative effect on you. For example, when you feel angry, you should be able to control yourself so that you don't hurt yourself or someone else.

Emotional growth is influenced mainly by your environment, especially by the adults with whom you interact. Parents and other family members set examples, and you are likely to learn their ways of dealing with emotions. If they can control their emotions, you probably will learn how to control yours too. If they cannot, you will have a more difficult time with this aspect of emotional growth.

During adolescence, you also grow mentally. You begin to think and reason in a different way. Your thinking becomes more logical and abstract. You are able to ask such questions as "Why is this correct?" or "Can this be done another way?"

You can deal with more complex problems. For example, you are able to consider the immense size of the sun and its constant chemical changes. As a child, you may have understood only that the sun provides light and heat.

Your improved mental abilities also allow you to make realistic plans, because you can imagine the consequences of actions and think about alternatives. You can evaluate the results of decisions and learn from your successes and mistakes.

You also grow socially during adolescence. You move away from being totally dependent on other people to being more independent. At the same time, you develop an increased awareness of the feelings of others.

Review

1. *Describe how puberty affects the male body.*
2. *Describe how puberty affects the female body.*
3. *Describe the nonphysical changes that occur during adolescence.*
4. ***Critical Thinking*** *How might the changes of puberty affect a person emotionally?*

ASSESS

Section Review

Have students answer the Section Review questions.

Alternative Assessment

What Would You Say?

Tell students to suppose a younger sister, brother, or friend is just entering puberty and is worried about the changes in his or her body. Ask how they would explain the changes to the younger child.

Closure

Which Change Is Most Difficult?

On the chalkboard, write the heading *CHANGES DURING PUBERTY* with these subheadings: *PHYSICAL, EMOTIONAL, THINKING ABILITY, SOCIAL.* Ask students which changes they think are most difficult to deal with, and why.

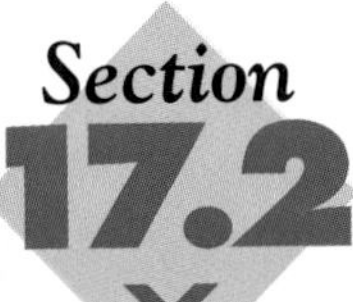

Section 17.2 Communicating Effectively

Objectives

- *Learn how to use "I" messages instead of "you" messages.*
  LIFE SKILLS: Communicating Effectively
- *Learn active-listening skills.*
  LIFE SKILLS: Communicating Effectively
- *Learn a method of verbally resisting pressure.*
  LIFE SKILLS: Communicating Effectively
- *Learn a method of resolving conflict.*
  LIFE SKILLS: Communicating Effectively

As a teenager, you are beginning to learn how to communicate in a more adult way. If you learn effective communication techniques now, you'll be much more successful in your interpersonal relationships throughout your life.

Levels of Communication

There are four levels of communication, each of which is appropriate for different situations:

1. Information giving
2. Directing or arguing
3. Exploring
4. Self-disclosing

An example of Level 1 communication, information giving, is talking about the weather. Another example might be telling someone what you plan to wear to the football game on Friday night. Most casual conversations are conducted at Level 1, the least risky level of communication.

You might use level 2 communication, directing or arguing, when you tell a driver not to switch lanes because a car is there, or when you disagree with a statement another person has made.

Level 3 communication, exploring, is a safe way to find out how someone feels about something. For example, you might ask how your boyfriend or girlfriend feels about your relationship. Since you have not told the other person how you feel, you do not risk exposing your feelings. If the other person says your relationship is great, you can agree. If the person says he or she doesn't see much future together, you can also agree. Level 3 communication provides you with a safe way to explore another person's feelings, but it is not completely honest. The other person may never know how you really feel.

Level 4 communication, self-disclosing, is the deepest and the riskiest way of communicating. When you self-disclose, you reveal your feelings before you know how the other person feels. You might tell a friend, for example, that you really like her and want to spend more time with her. Her response might be positive or negative—she may tell you she feels the same way, or she may tell you that she doesn't share your feelings. Either way, you should have a good idea of where you stand, as a result of risking Level 4 communication. Self-disclosing can be a very honest and open way of communicating.

Background

Communication Is Important

Leo Buscaglia, a well-known author of books on relationships, surveyed 1,000 adults to identify the most important qualities of relationships. The majority responded that the most essential ingredient of a relationship is *communication,* and the quality most destructive of relationships is *lack* of communication.

Section 17.2 Lesson Plan

MOTIVATE

Game

Communication Warm-Up

Have students play the following game as a warm-up activity. Divide the class into two teams. Have them write three statements for each of the four levels of communication. If necessary, provide these examples:

Level 1 (information)—The dance is tonight at eight.

Level 2 (direction)—You should ask Tina to the dance.

Level 3 (exploring)—Do you feel like going to the dance?

Level 4 (self-disclosing)—I don't feel much like going.

Have one team read their statements to the other team, which is to identify the level of each, and vice versa. Interrupt to discuss the interpretations as needed.

TEACH

Demonstration

Nonverbal Communication

Have students demonstrate nonverbal communication by having several volunteers listen to another student say a few words and then act out these statements without speaking: Feel sad. Feel angry. Feel happy. Strongly agree. Strongly disagree. Ignore the class. Feel bored. Be very interested in a

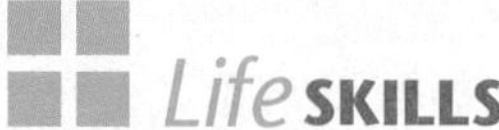

Sending "You" and "I" messages.

Have students complete the Life Skills feature, then ask volunteers to read their "I" messages aloud. Extend the concept by practicing "I" messages in the context of talking with parents and teachers. On the chalkboard, write these "you" messages:

Parent: *How many times must I tell you to take out the trash?*

Parent: *Your music is awful. Turn that thing down.*

Teen: *You never let me go out with anyone!*

Teen: *You always buy my sister what she wants, but never me!*

Teen: *You teachers are always picking on me!*

Teacher: *Is giggling the only thing you people can do?*

Then, ask students to create "I" messages for each sentence and discuss their likely effect on the recipient.

"You" and "I" Messages

A "you" message is a blaming or shaming message, which is likely to put the other person on the defensive. Unfortunately, most people use "you" messages without thinking when they are upset. Jeremy, for instance, sent a "you" message to Angelique when she forgot to call him.

Jeremy: *You are so inconsiderate! How could you forget to call me when you promised? I'm not going to sit around waiting for you to call ever again!*

Angelique is likely to respond negatively to this "you" message. The conversation will probably go downhill without much chance of getting better.

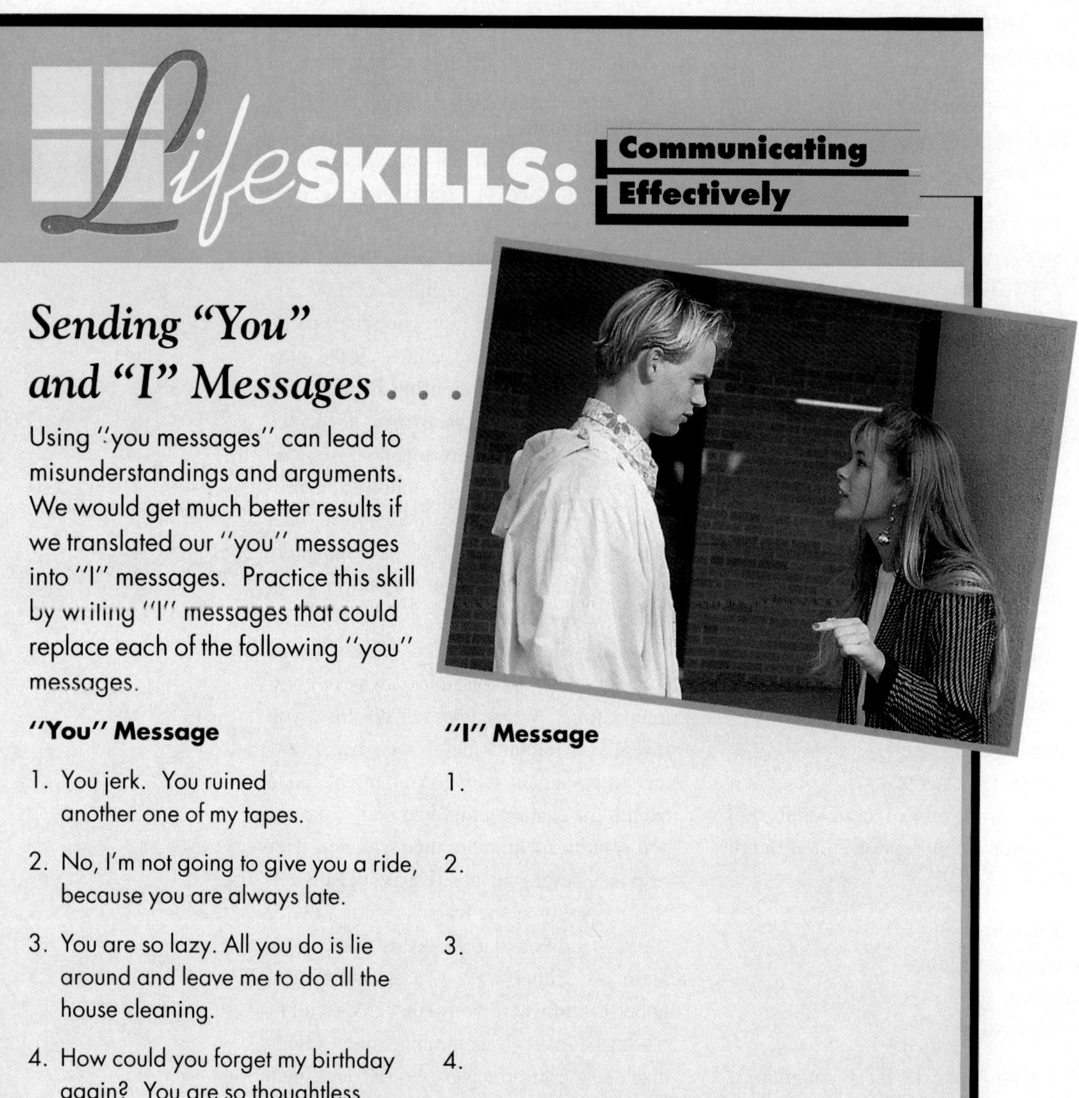

Sending "You" and "I" Messages . . .

Using "you messages" can lead to misunderstandings and arguments. We would get much better results if we translated our "you" messages into "I" messages. Practice this skill by writing "I" messages that could replace each of the following "you" messages.

"You" Message	"I" Message
1. You jerk. You ruined another one of my tapes.	1.
2. No, I'm not going to give you a ride, because you are always late.	2.
3. You are so lazy. All you do is lie around and leave me to do all the house cleaning.	3.
4. How could you forget my birthday again? You are so thoughtless.	4.

• • • TEACH continued

classmate in the front row. Ask students to describe what the actors' bodies, faces, and eyes do when communicating each emotion.

Role-Playing
Mixed Messages

Have students act out the following scenarios, paying attention to body language. Ask them to indicate which situations have mixed messages:

1. Boy asks girl out; she says yes and really wants to go out.

2. Girl asks boy out; he says yes to avoid hurting her feelings, but really isn't interested.

3. Student asks two classmates for some lunch money; both comply but one does so willingly and the other does not.

4. Student running for class secretary approaches several classmates for votes; all say they will, but inside some know they won't.

Cooperative Learning
Are You Actively Listening?

Divide the class into groups of four. Have each group select a reader, two active listeners, and a monitor. Provide each group with letters to the editor or opinion columns from newspapers. In each group, the reader chooses an item and reads it aloud as the active listeners practice listening—identifying the main concepts, and providing feedback to the reader. The monitor listens and suggests improvements.

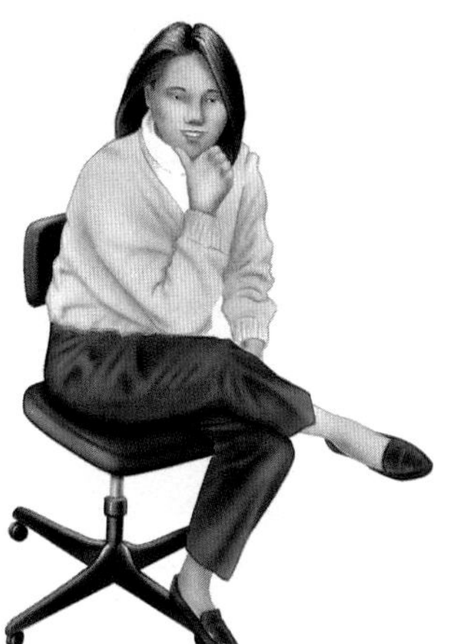

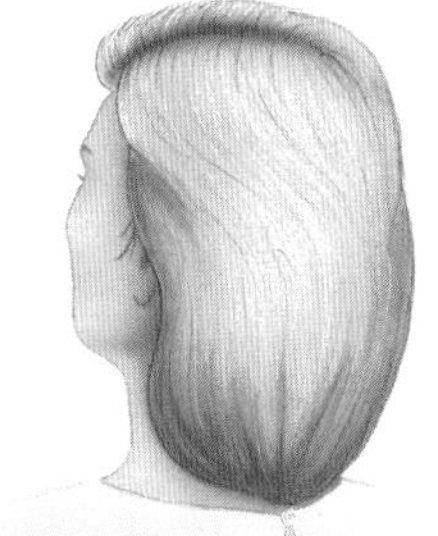

(FIGURE 17-4) **You send messages through your body language without even being aware of it. In the top drawing, the girl is very interested in what the other person is saying. In the bottom drawing, she is showing very little interest.**

An "I" message, on the other hand, is much more likely to be successful because it doesn't put the other person on the defensive. The "I" message has three basic parts: the event, the results of the event, and feelings about the event.

Jeremy could have sent the following "I" message when Angelique forgot to call.

Jeremy: *When you forgot to call me* (the event), *I wasted time waiting for you* (the result), *and I felt really angry with you* (feelings about the event).

Angelique is now likely to apologize to Jeremy, rather than snap at him defensively.

You can practice sending "I" messages by doing the Life Skills activity on page 358.

Nonverbal Communication

Words are important, but they are not the only messages we send. We also communicate through our behavior, through **nonverbal communication**. This kind of communication involves eye contact, facial expression, and body positions. Sometimes we communicate more with nonverbal communication than with verbal communication. If you are interested in something, you may lean forward in your chair and make direct eye contact. If you are bored, you may look around the room and lean back in your chair. You send messages about your feelings without even being aware of it.

If you pay attention to the nonverbal communication of your friends and family, you will have a better idea of how they are feeling. A friend, for example, may take his ring on and off when he is nervous. When you see him do this, you will know that he feels nervous.

nonverbal communication:

nonverbal behavior, such as eye contact, facial expression, and body position, that communicates information.

SECTION 17.2

Background
Nonverbal Communication

Nonverbal communication occurs through facial expressions, eye contact, and "body language." *Kinesics* is the study of the facial and body movements that accompany speech. *Proxemics* examines how different cultures use speaking distance, posture, and hand movements to silently communicate feelings and power. Generally, facial expressions communicate the same meanings worldwide, but eye contact and body language vary considerably among cultures. For example, in Arab culture, people may speak closely together and look intently into one another's eyes in a manner that would cause most Westerners discomfort.

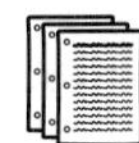

Life Skills Worksheet 17B

Nonverbal Communication

Assign the Nonverbal Communication Life Skills Worksheet, which asks students to describe an important conversation they had with someone and analyze the conversation for nonverbal cues.

Class Discussion
Active Listening

In what types of work is active listening especially important to people? *[Counselors, teachers, doctors, psychologists, psychiatrists, clergy, attorneys, hotline operators, diplomats, talk-show hosts, salespeople]* **In what family situations would active listening be especially helpful?** *[During disagreements, when someone is hurt or upset, and when someone is seeking advice]*

Journal 17C
Resisting Pressure Verbally

In the Student Journal, ask students to describe a situation in which they were under pressure to do something they didn't want to do. Suggest these possibilities: an invitation to drink, smoke, use drugs, have sex, or break the law; pressure from an abusive adult; or sales pressure to buy something. Have them write down how they could have verbally resisted the pressure, using the five-step method.

Role-Playing
Practice Resisting and Reasserting

Have students role-play the Li-Kirsten dialogue (*Resisting Verbally* feature) to practice resisting verbally, resisting nonverbally, and reasserting resistance. Focus students' attention on the nonverbal resistance (looking straight in the eyes, standing firmly, and speaking confidently), which must accompany

Background
Active Listening

Active listening is used in many contexts. Marriage counselors, doctors, and nurses use active listening to find out what they need to know from patients. Company personnel specialists are trained in active listening to identify the concerns of dissatisfied employees. Clergy use this technique to help people talk out their problems. Community volunteers are trained in listening skills so that they can help social workers in agencies and crisis intervention.

mixed message: *a message that is sent when the verbal and nonverbal communications do not match.*

A **mixed message** is sent when the verbal and nonverbal communications do not match. If Cynthia says she is interested in working with you on a project, but has a frown on her face and sits at the back of her chair with her arms crossed, she is sending a mixed message. When people receive mixed messages, they are more likely to believe the nonverbal communication than the spoken words.

Active Listening

Colleen was watching TV when her mom came home from work. Her mom asked Colleen about her day and continued talking to her. Colleen kept watching TV and didn't pay much attention, other than to grunt an occasional "ya" or "na." Finally her mom came into the room and asked Colleen if she had been listening. "Sure, Mom," Colleen answered.

Actually, Colleen was hearing the words her mother said, but she wasn't really listening to them. Consequently, her mother felt that Colleen didn't care about what she was saying.

active listening: *the process of hearing the words of the speaker and clarifying anything that is confusing.*

You can improve your communication skills by practicing **active listening.** Active listening is the process of hearing the words of the speaker and clarifying anything that you find confusing. Here is how to practice active listening.

- Give the speaker your full attention. This means that you should not think about something else or about what you are going to say next.
- Try to identify the main concepts and ideas that are being communicated.
- Make eye contact with the speaker.
- Indicate you are listening by nodding your head or saying "um-hmm."
- Provide feedback to the speaker. Ask questions, or repeat in your own words the speaker's comments to make sure you understand. For example, you might say, "If I understand you correctly, you are saying . . ."
- Wait until the speaker is finished before you start talking. Do not finish sentences for the speaker.

Resisting Pressure

The ability to resist pressure is extremely important to staying well. A person who cannot resist pressure to smoke cigarettes, for instance, or to take a ride with a drunk person, runs serious health risks. It is possible to resist pressure to do things that you don't want to do and still keep your friends.

Resisting Verbally Li's friend Kirsten got drunk last Saturday night and insisted that she drive Li home. Li knew she shouldn't ride with Kirsten, but she didn't know how to turn her down without looking stupid. Here is a five-step method of verbally resisting pressure that would have helped Li.

Step 1: Identify the problem.
Step 2. State your feelings about the problem.
Step 3: State what you would like to happen instead.
Step 4: Explain the results if the requested change is made.
Step 5: Explain the results if the requested change is not made.

Using this method, Li could have said to Kirsten:

When you want to drive me home after you've been drinking (identify the problem), *I'm afraid that we'll have a wreck* (state your feelings). *I'd like to drive you home or get someone else to take us home* (state what you would like to happen in-

• • • TEACH continued

the verbal resistance to avoid sending a mixed message. Alternatively, have students devise another scenario in which to practice resistance techniques, such as saying no to alcohol, tobacco, or drugs.

Role-Playing
Resolving Conflicts

On the chalkboard, write for reference:

- Recognize a difference of opinion.
- Eliminate your own thoughts for the time being.
- Scan other person's words.
- Paraphrase other person's words.
- Express what you want and why.
- Collect alternative solutions.
- Try the best one.

Divide the class into small groups. Ask students to think of a typical conflict between two people, and then act it out, applying the RESPECT method. Conclude with a class discussion of the advantages of the RESPECT method.

Extension
Body Language in Other Cultures

Have students interview people from different cultures to find out about nonverbal communication in those cultures and whether it includes unfamiliar body language.

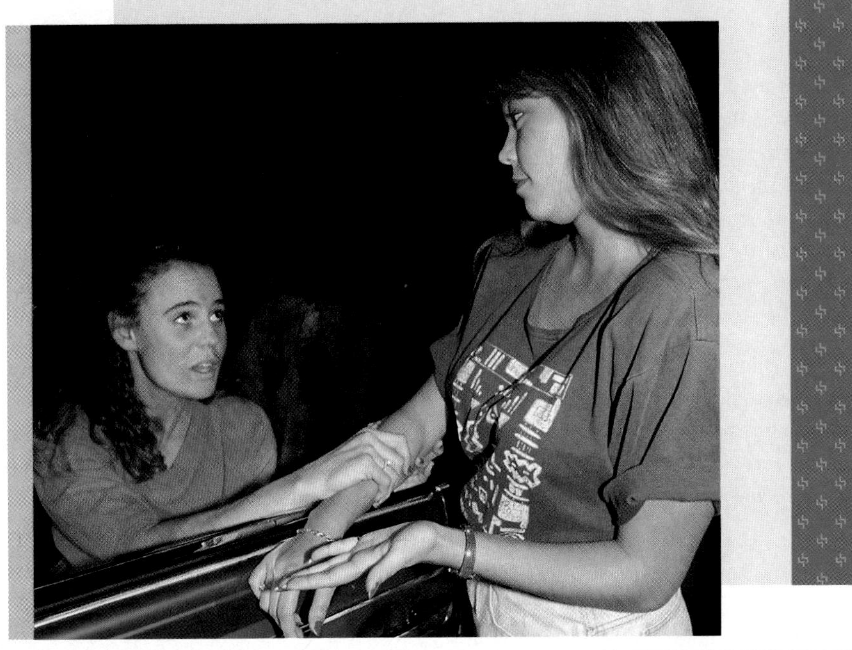

(FIGURE 17-5) **The best way to resist pressure to do something you don't want to do—like taking a ride with someone who has been drinking—is to state your feelings clearly and honestly.**

stead). *If you take my suggestion, I will feel good about going to other parties with you and I won't worry about you being hurt in a wreck—that's very important to me because I like you so much* (state results if change is made). *But if you insist on driving after you've been drinking, I won't ride with you and I'll think less of your judgment* (state results if change is not made).

In this way Li does not place herself in a dangerous situation, and she probably won't lose Kirsten's friendship either, because she let Kirsten know how much she cares about her.

Resisting Nonverbally If Li's nonverbal communication didn't reinforce what she said, Kirsten probably wouldn't take Li seriously. What if Li refused to look Kirsten in the eyes, shifted her weight back and forth, and laughed nervously as she spoke? Kirsten might feel that she could bully Li into doing what she wanted. To be effective in your resistance, you must look the other person directly in the eyes, stand straight and steady on both feet, and speak with confidence and sincerity.

Reasserting Your Resistance Sometimes people will continue to pressure you even after you've used the five-step method for resisting pressure. Then it's time to use other communication techniques. There are two that are particularly effective.

- The Broken Record—If the other person keeps pressuring, keep stating your resistance, like a broken record. Eventually, the other person may believe you are serious about resisting.

Section 17.2

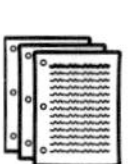

Section Review Worksheet 17.2

Assign Section Review Worksheet 17.2, which requires students to recognize when and how to use the four methods for effective communication presented in the section.

Section Quiz 17.2

Have students take Section Quiz 17.2.

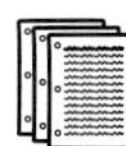

Reteaching Worksheet 17.2

Students who have difficulty with the material may complete Reteaching Worksheet 17.2, which requires them to choose the appropriate communication methods for specific situations.

Review Answers

1. Answers will vary. One "you" message might be, "You are so self-centered! You never listen to what I have to say." To change this message into an "I" message one might say, "When you don't pay attention to me while I'm talking to you (event), I feel that what I have to say is not important (the result), and my feelings get hurt (feelings about the event).

2. Active listening requires that you give the speaker your full attention and not think about what you are going to say next.

- Separating Issues—Imagine that Kirsten said, "If you were really a good friend, you'd let me drive you home." Li can counter by separating the "good friend" issue from the "driving home" issue. Li could say, *I think I am a good friend because I spend a lot of time with you, especially when you need someone to talk to. But I don't want to put myself in a dangerous position by letting you drive me home after you've been drinking.*

If nothing works and you are truly in danger, you may have to resist physically. If someone were trying to pull you into a car against your will, for instance, physical resistance would be entirely appropriate.

Resolving Conflicts

Conflicts are a natural part of life. It would probably be impossible to go for a week without some sort of conflict arising with someone. But conflicts can usually be resolved if people show respect for each other. The following is an example of how not to resolve a conflict. Trina and Ronnie have been dating for a long time, but sometimes their tastes in friends are not the same.

Trina: *Let's go to Jenny's party tonight. I hear it's going to be great.*

Ronnie: *Are you kidding? Jenny's friends are boring. No way I'm going to that party!*

Trina: *Oh come on. How can you say Jenny's friends are boring? You're not the most exciting person in school, you know.*

Ronnie: *Who do you think you're talking to? I don't have to take that from anyone. Go out with yourself tonight. In fact, don't bother calling me again.*

Trina: *Don't worry about me calling you. No chance!*

When this conflict began, Trina and Ronnie wanted to spend the evening together. When it ended, not only did they not want to spend the evening together, but they had decided never to see each other again. The couple's predicament resulted from a lack of conflict-resolution skills.

Trina and Ronnie could have used the following RESPECT method for resolving conflicts, which requires that you show respect for the other person and for yourself.

1. **Recognize** that there is a difference of opinion.
2. **Eliminate** from your mind any thought of what you want for the time being. You'll get back to it later.
3. **Scan and listen** to what is being communicated by the other person in words and feelings.
4. **Paraphrase** what was communicated in words and state the feelings you believe the other person is experiencing.
5. **Express** what you want and describe your reasons for wanting it.
6. **Collect** several alternative solutions that meet both your needs.
7. **Try** the best of the alternative solutions.

Imagine that Trina had used the RESPECT method:

Trina: *Let's go to Jenny's party tonight. I hear it's going to be great.*

Ronnie: *Are you kidding? Jenny's friends are boring. No way I'm going to that party!*

Trina: (She recognizes there is a conflict and eliminates her own desires for the moment). *You sound as though you wouldn't be comfortable with Jenny's friends and wouldn't have a good time.* (Trina scans Ronnie's words and paraphrases them. She also paraphrases any feelings she thinks he might have, even those that were not expressed verbally.)

Ronnie: *That's right! All those people ever talk about are the honors and scholarships they're getting and the places that they travel to over summer vacation. I always feel out of place when they do that.*

Trina: *I know what you mean. Sometimes I feel out of place, too. But I like parties where I can dance and listen to music. I had a rough week, and I need to wind down tonight.* (Trina expresses what she wants and why she wants it.) *Let's see how many alternatives we can think of in which you feel comfortable and I can wind down.* (They collect several alternative solutions.)

Ronnie: *Well, maybe we could stay just a little while at the party.*

Trina: *Or we could go to the party but stay to ourselves. We really don't have to talk to anyone there, except to say hello. That way I can listen to music and you can be more comfortable there.*

Ronnie: *And I guess another possibility is for us to do what you want this time and for me to get my way next time we disagree.*

After generating several other alternatives, they try one. Using RESPECT, Trina and Ronnie both get what they need. If you respect the other person's needs, that person will be more likely to respect your needs.

Review

LIFE SKILLS: Communicating Effectively *Write a "you" message you might use and then translate it into an "I" message.*

LIFE SKILLS: Communicating Effectively *During a debate, each debater is thinking about his or her reply while listening to the other debater. Explain why this is not an example of active listening.*

LIFE SKILLS: Communicating Effectively *A friend is pressuring you to go to a party where you will see the person who broke up with you last week. You feel that you are not yet ready to socialize with this person. Using the five-step method of verbally resisting pressure, write down the words you would use in talking with your friend.*

4. ***LIFE SKILLS: Communicating Effectively*** *Daniel and his buddy Josh get together every Tuesday night to watch their favorite television show. Then the show is canceled. Daniel wants to continue getting together on Tuesday, but to play pool instead. Josh wants to switch to Monday nights and watch a different television show. Suggest several alternatives that could resolve their conflict.*

5. ***Critical Thinking*** *Name one situation in which Level 1 communication, information giving, would be inappropriate. Explain your answer.*

Section 17.2

Answers to Questions 1 and 2 are on p. 362.

3. Answers will vary. Students might respond: "I don't want to go to the party because the person I just broke up with will be there and I'm not ready for that. I would like to do something else instead of going to the party. If you take my suggestion, I will go to other parties with you in the future. But if you insist on going to the party, I will not go with you and will find something else to do."

4. Answers will vary. Students might suggest that they alternate weeks—one week they can play pool on Tuesday and the next week they can watch a show on Monday. Accept any answers that show students' ability to recognize and resolve a conflict.

5. Answers will vary. Students may answer that level 1 communication would be inappropriate when trying to resolve a conflict because it is important to talk about what is causing the conflict instead of avoiding the issues by trying to talk about casual subjects.

ASSESS

Section Review

Have students answer the Section Review questions.

Alternative Assessment

Identify the Communication Skill Needed

On the chalkboard, write the following quotations:

1. That was rotten of you to make fun of me in front of my friends!

2. I made the team today!

3. If you like me, you'll go drinking with me.

4. We're out of here.
No! I want to stay.

Ask students to identify which communication skill is needed to reply in each case (*"I" message, active listening, resisting verbally, resolving conflicts with RESPECT*) Assess further by having students think of responses to each.

Closure

Applying Your Skills

Ask students to describe to a partner a conflict they experienced recently. Have them tell whether any of the methods presented in this section were used to resolve the conflict. If none were used, which ones do they feel would have helped?

Background
Quiet, Shy, or Nonassertive?

We call a person shy who is quiet, has difficulty talking to people, is anxious around others, and is nonassertive. But people are more complicated than that. *Quiet* people simply don't talk a lot; this is not a social handicap. *Shy* people are anxious and usually at a loss for words, a definite handicap. *Nonassertive* people generally converse well enough, but falter when they need to say "I want . . . ," "I disagree . . . ," or "No," because they can't assert themselves. Both shy and nonassertive people lack self-confidence and need encouragement and practice in dealing with others. About 40 percent of people consider themselves shy, including some famous people, such as TV personalities Barbara Walters and Jane Pauley.

Section 17.3 Relationships With Peers

Objectives

- *Describe how to make and keep a friend.*
- *Name three functions that dating serves.*
- *Name three actions you can take that will help you cope with a breakup.*
  LIFE SKILLS: Coping

relationship: *a connection between people.*

A **relationship** is a connection between people. It can be long-lasting and strong, such as a relationship between a parent and child, or it can be shorter and fairly superficial, such as a relationship between a supervisor and a summer employee. It can involve romance, as a dating relationship does, or it can be linked to friendship.

Each of us has a variety of relationships, including those with peers. Because you spend so much time with your peers, it is crucial for you to understand the nature of peer relationships.

Friendships

A friend is someone you know and like. Most friendships are based on common interests and values. You may have different friends for the different things you like to do. Perhaps one friend is fun to play basketball with, and another is good to talk with on the telephone. If you were going on a class field trip, another friend might come to mind. As friendships grow, they provide opportunities for emotional closeness.

How to Make a Friend Some people are able to make friends easily. If you are shy, however, you may have difficulty making and keeping friends. Especially if you've just moved to a new town or started attending a new school, you may find yourself feeling lonely. It is possible that you have *no* friends. If you would like to make some new friends, you will have to take some positive risks.

First, look at the people around you and think about a person you would like as a friend. Try to find someone you think you would feel comfortable with, someone you wouldn't have to impress. Think about someone you would like to spend time with that you could trust. You may notice someone who seems to be alone a lot; that person may also be shy and would be happy to have a new friend. Don't try to fit in with people who don't show much interest in you, no matter how popular they are. It isn't much fun to be one of the "hangers-on" of an "in" group.

No matter how shy you are, you can find people who really like you and want to be your friend. After you've looked around, decide on one person you think would make a good friend for you.

Then approach the potential friend. Yes, this is a frightening prospect. What if the person looks at you like you're an idiot? What if the person just ignores you? These are definite possibilities, but you must risk rejection if you want to make friends. You can make it easier on yourself by first talking casually with the person about a class or other activity you share, or about something else that is happening in school. If that con-

Section 17.3 Lesson Plan

MOTIVATE

Journal 17D
Potential Friends

This may be done as a warm-up activity. In the Student Journal, have students list the names of potential friends and what they think they can do to earn their friendships.

TEACH

Class Discussion
How Can You Make Friends?

Ask students to tell how they make friends in various situations, such as moving to a new place, changing to a new school, joining a new organization, or going to a party where they know hardly anyone. Then, solicit suggestions for how shy or nonassertive people might go about making a new friend.

Class Discussion
Six Rules for Keeping Friends

On the chalkboard, write the heading SIX RULES FOR KEEPING FRIENDS and list them as follows:

1. Be trustworthy.
2. Be honest but kind.
3. Show empathy.
4. Say "I'm sorry" when necessary.
5. Be tolerant of differences.
6. Don't pressure.

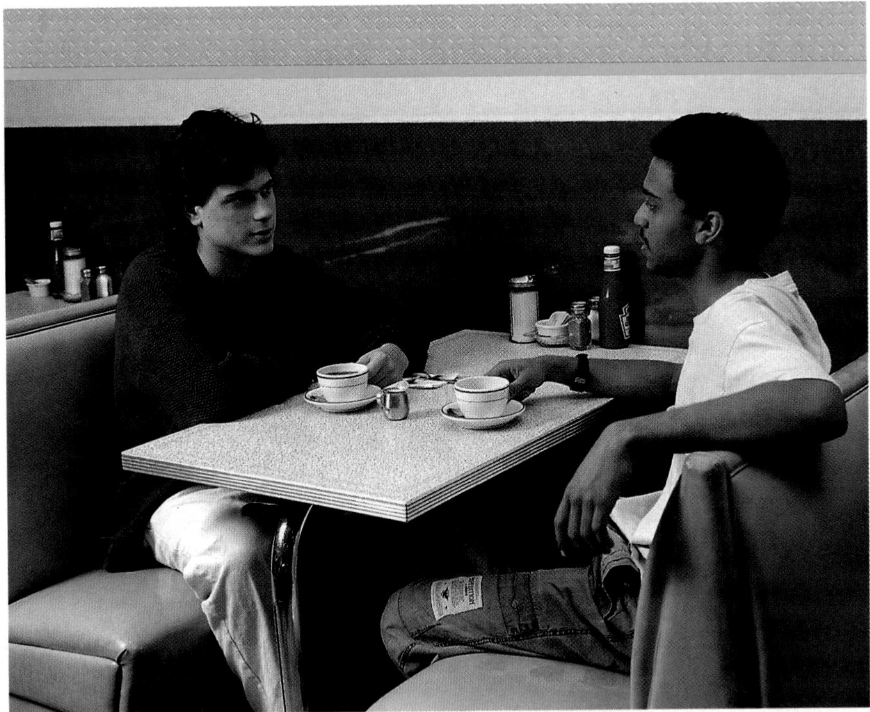

(FIGURE 17-6) **If you want to make new friends, you have to take some risks. After you've found someone you think would be a good friend, approach that person and start a conversation.**

versation goes fairly well, you can later invite your potential friend to do something with you—to go with a group of friends somewhere, for example, or to come over to your home to study.

If the person doesn't respond positively, don't take it too hard. Try not to think that you weren't "good enough." Everyone gets rejected sometimes. It is a fact of life that some people will like you and some people won't, no matter who you are. If you are rejected, just think to yourself, "It's their loss." If your first potential friend doesn't work out, try again with someone else, and keep trying until you find someone who responds positively. Eventually you'll find someone you like who also likes you.

How to Keep a Friend "You have to be a friend to have friends," goes an old saying. Different people require different qualities in friends, but there are some qualities that almost everyone values.

One of the most important qualities of a good friend is trustworthiness. It's very important that your friends know you won't tell other people personal things about them or any secrets that they have shared with you. It's also important that you don't criticize a friend to other people.

The way you talk with your friends is also critical to maintaining a friendship. Be honest, but temper your honesty with kindness. It would be better to tell someone that she looks best in blue, for example, instead of saying that she looks terrible in red.

Ask students to weigh their relationships with their friends against the six rules. Do they and their friends follow the rules? Then have them evaluate people they would like to have as friends against the six rules. Finally, ask them to weigh their relationships with family members. Ask: What were the problems? Did you see some areas where you can improve your own behavior in a friendship?

Cooperative Learning
Evaluating Relationships

On the chalkboard, draw the table shown, leaving a lot of vertical room.

IMPORTANCE OF QUALITIES IN RELATIONSHIPS

Qualities	Friendship	Dating	Crush
[Fun to be with	*3*	*2*	*1]*

Ask students what they look for in people, and write their ideas in the Qualities column. (Add as needed: humor, intelligence, common interests, responsibility, maturity, trust, honesty, tolerance, no pressure.) Divide the class into three groups. Have each group complete a column in the table. Tell them to evaluate each quality for their column with the appropriate number from the value scale. (0 = unimportant; 1 = not very important; 2 = pretty important; 3 = essential) Then, in a class discussion, have students compare the essential qualities in different relationships.

Background
Teens Need Peer Groups

Pre-teen children learn their rules from parents. But adolescence involves individual development and growing independence, so teens struggle to separate themselves from their parents. Because teens are going through this turbulent time together, they seek security with each other and form peer groups. These groups set their own values, standards, and define their own sense of "normal." Adolescents use each other to justify what they think, do, and like ("*Everyone* is doing it!"). To be a part of a group, one must conform, and anyone who does not is an outcast. Later in adolescence, each teen matures into a more individual self, and the importance of the peer group fades.

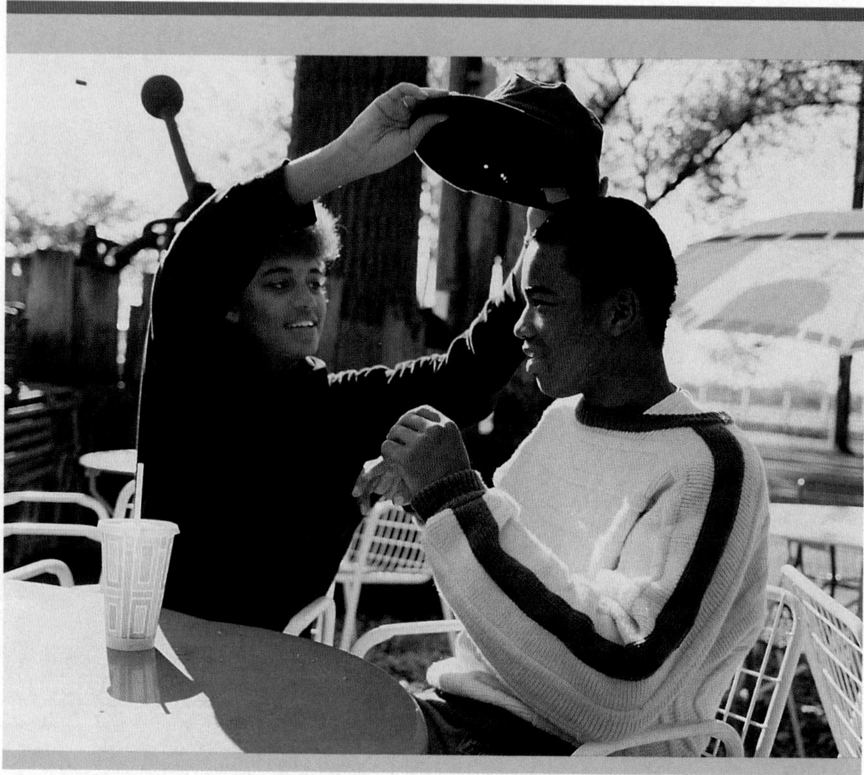

(FIGURE 17-7) **Besides just being fun, dating serves important functions in a person's social development.**

empathy: *the ability to understand how another person feels.*

Show **empathy** when talking with your friends. Empathy is the ability to understand how another person feels; it involves putting yourself in your friend's place. For example, if your friend just found out that he didn't get a part in a school play, you could show empathy by saying: "I'm really sorry you didn't get that part. I know how rotten that feels." On the other hand, be sure to show your support when your friend succeeds, too.

If you have hurt someone's feelings, don't be afraid to say, "I'm sorry." The ability to admit that you are wrong demonstrates that you are mature, more mature than many adults.

Try to be tolerant of any differences between you and a friend. The more tolerant you are of your friends, the more likely it is that they will be tolerant of you.

Finally, don't try to pressure someone else into doing something he or she feels uncomfortable doing. Just as you don't want to be pressured, others don't want to be pressured either.

Groups of Peers Peer groups provide you with a sense of belonging, support, and friendship. In a group of friends and acquaintances, you can learn how to present yourself to others and how to lead and follow others. You can talk about your values and what you believe is important. These experiences will allow you to compare your values and goals with others, as you decide what kind of adult you want to be.

• • • TEACH continued

Class Discussion
Importance of Dating

How is dating important to your social development? *[Learn how to talk and act with the other sex; learn skills such as talking easily with others, cooperating, and being considerate; discover with whom you are compatible; gain self-confidence]*

Demonstration
Breaking Up Is Hard To Do

Ask by show of hands how many in the class have experienced a romantic or nonromantic breakup and write the percentage on the chalkboard: ____% OF CLASS HAS BROKEN UP. Ask for reasons why they broke up and how they felt about the breakup. Finally, solicit students' advice on how to go about breaking up fairly and what mistakes should be avoided.

Extension
Writing About Relationships

Have students write a poem that expresses their feelings about a friendship that is, or was, particularly important to them. Ask volunteers to read their poems aloud in class.

Your contact with peer groups probably started when you were a preschooler with a circle of friends. You learned about the give-and-take of relationships and began to practice social skills, such as learning how to compromise.

Sometime between the fourth and sixth grades, cliques start to form. Cliques are small groups of three to eight people who exclude others from the group. If you are in a clique, you probably don't mean to be deliberately exclusive. The result, though, is that many people are left out of your group.

Teenagers often belong to a crowd, which is a loosely knit group of peers. A crowd starts to form when cliques begin to interact with each other. A crowd helps its members become familiar with different types of people. If the crowd is diverse—that is, if it includes people of different genders, ethnicities, cultures, and religions—it is beneficial to be in a crowd. Toward the end of high school, crowds begin to break up, as dating becomes more important.

Dating and Romantic Relationships

Dating is an important way for young men and young women to get to know each other. Many people begin dating in a group. In a group, there is a chance to develop social skills without the pressure that is sometimes found in a one-to-one dating situation.

Though dating provides positive, enjoyable experiences for many people, not all people begin dating as teens. Some teenagers find that other activities provide a full life without dating.

Friends or Dates? It is common in elementary school for close friends to be of the same sex. In the teen years, however, close friendships often form with members of the other sex. Two people may not be interested in each other romantically, but they still enjoy being together. For example, a boy may find that he can relax with a certain girl because the relationship doesn't have the demands of a romantic relationship. Friendships like these are said to be ''platonic'' relationships.

Crushes Whether they are called crushes, infatuations, or puppy love, the short-lived romantic feelings many teenagers experience can be intense. Someone experiencing a crush may daydream about the other person and become fascinated with details of his or her life. The other person, however, may not even know about the crush.

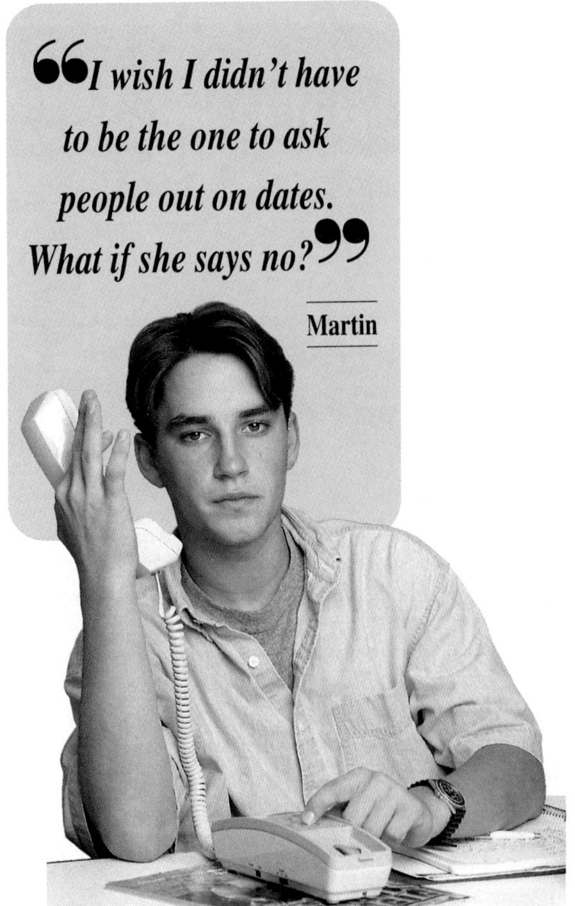

SECTION 17.3

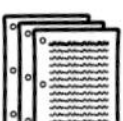

Section Review Worksheet 17.3

Assign Section Review Worksheet 17.3, which requires students to complete sentences about peer relationships, including friendships, group relationships, and dating.

Section Quiz 17.3

Have students take Section Quiz 17.3.

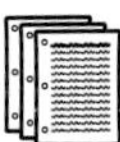

Reteaching Worksheet 17.3

Students who have difficulty with the material may complete Reteaching Worksheet 17.3, which requires them to explain whether certain advice is valid or not.

Such one-sided relationships are part of learning to love. Since the other person is not required to respond, a crush lets you explore romantic relationships in a safe way.

Beginning to Date It's normal to feel both excitement and fear about dating. And it's completely normal to be unsure about who to ask for a date. The qualities you look for in a friend are also good qualities to look for in a date.

In the past, it was almost always the boy who asked the girl out. But in recent years, it has become more common for girls to initiate dates.

As you begin to date, you learn how to talk and act with members of the other sex. You might feel as though others are judging every move you make. That is unlikely to be true; in fact, others are probably more concerned about how they appear to you.

Besides just being fun, dating serves important functions in a person's social development. It provides an opportunity to learn skills such as being able to talk easily with others, cooperate with them, and be considerate of them. Through dating, you learn what characteristics you like in others and what kind of people you are compatible with. And knowing that you are attractive to someone else helps you gain confidence.

As a dating relationship develops, you can share your thoughts and feelings. You can have a companionship that doesn't necessarily lead to a long-term commitment.

As in other relationships, communication is crucial for success. Clearly communicating your feelings and expectations gives you a better chance for understanding each other. See Figure 17-8 for other ways to make your dates more successful.

Two people sometimes decide to date only each other, which is called "going together" or "going steady." One advantage of going together is the opportunity to get to know the other person very well. But there are also some disadvantages. Going steady with someone limits a person's opportunity to meet other people, and if the relationship ends, it might be difficult to begin dating other people.

Suggestions for Successful Dating

Don't give up on yourself if you're rejected. It hurts if the person you like doesn't want to go out with you, but keep trying. You'll eventually find people you like who also appreciate you.

Have courage to date someone you like even if others don't agree with your taste.

Don't break a date unless you absolutely must. It is not acceptable to break a date just because something better came along.

Show up on time. If you must be late, call.

Don't expect every date to be wonderful.

Let your date know if you had a good time. Saying something like, "Thanks, you're fun to be with," is all it takes.

Don't accept bad treatment from your date. If your date is inconsiderate, don't go out with him or her again.

(FIGURE 17-8)

Breaking Up When two people are going together, they usually don't think about the relationship ending. Yet in reality, most romantic relationships developed during adolescence end by breaking up. Even though breakups are so common, they can be devastating.

Usually the first stage of a breakup is shock and numbness. A person who has been rejected may find it difficult to believe

Review Answers

1. To make friends, look at the people around you and think about who you would like as a friend. Decide on one person, approach the potential friend, and later suggest doing something together. To keep a friend, be trustworthy, be honest, show empathy, don't be afraid to say "I'm sorry," be tolerant of differences, and don't pressure anyone into doing something he or she doesn't want to do.

the other person really wants to break up. There is a tendency to deny the other person's words. It is easy to think the other person will want to get back together.

When the reality of a breakup is accepted, there may be anger. The other person's faults may be magnified. If the other person has started going with someone else, the anger may be directed at that person also, especially if the person was a friend.

A breakup can cause self-doubt, resulting in negative thoughts such as "If only I had been more fun" or "If only I were better looking." But it is better not to dwell on and give in to negatives. Instead, try to be very good to yourself.

If a relationship you were in has just ended, think of things you especially like to do and indulge yourself a little. Stay in contact with your friends. Remember that you are in the middle of a healing process and that the pain will end eventually. However, if you feel seriously depressed for more than a few weeks, seek help. Talk with a parent or guardian, or a school counselor, teacher, or coach.

Just remember that you will recover, that you will pick up your life and keep going. Although breaking up with someone is painful, it can also lead to personal growth. Your judgment about people becomes more reliable as you learn to evaluate people more realistically. Everything you have learned in this relationship will help you when you develop a deep and lasting relationship that doesn't break up. The suggestions in Figure 17-9 may help you cope with a breakup.

If you are the person who is ending the relationship, act with sensitivity and integrity. Tell the other person plainly that you want to break up. Don't just avoid the person and hope that the message is communicated. Be honest about your feelings, but don't say unnecessarily hurtful things.

Coping With a Breakup

Be very good to yourself. Indulge yourself by doing things you especially like to do.

When you start thinking or reminiscing about your ex-boyfriend or ex-girlfriend, command yourself to "Stop!"

Don't look at his or her photograph, reread old letters, or play "your song."

Ask trusted friends or family members if you may call them when you feel like calling your ex-boyfriend or ex-girlfriend.

If you are seriously depressed for more than a few weeks, seek help from a trusted adult.

Remember that you will recover from your loss.

Remember that you will find someone else.

(FIGURE 17-9)

Review

1. *Describe how to make and keep a friend.*
2. *Name at least three functions that dating serves in a person's social development.*
3. ***LIFE SKILLS: Coping*** *Name at least three actions you can take that will help you cope with a breakup.*
4. ***Critical Thinking*** *Look at your answer to Question 2 of this Review. What activities other than dating could serve each function you listed?*

Answer to Question 1 is on p. 368.

2. Answers may include: dating enables one to learn how to talk and act with a person of the opposite sex; provides an opportunity to learn skills such as being able to talk easily with others, cooperate with others, and be considerate of others; enables one to learn what he or she likes in people; and helps in gaining self-confidence.

3. Answers may include: be good to yourself and indulge yourself; try not to think about your ex-girlfriend or ex-boyfriend; don't look at photographs of your ex-girlfriend or ex-boyfriend; talk with trusted friends and family members; and remember you will recover from the loss and find someone else.

4. Answers may include making, developing, and keeping friendships; becoming an active member of a club; doing volunteer work.

ASSESS

Section Review

Have students answer the Section Review questions.

Alternative Assessment

Helping a Friend

In any group of teens, someone right now is having difficulty with a friendship, a peer group, dating, or breaking up. Ask students to think about friends who are having problems with relationships. Have students formulate a plan in which they can use their knowledge and skills in active listening, resisting pressure, and resolving conflicts to help their friends.

Closure

The Keys to Success and Failure

Ask students to summarize, while you write on the chalkboard, the keys to successful friendships and dating.

Background
Resources on Homosexuality

A high school-based organization that promotes tolerance for homosexual students, both male and female, is Project 10, Inc., Fairfax High School, 7850 Melrose Avenue, Los Angeles, CA 90046, 1-213-651-5200. Other organizations providing help include Dignity, 755 Boylston Avenue, Boston, MA 02116 and Out Youth-Austin, 2330 Guadalupe, Austin, TX 78705, Helpline 1-800-969-6884.

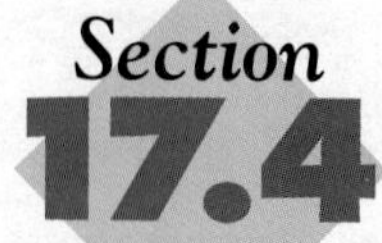

Section 17.4 Sexuality and Responsibility

Objectives

- *Describe the difference between sexual and emotional intimacy.*
- *Name three possible consequences of teenage pregnancy.*
- *Describe the advantages of sexual abstinence.*
- *Consider how a pregnancy now would affect your life goals.*
  LIFE SKILLS: Setting Goals

heterosexuals: *people who are sexually attracted to those of the other sex.*

homosexuals: *people who are sexually attracted to those of the same sex.*

The adolescent years are a time of emerging sexuality. During this time a person's interest in sexual matters increases dramatically. An increased interest in sexual matters is a completely normal part of becoming an adult. Another important part of maturing is making responsible decisions about sexual behavior. The ability to use good judgment about sexual matters is crucial not only to your romantic relationships, but to your health.

What Is Sexuality?

People often use the word "sexuality" as a synonym for "sexual activity." But sexuality is not just a physical act. It includes everything that makes someone a sexual person. Sexuality involves how we feel about our bodies, our desire for physical closeness with others, and all the thoughts and feelings we have about sexual intimacy. In fact, sexuality encompasses everything about being a male or female person. It isn't necessary to "have sex" to be a sexual person In fact, people who abstain from sexual intimacy are just as sexual as those who don't. Everyone has sexuality, and everyone is a sexual being.

Most people are **heterosexuals,** people who are sexually attracted to those of the other sex. Some people are **homosexuals,** people who are sexually attracted to those of the same sex. Homosexual men are also called gay men, and homosexual women are also called lesbians.

It is not unusual for adolescents to have sexual feelings for those of the same sex, and even act on those feelings, but be heterosexual as adults. Similarly, some people who are homosexuals as adults have had sexual feelings for members of the other sex. It is the predominant sexual attraction—to those of the other sex or those of the same sex—that determines whether a person is considered to be heterosexual or homosexual in orientation.

Much of the evidence from recent studies indicates that people don't choose whether they are heterosexual or homosexual, just as they don't choose whether to be tall or short, male or female, or brown-eyed or blue-eyed.

Everyone—regardless of his or her sexual orientation—deserves to be treated with respect and dignity and without discrimination.

Influences on Sexuality As you grow up, your sexuality is influenced to a large extent by the people around you and the things you see, hear, and read. The earliest influences come from your family. If the people who raise you are comfortable showing affection through touch, you have a

Section 17.4 Lesson Plan

MOTIVATE

Writing
Feelings About Sexuality

Have students write a paragraph that expresses their concept of what sexuality is. In a discussion afterward, ask them to provide examples to illustrate the complexity of sexuality—which includes feelings, actions, and decisions.

TEACH

Class Discussion
Myths and Facts About Sexuality

Refer students to Figure 17-10, "Myths and Facts About Sexuality." Discuss the first myth in the table, asking their opinions on what *really* indicates that a couple is in love. Encourage discussion of each myth. Myth number four raises the opportunity to invite questions on homosexuality.

Debate the Issue
Censorship of TV and Movies

Divide the class into two teams and ask students to debate this question: Because preteens and younger teens are so impressionable and easily misled, should explicit and unrealistic sexual behavior be banned from TV and the movies? Close with a discussion attempting to reach a compromise on this controversial issue.

Myths and Facts About Sexuality

Myth	Fact
Becoming sexually intimate shows a couple is really in love.	*Although sexual intimacy can be an expression of love, it doesn't really prove a couple is in love. Couples become sexually intimate for reasons other than being in love: curiosity, trying to hang on to a partner, proving to themselves that they are sexually normal, or because one partner wants to. It is possible for couples to express their love in ways that do not include sexual intimacy.*
If a person has been sexually intimate once, there's no reason to say no to being sexually intimate again.	*Many people are intimate once and decide there are many reasons not to do it again: fear of pregnancy or diseases, moral or religious beliefs, waiting for the right person, or wanting to wait until it can be a very satisfying experience.*
One way to keep a boyfriend or girlfriend is to be sexually intimate.	*Sexual intimacy doesn't guarantee a boyfriend or girlfriend will stay. Sometimes sex will keep a partner for a period of time because of a sense of duty or feelings of guilt. Sometimes a relationship will end after sexual intimacy because the challenge is gone or because a partner feels tied down and doesn't want to be.*
If a male is a virgin when he graduates from high school, he's probably homosexual.	*Many heterosexual men don't become sexually intimate until after high school because they believe they should wait for marriage. Many others have strong beliefs about when sex will be appropriate and control their sexual desire until then. Studies show that delaying sexual intimacy has most to do with religious beliefs and life goals.*
The best way to get to know someone is to be sexually intimate with him or her.	*Sexual intimacy is only one way of getting to know someone. There are many facets of a person's character one does not learn during sex. If sex replaces talking, spending time with mutual friends, and enjoying activities together, a couple may never truly get to know each other.*

(FIGURE 17-10)

Making a Choice 17A

Anti-Discrimination Measures

Assign the Anti-Discrimination card. The card directs students to research measures proposed to prevent discrimination based on sexual orientation and to summarize their findings in an oral presentation to the class.

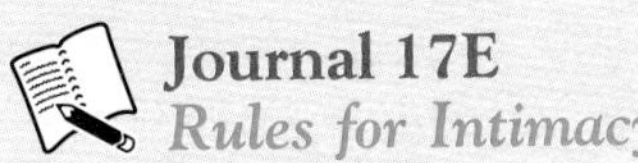

Journal 17E
Rules for Intimacy

On the chalkboard, write two headings, SEXUAL INTIMACY and EMOTIONAL INTIMACY. Ask students for definitions and examples of each, writing their comments beneath the headings. Explore with them how sexual intimacy makes one vulnerable. (Emotional risk, physical risk, pregnancy and STD risk) Then have them turn to the Student Journal and write their personal rule for sexual intimacy.

Demonstration
It Won't Happen to Me

Explain that 1 out of 10 teen girls becomes pregnant every year. Because each pregnancy requires a boy, too, this means that 1 out of every 10 teens—boys and girls—will be involved in a teen pregnancy this year. On the chalkboard, write the number of students in your school, followed by 10 percent of that number—for example:

817 STUDENTS IN OUR SCHOOL
82 STUDENTS POTENTIALLY INVOLVED IN PREGNANCY

Then have each student write on an index card "$2,000—IT WON'T HAPPEN TO ME!". Select 10 percent of your class to hold up their cards and tell students that this many of them are wrong, because it may happen to them, and it will cost them about $2,000 a year, the typical annual cost of baby care.

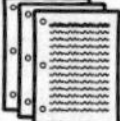

Section Review Worksheet 17.4

Assign Section Review Worksheet 17.4, which requires students to determine which phrases correctly complete sentences about sexuality and responsibility.

Section Quiz 17.4

Have students take Section Quiz 17.4.

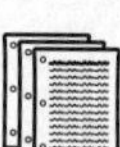

Reteaching Worksheet 17.4

Students who have difficulty with the material may complete Reteaching Worksheet 17.4, which requires them to explain why sexual abstinence is the best choice in each of four different situations.

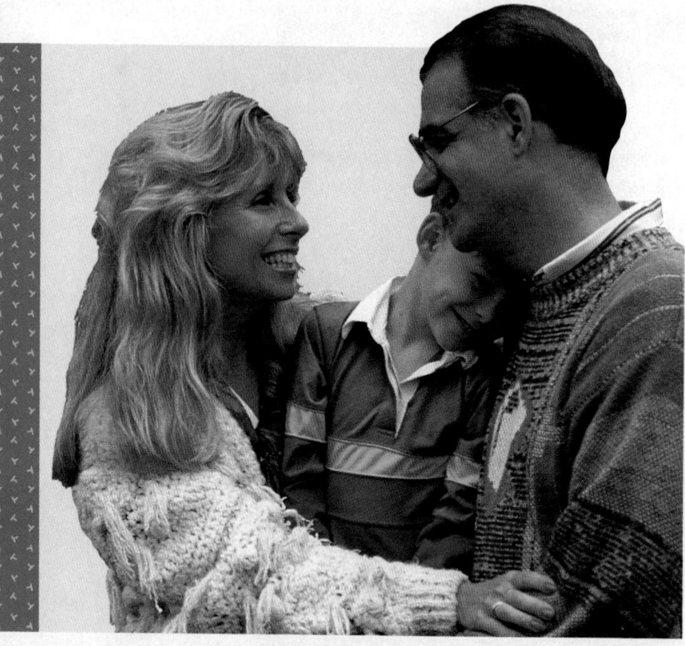

(FIGURE 17-11) **If the people who raise you are comfortable showing affection through touch, you are likely to feel comfortable with physical affection as well.**

sexual intimacy: *breast and genital touching and sexual intercourse.*

emotional intimacy: *sharing thoughts and feelings, caring for and respecting the other person, and gradually learning to trust one another.*

pretty good chance of growing into a person who can also show physical affection easily. If, on the other hand, your family has difficulty with physical displays of affection, you may also have a hard time with this aspect of sexuality.

How your family talks about sexuality also can influence your attitudes about the subject. In some families, sexuality is openly discussed, and in others, there is an unspoken rule that it should not be discussed at all. Most families fall somewhere in between.

As you get older and enter adolescence, your peers become more important as sources of information about sexual matters. You hear what they think about sexuality and what they say they do. However, teenagers often misrepresent their sexual activities to impress others, so peer information may not be the most reliable.

An increasingly important influence on your sexuality is mass media—television, movies, magazines, and newspapers. Most of the information you get from the media is designed to sell you something. The more viewers a television show gets, the more it can charge for advertising time. And the more movie tickets are sold, the more money a movie makes. That's why the sex scenes in television shows and movies are usually so unrealistic: the hotter and steamier the scenes are, the more money is made. Realistic sexual and emotional intimacy is rarely shown on the screen. What you see is what sells.

Sexual Intimacy Versus Emotional Intimacy Sexual intimacy and emotional intimacy are often confused. **Sexual intimacy** involves genital touching and intercourse. **Emotional intimacy** involves sharing thoughts and feelings, caring for and respecting the other person, and gradually learning to trust one another. It is entirely possible to have one kind of intimacy without the other.

"Casual sex" is an example of sexual intimacy without emotional intimacy. When people have casual sex, they are often using the other person for gratification without regard for the person's feelings. In this way they are treating the other person as an object rather than as a human being.

Sometimes a person who is lonely or uncomfortable around others will offer sexual intimacy in an effort to achieve emotional intimacy. This can be a painful experience and can be harmful to one's self-esteem.

When people are sexually intimate, they allow themselves to be vulnerable, and for that reason it is very important to trust the other person a great deal. Trust is established over a period of time and requires commitment. When two people love, trust,

• • • TEACH continued

Class Discussion

Reasons to Avoid Pregnancy

Write two headings on the chalkboard: REASONS TO GET PREGNANT and REASONS TO AVOID PREGNANCY. Solicit reasons for each and list them. Lead a discussion of the reasons. Conclude with these questions:

- Which of you think your parents would be upset if you were involved in a pregnancy right now?
- Which of *you* would be upset if you were involved in a pregnancy now?
- Which of you has plans for college or a job that would be disrupted by a pregnancy right now?
- Which of you has the money to pay for the birth of a baby and to care for it?

Class Discussion

Contraception

What methods of contraception do you know about? *[Abstinence, withdrawal, rhythm method, condom, pill, foam, sponge, diaphragm, IUD, vasectomy, and tubal ligation]* Write them on the chalkboard. **Which method is 100 percent effective?** *[Abstinence; all other methods risk pregnancy, as well as STDs and side effects.]*

Extension

More Facts on Teen Pregnancy

Suggest that students visit a public health facility, doctor's office, or organization such as Planned Parenthood to obtain pamphlets on teen pregnancy

and are committed to each other, sexual intimacy can be one of the best experiences in life.

Risks of Teenage Sexual Intimacy

Though sexual intimacy is a positive, pleasurable part of adult life, it can be harmful if engaged in prematurely. The risks of teenage sexual activity include conflicts with personal and parental values, sexually transmitted diseases, and unwanted pregnancy.

Conflicts With Personal and Parental Values Everyone must consider his or her own values—what he or she strongly believes—when making decisions about sexual behavior. Actions that conflict with one's own values can cause feelings of guilt and low self-esteem.

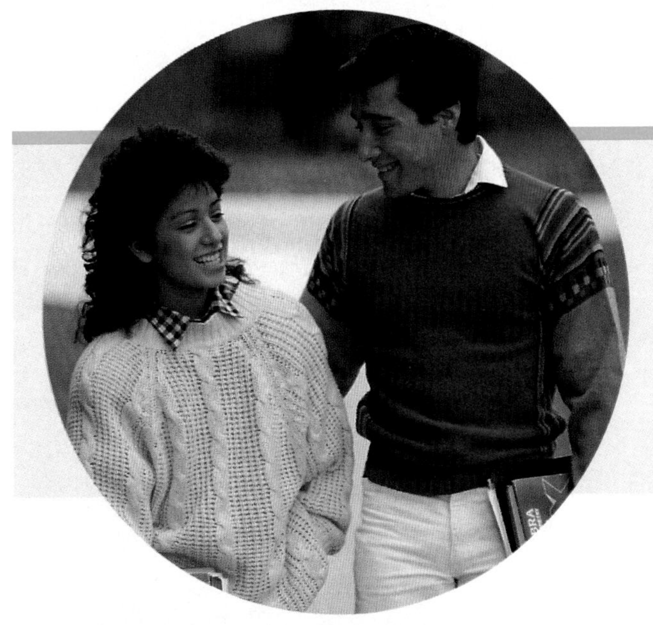

(FIGURE 17-12) **As people become emotionally intimate, they share their thoughts and feelings, care for and respect the other person, and gradually learn to trust one another.**

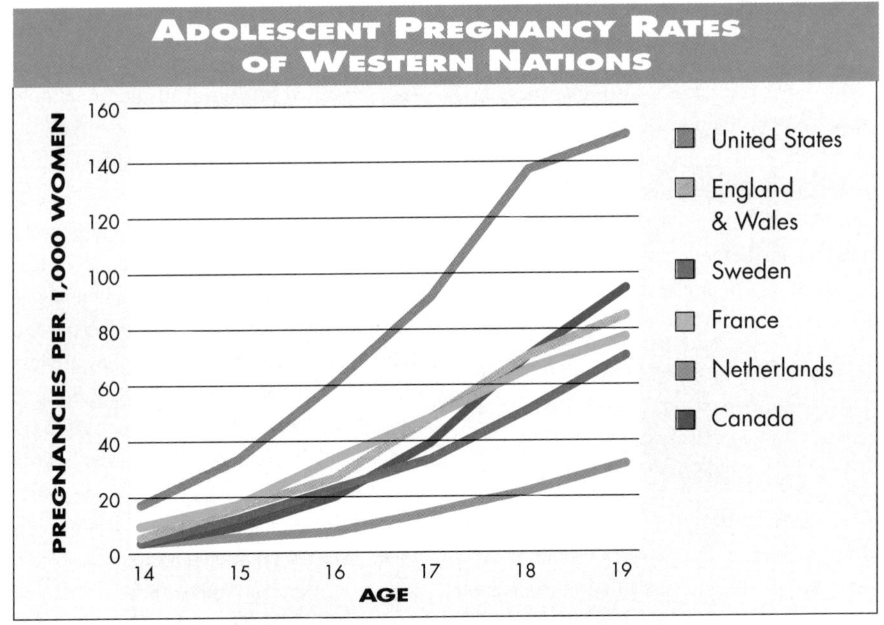

(FIGURE 17-13) **The United States has the highest teen pregnancy rate of any industrialized nation in the Western world.**

SECTION 17.4

Background

Teen Pregnancy

Each time a couple is sexually intimate without contraception, the girl has a 1-in-12 chance of becoming pregnant. About 1 out of 20 girls becomes pregnant from first-time unprotected sex. Twenty percent of pregnancies occur during the first month of sexual activity, and 90 percent occur during the first year. Teens become pregnant mainly because (1) they don't abstain or use proper contraception and (2) having a baby appeals to many. If any of your students are faced with teen pregnancy, refer them to the school counselor, school doctor, or the Blue Pages in the telephone directory under Human Services: Sex-Related concerns.

and display the pamphlets in the classroom. Alternatively, invite a representative from a family planning clinic to speak to the class.

Background
Cervical Cancer
In addition to pregnancy and STDs, another hazard of sexual intimacy that teenage girls face is cervical cancer, which is more frequent among those who have early and frequent sexual activity, multiple partners, and STDs such as venereal warts.

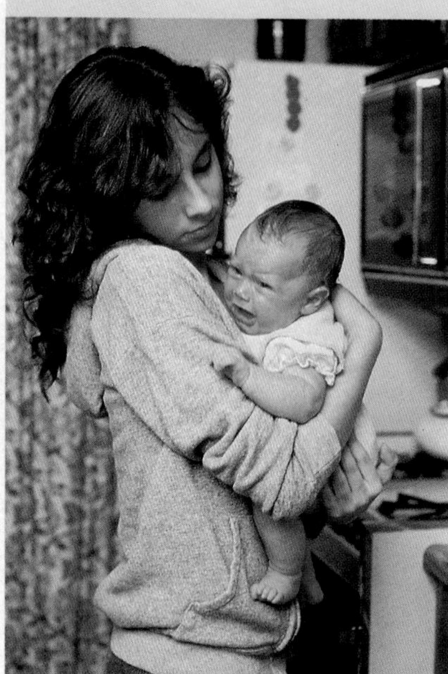

(FIGURE 17-14) **Caring for a child is a 24-hour-a-day responsibility. Teenage parents often find that they don't have time to do things they used to enjoy doing.**

Adolescents must also consider the values of their families. When you are part of a family, your decisions affect not just you, but other family members as well. If your parents believe, for example, that sexual intimacy before marriage is wrong, they would be disappointed and hurt if you became sexually active.

STDs are fully discussed in Chapter 22.

AIDS is the subject of Chapter 23.

Sexually Transmitted Diseases A sexually active person risks contracting sexually transmitted diseases (STDs), including AIDS. Chapters 22 and 23 deal with STDs.

Teenage Pregnancy Adolescence is a time of coming of age—of emotional, social, and intellectual growth—and all this can be jeopardized by a pregnancy. A person may not be able to reach his or her goals in life because of an unwanted pregnancy.

Many teenage pregnancies occur because teens tend to think: "It won't happen to me." But in fact, it does happen to about one million adolescent girls in the United States each year. This works out to 1 out of every 10 girls, the highest rate of teen pregnancy of any industrialized nation in the Western world.

A teenager facing an unwanted pregnancy must decide among three options: give the child up for adoption, raise the child, or have an abortion. Such a choice is difficult for anyone. It is especially hard for adolescents, who are still developing the ability to make responsible decisions.

Because teenagers often delay making a decision about their pregnancies, they may not get adequate prenatal care. Partly as a result of less prenatal care, teenagers are more likely than older women to have health problems during a pregnancy. In fact, the risk of death due to complications is 60 percent higher for girls younger than 15 than for mothers who are older than 20. Many of these deaths are caused by a condition called toxemia, which is characterized by high blood pressure and fluid retention. Teenage mothers are also more likely to give birth to premature babies and to babies who weigh less than normal.

In addition to suffering health problems, teenage mothers experience educational, economic, and social disadvantages. They are only half as likely to finish high school, and once out of school, they are less likely to become employed. In addition, half of the teen mothers who marry the fathers of their children are divorced within five years.

These dry facts, of course, do not begin to describe the emotional consequences to a teenager facing early parenthood. It can be very stressful to care for a helpless baby. The 24-hour-a-day responsibility, including middle-of-the-night feedings and diaper changing, takes its toll on a person's emotional resources.

Teenage parents may also find that they simply do not have enough time to do the things they previously enjoyed—going out with friends, for example, or dating, or going to the movies, or just relaxing at home.

Teenage mothers are not the only ones who suffer the emotional consequences of premature parenthood. Teenage fathers, too, may experience major difficulties. They often feel guilty and depressed. Like the others, they may find the sudden responsibility overwhelming. And like the mothers, teenage fathers are less likely to finish high school and are less successful financially than their peers who are not parents.

In addition, according to federal law the father must take financial responsibility for his child. This means that a boy who gets a girl pregnant must be prepared to pay for the child's needs. What if a boy who

Life SKILLS: Setting Goals

How Would a Pregnancy Affect Your Life Goals? . .

Take a few minutes to think about the consequences of becoming pregnant or having your girlfriend become pregnant. How would a pregnancy affect your goals—the personal, educational, and career plans you have made?

1. List the actions you would have to take within three months of finding out about the pregnancy.
2. Describe how the pregnancy would affect your goals over the next year.
3. Describe how the pregnancy would affect your goals over the next 10 years.

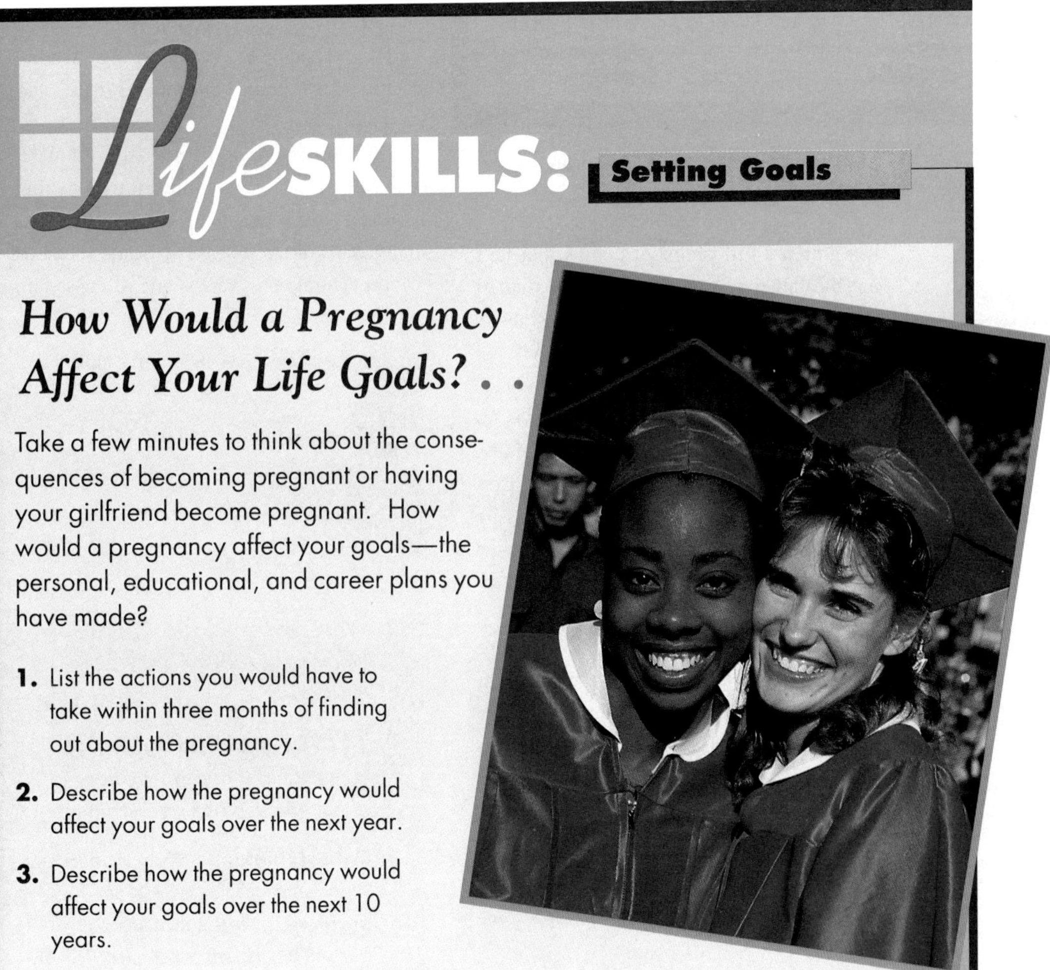

Life SKILLS

How Would a Pregnancy Affect Your Life Goals?

Have students do this exercise independently. Then summarize their responses on the chalkboard under the headings: IMMEDIATE ACTIONS, EFFECTS ON SHORT-TERM GOALS, and EFFECTS ON LONG-TERM GOALS.

Review Answers

1. Sexual intimacy involves genital touching and intercourse, whereas emotional intimacy involves sharing thoughts and feelings, caring for and respecting another person, and learning to trust another person.
2. Answers may include you avoid conflicts with personal and parental values, you avoid sexually transmitted diseases, and you avoid an unwanted pregnancy.

Answers to Questions 1 and 2 are on p. 375.

3. Answers would reflect the effect pregnancy would have on personal and educational plans. Students may also answer that they would not be free to do many activities with friends, and they may feel very stressed, guilty, and depressed.

4. Answers will vary. Students may answer that two people just meet, have sexual intercourse, and decide they love one another—all in one night. This is unrealistic. Love is a feeling that develops between two people over a period of time, as the two people get to know one another and have time to develop emotional intimacy. Sexual intimacy does not automatically lead to love.

Some Consequences of Teenage Pregnancy

Some Consequences of Teenage Pregnancy
Difficult choice among pregnancy options
Higher chance of suffering health problems during pregnancy
Higher chance of giving birth to premature babies who weigh less than normal
Stress of caring for an infant
Possible depression, guilt, and sense of isolation
Both mothers and fathers are less likely to finish high school
Both mothers and fathers are less successful financially

(FIGURE 17-15)

sexual abstinence: *delaying or refraining from sexual intimacy.*

has gotten a girl pregnant claims that he's not the father of the child? In most states the mother can take legal steps to establish the paternity—who the father is—of her child without the father's permission. Once the paternity is established, the father is legally bound to support the child financially.

A premature pregnancy affects different people in different ways. The Life Skills activity on page 375 will help you get an idea of how a pregnancy now would affect your life.

Though the consequences of teenage pregnancies are felt most deeply by the individuals directly involved, society as a whole also pays a cost. Teen pregnancies cost taxpayers an estimated $20 billion annually in public support.

A Positive, Responsible Decision

It is a positive, responsible decision to avoid teenage pregnancy, as well as sexually transmitted diseases. And it is responsible to act according to your own values and the values of your family.

The most responsible choice for a teenager is to delay sexual intimacy until he or she is in a stable, committed relationship such as marriage. A person who delays or refrains from sexual intimacy is practicing **sexual abstinence.** Teenagers who practice sexual abstinence grow by acting responsibly and by learning to develop relationships that are not based on sexual intimacy. And by practicing abstinence, they protect themselves from sexually transmitted diseases. As adults, they may be better prepared to build strong, lasting relationships based on mutual trust and respect.

If you decide to be sexually intimate, you must take responsibility for protecting yourself from unwanted pregnancy and sexually transmitted diseases. Some methods of preventing pregnancy are discussed in Chapter 18.

Review

1. *Describe the difference between sexual intimacy and emotional intimacy.*
2. *What are the advantages of delaying sexual intimacy until marriage?*
3. ***LIFE SKILLS: Setting Goals*** *How would a pregnancy now affect your life one year from now?*
4. ***Critical Thinking*** *Name one love scene in a movie, television program, or book that seems unrealistic to you, and explain why it is unrealistic.*

ASSESS

Section Review

Have students answer the Section Review questions.

Alternative Assessment

Three Reasons to Abstain

Ask students to write the three most important reasons for abstaining from sexual intimacy until they are in a stable, committed relationship.

Closure

What If?

Tell students to imagine that everyone stopped practicing abstinence, stopped using contraceptives, and focused upon sexual intimacy instead of emotional intimacy. What would happen to the pregnancy rate, disease rate, world population, and families?

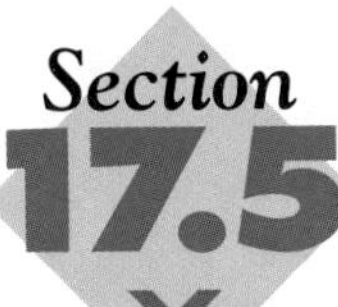

Section 17.5 Skills for Responsible Sexual Behavior

Objectives

- *Learn how to deal with internal pressures to become sexually intimate.*
  LIFE SKILLS: Coping
- *Learn how to resist pressure to become sexually intimate.*
  LIFE SKILLS: Resisting Pressure
- *Apply the decision-making model in this textbook to decisions about your own sexual behavior.*
  LIFE SKILLS: Making Responsible Decisions

Choosing not to engage in sexual intimacy is a sound, responsible decision. It doesn't help to decide to delay sexual intimacy, however, if you haven't developed the skills necessary to carry out your decision. In this section, you'll learn some valuable skills for responsible sexual behavior.

Dealing With Internal Pressures

A person must first acknowledge sexual feelings before he or she can deal with them. The sex drive can be especially powerful during the teen years, when hormonal changes occur rather suddenly, and an increased awareness of sexuality develops. Especially when you are in love, the natural sex drive can make sexual intimacy a very strong temptation.

The main way to deal with the internal pressures to be sexually intimate is by exercising self-control. You can also learn to express your romantic love for another person in ways other than sexual intimacy.

Practicing Self-Control We exercise power over our lives by practicing self-control. When you practice self-control, you make rules for yourself and act on them. It helps to think ahead about temptations and plan what you will do about them.

Sexual self-control is necessary not just for teenagers, or even adult single people, but for married people as well. Everyone must occasionally practice sexual abstinence. When a spouse is out of town, for example, a married person must practice abstinence: he or she must delay sexual intimacy until the spouse returns. Similarly, married people must practice self-control over their sexual impulses toward people other than their spouses. If they do not, they run the risk of ruining their marriages. Therefore, learning self-control now through sexual abstinence will help you later in life, in addition to now.

Other Ways to Show Love You can show your love for another person while delaying sexual intimacy. Showing consideration for another's feelings, doing special favors, hugging, kissing, and laughing together—all these show love.

A good way to think of ways to express love without sexual intimacy is to think of how you would want someone to show love to you. What could another person do that would make you feel cared for?

Background
On Sex Education
"Sex is too powerful to stay in the realm of superstition. Sex is too beautiful to be made ugly by ignorance, greed, or lack of self-control."
—Reverend Jesse Jackson

Background
"Everybody's Doing It!"
Aside from peer-group opinion, where does the notion of "everybody's doing it" come from? Some experts point to TV and movies. One study counted 20,000 sex scenes in a typical year of TV watching. Typically, these scenes are romanticized and overblown—and birth control is not brought up.

Section 17.5 Lesson Plan

MOTIVATE

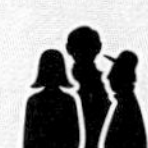

Cooperative Learning
Managing Internal Sexual Pressure

This may be done as a warm-up activity. Divide the class into four groups and appoint a recorder for each group. Have two groups brainstorm ways of self-control in resisting internal sexual pressure. Have the other groups brainstorm ways to show love besides sexual intimacy. Then ask the recorders to present their groups' ideas, and discuss their effectiveness.

TEACH

Class Discussion
Who Owns Your Body?

Draw an analogy between ownership of your body and ownership of anything else, such as a stereo: You own it and must keep control over how it is used. Ask the class to discuss the types of sexual pressure encountered in dating (lover's desires, friends' attitudes, stereotypes, media fantasies). Guide discussion to the conclusion that sexual intimacy is something each person must control and decide whether to use his or her body that way.

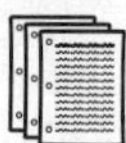 Life Skills Worksheet 17C

Sexual Abstinence

Assign the Sexual Abstinence Life Skills Worksheet, which helps students build self-esteem for making the decision to abstain from sex.

 Making a Choice 17B

Fun Date Ideas

Assign the Fun Date Ideas card. The card directs students to brainstorm fun ideas for dates that don't pressure people into sexual intimacy and to make a collage of such ideas for display in the classroom.

Dealing With External Pressures

External pressures come from outside you. They include pressures from your boyfriend or girlfriend, your friends, or from media messages. Sometimes the external pressures can become internal pressures. If, for instance, you get the idea from television programs that virtually everyone your age is sexually active, you might begin to put pressure on yourself, telling yourself that something is wrong with you if you have not yet experienced sexual intimacy.

Old-fashioned stereotypes of male and female sexual behavior can contribute to the external pressures. Young men may feel that they are expected to be the sexual aggressor, to push for a greater degree of sexual intimacy, whether or not they really want to. And a young woman may think that to please a boyfriend she must go further than she is emotionally ready to.

The most important thing to know is that you have a right to refuse sexual intimacy, anytime, for any reason. If you are not sure you are ready to be sexually intimate, you probably aren't. If someone tries to make you feel guilty or "no fun" because you don't want to do a certain thing with your body, that person probably doesn't respect you. Being pressured into sexual intimacy with someone who doesn't respect you is almost certainly going to be harmful to your self-respect, not to mention "no fun" for you.

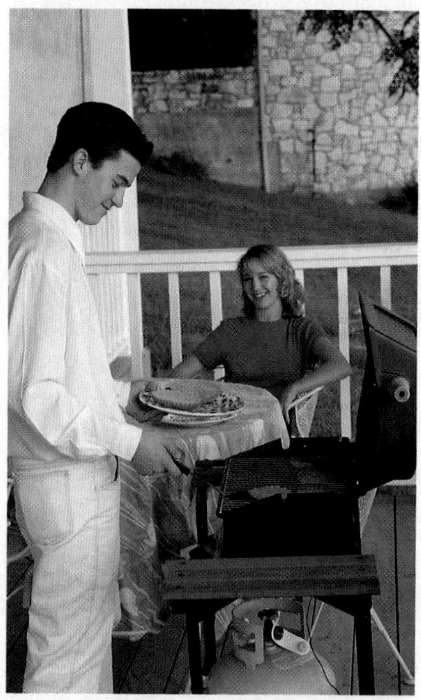

(FIGURE 17-16) **You can show you love someone in nonsexual ways. Doing favors for your loved one, such as cooking a meal, shows that you care.**

Resisting Sexual Pressure Lisa and Jamal have been going out for about two months. They spend a lot of time alone together, talking and kissing, and things have started to heat up. Lisa loves being with Jamal, and sometimes it's hard for her to keep from going further. Jamal, for his part, isn't even trying to restrain himself. He knows what he wants. He wants to have sexual intercourse, and the sooner the better. Though he hasn't tried to make Lisa feel bad about not going further, he has told her that he feels extremely frustrated. Lately he's become insistent, making it more and more difficult for Lisa to resist.

Lisa genuinely cares for Jamal and wants to continue seeing him, but she doesn't feel ready for sexual intimacy. Deep down, it just doesn't feel like the right thing to do at this time in her life. Plus, she doesn't want to jeopardize her future by becoming pregnant or getting a sexually transmitted disease.

The resistance skills discussed in Section 17.2 could help Lisa avoid a degree of sexual intimacy she doesn't want, in a way that won't make Jamal feel that he has been attacked.

• • • TEACH continued

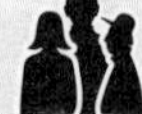 **Cooperative Learning**
What's on TV?

Have students conduct a survey about sexual intimacy on television. In small groups, students should compile a list of questions to ask, such as: Do you think too much sex is shown on TV? Does television influence your feelings about sexual intimacy? Suggest that students survey older adults, young adults, and teenagers, keeping their responses separate so that comparisons can be made. Have each group report its findings to the class.

Role-Playing
Resisting Sexual Pressure

Have student teams take turns acting out and observing a situation similar to Lisa's and Jamal's (*Resisting Sexual Pressure* feature), in which one partner wants more sexual intimacy than the other and is applying pressure. Have them vary details of the scenario, such as the length of time the couple has dated, future plans, fear that pregnancy would change the plans, and whether it's the girl or boy who is applying the pressure. Students are to apply the skills they have learned in this chapter: "I" messages, active listening, and nonverbal communication.

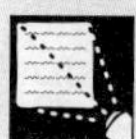 **Teaching Transparency 17B**
"First Kiss"

Use Teaching Transparency 17B to initiate a discussion of sexual feelings among teens and how to handle them.

The five-step method of verbally resisting pressure is:

1. Identify the problem.
2. State your feelings about the problem.
3. State what you would like to happen instead.
4. Explain the results if the requested change is made.
5. Explain the results if the requested change is not made.

Here is how Lisa could express her feelings to Jamal:

The problem is that I don't want to go as far sexually as you do (identify the problem). *I like you a lot, and I want to keep going out with you. I'm also sexually attracted to you and love what we've been doing together, but I feel uncomfortable about going any further* (state your feelings). *I'd like you to respect my feelings about this and not pressure me* (state what you would like to happen instead). *If you do respect my feelings and back off, I'll keep seeing you, because I think you're great* (state results if change is made). *But if you keep pressuring me, I won't go out with you anymore* (state results if change is not made).

Lisa has stated how she feels and what she wants in a way that leaves no doubt about what she means. To be certain that Jamal gets a clear message, Lisa must reinforce her verbal statements with her nonverbal communication. She must look him straight in the eyes and speak confidently.

Sometimes we are in a situation in which we don't know what we want. If someone is putting on the pressure, we might do what he or she wants because we think we have to answer yes or no on the spot. But actually, we don't have to make a decision at that moment. We can say, "Let me think about it." Learning how to say this simple sentence can be a lifesaver.

What Would You Do ?

What if You've Already Become Sexually Active?

Making Responsible Decisions

You finally did it. You had sexual intercourse with your boy/girlfriend Dylan. It seemed impossible not to—everything felt so good, and you thought you would be closer to Dylan as a result. But you find that you don't feel any closer. In fact, Dylan has been acting a little weird around you—sort of quiet and self-conscious. You've already made plans to be together this weekend, but you are starting to wonder if you want to continue the sexual intimacy.

As you make a decision about what to do, carefully consider your values and the values of your family. Also, when you do Step 6, don't forget to outline the steps you would take to implement your decision.

Remember to use the decision-making steps:

1. **State the Problem.**
2. **List the Options.**
3. **Imagine the Benefits and Consequences.**
4. **Consider Your Values.**
5. **Weigh the Options and Decide.**
6. **Act.**
7. **Evaluate the Results.**

What if you've already become sexually intimate with someone and then decide it was a bad decision? You are allowed to change your mind. Just because you've done something once doesn't mean you have to continue doing it. It is your right to say no even if you've already said yes.

Respecting Others Just as it is your right to resist pressure to do things with your body that don't feel right, it is also your ob-

What Would You Do ?

Have students apply the seven decision-making steps to determine whether to continue the sexual intimacy described in the situation.

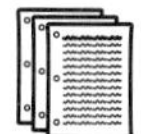

Section Review Worksheet 17.5

Assign Section Review Worksheet 17.5, which requires students to determine whether a situation would call for them to resist pressure or to practice self-control.

Section Quiz 17.5

Have students take Section Quiz 17.5.

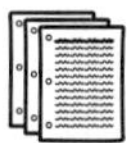

Reteaching Worksheet 17.5

Students who have difficulty with the material may complete Reteaching Worksheet 17.5, which requires them to apply the five-step method for verbally resisting pressure to a specific situation and then answer questions about the situation.

Reinforcement

Relationships Demand Respect

Refer students to the RESPECT method for solving conflicts in Section 17.2. Ask a volunteer to explain how this method could be used to resist sexual pressure. Tell students that in the best relationships, the couple balance their desire and respect for one another.

Extension

Date Rape

Direct students to the *Readers' Guide to Periodical Literature* to find articles about date rape. Have students write a report that explains what date rape is and summarizes information they read in the articles.

Review Answers

1. Exercise self-control and learn to express your romantic love for another person in ways other than sexual intimacy.

2. Identify the problem; state your feelings; state what you would like to happen instead; explain the results if the requested change is made; and explain the results if the requested change is not made.

3. Answers may include avoiding any activity that is high-risk for sexual intimacy, such as drinking and using drugs, avoiding being at home together when no one else is home, and becoming involved in group activities such as going to movies and sport events.

4. Answers may include that external pressures from the media, friends, and stereotypes dictate that adolescents should be sexually active. If you don't feel this way, those external pressures may lead you to feel uneasy about your own feelings toward sexual intimacy.

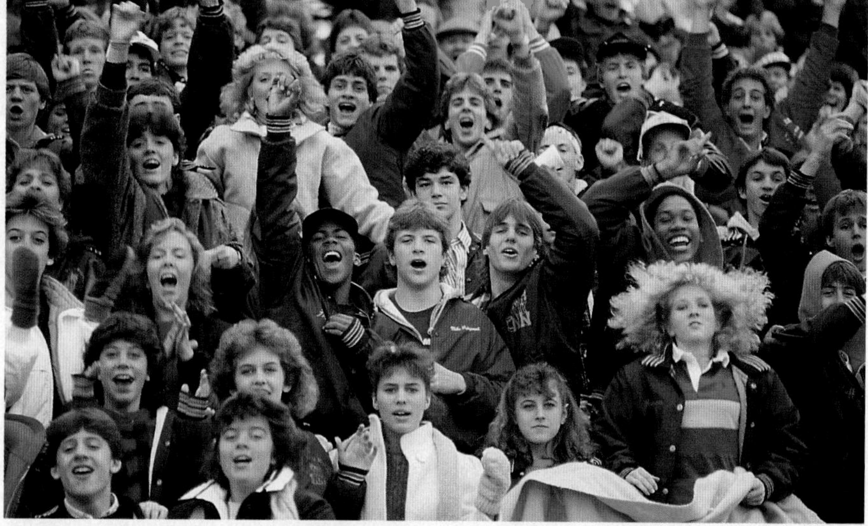

(FIGURE 17-18) **Group activities are best if you want to avoid sexual intimacy.**

ligation to respect the rights of others. People often don't realize when they are putting unfair pressure on others, especially in intimate situations when emotions run high.

If someone tells you that he or she doesn't want to do something sexually, believe it. If the person just acts reluctant but doesn't say anything, pay attention to the nonverbal signals. It's often difficult for people to admit that they feel uneasy about sexual intimacy. You might say something like, "You seem uncomfortable. Do you want to stop?"

High-Risk Situations If you have chosen to delay sexual intimacy, it will help to avoid situations that can make abstinence more difficult.

The main things to avoid are drinking alcohol or using drugs. These substances impair your judgment and self-control, making sexual activity more likely. Any party at which alcohol and drugs are present is a high-risk situation.

Spending all your time alone together is also risky. Avoid being at home together when no one else is there, as well as parking in cars in isolated spots. Group activities such as movies, shows, and sports are best if you want to avoid sexual intimacy.

Review

1. ***LIFE SKILLS: Coping*** *Describe how a person can deal with internal pressures to become sexually intimate.*
2. ***LIFE SKILLS: Resisting Pressure*** *Name the five steps of verbally resisting pressure.*
3. ***LIFE SKILLS: Making Responsible Decisions*** *If you made a decision to remain sexually abstinent, what steps would you take to ensure that you followed through on your decision?*
4. ***Critical Thinking*** *Why might it be difficult for a person to admit that he or she feels uneasy about sexual intimacy?*

ASSESS

Section Review

Have students answer the Section Review questions.

Alternative Assessment

Avoiding Risky Situations

Point out that good intentions to keep in control of one's sexual behavior can fall apart in special situations. Ask students to name some of these situations and write them on the chalkboard. *(Drinking, using drugs, parking, being home alone)* Discuss strategies for avoiding each situation.

Closure

Don't Create Sexual Pressure

This chapter has focused upon how to *resist* sexual pressure from others. Now, ask students to explain how they can avoid *creating* sexual pressure on someone else.

Highlights

Summary

- Adolescence, which is the gradual transition from childhood to adulthood, is a time marked by physical, emotional, mental, and social changes.
- Puberty is a period of physical development during which people become able to have children.
- Four types of communication are information giving, directing or arguing, exploring, and self-disclosing.
- Communication skills can be improved by using "I" instead of "You" messages, practicing active listening, and showing respect for the needs of others when conflicts arise.
- Most friendships are based on common interests and values. One of the most important qualities of a good friend is trustworthiness.
- Peer groups provide a person with a sense of support and friendship.
- The risks of teenage sexual activity include conflicts with personal and parental values, sexually transmitted diseases, and unwanted pregnancy.
- Pressures to be sexually intimate can be overcome by exercising self-control, learning to express romantic love in ways other than sexual intimacy, and avoiding high-risk situations.

Vocabulary

hormones chemical substances, produced by the endocrine glands, which serve as messengers within the body.

nonverbal communication nonverbal behavior, such as eye contact, facial expressions, and body position, that communicates information.

mixed message a message that is sent when the verbal and nonverbal communications do not match.

active listening the process of hearing the words of the speaker and clarifying anything that is confusing.

heterosexuals people who are sexually attracted to those of the other sex.

homosexuals people who are sexually attracted to those of the same sex.

sexual intimacy breast and genital touching and sexual intercourse.

emotional intimacy sharing thoughts and feelings, caring for and respecting the other person, and gradually learning to trust one another.

sexual abstinence delaying or refraining from sexual intimacy.

Chapter 17 Highlights Strategies

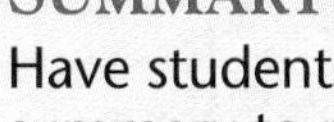

Summary

Have students read the summary to reinforce the concepts they learned in Chapter 17.

Vocabulary

Review the vocabulary words with students for understanding. Be certain all are clear on the distinction between sexual intimacy and emotional intimacy.

Extension

This chapter has discussed teen relationships in the United States. If you have students from other countries in the class, ask them to describe any differences they see between relationships among U.S. teens and among teens in their country.

Chapter 17 Assessment

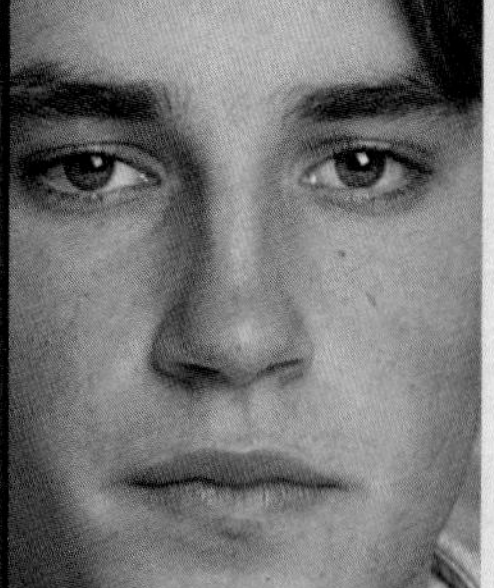

Chapter Review

Chapter Review

Concept Review

1. c.	4. c
2. a	5. d
3. b	6. a

Expressing Your Views

Sample responses:

1. Answers will vary with individual opinions. Students most likely will answer emotional growth, because emotions at this time may be more intense or the person may react to various familiar situations with different emotions than before. Adolescents may find that things will seem easier once they develop the ability to recognize and control emotions.

2. Some people may find it hard to make friends because they are shy or because they have low self-esteem. Some people may find it hard to maintain friendships because they do not know how to communicate effectively. They may not be trustworthy; they may use "you" statements instead of "I" statements; they may not be active listeners; they may try to pressure friends into doing what they want to do instead of compromising and doing what their friends want to do; they may not be tolerant of differences between themselves and their friends.

Concept Review

1. The period of physical development in which the body becomes able to produce children is called
   a. adulthood. b. childhood.
   c. puberty. d. adolescence.
2. Revealing your feelings before you know the feelings of another is the level of communication called
   a. self-disclosing.
   b. directing or arguing.
   c. information giving.
   d. exploring.
3. The process of hearing the words of the speaker and clarifying anything that is confusing is known as
   a. nonverbal communication.
   b. active listening.
   c. mixed messages.
   d. "you" and "I" messages.
4. The RESPECT method is used to
   a. resist pressure. b. listen actively.
   c. resolve conflicts. d. communicate nonverbally.
5. A friend is someone
   a. you feel comfortable with.
   b. who is trustworthy.
   c. who shows empathy.
   d. All of these.
6. Which of the following is not a high-risk situation if you have decided to delay sexual intimacy?
   a. group activities, such as movies and sports
   b. parties where alcohol is served
   c. using drugs on a date
   d. studying at home alone with your boyfriend or girlfriend

Expressing Your Views

1. In your opinion, what is the most difficult thing about adolescence? What would make it easier?
2. Some people find it hard to make and maintain friends. Why do you think this is true?

Life Skills Check

Sample responses:

1. I would tell him not to worry and that people develop at different rates. The age at which puberty begins varies from as young as 8 years to as old as 16 years.

2. Renew or make new acquaintances with cousins or other family members that are near your own age.

Chapter 17 Assessment

Life Skills Check

1. **Communicating Effectively**
   Your younger brother is 14 years old and still looks like he did when he was 12. He seems to be concerned about this. What advice would you give him?

2. **Coping**
   Your family is planning to attend the yearly family reunion. You can't imagine anything more boring than listening to the same old family stories. All you can think about is the upcoming school dance and whether your new friend will ask you out. You feel as if you must go to the reunion. What could you do to make your family day pleasant?

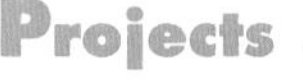

Projects

1. Select a biography or historical story about someone and note what you can about this person's teenage years. Look for events, circumstances, and behaviors that were different from the experiences of your adolescent years. Report your findings in writing.

2. Write *age 5*, *age 9*, and *age 14* across the top of a poster board. Under each age, list games and activities you enjoyed as well as any responsibilities you might have had at that particular time in your life. Evaluate why the list changed from age to age and report this information to the class.

3. Choose three letters from an advice column dealing with teenage relationship problems. Without looking at the advice offered, write your own responses to the problems. Then compare your responses to the ones given in the paper. Bring the letters and both sets of responses to class for discussion.

Plan for Action

The period between childhood and adulthood is an intense time of change that can be very difficult. Create a plan to help you cope with this period of transition.

Projects

Have students complete the projects on adolescence.

Plan for Action

Students now need to apply the valuable skills they've learned in communicating and resisting pressure. Ask them to describe upcoming situations in which they will need these skills, such as a problem at home or in a relationship, or a special date. In each case, have the class formulate an action plan to handle the problem.

Assessment Options

Chapter Test

Have students take the Chapter 17 Test.

Alternative Assessment

Have students do the Alternative Assessment activity for Chapter 17.

Test Generator

The Test Generator (Macintosh® or IBM® format) contains an additional 50 assessment items for this chapter.

CHAPTER 18

ADULTHOOD, MARRIAGE, AND PARENTHOOD

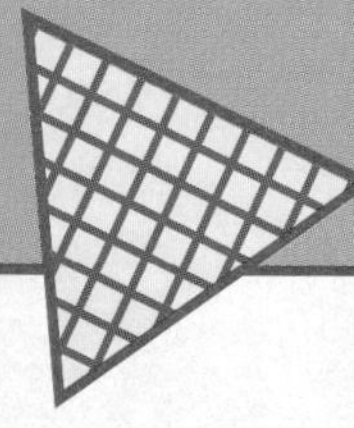

PLANNING GUIDE

TEXT SECTIONS	OBJECTIVES	TEXT FEATURES	OUTSIDE RESOURCES	NOTES
18.1 **Adulthood** pp. 385-392 2 periods	• Know the three stages of adulthood. • Define emotional maturity. • Name three concerns an elderly person might have. ■ Identify the difficulty of coping with a grandparent who has Alzheimer's disease.	■ LIFE SKILLS, Coping, p. 388 **ASSESSMENT** • Section Review, p. 392	**TEACHER'S RESOURCE BINDER** • Lesson Plan 18.1 • Personal Health Inventory • Journal Entry 18A • Life Skills 18A, 18B • Section Review Worksheet 18.1 • Section Quiz 18.1 • Reteaching Worksheet 18.1 **OTHER RESOURCES** • Transparency 18A • Making a Choice 18A	
18.2 **Marriage and Parenthood** pp. 393-398 2 periods	• Name two reasons why people get married. • List three ingredients that can help a marriage be successful. • Name three difficulties teenagers who marry may face. • Name three responsibilities of parenthood.	• Check Up, p. 397 **ASSESSMENT** • Section Review, p. 398	**TEACHER'S RESOURCE BINDER** • Lesson Plan 18.2 • Journal Entry 18B • Life Skills 18C • Section Review Worksheet 18.2 • Section Quiz 18.2 • Reteaching Worksheet 18.2 **OTHER RESOURCES** • Making a Choice 18B	
End of Chapter pp. 399-401		**ASSESSMENT** • Chapter Review, pp. 400-401	**TEACHER'S RESOURCE BINDER** • Chapter Test • Alternative Assessment **OTHER RESOURCES** • Test Generator	

■ Denotes LIFE SKILLS objectives

• Items in blue are also part of the *Holt Health Activity Book*.

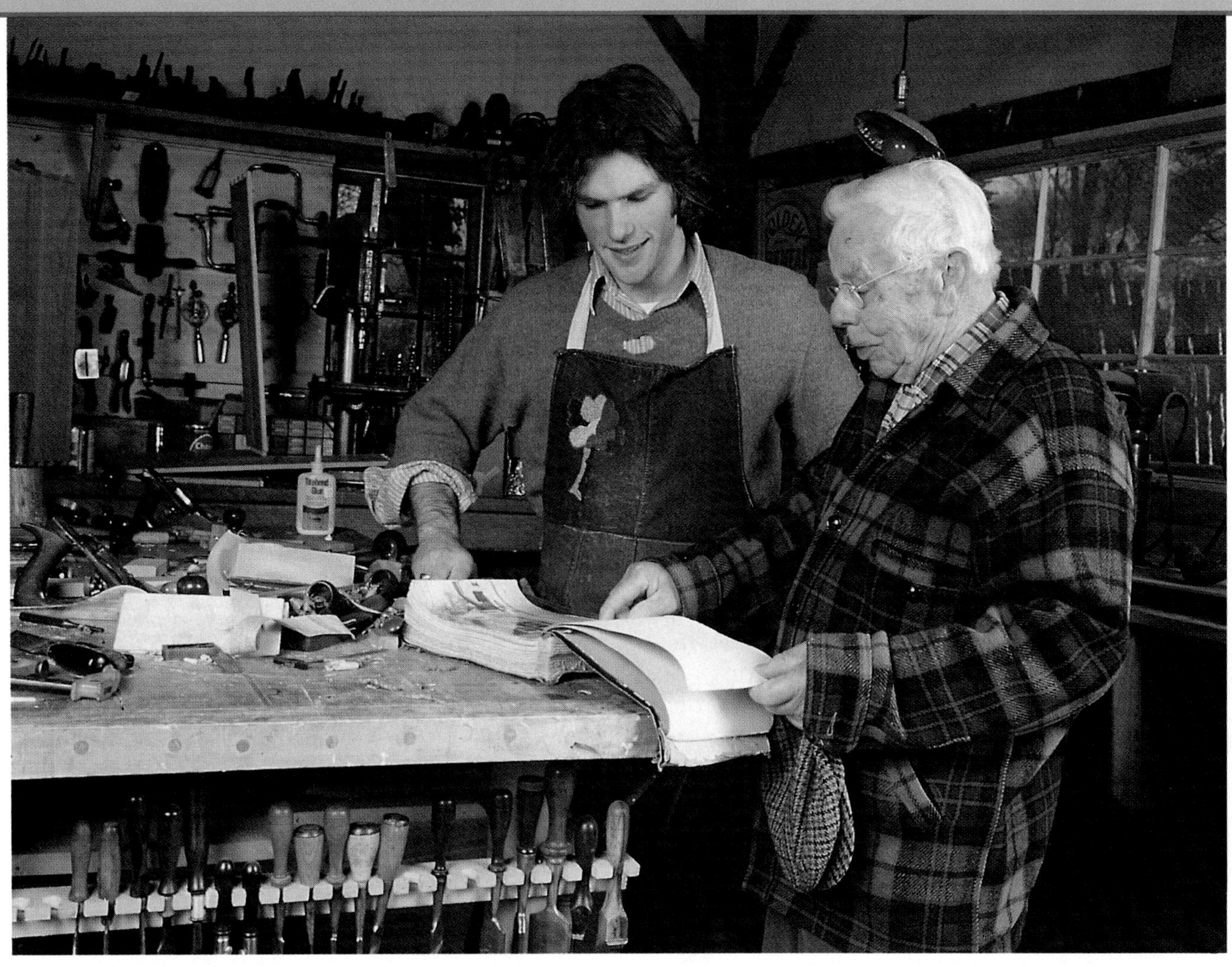

CONTENT BACKGROUND Social Costs of Ageism

AGEISM IS THE TERM USED TO REFER TO prejudice against older people. As with any type of prejudice, a certain amount of slang and euphemism has been created. The use of euphemisms for old age has increased over the last few years. Political correctness dictates the use of the terms "senior citizen" and "the golden years" instead of terms such as "old people" and "old age." The use of derogatory terms like "old maid" and "old fogey" is declining but not gone. The use of euphemism and slang indicates discomfort with the concept of aging. There is a fear that sexuality is only for the young. Patronizing adjectives such as cute, little, spry, adorable, and precious—some of the same words used for children—are applied to the elderly. This suggests that they are somehow not complete people.

The fears of old age are often unfounded, based on ignorance and stereotypes. Prejudice stems in part from a natural fear of getting old and dying. But the view of old age as lonely, intellectually uninteresting, emotionally rigid, and asexual frightens people unnecessarily. In fact, most people over the age of 65 are relatively independent: only 5 percent are in nursing homes. And older people usually retain their personalities, not becoming conservative and inflexible, as stereotypes suggest. Even older people may feel that, though they themselves are independent and energetic, they are the exception. In fact, they are the rule.

Misconceptions about aging are largely the result of the lack of contact between young and old. In part this is because nuclear families often live apart from the grandparents and do not have daily knowledge of them. It is also because, for economic and political reasons, people are forced to retire from work earlier than they otherwise might.

Should an individual retire automatically at the age of 65? Is it best for the employee? Is it in the best interest of our economy to have our work force leaving active income production at a preset age? Sometime between 2010 and 2020 the amount of money being paid into the social security system by wage earners will slip below the necessary amount needed to pay benefits. In 1983, Congress tried to prepare for this by passing a tax increase designed to create a surplus of $2.5 trillion to be placed in a trust fund by the early part of the next century. However, that money is now used for the operation of government. The trust consists of IOUs or government bonds. Taxes will need to increase again in order to pay the IOUs. Some estimates say that if mandatory retirement were gradually increased to age 72 by the year 2060, the system could be kept in balance without any tax hike.

Another reason for increasing the retirement age has to do with the decline in population growth. It is a misconception that retiring older workers make room for the young. The pool of young people entering the work force is shrinking, and the demand for higher skilled and experienced workers is rising. By the year 2000 there will be 15 million fewer young people to fill 21 million new jobs. Add to this an overall shortage of skilled workers and a clear problem in this country's future emerges.

In addition to their numbers, older people contribute skills and experience to the workplace. The demand for highly skilled workers is increasing; jobs are becoming more complex technologically and require stronger reading and communications abilities. Sixty percent of the new jobs will require strong skills, while only 25 percent of young workers will have the skills to compete for them. The number of low-skilled jobs is declining, while 75 percent of the work force compete for them.

It does not make sense to retire highly skilled workers at a time when they are needed. There are signs that the retirement age is indeed moving up. Extending the active participation of older people in the economic realm of the country may influence the way younger people see and speak of them. Ageism is a product of many misconceptions, some of which are being changed.

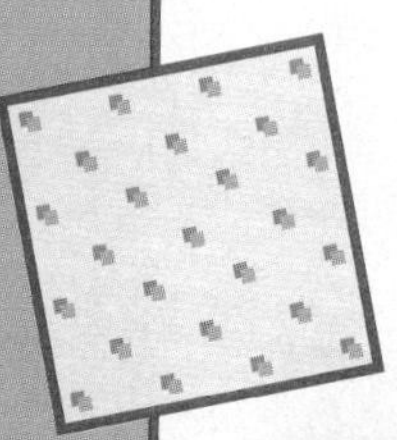

PLANNING FOR INSTRUCTION

KEY FACTS

- **People continue to change throughout their lives; adulthood is a time for gaining emotional maturity, making important life decisions, becoming reconciled to changes and losses, and accepting the aging process.**
- **The elderly face problems with mandatory retirement, ageism, finding appropriate housing, and the many adjustments that physical changes can bring.**
- **A successful marriage requires emotional maturity, mutual love and respect, and the ability to compromise and communicate.**
- **The demands of parenthood include the financial and emotional support of another human being.**
- **Marriage and parenthood are even more challenging for teenagers, who are likely to lack the necessary maturity and financial resources to meet the additional responsibilities.**
- **Many couples defer the responsibilities of parenthood by using various contraceptive methods, such as birth control pills, condoms, and diaphragms.**

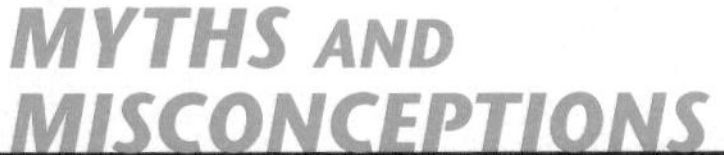

MYTHS AND MISCONCEPTIONS

MYTH: Memory loss is inevitable with aging.

Short-term memory changes very little, if at all, with aging. Long-term memory begins to decline before the middle years, but not for everyone and not at any set rate.

MYTH: In old age, health problems are inevitable.

In fact, many of the health problems associated with old age are preventable or can be controlled. Some of the conditions that were once thought to result from the aging process are now believed to be due largely to poor diet and a sedentary lifestyle.

MYTH: People fall in love and stay in love—their feelings for each other won't change if it's really love.

Healthy relationships encompass many envolving dynamics. If a couple's relationship develops as they go through life, they will fall in love in different ways many times over the course of many decades. Romantic love or physical attraction may be the strongest first attachment. However, mutual respect, shared experiences, children, appreciation for unique qualities, commitment, and personal growth change the nature of people's love for one another as they themselves change.

VOCABULARY

Essential: The following vocabulary terms appear in boldface type.

young adulthood	Alzheimer's disease
emotional maturity	Parkinson's disease
middle adulthood	divorce
older adulthood	contraception

Secondary: Be aware that the following terms may come up during class discussion:

ageism	separation
menopause	diaphragm
mandatory retirement	rhythm method

FOR STUDENTS WITH SPECIAL NEEDS

Visual Learners: Have students create a time line of their own showing the three stages of adulthood as they hope to experience them. Encourage students to illustrate important life events they may anticipate, such as career, marriage, family, new home, losses, etc. For example, students might draw pictures of themselves at different ages, and write articles or letters to show possible achievements or experiences.

At-Risk Students: Have students interview school counselors and any teenagers who are married and/or parents to learn about the special needs and problems of teen marriage and parenthood. They can present their findings in a panel, and take questions from the audience afterward.

ENRICHMENT

- Students can create a set of feature articles on the topics of marriage, parenthood, and aging. They may want to explore recent trends, research case studies, or write from their own experience. They could use the lifestyle section of a newspaper for inspiration or models.
- Students may enjoy reading Gail Sheehy's *Passages: Predictable Crises of Adult Life* (NY: E. P. Dutton, 1974). It follows adult development through the twenties, thirties, and forties, describing changes as well as the inner and outer forces that act upon us. Have students work together to create a presentation on passages for the rest of the class.

Chapter 18 Chapter Opener

GETTING STARTED

Using the Chapter Photograph

Have students speculate about the decisions they think this couple made before taking this step. What skills and qualities do they think are needed to make a marriage work? When do students think they might be ready for marriage, and why?

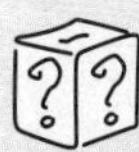

Question Box

The Question Box provides students with an opportunity to ask questions anonymously. To ensure that students with questions are not embarrassed to be seen writing, have those who do not have questions write something else—such as something they already know about marriage, parenthood, or aging—on the paper instead.

Preview the questions and then answer them at appropriate points in the chapter. You may wish to allow students to write additional anonymous questions as they go through the chapter.

Personal Issues *ALERT*

Many of your students will be affected by divorce and the special concerns of caring for an older relative. Some students may be coping with parenthood themselves. By creating a caring but direct approach to the topics of this chapter and fostering frank, open discussion, you may help these students feel at ease and willing to offer valuable insights.

Chapter 18

Adulthood, Marriage, and Parenthood

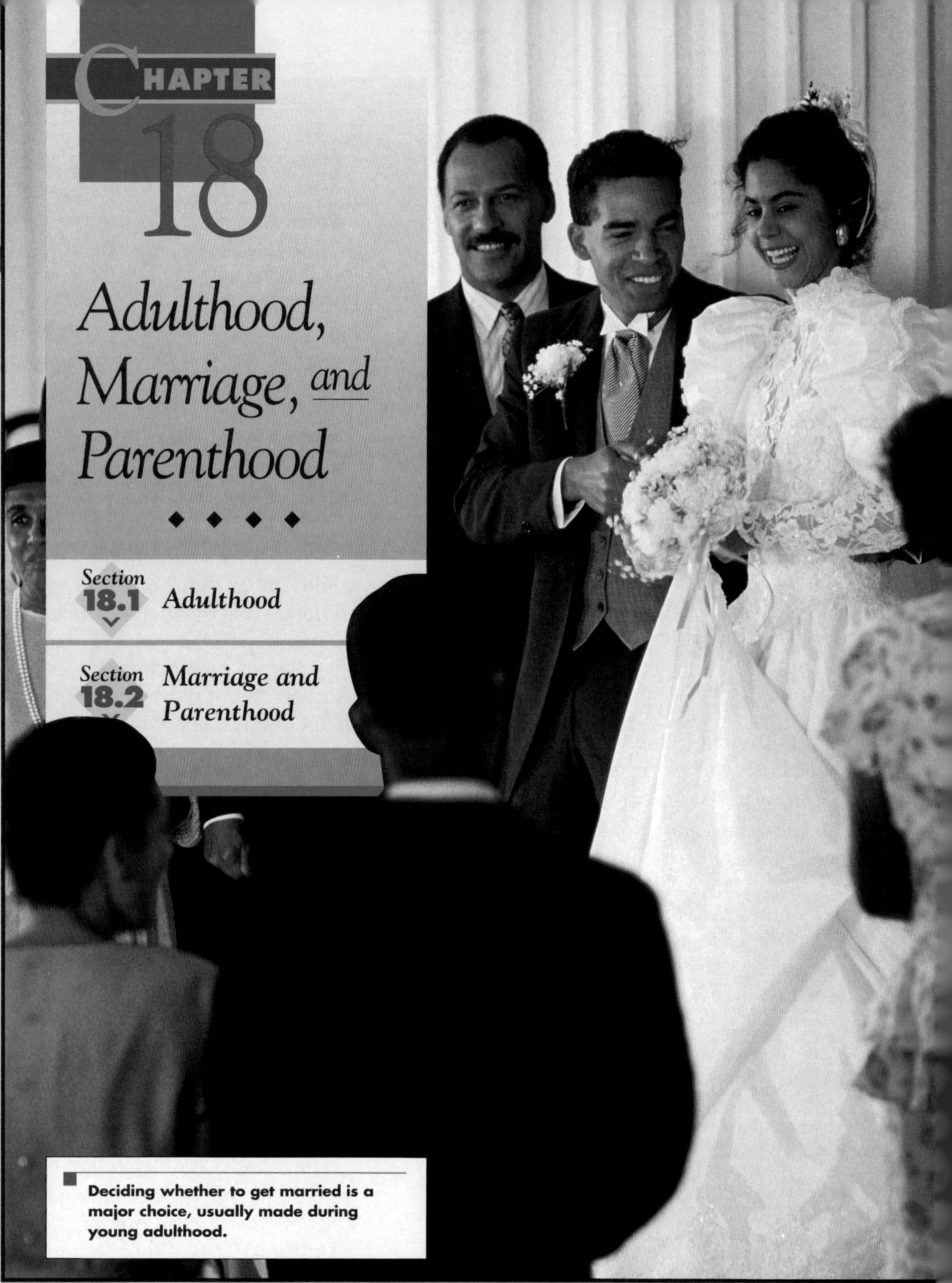

Deciding whether to get married is a major choice, usually made during young adulthood.

Carmen had a pretty strange dream last night. She dreamed it was her wedding day but she hadn't bought a dress. She also hadn't chosen a place to live, a job she wanted to do, or even the person she was going to marry. When she awoke, Carmen laughed out loud. But she also had to admit that she was relieved she would not have to make those kinds of decisions for several more years. Being an adult, she thought to herself, can't be all that easy.

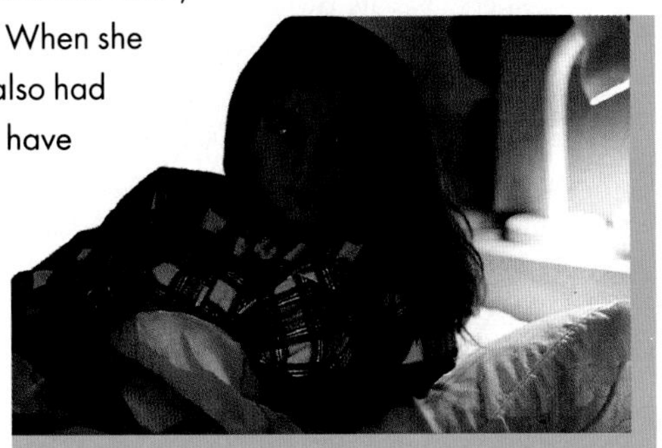

Section 18.1 Adulthood

Objectives

- *Know the three stages of adulthood.*
- *Define emotional maturity.*
- *Name three concerns an elderly person might have.*
- *Identify the difficulty of coping with a grandparent who has Alzheimer's disease.*
  LIFE SKILLS: Coping

It may seem as though you'll be young forever. The thought of being an adult might bring a mixture of excitement and anxiety. How will you know what choices to make? Will you want to get married, or remain single? What kind of parent will you be? As you leave your teenage years and enter your twenties, many of these questions will become clearer to you. Even so, every day of your adult life you will be faced with decisions—some obvious, others more difficult.

In that way, adulthood doesn't differ that much from adolescence. Life never becomes easy for anyone, but your adult years will offer you opportunities to accomplish goals, and the freedom to pursue the dreams, you are setting for yourself now.

The Stages of Adulthood

How will you know when you're an adult? Will you wake up one morning and just feel different? In the United States, a person is legally an adult when he or she turns 18. That doesn't mean, of course, that the person you are on your 18th birthday is the person you'll be for the rest of your life. In fact, you are likely to change just as much during your adulthood as you do during your teenage years. Adulthood is divided into three stages: young adulthood, middle adulthood, and older adulthood.

Young Adulthood Even though Americans are considered legal adults at the age of

Background
Aging Population
From 1900 to 1990, the number of Americans over age 65 grew 900 percent. From 1990 to 2030, the American population over 65 will increase another 75 percent. Persons over 85 are now the fastest-growing segment of the U.S. population.

Section 18.1 Lesson Plan

MOTIVATE

Class Discussion

As a warm-up activity, have students respond to these questions: When does a person become an adult? Is the meaning of adulthood different for a parent? a grandparent?

TEACH

Class Discussion
Kinds of Maturity

Write on the chalkboard "An adult is mature." Ask students what this statement means to them. Organize the following information to illustrate the aspects of maturity they discuss.

An adult is mature physically when:
- sexually mature
- physiologically mature

An adult is socially mature when:
- responsible for self
- accepts responsibility for others

An adult is emotionally mature when:
- independent
- capable of sustained relationships

How is maturity a lifelong process?
[As people grow and develop new relationships, their responses to various types of people, situations, and challenges all affect their emotional development.]

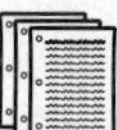

Personal Health Inventory

Have students complete the Personal Health Inventory for this chapter. The inventory helps them assess their emotional maturity at this time in their lives.

Making a Choice 18A

Emotional Maturity

Assign the Emotional Maturity card. The card directs students to read about a conflict situation and come up with three ways to handle the conflict in a way that demonstrates emotional maturity.

young adulthood: *the period of adulthood between the ages of 20 and 40.*

middle adulthood: *the period of adulthood between the ages of 41 and 65.*

emotional maturity: *the capacity to act independently, responsibly, and unselfishly. Being emotionally mature requires having compassion, integrity, and self-esteem.*

18, a person who is 18 is still technically a teenager. According to most guidelines, a person is in the stage of **young adulthood** between the ages of 20 and 40. Young adulthood has its own series of decisions and challenges. Most people who marry, for example, do so during this stage of adulthood. You will most likely choose the career you want to pursue early in your adulthood as well. In addition, the friends you choose during your young adult years may be the longest lasting of your life.

Decisions such as these require a certain degree of maturity. There are two types of maturity. The first of these, physical maturity, is usually an automatic part of growing up. Being physically mature simply means being fully developed and fully grown. This happens to most people by the time they are in their early twenties. The second type of maturity, **emotional maturity**, is not quite as automatic. People who are emotionally mature have the capacity to form close relationships yet act independently, and to make decisions that are responsible and unselfish. Being emotionally mature requires having the self-esteem to appreciate your talents when you perform well, and to forgive and like yourself when times are hard.

No one can be emotionally mature all the time—everyone makes mistakes. But being equipped with a proper amount of emotional maturity will make the decisions you face during your entire adulthood a lot easier to make. For that reason, emotional maturity is a major goal to attain during young adulthood.

Middle Adulthood The **middle adulthood** years, the period between the ages of 41 and 65, are for some people the most enjoyable time of adult life. Some of life's most difficult choices—marriage, career, and parenthood, for example—have been made during the young adult years. Middle age can present a time to savor and appreciate those experiences.

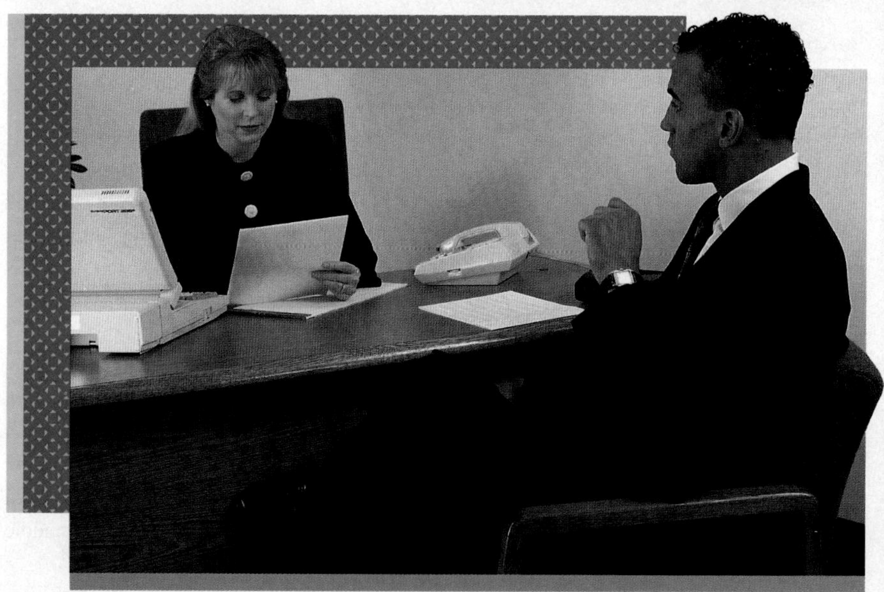

(FIGURE 18-1) **Finding the right job is one of the most important decisions young adults face.**

• • • TEACH continued

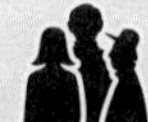

Cooperative Learning

Stages of Adulthood

Have students work in small groups to list experiences and characteristics they associate with the three phases of adulthood. Each group can clip or draw pictures and find quotes to create a collage, poster, or other visual impression of one of the phases.

Journal 18A

What Makes Romance in Middle Age?

Ask students to refer to Figure 18-2 and read its caption. How might this couple's marriage have changed over the years? Have them write in the Student Journal in the Student Activity Book their thoughts about the physical and emotional changes that may affect a good marriage by the time partners reach middle age.

Class Discussion

Debunking the Myths

Have students refer to Myths and Facts About Aging and point out the facts that most surprised them. **What might account for the increase in knowledge of the elderly?** *[Life experience—most older people not only retain their mental ability, they continue to learn and grow, and are frequently more creative and flexible in their approaches to problem solving than their younger counterparts.]*

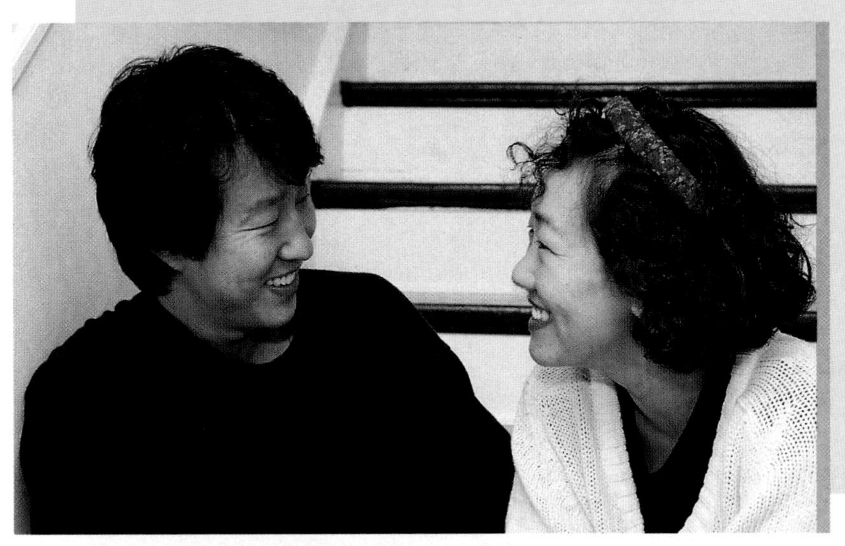

(FIGURE 18-2) **Middle adulthood is often a time to savor the romance of a good marriage and the satisfaction of a happy life.**

Middle adulthood does involve a series of physical and emotional changes. Hair may turn gray, some wrinkles will develop, a few pounds will probably be gained. In addition, most women stop menstruating during the middle adult years. Once a woman permanently ceases to menstruate, she can no longer bear children. Some women find this occurrence, known as menopause, disheartening. Others welcome the end of their menstrual cycle. Middle-aged men and women who are unhappy in their career may start to question whether the choices they made during young adulthood were the right ones. In addition, middle-aged adults often find themselves confronting death for the first time. Losing a spouse, a parent, or a close friend is very painful and is a reminder that life must end for everyone.

Parents in the middle-adult stage may also experience feelings of sadness when their children become adults and leave home. Although a change like this requires adjustment, married parents sometimes find that it brings romance to their relationship.

Older Adulthood The **older adulthood** stage, which begins at the age of 65, was once an almost miraculous feat to accomplish. A person born in the year 1900 had a life expectancy of no more than 47 years. Today, more people than ever can expect to reach the stage of older adulthood.

older adulthood:

the period of adulthood past the age of 65.

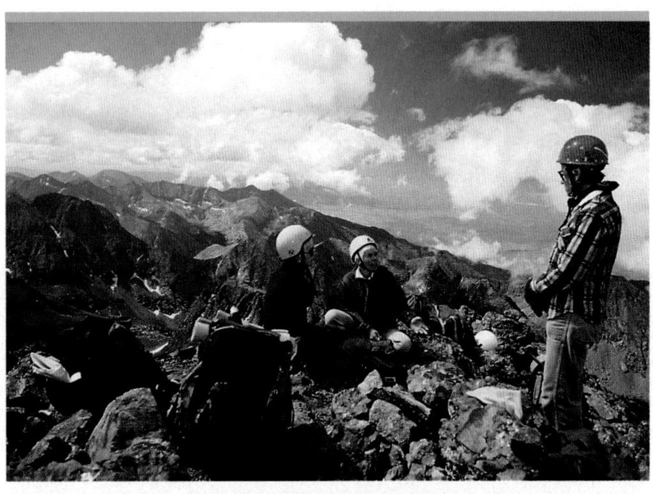

(FIGURE 18-3) **Older adults often find that they have more time for leisurely and healthy activities, such as exercise.**

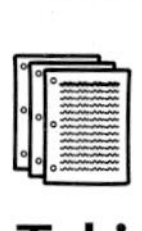

Life Skills Worksheet 18A

Taking Steps to Meet Future Goals

Assign the Taking Steps to Meet Future Goals Life Skills Worksheet, which requires students to list goals they want to reach in adulthood and to describe steps they can take now to reach those goals.

Role-playing

What About Grandparents?

Have small groups of students create a scenario for an extended family that wants to convince an ailing grandparent to make an important life change (give up driving, live with children, move to a retirement home). Have each group create a dialogue among family members; students can switch roles, so that each has a chance to consider the effects of the decision on child, parent, and grandparent.

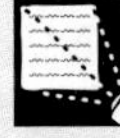

Teaching Transparency 18A

The Healthy Older Adult

Show students the transparency of a healthy older person. Have them list things the person does to maintain each of the following: physical health (brushes and flosses teeth daily; has regular physical exams; exercises regularly; wears sensible shoes), mental health (reads and enjoys intellectual activities), and emotional health (has an active social life; has warm, caring relationships with family, friends, and pets; feels satisfied with life; proud of gray hair).

Encourage students to talk about older people they know who are healthy and about the things they do to stay healthy.

Case Study

Gray Panthers Fight Ageism

Have students put together a case study on the actions of the Gray Panthers, or on the work of the American

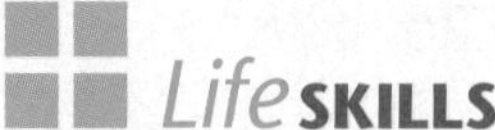

A Family Member With Alzheimer's Disease

Have students read the feature about a family member with Alzheimer's disease. Then have volunteers role-play scenes in which Nate talks to friends or family members about his grandfather.

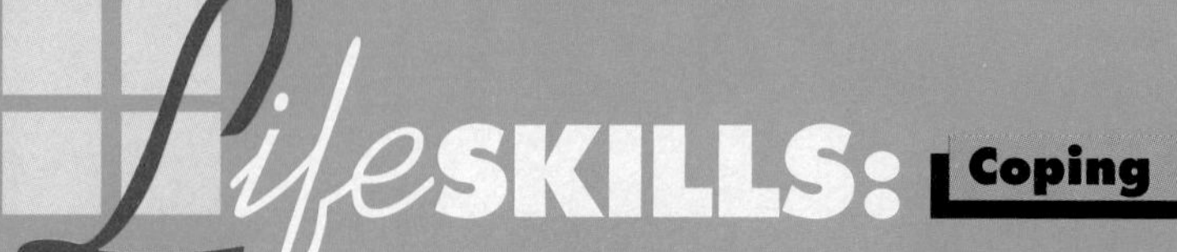

A Family Member With Alzheimer's Disease . . . .

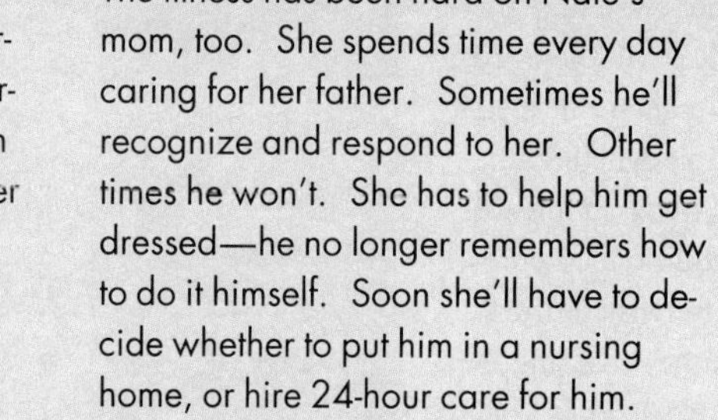

At first Nate wasn't especially upset by his grandfather's forgetfulness. That just happens when people get old, he thought to himself. Then one night Nate's mother got a call from the police. Nate's grandfather had been found wandering around his neighborhood, lost. "How could Grandpa be lost in his own neighborhood?" Nate asked his mom, who was equally puzzled.

Nate's mom took his grandfather to a doctor. After doing some tests, the doctor asked Nate's family to come in for a meeting.

The news wasn't good. Nate's grandfather has Alzheimer's disease, an incurable illness that gradually destroys a person's memory. Eventually a person with Alzheimer's will not be able to remember how to do things that once came naturally—like reading and writing. The names of family members may be forgotten—many Alzheimer's sufferers don't recognize their own spouses or children.

In the several months since he was diagnosed, Nate's grandfather has gotten progressively worse. Sometimes he stares at Nate for long periods of time without speaking. Other times he'll yell at him for no reason.

The illness has been hard on Nate's mom, too. She spends time every day caring for her father. Sometimes he'll recognize and respond to her. Other times he won't. She has to help him get dressed—he no longer remembers how to do it himself. Soon she'll have to decide whether to put him in a nursing home, or hire 24-hour care for him.

Nate spends time every day thinking about his grandfather. He's also shared some memories of his grandfather with his friends from school. His friends know that Nate needs to talk about his grandfather, but they're not always sure what they should say to him. What would *you* say?

• • • TEACH continued

Association of Retired Persons and the National Council on Aging. The Gray Panthers, for instance, founded in 1970, work to end mandatory retirement, age discrimination, and negative stereotyping. How have these organizations changed public responses to the elderly? What changes have they effected in services such as Social Security, Medicare and Medicaid, and housing and job discrimination laws?

Extension

Contributions of the Elderly

The image of the elderly as sick, senile, and sedentary doesn't fit today. More and more people are remaining vital and productive into their 80s and 90s. Some students may enjoy researching and reporting on the late-life contributions of Pablo Picasso, Michelangelo, George Bernard Shaw, Agatha Christie, Georgia O'Keefe, and others.

Young Adulthood: Making Decisions

Have students interview a young adult about job and family decisions and ways his or her perspectives have changed since adolescence.

Many people think of older adulthood as a time characterized by physical and mental deterioration. It's true that the older a person is, the more likely he or she is to get certain illnesses and conditions. Someone who is 65 is much more likely to suffer cancer, heart disease, and arthritis, for example, than a person who is 21. Cancer, heart disease, and arthritis are discussed in greater detail in Chapter 24. **Alzheimer's disease**, an incurable illness characterized by a gradual and permanent loss of memory, and **Parkinson's disease**, which causes a gradual loss of muscle function, are two other serious diseases that most commonly affect the elderly.

Even so, many elderly adults can remain happy and healthy for many years. For these individuals, older adulthood provides an opportunity for family, relaxation, and happy reflection on what have been rich, fulfilling lives.

Aging

To a very large extent, the choices that you make now will influence how healthy you will remain as you grow older. For example, a person who exercises and eats regular, nutritious meals is much less likely to suffer heart disease than an inactive person who eats foods high in fat and cholesterol.

Common Concerns Physical well-being is an essential concern of aging, but it is not the only one. Jesse's grandparents, for example, had a happy life together for 40 years. But when Jesse's grandfather died last year, his grandmother was left alone. During the past year her health has gotten progressively worse. Jesse's parents are worried about her and have asked her to move in with them. But whenever they bring the subject up, Jesse's grandmother gets angry and defensive. "You don't trust me to take care of myself," she says.

Cancer, heart disease, and arthritis are discussed in greater detail in Chapter 24.

Alzheimer's disease: *an incurable illness characterized by a gradual and permanent loss of memory. Alzheimer's disease most commonly affects the elderly.*

Parkinson's disease: *an incurable disease characterized by a gradual loss of control of muscle function. Parkinson's disease most commonly affects the elderly.*

Myths and Facts About Aging

Myth	Fact
Most older people are sickly and unable to take care of themselves.	*Only 5 percent of elderly people live in nursing homes. The remainder are fairly healthy and self-sufficient.*
Intelligence declines with age.	*Most people actually become more knowledgeable as they get older.*
Older people should stop exercising and get a lot of rest.	*Exercise at any age strengthens heart and lung function. Older people can benefit as much from exercising as anyone else.*
People's personalities change as they get older.	*People's circumstances may change when they become older adults, but their personalities don't.*

Background

Alzheimer's History and Facts

In 1906, Dr. Alois Alzheimer, a German neuropathologist, studied the brain tissue of a patient who had died after suffering loss of memory and reason. Under the microscope, he saw the two brain tissue abnormalities typical of Alzheimer's disease: tangled nerve fibers and plaque buildup around nerves. An absolutely certain diagnosis of Alzheimer's is still only possible from brain-tissue biopsy or autopsy. Diagnosis comes after thorough physical, neurological, and psychological examination. Over time, an Alzheimer's sufferer experiences changes in memory, thought, personality, and language; the condition gradually worsens until death comes, usually brought on by a secondary infection. A progressive, degenerative disease, its cause and cure are at present unknown. Very rare in people under 40, Alzheimer's is more common as people get older. It occurs in 20 to 30 percent of people age 85 and older.

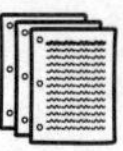

Life Skills Worksheet 18B

Caring for an Older Person

Assign the Caring for an Older Person Life Skills Worksheet, which asks students to imagine an older person they care about becoming ill and needing extra care. It also asks them to assess their feelings about aging and older people.

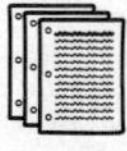

Section Review Worksheet 18.1

Assign Section Review Worksheet 18.1, which requires students to identify characteristics of younger, middle, and older adulthood, and to discuss ways to help the elderly with some of their most difficult concerns.

One afternoon after school when Jesse stops by to say hello to his grandmother, she tells him that she's beginning to worry about finances. Her utility bills keep rising, and she's concerned that if she were to become very ill she wouldn't be able to afford good medical care.

"Why don't you move in with us?" Jesse asks her. "We'll take care of you." But his grandmother worries about that too. She doesn't want to burden her children. "You and your family have your own home and your own life," she tells Jesse. "You're not going to want to take care of a helpless old woman."

Jesse's grandmother's concerns are not at all unusual. Elderly people must consider and cope with circumstances that younger people don't have to worry about. For example, many companies have mandatory retirement policies, which means that once a person reaches a certain age, he or she must stop working for that company.

Filling the sudden increase of leisure time with fulfilling activities can be a challenge. Some elderly people rise to this challenge admirably, and pursue options such as volunteer work or travel with enthusiasm. Others, though, find the sudden freedom overwhelming and depressing.

Cultural DIVERSITY

Growing Old in China

"I dread getting old," you hear people say. It seems that in our society, getting old often means losing much of what we value. But in other cultures, growing old can have an entirely different meaning.

In many cultures, the older people are the most knowledgeable about the things that make life possible. They know how the weather affects the crops, for example, and they know the habits of the domesticated animals. They are the repositories of knowledge. To exclude old people in these cultures would be akin to destroying libraries in our own society.

Though many cultures have shown great respect for the old, ancient China was extreme in this characteristic. Respect for older people was one of the

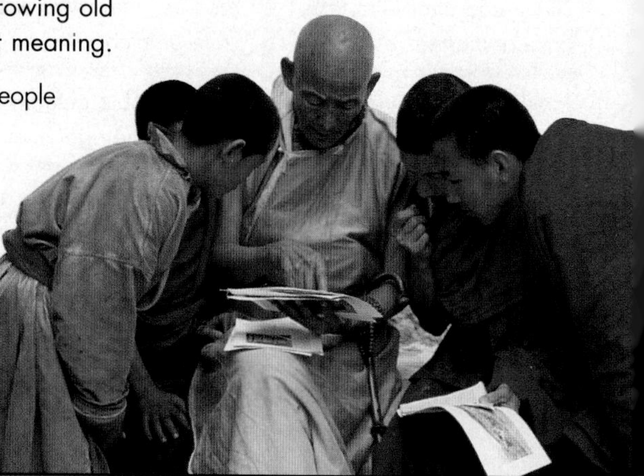

Loneliness can also be a problem for elderly people. Jesse's grandmother is luckier than many older adults—even though she has lost a spouse, she has a loving family who wants her to move in with them. The death of a spouse can leave some elderly people completely alone and isolated.

Another problem elderly people sometimes face is age discrimination. Also called "ageism," age discrimination occurs when a person is judged solely on the basis of his or her age. If, for example, a company chooses to hire a young person rather than an older person who is more qualified for the job, that company is practicing age discrimination.

Like all prejudices, age discrimination results from ignorance. It is important to know that judging a person on the basis of age is as wrong as deciding not to like someone because of his or her race, religion, or physical impairment.

Needs of the Elderly Jesse's grandmother used to love to cook. Recently, however, she has lost interest in preparing foods. She doesn't even enjoy eating any-

most important tenets of the Confucian system of ethics. The tradition of revering the elderly was so strong that, in large measure, it survived the communist revolution of the 1940s and the Cultural Revolution of the 1960s.

The respect that Chinese people owed their parents was called *xiao*. To show *xiao* meant to obey one's parents, to be extremely polite to them, and to care for them in their old age. It was thought that nothing could repay parents for the gift of life, but *xiao* was at least a meager attempt.

Older people were considered so special that only they could have birthday celebrations. A birthday was not considered to be noteworthy unless it was a 60th, 70th, 80th, 88th, or 100th birthday.

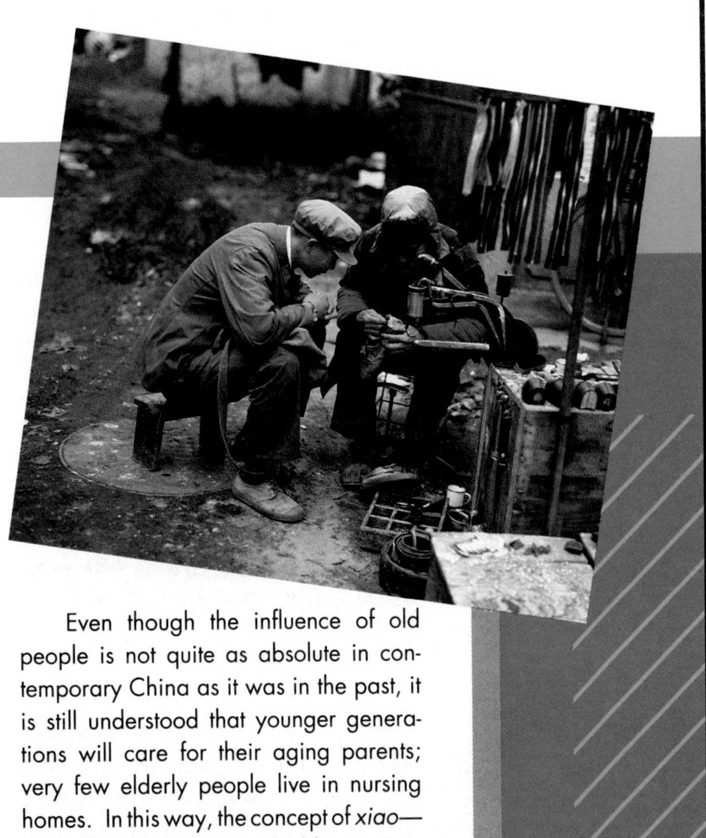

Even though the influence of old people is not quite as absolute in contemporary China as it was in the past, it is still understood that younger generations will care for their aging parents; very few elderly people live in nursing homes. In this way, the concept of *xiao*—a feeling of respect and obligation toward the aged—remains to tie the generations together.

Section Quiz 18.1

Have students take Section Quiz 18.1.

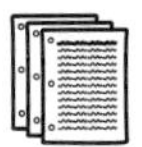

Reteaching Worksheet 18.1

Students who have difficulty with the material may complete Reteaching Worksheet 18.1, which requires them to read quotes from people in different stages of adulthood and to identify the stage.

Review Answers

1. Young adulthood, middle adulthood, older adulthood

2. Having the capacity to form close relationships yet act independently, responsibly, and unselfishly. Being emotionally mature requires having the self-esteem to appreciate your talents and to like yourself. Physical maturity happens to a person's body automatically.

3. Answers may include physical well-being; finances; becoming a burden to their family; mandatory retirement policies; age discrimination; alternative housing; nutrition.

4. Accept any response that shows students' understanding and empathy in dealing with a person who has a loved one with a debilitating disease.

5. Students may answer that Jesse's grandmother still wants to remain independent; by responding the way she did, she may be trying to cover up the problems she is experiencing. Also, she may not want to burden her family with her problems. Students may answer that they would have reacted in the same way.

Stress-management techniques are discussed in detail in Chapter 9.

more. Jesse's grandmother might be losing her sense of taste, which sometimes happens as a person gets older. She may need to eat specially prepared foods that are highly seasoned in order to enjoy meals again. Some organizations, such as Meals on Wheels, serve hot, specially prepared foods to people such as Jesse's grandmother, who are confined to their homes.

Another common need among elderly people is appropriate housing. Like Jesse's grandmother, most older adults prefer to live in their own homes for as long as they can. Modifications and adjustments can be made to make this possible. Special ramps, lighting, and wider doorways, for example, can make it possible for a person in a wheelchair to be mobile around the house.

If living at home becomes too difficult, though, a choice must be made. People who can afford to do so may choose to live in retirement communities, which offer special care and companionship.

Another option for people in this situation is to move in with family. Jesse's grandmother finally decided to do this. At first Jesse was surprised at how many adjustments had to be made. He could no longer listen to his radio late at night—it kept his grandmother awake. Sometimes he had to come straight home from school to care for her when no one else was around. But eventually Jesse grew to love living with his grandmother. She had great stories to tell, and she always had time to listen whenever something was troubling him.

Sometimes an elderly person can lose almost complete mental and physical functioning. When this happens, a nursing home may be recommended. A nursing home is a facility that offers special attention and long-term care for those who require it. Only about 5 percent of elderly people in the United States live in nursing homes.

Tips for Healthy Aging The most important thing you can do now to stay healthy in the years to come is to practice good health habits. You learned earlier that getting regular exercise and eating a healthy diet decrease your risk of suffering certain diseases when you get older. Getting regular physical checkups, seeing a dentist regularly, and practicing good hygiene are some other things you can do to help yourself remain healthy during the years to come.

Avoiding tobacco, alcohol, and other drugs can also help you stay healthy throughout your life. Some people turn to these drugs to help them handle stress. When not managed properly, stress can cause physical disease, but there are better ways to manage stress than to use drugs. The techniques discussed in Chapter 9 can help you do this.

Review

1. *Name the three stages of adulthood.*
2. *Define emotional maturity. How does it differ from physical maturity?*
3. *Describe three things an elderly person might be concerned about.*
4. ***LIFE SKILLS: Coping*** *What could you say to a friend who has just found out that his or her grandfather has Alzheimer's disease?*
5. ***Critical Thinking*** *Why do you think Jesse's grandmother reacted the way she did when Jesse's parents asked her to live with them? How do you think you would react?*

ASSESS

Section Review

Have students answer the Section Review questions.

Alternative Assessment

Jesse's Point of View

Ask students to write a two-minute monologue in which Jesse speaks. It should reveal Jesse's understanding of his grandmother's situation and feelings, and his own mixed emotions about her living with his family.

Closure

Maturity vs. Aging

Draw two large, overlapping circles on the chalkboard. Label one MATURITY and one AGING. Have students take turns coming to the board and writing a characteristic of aging or of maturity in the appropriate area. If a characteristic belongs to both, they should write it in the area of overlap.

Section 18.2 Marriage and Parenthood

Objectives

- *Name two reasons why people get married.*
- *List three ingredients that can help a marriage be successful.*
- *Name three difficulties teenagers who marry may face.*
- *Name three responsibilities of parenthood.*

Carmen, the girl discussed in the beginning of this chapter, has been seeing Danny for about two months. They really like being together—Carmen has feelings for Danny she's never had for anyone else. For that reason, she was kind of disturbed that Danny wasn't in her dream about getting married.

But the more she thought about it, the more she realized that it was pretty silly to think about marrying Danny—or anyone else, for that matter—at this time of her life. In fact, she wasn't all that sure she ever wanted to get married. As for having children—well, that can wait a while, too.

Why People Get Married

Carmen isn't certain how she feels about it yet, but when she gets older she may very well decide that she does want to get married. More than 90 percent of American adults have made that decision. There are several different reasons why people get married. Some people may get married for financial security. Others may do so because they want to have children, or because they seek the close companionship marriage can provide. Still others get married because it is expected of them, or because they are scared they will end up alone.

Perhaps the best reason why people get married is that they want to make a lifelong commitment to be with a person they love and respect.

Successful Marriage

The most important ingredients two people can bring to a marriage are love and respect. Marriage often involves putting the other person's needs before your own and making difficult sacrifices for the sake of your spouse's happiness. It takes a great deal of love and respect to do these things.

A third factor needed for a successful marriage is emotional maturity. The decisions you make when you are married affect not only yourself, but your spouse as well. What if a certain job you want involves moving across the country? What if you want to have children, but your spouse doesn't know if he or she wants them? The ability to compromise is one of the most important tools anyone can bring to a marriage. A person who is not emotionally mature would probably have a very hard time making these kinds of compromises.

One more ingredient that makes marriage successful is the ability to communicate effectively. Two people who are in a

Background

More on Contraception

Students may be curious about intrauterine devices (IUDs), which are implanted in the uterus to prevent conception. They are not recommended for adolescents, women who have not had children, or women who have had more than one sexual partner. Tubal ligation and vasectomy—operations that effectively sterilize women and men, respectively—are options for people who do not wish to have children at all or who have had all the children they plan to have. The following "methods" do not work:

- withdrawal (removal of penis just before ejaculation)
- douching (flushing the vagina with a solution after sex)
- having sex while the woman is menstruating

Section 18.2 Lesson Plan

MOTIVATE

Journal 18B

Marriage: Dream or Nightmare?

Ask students to put themselves in Carmen's place. Would it be a dream come true or their worst nightmare to marry now? Have students write their feelings in the Student Journal in the Student Activity Book.

TEACH

Class Discussion

Preparing for Marriage

Have students name and prioritize reasons why people get married. Let them discuss their points, then list the reasons on the board in order from most important to least important. Then ask: **What are you doing now that will prepare you for marriage?** *[Socializing and dating, taking on responsibilities at home, working and handling finances, making decisions; some may take classes or receive counseling just prior to marriage.]* Then discuss the following questions with students: How do you think young men and women should prepare for marriage? What qualities would make a person "the perfect date"? How do they differ from the qualities you would list for "the ideal mate"?

Background
Failure Rates of Contraceptive Methods
The following percentages of women become pregnant during the first year of continuous use of each type of contraceptive method:

vasectomy	0.2 %
tubal ligation	0.4 %
condom without spermicides	2 %
birth control pill	3 %
IUD	3 %
diaphragm with spermicides	18 %
sponge (female has not had baby)	18 %
(female has had baby)	28 %
periodic abstinence (rhythm)	20 %
spermicides alone	21 %
no contraception	85 %

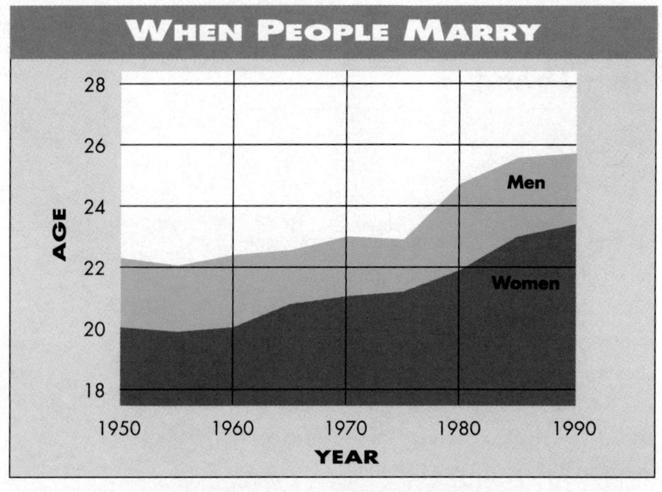

(FIGURE 18-5) **Studies show that men and women are getting married at an older age than they once did.**

lifelong partnership must be able to tell each other how they are feeling and what they are thinking. As they do in all relationships, conflicts will inevitably arise in marriage. People who are in a good marriage are able to resolve these conflicts through communication and respect. Conflict-resolution skills are discussed in some detail in Chapter 17.

Conflict-resolution skills are discussed in Chapter 17.

When two people are willing to make the commitment marriage requires, the result can be a rewarding, fulfilling relationship, well worth the work and compromise it requires.

Reasons People Don't Get Married

Like all of life's choices, marriage is not for everyone and is not right for every partnership. Two people who enjoy being together but are not willing to make necessary compromises, for example, probably would not be happy married to each other.

People who have very busy jobs that require extensive travel or whose jobs require that they move often may also choose not to marry. It's not always easy to juggle a busy, demanding career with marriage, although it can be done.

Some people decide not to get married simply because they prefer to remain single. The decision to remain single is the right one for many people. Those who don't marry usually have more time for friends and career and are generally able to be completely independent and self-sufficient. Marriage, they may feel, would jeopardize these freedoms.

Teen Marriage

In addition to the challenges of every marriage, teenage marriage has its own set of difficulties. It may be difficult for teenagers who are still in school to support each other financially. In order to make ends meet, married teenagers may find that they have to work full time and leave school to do so.

Having enough money to live on becomes more important—and more difficult to accomplish—if the married couple has a child to support. Married teenagers who are also parents will find it difficult to find the time and energy to do the things they once took for granted—such as going to the movies, eating out, or just being with friends.

The emotional responsibilities of marriage can also take their toll on teenagers. No one finds it easy to make the compromises and selfless decisions required for a successful marriage. But it can be especially difficult for teenagers, who are still developing emotionally and may not be ready to put another person's needs before their own.

• • • TEACH continued

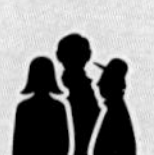

Cooperative Learning
Marriage—Think Before You Leap

Have students meet in small groups to brainstorm a list of factors they think two people should consider before they marry. Provide the following list and have students phrase questions to be answered by the couple: values, goals and interests, communication, finances, sexuality, extended family, children, conflict resolution. You might have pairs of students role-play scenes in which couples work through the issues involved in these questions.

Class Discussion
When People Marry

Ask a volunteer to interpret the trend represented in Figure 18-5. Encourage students to give reasons why young adults might be waiting longer to marry. Ask students to think about themselves 10 years from now, as young adults. What will they be doing? Will they be married? How will they prepare for the future?

Debate the Issue
Teenage Marriages

Have student teams debate the topic: Young people should not marry as teenagers. You may wish to allow some out-of-class time for research and preparation of arguments. Debaters should be ready to present their arguments, give counterarguments, and take questions from the class.

Divorce and Remarriage

Unfortunately, not all marriages are successful. When a marriage falters, some couples try living apart for an agreed period of time. Such an arrangement is called a separation. If one or both partners decide that the marriage has failed, a divorce will usually result. A **divorce** is the legal end of a marriage.

A divorce can be very painful, not only for the two people going through it, but also for their sons and daughters. Sometimes divorced people decide to marry again. Remarriage can also be difficult, particularly when there are children involved. Chapter 19 examines divorce and marriage in greater detail and offers some advice on ways to cope if your parents should divorce.

Parenthood

The decision to have children may be the most important one you will ever make. A commitment to a child is a lifelong commitment. Parenthood is rewarding and exciting. But it isn't easy. In fact, being a parent is a job that requires care and attention 24 hours each day, 7 days each week.

Family Planning Married couples often want to wait a little while before beginning a family. They can do this by using proper **contraception** every time they have sexual intercourse. Contraception is a device or method that prevents the fertilization of a woman's egg. Some methods of contraception are more reliable than others. Using a condom with spermicidal foam, for example, is a more effective method of contra-

Chapter 19 discusses the effects of divorce and remarriage on teenagers.

divorce:

the legal end to a marriage.

contraception:

a device or method that prevents the fertilization of a woman's egg.

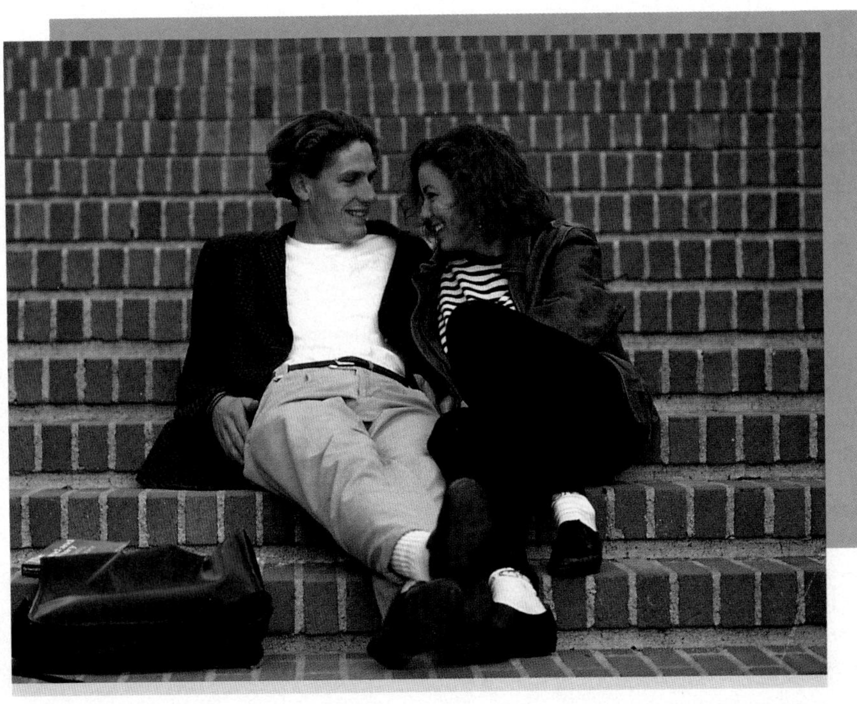

(FIGURE 18-6) **Dating is an exciting and pleasurable activity for many teenagers. But teenagers who decide to get married must contend with some very difficult circumstances.**

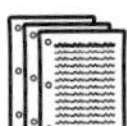

Life Skills Worksheet 18C

Obtaining Contraception

Assign the Obtaining Contraception Life Skills Worksheet, which helps students learn about and evaluate services at physicians' offices, clinics, and pharmacies where they can obtain contraceptive devices and information about using contraception.

Class Discussion

Contraception Issues

Discuss with students the issues involved in selecting a suitable means of contraception: religious beliefs or personal values, age, state of health, what partners are comfortable with, and effectiveness of the device or method.

Extension

More on Parenthood

Suggest that students visit local child-care facilities to observe small children. What are they like? What demands do they probably make on parents?

Making a Choice 18B

Parenthood: Doing It Right

Assign the Parenthood: Doing It Right card. This card encourages students to discuss with a partner three things their parents or guardians have done right and three things they could improve upon.

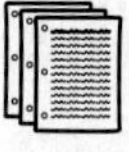

Section Review Worksheet 18.2

Assign Section Review Worksheet 18.2, which requires students to complete a diagram listing reasons for getting married, ingredients for success in marriage, difficulties of teen marriages, and the responsibilities of parenthood.

For information on fertilization and conception, see Chapter 16.

ception than using the rhythm method. For definitions and reliability of different forms of contraception, see Figure 18-7.

Responsibilities of Being a Parent Being a parent means caring for another human being completely. It means putting the welfare of your children before everything else. It means being able to support your children both financially and emotionally. It means feeding your children when you would rather be sleeping, laughing at their jokes when you've heard them thousands of times before, and letting them know you love them when they are convinced they are unlovable.

In other words, being emotionally mature is the most important key to being a

Actions and Effectiveness of Some Contraceptives

Method	Action	Effectiveness
Birth Control Pill	*Temporarily stops a woman from ovulating and prevents the implantation of an ovum onto uterus lining. Women taking the pill must adhere to a 4-week cycle. One pill is taken daily for 21 days, then nothing for 7 days, until the cycle begins again.*	*95–99%*
Condoms	*Thin rubber sheath that fits over penis and collects sperm. Most effective when used with spermicide.*	*88–98%*
Diaphragm	*Rubber cup that covers cervix and prevents sperm from reaching egg. Most effective when used with spermicide. Requires prescription and is specially fitted by a doctor.*	*70–94%*
Spermicidal Foams, Creams, Jellies, Vaginal Suppositories	*Chemicals that are inserted inside the vagina to kill sperm and also prevent sperm from entering the uterus.*	*79–97%*
Sponge	*Soft, synthetic material that is inserted into the vagina. Releases spermicide, and acts as partial barrier preventing sperm from entering the uterus.*	*72–94%*
Levonorgestrel Implants (Norplant ®)	*Six small capsules injected into the skin of a woman's arm. Releases a contraceptive hormone called progestin. Effective for up to five years.*	*91–99%*
Rhythm Method	*Requires couple to abstain from sexual intercourse while the woman is ovulating.*	*60–86%*

(FIGURE 18-7) **Contraceptives are most effective when they are used correctly. A woman taking birth control pills, for example, must remember to take a pill every day it is required.**

Check Up

How Good a Parent Would You Be?

Answer the following questions to determine how ready you are to be a parent.

1. Could you handle a child and a job at the same time? Would you have time and energy for both?
2. Would you be willing to give up the freedom to do what you want to do, when you want to do it?
3. Would you be willing to decrease the time spent on your social life and spend more time at home?
4. Could you afford to support a child?
5. Would you want to raise a child where you now live? If not, can you afford to move? Are you willing to move?
6. Would a child fit into your career plans or educational plans for the future?
7. Are you willing to devote about 18 years of your life to the complete care of a child?
8. Is demonstrating your love easy for you? Could you demonstrate that love for a child?
9. Do you have the patience to cope with the noise and confusion that comes with caring for a child?
10. Are you able to control your anger so that you won't take it out on a child?
11. Would you be able to discipline a child without being too strict?
12. Are you willing to take responsibility for a child's health and safety?
13. Would you be able to accept a child who developed values and ideas that are different from your own?
14. Would it matter to you whether the child you have is male or female?
15. Would you be as loving and accepting of an unhealthy child as you would be of a healthy child?

The more "Yes" answers you gave, the better parent you would probably be. Remember that becoming a parent is a serious responsibility. It is unfair—to you and to the child—to conceive a child without having considered your reasons for wanting to become a parent. Having a child doesn't make you "adult"; acting responsibly does.

Check Up

Have students answer the Check Up questions independently. Encourage them to discuss areas in which they feel least prepared for parenthood. What, in the next 10 years, might help them become more competent in these areas?

Section Quiz 18.2

Have students take Section Quiz 18.2.

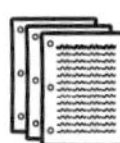

Reteaching Worksheet 18.2

Students who have difficulty with the material may complete Reteaching Worksheet 18.2, which has them rate reasons why people get married, list reasons why they may not marry, evaluate the ingredients for a successful marriage, and rate the responsibilities of parenthood according to difficulty.

Review Answers

1. Answers may include they want financial security, they want to have children, they seek close companionship, it is expected of them, they don't want to end up alone, they want to make a lifelong commitment to be with a person they love and respect.

2. Answers may include love and respect, sacrifice, emotional maturity, and the ability to communicate effectively.

3. Answers may include meeting financial responsibilities, finding the time and energy to do the things they want to do, not being emotionally mature.

4. Answers may include putting the welfare of children before everything else, supporting your children financially and emotionally, meeting the physical and emotional needs of your children before your own, discipline with compassion and love.

5. Answers will vary. Students may answer emotional maturity because this enables the parent to meet the needs of the child with love, unselfishness, and compassion.

(FIGURE 18-8) **Parenting requires time, patience, love, and a great deal of emotional maturity. But the rewards it offers are plentiful.**

successful parent. As you now know, emotional maturity is not a quality you can acquire overnight. It takes years of growth and experience to become a mature adult. This is one reason why teenage parents, who are still growing physically and emotionally, so often find their responsibilities overwhelming. The difficulties of being teenage parents are discussed in greater detail in Chapter 17.

Chapter 17 discusses the difficulties of teenage parenting.

Being financially secure can also make the job of parenting more manageable. Every state requires parents to support their children financially until the age of 18 (in some states it is 21). Clothing, feeding, and educating a child for 18 years can be very expensive.

It is also important for good parents to provide discipline. It is not easy to reprimand or punish a child for making mistakes. Some parents may remember making the same mistakes when *they* were younger. On the whole, discipline that is accompanied by compassion and love is the surest way to help a child understand what is right and what is wrong.

For all its difficulties and challenges, being a parent is one of life's most satisfying experiences. How good a parent do you think you'd be? Read the Check Up feature on page 397 to find out.

Review

1. *What are two possible reasons why people get married?*
2. *Name three ingredients that can help a marriage be successful.*
3. *What are three difficulties teenagers who marry may face?*
4. *Name three responsibilities of parenthood.*
5. ***Critical Thinking*** *What do you think is the most important quality a parent can have? Explain your answer.*

ASSESS

Section Review

Have students answer the Section Review questions.

Alternative Assessment

Successful Marriages

Have students work in small groups to prepare a visual or verbal summary of what they think goes into a successful marriage. Visual forms could include formulas, diagrams, and illustrations; verbal forms might be songs, dialogues, essays, or letters between spouses.

Closure

Marriage, Parenthood, and You

Have students write a few sentences describing the personal qualities they either already have or would like to develop that will help them in marriage and parenthood.

Highlights

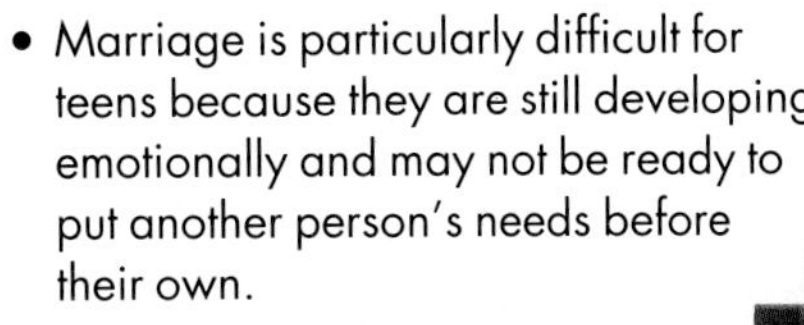

Summary

- Adulthood is divided into three stages: young adulthood, middle adulthood, and older adulthood.
- Decisions made during your adulthood require a certain degree of emotional maturity. For that reason, emotional maturity is a major goal to attain during young adulthood.
- Some middle-aged people may experience feelings of sadness when their children leave home, but middle adulthood also presents an opportunity to savor happy experiences.
- Common needs among elderly people include obtaining proper meals and appropriate housing. People in this situation may elect to modify their own homes, move in with family, or live in retirement communities or nursing homes.
- The most important ingredients two people can bring to a marriage are love and respect.
- Marriage is particularly difficult for teens because they are still developing emotionally and may not be ready to put another person's needs before their own.
- Being emotionally and financially secure are important keys to being a successful parent. Good parents should also provide discipline accompanied by compassion and love.

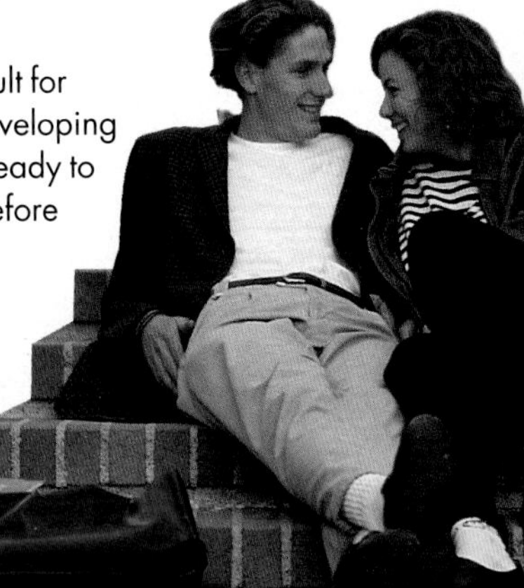

Vocabulary

young adulthood the period of adulthood between the ages of 20 and 40.

middle adulthood the period of adulthood between the ages of 41 and 65.

emotional maturity the capacity to act independently, responsibly, and unselfishly. Being emotionally mature requires having compassion, integrity, and self-esteem.

Alzheimer's disease an incurable illness characterized by a gradual and permanent loss of memory. Alzheimer's disease most commonly affects the elderly.

Parkinson's disease an incurable disease characterized by a gradual loss of control of muscle function. Parkinson's disease most commonly affects the elderly.

contraception a device or method that prevents the fertilization of a woman's egg.

Chapter 18 Highlights Strategies

Summary

Have students read the summary to reinforce the concepts they learned in Chapter 18.

Vocabulary

Have students write a paragraph about adulthood and its events, using the vocabulary words correctly.

Extension

Have students work in small groups to search the Yellow Pages and local community guides for agencies and services that help people make and carry out decisions about their lives at various stages of adulthood. These may include marriage counseling, family planning, and child care; financial planning, job retraining, vocational or professional education and career planning; single-parent, divorce, and surviving spouse support groups; and housing, food service, and medical assistance for the elderly. The class can organize the information into a community services directory.

CHAPTER 18 ASSESSMENT

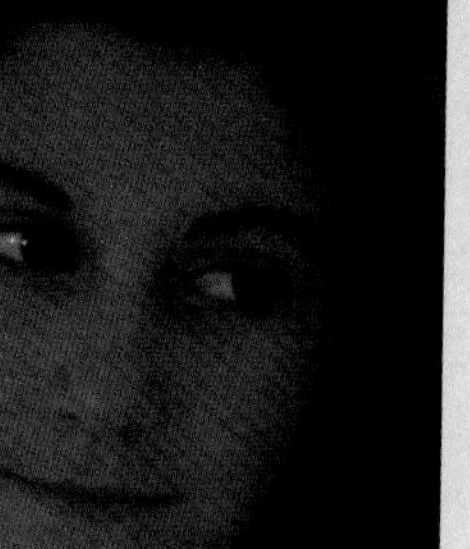

Chapter Review

Concept Review

1. The period between the ages of 20 and 40 is known as ________.
2. Age does not necessarily reflect ________ maturity.
3. Menopause occurs during ________.
4. ________ and ________ are two incurable diseases that affect the elderly.
5. ________ occurs when a person is judged solely on the basis of his or her age.
6. A ________ may be recommended as housing for elderly people who lose almost complete mental and physical functioning.
7. Perhaps the best reason people get married is that they want to make a ________ to someone they love and ________.
8. An important ingredient that makes a marriage successful is the ability to ________ effectively.
9. If one or both partners decide that the marriage has failed, a ________ will usually result.
10. Discipline that is combined with ________ and ________ is the best way to help a child understand what is right and what is wrong.

Expressing Your Views

1. Your grandparents are close to retirement age. You have always enjoyed going out to their farm on holidays to visit them, but now they want to move to a community where mostly older adults live. They have asked for your advice. What would you say?
2. What are some advantages of being middle-aged? What are some disadvantages?
3. Your friend Jed is planning to drop out of school and get married. He has asked you for your opinion of his decision. Explain how you would answer your friend.
4. Explain why you think compromise plays such an important role in the success of a marriage.

CHAPTER REVIEW

Concept Review

1. young adulthood
2. emotional
3. middle adulthood
4. Alzheimer's disease, Parkinson's disease
5. age discrimination
6. nursing home
7. lifelong commitment, respect
8. communicate
9. divorce
10. compassion and love

Expressing Your Views

Sample responses:

1. I would be honest with them and tell them that I would miss visiting them on the farm, but I also understand that the farm may be too much for them to care for at this stage of their lives. If necessary modifications cannot be made to accommodate their needs, then moving to a retirement community is the most appropriate choice.

2. Middle age can offer a time to benefit from the experiences you gained during young adulthood. It can be a time of peak professional ability. Married parents may find that it is a time to renew their romantic relationship. Middle age also involves physical changes such as gray hair, wrinkles, and menopause. Middle-aged adults may also have to confront death for the first time and may experience feelings of sadness when their children leave home.

3. I would tell Jed that I felt it would be best if he waited awhile before getting married and that he should finish school before he considers marriage. It will be difficult to get a well-paying job without a completed education. Without a job that pays well it will be hard to meet the financial obligations of marriage. Also, it is not easy for teenagers to make the compromises and selfless decisions that are required for a successful marriage. With marriage comes the possibility of having children. Having children when you are not financially or emotionally ready can be difficult on the parents and the marriage.

4. Because marriage is a partnership it is important to consider the needs and wants of the other person. The best way to meet your needs and those of your partner is through compromise. Marriage will not work if one partner is emotionally immature and always wants things his or her way.

Chapter 18 Assessment

Life Skills Check

1. Setting Goals
Think of two long-range goals you have for the next five years. Then list ways these goals would be affected by marriage and by parenthood. How can you help yourself stay on track and achieve your goals? Share your thoughts about the impact of marriage and parenthood on one's life with the class.

2. Coping
Your grandmother has just been placed in a nursing home. You know it is the best place for her because she is too sick to stay at home. You have always been close to your grandmother and want to continue the close relationship; however, you feel reluctant to visit her in the nursing home. What should you do? How can you maintain a strong relationship with her?

Projects

1. Develop a questionnaire for adults. Interview three adults, one from each of the three age groups. Include the following questions: What are your goals now? How are they different from the goals you set during your teenage years? Share your results with the class.
2. Write a creative essay in which you describe yourself and your life at age 35 and at age 70. Include a discussion of your work, your family life, and your leisure time.
3. Work with a group to plan a budget for a newlywed couple. Include expenses such as rent, utilities, food, clothing, insurance, transportation, and entertainment. Consider who would be responsible for paying the bills and what would be done to cover emergency expenses.

Plan for Action

Marriage and parenthood are two of the most life-changing events that you can experience. Create a plan that you think would help you become better prepared for decisions regarding these actions.

Life Skills Check

Sample responses:

1. Goals and the effect that marriage and parenthood will have on these goals will vary with each student.

2. I should overcome my reluctance and make time to visit her. When I am not visiting her, I could call her on the telephone and send her notes, cards, and even flowers to let her know that I care about her and I am thinking of her.

Projects

Have students complete the projects on adulthood, marriage, and parenthood.

Plan for Action

Have each student submit a card with a summary of an important decision unique to a stage of adulthood. For example: Young Adulthood—couple decides when to start a family, or Middle Adulthood—man decides whether to retrain for new career or retire early. Divide the class into groups and have each group draw a card, make up characters for the situation it describes, and prepare to role-play the decision-making process.

Assessment Options

Chapter Test

Have students take the Chapter 18 Test.

Alternative Assessment

Have students do the Alternative Assessment activity for Chapter 18.

Test Generator

The Test Generator (Macintosh® or IBM® format) contains an additional 50 assessment items for this chapter.

FAMILIES

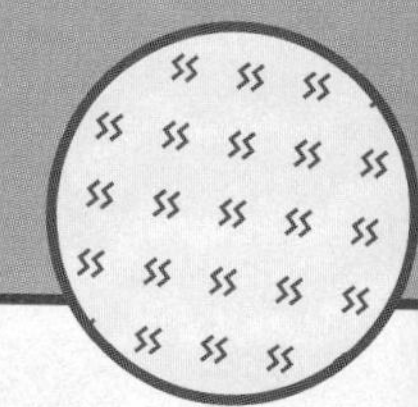

PLANNING GUIDE

TEXT SECTIONS	OBJECTIVES	TEXT FEATURES	OUTSIDE RESOURCES	NOTES
19.1 Understanding Family Relationships pp. 403-410 2 periods	• Name the three main functions of healthy families. • Explain how families have changed in recent years. • Name the characteristics of healthy families. ■ Consider what your own family will be like when you are an adult.	■ LIFE SKILLS: Setting Goals, p. 409 **ASSESSMENT** • Section Review, p. 410	**TEACHER'S RESOURCE BINDER** • Lesson Plan 19.1 • Personal Health Inventory • Journal Entries 19A, 19B • Section Review Worksheet 19.1 • Section Quiz 19.1 • Reteaching Worksheet 19.1 **OTHER RESOURCES** • Transparency 19A • Making a Choice 19A, 19B	
19.2 Coping With Family Problems pp. 411-414 2 periods	• Describe the common emotional reactions of a child to parents' divorce. ■ Name two actions a person can take to cope with parents' divorce. • Describe the effects on a child of growing up in a dysfunctional family. ■ Name two actions that could help a teenager cope with living in a dysfunctional family. ■ Apply the decision-making model to a family problem.	• What Would You Do?, p. 412 **ASSESSMENT** • Section Review, p. 414	**TEACHER'S RESOURCE BINDER** • Lesson Plan 19.2 • Journal Entries 19C, 19D • Life Skills 19A • Section Review Worksheet 19.2 • Section Quiz 19.2 • Reteaching Worksheet 19.2	
End of Chapter pp. 415-417		**ASSESSMENT** • Chapter Review, pp. 416-417	**TEACHER'S RESOURCE BINDER** • Chapter Test • Alternative Assessment **OTHER RESOURCES** • Test Generator	

■ Denotes LIFE SKILLS objectives

• Items in blue are also part of the *Holt Health Activity Book*.

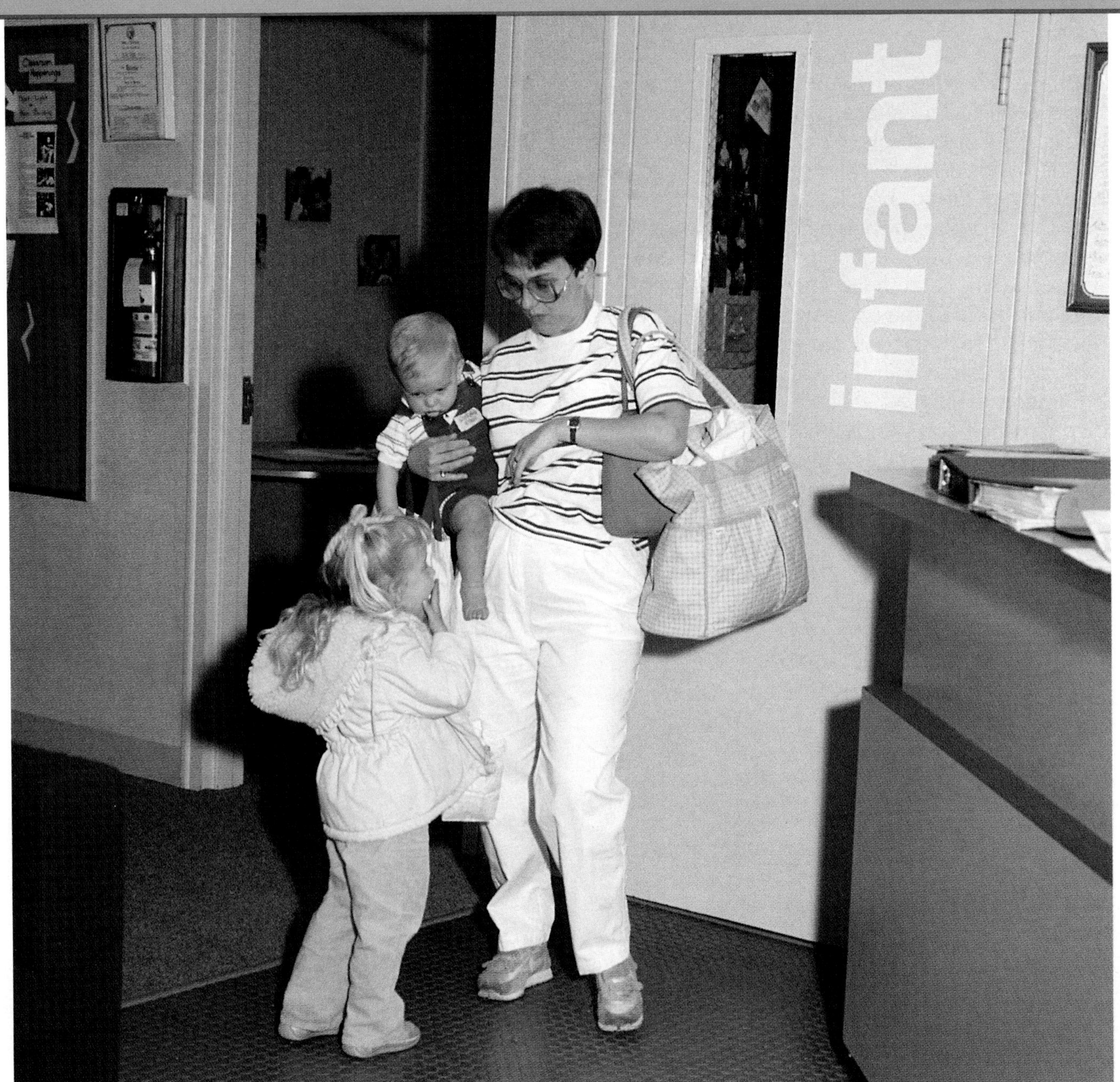

Content Background

Family Responses to Economic Distress

Families in the United States come in many configurations, from the single-parent unit, to the nuclear family, to the extended network of relations. Each one of these can be a stable, harmonious system that meets the economic and emotional needs of its members. One, two, or many incomes can contribute to the family's support. Economic instability introduces to family dynamics the elements of unemployment and job insecurity. These economic factors require changes in family roles that were once made by choice. For example, parents who once chose not to work outside the home may now have to seek employment. An unemployed parent may become the primary care-giver at home. Single-income families may experience particular hardship.

Changes in roles have sometimes added emotional conflicts to the economic stresses families are facing. For example, parents must balance the demands of work, child care, and a marriage relationship. Often they are not getting the support they need from their partners. Feelings of guilt may result as parents spend less time with their children. Later in life, the career paths of men and women may diverge and conflict. While one spouse may settle down for retirement, the other spouse may join the work force.

Sometimes such a decision is necessitated by a divorce: one parent finds he or she must support the children. If the person has not prepared to work outside the home, he or she may lack marketable skills. The job he or she finds may be low paying. The toll in fatigue and stress can be costly to the parent and children. The family's income is likely to drop dramatically. For this reason, many children fall below the poverty line.

Studies indicate that adaptability, shared family work, and family cohesion facilitate effective coping with economic distress. Strong bonds between partners prior to economic distress reduce the negative impact on family relationships. Economic distress can, however, result in dysfunctional behaviors. For example, parents who have lost their jobs appear to nurture their children less and to discipline them arbitrarily and less consistently than do parents who are fully employed. Children in these families are more likely to show signs of distress such as temper tantrums.

Families are faced with so many pressures today that maintaining a balance is difficult. Helping students become aware of the strains caused by economic distress and by changing work roles can help to lessen their tendency to blame themselves for tensions that are a result of these changes. Good communication within the family, including frank talks about finances and ways all family members can contribute to the family's welfare, helps every member feel emotionally secure even when times are insecure financially.

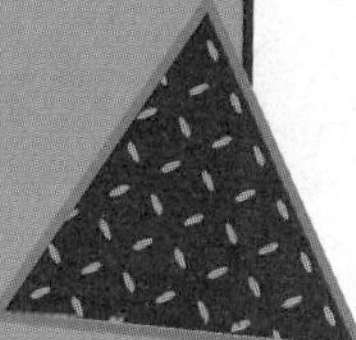

PLANNING FOR INSTRUCTION

KEY FACTS

- **Families help meet our basic physical needs, provide emotional support, and give structure to our lives.**
- **The traditional family type is the nuclear family; other family types include extended families, couple families, single-parent families, blended families, and other arrangements.**
- **The high rate of divorce, large number of working mothers, and high cost of raising children have helped change the American family structure dramatically.**
- **Within healthy families, members respect one another, share responsibilities, communicate effectively, support one another emotionally, and adapt well to changes.**
- **A young person may cope with divorce by working through the grieving process, seeking support and open lines of communication, and getting involved in activities.**
- **The remarriage of a parent can create feelings of loss and require a period of adjustment.**
- **Dysfunctional families do not meet the needs of members, usually because parents are overwhelmed by their own problems.**

MYTHS AND MISCONCEPTIONS

MYTH: The healthy, happy, normal family is without problems.

All families must cope with problems. Some experts feel that up to 95 percent of our population comes from families in some way dysfunctional—that is, not in the best working order. The family that appears perfect outwardly may in fact be in deep trouble, for its members may be denying problems rather than trying to solve them. What matters is not the appearance of the family's situation but how its members meet and deal with their problems together.

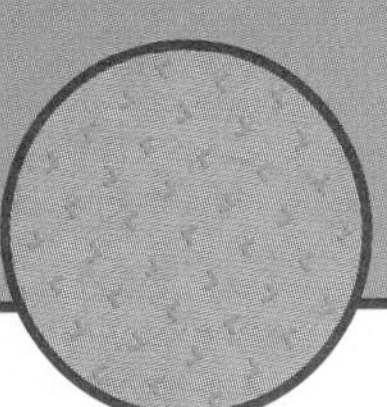

MYTH: You can create a healthy family by modeling your family after one you admire, such as a family you see on television.

Television family situations are artificial and resolve situations without going through the extensive emotional and communication work that go into resolving conflicts. They are based on story lines that must be resolved in 20 minutes; this has little to do with real conflict resolution.

MYTH: Problems with the American family would be solved if we returned to nuclear families.

To believe that profound emotional, financial, and social problems can be solved merely by placing children in a home with their natural parents is simplistic and wrong. An intact nuclear family suffering from alcoholism, for example, may be much more harmful to children than an alternative family structure. What family members need is a nurturant support system that can be relied upon.

VOCABULARY

Essential: The following vocabulary terms appear in boldface type:

nuclear family	**single-parent family**
extended family	**blended family**
couple family	**dysfunctional family**

Secondary: Be aware that the following terms may come up during class discussion:

empty-nest stage   stepparent

FOR STUDENTS WITH SPECIAL NEEDS

Less-Advanced Students: Create a bulletin board titled "Coping With Change in the Family." In the center of the display, pin a phrase describing a change that affects family dynamics (such as "Serious Illness," "Divorce and Remarriage," "New Baby," or "Unemployment"). Have students fill the board with illustrations and written suggestions for how family members support each other, communicate, and adapt responsibilities to cope with this change. Pin up new phrases and solicit new student contributions as chapter study progresses.

At-Risk Students: Have students write fantasy stories about living in their ideal families. Where would they live? Who would live with them? What kinds of activities would the family members share? What would be unique about their relationship with each member of the family? Then have them write a few sentences telling how they might make choices and plans to realize some of their ideals about family living.

ENRICHMENT

- Encourage students to read a book on the family and explain to the class what they learned about the evolution, current problems, or dynamics of the family. You may want to suggest the following books:

  Bradshaw On: The Family, John Bradshaw (Deerfield Beach, FL: Health Communications, 1988)

  "It Will Never Happen to Me!" Claudia Black (NY: Ballantine, 1981)

  The Measure of Our Success: A Letter to My Children and Yours, Marian Wright Edelman (Boston: Beacon Press, 1992)

  Traits of a Healthy Family, Delores Curran (Minneapolis: Winston Press, 1983)
- Arrange for a family services counselor to speak to the class and answer questions. Have students prepare questions about coping with divorce and other family problems.
- Have students write articles, stories, poems, features, columns, and editorials for a family magazine. Students may explore the history of the family, current statistics, effects of problems such as divorce or drug addiction, and advice that may help solve problems.

Chapter 19
Chapter Opener

Getting Started

Using the Chapter Photograph

Ask students how the group in the picture fits their idea of family. How does it differ? Discuss the ways that our image of the ideal family is affected by how we feel about our own family.

Question Box

The Question Box provides students with an opportunity to ask questions anonymously. To ensure that students with questions are not embarrassed to be seen writing, have those who do not have questions write something else—such as something they already know about different types of families or dysfunctional families—on the paper instead.

Preview the questions and then answer them at appropriate points in the chapter. You may wish to allow students to write additional anonymous questions as they go through the chapter.

Personal Issues *ALERT*

All families have problems, but many young people believe that there is something wrong with a family that has problems. It's safe to say that most students will be anxious about some aspect of their family situation; a number of them may be going through the pain of a divorce or come from dysfunctional families. Alleviate anxiety and establish a healthy climate for discussion by dispelling myths, respecting each student's right to privacy, and fielding questions honestly and objectively.

Chapter 19

Families

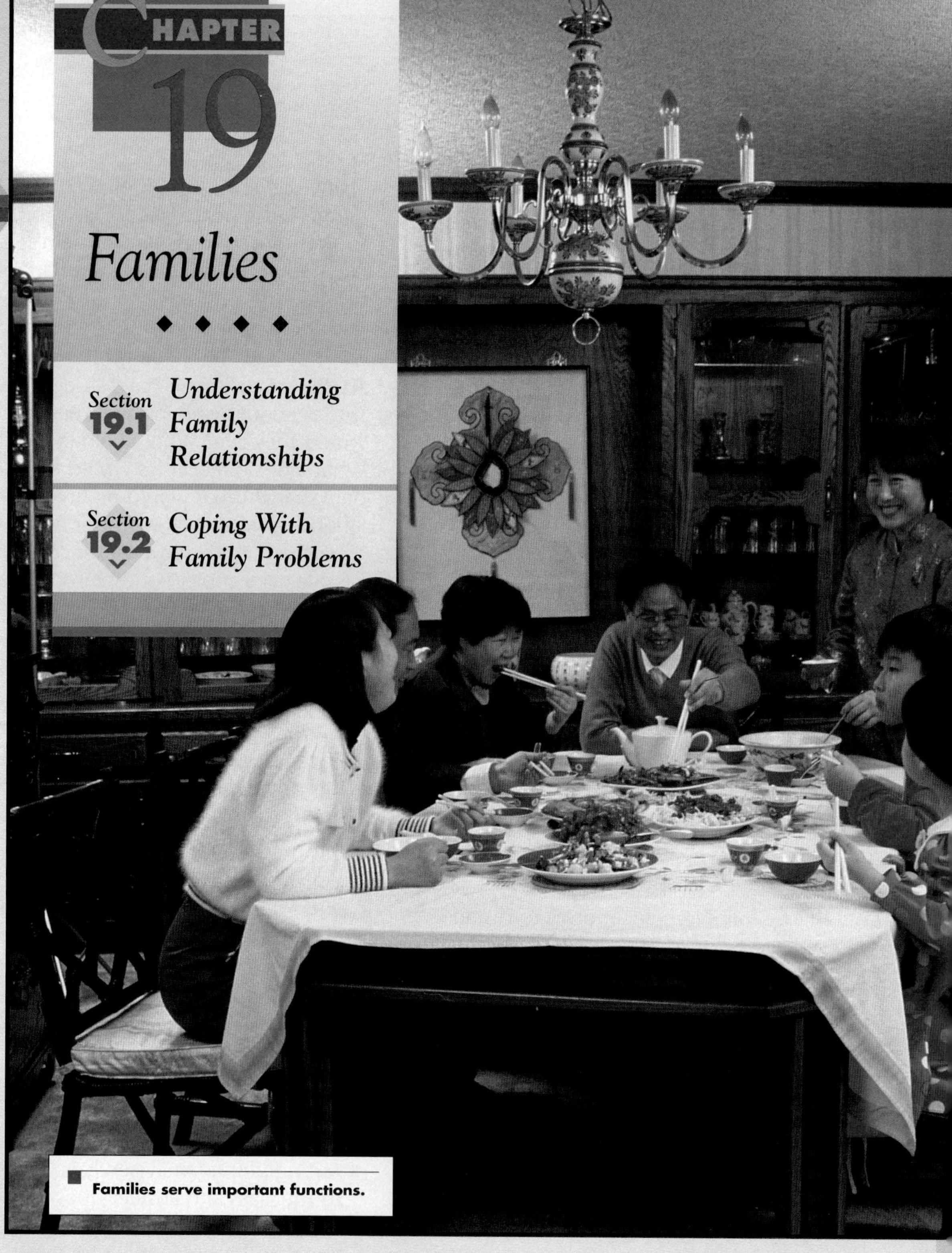

Families serve important functions.

After Braylon's mother died he moved in with his grandparents. He got to see his father only a few times a year because he lived thousands of miles away. It was a rough time. Braylon loved his grandparents, but he also missed his mother and father. His grandparents took good care of him though; they were always ready to listen when he had something on his mind.

Things gradually started to settle down, and Braylon was able to concentrate on school again. Then his Uncle Weldon moved back home and Braylon had to share a bedroom with him! Weldon was in his twenties—what right did he have to move back home and mess up Braylon's bedroom with all of his stuff? Braylon decided to talk with his grandfather about how he was feeling. Maybe he could help Braylon cope with all the changes.

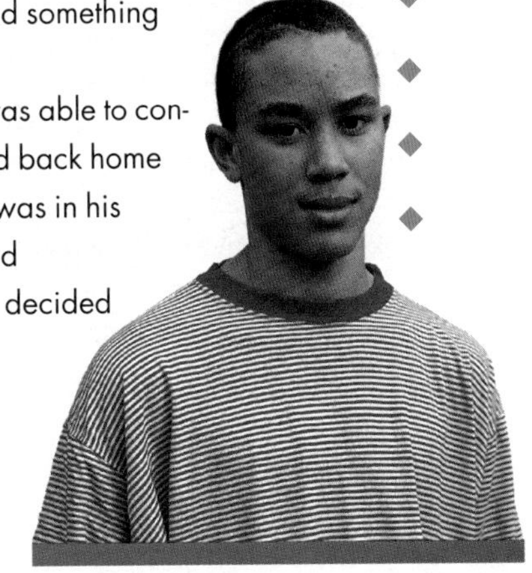

Background
Changing Households
In 1960, 60 percent of U.S. households were made up of a working parent, a homemaker parent, and one or more dependent children. By 1988, the estimate was 4 percent. Today, the average size of the U.S. household is just over two people.

Background
Young Families in Trouble
Since the early 1970s, young families' earnings have decreased (between 1973 and 1989 the median income of young families with children fell 26 percent), the number of births to unmarried women has doubled, and the number of single-parent families has increased dramatically. Forty percent of the children in households headed by someone under 30 are poor. If current trends continue unchecked, by the year 2000, one of every four children will be poor.

Section 19.1 Understanding Family Relationships

Objectives

- *Name the three main functions of healthy families.*
- *Explain how families have changed in recent years.*
- *Name the characteristics of healthy families.*
- *Consider what your own family will be like when you are an adult.*
  LIFE SKILLS: Setting Goals

Most of us grow up in some type of family. Your family may be the traditional kind, composed of a father, a mother, and one or more children. Or like Braylon's family, it may be less traditional.

Whatever kind of family you have, it probably means a lot to you. Healthy families provide us with love and support. They also teach us lessons about family relationships, which we use when we establish our own families. When people begin their own families, they tend to model them after the family relationships they experienced when they were children. If you grew up in a healthy family, this tendency to reproduce your childhood experience can have very positive effects.

Functions of Healthy Families

Although there is great diversity among families, all healthy families have similar functions. Whether a healthy family consists of just a parent and child, or if it also includes grandparents, a stepparent, and

Section 19.1 Lesson Plan

MOTIVATE

Cooperative Learning
Braylon's Situation
Have students form small groups and discuss Braylon's situation. Have them make suggestions for how he might cope with the changes. Have students imagine the conversations Braylon might have with Weldon, his grandfather, and his father.

Journal 19A
Family Relationships
Have students complete the statement "The most important relationship in my family is . . ." in the Student Journal in the Student Activity Book.

TEACH

Class Discussion
Functions of Family Life
Have students name the three functions of any family. Discuss different ways families meet these needs. Do any of the family structures make it more difficult to fulfill the functions? For example, how is caring for a sick child different in a single-parent family from an extended family?

Reinforcement
Stages of Family Life
On the chalkboard, draw a model (such as the one that follows) for the stages of the family.

SECTION 19.1

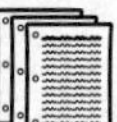

Personal Health Inventory

Have students complete the Personal Health Inventory for this chapter. The inventory helps them assess their own behavior with respect to other family relationships.

halfbrothers and sisters, it serves three basic functions.

First, families help provide basic physical needs such as food and shelter. When a family member is ill, the family provides the necessary care.

Second, families provide emotional support. The members of a supportive family know they can turn to each other when they have problems. Emotional bonding occurs in healthy families through shared experiences and close communication.

Third, families help provide structure for our lives. Your family helps you organize your activities and schedule your time. You might want to stay up late at night, for example, but your parents or guardians probably require that you go to bed early so you will be rested the next day. A healthy family looks out for your best interests by providing structure.

Types of Families

The great variety of family types makes it difficult to describe a "typical" family. Yet, regardless of type, any family can be healthy and happy.

The traditional family of a mother, father, and one or more children is known as

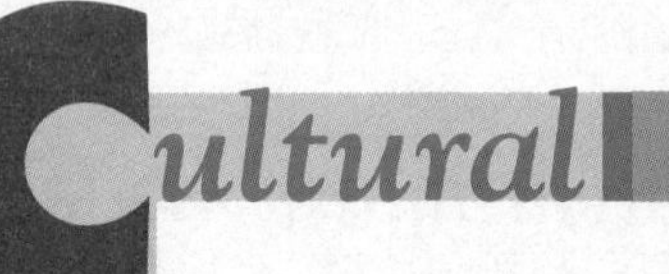

Cultural DIVERSITY

Extended Families of Hispanic Americans

Hispanic Americans are the second largest ethnic minority group in the United States. Immigrants and their descendants from Mexico, Cuba, Puerto Rico, Central and South America, and other Spanish-speaking areas make up this culturally diverse group. Despite their differences, Hispanic cultures share one important characteristic—the importance of family.

In Hispanic cultures, the word *familia* means not just the nuclear family but an extended network of parents, brothers and sisters, grandparents, aunts, uncles, cousins, and in-laws. Godparents, too, are considered to be members of the extended family. Through the custom called *compadrazgo*, a *compadre* (godfather) or *comadre* (godmother) has real responsibility for the spiritual, emotional, and material welfare of the godchild.

• • • TEACH continued

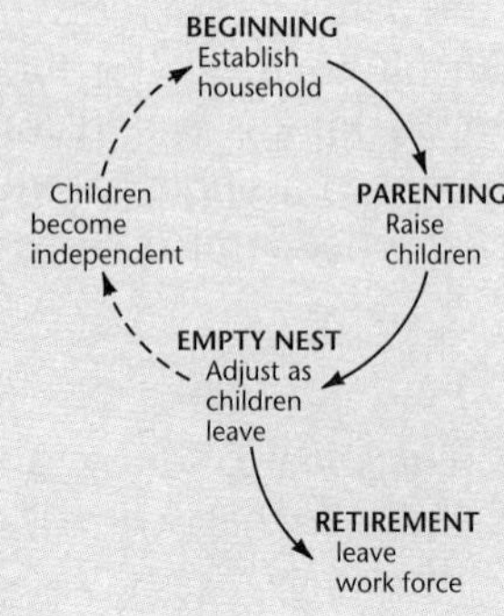

Ask students to explain how the model might differ for a couple family, adoptive family, extended family, foster family, single-parent family, or blended family. Add modifications or create new models to represent each of these family types.

Teaching Transparency 19A
Living Arrangements of Children Under 18 Years Old

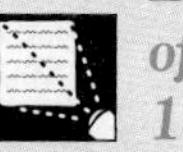

Use this transparency to help students become aware of the makeup of modern families.

Debate the Issue
Moving Back Home

Have students debate the issue: Should young adults be allowed to live with their parents for as long as they want?

the **nuclear family.** At one time the father typically worked outside the home, and the mother worked inside the home and took care of the children and the household. These days, that pattern is becoming less and less common as more women work outside the home.

The nuclear family tends to go through the following four stages: beginning stage, parenting stage, empty-nest stage, and retirement stage.

The focus of the beginning stage is the establishment of the household by the new couple. They are adjusting to each other and are determining the things that will be important to them in their life together.

The parenting stage lasts until the youngest child leaves home. During this stage, the parents do their best to raise their children to be responsible and productive adults.

The empty-nest stage takes place when the children leave home, which used to be when the parents were middle-aged. It may now be later than middle age for parents who have children later in life, or whose children live at home for awhile as adults. Some parents experience adjustment problems when the children leave home, especially if the children were the center of their

nuclear family:

a family in which a mother, a father, and one or more children live together.

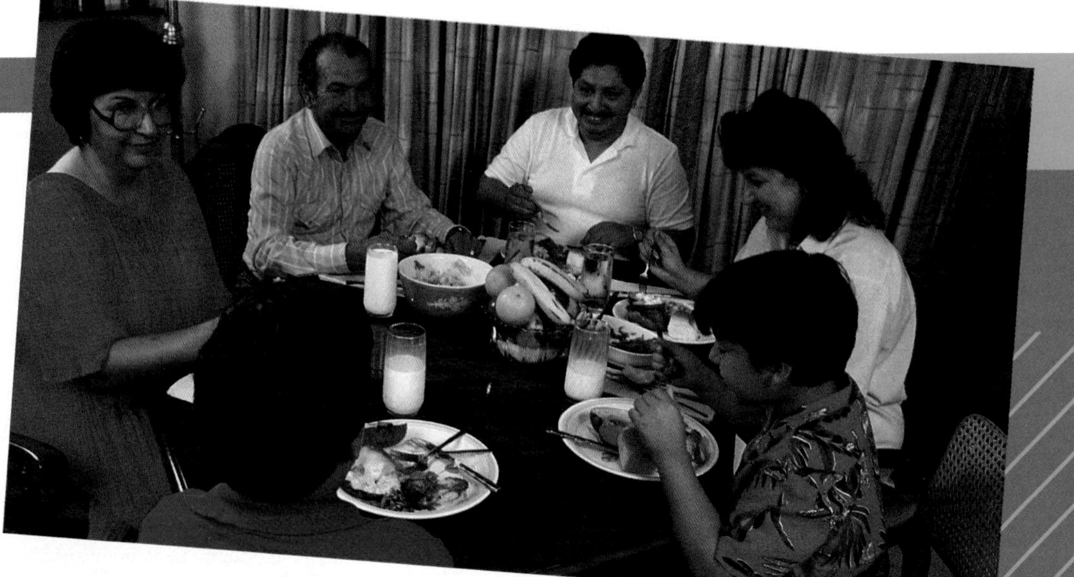

A child who grows up in such a family therefore has the benefit of a great deal of social support.

Grandparents in many traditional Hispanic families are highly respected by younger family members. As esteemed authority figures, they play a large role in family decisions. The elders also make significant contributions by helping with household tasks and child care.

A strong family system like this promotes good health by providing social support and by serving as a buffer against everyday stress.

SECTION 19.1

Background

Teenage Mothers and the Changing Family Structure

The United States has the highest teenage pregnancy rate among the industrialized nations of the world. Every day 40 American teenage girls give birth to their third child. It is estimated that as many as 90 percent of unwed mothers keep their babies, giving rise to a form of extended family that takes on what has become known as skip-generation parenting. Often, the mother's parents or siblings give primary care to the child, while she works. Grandparents, uncles, aunts, cousins, and a broad range of unrelated people rear the children.

After both sides are presented, list possible compromise arrangements on the chalkboard (grown child living at home must pay rent; parents and child must work out acceptable schedules and rules, and so on).

Class Discussion

Changing Family Structures

Are there other family structures not mentioned in the text? *[gay families, adoptive families, foster families]* **What is implied about the family in America by the many different types of structures?** *[The family unit is fluid, constantly changing, and often under great economic and emotional stress.]* Ask students to discuss some of the problems a blended family may face—such as children who spend only part of the time in the family, and conflicts between children of different parents. Have they seen these problems on television programs? Have they seen these problems in life? Are the TV solutions realistic?

Reinforcement

Evolution of the Family

Today, families have fewer children than they did years ago, thanks in part to better methods of birth control. Have students explore their family history and record the number of children their parents, grandparents, and great grandparents had. Graph these data and derive an average number of children per family for three generations.

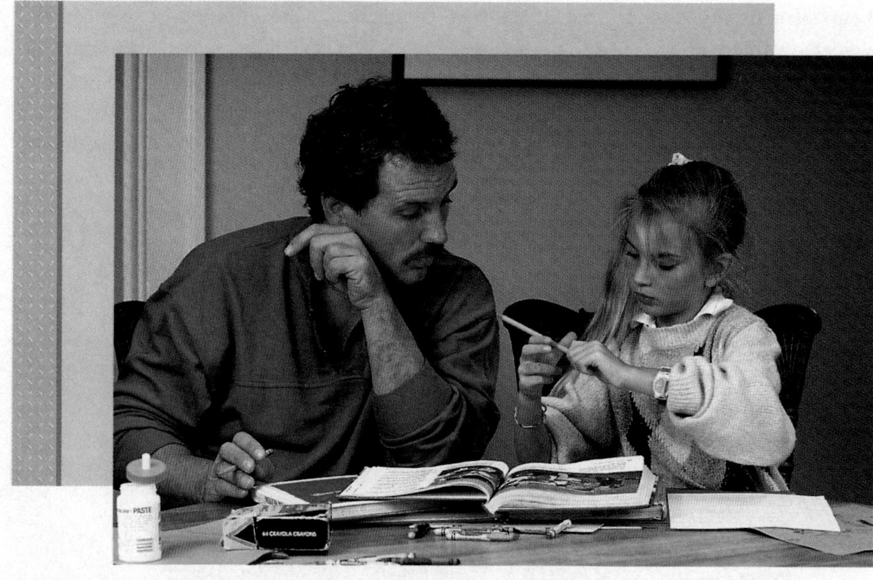

(FIGURE 19-1) **Single-parent households are becoming increasingly common.**

couple family:

a family in which only a husband and a wife live together in the home.

single-parent family:

a family in which only one parent lives with the children in the home.

extended family:

a family in which relatives outside the nuclear family live in the same home with the nuclear family.

activities. Others manage perfectly well and, in fact, welcome the freedom to make decisions and to use their time without having to consider their children at home.

It is becoming more common for grown children to live at home with their parents. Many young adults cannot afford to live on their own, so they continue to live with their parents until they have the money to move. Others move out, find out they can't afford their own place or miss the emotional support of home, and move back in with their parents.

In the retirement stage, people adjust to changes associated with leaving the work force. They also deal with the changes that are part of aging.

An **extended family** includes relatives who are not part of the nuclear family but who live in the same home. They may be grandparents, grandchildren, aunts, uncles, or cousins. The extended family was a very common living arrangement years ago, but it is less common now.

A **couple family** has only the husband and wife living at home. Some couples never have children. They may choose not to have children, or they may be unable to reproduce or to adopt children. Others may have children who are living with someone else—a former spouse, a grandparent, or another relative.

A family in which only one parent lives with the children is called a **single-parent family.** The single parent may be divorced, never married, or widowed. Most single-parent families are headed by women, although many are headed by men. The single parent manages all aspects of the household alone, which can be extremely difficult if the parent also works outside the home. Juggling home and work responsibilities is not easy.

Sometimes divorced parents spend equal amounts of time with their children. In one arrangement, the children may spend one week with one parent and the next week with the other. Or the children may spend

• • • TEACH continued

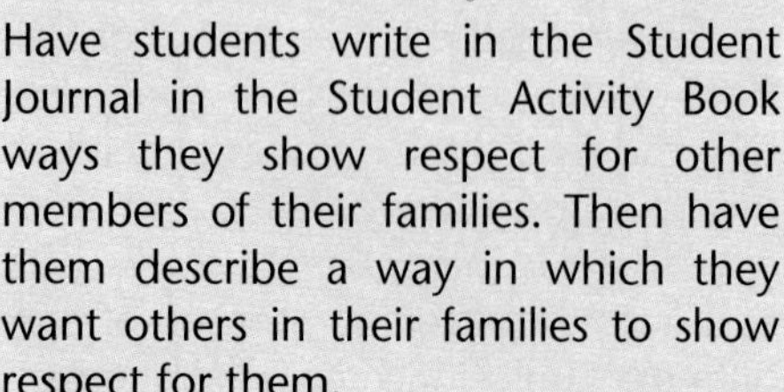

Journal 19B
Respecting Others in Your Family

Have students write in the Student Journal in the Student Activity Book ways they show respect for other members of their families. Then have them describe a way in which they want others in their families to show respect for them.

Demonstration
Healthy Families

Have students each write on an index card a line or two of dialogue that suggests poor family dynamics (*I haven't time for that now; you'll do fine without my advice; you'll never learn to do that right*). Shuffle the cards. Have each student draw one, read it aloud, and suggest a line of dialog that would address the problem (*I would like to discuss that later, when can we talk?*).

Class Discussion
How Much Responsibility?

Ask the class to discuss the kinds of responsibilities they think are appropriate for a teenager. What happens when teens do not have enough responsibility? When they have too much?

Reinforcement
Communication Skills

Remind students of the communication skills they learned in Chapter 17. Have them practice effective family communication by changing "you"

three or four days with one parent, then three or four days with the other parent. The important consideration in making arrangements is what is best for the child.

A **blended family** results when divorced parents remarry. The parents and their children from previous marriages combine to form the blended family. The parents may then have more children together. The parent who is not a child's biological father or mother is known as a stepparent. Some stepparents will adopt their new spouse's children.

The members of a blended family face unique problems. They often must deal with changes in the family rules, for example, or they must work out arrangements in which unrelated children share a bedroom. These problems can usually be worked out, but not always in the amusing ways shown in television programs such as "The Brady Bunch."

Some families don't fit any of the descriptions but are families nevertheless. A grandparent may take care of one or more grandchildren, for instance, or a child may live with a foster family.

How Families Have Changed

In recent years families have changed a great deal. The typical family of the 1950s and 1960s was defined as a working father, a mother who stayed home, and two children. Today only about 6 percent of families in the United States fit that description.

Years ago women were expected to stay at home, care for their children, and do the household chores. But circumstances have changed. Today most women with children work outside the home. Many women work primarily because of the satisfaction they receive from their accomplish-

blended family: *a family that results when divorced parents remarry; the parents and their respective children from previous marriages live in the home together.*

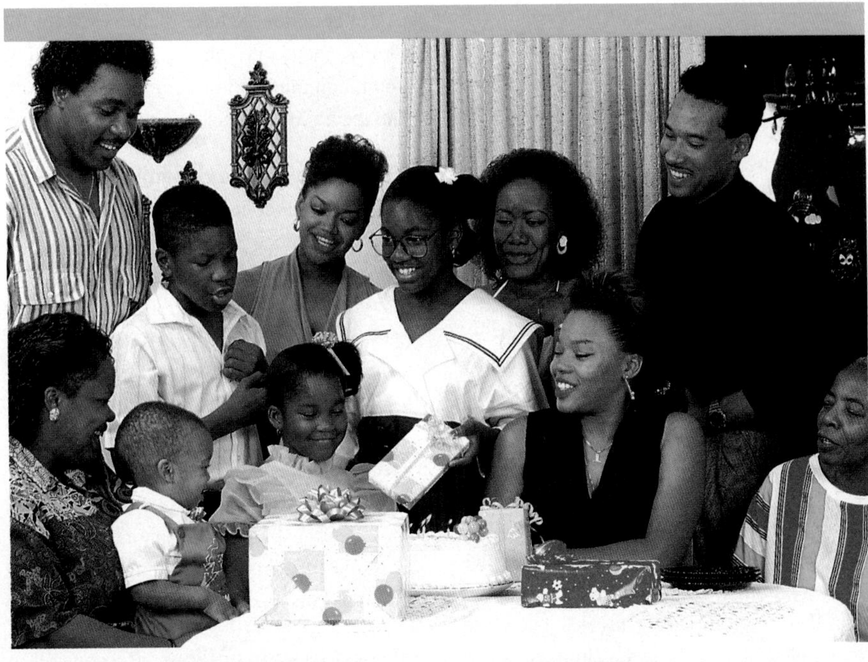

(FIGURE 19-2) **Blended families bring two households together.**

SECTION 19.1

Making a Choice 19A

Sharing Family Responsibilities

Assign the Sharing Family Responsibilities card. The card requires students to assign household chores for an extended family in a logical manner that encourages appreciation among family members for each other.

Making a Choice 19B

Discovering How Families Have Changed

Assign the Discovering How Families Have Changed card. The card requires students to compare characteristics of today's families with those of the past.

messages (condemning) into "I" messages (revealing how you are affected by someone else's behavior). The following sentence can be a model for constructing "I" messages:

"When you *(state behavior),* I feel *(name the feeling)* because *(state results of behavior).*"

Extension

Families Around the World

Have students research and report on the structure of families they are familiar with. Each student should draw a simple family tree for five different families. Duplicates should be eliminated. Then class statistics should be compiled and percentages of each type computed. What's the most common type in this sample? How many types are there?

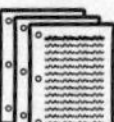

Section Review Worksheet 19.1

Assign Section Review Worksheet 19.1, which requires students to identify the different kinds of families and to describe the functions, characteristics, and ways families have changed since the 1950s and 1960s.

Section Quiz 19.1

Have students take Section Quiz 19.1.

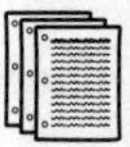

Reteaching Worksheet 19.1

Students who have difficulty with the material may complete Reteaching Worksheet 19.1, which requires them to identify characteristics of families of the past, present, or both.

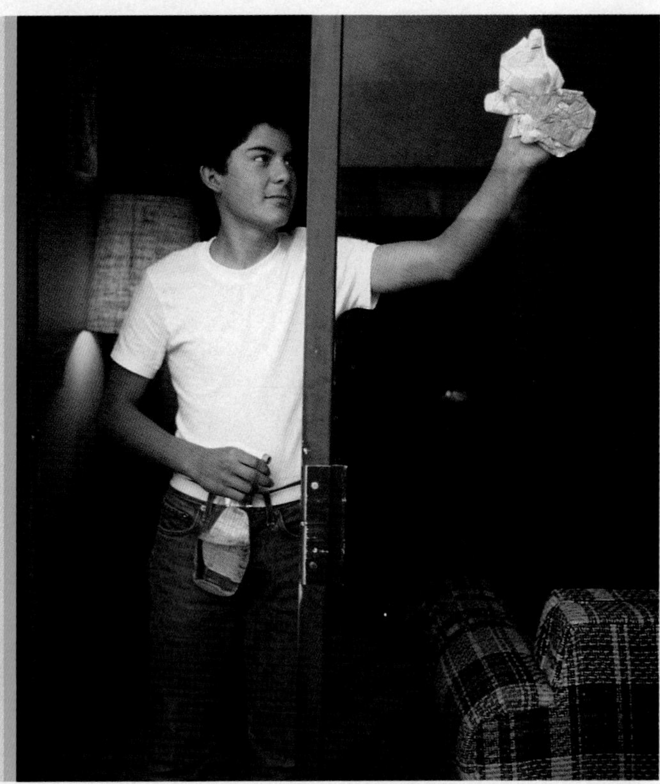

(FIGURE 19-3) **It is important for all family members to have responsibilities.**

ments in the workplace. Others would prefer not to work outside the home but must do so to support themselves and their families. Still other women prefer to stay at home and are able to do so. They find it rewarding and challenging to care for their families and their homes. One of the benefits of recent changes in society is that many options are available to women and each can be very satisfying.

Another major difference between today's families and those of the past is the number of single-parent families. Mostly as a result of the high divorce rate, single-parent families are much more common than they were in earlier times. There are also many more blended families, since most divorced people remarry.

Today's families are smaller in comparison with the families of the past. Before, having many children was beneficial if a family owned a farm or business; the children contributed to the material success of the family by working from an early age. Now, very few people in this country rely on their children for the family's economic survival. Even people who own a farm or business do not depend on their children as they did years ago. They usually hire other people to work in the business or on the farm and expect their children to help out only occasionally. Another reason for smaller families today is the high cost of raising children. It now costs a minimum of $85,000 to raise and educate one child through high school.

Characteristics of Healthy Families

Healthy families have certain characteristics in common. These include respect for family members, shared responsibilities, good communication, emotional support, and the ability to manage change.

Respect for Family Members Respect for family members is essential to a healthy family—respect for their privacy, their property, and their feelings. Respect means that you value what is important to the other person. A brother might show respect for a sister, for example, by controlling his desire to read her diary. In this way he is respecting her privacy. A father might show respect for a teenage son by not making fun of his friends. In this way he is respecting his son's feelings. If family members are not treated with respect, they might withdraw from the family.

Shared Responsibilities Responsibility helps us feel important and valuable. It is important that all family members have responsibilities, though they should be appropriate to each person's age and abilities. The responsibilities of a 4-year-old should be different from those of a 14-year-old, which should be different from those of a 40-year-old.

Good Communication Good communication is a vital ingredient of successful family relationships. People need to be able to express their feelings in an open and supportive environment. One of the most important communication skills is listening. Sometimes the best thing you can do for someone is simply to listen.

Effective communication can go a long way toward helping families work through their problems. Without it, the problems will probably get worse.

Communication skills are discussed in Chapter 17.

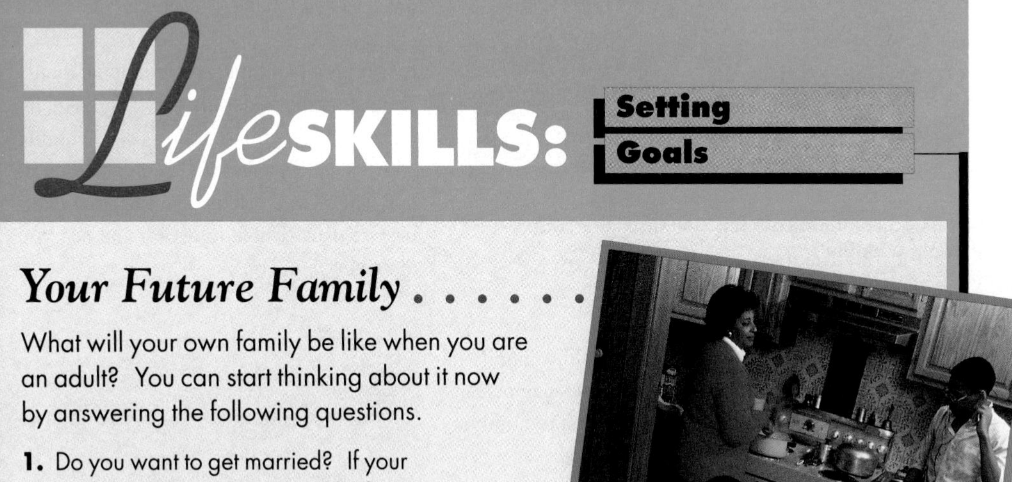

Your Future Family

What will your own family be like when you are an adult? You can start thinking about it now by answering the following questions.

1. Do you want to get married? If your answer is yes, when do you think you will be ready for marriage?
2. Will you work outside the home? Explain.
3. Will you want your spouse to work outside the home? Explain.
4. Do you want to have children? Explain.
5. If you want to have children, how many would you like?
6. Who will watch your children before they enter kindergarten? You? Your spouse? Another family member? A day-care center? Someone else?

Life SKILLS

Your Future Family
Have students answer questions 1–6 independently and turn in their answers anonymously (but indicate gender). Poll the yes and no answers for 1–4, separate responses of males and females, and place results on the chalkboard. What trends are shown? Discuss students' responses including their responses to Questions 5 and 6. Ask students what their ideas suggest about future changes in family structure.

Review Answers

1. Meet basic physical needs, provide emotional support, provide structure
2. An extended family is less common now, more mothers work outside of the home, increase in number of single-parent families and blended families, smaller size of family
3. Respect for family members, shared responsibilities, good communication, emotional support, and the ability to manage change
4. Answers will vary. Students' plans should reflect an understanding of the needs families meet for physical and emotional support and structure. They can practice good communication skills, lay the educational basis for a career, and make responsible decisions about sexual behavior.
5. Answers may include that women have been encouraged to pursue careers, and women need to work to support themselves and their families or because they are divorced. Society has changed so that many options are available to women.

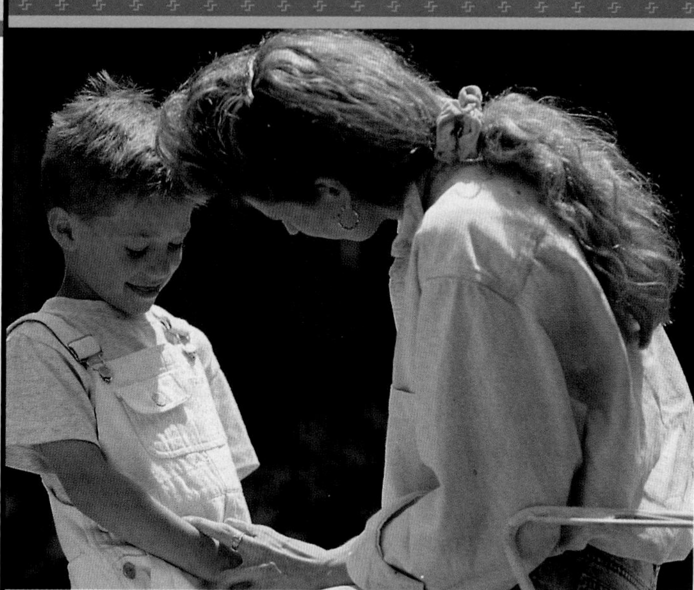

(FIGURE 19-4) **Good communication is an important characteristic of a healthy family.**

Emotional Support A healthy family provides emotional support to its members. For example, a teenager in a healthy family could turn to the family for support if he or she didn't make the track team or failed a test. A husband or wife can seek support from a spouse when going through a difficult time at work.

Ability to Manage Change Changes occur frequently in families. A healthy family can manage the variety of changes that occur during its members' lifetimes.

When family members are added to a household, the relationships among members become more difficult, just because there are more people. Additions to families occur when a baby is born, a grandparent moves in, a parent remarries, or when grown children move back home after living on their own for a while. These changes aren't bad; they just mean the family has to work harder to maintain good relationships. Space must be shared, new responsibilities must be assumed, and the family rules might have to be changed.

If a family member becomes disabled, the family must change to accommodate the disability. The physical structure of the apartment or house may have to be altered, and other family members may be called on to assist the disabled person, and to help him or her adapt to a new situation.

Disability and the addition of new family members are examples of dramatic changes that a family must adjust to. Most changes are less dramatic and occur over a longer period of time. As individual family members grow older, they develop new interests and begin to follow different life paths. Such changes are a completely normal part of life. Members of healthy families are usually able to accept and adapt to these new situations.

Review

1. *Name the three main functions of healthy families.*
2. *Explain how families have changed in recent years.*
3. *Name the characteristics of healthy families.*
4. ***LIFE SKILLS: Setting Goals*** *Describe the kind of family you would like to have when you are an adult. What actions can you take now to help your plans succeed?*
5. ***Critical Thinking*** *What social changes have caused the shift in attitudes about women working outside the home?*

ASSESS

Section Review

Have students answer the Section Review questions.

Alternative Assessment

Families in All Shapes and Sizes

Have students write a few sentences expounding on this thought: "The healthiness of a family has less to do with its size than with quality."

Closure

Family Problems and Solutions

As a whole class activity, have a student describe an imaginary family's problem to a classmate. The classmate supplies a satisfactory solution showing how the family could adapt. That person then initiates the next imaginary problem, and a third classmate supplies a solution.

Section 19.2 Coping With Family Problems

Objectives

- *Describe the common emotional reactions of a child to parents' divorce.*
- *Name two actions a person can take to cope with parents' divorce.*
  LIFE SKILLS: Coping
- *Describe the effects on a child of growing up in a dysfunctional family.*
- *Name two actions that could help a teenager cope with living in a dysfunctional family.*
  LIFE SKILLS: Coping
- *Apply the decision-making model to a family problem.*
  LIFE SKILLS: Making Responsible Decisions

Though it would be wonderful if all families lived happily ever after, we all know that is not the case. All families have problems. Some of the problems are temporary; the family copes and adjusts, and eventually rights itself. Other family problems are more serious and long lasting. As a teenager, you are not in a position to solve your family's problems, but you can find ways of coping with them.

If Your Parents Divorce

Divorce is a shattering experience for all members of a family, yet it is an extremely common experience. Each year, more than one million children experience their parents' divorce. If your parents divorce, you

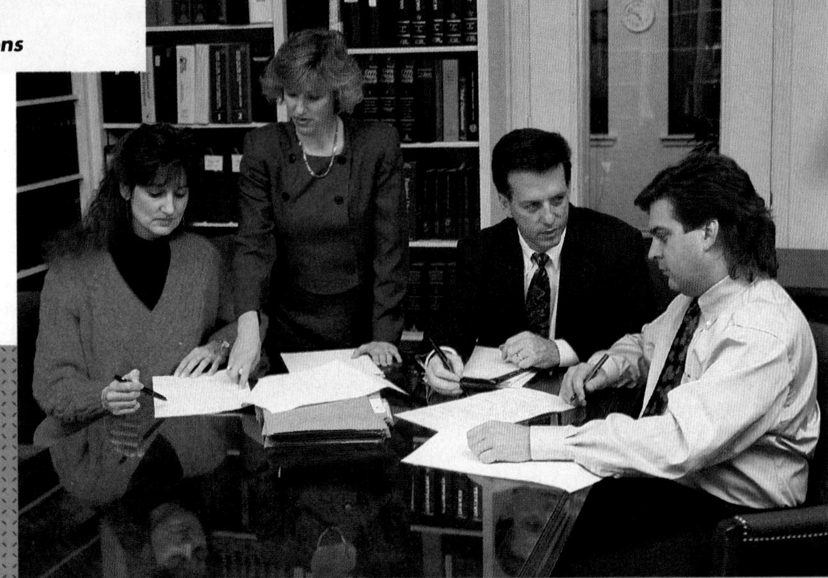

(FIGURE 19-5) **If your parents divorce, you must make major adjustments to cope with the losses that result.**

Background

Co-Dependency and Dysfunctional Families

In healthy family relationships, members are interdependent; in dysfunctional families, members are often codependent. When emotional needs are not met, a child or spouse may become so dependent upon another family member that he or she loses personal identity and allows that person to control the relationship completely—usually in destructive ways. Co-dependent relationships are common in families with alcohol, drug, physical, sexual, and mental abusers.

Section 19.2 Lesson Plan

MOTIVATE

Role-Playing

Divorce Dialogue

What do students think brought the couple in Figure 19-5 to this point? Ask volunteers to role-play the couple and their children. What does each parent say to each child? What do the children say to their parents?

Journal 19C

Unhealthy Families

No families are totally healthy all the time, and some families fail completely to meet the needs of their members. What do students consider to be abuse or neglect within a family? Have them write their thoughts in the Student Journal in the Student Activity Book.

TEACH

Writing

Reacting to Divorce

Have students respond as advice columnists to questions such as the following (which might be posed as letters from teens): Why was my mother/father so cruel? Why can't my parents just get back together? Did I cause my parents' divorce? What if we can't pay the bills? What if I have to

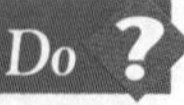

Should You Move Back Home?

Have students list options and decide what to do, then form small groups to discuss their solutions.

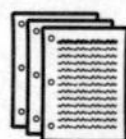

Life Skills Worksheet 19A

How Can a Counselor Help a Family?

Assign the How Can a Counselor Help a Family? Life Skills Worksheet, which requires students to compare community counseling services by conducting interviews.

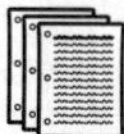

Section Review Worksheet 19.2

Assign Section Review Worksheet 19.2, which requires students to recognize family problems and ways of coping with them.

must make major adjustments in order to cope with the losses that result.

Emotional Reactions After parents divorce, children often see less of the parent who moved out. Sometimes they see the parent only on holidays or during the summer. Sometimes they never see the parent again. This creates a tremendous sense of loss for children who were close to the parent they no longer live with. It is natural to have strong emotional reactions, which are part of the grieving process.

At first there may be anger at the parent who left—a feeling of betrayal and abandonment. There may be anger at the parent who stays, for causing the other parent to leave. It is common to feel like taking sides with one parent or the other. But rarely does either parent deserve all the blame for a divorce. Because marriage is a very personal relationship, others outside the relationship cannot know all the underlying reasons for the divorce.

Sometimes children and teenagers feel guilty after a divorce, blaming themselves for their parents' decision. A person whose parents are divorcing may think, "If I had only been better, this would never have happened." If you feel this way, realize that getting married is a decision for adults and that ending the marriage is also a decision for adults. Children are not responsible for their parents' divorces, although they may feel that way.

Children of divorced parents may also experience anxiety about the future. Often there is anxiety about money, or whether the family will have to move, or other major concerns. Again, this is a matter for adults. You are not responsible for your family's financial situation. You may, however, have to make some sacrifices to help make ends meet, especially during the initial adjustment period.

Another emotional reaction may be depression. If your parents divorce, you may find it harder to concentrate in school or you may have problems sleeping. You may have a poor appetite or just generally

What Would You Do?

Making Responsible Decisions

Should You Move Back Home?

Imagine that you graduated from college a year ago, and got a job as a copywriter at a small advertising company. You hope to work your way up the ladder there. In the meantime, you bought a used car and began sharing an apartment with two of your friends.

Then you discover that you never have enough money to make it from one paycheck to the next. You're constantly having to borrow money from your parents. Finally your father suggests that you just move back home until you make enough money to live on your own.

In a way, his idea is tempting; you have missed the refrigerator full of food and a washer and dryer in the house. But on the other hand, your younger brother drives you crazy. He was always a pain, and you know that if you moved back home he would tease you about it relentlessly. You don't know if you can stand to live in the same house with him again. What would you do? What are your options?

Remember to use the decision-making steps:

1. **State the Problem.**
2. **List the Options.**
3. **Imagine the Benefits and Consequences.**
4. **Consider Your Values.**
5. **Weigh the Options and Decide.**
6. **Act.**
7. **Evaluate the Results.**

• • • TEACH continued

move to a different home/neighborhood/school? Can I still love both my parents? Should I? When will this misery go away? Ask volunteers to read their responses aloud in class.

Cooperative Learning
Stepsister, Stepbrother

Allow students to work in small groups to discuss conflicts that might arise between children in a blended family. How can they be resolved? Remind students what they have learned about active listening, problem solving, and conflict resolution.

Class Discussion
Defining Dysfunctional

Draw a continuum on the chalkboard. Label the left end "Healthy Family Relationships—all needs met" and the right "Dysfunctional Family Relationships—no needs met." Explain that just as most healthy families fall somewhere to the right of the ideal (represented by the extreme left), most dysfunctional families fall in a range to the left of total failure. There are many different degrees of dysfunction. **What are some problems that can cause families to become dysfunctional?** *[Alcoholism, drug addiction, emotional or mental illness, abusive parents]* **In what ways does the problem show itself outwardly?** *[Behaviors of children whose needs are not met; overt physical or emotional abuse of spouse or children; depression, anger, and low self-esteem of children]*

feel listless and down. Again, realize that it is normal to experience depression when parents divorce. If your depression continues for more than a few weeks, seek professional help. You might start by talking with one of your parents or with your school counselor, who can refer you to a therapist or support group.

One good way to deal with the emotions you feel is to communicate them to people you trust. You might want to spend more time talking with your friends, especially those who have been through a divorce in their family.

Another thing you can do is get involved with a new hobby or sport. Find something that absorbs your interest and takes your mind off problems that you cannot solve. Get excited about your new activity, and by the time you focus again on your family situation, you may find that it isn't as bad as you thought. Perhaps worry caused you to exaggerate some aspects of it.

When you have managed to accept your parents' divorce, you will be able to look at it and evaluate it more objectively. You may find that a happy single-parent family suits you better than an unhappy two-parent family. The calmer atmosphere may make it easier to concentrate on school and other activities.

Remarriage At some point, divorced parents may begin dating and then remarry. Though a happy occasion, the remarriage of a parent can create new feelings of loss for the children. A stepparent may take away some of the attention a child was used to receiving from a parent. The stepparent may have children, or there may later be half-siblings, all of whom may present a threat of loss in terms of time and where money is spent.

It will take some time to build the new family and weld together all the pieces. Be realistic and recognize that adjustments may be difficult. But also be aware that second marriages are usually more successful than first marriages and that a happy, united family can emerge. Do your part to bring this about—be patient and understand that all family adjustments take time to be successful—and you may find that rather than losing a parent, you have gained valuable family members.

Dysfunctional Families

A family that fulfills the basic functions of a healthy family—to meet the basic physical needs of family members, to provide emotional support, and to provide structure—can be thought of as a functional family. A family that does not fulfill these basic functions is known as a **dysfunctional family.**

dysfunctional family: *a family that does not fulfill the basic functions of a healthy family.*

In some dysfunctional families, children may not be physically cared for. They may not be fed, clothed, or sheltered properly. In most dysfunctional families, however, the basic physical needs of children are met, but their emotional needs are not. Children might be neglected or abused. In some dysfunctional families children are rigidly controlled, while in others very little structure is provided.

Most dysfunctional families are a direct outgrowth of troubled parents. The parents may have an unhappy marriage, alcohol or drug problems, or emotional problems. Usually, the parents grew up in troubled families. These parents rarely intend to be inadequate parents; they are simply overwhelmed by their own problems and are therefore incapable of meeting their children's needs.

But regardless of their intentions, parents' behaviors have a profound and lasting effect on their children. Children who do not receive adequate parenting may grow up with low self-esteem, ashamed of their families and themselves. They often feel that

Section Quiz 19.2

Have students take Section Quiz 19.2.

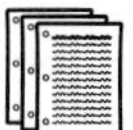

Reteaching Worksheet 19.2

Students who have difficulty with the material may complete Reteaching Worksheet 19.2, which requires them to complete sentences concerning children's reactions to divorce and the effects of dysfunctional families.

Review Answers

1. Anger—a feeling of betrayal and abandonment; guilt—blaming oneself; anxiety—worries about having enough money or that the family will have to move
2. Answers may include: talk with a trusted adult and/or seek professional counseling; become involved with a new hobby or sport.
3. Children may not be physically cared for; children may be neglected or abused; emotional needs may not be met; children may have low self-esteem, feel ashamed of their families and themselves, or feel as if they don't belong; children may feel angry or depressed.

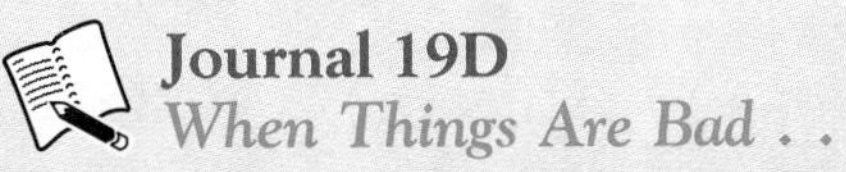

Journal 19D
When Things Are Bad . . .

Have students write in the Student Journal three positive actions a teenager in a dysfunctional family can take to meet his or her needs or to gain a sense of personal worth.

Debate the Issue
A Child's Right to Divorce Parents

Have students debate the topic: Should a child have the right to divorce his or her parents? After both sides present arguments and counterarguments, have a class vote.

Extension
Researching the Divorce Epidemic

Have students explore the card catalog, periodicals, and pamphlets of counseling and family services agencies for the most recent statistics on divorce and its effects on children.

Answers to Questions 1–3 are on p. 413.

4. Seek counseling for the family or just for himself or herself; get emotional support from other adults who are able and willing to give such support; remember that he or she is a valuable and lovable person, that it is not the child's fault that a family is dysfunctional, and that he or she will have more control over life as an adult

5. Answers will vary. Students might cite emotional support and having physical needs met. Disadvantages may include still having to follow household rules or dealing with siblings.

6. Answers will vary. Students may answer that through counseling, the person may recognize the source and cause of the mistakes and how those mistakes affected his or her self-esteem, as well as how to change behaviors in order not to repeat the behaviors of the parents.

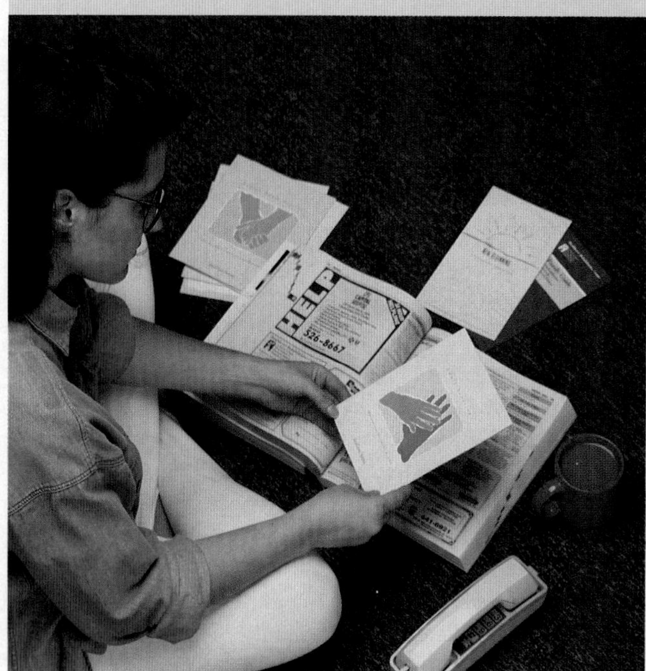

(FIGURE 19-6) **Many forms of help are available for troubled families.**

Emotional, physical, and sexual abuse are discussed in Chapter 20.

they don't belong anywhere and that they are not "good enough." As a result, they may be angry or depressed.

If Your Family Is Dysfunctional If you have grown up in such a family, know that help is available. Talk with an adult you trust about getting counseling. It would be most helpful if your entire family received counseling, but if that is not possible, don't hesitate to go by yourself.

It will also help to seek out adults who care about you and who will give you some of the emotional support you are missing. Do you have a relative—a grandparent, an aunt or uncle, or a brother or sister—that you can turn to for support? Perhaps there is a teacher, a religious leader, or another adult who would be willing to listen to you and help you.

After you have done what you can to improve your situation, remember that you are a valuable person, even if your parents don't treat you that way. Remember that you are lovable, even if it seems that your parents don't love you. It isn't your fault that you grew up in a troubled family.

When things seem especially bad, remind yourself that when you reach adulthood, you will have much more control over your life. You will be in a position to heal the old hurts and create the kind of life you want for yourself.

Review

1. *Describe the common emotional reactions of a child to parents' divorce.*
2. ***LIFE SKILLS: Coping*** *Name two actions a person can take to cope with parents' divorce.*
3. *Describe the effects on a child of growing up in a dysfunctional family.*
4. ***LIFE SKILLS: Coping*** *Name two actions that could help a teenager cope with living in a dysfunctional family.*
5. ***LIFE SKILLS: Making Responsible Decisions*** *What are the advantages and disadvantages of continuing to live at home after high school graduation?*
6. ***Critical Thinking*** *How could a person who grew up in a troubled family avoid making the same mistakes with his or her own family?*

ASSESS

Section Review

Have students answer the Section Review questions.

Alternative Assessment

Comparing Divorced and Dysfunctional Families

Have students decide which they think is less desirable: being part of a family split by divorce or belonging to a dysfunctional family. Ask them to write an explanation, including the way they see human needs being met in each circumstance.

Closure

Family Problems

Have students explain in their own words the differences between a family that copes with its problems and one that disintegrates or is dysfunctional. Have each student contribute his or her ideas to a class consensus.

Highlights

Summary

- Families help meet basic physical needs and provide emotional support and structure for our lives.
- There are a variety of family forms, including nuclear families, extended families, single-parent families, and blended families. Some families don't fit into any of these categories.
- In recent years the number of nuclear families has decreased, while the number of single-parent and blended families has increased.
- Healthy families have certain characteristics in common: respect for family members, shared responsibilities, good communication, emotional support, and the ability to manage change.
- A family that does not fulfill the basic functions of a healthy family is known as a dysfunctional family. In most dysfunctional families, physical needs are met, but emotional needs are not.
- Children who grow up without adequate parenting may have low self-esteem, be ashamed of their families and themselves, or be angry or depressed.
- Children of dysfunctional families can be helped through counseling or by seeking emotional support from other trusted adults.

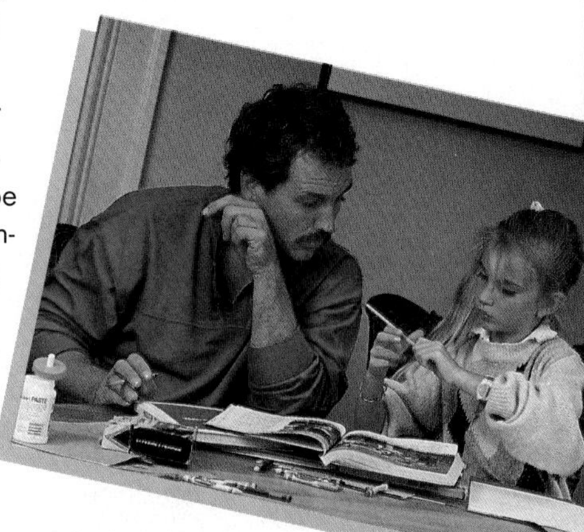

Vocabulary

nuclear family a family in which a mother, a father, and one or more children live together.

extended family a family in which relatives outside the nuclear family live in the same home with the nuclear family.

couple family a family in which only a husband and a wife live together in the home.

single-parent family a family in which only one parent lives with the children in the home.

blended family a family that results when divorced parents remarry; the parents and their respective children from previous marriages live in the home together.

dysfunctional family a family that does not fulfill the basic functions of a healthy family.

Chapter 19 Highlights Strategies

Summary

Have students read the summary to reinforce the concepts they learned in Chapter 19.

Vocabulary

Have students make an imaginary family tree that includes all the family types mentioned in the chapter. They should label each configuration appropriately and label the whole diagram "extended family."

Extension

Have students write a newsletter on the American family. They might include explanations of changes in the family, important qualities for healthy families, and how to get help for dysfunctional families.

Chapter 19 Assessment

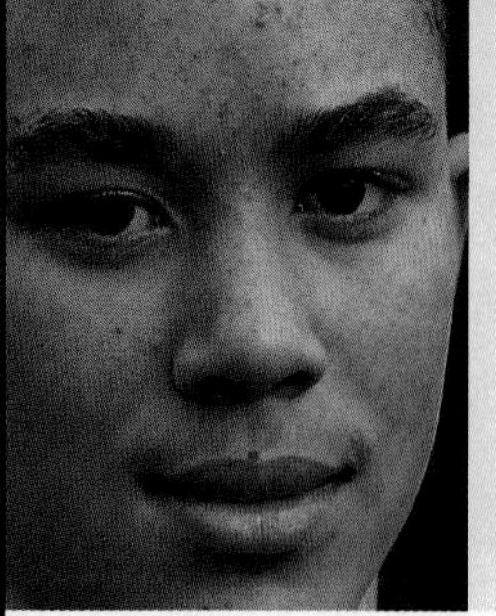

Chapter Review

Concept Review

1. When people begin their own families, they tend to model them after the family relationships they experienced as ________.
2. Emotional bonding occurs in healthy families through shared ________ and close ________.
3. A nuclear family tends to go through stages. The ________ stage takes place when the children leave home.
4. Grandparents, uncles, aunts, and cousins make up an ________ ________.
5. A ________ family is a household in which only one parent lives with the children. Most of these families are headed by ________.
6. Today, most women with children work ________ the home. Also, today's families are ________ in size.
7. ________ for family members, which is essential to a healthy family, means that you value what is important to the other person.
8. It is important that all family members have ________, but they should be appropriate to each person's age and abilities.
9. One of the most important communication skills for a successful family is ________.
10. ________ and ________ are examples of changes that a family must adjust to.
11. In most dysfunctional families, the ________ needs of the children are met, but their ________ needs are not.
12. Most dysfunctional families are the result of ________, ________, or the emotional problems of the parents.

Expressing Your Views

1. How are your family responsibilities helping you prepare for independent life?
2. How can teenagers whose parents have divorced help other family members cope? How could they help friends experiencing a family breakup?
3. Many family problems are worked out through communication. Why do you think it is sometimes difficult for family members to communicate with each other?
4. What are some advantages of living within an extended family structure? What are some disadvantages?

Chapter Review

Concept Review

1. children
2. experiences, communication
3. empty-nest
4. extended family
5. single-parent, women
6. outside; smaller
7. respect
8. responsibilities
9. listening
10. disability, addition of new family members
11. physical, emotional
12. unhappy marriage, alcohol or drug problems

Expressing Your Views

Sample responses:

1. As I get older, I assume more and greater responsibilities. Assuming these responsibilities now under my parent's guidance will help me become more capable and efficient at dealing with these and similar responsibilities when I am on my own.
2. They can talk with other family members and help them share what they are feeling about the divorce. Teenagers can also help get younger siblings involved in activities so that they will not dwell on the divorce so much. Teenagers can help their friends who are experiencing a family breakup by giving emotional support, sharing how they felt when their parents divorced, or listening to how their friends are feeling and letting their friends know that they understand.
3. Some family members may not be emotionally mature or may not have developed good communication skills. Some family members may not have good listening skills. Some family members may find it difficult to express their feelings, especially if the family setting is not an open and supportive environment.
4. An advantage of an extended family is that there are more people to share in the household responsibilities. A disadvantage is that someone may have to give up a room or share a room with the person moving in.

Chapter 19 Assessment

Life Skills Check

1. Setting Goals
Sometimes just listening to someone is the most helpful thing you can do. How good are your listening skills? For a week, try to practice really listening to at least one person every day. Then evaluate your efforts. Set a goal to increase the amount of time you spend listening to people who are important to you.

2. Coping
Simira's mother is planning to remarry, and her mother's future husband has two small children. Simira and her mother have lived alone for almost all of Simira's life. Now Simira is afraid that she will never get to spend time with her mother, and she's worried that her new stepbrothers will complicate her life. What could you say to Simira to help her adjust to the change?

Projects

1. Working with a partner, research and compare the family structures of two different cultures. Give an oral report on your findings.
2. Work with a group to prepare a skit involving a family with two working parents, one teen, and one eight-year-old child; the family is trying to set up a schedule for household responsibilities and tasks. After presenting your skit, evaluate how successful and fair the family was with the schedule.
3. Work with a group to create a bulletin-board display entitled "Healthy Families." Include family photographs, magazine pictures, or original art showing a variety of family types.

Plan for Action

A strong society depends on healthy family structures. Healthy families develop skills to work through problems. Devise a plan to help your family work out its problems and to help promote your family's health.

Life Skills Check
Sample responses:
1. Evaluations and goals for listening skills will vary with each student.
2. I might suggest that she talk with her mother about how she is feeling. Simira might also talk with her mother about what the new family rules and responsibilities will be as well as the living arrangements. I would assure Simira that, with compromise, all of the problems can be worked out to everyone's satisfaction.

Projects
Have students complete the projects on families.

Plan for Action
Have students work in small groups to create an imaginary case study of a dysfunctional family. After they have invented the family's difficulties, have students use what they have learned to make suggestions for the family's recovery.

Assessment Options

Chapter Test
Have students take the Chapter 19 Test.

Alternative Assessment
Have students do the Alternative Assessment activity for Chapter 19.

Test Generator
The Test Generator (Macintosh® or IBM® format) contains an additional 50 assessment items for this chapter.

CHAPTER 20

PREVENTING ABUSE AND VIOLENCE

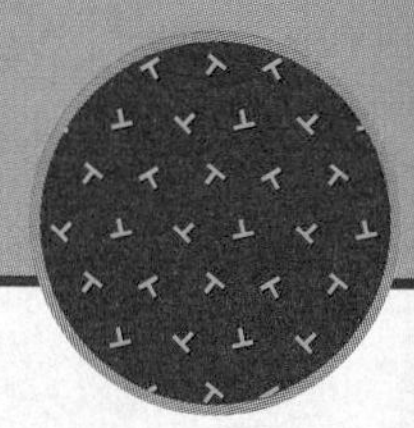

PLANNING GUIDE

TEXT SECTIONS	OBJECTIVES	TEXT FEATURES	OUTSIDE RESOURCES	NOTES
20.1 Abusive Families pp. 419-423 2 periods	• Name four different types of child abuse. • Define spouse abuse. • Define elder abuse. ■ Use a decision-making model to decide what you would do if you suspected child abuse. ■ Know at least two ways you could report an abusive situation.	• Check Up, p. 420 • What Would You Do?, p. 422 **ASSESSMENT** • Section Review, p. 423	**TEACHER'S RESOURCE BINDER** • Lesson Plan 20.1 • Personal Health Inventory • Life Skills 20A, 20B • Section Review Worksheet 20.1 • Section Quiz 20.1 • Reteaching Worksheet 20.1 **OTHER RESOURCES** • Making a Choice 20A • English/Spanish Audiocassette 5 • Parent Discussion Guide	
20.2 Sexual Assault pp. 424-428 2 periods	• Define sexual assault. • Define acquaintance rape. • Discuss how young men can avoid committing acquaintance rape. ■ Know who a victimized person should contact after a sexual assault.	**ASSESSMENT** • Section Review, p. 428	**TEACHER'S RESOURCE BINDER** • Lesson Plan 20.2 • Journal Entry 20A • Life Skills 20C • Section Review Worksheet 20.2 • Section Quiz 20.2 • Reteaching Worksheet 20.2 **OTHER RESOURCES** • Transparencies 20A, 20B	
20.3 Preventing Violent Conflict pp. 429-432 1 period	• Name the three major risk factors associated with homicides. • Discuss the reasons why some teenagers join gangs. ■ Know how to prevent your anger from turning into violence. ■ Know how to resolve conflicts without violence.	• LIFE SKILLS: Solving Problems, p. 431 **ASSESSMENT** • Section Review, p. 432	**TEACHER'S RESOURCE BINDER** • Lesson Plan 20.3 • Journal Entry 20B • Life Skills 20D • Media Worksheet • Section Review Worksheet 20.3 • Section Quiz 20.3 • Reteaching Worksheet 20.3 **OTHER RESOURCES** • Making a Choice 20B • Transparency 20C	
End of Chapter pp. 433-435		**ASSESSMENT** • Chapter Review, pp. 434-435	**TEACHER'S RESOURCE BINDER** • Chapter Test • Alternative Assessment • Personal Pledge **OTHER RESOURCES** • Test Generator	

■ Denotes LIFE SKILLS objectives

• Items in blue are also part of the *Holt Health Activity Book*.

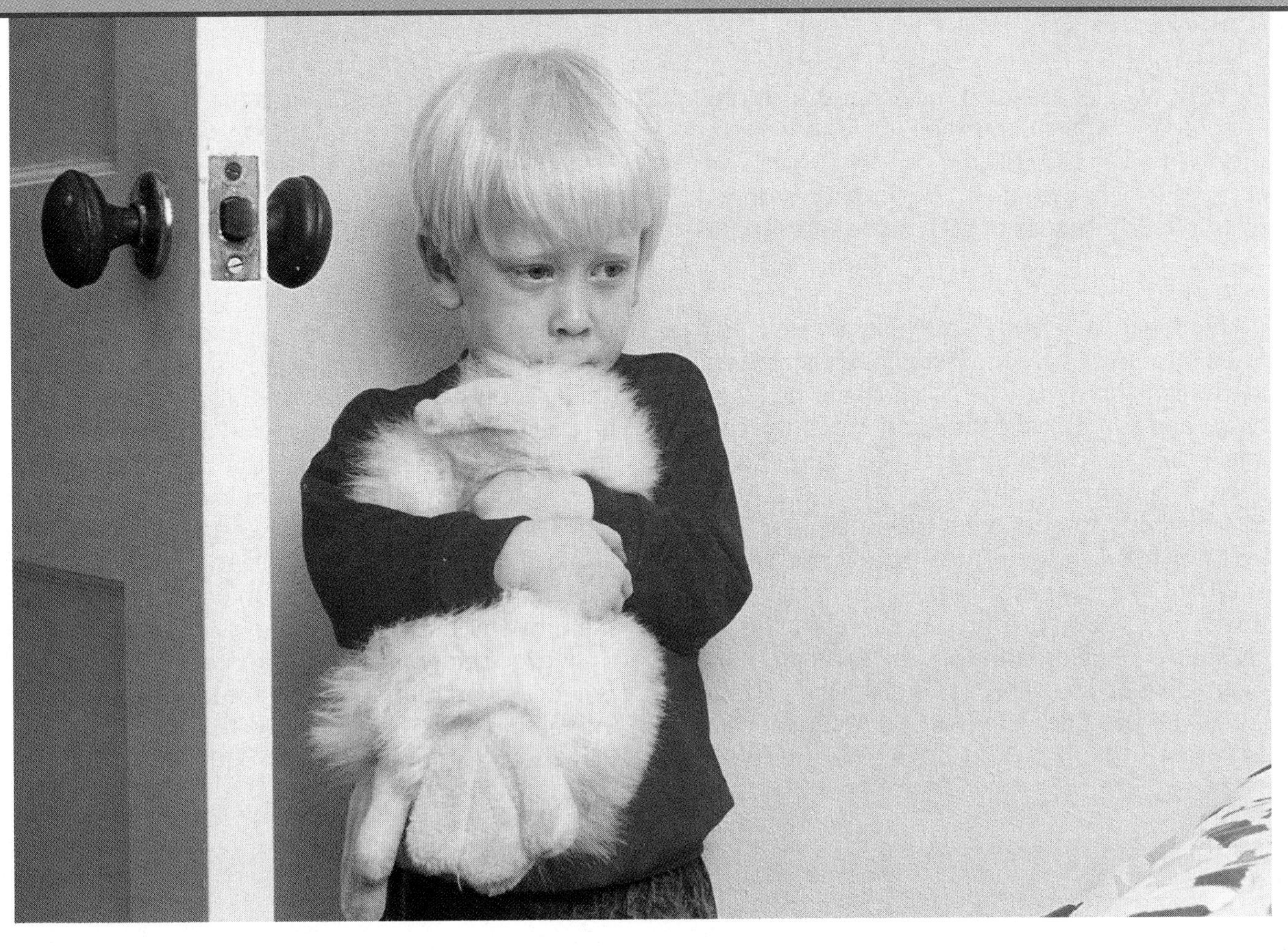

Content Background: Emotional Child Abuse

Every 26 seconds, a young person runs away from home in the United States. Fifty percent of these young people never return. Every year 100,000 children enter psychiatric hospitals, and 30,000 are in residential treatment centers. Why? A significant factor is emotional child abuse.

Emotional abuse involves a continual pattern over time in which the child develops a chronic feeling of worthlessness, rejection, and guilt. The infrequent or occasional parental mistakes that make a child feel bad about himself or herself are not defined as emotional abuse. Rather, the emotionally abusive adult continually exposes the child to negative emotions, with destructive results. Emotional abuse can take place without sexual or physical abuse occurring; however, it is a natural consequence of other types of abuse. Some specific indicators that a child has been emotionally abused are depression; an inability to concentrate; speech disorders; a lag in physical development; and habits like rocking, sucking, and biting.

What kind of parents treat their children in such a way as to cause this type of disturbance? Emotionally abusive parents are not monsters. Most were abused themselves as children. Abused children and the adults they become are plagued by shame and guilt. Parents control children with shame, that is, by labeling them as evil, defective, worthless, and so on. Guilt is deep seated and long lasting; it becomes an aspect of the child's conscience. The emotionally abused child experiences guilt about personal thoughts and feelings or about things he or she has not done or is not responsible for. It is natural for the child to respond to this inescapable guilt by focusing on pain, hatred, hostility, ways of getting even, or ways of escaping further abuse. Running away and lying are common. The legacy of abuse is passed on to the children of adults who have to cope with their own guilt. When parents do not realize the root cause of their own guilt and the inadequacy of their upbringing, they will abuse their children.

Emotional abuse and discipline often are confused by abusive parents. Discipline assists the child in learning appropriate behavior. Discipline at home and in the classroom also nurtures the child's intellectual and moral growth, self-image, and confidence. Punishment, shaming, guilt, and control of the child's thinking have the opposite effect. The best way to teach discipline is by example.

What preventive measures can be taken to stop the chain reaction of emotional abuse before it causes permanent harm to a child? A parent who is afraid he or she will abuse a child can call a hotline when emotions flair (Parents Anonymous 1–800–421–0353). Child protective services, in addition, are available to help the child. Sometimes they are able to reunite the family in a healthy setting. Eighty to eighty-five percent of abusive parents become nonabusive if they get the proper help. Controlling language is very important in stopping emotional abuse. Parents should avoid using such words as *worthless, jerk, dummy, stupid,* and *you always* and *you never* in a negative context. Instead, they should remind children of their value, worth, talents, skills, abilities, and appeal, and when giving criticism, parents should always make a clear distinction between the behavior and the child. The manner of speaking is also key. They should avoid a loud voice and belligerent or aggressive language.

Increased prevention, recognition, and treatment of emotional abuse are more necessary now than ever before. It is important for parents to practice good manners and mutual respect when interacting with their children. This can go a long way toward stopping abusive patterns.

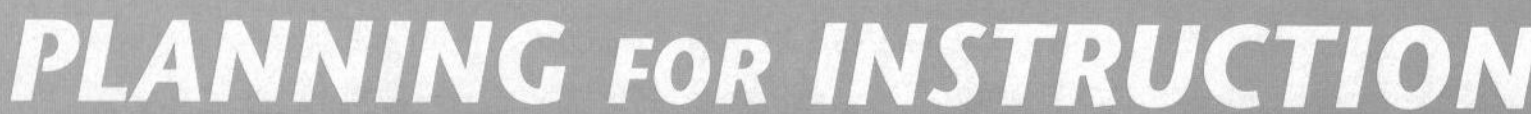

PLANNING FOR INSTRUCTION

KEY FACTS

- **Children and adolescents are abused most often by members of their family. They may be neglected or mistreated physically, sexually, or emotionally.**
- **Many abused children go on to become abusive parents unless they are taught appropriate parenting skills.**
- **Children and adolescents have the right to take action to stop sexual abuse, which is against the law.**
- **Abused or battered spouses are usually women with low self-esteem and few financial resources.**
- **Abusive families can be helped, but only if abuse is reported. Police, 911, hotlines, community health agencies, and trusted adults can help parents and children deal with reports of abuse.**
- **Sexual assault, which is most often committed by people who know their victims, expresses a desire to dominate and humiliate.**
- **The victim of a sexual assault is never at fault, but by taking precautions and actively resisting assault, a potential victim can sometimes prevent assault.**
- **Solving the problem of acquaintance rape will require changing the male view that sexual intimacy is a game of aggression, competition, and control.**
- **Substance abuse, possession of a gun, and violent arguments drastically increase the odds that a conflict will end in a homicide. Learning to recognize and channel anger and to compromise helps control violence.**
- **Many disaffected teens join gangs to get money, status, and the feeling of belonging to a "family"; however, their ultimate reward is often violence, crime, and death.**

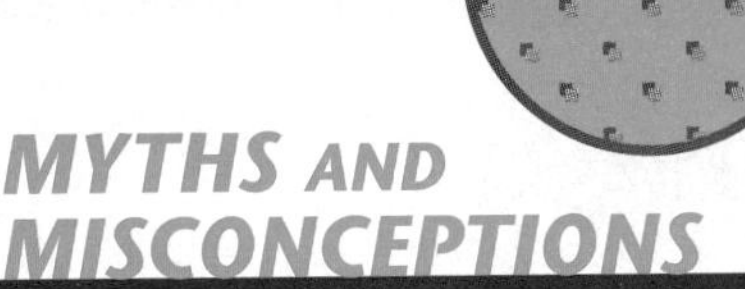

MYTHS AND MISCONCEPTIONS

MYTH: No one should interfere in what goes on within a family.

The abuse of a spouse or child is against the law. No one has the right to abuse another person. The home belongs to all the members of the family, and all deserve to live without fear and abuse.

MYTH: Women who stay with a physically abusive husband or lover must like to be beaten.

Beatings hurt and humiliate; no one likes them. Women sometimes stay in such situations out of fear of worse reprisals, financial hardship, emotional attachment to the man, and the belief that the family should stay together.

MYTH: Child abuse means physical and sexual mistreatment only.

Withholding love, tearing children down verbally, and neglecting their needs are serious forms of abuse. The wounds are not as visible, but they are just as real as those from beatings, incest, and other physical forms of abuse.

MYTH: Rape is a woman's fault if she first says yes and then changes her mind, or if she dresses provocatively.

Rape is never the victim's fault. A woman has the right to say no, even if she said yes earlier. What you wear and do on a date does not give your partner the right to sexual intercourse.

VOCABULARY

Essential: The following vocabulary terms appear in boldface type:

child abuse	**sexual abuse**
physical abuse	**neglect**
emotional abuse	**sexual assault**
spouse abuse	**acquaintance rape**
elder abuse	**homicide**

Secondary: Be aware that the following terms may come up during class discussion:

battering
cults
affiliation

FOR STUDENTS WITH SPECIAL NEEDS

At-Risk Students: Have students find information and statistics on gangs in your area or state. Supply a list of possible sources for data (police department, family services agencies, and so on). Suggest that students gather information on crimes and deaths related to gangs, as well as what happens to gang members over time. They can communicate to the class what they learn from their research through an oral presentation or a visual display.

Visual/Auditory Learners: Have students write skits about and act out conflict situations that could lead to violence or abuse. Have them act out the scenes a second time, showing how communication skills and appropriate reaction could defuse the situation. You may want to suggest that students use the RESPECT method for resolving conflicts (described in Chapter 17). If possible, have students videotape and narrate the skits, using a student narration followed by a class viewing and discussion.

ENRICHMENT

- Have students create public service advertising campaigns to educate people about different types of abuse and violence and to convince them to report these illegal, harmful behaviors. Students should create TV ads, posters, brochures, or letters to convey their message.
- Have a psychologist, social worker, or other counselor from a family services agency or private clinic speak to the class about abusive families. Encourage the speaker to tell about patterns of abuse in families he or she has helped and explain how and when such families are helped.

CHAPTER 20
CHAPTER OPENER

GETTING STARTED

Using the Chapter Photograph

Ask students to describe what the children in the photograph are watching. How common is this exposure? What effect does it have on American children?

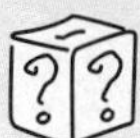

Question Box

Have students anonymously write out any questions they have about abuse and violence and put them in the Question Box. To ensure that students with questions are not embarrassed to be seen writing, have students who do not have questions write a fact they already know about sexual assault, gang violence, or abuse instead.

Preview the questions and then answer them at appropriate points in the chapter. You may wish to allow students to write additional questions as they go through the chapter.

Personal Issues *ALERT*

This chapter deals with sensitive, difficult subjects. Teenagers may be embarrassed to discuss sexual abuse and assault; some students may be victims of rape or child abuse. A tone that is sensitive, serious, and calm will help create an atmosphere in which meaningful discussion can emerge. Acknowledge that the subject is hard to talk about and makes many people uncomfortable. However, it is too important a topic to ignore. Make it clear that jokes will not be tolerated.

CHAPTER 20

Preventing Abuse and Violence

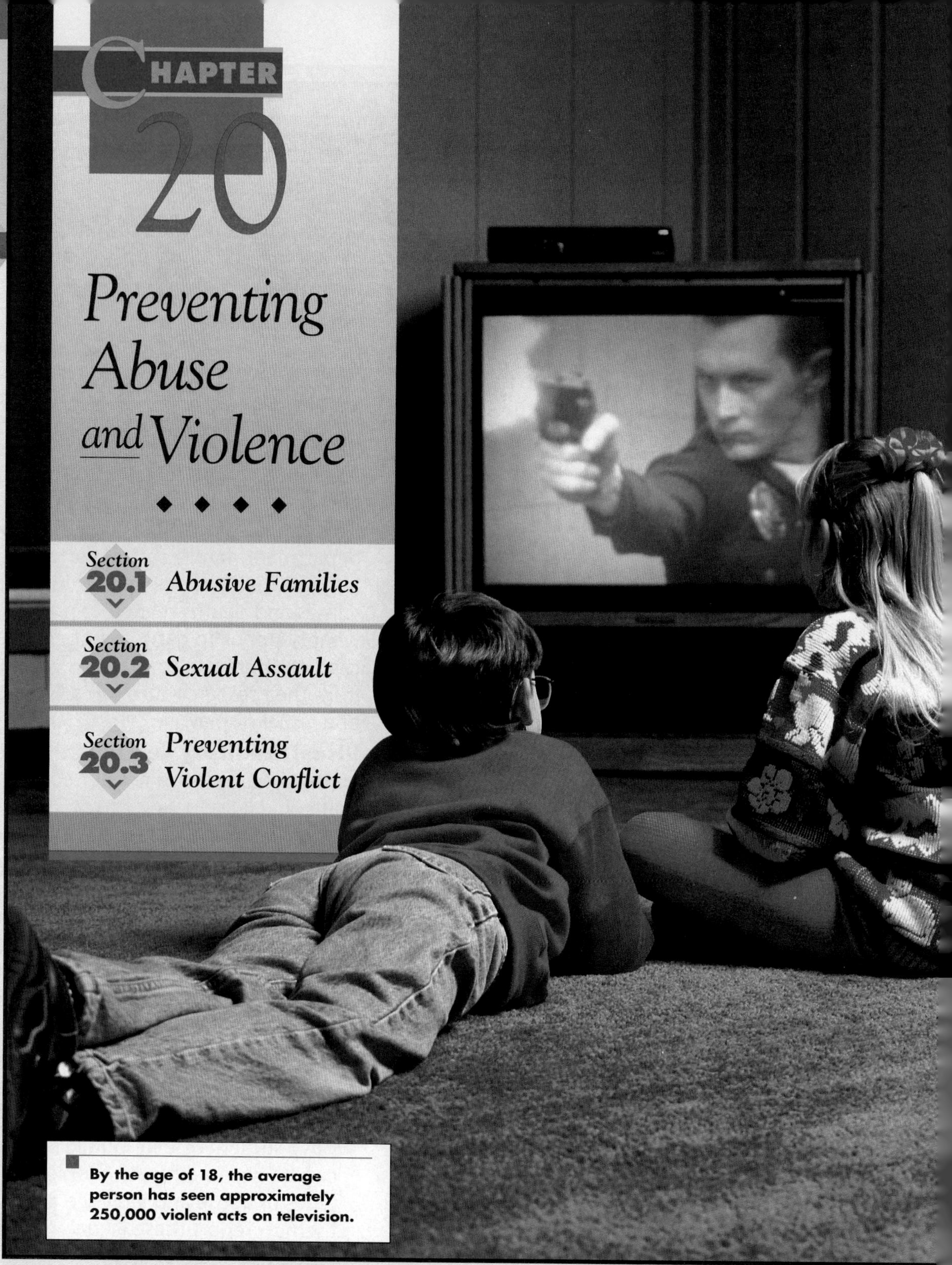

By the age of 18, the average person has seen approximately 250,000 violent acts on television.

Naomi and her family live next door to the Stones, a young couple with a little boy. The Stones always seem to be arguing—sometimes Naomi can hear Mr. Stone shouting at his wife and son late at night. At first Naomi's family tried not to listen; they figured that whatever the Stones said to each other was none of their business. But lately Naomi has become concerned about the Stones' son, Steve. He's a very withdrawn little boy who never smiles or laughs when Naomi tells him a joke.

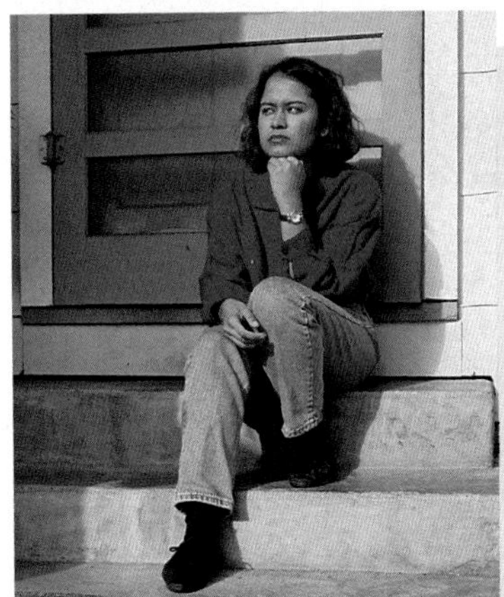

Yesterday Naomi noticed that Steve had a swollen lip and some bruises on his leg. It's not the first time Naomi has seen him with bruises. Steve always says that he got hurt falling off his bike, but Naomi thinks he's being abused. After talking to her parents, Naomi has decided to call the police and tell them about the Stones.

Section 20.1 Abusive Families

Objectives

- *Name four different types of child abuse.*
- *Define spouse abuse.*
- *Define elder abuse.*
- *Use a decision-making model to decide what you would do if you suspected child abuse.*
  LIFE SKILLS: Making Responsible Decisions
- *Know at least two ways you could report an abusive situation.*
  LIFE SKILLS: Using Community Resources

In too many families, members are treated with little respect. Sometimes this can take the form of abuse. In this section you will learn about the various types of abuse and what you can do if you or someone you know is the victim of abuse. Remember that physical abuse, sexual abuse, and neglect are all against the law, which means that authorities can intervene. They can arrest the offender or otherwise make sure that the abuse does not continue.

Child Abuse

The term **child abuse** refers to the mistreatment of children or adolescents. Child abuse can take the form of physical, emotional, or sexual abuse, as well as neglect. Though some children and adolescents are

child abuse:
mistreatment of a child or adolescent.

Section 20.1

Background
Domestic Violence in America
Domestic violence cuts across age, race, religious, income, and class lines. About three million households in the United States experience one or more violent episodes a year. Spouse abuse and child abuse often go hand-in-hand in a family. It is likely that over three million children witness family violence each year. Children who try to stop battering between their parents often end up injured. Even the unborn are affected: one in four abused women is pregnant, and many miscarry because of abuse. Violence between parents often escalates, and children are abused. However, simply witnessing such violence also scars children emotionally for life. Finally, children learn that violence is acceptable and perpetuate the pattern as adults.

Background
Sexual Violence in the Home
In many states, it is now unlawful for a man to force his wife to have sexual intercourse with him against her will.

Section 20.1 Lesson Plan

MOTIVATE

Class Discussion
What Is Child Abuse?
Ask students to give examples of acts by parents that they consider child abuse. What rights do parents have to discipline their children? Where do you draw the line between discipline and abuse? Is abuse always physical?

TEACH

Class Discussion
The Roots of Child Abuse
Why do some parents abuse their children? *[It's a pattern they learned as children. They don't understand children or parenting. Usually, they lack the resources to work out their problems, so they take their frustrations out on children.]* **If child abuse is passed on from generation to generation, how can it be stopped?** *[Adults can learn new responses and skills so that they don't repeat their own parents' mistakes.]* **What do you think abused children can do to stop abuse?** *[Call a hotline; talk to a trusted adult; call 911. Keep talking until someone listens and takes action. Running away may stop the abuse, but causes worse problems for the child.]*

Check Up

Have students answer the questions independently and turn them in anonymously. Tally their answers on the chalkboard, and focus on questions often missed.

Check Up

How Much Do You Already Know About Abuse and Violence?

1. Is it a crime to have sex with a child?
2. Are most batterers under the influence of alcohol or other drugs when they assault their spouses?
3. Are most rapes committed by someone who is a stranger to the victim?
4. Is it common for a woman to falsely accuse a man of rape?
5. Are most homicides committed by someone who is known to the victim?
6. Do most homicides occur between people of the same race?
7. Who is more often assaulted by gang members: members of other gangs, or people with no gang affiliation?

1. yes 2. yes 3. no 4. no 5. yes 6. yes 7. people with no gang affiliation

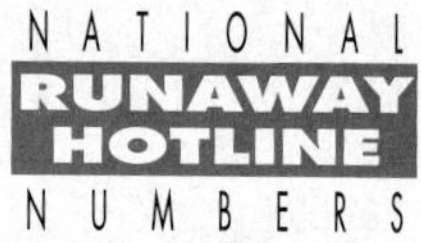

1-800-231-6946

sexual abuse: *sexual behavior between an adult and a child or adolescent.*

abused by people outside the family, more than 90 percent of child abuse is inflicted by family members.

Many abused children and adolescents run away from home to escape the abuse. They hope that living on the streets will be better than living at home. But tragically, many runaways survive by prostitution and other behaviors that endanger their lives. They also run the risk of being victims of a violent crime. Anyone who is thinking of running away from home should call the hotline shown at the left to learn about better options. The person who answers the hotline number can also help a teen who has already run away from home.

There are many reasons why parents abuse children. Personal problems such as lack of money, unemployment, or alcohol or drug abuse can make a parent angry and frustrated. Some parents take out their frustrations on their children.

Abusive parents may not understand child development; they may expect more mature behavior from a child than is reasonable. When the child isn't able to perform as the parent expects, the parent may become abusive.

People who were abused as children are more likely than others to abuse their own children when they become parents. They may not even realize what they are doing. To them abuse may seem normal, just a form of discipline. It's important to remember, however, that people who were abused as children will not necessarily repeat the abuse with their own children. They can stop the destructive patterns by learning appropriate parenting skills before they have children.

Physical Abuse **Physical abuse** occurs when an adult inflicts bodily harm on a child or adolescent. Physical abuse is physical punishment that goes far beyond normal discipline. The child may suffer scratches, bumps, bruises, broken bones, burns, or chipped teeth.

Though some cases of physical abuse are obvious, others may be hard to detect. The abusing parent may be careful to hit the child in areas that are usually covered by clothing, or may try to attribute the injury to an accident the child had. The child may also try to conceal the evidence of mistreatment, which can make abuse even more difficult to detect.

Sexual Abuse **Sexual abuse** is sexual behavior between an adult and a child or adolescent. Sexual abuse is most often inflicted upon girls between the ages of 12 and 14 by a father, stepfather, other relative, or friend of the family.

• • • TEACH continued

Writing
Keeping Child Abuse a Secret

Gena is a 13-year-old whose parents are abusing her physically, emotionally, and sexually. Have students write a paragraph telling why Gena might not report the abuse to other adults.

Cooperative Learning
Teach Your Children Well

After students discuss the bulleted list of principles, have them imagine that they are parents of young children or have a young brother or sister they want to protect from abuse by strangers. Have students work in groups to develop a plan for educating youngsters about protecting themselves from abuse. Plans should be frank and honest, without inducing fear.

Class Discussion
It Isn't Only Physical

Why are neglect and emotional mistreatment considered abusive? *[Neglect means a child's most basic needs are not met, thereby endangering his or her life; failing to love and destructively criticizing a child cause devastating psychological and emotional damage that lasts a lifetime.]* **What is an indicator that a child is neglected or emotionally abused?** *[Low self-esteem]*

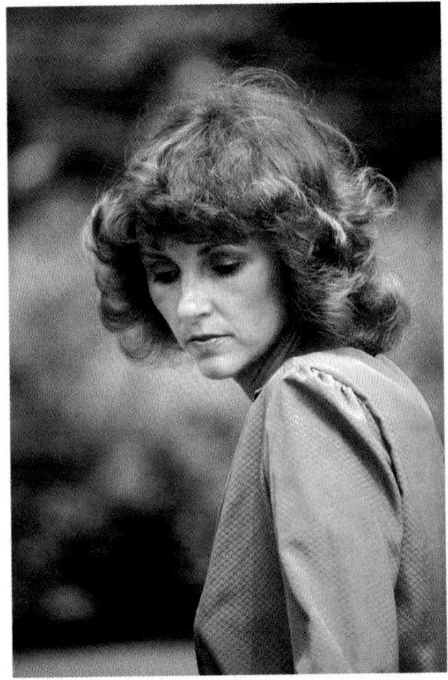

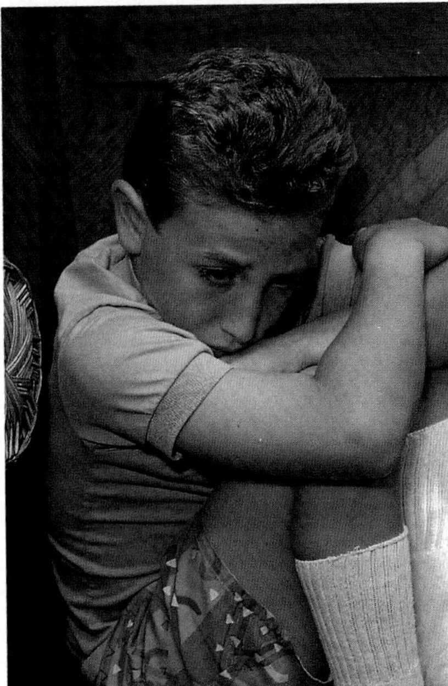

(FIGURE 20-1) **One of these people appears to be a abuser and the other a victim. In reality, however, most adults who abuse children were also the victims of child abuse.**

Though young girls are the most common victims of sexual abuse, boys are also frequently sexually abused. It is difficult to estimate how many boys are sexually abused, because they are less likely to tell anyone about the abuse.

It is rare for children to report sexual abuse. As a result, it is very difficult to get an accurate estimate of the extent of sexual abuse. However, some experts estimate that as many as 40 million people in the United States have been sexually abused.

Programs have been developed in schools and other community settings to make sure that children and adolescents understand several important principles:

- Sexual abuse is against the law.
- Children and adolescents have the right to refuse any sexual contact, and to run away or yell if they are being abused.
- Children and adolescents should tell a trusted adult if they are being abused.
- If that adult does nothing to stop the abuse, the child or adolescent should keep telling adults until someone helps.
- Even if they did nothing to stop the abuse, children and adolescents should not blame themselves for what happened.

People who have experienced sexual abuse often have emotional problems. They may have great difficulty forming close friendships and becoming part of a peer group. It is extremely important that sexually abused children and adolescents who have been sexually abused receive counseling and assurance that the abuse was not their fault.

Neglect Few people realize that **neglect** is a form of abuse. Neglect is the failure of a parent or guardian to provide for a child's

physical abuse:

to cause bodily harm to a child or adolescent.

neglect:

failure of a parent or guardian to provide for a child's basic needs.

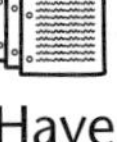

Personal Health Inventory

Have students complete the Personal Health Inventory for this chapter. The inventory helps them assess their knowledge about abuse and about healthy ways to handle anger.

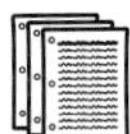

Life Skills Worksheet 20A

Making Daily Affirmations

Assign the Making Daily Affirmations Life Skills Worksheet, which directs students to say an affirmation to themselves every day for a week as an exercise for building self-esteem.

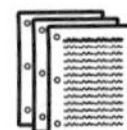

Life Skills Worksheet 20B

Help for Abusive Families

Assign the Help for Abusive Families Life Skills Worksheet, which directs students to choose a community resource that helps abusive families and find information about the services that resource offers.

Class Discussion

Reporting Abuse

Many people who suspect or know about child abuse fail to report it, although it is a crime. Ask students to list reasons why adults might fail to intercede *(feeling it's not their business, fear of retaliation)*. Also have them give reasons why a child might not report abuse he or she had witnessed *(fear that no one would listen, fear that things would get worse for the abused child)*. List these reasons on the chalkboard. For every reason listed, ask students to think of a reason why abuse should be reported.

Class Discussion

Linking Spouse and Child Abuse

In many families experiencing spouse abuse, child abuse is also occurring. **Why do you think spouse and child abuse so often occur together?** *[A dysfunctional adult who has learned violence as a response to frustration or a means of getting what he or she wants will likely strike out at an adult as well as a child.]*

Debate the Issue

Media Messages

Have students debate the topic: American culture and role models are responsible for much of the abuse of women and children. You may want to initiate a discussion before the debate by asking, **What messages do we often get from the media and society**

What Would You Do?

A Case of Child Abuse?

Have students write their responses; compare the responses to collect a range of options. Discuss the possible outcomes for each option.

Making A Choice 20A

Emergency Phone Numbers for Abuse

Assign the Emergency Phone Numbers for Abuse card. The card directs students to compile a list of phone numbers of various types of agencies in their community that people can call for help in abusive situations.

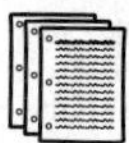

Section Review Worksheet 20.1

Assign Section Review Worksheet 20.1, which requires students to define and answer questions about different kinds of abuse that occur among family members.

Section Quiz 20.1

Have students take Section Quiz 20.1.

What Would You Do?

Making Responsible Decisions

A Case of Child Abuse?

You baby-sit to make extra money, and it is not unusual for you to get calls from people asking you to baby-sit at the last minute. Tonight you get such a call from someone you don't know very well. You can use the money, so you agree to baby-sit.

When you get to the couple's house, you are told that their three-year-old son is asleep and shouldn't give you much trouble. But shortly after the couple leaves, the child starts screaming. You decide to pick him up and walk with him until he goes back to sleep. As you are lifting him out of bed you notice very large black-and-blue marks on both arms, and on looking further, you see huge welts on the child's back. You don't know what could have caused the injuries, but you are sure the boy is in a lot of pain.

You've just learned about child abuse in school. You think this child may have been beaten, but you aren't sure. What would you do?

Remember to use the decision-making steps:

1. State the Problem.
2. List the Options.
3. Imagine the Benefits and Consequences.
4. Consider Your Values.
5. Weigh the Options and Decide.
6. Act.
7. Evaluate the Results.

basic needs. Failure to feed a child or provide adequate supervision are examples of neglect. You can help prevent the consequences of neglect by reporting such cases to the proper authorities.

emotional abuse: *emotional mistreatment of a child or adolescent.*

Emotional Abuse **Emotional abuse** is emotional mistreatment of a child or adolescent. A parent may continually criticize a child or fail to show love and affection. Although the effects of emotional abuse aren't as visible as those of physical abuse, they can be just as devastating. One of the worst effects of emotional abuse is low self-esteem. Children or adolescents who are emotionally abused can report the abuse to a trusted adult or call the Child Abuse Hotline shown on page 423 for help.

Spouse Abuse

Physical abuse of one's husband or wife is known as **spouse abuse.** Spouse abuse is also called spouse battering. When violence occurs between spouses, it is usually the woman who suffers injuries because of differences in strength.

The male abuser is usually a controlling person who becomes easily frustrated. Male abusers were often victims of abuse as children. In the majority of battering cases, the man had been drinking or using other drugs.

It may be difficult for someone to understand why an abused woman would stay with her spouse. Experts think that many abused women have low self-esteem and believe they deserve the abuse. They may feel that abuse is normal in marriage, especially if they observed their own mothers being abused. Another reason abused women stay in the relationship is that they often don't have enough money to move out and live on their own. But the most common reason is that battered women are often more afraid to leave than to stay. In many cases the batterer has threatened to kill her or the children, to kidnap the children, or to harm himself if she leaves.

Abused spouses may finally reach the point where they can no longer tolerate the mistreatment. They feel that they have to get out at any cost. Many communities have established shelters for such people.

• • • TEACH continued

about what it takes to be a real man? *[Real men are often portrayed as tough, strong, aggressive, financially successful, never-failing, and inexpressive.]* **In what ways do movies, television, books, and music appear to connect male sexuality with aggression and female sexuality with submission?** *[Much violence of men toward women is shown; some images even suggest that women deserve this or enjoy it. These messages appear to give social permission for force or violence.]*

Role-Playing

Helping Victims of Abuse

Discuss several observations that might alert students to a case of abuse, including suspicious marks and behaviors, witnessing abuse, or having someone confide that he or she has been abused. Brainstorm a situation in which several teenagers suspect abuse. Have volunteers role-play the situation, presenting different opinions about what should be done and taking action to help the victim(s). Continue the role-playing with other situations.

Extension

Information on Advocates for Abuse Victims

Encourage students to visit local mental health clinics, family service agencies, or the police department to get pamphlets and brochures describing the advocacy groups in your area that help victims of abuse. Allow students

The shelters provide a temporary home and help people find jobs or other means of financial support. In most communities shelters for abused spouses are listed in the white pages of the telephone book under "Battered Women."

Elder Abuse

Elder abuse is physical abuse of an elderly person. As with other kinds of abuse, family members who abuse elders are often frustrated with their lives and take their frustrations out on someone else. When a case of elder abuse is reported, trained professionals will probably require that the family participate in some type of counseling. The elderly person may be placed in another living arrangement if the counseling does not end the abuse.

Help for Abusive Families

No one should ever be abused, whether the abuse is physical, emotional, sexual, or in the form of neglect. It is important to report abuse immediately. You could report the abuse to a trusted adult or the police. You could also call 911 or one of the hotline numbers shown in this book. If a child or adolescent is being abused, you can call the National Child Abuse Hotline shown at the right.

Families in which abuse and violence occur need professional help to break the cycle of abuse. It is best if help is sought voluntarily, but it can be mandated by law.

Many victims feel responsible for the abuse. They believe that they are bad people who did something to deserve the abuse. Counseling will help them realize that they are not responsible for what has happened to them.

Counseling is available at many community health agencies for parents and children. The fees for counseling are usually based on ability to pay; the more money you have, the more money you pay. If you have very little money, you pay very little or nothing for the counseling. Counseling with a private therapist will usually involve a set fee, but sometimes an agreement based on ability to pay can be arranged.

People who abuse children or fear they will do so can also be obtained through Parents Anonymous, a national organization that helps parents cope without using violence. Many cities have local chapters of Parents Anonymous.

Parents can call the Parents Anonymous hotline number shown at the right when they feel they are losing control. The people who answer the phones at the hotline number are trained to defuse the immediate situation and encourage parents to get ongoing help.

Review

1. *Name four different types of child abuse.*
2. *Define spouse abuse.*
3. *Define elder abuse.*
4. ***LIFE SKILLS: Making Responsible Decisions*** *If you knew that a two-year-old child was frequently left alone for hours at a time, what would you do?*
5. ***LIFE SKILLS: Using Community Resources*** *To whom could you report a case of elder abuse?*
6. ***Critical Thinking*** *Why do you think sexually abused children often have trouble making friends?*

elder abuse:
physical abuse of an elderly person.

spouse abuse:
physical abuse of one's husband or wife.

NATIONAL
PARENTS ANONYMOUS
NUMBERS
1-800-421-0353

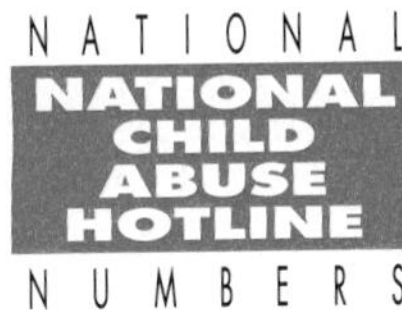

1-800-422-4453

SECTION 20.1

Reteaching Worksheet 20.1

Students who have difficulty with the material may complete Reteaching Worksheet 20.1, which requires them to match different forms of abuse with the definitions and complete sentences that list reasons for, results of, and help for the different forms of family abuse.

Review Answers

1. Physical abuse, sexual abuse, neglect, and emotional abuse
2. Physical abuse of one's husband or wife
3. Physical abuse of an elderly person
4. Students might talk with a trusted adult, call and talk with someone on the Child Abuse Hotline, or report the information to the police.
5. Students might talk with a trusted adult, call 911, or report the information to the police.
6. Students might answer that these children have difficulty making friends because they have low self-esteem and/or because these children feel that they brought about the abusive behavior and are bad people whom no one likes.

to report on these centers and explain how they work.

ASSESS

Section Review

Have students answer the Section Review questions.

Alternative Assessment

Why Abuse Is Hard to Stop

Have students write a brief essay explaining several reasons why abuse may be hard to detect and report, and why abusers and abused tend to perpetuate the problem rather than seek help.

Closure

Expressing Your Outrage

Have students create a poem, story, or artwork that expresses their feelings about child abuse.

Background
Profile of the Rapist

Most rapists are males between 15 and 35 years of age; they look and act normal. In most cases, the rapist already has a sexual partner, so he is not sexually deprived. Rapists come from every social, economic, and religious group and may have any intelligence level. The rapist wants to control, overpower, and humiliate someone. He doesn't accept blame or see the harm in what he does; in fact, he blames the victim. He may be a loner or have few close friends. He may have been abused as a child. Without treatment, the rapist is likely to continue the pattern of sexual assault with others.

Section 20.2 Sexual Assault

Objectives

- *Define sexual assault.*
- *Define acquaintance rape.*
- *Discuss how young men can avoid committing acquaintance rape.*
- *Know what a victimized person should do to get help after a sexual assault.*

LIFE SKILLS: Using Community Resources

sexual assault: *any sexual contact with a person without his or her consent.*

Sexual assault is defined as any sexual contact with a person without his or her consent. Sexual assaults include sexual abuse of children, forced sexual intercourse (rape), and all other kinds of forced sexual contact. Most sexual assaults—approximately 75 percent—are committed by people known to the victim.

It is estimated that at the current rates, one out of every four women in the United States will be sexually assaulted in her lifetime. In fact, every 46 seconds a woman is raped in this country.

Rapists do not discriminate on the basis of age, marital status, or physical appearance. Rape victims can be young or old, married or single. Research has shown that sexual assault is not a sexual act, but a violent way to show dominance or anger. Though most victims are female, males are also sexually assaulted, usually by heterosexual men.

Taking Precautions Against Sexual Assault

A person who is sexually assaulted is never responsible for what happened. Even if the assaulted person left the doors or windows unlocked, or wore ''provocative'' clothing, or hitchhiked, or went out on a date with the assailant, the victim was not responsible for the assault.

Even so, every woman should be aware of the potential danger and should do whatever she can to minimize her chances of being assaulted. Here are some recommended precautions you can take to reduce the risk of assault.

- Avoid walking alone in deserted areas.
- Have your keys ready for the car or the front door.
- Make sure that no one is in the rear seat of the car before getting in.
- Keep entrances and doorways to your house or apartment brightly lit.
- Use deadbolt locks on the doors of your house or apartment.
- Keep all windows and doors locked.

Sex offenders are often not instantly recognizable; most people who commit these crimes look like everyone else. There are, however, some behaviors that are known to be associated with sex offenders. Be wary if someone does the following:

- acts as if he knows you better than he does
- stands too close to you and seems to enjoy your discomfort
- blocks your way
- grabs or pushes you

Section 20.2 Lesson Plan

MOTIVATE

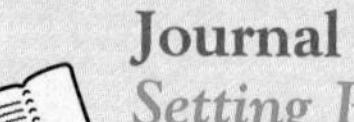

Journal 20A
Setting Personal Limits for Sex

This may be done as a warm-up activity. Have students privately consider their beliefs about sexual behavior on dates. Ask them to write in the Student Journal in the Student Activity Book what they would say to a date to make it clear what they expect and will or will not do.

Class Discussion
Sexual Assault

Write on the chalkboard "No one deserves to be sexually assaulted or abused." Explore students' conceptions of sexual assault by asking questions such as: What is sexual assault? What is the typical rapist like? Why would anyone sexually assault another person? What is the typical victim like? How are victims of sexual assault hurt?

TEACH

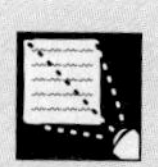

Teaching Transparency 20A
Myths and Facts About Rape

Show the transparency called "Myths and Facts About Rape" (Figure 20-2) and have students point out facts about rape that surprised them, and myths they previously believed were

Myths and Facts About Rape

Myth	Fact
Only young, beautiful people are raped.	*Rape victims include people of all ages and appearances.*
People who hitchhike or wear sexy clothing are asking to be raped.	*Rape is a humiliating crime that inflicts long-lasting damage on its victims. No one asks to be hurt in this way.*
Most rapes occur in dangerous places.	*More than half of all rapes occur in the home. The next most common place is in an automobile.*
Most rapes occur because the rapist is sexually starved.	*Most rapes occur because the rapist has a desire to overpower and humiliate someone else.*
Most rapes are committed by someone unknown to the victim.	*Most rapes are committed by a person known to the victim.*
It is common for a woman to falsely accuse a man of rape.	*There are no more false reports of rape than of any other crime. Most victims do not even report the rape.*
Men are never raped.	*Men are raped, usually by heterosexual men. However, men are less likely to report a rape.*

(FIGURE 20-2)

The best protection is to act quickly when someone's behavior seems strange. It might require causing a scene in public, but that's better than being assaulted. Begin with a loud yell, which can intimidate the aggressor and give you confidence.

Physical resistance, including yelling, running, or fighting, is entirely appropriate if you are in danger of being assaulted. It is also important to know, however, that a person who has been sexually assaulted and did not try to resist or run away has also acted appropriately. Anything a person does to stay alive during such an attack is absolutely acceptable and is nothing to be ashamed of.

Many people take self-defense classes to learn how to protect themselves. If you would like to do this, choose a class that deals specifically with self-defense in real-life situations, not martial arts such as judo and karate. Martial arts are good sports and give a person confidence, but they don't provide the kind of experience a person needs to defend against a sexual assault.

Background
Helping a Friend Who's Been Assaulted

Rape victims have been physically and emotionally traumatized; they need help and support. If a friend confides that she or he has been raped, the listener should:

- Practice active listening. (Don't interrupt; respond to what the person says, not to what you think she or he needs; nod to show you are listening; repeat if the person has trouble going on.)
- Show caring and compassion. (Give support, not blame; express sympathy in a way natural to yourself; don't say "You'll soon get over it.")
- Believe the victim. (People almost never invent sexual assaults.)
- Help the victim get immediately needed help. (Encourage reporting the incident; offer to accompany the victim for a medical exam or police interview.)

true. How do you think these myths became part of our culture? Do the media and advertisers affect your view of acceptable sexual behavior? What other factors influence your beliefs?

Reinforcement
Sexual Assault—Whose Fault Is It?

Emphasize that the victim of sexual assault is never at fault for being assaulted. The crime is not one of passion but of force and violence. Ask students to respond to the double message often conveyed by our culture: "Nice women don't say 'yes' and real men don't listen to 'no.'"

Reinforcement
Precautions Against Sexual Assault

Emphasize the importance of taking precautions and responding actively to avoid putting yourself at risk of sexual assault. Review the bulleted suggestions listed on page 424.

Teaching Transparency 20B
A Case of Acquaintance Rape

Show the transparency "A Case of Acquaintance Rape" (Figure 20-3). Have students pick out statements and actions that caused miscommunication between Ann and Jim. Compare Ann's and Jim's thoughts at each stage of their date, writing them on the chalkboard side by side. Encourage students to add more statements to the list that

Background
When the Victim Is Male
Males are sexually assaulted, too. National statistics say one in seven young men is sexually assaulted (the number for young women is one in four). Most often, the attacker is an adult heterosexual male. (This statistic reinforces the notion that rape is about power and humiliation, not sexuality.) Very young males are most often assaulted by caretakers or family members; young teenage boys are most often assaulted by authority figures such as coaches, teachers, or youth leaders; and older teenage boys are most often assaulted by peers and adults. Very few males report the assault, but these attacks are just as hurtful and criminal as assaults on females.

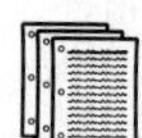 **Life Skills Worksheet 20C**

Preventing Sexual Assault
Assign the Preventing Sexual Assault Life Skills Worksheet, which requires students to rewrite Ann's story of sexual assault, having Ann use any methods of resistance that seem appropriate.

A Case of Acquaintance Rape

How Ann Described What Happened	How Jim Described What Happened
I first met Jim at a party. He was really good-looking and he had a great smile. I wanted to meet him but I wasn't sure how. I didn't want to appear too forward. Then he came over and introduced himself. We talked and found we had a lot in common. I really liked him. When he asked me over to his place for a drink, I thought it would be okay. He was such a good listener, and I wanted him to ask me out again. *When we got to his room, the only place to sit was on the bed. I didn't want him to get the wrong idea, but what else could I do? We talked for a while and then he made his move. I was so startled. He started by kissing. I really liked him so the kissing was nice. But then he pushed me down on the bed. I tried to get up and I told him to stop. He was so much bigger and stronger. I got scared and I started to cry. I froze and he raped me.* *It took only a couple of minutes and it was terrible, he was so rough. When it was over he kept asking me what was wrong, like he didn't know. He had just forced himself on me and he thought that was okay. He drove me home and he said he wanted to see me again. I'm so afraid to see him. I never thought it would happen to me.*	*I first met her at a party. She looked really hot, wearing a sexy dress that showed off her great body. We started talking right away. I knew that she liked me by the way she kept smiling and touching my arm while she was speaking. She seemed pretty relaxed so I asked her back to my place for a drink. When she said yes, I knew that I was going to be lucky!* *When we got to my place, we sat on the bed kissing. At first, everything was great. Then, when I started to lay her down on the bed, she started twisting and saying she didn't want to. Most women don't like to appear too easy, so I knew she was just going through the motions. When she stopped struggling, I knew that she would have to throw in some tears before we did it.* *She was still very upset afterwards, and I just don't understand it! If she didn't want to have sex, why did she come back to the room with me? You could tell by the way she dressed and acted that she was no virgin, so why she had to put up such a struggle I don't know.*

(FIGURE 20-3) **These are two accounts of an acquaintance rape that occurred at a college. Notice that Jim has no idea he raped Ann. Whenever someone's protests against sexual intercourse are ignored, a rape has occurred.**

• • • TEACH continued

describe other possible misunderstandings that may occur during a date.

 **Cooperative Learning**
Miscommunication
Have students work in small groups to create a comic strip that illustrates one or more miscommunications during a date. Then have them prepare a second comic strip that shows good communication and an alternative outcome.

Class Discussion
Setting Limits
Write on the board "Your date doesn't have ESP!" Around the statement, draw balloons with thoughts such as "I wonder if it's okay to kiss him?" "Will she think I'm a wimp if I don't go all the way?" "All I have to do is push a little, and she'll do it." "How do I get him to stop with just kissing?" Have students suggest other balloon thoughts and add them to the board. Ask students to come up with a set of "Daters' Communication Laws" that will clear up all this confusion. *(Possible responses might include thinking through your limits before the date, talking to your date about your feelings, limits, and expectations; and listening to your partner's limits and respecting them.)*

Role-Playing
Tell It Like It Is
Have students write descriptions of dating situations on index cards. (A couple are going with a large group to a party where liquor may be served

Preventing Acquaintance Rape

Acquaintance rape, which is sometimes called "date rape," occurs when a woman is forced or coerced into sexual intercourse by an acquaintance or date. The force or coercion may be verbal pressure, threats, physical restraint, or physical violence. Any time a woman's protests against engaging in sexual activity are ignored by the man, a rape has occurred.

Acquaintance rape is partly the result of the way many men think they are supposed to behave with women. Many men think they should always be aggressive and in control.

Some men see sexual intimacy as a competition between the man and the woman, almost like a sport. As in playing sports, some young men might feel that they should "win" at any cost. Even the slang of sexual conquest is similar to that of sports: men speak of "scoring" with a woman. One young man described the situation this way: "A man is supposed to view a date with a woman as a premeditated scheme for getting the most sex out of her. . . . He's supposed to constantly pressure her to see how far he can get. She is his adversary, his opponent in a battle . . ."

Most young women, however, have not been socialized into thinking of sexual intimacy as a contest. Neither have they been encouraged to be assertive in resisting things they don't want to do. As a result, they may be unprepared to resist aggression.

Read the two accounts of an acquaintance rape in Figure 20-3. The account on the left was given by a female college student who was raped. The one on the right is the account given by the male college student who committed the rape. Notice how differently the two saw the events.

As with any sexual assault, the burden of responsibility for preventing acquaintance rape lies with the offender, not the potential victim. It requires a fundamental change in the way many men view sexual encounters.

Young men can avoid committing acquaintance rape by remembering that if someone says "no" at any point, they are

"I know that when girls say no they really mean it—and guys who don't listen are jerks."

Rick

acquaintance rape:
the forcing or coercion of a woman into sexual intercourse by an acquaintance or date.

SECTION 20.2

Section Review Worksheet 20.2

Assign Section Review Worksheet 20.2, which requires students to recognize behaviors associated with sexual offenders and precautions to reduce the risk of assault.

Section Quiz 20.2

Have students take Section Quiz 20.2.

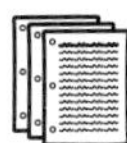

Reteaching Worksheet 20.2

Students who have difficulty with the material may complete Reteaching Worksheet 20.2, which requires them to read about a situation involving an acquaintance rape and answer questions about it.

and adult supervision may be lax; a couple are going on a hayride.) Each situation should present an opportunity for partners to communicate clearly what they want. Have volunteers role-play each situation, focusing on skill building in these areas:

- Communicating limits
- Noticing power-play behavior
- Being assertive

Class Discussion

Help for Victims of Sexual Assault

Many victims of sexual assault choose not to report the crime. Discuss reasons why this occurs. *(Victims may assume wrongly that they are at fault, want to avoid public shame or attention, fear reprisal by the criminal, want to put it out of their mind, feel they won't be believed, fear punishment because they were breaking rules when it happened.)* Stress the positives of reporting:

- Victims will receive medical and counseling care.
- The criminal should not be able to hurt others.
- Victims can receive needed protection and support.
- Police and other advocacy groups are trained to help the victim.
- Victims need to know if disease was transmitted during the assault.

Review Answers

1. Any sexual contact with a person without his or her consent
2. The forcing or coercion of a woman into sexual intercourse by an acquaintance or date
3. Men have to change the way they view sexual encounters and they must remember that if someone says no at any point, they are obligated to accept no as the answer to further sexual behavior.
4. They could contact the police and/or the local rape-crisis hot line.
5. Just because Ann said yes to going to Jim's place, Jim assumed that Ann was also saying yes to sexual intercourse. When Ann told Jim to stop his sexual advances, Jim ignored her, feeling that Ann really wanted to have sex but didn't want to appear too easy.

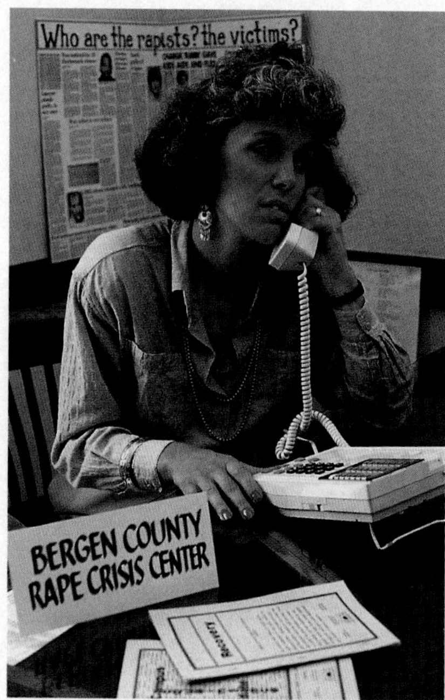

(FIGURE 20-4) **Help for victims of sexual assault can be obtained by calling a local rape-crisis hotline.**

obligated to accept "no" as the answer. Even if a young woman voluntarily engages in some degree of sexual intimacy, it is not the same as agreeing to intercourse. One thing does not necessarily lead to another. No matter how quietly a young woman objects, she still means "no."

It is important that young women communicate their limits clearly and assertively to the other person. It will help to review the discussion about resisting pressure on pages 378–379 in Chapter 17. As in any kind of sexual assault, running away or physically resisting is entirely appropriate.

After a Sexual Assault

After any sexual assault, a victimized person should contact the police as soon as possible. It is also helpful to call the local rape-crisis hotline, which can provide counseling and emotional support, as well as assistance with the judicial system. In addition, a medical examination will probably be necessary to collect legal evidence of the assault and to screen for possible sexually transmitted diseases and pregnancy. A worker from the rape-crisis center can accompany the person throughout this crisis and can provide assistance even if the person chooses not to report the crime to the police.

Unfortunately, most rapes are not reported. It's not always easy to report a rape—victims of sexual assault often feel humiliated and ashamed. Reporting the crime, they may feel, might prolong their feelings of anguish. It may be better to try to forget what happened and get on with life. These feelings are completely understandable, but it is also important to know that rape is a serious crime. No matter whether the rape occurred between strangers, acquaintances, or even friends, the person who committed the rape is a criminal and deserves to be punished.

Review

1. *Define sexual assault.*
2. *Define acquaintance rape.*
3. *Discuss how young men can avoid committing acquaintance rape.*
4. ***LIFE SKILLS: Using Community Resources*** *What can a victimized person do to get help after a sexual assault?*
5. ***Critical Thinking*** *Review the two accounts of a rape in Figure 20-3. What were the fallacies in Jim's thinking that led to his committing an acquaintance rape?*

• • • TEACH continued

Extension

What Happens After Sexual Assault?

Have students visit or phone local sexual assault, rape crisis, or mental health centers as well as the police department to find out about procedures and victims' rights in each of the following areas: medical care, criminal justice procedures, prosecution, and emotional recovery.

ASSESS

Section Review

Have students answer the Section Review questions.

Alternative Assessment

Who Is the Villain?

Have students write an essay explaining their point of view about who is responsible when an acquaintance rape occurs. They should defend their opinions as persuasively as possible.

Closure

Ideas About Sexual Assault

Ask students to mention something they have learned about sexual assault that was entirely new to them or contradicted a previous belief.

Section 20.3 Preventing Violent Conflict

Objectives

- *Name the three major risk factors associated with homicides.*
- *Discuss the reasons why some teenagers join gangs.*
- *Know how to prevent your anger from turning into violence.*
  LIFE SKILLS: Coping
- *Know how to resolve conflicts without violence.*
  LIFE SKILLS: Solving Problems

It is estimated that by age 18, the average youth has watched 250,000 acts of violence and 40,000 attempted murders on television. These figures don't even include the violent acts depicted in movies, books, and magazines. Violence in the media often appears exciting and glamorous. Even grisly cult murders are presented in gory detail. It seems that violence has become so commonplace that we hardly react to it anymore. The lesson that many learn from all this is that if you have a problem, you solve it with violence.

What we know about violence in our society seems to indicate that too many people are attempting to solve their problems with violent acts. **Homicide**—a violent crime that results in the death of another person—is the second leading cause of death of all people aged 15 to 24.

One of the major risk factors related to homicide is the use of alcohol or other drugs. Substance abuse is a factor in almost half of all homicides in this country. Alcohol alone is involved in more than half of all violent crimes committed in the United States.

Another major risk factor is possession of a gun, since the most common weapon used to kill people is a firearm. A recent survey of high school students showed that approximately one out of 20 students had carried a gun at least once during the 30 days preceding the survey. Clearly, many deaths of young people could be prevented if people did not carry guns.

Arguments are also a major risk factor associated with homicide. As you can see in Figure 20-5, the most common event associated with a homicide is an argument. If

homicide: *a violent crime that results in the death of another person.*

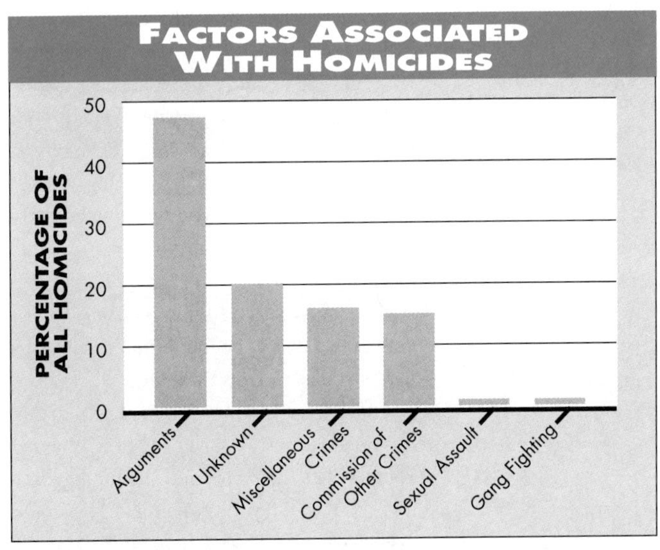

(FIGURE 20-5) **The most common event associated with a homicide is an argument.**

Background
Gun Control

In the late 1980s, about 33,000 people died in the United States annually from gunshot wounds. Thousands of federal, state, and local laws control the use of firearms. For example, some laws prohibit the ownership of guns by people who are mentally impaired or have a criminal record. However, these laws are difficult to enforce because guns are so widely available. A survey conducted in 1990 showed that 43 percent of the respondents had firearms in their homes. White men are most likely to own a gun. The less educated, the more likely a person is to own a gun.

Section 20.3 Lesson Plan

MOTIVATE

Journal 20B
Feeling Your Anger Pulse

This may be done as a warm-up activity. Ask students to think about things that make them angry or upset. When have they been angry enough to hit someone? What did they do? Have them describe in the Student Journal in the Student Activity Book an experience they had recently that required them to deal with their anger.

TEACH

Class Discussion
Acceptance of Violence

Ask students to name TV shows, videos, and movies that depict violence; list these on the chalkboard. Have students describe their reaction to seeing violent acts on the screen. Discuss the effects of this constant exposure. *(Viewers become desensitized, cynical, and more accepting of violence; some may be persuaded to use violence themselves, either to get what they want or to resolve conflicts.)*

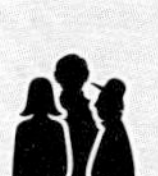

Cooperative Learning
Violence in Popular Culture

Divide the class into small groups and give each group a list of television programs and several super-hero comic books to analyze for violence. With the

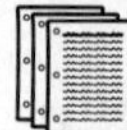

Life Skills Worksheet 20D

Managing Anger

Assign the Managing Anger Life Skills Worksheet, which requires students to set goals for managing anger and channeling it in positive ways.

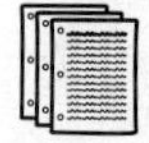

Evaluating the Media Worksheet

Have students complete the Evaluating the Media Worksheet for Unit 5.

Making A Choice 20B

Resolving Conflict Without Violence

Assign the Resolving Conflict Without Violence card. The card directs students to describe a conflict that had a violent resolution, discuss possible nonviolent resolutions to the conflict, and role-play the different nonviolent solutions.

we can prevent violent arguments, especially when they occur between people who have been abusing drugs and who are carrying guns, many homicides can be avoided.

Controlling Anger

Violence often occurs when people who know each other become uncontrollably angry. Therefore, we can prevent many injuries and deaths by learning to deal with and to control angry feelings before they become overwhelming.

The first step is to recognize that anger is a perfectly normal emotion. We all feel angry from time to time, and we will continue to do so all our lives. It doesn't help much to try to keep from getting angry. What matters is stopping the anger, which is an emotion, from turning into violence, which is a behavior.

Many people don't even realize they are angry until the feeling is out of control. They need to learn how to recognize the early signs of anger, which are usually felt in the body before the mind is aware of them. Think back to a time when you were extremely angry. Try to remember how your body felt. Did your heart beat faster? Were you breathing rapidly? Did your muscles tense up? If so, these were physical clues that you were getting angry. Remember them so that you will immediately recognize the next time you begin to feel anger.

As soon as you know you are beginning to feel angry, get out of the situation as fast as you can. Don't wait until it's too late and the damage is done. It may help to talk to someone about your anger or to channel your physical response into something positive, like walking or running. You could even hit a pillow or a punching bag. Do whatever works to keep you from damaging people or property.

Resolving Conflicts Without Violence

The best way to deal with potentially violent conflicts is to avoid them. If someone seems to be picking a fight with you, just walk away if you can.

If you cannot avoid the conflict, do what you can to keep the conflict from becoming violent. Take some deep breaths, stay calm, and do not raise your voice. Try to think of a way to compromise with the other person.

It will help you prepare to resolve conflicts without violence if you review the RESPECT method of resolving conflicts presented on pages 362–363 in Chapter 17.

Gangs

Gang-related violence is increasing in this country, and more and more teenagers are becoming involved. Though many gang-related crimes are directed at enemy gang members, these do not constitute the majority of gang incidents. More than half the time, people with no gang affiliation are the ones who are killed or assaulted.

Why do teenagers join gangs? Certainly, poverty and poor job prospects contribute to the proliferation of gangs.

Gangs also provide a sense of family and a feeling of belonging that is lacking in many young people's lives. Michael, another former gang member who is serving time in prison, said that after his parents split up he didn't get the attention he needed. Then he joined a gang. "There I got a little attention—from the other gang members," Michael said. "I felt they loved me and they were a family."

The desire to belong to a family is also a major reason some people join cults. Although not as violent as gangs, cults can be just as dangerous—particularly ones that involve occult or satanic practices.

• • • TEACH continued

whole class, design an evaluation form. (It may include spaces for the program or comic book's name, types of violence shown, frequency of violent episodes, and motivation for violence.) Then have each group review the evaluations. They should assign a numerical violence rating to each program or comic book. How violent are the programs and comics they reviewed? Are there any general differences between the two media?

Class Discussion
The Physical Effects of Anger

Remind students that anger is a normal emotion everyone experiences. Have students list things that make them angry. Ask them to describe physical changes they experience when angry. *(Increased heart rate, faster breathing, muscle tension, flushed face, clenched fists, and so on)* Explain that anger creates physical reactions that require release.

Cooperative Learning
Dealing with Anger

Have students work in small groups to list situations that they feel are anger inducing and a number of different nonviolent responses to anger. *(Some suggestions include deep breathing, leaving the situation, exercising, hitting something soft, talking to a friend or teacher or counselor, finding the humor in the situation, talking to the person you are angry at, or giving the other person an out.)* Have each group take a

There are many good clubs and organizations for teens that can also provide a feeling of belonging to a family without the goal of violence. Recreation centers, for example, generally sponsor youth groups, and many schools have athletic, academic, or social clubs for interested students. Check your phone book or with your school guidance counselor for possible options.

The desire for status is another reason some people join gangs. Gang members may get "respect" from others. The media may also contribute to the appeal of gangs. A radio ad for a malt liquor, for example,

LifeSKILLS: Solving Problems

Nonviolent Conflict Resolution

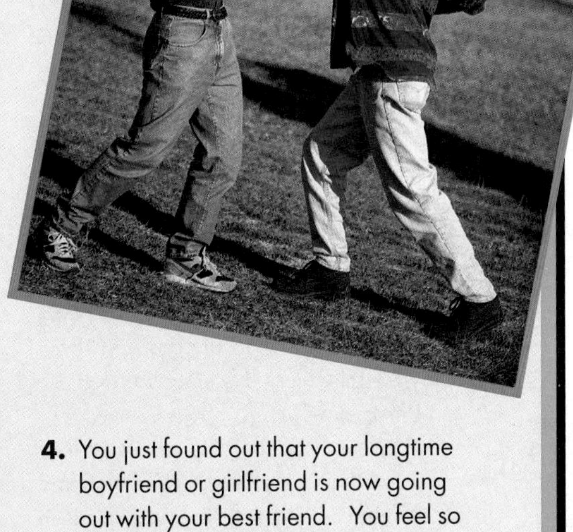

For each of the situations described below, explain how you might prevent a violent conflict.

1. You've just moved from another region of the country and started attending a new school. Two other students begin making fun of your accent and tell you to meet them after school so they can "teach you how to talk right."
2. Another student has borrowed money from you repeatedly but never pays it back. You see him in the hall with a group of his buddies, staring and laughing at you. They walk over to you and demand all your money.
3. A student at your school accused you of covering a wall with graffiti. But you didn't do it. You have an idea who *did* do it, but you aren't sure. The more you think about it, the angrier you get. What would you do?

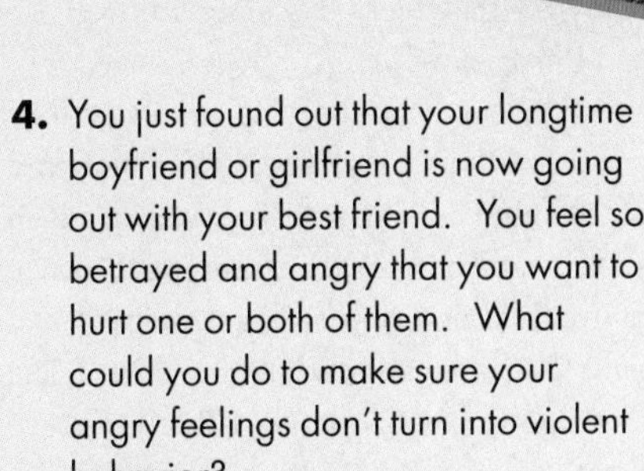

4. You just found out that your longtime boyfriend or girlfriend is now going out with your best friend. You feel so betrayed and angry that you want to hurt one or both of them. What could you do to make sure your angry feelings don't turn into violent behavior?

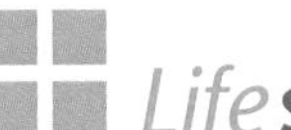

Life SKILLS

Nonviolent Conflict Resolution

You may want to divide the class into four groups and have each one work out a nonviolent resolution to one of the conflicts featured. Which solutions seemed to work best?

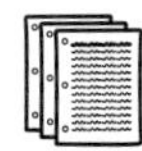

Section Review Worksheet 20.3

Assign Section Review Worksheet 20.3, which requires students to fill in charts on risk factors associated with homicide, steps to prevent anger from turning to violence, and steps to resolve conflict without violence.

Section Quiz 20.3

Have students take Section Quiz 20.3.

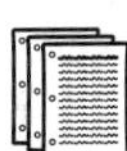

Reteaching Worksheet 20.3

Students who have difficulty with the material may complete Reteaching Worksheet 20.3, which requires them to answer true-false questions about violence and order steps used to prevent anger from turning to violence.

situation from another group and decide how to respond, using their list of nonviolent responses. Students may wish to role-play their solutions. Discuss which responses worked best for each situation.

Reinforcement

Who Suffers Most from Gang Violence?

Remind students that many of the victims of gang violence are innocent people who got in the line of fire. In over half of gang-related incidents, the people who are injured or killed are not gang members.

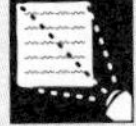

Teaching Transparency 20C

People in Conflict

In this transparency, students should discuss what the cartoon characters who are in conflict might be saying. Have students provide a possible dialog for the people in the cartoon.

Extension

Nonviolent Conflict Resolution in History

Encourage students to research and report on famous figures—such as Mohandas K. Gandhi and Martin Luther King, Jr.—who have led by nonviolent example.

Review Answers

1. Use of alcohol and/or drugs, possession of a gun, and arguments

2. Poverty and poor job prospects, access to money, glorification by media, desire for status, sense of a family and a feeling of belonging

3. Answers will vary. Some students may answer that they would get out of the situation as soon as they began to feel angry and then channel that anger into some positive action, such as exercise. Students may also suggest that they try to resolve the differences that are causing the anger by compromising.

4. Answers will vary. Students may answer that they would ask for the jacket back and resolve any conflicts using the RESOLVE method.

5. Answers will vary. Most people join satanic cults for many of the same reasons that people join gangs. They may join satanic cults because the media glorify such behavior, for a feeling of status and power, or for a feeling of belonging to a family and being accepted.

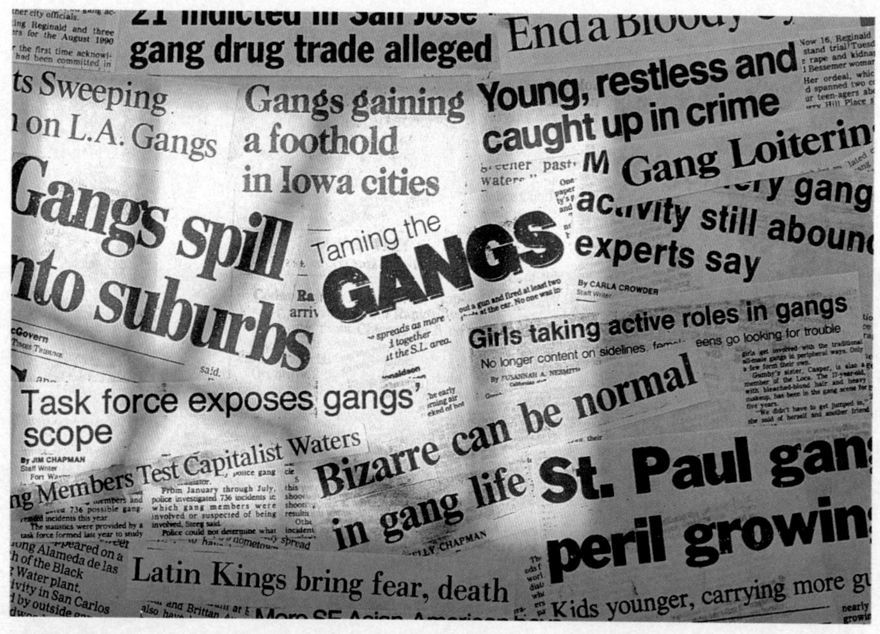

(FIGURE 20-6) **In recent years, drive-by shootings and other incidents of gang violence have become more common on the streets of our cities.**

referred to a gang tradition and compared the drink to a certain type of gun.

Unfortunately, the status that members get from gangs is often short-lived. Gang members are extremely vulnerable to homicide. A teenage gang member who was locked up in a juvenile security camp in Los Angeles County described his brief life: "I've been stabbed four times, shot three times, and locked up and beaten up so many times that it's hard to keep count. The only thing left for me is to die, but I've been ready for that every day since I turned 13, and I'm 16 now."

There is hope for gang members; they can leave their gangs and make a new life for themselves. After losing five friends in street warfare, Michael is learning the trade of welding and hopes to get married and have kids when he gets out of prison. "The guys in my neighborhood, I'll always love them . . . . But I don't want that life anymore."

Review

1. *Name the three major risk factors associated with homicides.*
2. *Discuss the reasons why some teenagers join gangs.*
3. ***LIFE SKILLS: Coping*** *If you felt yourself becoming extremely angry with a stranger, what could you do to prevent your anger from turning into violence?*
4. ***LIFE SKILLS: Solving Problems*** *If a fellow student stole your jacket, what could you do to resolve the conflict without violence?*
5. ***Critical Thinking*** *Discuss some possible reasons why people join satanic cults.*

ASSESS

Section Review

Have students answer the Section Review questions.

Alternative Assessment

Reducing the Risk of Homicide

Have students make a collage featuring one factor that increases the risk of violent death. Each collage should also include a visual representation of how the violence might be prevented.

Closure

Joining a Gang

Ask students to consider what, if anything, could change in people's lives that might make them seriously consider joining a gang. *(They may mention changes in family circumstances, encounters with gang members, or the need to make a lot of money.)*

Highlights

Summary

- Child abuse can take the form of physical, emotional, and sexual abuse, as well as neglect. Most child abuse is inflicted by family members.
- People who were abused when they were children are more likely to abuse their own children.
- Alcohol and other drug abuse is a factor in most cases of spouse abuse. When violence does occur between spouses, it is usually the woman who suffers injuries, because of differences in size and strength.
- Many abused women who stay in abusive marriages do so because they have low self-esteem.
- It is important to report abuse immediately. Families in which abuse and violence occur need professional help to break the cycle of abuse.
- Sexual assault is less a sexual act than a way to show dominance or anger toward the victim. Most sexual assaults are committed by someone the victim knows.
- To avoid acquaintance rape, men should accept that when a woman says "no" she means "no." It's also a good idea for women to communicate their limits clearly and assertively.
- The best way to deal with potentially violent conflicts is to avoid them.
- Poverty, poor job prospects, the desire for status, and the need to belong are factors that cause youths to join gangs.

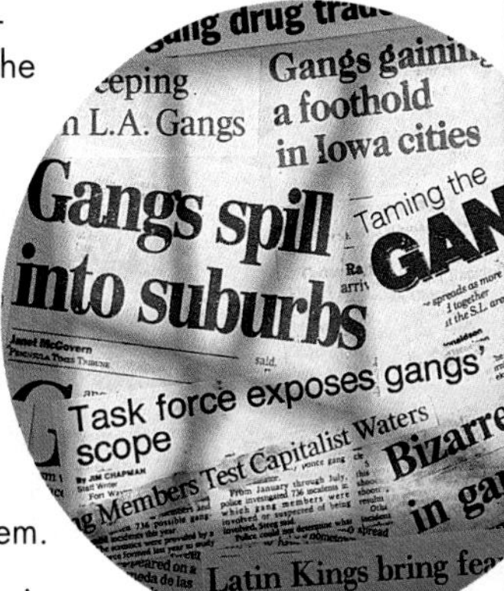

Vocabulary

child abuse mistreatment of a child or adolescent.

physical abuse to cause bodily harm to a child or adolescent.

sexual abuse sexual behavior between an adult and a child or adolescent.

neglect failure of a parent or guardian to provide for a child's basic needs.

emotional abuse emotional mistreatment of a child or adolescent.

spouse abuse physical abuse of one's husband or wife.

elder abuse physical abuse of an elderly person.

sexual assault any sexual contact with a person without his or her consent.

acquaintance rape the forcing or coercion of a woman into sexual intercourse by an acquaintance or date.

homicide a violent crime that results in the death of another person.

Chapter 20 Highlights Strategies

Summary

Have students read the summary to reinforce the concepts they learned in Chapter 20.

Vocabulary

Have students make a violence wheel, dividing a circle into eight sections. In each section, they place their own definition of one vocabulary word. Below the wheel, students can explain what all these forms of violence have in common.

Extension

Encourage students to locate and read books and current articles on abuse, sexual assault, or violent crime in America. They can share what they learn from reading in a panel presentation.

CHAPTER 20 ASSESSMENT

CHAPTER REVIEW

Concept Review

Sample Responses:

1. Child abuse is the mistreatment of a child or adolescent. Abuse can be physical, emotional, or sexual. Neglect is the failure of a parent or guardian to provide for a child's basic needs.

2. Parents were abused as children; personal problems, such as lack of money, unemployment, and alcohol or drug abuse can make parents angry and frustrated and cause them to take their feelings out on their children; parents may not understand child development.

3. They may be embarrassed, afraid the abuser will harm them further, or may not want the abuser to be jailed.

4. Child abuse, spouse abuse, and elder abuse

5. They have low self-esteem, they believe they deserve to be abused, and they may feel that they cannot make it on their own financially.

6. Acts as if he knows you better than he does, stands too close to you and seems to enjoy your discomfort, blocks your way, or grabs or pushes you

7. In order to collect legal evidence and to screen for sexually transmitted diseases and pregnancy.

8. One that teaches a person how to protect and defend himself or herself in real-life situations.

9. Very prevalent; homicide is the second leading cause of death for all people ages 15 to 24.

10. Your heart beats faster, you breathe more rapidly, and your muscles tense up.

11. They provide a sense of belonging by giving the attention and "love" that may be lacking in a family.

Expressing Your Views

Sample responses:

1. Yes. Sexual assault is against the law. When sexual assault is reported, the person committing the assault has a better chance of getting help to prevent him or her from doing the same thing again. Also, by reporting the assault, the victim can get the help he or she needs in dealing with the experience.

2. Emotional abuse can lead to low self-esteem. People with low self-esteem are

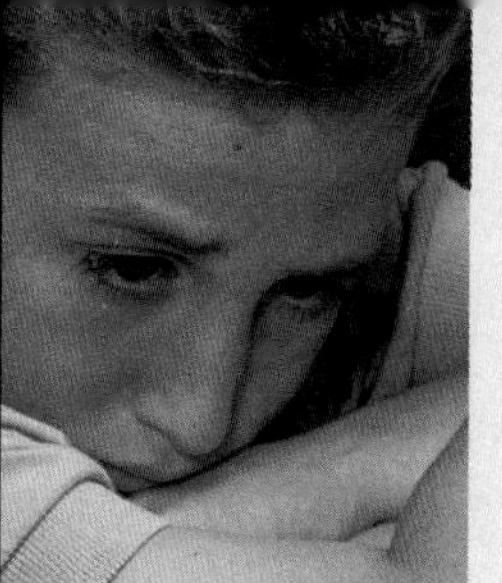

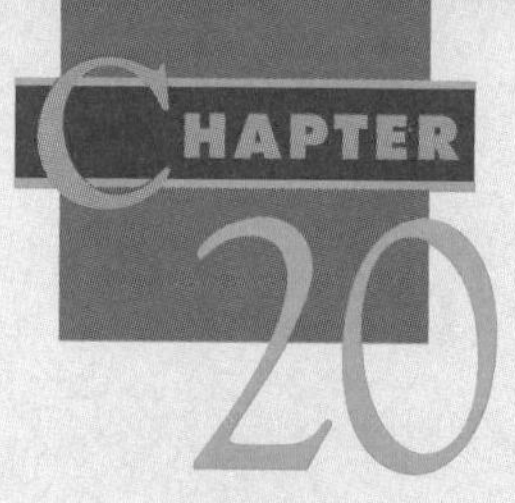

Chapter Review

Concept Review

1. Compare child abuse and child neglect.
2. What are three reasons why parents abuse children?
3. Why is it unlikely that a sexually abused child will report the abuse?
4. Describe three kinds of family violence.
5. Why do abused wives have trouble leaving their spouses?
6. List three behaviors that are known to be associated with sex offenders.
7. Why is a medical examination necessary after a sexual assault?
8. Which type of self-defense class is recommended for people wanting to learn how to protect themselves?
9. How prevalent is homicide in our society?
10. What signs does your body give you when you are getting angry?
11. How do gangs provide a sense of family?

Expressing Your Views

1. Do you think all forms of sexual assault should be reported? Explain.
2. Why do you think emotional abuse should not be ignored even though the effects aren't visible?
3. Your friend confides to you that her uncle has been sexually abusing her for over a year. She refuses to tell her parents because she thinks it was her own fault for being too friendly with her uncle. How could you help her?
4. Patty works late three nights a week and must walk across a large parking lot to her car. What precautions would you encourage her to take?

Life Skills Check

1. **Using Community Resources**
   Your cousin confided that she often feels as if she is losing control with her children and that she is afraid she might hurt them. What could you advise her to do?

2. **Making Responsible Decisions**
   Katie's parents seem to criticize everything she does. They are hardly ever at home, and when they are, Katie never hears one kind or encouraging word from them. The situation has gotten so bad that she is thinking about running away. What alternatives does Katie have?

3. **Coping**
   You like Ray a lot and enjoy some degree of sexual intimacy, but you do not want to have intercourse with him. The last time you were on a date, he assumed that because you enjoyed kissing him, you didn't want him to stop—you had to be really firm. The two of you are supposed to go out tonight. What should you do?

Projects

1. Most child-care centers are very reliable. However, child abuse does occasionally occur at these facilities. Interview a parent whose child attends a child-care center. How did the parent choose the center? What does the parent do to make sure no abuse is taking place? What would he or she do if child abuse were suspected? Share your findings with the class.

2. Work with a group to develop a puppet show to teach young children about child abuse and how to report it. Try to obtain permission to present the show to first- or second-graders in your school district.

Plan for Action

Crime is one of the major health problems facing Americans today. List 10 ways to reduce your risk of becoming a victim of violent crime.

Chapter 20 Assessment

not as successful in school and jobs, and are at a higher risk for self-destructive behaviors, such as eating disorders and suicide.

3. I would encourage her to call the Child Abuse Hotline or to talk with a trusted adult, such as a teacher, school counselor, or religious leader.

4. Walk out with a friend or have the security guard escort her to her car, be alert to her surroundings, have her keys ready for the car, and make sure that no one is in the rear seat of the car.

Life Skills Check

Sample responses:

1. Call the Parents Anonymous Hotline.

2. Katie can call the Child Abuse Hotline to learn about better options. She may also talk to a trusted adult, such as a teacher, school counselor, or religious leader.

3. Before we even leave on the date I should communicate my limits clearly and assertively to Ray.

Projects

Have students complete the projects on abuse and violence.

Plan for Action

Have the class suggest communication skills that should be taught to children to help them learn to manage anger, resolve conflicts, and make their feelings and needs known.

Personal Pledge

Have students read and sign the personal pledge for Chapter 20.

Assessment Options

Chapter Test

Have students take the Chapter 20 Test.

Alternative Assessment

Have students do the Alternative Assessment activity for Chapter 20.

Test Generator

The Test Generator (Macintosh® or IBM® format) contains an additional 50 assessment items for this chapter.

Issues in Health

EVALUATING MEDIA MESSAGES

Violence and the Media
Have students read the Evaluating Media Messages feature. Ask them for their reactions. Do they think they are being influenced in any way when they see violence on TV or in a movie? Do they agree with the feature's contention that people who buy albums advocating violence or who watch violent movies or shows are "endorsing the destructive messages they contain"?

Hold a class debate on that question. Those who oppose the argument presented in the feature might suggest that violence experienced vicariously discharges emotions that might otherwise get out of control. Students might do research to find out whether such arguments are valid.

Evaluating Media Messages

Violence and the Media

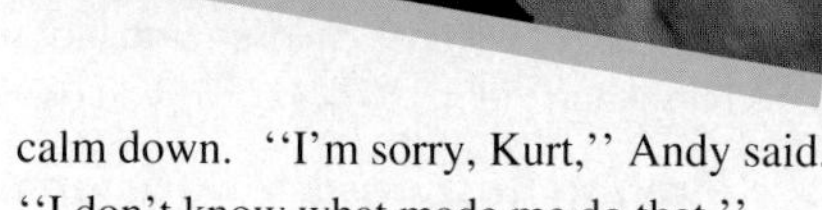

Andy couldn't believe it. Ten extra laps! What had he done this time? It didn't seem to matter; no matter what he did, the coach always managed to find something wrong. Kurt, on the other hand, could get away with anything. Andy didn't really blame Kurt—after all, they were good friends—but it did seem completely unfair. The more Andy thought about it, the angrier he got. By the time he started to step into the shower, he was ready to explode. At that moment, Kurt showed up and, with a grin, popped Andy with a towel. It took Andy only a split second to react. His arm shot up, and without thinking, he shoved Kurt against the wall.

Andy and Kurt were both stunned. Andy slowly lowered his hand, struggling to calm down. ''I'm sorry, Kurt,'' Andy said. ''I don't know what made me do that.''

When people see acts of violence used over and over again, they lose their natural horror of cruelty and gore.

Andy is not the only teenager who has reacted violently to frustration and anger. Over the past several years, the incidence of violence has increased among young people to the point that homicide is now the second leading cause of death for people 15 to 24. Although aggressive and violent behavior can result from a number of factors, many psychologists and educators believe that mass media have had an enormous effect on the increase in these behaviors. From television programs to rock concerts, mass media too often depict people taking violent actions. It is possible, therefore, that Andy's behavior in the locker room could be linked to the amount of violence he has witnessed through mass-media channels.

One of the most powerful ways that mass media influence people is by providing role models. Like many living things, people learn much of their behavior by copying what they see. Someone whose behavior is copied is a role model. If the role model is an admired person, like a popular actor or athlete, association makes the role model an even more powerful factor in influencing behavior. Therefore, when a person (receiver) sees a role model coping with a problem by asking for help and talking about it calmly, he or she is likely to behave this way. And studies have shown that when people watch others using violence in movies or on television, their behavior tends to become more aggressive.

Another way media messages influence people is by attempting to teach attitudes and values. Unfortunately, too few of the situations used to teach values are based in reality. For instance, a Harvard University study found that many of today's cartoons represent the world as a very fearful place, where the criminals are so evil that the only way to deal with them is to destroy them completely. Even though the heros usually win, the world they live in and the solutions they use are not realistic. As a result, viewers cannot easily apply the values presented in these cartoons to real-life situations. In addition, the pain and humiliation that real victims of violence experience is generally missing from the media's treatment of violence. By not showing the negative consequences of violence, the source of a media message omits an important part of the values lesson—a reason for not using violence.

Seeing violence in the media also affects viewers in another, more subtle, way. When people are repeatedly exposed to stressful events, especially while in pleasant surroundings, the stress reaction is reduced. Consequently, when people see acts of violence over and over again, they lose their natural horror of cruelty and gore. Even news programs have this effect.

It is possible to reduce the amount of violence seen in mass media if you remember that receivers of media messages have power over the sources of those messages. Most media experts agree that violence is prevalent in the media because it attracts attention and sells products. But in a way, people who buy albums that advocate violence or who watch violent movies and television programs are endorsing the destructive messages they contain.

As members of a major consumer group, teenagers have more power to affect the media than they realize. To help reduce the use of violence in the media and in society, recognize when it is being used to attract your attention and do not buy products that promote violence.

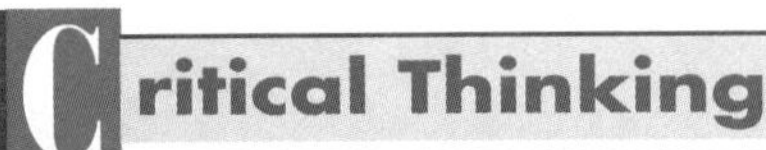

Critical Thinking

1. Think about how you usually react when someone makes you angry.
   - Have you always reacted this way?
   - Do people you admire behave this way? Who?
   - What kinds of things have influenced your behavior?
2. When you watch your favorite television programs tonight, take notes on how many times disagreements are handled with nonviolent solutions.
3. Analyze a movie or television program that contains violence by answering the following questions.
   - What is the source of the message to use violence?
   - What was the reason for making this movie or television program?
   - How do I benefit from the messages in this show?
4. Automobile accidents are the leading cause of death for teenagers. How do you think the scenes of car chases in movies and television programs might contribute to reckless driving and accidental deaths among teenagers?
5. Homicide is the second leading cause of death for people 15 to 24. How do you think media messages might affect violent behavior among teenagers?

UNIT 6

DISEASES AND DISORDERS

CHAPTER OVERVIEWS

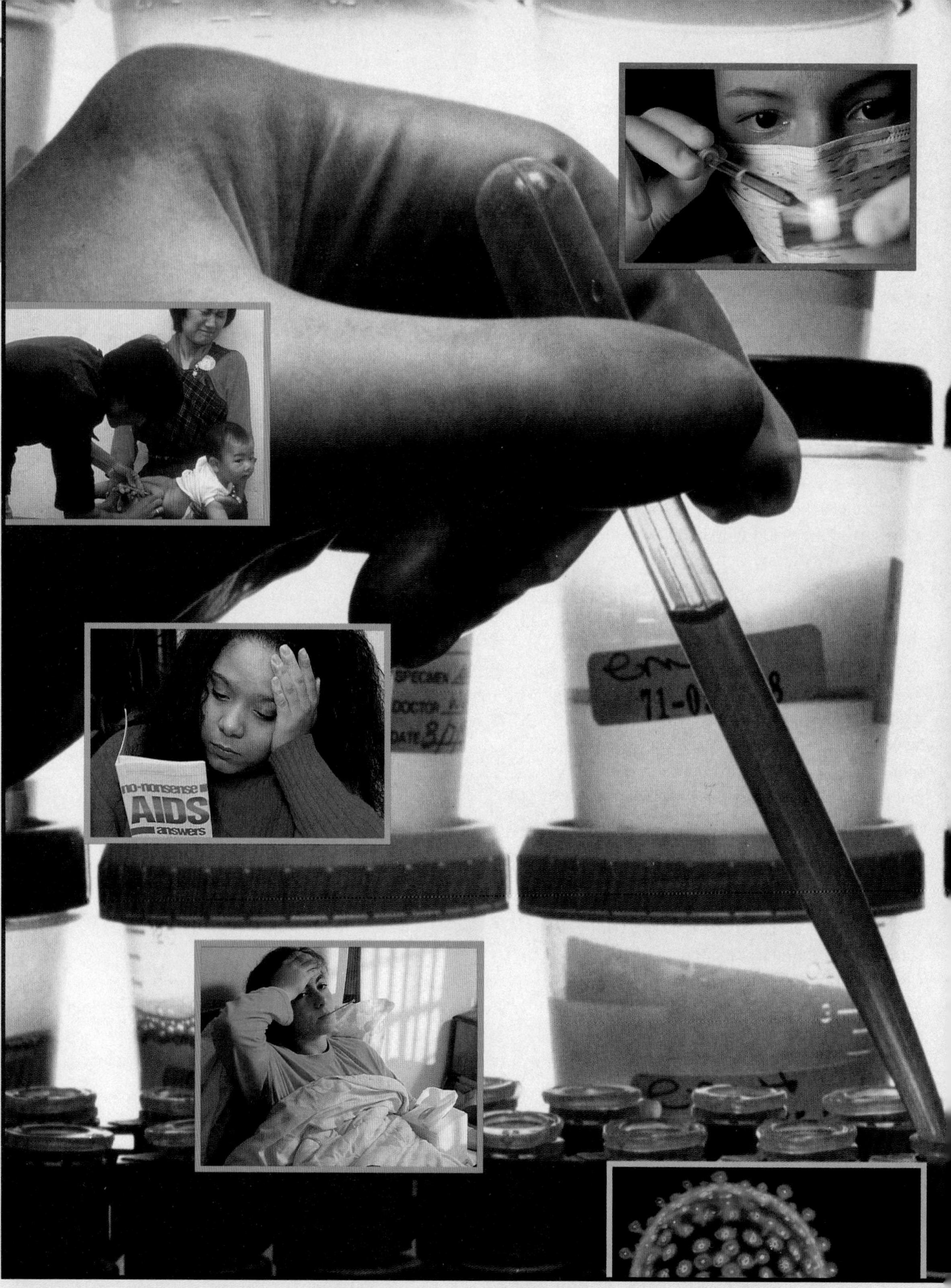

CHAPTER 21

INFECTIOUS DISEASES

A general discussion of infectious diseases, including their causes, methods of transmission, and the body's defenses against them opens the chapter. This is followed by specific information about the symptoms, treatment, and prevention of the most common viral and bacterial diseases. Conditions and diseases caused by protists, animal parasites, and fungi are also described.

CHAPTER 22

SEXUALLY TRANSMITTED DISEASES

For each sexually transmitted disease (STD) described, students learn how it is spread, its symptoms, and the consequences of leaving it untreated. Ways of preventing STDs are discussed, particularly sexual abstinence. Students are also given information about where to go for help if they suspect infection.

CHAPTER 23

HIV INFECTION AND AIDS

This chapter describes the phases of HIV infection and emphasizes the difference between being HIV-positive and having AIDS. Students learn how HIV is transmitted and how they can protect themselves from infection. Sexual abstinence is emphasized as a means of prevention. HIV-related concerns for teenagers, including risky behaviors and peer pressure, also are addressed. The chapter explores a number of social issues, such as the rapidly rising incidence of AIDS, reasons for anonymous testing, and discrimination against those who are HIV-positive.

CHAPTER 24

NONINFECTIOUS DISEASES AND DISORDERS

Hereditary, congenital, autoimmune, and degenerative diseases and ailments are described in this chapter. The difference between autoimmune diseases and AIDS is stressed. Students learn about lifestyle choices they can make to protect themselves from developing certain diseases in the future.

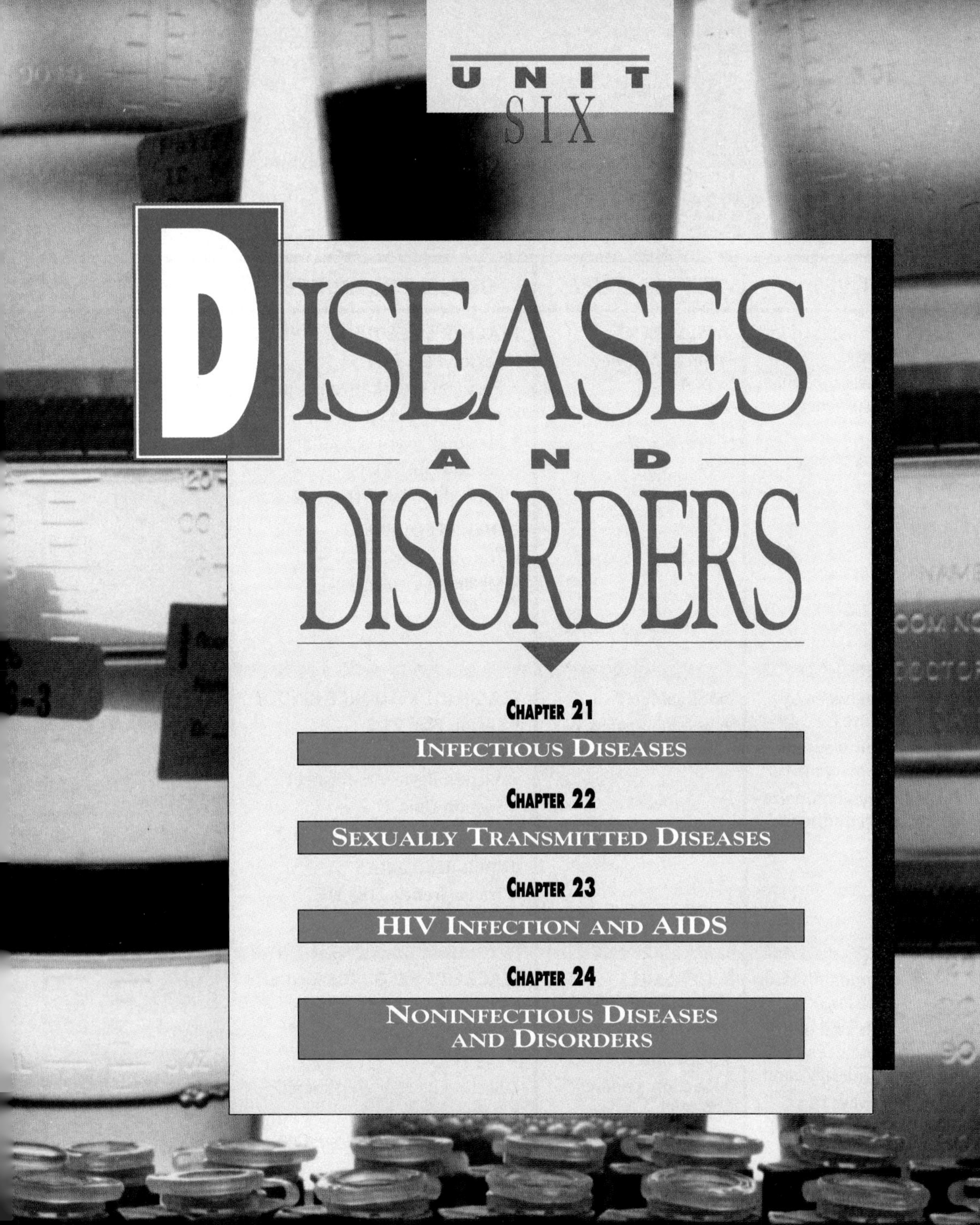

UNIT PREVIEW

Understanding diseases and the disease process helps students make the right choices to stay healthy. This unit provides information about various diseases and disorders of particular importance to students. Besides learning about the causes and symptoms, students examine ways they can reduce their risk of contracting or developing the diseases. Recent medical advances in the prevention and treatment of diseases are also discussed. The five major health themes are emphasized throughout the unit, as indicated in the chart below.

THEMES TRACE

	WELLNESS	BUILDING SELF-ESTEEM	DECISION MAKING	DEVELOPING LIFE-MANAGEMENT SKILLS	ACCEPTANCE OF DIVERSITY AMONG PEOPLE
Chapter 21				p. 456	
Chapter 22			pp. 475–476	pp. 476, 478	
Chapter 23			p. 485	pp. 488–489, 495, 499–500	pp. 503–504
Chapter 24	p. 527			pp. 528–530	p. 517

CHAPTER 21

INFECTIOUS DISEASES

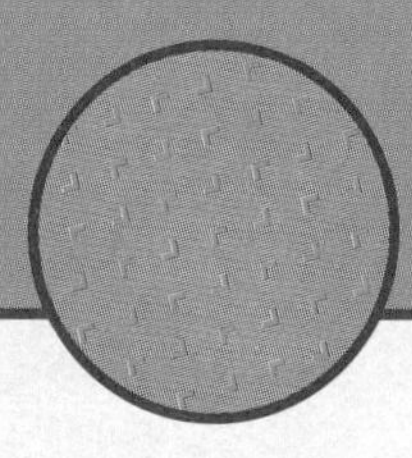

PLANNING GUIDE

TEXT SECTIONS	OBJECTIVES	TEXT FEATURES	OUTSIDE RESOURCES	NOTES
21.1 What Are Infectious Diseases? pp. 441-444 1 period	• Describe the causes of infectious diseases. • Identify the ways in which diseases are spread.	**ASSESSMENT** • Section Review, p. 444	**TEACHER'S RESOURCE BINDER** • Lesson Plan 21.1 • Personal Health Inventory • Journal Entries 21A, 21B • Section Review Worksheet 21.1 • Section Quiz 21.1 • Reteaching Worksheet 21.1 **OTHER RESOURCES** • Transparency 21A • Making a Choice 21A	
21.2 Fighting Disease pp. 445-451 1 period	• Distinguish between infection and disease. • Name the four ways the body resists infection. • Explain how an immunization can prevent disease.	**ASSESSMENT** • Section Review, p. 451	**TEACHER'S RESOURCE BINDER** • Lesson Plan 21.2 • Journal Entry 21C • Section Review Worksheet 21.2 • Section Quiz 21.2 • Reteaching Worksheet 21.2 **OTHER RESOURCES** • Transparency 21B, 21C	
21.3 Common Infectious Diseases pp. 452-458 2 periods	• List four common diseases caused by viruses. • Explain which kind of diseases antibiotics can cure, and which kind they can't. ■ Know some ways to decrease your chances of getting an infectious disease.	■ LIFE SKILLS: Practicing Self-Care, p. 456 **ASSESSMENT** • Section Review, p. 458	**TEACHER'S RESOURCE BINDER** • Lesson Plan 21.3 • Journal Entry 21D • Life Skills 21A • Section Review Worksheet 21.3 • Section Quiz 21.3 • Reteaching Worksheet 21.3 **OTHER RESOURCES** • Making a Choice 21B	
End of Chapter pp. 459-461		**ASSESSMENT** • Chapter Review, pp. 460-461	**TEACHER'S RESOURCE BINDER** • Chapter Test • Alternative Assessment **OTHER RESOURCES** • Test Generator	

■ Denotes LIFE SKILLS objectives

• Items in blue are also part of the *Holt Health Activity Book.*

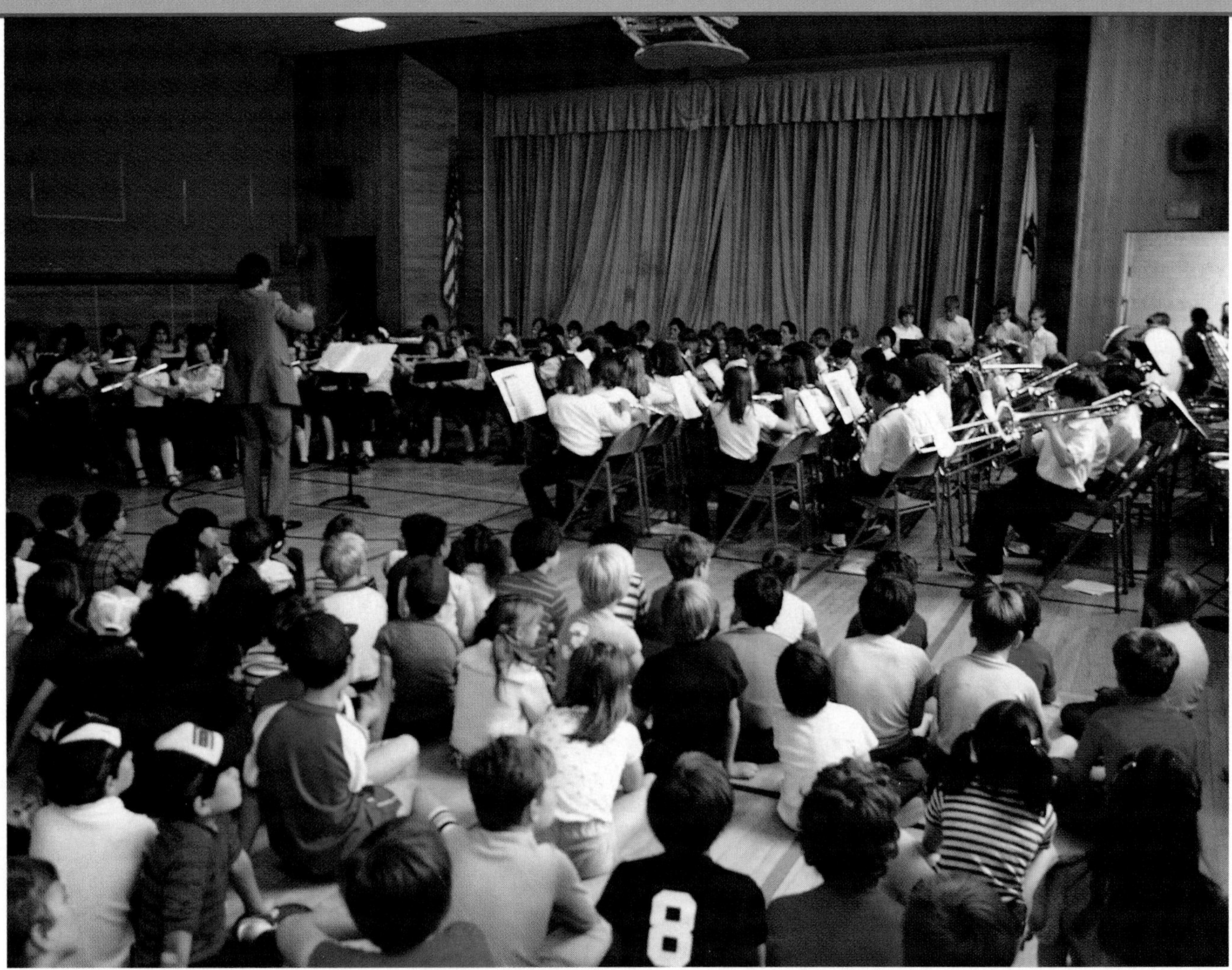

CONTENT BACKGROUND Some Common Communicable Diseases

MEASLES

The measles vaccine was introduced in 1963 in an attempt to save thousands of people who died of measles every year. The vaccine was so effective that, until the 1980s, health officials believed the disease was under control in the United States. As the disease became rare, those who were vaccinated were given one dosage only, which did not ensure immunity. As a result, the number of cases of measles in the United States has risen steadily since 1981.

Complications of this infectious disease increase with the age of the person and include lung infection, hearing loss, pneumonia, and damage to the brain. They even lead to death.

The American Academy of Pediatrics recommends a two-dosage immunization schedule against measles. The first dose is to be given when a child is 15 months old, and the second dose should be administered between the ages of 11 and 12.

INFLUENZA

Epidemics of influenza are estimated to cause about 20,000 deaths annually in the United States. With the many strains of influenza that exist, how is it possible to develop vaccines to prevent people from getting the flu—especially those who are at high risk?

The Centers for Disease Control and Prevention

continually work with health services of many countries to assist in the development of vaccines against the various types of influenza. Then, to determine the type of vaccine that should be used in a given year, the CDC evaluates what types of influenza strains are causing the disease in the cases that are reported to the center for the first few months of a particular year. This early evaluation and identification of the strain allows the manufacture and testing of the more than 30 million doses of the right vaccine before the flu season begins.

THE COMMON COLD

The rhinoviruses responsible for the common cold can survive in the air or on surfaces for several hours or even days. But the exact modes of transmission of the viruses that cause most colds are unclear. Studies done in the early 1970s by researchers at the University of Virginia suggest that colds are transmitted when a person touches a surface that has been contaminated with the virus(es) and then touches his or her eyes or nose. Researchers at the University of Wisconsin, however, disagree with this hypothesis. Their studies show that the virus(es) must be inhaled in order to produce cold symptoms. Research toward a cure for the cold is ongoing. Unfortunately, the 100 or so strains of rhinoviruses easily mutate, which can cause antibodies in the immune system to fail to recognize them.

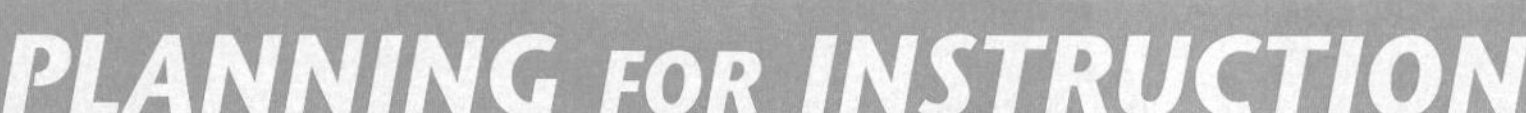

PLANNING FOR INSTRUCTION

KEY FACTS

- **An infectious disease, also known as a communicable disease or contagious disease, can be passed to a person via another person, an animal or object, food, air, or water.**
- **Infectious diseases are communicated by five types of pathogens: bacteria, viruses, protists, fungi, and parasitic worms.**
- **Pathogens are spread in five ways: through the air, person-to-person contact, contact with a contaminated object, contact with an animal, and through food and water.**
- **The body's defenses include the skin, sweat, oils, tears, saliva, mucous membranes, strong stomach acids, helpful microorganisms that crowd out the disease-causing ones, and inflammation.**
- **The body's immune system responds to invading pathogens with T-cells, which attack and remember the invaders, and B-cells, which produce antibodies that engulf them.**
- **Immunity is protection against developing a certain disease. The three immunity types are *innate, active,* and *passive.***
- **The most common viral diseases in the United States are colds, flu, chickenpox, measles, mononucleosis, and hepatitis. No drugs exist to cure viral diseases.**
- **Bacterial diseases include strep throat, tuberculosis, and sinus infections. They should be treated promptly with antibiotics.**

MYTHS AND MISCONCEPTIONS

MYTH: You'll catch a cold if you run outside with your hair wet or don't wear a jacket when it is cold.

Getting wet and feeling cold are unpleasant, but they have nothing to do with the viral infection of the respiratory tract that we call a cold.

MYTH: The cold sores around my lips were caused by a cold.

Cold sores have a misleading name, for they have no connection with colds. They are caused by the herpes simplex type 1 virus, which thrives in saliva. The sores are unpleasant and unsightly but harmless in themselves, although fluid from them, if transferred to the eyes, can cause serious eye infections and can lead to blindness.

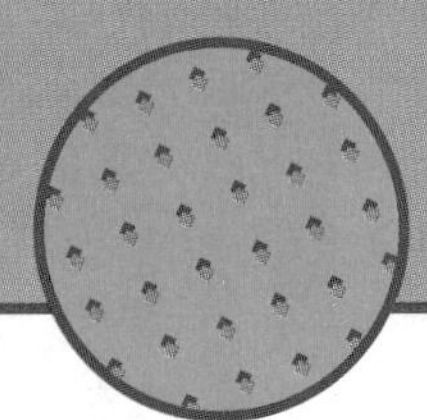

MYTH: I feel much better, so I can stop taking the medicine that the doctor prescribed.

If a doctor prescribes a medicine for 10 days, the entire prescription must be taken, on schedule, to assure that the proper level of medication is in the body long enough to kill all the pathogens. Not taking the entire prescription may allow the disease to return when medication stops.

MYTH: I don't feel well, so I'll just take the antibiotics my sister had left over from when she was sick.

Treating an unknown disease with medicine that happens to be handy usually doesn't work and can be dangerous. The disease might be caused by a virus, against which the antibiotic would be useless. Or, the antibiotic might be the wrong one for the disease and do nothing while a person becomes sicker.

VOCABULARY

Essential: The following vocabulary terms appear in boldface type:

infectious disease
communicable disease
bacterium
microorganism
pathogens
mucous membranes
T-cells
B-cells
antibodies
immune system
immunization
virus
antibiotics

Secondary: Be aware that the following terms may come up during class discussion:

influenza/flu (alternate names)
bacterium/bacteria (singular and plural)
immunity—innate, active, passive
immunization/vaccination (alternate names)
protist
infection
inflammation
mononucleosis (mono)
tuberculosis (TB)

FOR STUDENTS WITH SPECIAL NEEDS

Auditory Learners: Prepare cards containing the following information. Card 1: names of the five types of pathogens (for Section 21.1), Card 2: the five ways in which diseases are spread (21.1), Card 3: the body's six defenses (21.2), Card 4: the three immunity types (21.2), and Card 5: the nine diseases headlined in the text (21.3). Have pairs of students use the cards to query each other to define each term.

Visual Learners: Have students find appropriate pictures and ads to construct a scrapbook on infectious diseases. This might include photos of people from various nations.

ENRICHMENT

- The Centers for Disease Control and Prevention (CDC) in Atlanta, Georgia, is a division of the U.S. Public Health Service. It studies and tries to control infectious diseases to prevent epidemics, if possible. Assign a pair of students to discover what this government agency does and report to the class.
- Have students obtain free literature on infectious diseases from clinics, hospitals, emergency rooms, and offices of health-care professionals (doctors, dentists, eye specialists, skin specialists, and others) and organize an informative resource library for classroom use.
- Have students who are interested in history do research on the effect of one of the infectious diseases, such as the bubonic plague, on the populations of the world during the Middle Ages. They could describe the symptoms of the disease, how it is spread, and how the epidemic affected the population.

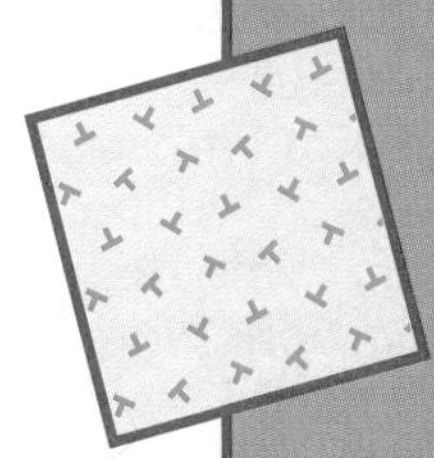

CHAPTER 21
CHAPTER OPENER

GETTING STARTED

Using the Chapter Photograph

Call students' attention to the photo, and ask: **How could each person be spreading a disease without realizing it?** *[Touching, sneezing, coughing, sharing a drink or food]* **What are some diseases they might spread?** *[Cold, flu, virus, strep throat]* **What are some ways they could prevent spreading these diseases?** *[Covering their mouths when they cough or sneeze, washing hands carefully, not sharing food or drinks]*

Explain to students that in this chapter they will study the causes of infectious diseases, how such diseases spread, and how they can be prevented.

Question Box

Have students write out any questions they have about infectious diseases and put them in the Question Box. The Question Box provides students with an opportunity to ask questions anonymously. To ensure that students with questions are not embarrassed to be seen writing, have students who do not have questions write something else—such as something they already know about infectious diseases—instead.

Preview the questions and then answer them at appropriate points in the chapter. You may wish to allow students to write additional anonymous questions as they go through the chapter.

Note: STDs and AIDS are also infectious diseases, but are covered in Chapters 22 and 23.

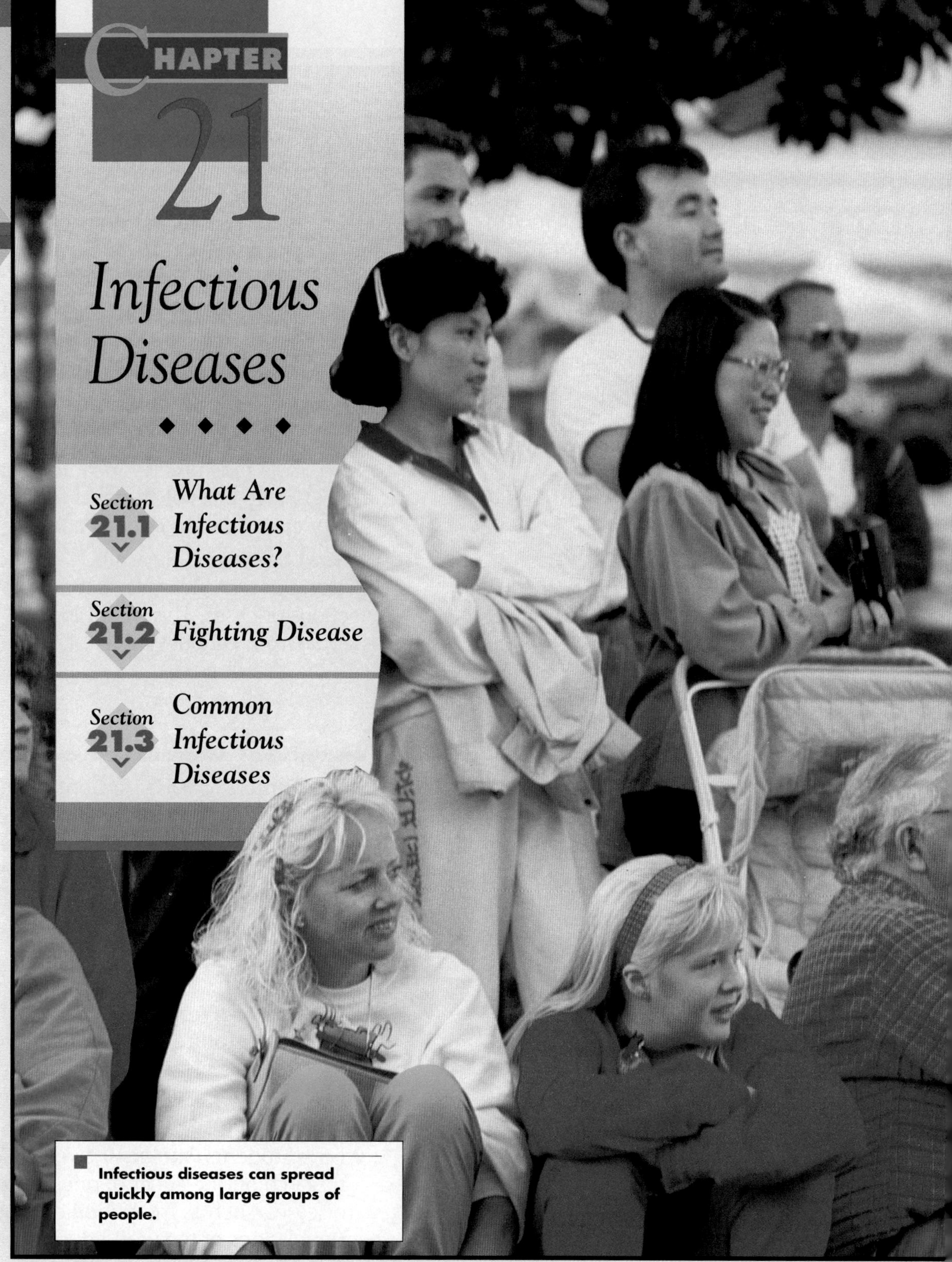

CHAPTER 21 Infectious Diseases

Infectious diseases can spread quickly among large groups of people.

Personal Issues *ALERT*

Discussion of infectious diseases may make some students uncomfortable, particularly if they have visible signs such as cold sores, a rash, or severe cough. Some students may have questions they feel are too personal—or even too simple—to bring up before the class, so provide opportunities for them to ask anonymous questions by using the Question Box.

The clock radio beside Tanita's bed suddenly blares out rock music, as it does every school morning at 6:30. But as she reaches out to turn down the volume, she realizes something is wrong. When she went to bed the night before, she thought she felt more tired than usual. She feels more than tired now. Her throat hurts and she feels feverish.

Tanita's best friend, Clarissa, has been out of school the past two days with the flu. Now it's Tanita's turn. She spends most of the day sleeping. When she's awake she drinks a little water and lies still, feeling queasy. Over the next several days, she gradually feels better. She's able to eat some soup and crackers, to watch TV, and to read a magazine.

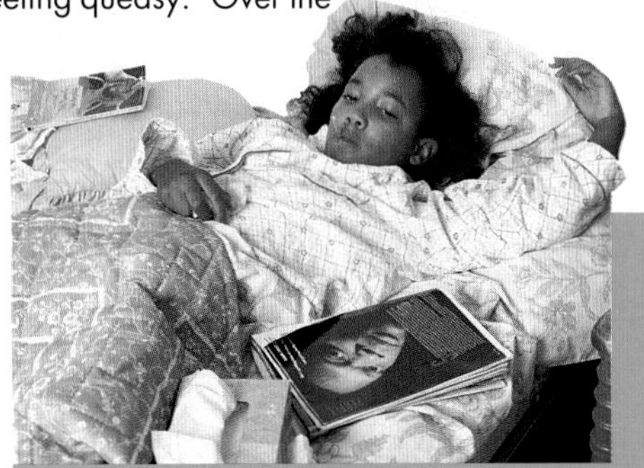

Finally Tanita is well enough to go back to school. There's a history test to make up and she's way behind in her homework, not to mention the dance she missed last Friday. Being sick is no fun.

Background
Safe Sneezing
Covering the mouth during a sneeze reduces the spray but concentrates pathogens on the hand; from there they are easily transferred to another person by handshake or by handling food, doorknobs, and so on. Covering the mouth with a tissue during a sneeze and then promptly disposing of it is probably the most effective way to reduce the spread of pathogens during a sneeze.

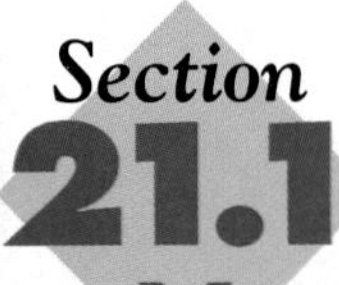

Section 21.1 What Are Infectious Diseases?

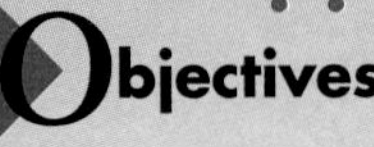

Objectives

- *Describe the causes of infectious diseases.*
- *Identify the ways in which diseases are spread.*

The disease that Tanita had is influenza, which is often called "flu" for short. If you have had influenza, you know that it makes you feel pretty miserable for a few days. But after resting and taking care of yourself, you soon feel like your old self again.

Influenza is an example of an **infectious disease.** An infectious disease is an illness that can pass from one organism to another. Influenza is also a contagious or **communicable disease**, which is an infectious disease that is passed from one person to another. Tanita feels sure that she "caught" the flu from Clarissa, and most likely she is right.

Not all diseases are infectious diseases. Illnesses like cancer and heart disease are not spread from one person to another. No one knows exactly why one person gets cancer or has a heart attack and another person does not. Researchers have found that certain things—like smoking, a high-fat diet, or not getting exercise—can increase your chances of getting these kinds of diseases. But you don't "catch" these diseases from another living thing.

communicable disease: *an infectious disease that is passed from one person to another.*

infectious disease: *a disease caused by an agent that can pass from one living thing to another.*

Section 21.1 Lesson Plan

MOTIVATE

Journal 21A
Diseases You Have Had

This may be done as a warm-up activity. In the Student Journal in the Student Activity Book, ask students to list diseases they can remember having, what the symptoms were, and what was done to treat the disease.

TEACH

Class Discussion
Infectious and Noninfectious

On the chalkboard, write the headings INFECTIOUS and NONINFECTIOUS. Discuss the distinction between these two types of disease, and write some key ideas and some sample diseases beneath the headings.

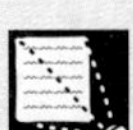

Teaching Transparency 21A
Four Pathogens

Show the transparency illustrating four of the pathogens of infectious diseases (Figure 21-1). Emphasize the tiny size of these microorganisms: one drop of saliva contains millions of bacteria and even more viruses. Viruses are so small that they can be seen only with an electron microscope. Some worms are large enough to be visible without a microscope. Also, point out that

Background
Animals Spreading Disease

Animals that spread diseases are called *vectors,* from a Latin word meaning "to carry." Some vectors, the diseases they carry to humans, and the type of pathogen are: dogs and cats (ringworm—fungus); dogs, raccoons, bats, and squirrels (rabies—virus); mosquitos (malaria—protist, encephalitis—virus); snails and sheep (liver fluke—parasitic worm); deer ticks (Lyme disease—virus); wood ticks (Rocky Mountain spotted fever—viruslike organism); rats and fleas (bubonic plague—bacteria); rabbits and squirrels (tularemia or rabbit fever—bacteria); birds (psittacosis or parrot fever—viruslike organism).

microorganism:

a living thing that can be seen only with a microscope.

bacterium:

a type of microorganism that can cause disease.

What Causes Infectious Diseases?

In the United States, the most common infectious diseases are caused by bacteria and viruses. Sometimes disease-causing bacteria and viruses are all simply called "germs." However, it is important to remember that bacteria and viruses are two different things.

Infectious diseases can also be caused by fungi, protists, or other types of organisms, such as parasitic worms. Bacteria, protists, and many fungi are too small to be seen without a microscope. For this reason, they often are called **microorganisms**. Some of the organisms that can cause disease are shown in Figure 21-1.

Bacteria Bacteria are very simple living things. Each **bacterium** is a single cell, much smaller than the cells that make up your body. The vast majority of bacteria are harmless.

A few types of bacteria, however, are a real problem for people. They can spoil food or cause diseases. Common diseases caused by bacteria are strep throat, food poisoning, and urinary tract infections.

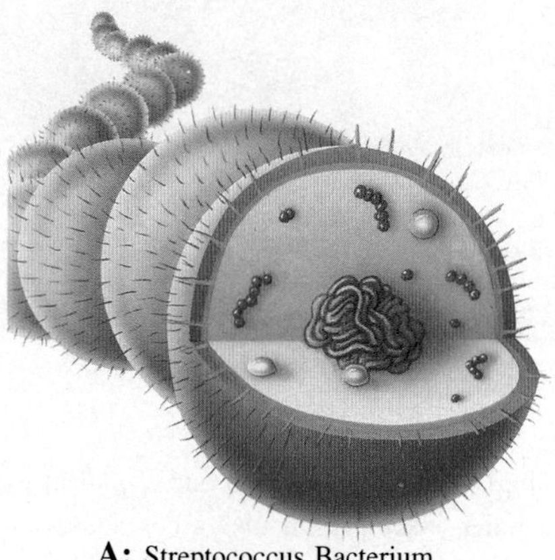

A: Streptococcus Bacterium
Causes strep throat

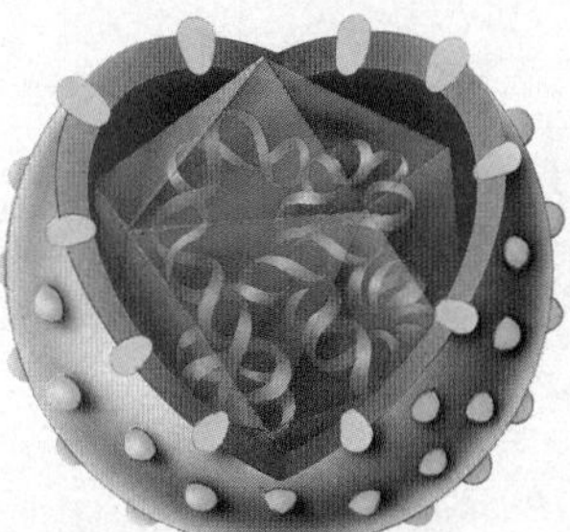

B. Herpes Virus
Causes chicken pox, herpes, and shingles

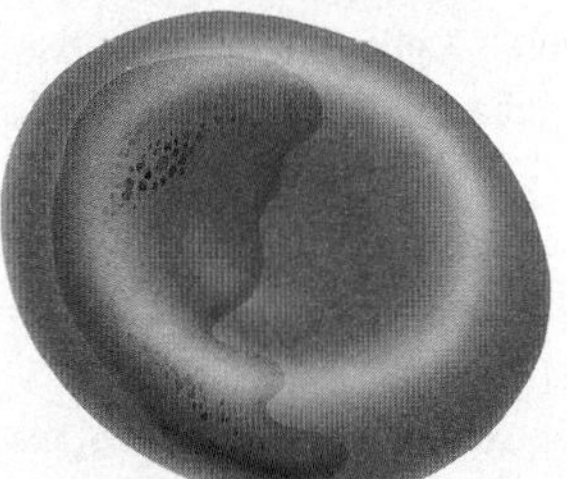

C. Plasmodium
(in red blood cell)
Causes malaria

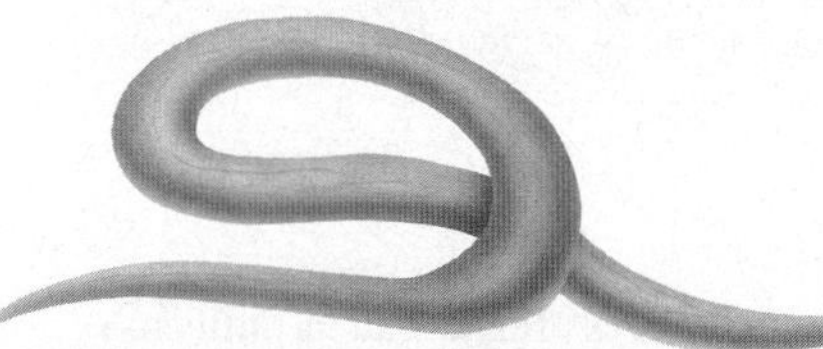

D. Roundworm Parasite

(FIGURE 21-1) **Four causes of infectious diseases are bacteria, viruses, protists, and parasitic worms. Any agent that can cause an infectious illness is called a pathogen.**

• • • TEACH continued

viruses reproduce very rapidly and mutate often.

Reinforcement
Word Origins

Write on the chalkboard:

pathos (suffering) + genes (to produce) = pathogen

Explain to students that knowing the etymology of a word will help them remember its meaning.

Journal 21B
Person to Person

Have students turn to the Student Journal in the Student Activity Book and list all the person-to-person contacts they can remember having had yesterday. Tell them to include handshakes, contact sports, hugs, playful shoves, accidental bumps, or helping someone with their hair or clothing. Explain that no one will see their list—the purpose is to help them realize how many opportunities occur each day for them to exchange pathogens with someone else.

Game
Disease Detective

Have students work in small groups. One person is It. He or she chooses a disease, a pathogen, and a method of transmittal (food poisoning, bacteria, potato salad). Other students question the person with the disease, who can only answer yes or no. Have you been on a picnic lately? Have you been camping? Did you boil the water? Do

Viruses Viruses also cause infectious diseases. They are even smaller than bacteria. When a **virus** enters a cell, its genetic material acts as a program that directs the cell to make more viruses. After the cell makes new viruses, it often dies and releases the viruses. These viruses spread to new cells, which also die.

Viruses are specialized to infect only certain types of cells. For example, some viruses attack only plant cells, while other viruses attack certain animals. If you have a dog, you know your pet needs to be immunized against certain diseases that affect only dogs. You also have your pet immunized against rabies, a viral disease that both humans and dogs can get.

Some common diseases caused by viruses include the common cold, flu, cold sores, and measles.

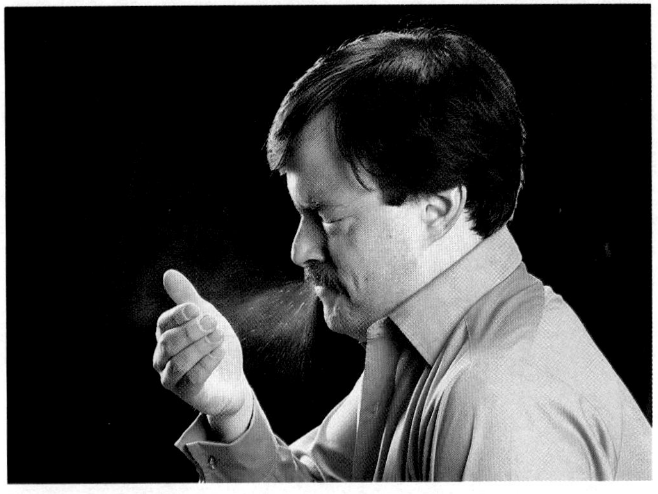

(FIGURE 21-2) **The viruses that cause influenza are spread through droplets in the air.**

How Are Infectious Diseases Spread?

You have seen that all infectious diseases are caused by agents that can be passed from one organism to another. All agents that cause disease are known as **pathogens** (PATH uh junz). In order for you to catch an infectious disease, a pathogen must first leave the body of a living thing, and then enter your body. There are several ways that this can happen.

Through the Air Clarissa was sick with the flu because influenza viruses were invading cells in her respiratory system, mainly in her nose and throat. The viruses then moved from Clarissa to Tanita, and Tanita got sick.

How did the viruses get from Clarissa to Tanita? Influenza viruses usually travel through droplets in the air. When you sneeze, thousands of tiny drops of mucus and saliva are sprayed into the air, as shown in Figure 21-2. If your nose and throat are infected with viruses, some viruses are carried out into the air in the droplets. Someone nearby who breathes in the droplets can then become infected with the viruses.

Contact With Contaminated Objects A person who is sick may leave bacteria or viruses on objects like doorknobs, drinking glasses, toothbrushes, towels, or combs. Some agents of disease do not live for long outside of the human body, but other pathogens are tougher. These types of pathogens may be passed from one person to another when the second person opens the same door, shares a glass, or uses the sick person's toothbrush.

Person-to-Person Contact Sometimes the agents of disease are spread by direct person-to-person contact. For example, you can get some illnesses by shaking hands, kissing, or touching the ulcers or sores of a sick person. Some infectious diseases are spread by sexual contact. These diseases are discussed in more detail in Chapters 22 and 23.

virus:

a type of agent that can cause disease.

pathogens:

agents that cause disease.

Sexually Transmitted Diseases are discussed in Chapter 22. AIDS is discussed in Chapter 23.

SECTION 21.1

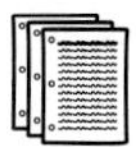

Personal Health Inventory

Have students complete the Personal Health Inventory for this chapter. The inventory helps students evaluate the health risks tobacco and tobacco products pose to their health.

Making a Choice 21A

What's Going Around?

Assign the "What's Going Around?" card. The card requires students to identify infectious diseases going around the school and to keep a record of one of the diseases.

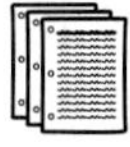

Section Review Worksheet 21.1

Assign Section Review Worksheet 21.1, which requires students to identify infectious diseases, their causes, and the ways in which they are spread.

you feel queasy? Students must determine the disease, pathogen, and methods of transmittal.

Reinforcement

Diseases and Their Pathogens

On the chalkboard, make a chart as shown. Allow room for about 10 diseases to be entered.

INFECTIOUS DISEASE	MICRO-ORGANISM (PATHOGEN)	HOW SPREAD
Influenza	Virus	Through the air

Then have students name infectious diseases for you to enter, the pathogen that causes the disease, and how the disease is spread (influenza is shown as an example).

Extension

Epidemics Around the World

Have students scan recent newspapers and magazines for articles on epidemics anywhere in the world. Have them photocopy the articles and post them on the bulletin board so classmates can read them. A geography and social studies link can be made by having students mark the locations of epidemics on a world map.

Section Quiz 21.1

Have students take Section Quiz 21.1

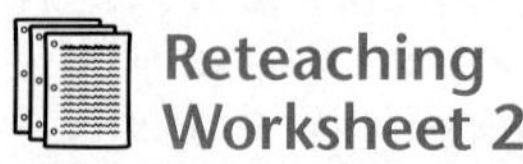

Reteaching Worksheet 21.1

Students who have difficulty with the material may complete Reteaching Worksheet 21.1, which requires them to identify pathogens, the ways in which they spread, and the diseases they cause.

Review Answers

1. Answers may include bacteria, viruses, fungi, protists, and parasitic worms.
2. Answers may include through the air, person-to-person contact, contact with contaminated objects, animals, and food and water.
3. Answers will vary. Tanita would not have gotten the flu from Clarissa if she had stayed away from her friend totally while Clarissa was ill. If Tanita attended any classes with Clarissa she would have had a hard time avoiding the flu, since it is spread through the air, person-to-person contact, and touching anything the infected person touched.

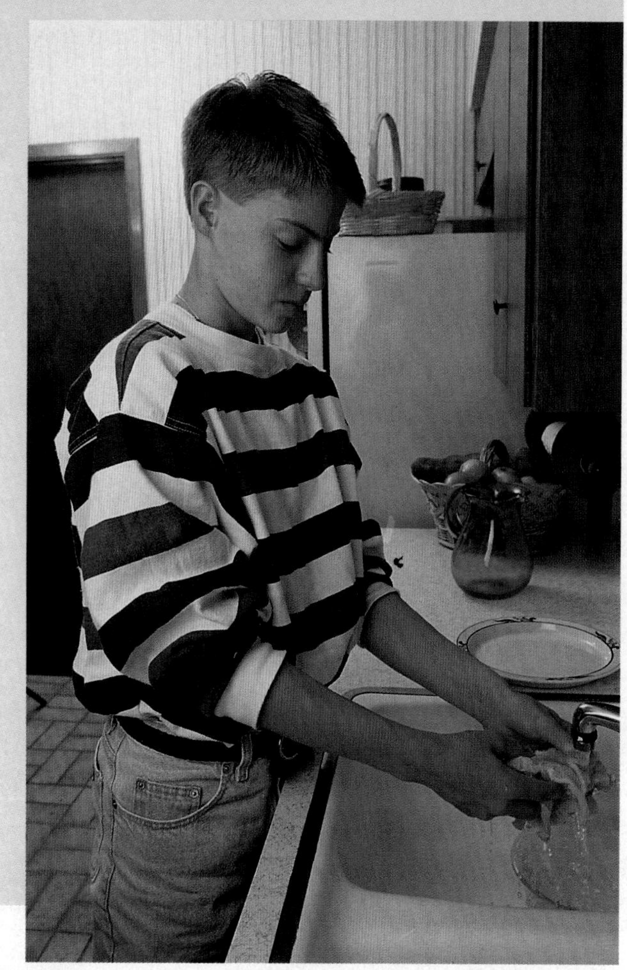

(FIGURE 21-3) **To help protect against *Salmonella*, a bacterium found on meat and eggs that causes food poisoning, make sure to wash and cook all poultry products thoroughly.**

Animals That Spread Disease Some infectious diseases are spread by animals. For example, humans can get ringworm from handling an infected dog or cat. It is also possible for people to get rabies from the bite of an infected animal. A type of encephalitis, or swelling of the brain, is spread from human to human by mosquitoes.

Food and Water Eating contaminated food or drinking contaminated water can also spread disease. Diseases that affect the digestive system are often spread when feces from an infected person contaminates food or water. This is why people who work with food are required by law to wash their hands thoroughly after every trip to the bathroom. For the same reason, fresh fruits and vegetables, particularly those that grow on the ground, should be washed thoroughly or cooked before they are eaten.

Large numbers of bacteria growing in food can also cause food poisoning. Symptoms of food poisoning include nausea, vomiting, and abdominal pain. The best way to prevent this type of infection is to refrigerate food except while it is actually being prepared or served, keep hands and utensils clean while preparing foods, and cook food thoroughly to kill any bacteria present.

In the United States, drinking tap water is safe. But campers and hikers who drink water from streams must purify the water first, either by boiling or by using water purification tablets or special filtering systems, to protect themselves from disease.

Review

1. *Name four causes of infectious diseases.*
2. *What are three ways in which infectious diseases can be spread?*
3. ***Critical Thinking*** *Is there anything that Tanita could have done to avoid catching the flu from Clarissa?*

ASSESS

Section Review

Have students answer the Section Review questions.

Alternative Assessment
What's the Pathogen?

For each incident listed, ask what the disease could be, what the pathogen is, how it was communicated, and how it might be prevented. **(1) Anita ate some unrefrigerated potato salad and now has stomach cramps and diarrhea.** *[Food poisoning; bacterium; food; refrigerate the food]* **(2) Jessie has a runny nose and sneezed several times during her last study session, and now her boyfriend has the same signs.** *[Cold; virus; through the air; avoid close contact and cover sneezes with a tissue]* **(3) Several people in Consuela's class have been out sick and now Consuela has a fever and feels achy.** *[Flu; virus; person-to-person contact; avoid contact]*

Closure
Risks of Infection

Ask students to think about all the activities they are involved in today. Ask them which activities will most expose them to infectious diseases.

Section 21.2 Fighting Disease

Objectives

- *Distinguish between infection and disease.*
- *Name four ways the body resists infection.*
- *Explain how an immunization can prevent disease.*

Bacteria, viruses, and other agents of disease are everywhere around us. They are found in the air you breathe, on surfaces you touch, and even on your own skin. So why aren't you sick all the time?

Remember that in order for you to get sick, a pathogen must not only leave another organism, but also enter your body. Even if it enters your body, it cannot make you sick unless it survives, multiplies, and somehow causes damage to your system. Most of the time, pathogens are quickly destroyed or swept away before they have a chance to multiply in your body.

Infection and Disease

If pathogens do enter your system and begin to spread and reproduce, then you are infected. Being infected is not the same as having a disease, or actually being sick. Even after pathogens begin to multiply, your body can mount such a good defense against them that they can be destroyed or made harmless before they cause any actual damage. If this happens, you will probably never know that you have been infected. But if you are infected with certain disease-causing agents, you *can* pass them to someone else.

Disease If your defenses fail or do not act quickly enough, you may begin to feel sick. A disease is any harmful change in your body's normal activities. A pathogen can cause disease when it is able to multiply in your body and cause damage to your cells and tissues.

Signs and Symptoms The effects of a disease are called signs and symptoms. A sign of a disease is something another person can see or detect. Tanita had a fever,

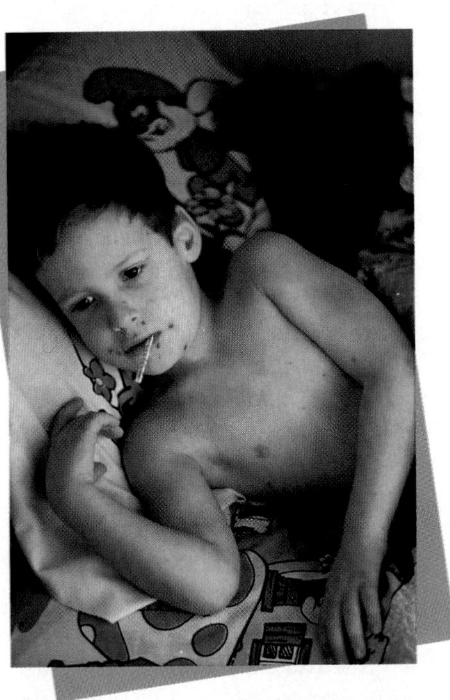

(FIGURE 21-4) **The effects of a disease are called signs and symptoms. One sign of the chickenpox is a red rash.**

Background

Body Temperature

Body temperature averages 98.6°F but can vary from person to person and with time of day, so that readings a few tenths lower or higher can be normal for an individual. When a virus attacks, the immune system signals the brain to raise body temperature to help fight the disease. This may cause a chill, compelling one to wrap up in a sweater or blanket, which insulates the body and helps drive up body temperature. Once a fever has done its job, body temperature returns to normal, sometimes accompanied by profuse sweating. Colds usually lack a fever in adults (although there often is a fever in children). Flu starts with a 100°F or higher fever. Temperatures above 104°F can be dangerous, especially to the elderly and those with heart problems. Fevers this high need prompt medical attention.

Section 21.2 Lesson Plan

MOTIVATE

Writing

Defective Immune Systems

This may be done as a warm-up activity. Tell students that some children are born with a defective immune system and have to live in a plastic bubble, away from all physical human contact. Ask them to write a few sentences explaining why they think the children must be isolated to survive. Explain that they will learn in this section how our bodies fight disease.

TEACH

Role-Playing

Signs and Symptoms

Pair off students to act out some signs of disease that reflect the symptoms they feel. For example, one student acts out the symptom of painful swallowing, which the student's partner interprets as a sign of sore throat. Have students take turns acting out symptoms and interpreting signs.

Outward Signs	Symptoms
1. painful swallowing	1. sore throat
2. arms wrapped around self	2. chills
3. listless posture, sighing	3. tiredness, weakness
4. holding stomach, distressed face	4. upset stomach
5. painful movements	5. achiness
6. feeling forehead	6. fever

Background
The Price of a Cold

In the United States, colds cost about $5 billion each year, which includes the cost of medical bills, symptom relievers, 60 million lost school days, and 50 million lost working days. The United States space program lost half a million dollars when a launch had to be postponed for a week because all three astronauts came down with colds!

which is a sign of influenza. Other diseases might have signs like sneezing, coughing, looking pale or flushed, or having a rash like the one shown in Figure 21-4.

A symptom is any feeling of pain or discomfort that you experience when you are sick. Tanita's sore throat, tiredness, and queasy stomach are all symptoms of influenza. Other symptoms of disease might include itching, tenderness, cramps, headache, or dizziness.

Defenses Against Infection

Your body has many ways of coping with disease-causing bacteria, viruses, and other pathogens.

Skin One of the functions of your skin is to protect the rest of your body from invasion by agents of disease. The outer part of your skin is very well designed for this job. The lower layers of this part of the skin are tightly joined so that it is difficult for anything to penetrate the skin and enter the tissues beneath it.

The upper layers of the skin are made of dead skin cells filled with a tough waterproof protein. Every day, millions of dead skin cells are shed from the surface of your skin and are replaced by new cells from the layers below. When you shower or bathe, you wash off even more skin cells. As the dead cells come off, they take any bacteria, viruses, or other pathogens that have settled on your skin with them.

mucous membranes: *the tissues that line the openings into your body; pathogens can enter the body through the mucous membranes, although many are trapped there.*

Chemical Warfare on Germs Many of the chemical substances your body makes for its activities also act to destroy pathogens. For example, sweat and oils produced by your skin contain acids that can kill bacteria. Enzymes in tears and saliva also kill bacteria.

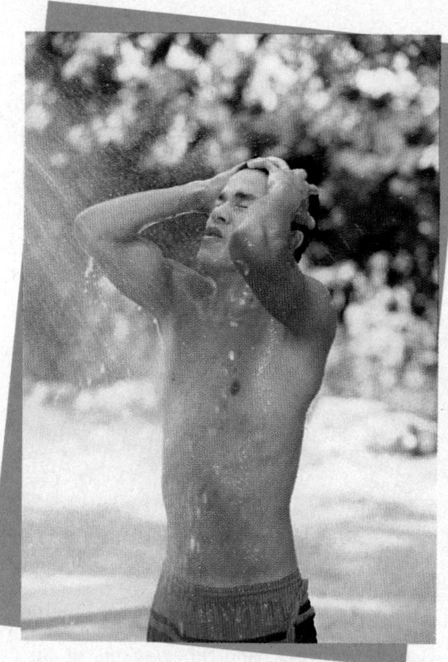

(FIGURE 21-5) **Every time you shower you remove dead skin cells from your body. Any agents of disease that have formed on these cells are washed away as well.**

Mucous Membranes The tissues lining the openings into your body, such as your mouth and nose, are different from the skin on the outside of your body. These tissues are called **mucous membranes** because cells in these tissues secrete a coating called mucus.

When you breathe through your nose, pathogens in the air are trapped in the sticky mucus that coats the passages of your respiratory system. The cells that line these passages have tiny projections on their surfaces called cilia, shown in Figure 21-6. In your nasal passages, the cilia sweep the mucus downward. In the tubes that lead to your lungs in the lower part of your respiratory system, the cilia sweep the mucus upward.

All of the mucus ends up in your throat and is swallowed, along with saliva from your mouth. This is a natural cleansing

• • • TEACH continued

Journal 21C
Symptom Awareness

In the Student Journal, ask students to record any symptoms they may have felt recently and any signs they may have observed in family members and friends. Explain that the purpose is to make them more aware and observant of signs and symptoms of diseases.

Cooperative Learning
Defenses

Divide the class into six groups, one for each defense (skin, chemical warfare, mucous membranes, stomach acid, helpful microorganisms, inflammation). Allow each group a few minutes to discuss the text information on how their defense guards against invasion by microorganisms. Then, ask each group to explain to the class how their defense works when a pathogen tries to invade the body.

Class Discussion
Immune Cells

Ask everyone in the class who has keys to hold them up. Have students note how the keys are all different, each shaped to fit its own lock. **How are the keys similar to immune cells?** *[Just as a key fits only the lock it is designed for, an immune cell recognizes only one type of invading molecule.]*

process that helps keep your respiratory passages free of microorganisms that might cause disease. Unless you have a disease that causes you to produce extra mucus, like a cold, you might not even be aware of it.

Stomach Acids Not all microorganisms enter your body through your respiratory system. A pathogen might get into your system through your mouth when you touch your fingers to your lips, breathe through your mouth, or bite your nails. All microorganisms that enter your body in these ways are swallowed, and eventually they end up in your stomach.

Most of the microorganisms that reach the stomach are destroyed there. This is because your stomach contains acids that are 10 times stronger than the acid in pure lemon juice. The acids not only help digest your food, but they also help protect you from disease.

Helpful Microorganisms Remember that most microorganisms are harmless to humans. Many of these microorganisms, especially bacteria, live on the skin and mucous membranes of every normal, healthy person. Within minutes after you were born, these microorganisms began to make themselves at home both on you and in you.

These microorganisms actually help protect you from pathogens. The harmless bacteria living in your mouth, for example, take up all of the space and use up all of the food available. When a pathogen is breathed in or eaten with a bite of food, it cannot multiply because there is simply no room for it.

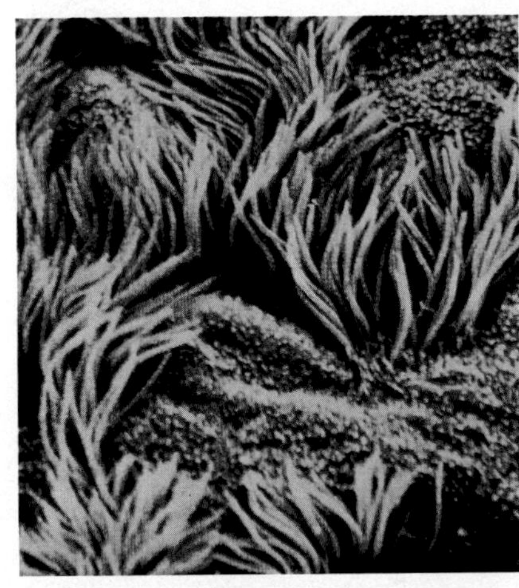

(FIGURE 21-6) **The cells that line the passages of your respiratory system contain tiny projections called cilia, which help sweep disease-causing agents out of your body.**

Inflammation If you have ever had an infected cut, you may have noticed that it was swollen, red, painful, and warm to the touch. These are the signs of inflammation, which is caused by the body's defense reaction to the invasion by pathogens.

Your skin and mucous membranes are very effective at protecting the tissues underneath them from infection by pathogens. However, when you cut or burn yourself, pathogens are sometimes able to cross these protective barriers.

Fortunately, another set of defenses against pathogens is waiting in the tissues underneath the skin and mucous membranes. Any damage to these tissues results in the release of several different kinds of chemicals. The purpose of these chemicals is to act as signals for mobilizing the disease-fighting defenses.

First, small blood vessels expand to bring more blood to the injured area. Fluids from the blood and white blood cells, called phagocytes, pour out of the blood and into the surrounding tissues. Then the phagocytes attack, eat, and destroy any microorganisms that they find in the vicinity. The extra blood and fluid cause the injured area to become swollen and (except in people with very dark skin) appear red.

Background
Rabies

Rabies is an old disease, but it has recently become a problem in some Eastern states. The virus is carried and spread by raccoons, foxes, bats, and other wild animals. These animals can communicate the virus to a dog or cat, and any of these animals can infect humans. Although people are rarely bitten and infected, rabies is fatal unless passive immunity is provided. Dogs and cats can be vaccinated against rabies, and many cities have ordinances requiring vaccination.

Reinforcement
Your Body's Watchdog

Compare the immune system to a watchdog. Explain that a watchdog always watches for intruders, and so does the body's immune system. As long as no strangers come along, the dog is quiet, and as long as no pathogens enter the body, the immune system is quiet, too. But if an intruder tries to get past the dog, it attacks (like killer T-cells), it barks to call for help (like helper T-cells), other dogs hear the noise and come running to help attack the intruder (like antibodies from B-cells), and the dog remembers the intruder if it ever returns (like memory T-cells). Ask students to draw a cartoon strip showing the immune system as a watchdog.

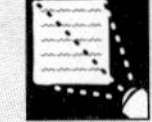

Teaching Transparency 21B
The Immune System

Use this transparency to help students visualize how the immune system works to destroy pathogens and to create immunity to a disease.

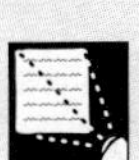

Teaching Transparency 21C
"Waging Battle Against Infection"

Use this transparency to explain to students how the immune system defends the body against pathogens.

Extension
Computer Viruses

Computer viruses are similar to human viruses. Have students research introductory computer books and articles

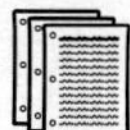

Section Review Worksheet 21.2

Assign Section Review Worksheet 21.2, which requires students to fill in a chart that shows all the different things that could happen when a person comes in contact with a pathogen.

Section Quiz 21.2

Have students take Section Quiz 21.2.

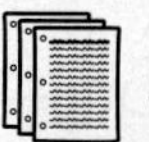

Reteaching Worksheet 21.2

Students who have difficulty with the material may complete Reteaching Worksheet 21.2, which requires them to distinguish between infection and disease and among innate, active, and passive immunity.

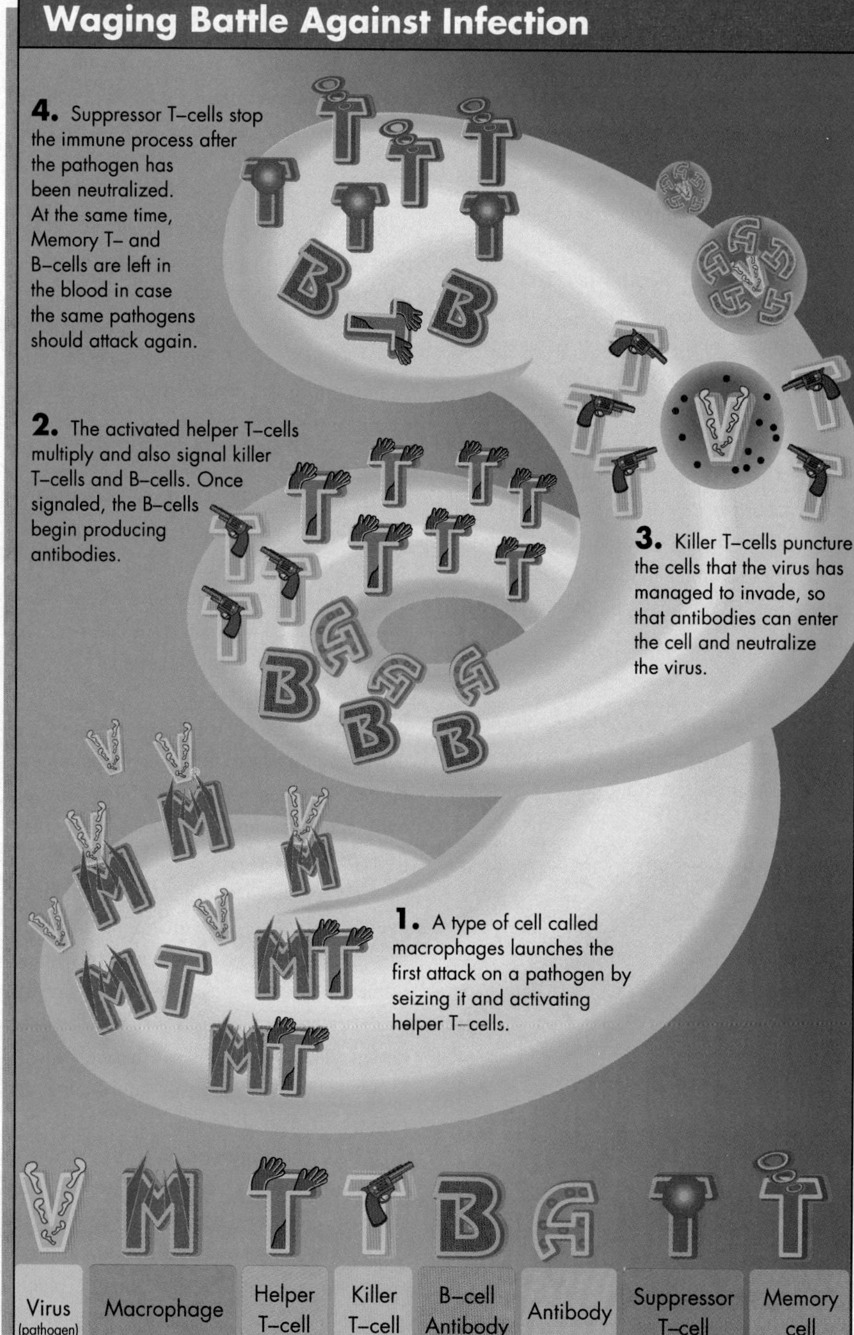

(FIGURE 21-7) **Your immune system launches an all-out war every time a pathogen invades your system.**

• • • TEACH continued

in computer magazines and report to the class on how computer viruses work, how they are like human viruses, how they are described in similar terms, and how they can be prevented.

The Immune System All of the defenses that you have learned about so far will attack and destroy any and all possible agents of disease. In addition, your body has a complex system of fighting specific invaders. For example, if a measles virus gets past your other defenses, your body will launch an all-out war on measles viruses throughout your body.

The weapons your body is using to fight the measles virus work only on measles viruses. They have no effect on any other kind of pathogen. When the body mobilizes its defenses to fight one specific type of invader, the process that is activated is called the immune response. The cells and organs that fight the war against specific invaders are called the **immune system.**

Weapons of the Immune Response

Before a baby is born and during the first years of its life, the immune system produces millions of different kinds of immune cells. Each of these cells can attack a molecule of a certain shape. Such a molecule might be a protein in the outer coat of a virus or a poison molecule made by a bacterium. When an immune cell comes into contact with a molecule that is the right shape, biologists say that the immune cell "recognizes" that molecule.

There are millions of different kinds of these cells, and each kind recognizes a different shape of molecule. So no matter what kind of pathogen might invade your body, there are some immune cells ready to fight it. There are two main types of immune cells that are able to fight any pathogen that might come along.

T-Cells One type of immune cell is called **T-cells.** Certain T-cells mobilize to fight pathogens directly. These T-cells are called killer T-cells. When a pathogen invades your body, its molecules will be recognized by some of your killer T-cells. These cells will divide into many cells that then kill the invaders.

Another class of T-cells, called helper T-cells, get the immune response going by activating killer T-cells, phagocytes, and other immune cells. Helper T-cells are activated by macrophages, which are cells that form the first line of defense against a pathogen. Suppressor T-cells turn off the immune response after the pathogen has been defeated.

Antibodies The other main type of immune cell is called **B-cells.** Their job is to produce antibodies. **Antibodies** (AN tee bahd eez) are Y-shaped molecules that stick to and cover foreign molecules in the body. When a pathogen invades, the B-cells that recognize that pathogen divide rapidly and produce thousands of antibody molecules apiece. When a bacterium or virus is covered with antibodies, it has great difficulty attacking body cells.

Immunity

You may know that after you have had certain diseases, you can't catch them again. For example, after a person has had the mumps, that person doesn't have to worry about getting the mumps a second time.

You probably never had the mumps, however. Most people your age have been immunized against mumps and so never get this disease even once.

In other cases, it doesn't seem to count for anything if you've already had a disease. You may have had two colds this year alone, not to mention the one you had last year, and the one two years before that.

Why the difference? How can you be protected against some diseases entirely by an immunization, get other diseases only once, and get still others over and over?

B-cells:

cells in the immune system that produce antibodies against infection.

antibodies:

substances that stick to the surface of pathogens, slowing their action.

immune system:

the system that protects the body from disease.

T-cells:

cells that regulate the action of the immune system.

Background

Passive Immunity

The key difference between active immunity and passive immunity is the source of the antibodies. In active immunity, one's own body develops the antibodies in response to a pathogen, and "remembers" the invader. In passive immunity, a person is given antibodies from another person or animal, and they remain active in the body long enough to fight off the pathogen. Since the body did not generate these antibodies, it doesn't remember them, so the temporary immunity is lost. This is why immunity received from one's mother fades a few months after birth and why some vaccines are only temporary.

immunization: *injection of a small amount of a pathogen that will provide protection against an infectious disease.*

Protection against developing a certain disease is called immunity. There are three basic types of immunity.

Innate Immunity You are immune to certain diseases just because you are who you are. First of all, you are a human being. You will never have to worry about diseases that affect only fish or rose bushes or horses. In addition, some people seem to inherit resistance to certain human diseases.

Active Immunity Once your body has launched an all-out war against a specific invader, it remains armed and ready to fight that same invader much more quickly and effectively if that same invader should ever show up again.

This happens because when the B- and T-cells that fight a specific invader multiply while they are fighting a pathogen, some of these cells are set aside as ''memory cells.'' The second time that specific pathogen tries to invade your body, your immune system is ready for it. Memory cells multiply quickly and produce huge numbers of antibodies in a very short time. The invaders are defeated and destroyed so quickly that they don't have time to make you sick. You never even know that they were ever present in your body.

There are two ways that you can acquire active immunity. One way is by actually having the disease. For example, the cells of Tanita's respiratory system were attacked by an influenza virus. Some of her immune cells recognized the proteins on the outside of the viruses. Those T-cells and the B-cells then began to divide and fight the infection.

At the same time, Tanita's immune system set aside memory T- and B-cells that recognize this flu virus. If that exact same influenza virus ever attempts to invade Tanita's body again, her immune system will fight it off before she even knows it.

But people sometimes get the flu more than one time in their lives. Why is that? Influenza viruses slowly change over time. After a while, a strain of flu may come along that is very different from the one Tanita is immune to. Her memory cells won't recognize this new flu virus, and she could get sick with the flu again.

Another way to acquire active immunity is through **immunization**. Sometimes called vaccination, immunization is a way of tricking your body into thinking that it has already had a disease. When you are immunized, dead or weakened pathogens, or sometimes just parts of a pathogen, are injected into your body. These pathogens can't multiply and cause damage to your body, so they don't make you sick. However, your immune system recognizes them as foreign invaders and mobilizes the immune response to the pathogen.

You may be able to feel your immune system at work. For example, your immune system causes your temperature to go up when it is working hard. A slight to moderate fever seems to make the immune system work better. When fever goes over a temperature of about 104°F, it may begin to do more harm than good. Some people get a little feverish and achy after an immunization—for example, after a diphtheria booster. This does not mean, however, that they got diphtheria from the immunization. It just means that they can feel their immune system going to work.

Just like actually having a disease, an immunization can leave memory cells behind. If you are effectively immunized against polio viruses, you cannot get polio. If polio viruses enter your body, your memory cells destroy them without your even knowing that you have been infected.

Many serious pathogens do not change much over time. Having the disease or being immunized against it, like the person shown in Figure 21-8, will give many years of protection, although periodic boosters are sometimes needed. It is also possible to be immunized against diseases that do change, like influenza. However, every time a new strain of flu virus appears, a new vaccine must be developed to protect against it.

Why isn't there a vaccine for the common cold? The virus that causes the common cold changes even more rapidly than the influenza virus. There may be several different cold viruses being passed around at any one time, and they are changing all the time. Plus, the common cold is not a very serious disease. A vaccine for the common cold would be a waste of time and money. By the time it was ready, the strain going around would have changed so much that the vaccine would be useless. Research into new vaccines is much more useful if it is focused on preventing really serious diseases like hepatitis and AIDS.

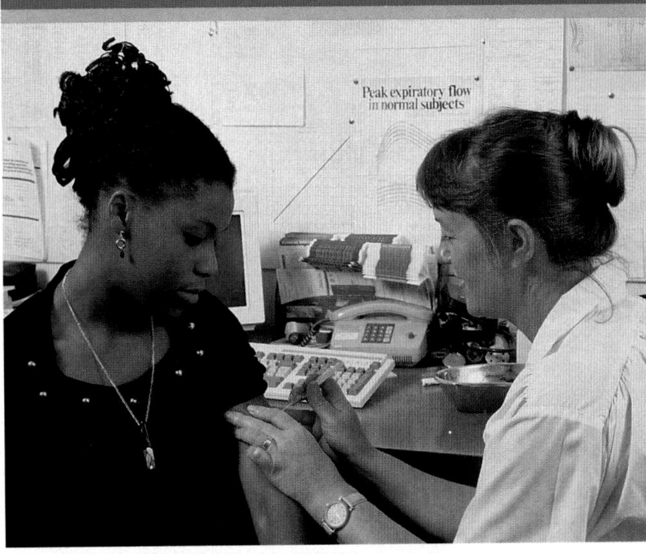

(FIGURE 21-8) **Immunizations, such as this one for tetanus, trick the body into thinking it already has had a specific disease. When this happens, the body produces memory cells that will automatically destroy the pathogens that cause that illness.**

Passive Immunity A third type of immunity to disease is called passive immunity. If you have passive immunity to a particular disease or infection, it means you have received antibodies from another person—or sometimes an animal—that have made you resistant to disease or infection.

Before you were born, some of your mother's antibodies passed from her to you. These antibodies gave you passive immunity that helped protect you from disease in the first few months of your life, until your immune system was mature enough to take care of your own body.

Antibodies are also injected into people who have been exposed to certain serious diseases. These antibodies may be extracted from the blood of human blood donors or from the blood of animals such as horses and sheep. For example, people bitten by a dog with rabies are treated by injections of rabies antibodies. Bites from poisonous snakes are treated by giving antibodies to snake venom.

Passive immunity lasts for only a short time. Eventually the antibodies break down and are removed from your bloodstream.

Review

1. *What's the difference between being infected and having a disease?*
2. *Name four ways that the body resists disease.*
3. *How does an immunization work to prevent disease?*
4. ***Critical Thinking*** *Is it always a good idea to take a medication that lowers fever? Why or why not?*

Review Answers

1. A person can be infected, or be invaded by a pathogen, and he or she will not develop any signs of symptoms. The person has a disease when a pathogen infects, or invades, a person's body and then that person develops signs and symptoms.
2. Skin, mucus and cilia in the respiratory system, stomach acids, immune system
3. An immunization injects weakened pathogens or parts of pathogens into the body. The immune system then mobilizes the immune response to destroy these harmless pathogens. The immunization leaves memory cells behind. When an active form of the same pathogen invades, or infects, the body, the memory cells multiply quickly to destroy the active pathogen.
4. No. A mild fever causes the immune system to work better. However, medical treatment may be needed for fevers of 104°F and higher, or if a temperature of 101°F lasts for more than three days.

ASSESS

Section Review

Have students answer the Section Review questions.

Alternative Assessment

Microorganisms Everywhere

We are surrounded by microorganisms that constantly try to infect us. Have students write an explanation of why we are sick only occasionally, instead of all the time.

Closure

Living in Isolation

Encourage students to imagine they are living in an isolated room, shut off from people. There is a window for air, and someone supplies them with food, water, and clean clothing through a small door. **Would you be completely safe from infectious diseases? Why or why not?** *[You would not be safe, because bacteria, viruses, protists, fungi, and parasites can travel in the air, water, food, and clothing.]*

Background
Meningitis
Meningitis is a serious bacterial infection of the brain or spine that can be fatal. Thus, meningitis immunization is recommended by the United States Public Health Service. A 1992 outbreak in Canada led to that nation's largest immunization program since a polio epidemic in the 1950s.

Background
Polio Immunization
Polio immunization has been a success. In 1952, the United States reported 21,000 cases of polio. In 1953 and 1955, polio vaccines were introduced. By the 1980s, fewer than 10 cases of polio were being reported annually in the United States.

Section 21.3 Common Infectious Diseases

Objectives

- *List four common diseases caused by viruses.*
- *Explain which kind of diseases antibiotics can cure, and which kind they can't.*
- *Know some ways to decrease your chances of getting an infectious disease.*

LIFE SKILLS: Practicing Self-Care

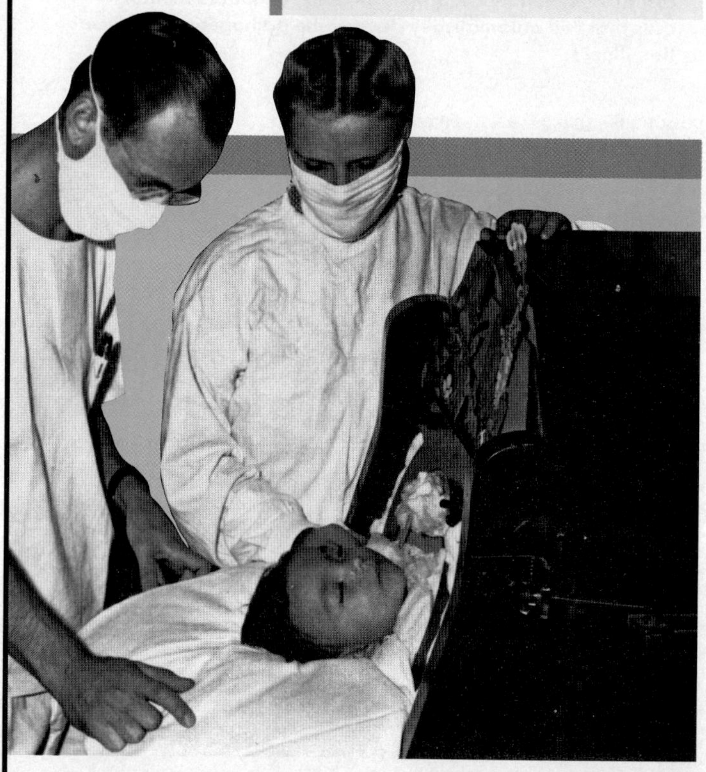

(FIGURE 21-9) **Polio, a viral disease that reached epidemic proportions during the 1940s and 1950s, left thousands paralyzed and unable to breathe without the help of an iron lung.**

You know now that diseases are caused by bacteria, viruses, fungi, protists, and other parasites. It's not always easy to avoid some infectious diseases, particularly those that are easily spread. But in general, the more you know about preventing an individual illness, the better your chances are of avoiding it. When you are sick, it's always a good rule of thumb to see your doctor. Keep in mind that even diseases that are not serious can have complications.

Viral Diseases

Some of the most common infectious diseases in the United States are caused by viruses. These include the common cold, influenza, cold sores, warts, mononucleosis, and chickenpox.

Preventing Viral Disease A number of viral diseases that were common when your parents and grandparents were young are now quite rare in the United States. In the 1940s and early 1950s, a polio epidemic left many children paralyzed. Some polio victims were unable to breathe on their own, like the child shown in Figure 21-9. Until the 1960s, almost everyone got measles, mumps, and rubella (sometimes called German measles) when they were children.

Today, almost all children are immunized against these diseases, which are now rarely seen. One exception is measles. Recently there have been several outbreaks of measles among high school- and college-aged young adults. Because of this, many people in this age group have had to get extra booster immunizations. In contrast,

Section 21.3 Lesson Plan

MOTIVATE

Journal 21D
Personal Experience With Disease

This may be done as a warm-up activity. On the chalkboard, write the heading DISEASES and vertically list the following: cold, flu, chickenpox, measles, mononucleosis, hepatitis, strep throat, sinus infection, mumps, tonsillitis, ear infection. In the Student Journal, have students describe a personal experience involving one of these diseases. Suggest that students describe any signs and symptoms they experienced. Record the number of cases beside each disease on the chalkboard. This shows the frequency of occurrence in your class and provides a reference for today's discussions.

TEACH

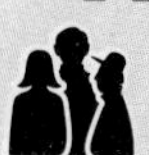

Cooperative Learning
Folk Medicine

Have students form small groups to discuss and prepare a list of folk "cures" for the cold. Have the groups present their list and let the class comment on each cure. Make sure students understand that such cures may relieve symptoms but cannot halt the reproduction of viruses in the respiratory tract. Point out that herbs, po-

the immunization campaign against smallpox, a disease that killed thousands of people several centuries ago, was so successful that smallpox has been eliminated.

The most serious viral disease in the United States today is AIDS. So far, there is no vaccine to prevent AIDS, but researchers in many laboratories are working hard to develop one.

Curing Viral Diseases There are only a few drugs that can cure viral diseases. Most of the time when you recover from a viral disease, it is because your immune system has destroyed the viruses in your body, or made them harmless.

Antibiotic (an tee by AHT ik) drugs like penicillin and tetracycline work by preventing the growth and cell division of living bacterial cells. Eventually the bacteria die. Viruses, however, cannot be killed by antibiotics.

What follows is a list of the most common viral infections you may come across. For symptoms, vaccine information, and treatment suggestions for each type of infection, see Figure 21-11.

The Common Cold The common cold should really be called the common colds. That is because more than 200 different viruses can cause the cold. A cold may make you feel really miserable, but it usually lasts only two or three days.

Each year, Americans spend more than $500 million on cold remedies. None of these remedies can actually cure a cold, but they can make you feel better while you are waiting to get well. Some over-the-counter drugs can help clear a stuffy nose or ease aching muscles.

Although there is no way to cure the common cold, there are some things you can do to reduce your chances of getting one. For one thing, try to avoid people who are sick with a cold. Colds are very contagious, especially through person-to-person contact. In addition, washing your hands often when colds are going around greatly improves your chances of not being infected yourself.

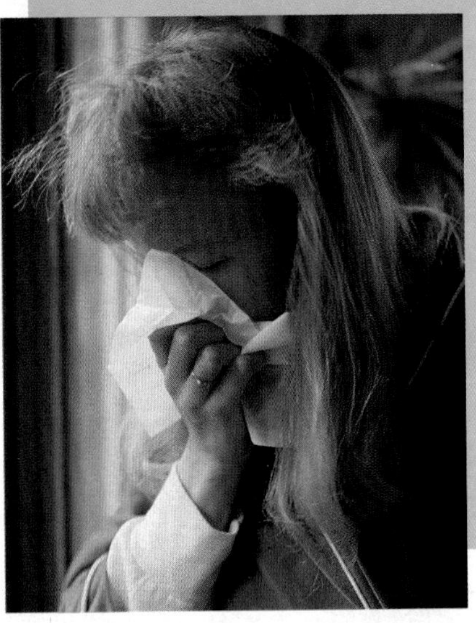

(FIGURE 21-10) **There is no immunization against the common cold. Fortunately, most colds last for only a few days.**

If you do get a cold, take care of yourself. Rest and drink plenty of fluids. The water you drink replaces body fluids lost to perspiration caused by fever.

Influenza Like the common cold, influenza is caused by a viral infection of the respiratory tract. The flu usually lasts longer than an ordinary cold. A cold usually lasts only two or three days, while it may take 7 to 10 days to feel like your old self again after having the flu.

Most people who are basically healthy recover from the flu without any serious problems. However, influenza may have serious complications and can be life-threatening for the elderly and people with respiratory problems. People at high risk should be immunized against influenza. If

antibiotics:

drugs that kill or limit the growth of bacteria.

SECTION 21.3

Background
Widespread Diseases
When an infectious disease affects many people, it is called an *epidemic.* If epidemics occur simultaneously at multiple locations in the world, they form a *pandemic.* Infectious diseases that occur continually in a particular region—such as malaria in parts of Africa—are called *endemic.*

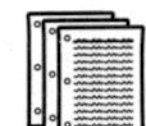

Life Skills Worksheet 21A

Being a Wise Consumer
Assign the Being a Wise Consumer Life Skills Worksheet, which requires students to analyze an advertisement for a cold remedy for false claims.

tions, and poultices used among some groups of people may bring symptomatic relief and comfort. In some cultures, a folk healer is a very trusted person in the community.

Class Discussion
Colds and Flu
Ask the following questions and have students answer and discuss them. **Why is it so difficult to develop vaccines against the many common cold viruses and the various flu strains?** *[Because there are so many viruses involved]* **Are the symptom-relieving drugs of value even though there are no cures for the flu and colds?** *[Yes, they may make you feel better.]* **What is proper treatment for these diseases and when is it necessary to get medical help?** *[Rest and drink fluids. You should see a doctor if your symptoms become severe.]*

Debate the Issue
Immunization
Remind students that vaccines sometimes have side effects that are harmful. If too many people in a population decide against being vaccinated for a disease, that disease rebounds. Schools commonly require students to be vaccinated for certain diseases. Have students debate the question: Should individuals have the right to refuse vaccinations that might harm them personally but that keep the population as a whole healthier? The DPT immunization (diphtheria, pertussis, tetanus) is a good example for students to use.

Making a Choice 21B

Common Infectious Diseases

Assign the Common Infectious Diseases card. The card requires students to find out more about common infectious diseases discussed in the chapter and to present the information to the class.

Common Viral Diseases

Disease	Signs and Symptoms	Treatment
Common Cold	*Sneezing, runny nose, sore throat, headache, fever, fatigue*	*Rest*
Influenza	*Sneezing, runny nose, sore throat, headache, fatigue, sometimes nausea and vomiting*	*Rest*
Chickenpox	*Skin rash, fever, muscle soreness*	*Rest*
Mononucleosis	*Swollen lymph nodes, swollen glands*	*Rest*
Hepatitis A, Hepatitis B, Hepatitis C	*Fever, weakness, loss of appetite, nausea, jaundice (yellowing of skin)*	*Gamma globulin injection, rest*
Measles	*Rash, high fever, sore throat, conjunctivitis, swollen lymph nodes*	*Gamma globulin injection, rest*

(FIGURE 21-11) **The best way to treat most viral diseases is to get plenty of rest and to drink lots of fluids.**

you do get the flu, check with your doctor if your symptoms become severe—for example, if you experience difficulty breathing or have a high fever.

Chickenpox There is no vaccine to prevent chickenpox (although one is under evaluation at this writing), so most people get this disease when they are children. The first signs of the disease are generally a skin rash, fever, and muscle soreness. The name ''pox'' comes from the characteristic blisters and scabs that form on the skin during the disease.

Like some other viruses, the chickenpox virus continues to live in cells in your body after you have recovered from the disease. Usually the virus causes no further problems, but occasionally it flares up again and causes a different disease, called shingles.

Measles One of the most serious viral diseases is measles. Without proper care, measles can lead to complications such as encephalitis and meningitis (an infection of the brain and spinal cord).

Like influenza, measles can spread through droplets in the air that can enter the body through the eyes, nose, and throat.

Mononucleosis Mononucleosis, often called mono for short, is caused by the Epstein-Barr virus. This virus is usually spread by contact with the saliva of an infected person. For this reason, the most common way of contracting the virus is

• • • TEACH continued

Reinforcement

Reduce Your Chance of Infection

Stress that mononucleosis, colds, flu, and other diseases are spread by sharing drinks, sharing food, sharing personal items, and personal contact. Have students think about anything they have done today, or may do later today, that might expose them to an infectious disease. Then, remind them to avoid such contacts when possible.

Game

Defenders

Divide the class into Team A and Team B to play "Defenders." Write this list of diseases on the chalkboard: cold, flu, chickenpox, measles, mono, hepatitis, polio, diphtheria, tetanus, whooping cough, strep throat, TB, sinus infection, trichinosis, mumps, and rabies. Use a harmless object (sponge, styrofoam ball, balled-up sheet of paper, etc.) for the "pathogen." Start with anyone on Team A calling out a pathogen ("Measles!") and tossing the object to the other team. Whoever catches it must call out a defense before tossing it back, such as, "I'm vaccinated!" or "I've already had it!" (Other defenses include: "I avoid contact with others," "I don't share drinks," "I'll take an antibiotic," and so on.) Whoever finally "becomes sick" with the pathogen (runs out of defenses) then calls out a different pathogen and tosses it toward the

through kissing or by sharing items like soft drink cans and cigarettes. These behaviors are most common among young adults aged 15 to 24. This is exactly the age group that gets mononucleosis most frequently.

The signs and symptoms of mononucleosis can last from two to eight weeks, but full recovery may take several months.

Hepatitis Hepatitis is a viral disease that can cause serious damage to the liver. There are three different types of hepatitis—Type A, Type B, and Type C hepatitis. These three diseases are caused by three different viruses. Type A hepatitis is usually spread by food contaminated with feces. It is more common than other forms of hepatitis, less severe, and usually more easily prevented. The most effective way to prevent hepatitis A is to wash your hands frequently when you prepare or serve food.

Hepatitis B is more serious than hepatitis A. It is usually spread through infected blood, semen, or saliva. It can also be spread through intravenous drug use, sexual contact, or tattoo needles and ear-piercing equipment that are not sterile. Hepatitis C is most often spread through blood transfusions. It is also very serious. Studies show, though, that hepatitis C can be treated with an antiviral agent called interferon.

A vaccine for Type B hepatitis has recently been developed. In addition, people exposed to hepatitis are often treated with an injection of gamma globulin, which is a fraction of blood that contains antibodies. Therefore, gamma globulin injections can provide some temporary passive immunity for hepatitis.

Common Bacterial Diseases

Immunization can prevent several serious bacterial diseases. In addition, antibiotics are very effective against bacterial diseases. If left untreated, however, bacterial diseases can be serious. That's why it's a good idea

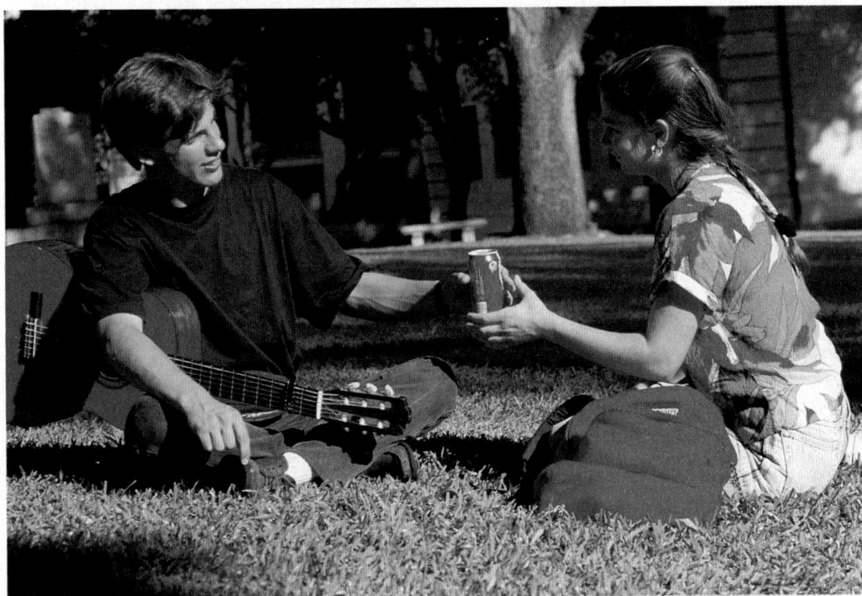

(FIGURE 21-12) **Mononucleosis is spread through contact with the saliva of an infected person. To avoid spreading disease, don't share partially eaten food.**

SECTION 21.3

Background
Tuberculosis

Tuberculosis is rapidly returning as a problem disease, mostly in the inner cities. About 10 to 15 million Americans carry the disease all the time, but their immune systems keep them from becoming ill. However, people who have impaired immune systems (people with AIDS and others) and those who are malnourished (people who cannot afford healthy diets or who are abusers of alcohol and drugs) are vulnerable to the TB bacterium. Although antibiotics can usually control tuberculosis, the poor often lack the money for treatment. In 1988, nearly 2,000 people died of TB in the United States.

other team to defend against, and so on. Award one point for each successful defense; the team with the most points wins.

Role-Playing
What Do I Have?

Divide the class into groups of three or four and have them role-play a situation in which a member shows disease signs and complains of symptoms from the text ("I have a skin rash, fever, and muscle soreness."). Other group members try to identify the disease (chickenpox) and inform the person of the necessary treatment (rest, fluids, seek a doctor). Have students take turns with different diseases.

Extension
Diseases Arriving With the Europeans

It is often pointed out that more Native Americans died from diseases introduced by Europeans than from warfare with them. Have students research this topic and report on it to the class.

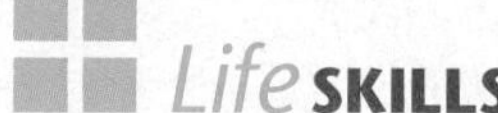

Tips on Preventing Infectious Diseases

Have students write an evaluation of their personal self-care, using steps 1–6. For example, if they are associating with someone who has an infectious disease, are they avoiding close contact and washing their hands often? Point out that this will help make them aware of things they might do to improve their own self-care.

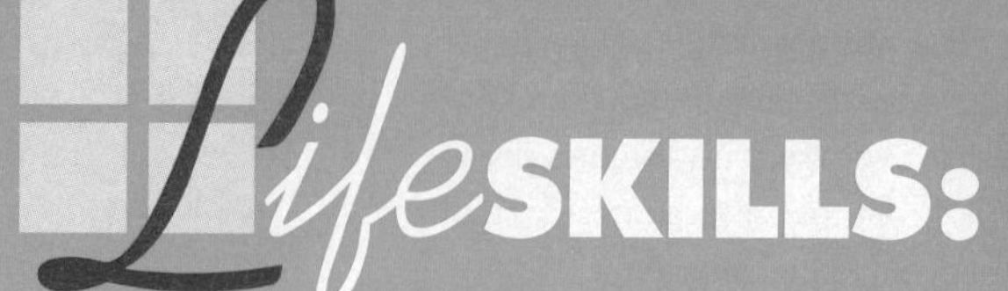

Practicing Self-Care

Tips on Preventing Infectious Diseases . .

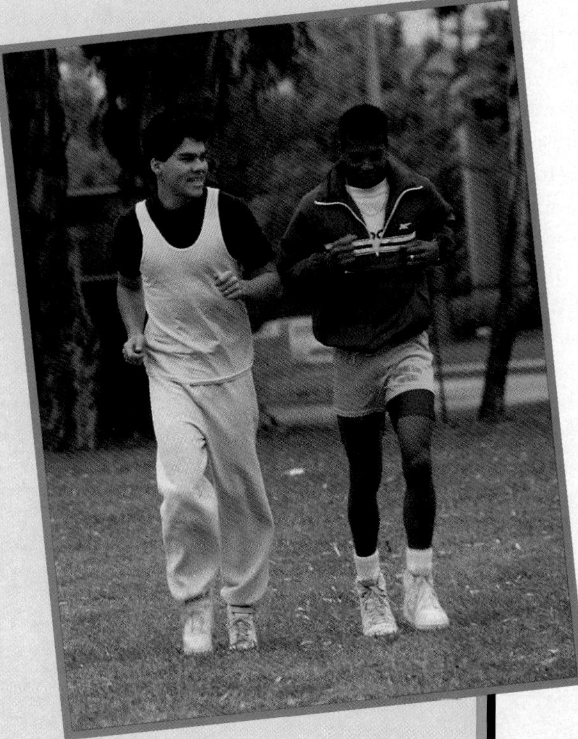

To decrease your chances of getting an infectious disease and increase your chances of staying healthy, you can do the following things:

1. Try to avoid close contact with people who have highly contagious diseases, like colds or flu. When "something is going around" or you must help care for someone who is sick, wash your hands often.
2. Keep your immune system working in top form by keeping your whole body healthy. Eat right, get enough sleep, and exercise regularly. High levels of stress can decrease the efficiency of your immune system. Try to manage your time so that stress doesn't get out of hand. Make time for some relaxing activities that you enjoy.
3. Do not share personal items like drinking glasses, soft drink cans or bottles, toothbrushes, hairbrushes, and combs.
4. Make sure you are up to date on your immunizations and boosters. When you have children of your own, make sure that they receive their immunizations on schedule.
5. Get regular checkups by doctors and dentists.
6. In spite of the best precautions, most people get sick once in a while. When it happens to you, rest and take care of yourself.

to see a doctor if you think you have a bacterial disease.

Strep Throat A sore throat caused by the *Streptococcus pyrogenes* bacterium is not a very serious disease in itself, but it can have serious complications. These complications include permanent heart and kidney damage. Unlike sore throats caused by the cold or flu viruses, strep throat can be easily cured by taking antibiotics.

Any severe sore throat, or a sore throat that lasts more than two days, should be checked by a doctor. A simple test that takes only a few minutes in a doctor's office can show if your sore throat is caused by a *Streptococcus* bacterium. If so, you will need to take antibiotics to avoid serious complications.

Tuberculosis The bacteria that cause tuberculosis, or TB, attack the lungs and cause fluid to build up there. Not surprisingly, people with tuberculosis suffer severe coughing spells. Other symptoms of TB include high fever, weakness, and loss of appetite.

Tuberculosis is another disease spread through droplets in the air. Fortunately, it is not easy to become infected, even if you inhale these droplets. Unless you are in close contact for a prolonged period of time with a person who has TB, chances are you won't catch the disease. In recent years tuberculosis cases have increased dramatically, partly because people with the AIDS virus are very vulnerable to it. Other factors that have contributed to the increase of tuberculosis include malnutrition and

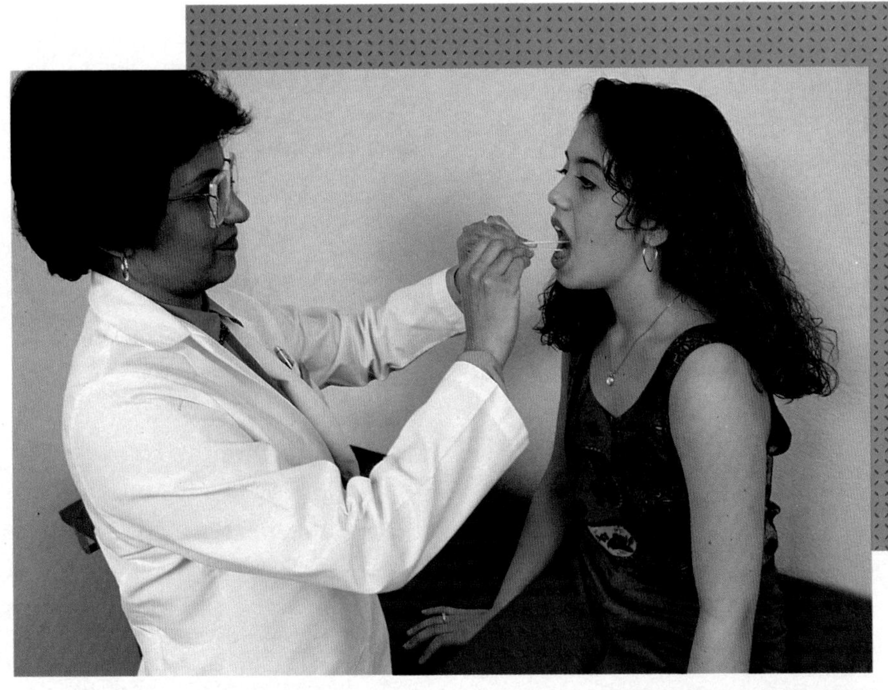

(FIGURE 21-13) **A teenager gets tested for strep throat. If you have a sore throat that lasts for more than two or three days, see your doctor. Strep is easily cured with antibiotics, but it can have serious consequences if left untreated.**

SECTION 21.3

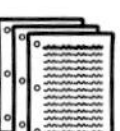

Section Review Worksheet 21.3

Assign Section Review Worksheet 21.3, which requires students to fill in a chart that lists the characteristics of a number of common infectious diseases.

Section Quiz 21.3

Have students take Section Quiz 21.3.

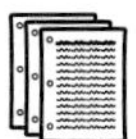

Reteaching Worksheet 21.3

Students who have difficulty with the material may complete Reteaching Worksheet 21.3, which requires them to diagnose and give treatments for common infectious diseases and discuss prevention and complication for some of the diseases.

Review Answers

1. Answers will vary. Students may answer chickenpox, common cold, influenza, measles, mononucleosis, hepatitis.

2. Bacterial; viral

3. Answers will vary. Students may answer getting immunizations; reducing person-to-person contact; not sharing items like soft-drink cans or bottles; washing hands before preparing or serving food; not sharing tattoo needles or ear-piercing equipment; keeping your whole body healthy; getting regular checkups.

4. Polio and AIDS are both caused by viruses. Polio is now preventable through immunizations, or vaccines. There is no immunization for the virus that causes AIDS.

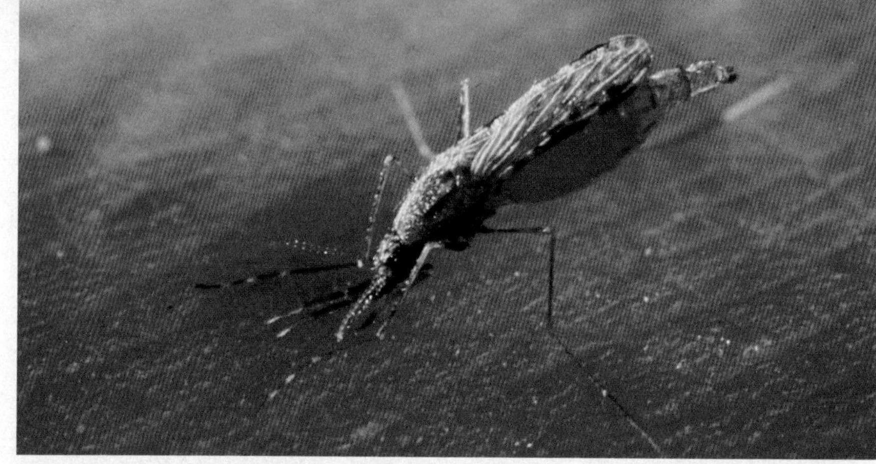

(FIGURE 21-14) **Malaria, which strikes 200 million people every year, is spread from person to person by mosquitoes.**

alcohol and drug abuse. Tuberculosis can be effectively treated with antibiotics, although some strains of the disease have proven to be resistant to treatment.

Sinus Infections A cold, flu, or allergy that leads to heavy mucus production can lead to a bacterial infection in your sinuses. The most common signs and symptoms of a sinus infection are thick, greenish mucus and sinus pain. A doctor can determine if you have a bacterial infection that needs to be treated with an antibiotic.

Other Diseases

Remember that there are diseases caused by pathogens other than bacteria and viruses. Fungi, protists, and animal parasites may also be agents of disease.

Three common conditions caused by fungi are athlete's foot, jock itch, and ringworm. These are discussed in Chapter 6.

Diseases caused by protists (which are complex, one-celled organisms) are not widespread in the United States, although they are common in other parts of the world. The most widespread and serious of these diseases is malaria. Each year, as many as 200 million people suffer from malaria, and one to two million people die from it. Malaria is caused by a protist that is carried from one person to another by mosquitoes.

Diseases can also be caused by animal parasites. Animals like hookworms, flukes, pinworms, and tapeworms can live inside the human body and cause disease. One kind of parasitic roundworm causes a disease called trichinosis. This roundworm can be found in the muscle tissue of pigs. For this reason, pork must always be cooked thoroughly before it is eaten.

Review

1. *What are four common diseases that are caused by viruses?*
2. *What kind of diseases can antibiotics cure? What kind can't they cure?*
3. ***LIFE SKILLS: Practicing Self-Care*** *Name four ways you can lower your chances of getting an infectious disease.*
4. ***Critical Thinking*** *What do polio and AIDS have in common? How are they different?*

ASSESS

Section Review

Have students answer the Section Review questions.

Alternative Assessment

When Do Antibiotics Work?

Ask students to imagine that several students and teachers have become sick with fever and sore throat, and are feeling weak. All are treated with antibiotics. Soon half of them improve, but the other half remain sick with the same signs and symptoms. **How could this happen? Is it one disease or two? What could the diseases be?** *[The half made well by the antibiotics had a bacterial infection, possibly strep throat. The other half have a viral infection, possibly flu.]*

Closure

Remembering

Have students write a paragraph describing an infectious disease, such as chickenpox, they remember having. Do they know where they got the disease? Did they pass it on to anyone else? How did they treat the symptoms? Did they see a doctor? Can they remember anything positive or humorous about the experience?

Chapter 21 Highlights

Summary

- Infectious diseases are diseases that pass from one organism to another. Communicable, or contagious, diseases are infectious diseases that pass from one person to another.
- In the United States, the most common infectious diseases are caused by bacteria and viruses. Other disease-causing pathogens are fungi, protists, and parasitic worms.
- A sign of a disease is something another person can observe, such as a fever, cough, sneeze, or rash. A symptom of a disease is any feeling of pain or discomfort a person experiences with a disease.
- Some of the body's defenses against disease are skin, mucous membranes, stomach acids, and body chemicals.
- The immune system is a complex system of organs and cells that fight specific agents of disease.
- A person can acquire active immunity to a disease by having the disease or by getting immunized, or vaccinated, against it.
- The common cold, influenza, hepatitis, mononucleosis, chickenpox, and AIDS are diseases caused by viruses.
- Strep throat, tuberculosis, and sinus infections are common bacterial diseases.

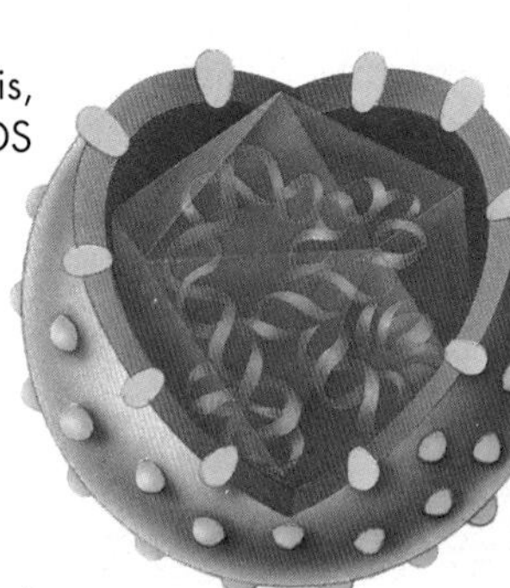

Vocabulary

infectious disease a disease that is passed from one living thing to another.

communicable disease an infectious disease that is passed from one person to another.

microorganism a tiny living thing that can be seen only under a microscope.

bacterium a microorganism that can cause disease.

virus an agent that can cause disease.

pathogens (PATH-uh-juhns) agents that cause disease.

immune system the system that protects the body from disease.

immunization injection of a small amount of a pathogen that will provide protection against a communicable disease.

antibodies substances that stick to the surface of pathogens, slowing their action.

antibiotics drugs that kill or limit the growth of bacteria.

Chapter 21 Highlights Strategies

Summary

Have students read the summary to reinforce the concepts they have learned in Chapter 21.

Vocabulary

Discuss the definitions of *infectious disease, pathogen, virus, bacterium, immune system,* and *immunization* and briefly review the relationships among them.

Extension

Rejection is a major problem with organ transplants, because the immune system sees the transplanted organ as a pathogen and attacks it. Have students research this topic and present a report to the class.

CHAPTER 21 ASSESSMENT

CHAPTER REVIEW

Concept Review

1. bacteria
2. ringworm, rabies
3. refrigerated, cooked
4. skin
5. infection
6. immune system
7. innate, active, passive
8. immunization
9. viruses
10. antibiotic
11. malaria

Expressing Your Views

Sample responses:

1. Yes. Foreign countries with poor living conditions often have "breeding grounds" for infectious diseases. These breeding grounds include open garbage pits and areas, open sewers, and untreated water. Also many people living in these countries have not received vaccinations against many preventable infectious diseases and therefore could infect others.

2. No. Buddy may still be contagious—he can spread the flu to others at work. Also, the throat lozenges may cover up Buddy's symptoms and the sore throat, if a bacterial infection, may only get worse.

3. Throw it away. Food that should have been refrigerated may now be contaminated with so much bacteria that it could cause food poisoning if eaten.

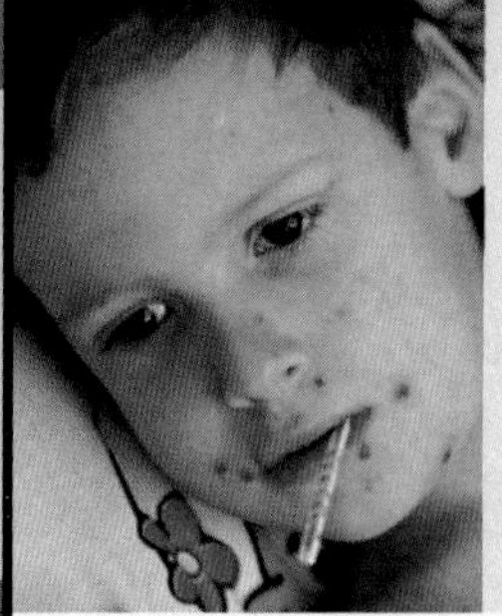

Chapter Review

Concept Review

1. Food poisoning and urinary tract infections are diseases caused by ________.
2. ________ and ________ are two diseases that affect humans but are spread by animals.
3. To prevent bacteria from growing in food, the food should be ________ and ________ thoroughly.
4. The ________ acts as a barrier to protect the rest of your body from pathogens.
5. If an infected cut is swollen, red, painful, and warm to the touch, it is a sign of ________.
6. The ________ ________ is the body's last line of defense against pathogens.
7. The three basic types of immunity are ________, ________, and ________.
8. Sometimes called a vaccination, ________ is a way of artificially acquiring immunity.
9. Measles and influenza are diseases caused by ________.
10. Bacterial infections can be cured with ________ drugs.
11. ________ is the most serious and widespread disease caused by a protist.

Expressing Your Views

1. Dion and Sam are planning to visit a foreign country that has poor living conditions. Do you think they will be at an increased risk of getting a disease? Why or why not?
2. Buddy is home with a sore throat. He says he can't afford to miss any more work, so he plans to stock up on throat lozenges and go back to work. Do you think that is a wise thing for Buddy to do? Why or why not?
3. Last night you had a party and had a lot of leftover food. You were too tired to put all the food away so you left most of it out all night on the counter. What should you do with the leftover food now? Explain.

Life Skills Check

Sample responses:

1. I would either inform the manager of the situation before the food was served and insist that the waiter wash his hands before serving any food or I would refuse the food when it was served.

2. I would talk with the school nurse or my doctor to see if I need to be immunized again.

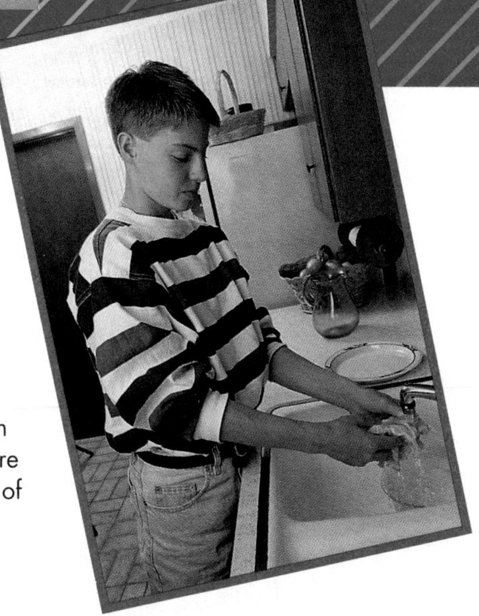

Life Skills Check

1. **Practicing Self-Care**
   While washing your hands in a restaurant restroom, you see your waiter leave the restroom without washing *his* hands. What should you do when your waiter comes to your table to serve your food?

2. **Practicing Self-Care**
   You were immunized against measles and mumps when you were an infant. You thought the immunizations were good for life, but you just read that there is an outbreak of measles at the local college. What should you do?

Projects

1. Choose a common infectious disease and create a poster containing information about it. Show the causes, symptoms, method of transmission, long-term effects, and treatments of the disease. Display your poster at a suitable place in your school.
2. Contact your doctor or school nurse and ask for a copy of your immunization record. The record should have vaccinations you have received during your life and the date when each was given. Make a list of diseases you have been vaccinated against, and record the date when your next booster shots, if any, are due.
3. Work with a partner to collect newspaper and magazine advertisements for cold remedies. On one side of a poster board, arrange the ads into a collage. On the other side, design your own ad for cold prevention, with suggestions for getting rest, drinking plenty of fluids, and continuing good nutrition and health habits. Display your poster in the classroom.

Plan for Action

There are several strategies a person can take to control the spread of infectious diseases. What are some things you can do to help keep infectious diseases from spreading?

Projects

Have students plan and carry out the projects on infectious diseases.

Plan for Action

On the chalkboard list the barriers to infection as students supply them, in the proper order. Have students discuss how each barrier operates and what they can do, if anything, to enhance the barriers' effectiveness.

ASSESSMENT OPTIONS

Chapter Test

Have students take the Chapter 21 Test.

Alternative Assessment

Have students do the Alternative Assessment activity for Chapter 21.

Test Generator

The Test Generator (Macintosh® or IBM® format) contains an additional 50 assessment items for this chapter.

SEXUALLY TRANSMITTED DISEASES

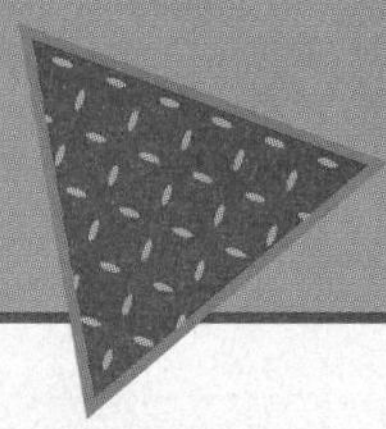

PLANNING GUIDE

TEXT SECTIONS	OBJECTIVES	TEXT FEATURES	OUTSIDE RESOURCES	NOTES
22.1 What Are Sexually Transmitted Diseases? pp. 463-474 2 periods	• Define sexually transmitted disease. • Know the names of four common sexually transmitted diseases. • Know how sexually transmitted diseases are spread from one person to another. • Know the signs and symptoms of sexually transmitted diseases.	**ASSESSMENT** • Check Up, p. 464 • Section Review, p. 474	**TEACHER'S RESOURCE BINDER** • Lesson Plan 22.1 • Personal Health Inventory • Journal Entries 22A, 22B, 22C, 22D, 22E, 22F • Life Skills 22A • Section Review Worksheet 22.1 • Section Quiz 22.1 • Reteaching Worksheet 22.1 **OTHER RESOURCES** • Transparencies 22A, 22B • English/Spanish Audiocassette 6	
22.2 Preventing Sexually Transmitted Diseases pp. 475-480 2 periods	• Know what you can do to decrease your chances of getting an STD. ■ Name 10 ways you can show love for someone without sexual intercourse. ■ Know where to go for testing and treatment for STDs.	■ LIFE SKILLS: Communicating Effectively, p. 476 **ASSESSMENT** • Section Review, p. 480	**TEACHER'S RESOURCE BINDER** • Lesson Plan 22.2 • Journal Entries 22G, 22H, 22I • Section Review Worksheet 22.2 • Section Quiz 22.2 • Reteaching Worksheet 22.2 **OTHER RESOURCES** • Transparency 22C • Making a Choice 22A, 22B	
End of Chapter pp. 481-483		**ASSESSMENT** • Chapter Review, pp. 482-483	**TEACHER'S RESOURCE BINDER** **OTHER RESOURCES** • Chapter Test • Alternative Assessment • Personal Pledge • Test Generator	

■ Denotes LIFE SKILLS objectives

• Items in blue are also part of the *Holt Health Activity Book.*

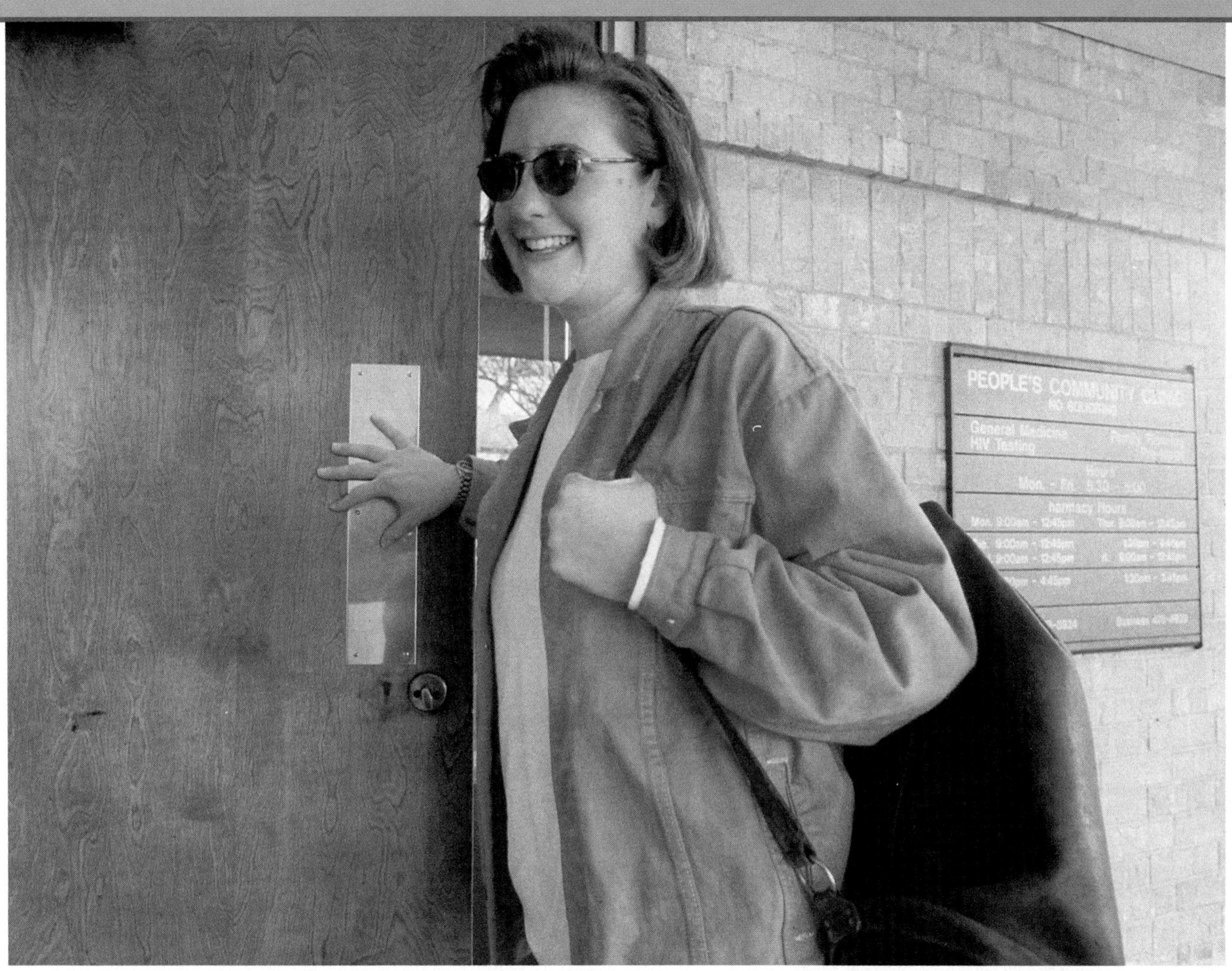

CONTENT BACKGROUND *Sexually Transmitted Diseases*

THE NATIONAL SURVEY OF FAMILY growth and the Urban Institute have discovered that more of today's teens in metropolitan areas are becoming sexually active. According to a survey done in 1979, 22 percent and 27 percent, respectively, of girls aged 15 and 16 were sexually active. By 1988, the sexual activity of girls of the same ages had increased to 27 percent and 34 percent, respectively. The survey did not include statistics for 15- and 16-year-old males in 1979; however, nearly a decade later 33 percent and 50 percent, respectively, of those same aged males reported being sexually active. In the 1988 survey the sexual activity of 17- and 18-year-old males and females ranged from 52 to 72 percent as opposed to 47 to 66 percent in 1979. Not surprisingly, STDs among sexually active teenagers are rising at alarming rates.

Chlamydia is probably the most commonly transmitted bacterial STD. Exact statistics on chlamydia are not known; however, some medical experts estimate that anywhere from 7 percent to 40 percent of female adolescents have contracted the disease and that females aged 15 to 19 have the highest infection rates among all women. Chlamydia is not routinely checked on a pap test. For this reason, all sexually active female adolescents should be advised to request this test when they visit their doctor or clinic.

According to the Centers for Disease Control and Prevention (CDC) in Atlanta, gonorrhea has declined over the past 15 years among most groups of teenagers because of a nationwide prevention program that began in the 1970s. On the other hand, syphilis among teenagers aged 15 to 19 has increased 67 percent since 1985.

In a recent study, doctors at the University of Washington found that genital herpes was extremely common among their female patients even though most of the women showed no outward signs of the disease. Nearly 66 percent of the cases were misdiagnosed when doctors only looked for herpes lesions and asked patients about past symptoms.

Genital warts are estimated to afflict as many as one-third of all sexually active teenagers. The warts can be treated by topical medication prescribed by a physician, lasers, electrical heat, or freezing with liquid nitrogen, but an estimated 20 percent of treated warts grow back.

The most serious sexually transmitted disease, acquired immune deficiency syndrome (AIDS), afflicted nearly 872 teenagers by June, 1992, according to the CDC. Teenagers are among the fastest growing groups of people contracting AIDS. Furthermore, researchers have found that more teenagers contract the virus that causes AIDS through heterosexual contact than do their adult counterparts. Teenagers at highest risk for contracting this disease are inner-city adolescents.

The increasing rates of STDs among adolescents only emphasizes the important role of educators in providing information to students. Many teens view themselves as invulnerable and feel that they just won't catch any diseases. It is crucial that today's teens be informed of the symptoms, treatment, and long-term effects of STDs.

PLANNING FOR INSTRUCTION

KEY FACTS

- **A sexually transmitted disease is passed from one person to another during sexual contact.**
- **The most dangerous STD is AIDS, which cannot be cured and is eventually fatal.**
- **Gonorrhea attacks the mucous membranes of the sex organs, throat, or rectum. This disease can lead to infertility.**
- **Chlamydia is the most common STD in the United States. It may cause infertility and problems during pregnancy.**
- **Genital herpes is an STD that causes sores on the genitals. The symptoms clear up, but the disease cannot be cured.**
- **Syphilis is a serious STD that has three stages. The tertiary stage of the disease can cause blindness, brain damage, paralysis, and death.**
- **The safe ways to express sexual affection for someone include talking, hugging, and holding hands.**
- **If you cannot accept sexual abstinence, there are some things you can do to make sex safer, although not completely so.**
- **Persons who think they have an STD have an obligation to get treatment immediately and to notify their recent sex partners. They should not engage in sexual activities until they are cured.**

MYTHS AND MISCONCEPTIONS

MYTH: Nice people don't contract or transmit STDs.

Anyone can contract or transmit STDs.

MYTH: A person cannot get an STD by having sex only once.

It takes only one sexual encounter with an infected person to get an STD.

MYTH: Using condoms provides complete protection against STDs.

The only behavior that provides absolute protection against an STD is abstinence.

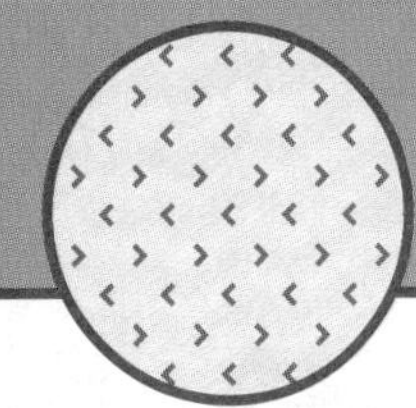

MYTH: Sexual contact is the only way for a person to get an STD.
Some STDs can be transmitted through blood contact. Others can be transferred from infected clothing or bed linens.

VOCABULARY

Essential: The following vocabulary terms appear in boldface type:

sexually transmitted disease (STD)	**genital herpes**
gonorrhea	**syphilis**
pelvic inflammatory disease (PID)	**genital warts**
chlamydia	**condom**

Secondary: Be aware that the following terms may come up during class discussion:

pelvic cavity	infectious
uterus	lymph nodes
Fallopian tubes	mucous membranes
microorganisms	sexual abstinence
vaginal discharge	monogamy
infertility	spermicide

FOR STUDENTS WITH SPECIAL NEEDS

Visual Learners: For students who learn best visually, show a film or video about STDs, such as *V.D.-Attack Plan,* film (Disney), or *Sexually Transmitted Diseases: Causes, Prevention and Cure,* video (Guidance Associates). Discuss the film afterwards to find out what areas students have problems with. Have them write any positive or negative thoughts they had about the film.

Auditory and Kinetic Learners: Form small groups of students who learn best from listening and performing. Have students make up a skit about a teenage star athlete who boasts that he has had sexual relationships with many girls and that he believes in having multiple partners. The other students should react to his boasting by telling him how dangerous his behavior is to himself and to everybody who has unprotected sexual intercourse with him.

ENRICHMENT

- Arrange for the school nurse or a health-care worker at an STD clinic to talk to students about STDs. Ask the speaker to provide case histories of people who have contracted STDs rather than simply an account of what STDs are and how they can be avoided. Have students prepare anonymous questions that the speaker can screen before talking. Ask the health-care worker and students to role-play a typical situation at a clinic. The health-care worker could interview students so they could experience the type of questions they would be asked if they were to visit a clinic.
- Have students write articles for the school newspaper that express how knowledge of STDs will affect their relationships. Tell them to sign their articles with a pen name to avoid possible embarrassment.

CHAPTER 22
CHAPTER OPENER

GETTING STARTED

Using the Chapter Photograph

Discuss why it was a good idea for the two girls to ask Vanessa's mother about sexually transmitted diseases. Ask students what surprised them most in what Vanessa's mother said about the effects of sexually transmitted diseases. Tell them that the chapter will discuss important facts about STDs as well as some of the misconceptions people have about the diseases.

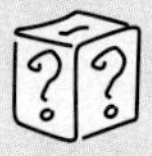

Question Box

Have students write out any questions they have about STDs and put them in the Question Box. The Question Box provides them with an opportunity to ask questions anonymously. To ensure that students with questions are not embarrassed to be seen writing, have those who do not have questions write something they already know about STDs on the paper instead.

Preview the questions and then answer them at appropriate points in the chapter. You may wish to allow students to write additional anonymous questions as they go through the chapter.

CHAPTER 22

Sexually Transmitted Diseases

Section 22.1 What Are Sexually Transmitted Diseases?

Section 22.2 Preventing Sexually Transmitted Diseases

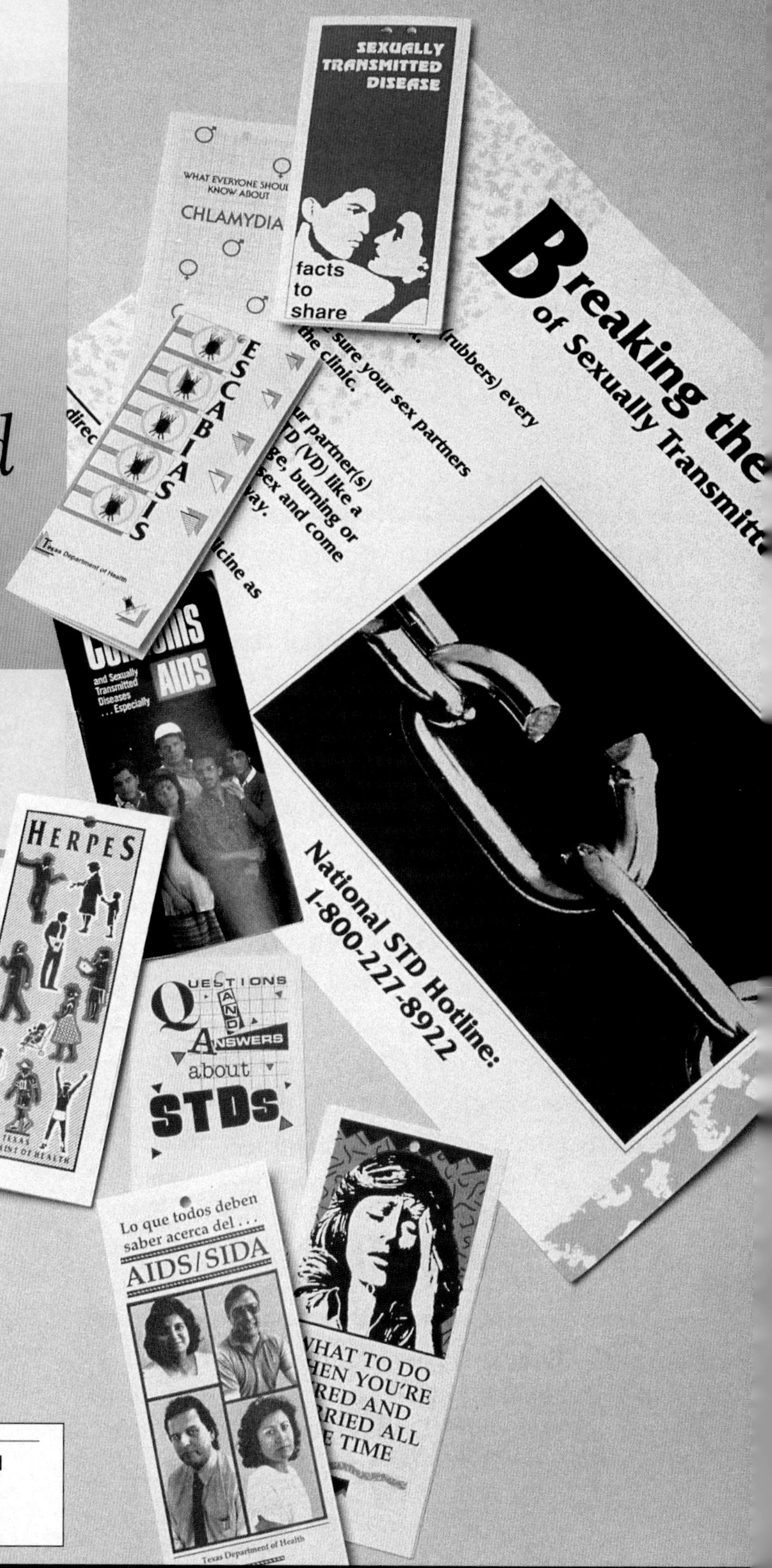

Education is the first step toward preventing sexually transmitted diseases.

Personal Issues *ALERT*

The discussion of STDs may make students uncomfortable for several reasons. For some, discussing diseases caused by sexual activity may be embarrassing. For others, it may be a difficult topic because they are concerned that their behavior may have put them at risk. Prepare the class to be respectful of others' privacy and sensitive to their feelings. Mention the importance of learning about STDs for their own protection.

Vanessa and her best friend, Han, agree that sometimes it seems like everybody takes it for granted that all teenagers are sexually active. In movies and on TV sitcoms the teenage characters joke about birth-control pills and losing their virginity. The songs on the radio are pretty explicit. It all adds up to a lot of pressure to have sex. At the same time, worrying about diseases that you could get makes sex seem pretty scary.

One evening Han was having supper with Vanessa and Vanessa's mother at their apartment. Han was surprised when Vanessa asked her mother about these diseases. Vanessa's mom is a nurse, so she was able to tell the girls a lot of what they wanted to know. Vanessa's mom said that AIDS is probably the worst disease you can get through sexual activity, but that there are others that are also dangerous. Some of them can cause infertility, the inability to have children. Vanessa didn't intend to get pregnant any time soon, but she had always assumed that some day she would have children. Finding out that a disease might make it impossible to have children made her realize that these diseases are serious.

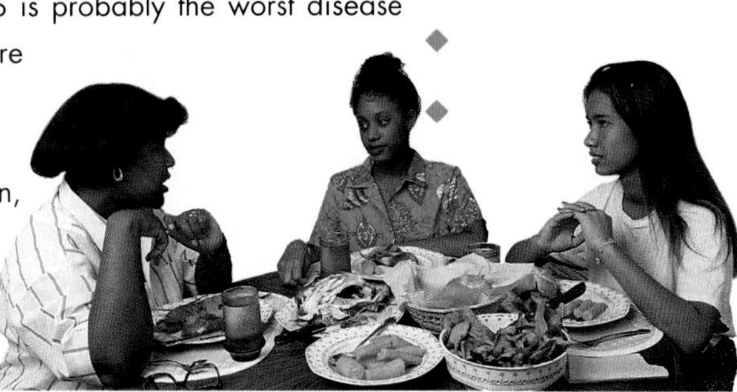

Section 22.1 What Are Sexually Transmitted Diseases?

Objectives

- *Define the term sexually transmitted disease.*
- *Know the names of four common sexually transmitted diseases.*
- *Know how sexually transmitted diseases are spread from one person to another.*
- *Know the signs and symptoms of sexually transmitted diseases.*

Each year, about 2.5 million teenagers are infected with sexually transmitted diseases. A **sexually transmitted disease,** or **STD** for short, is a disease that is passed from one person to another during sexual contact. These diseases used to be called venereal diseases (VD). Some of these diseases are merely uncomfortable, while others can be quite serious.

The most dangerous STD is AIDS. It cannot be cured and is eventually fatal. Because AIDS is such a serious threat, the next chapter will be devoted entirely to AIDS and the virus that causes it. This chapter will tell you about other diseases that are spread by sexual activity.

sexually transmitted disease (STD):
a disease that is passed from one person to another during sexual contact.

HIV infection and AIDS are discussed in Chapter 23.

Background
STDs in History

STDs are not a modern affliction. Many historical people have suffered from STDs: Julius Caesar, Henry VIII of England, Cleopatra, Napoleon Bonaparte, Franz Schubert, Adolf Hitler, and Al Capone, to mention a few. The search for a cure has an equally long history. Not until the advent of antibiotics was there a proper way to cure these diseases.

Background
Vaccines and STDs

Over the years, the dosage of penicillin needed to cure gonorrhea has had to be increased because the germs have become more and more resistant to the antibiotic. Researchers would like to develop a vaccine against gonorrhea. There is a problem with this, however, since vaccines work when they stimulate the production of antibodies in the bloodstream. Since gonorrhea bacteria do not go to the bloodstream until the disease has been in the body for a long time, its damage has been done before the antibodies would be able to affect it.

Section 22.1 Lesson Plan

MOTIVATE

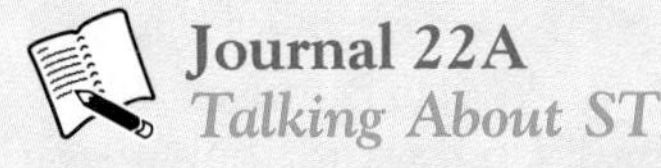

Journal 22A
Talking About STDs

This may be done as a warm-up activity. Encourage students to write down in the Student Journal in the Student Activity Book the names of any STDs they have heard about. Have them write why it was easy for the girls to talk to Vanessa's mother.

TEACH

Class Discussion
Staying Informed

Discuss the meaning of the term *sexually transmitted diseases.* Mention that these diseases are sometimes called venereal diseases. Tell students that, even though this is an uncomfortable topic, it is important for them to receive all the information they need to avoid these diseases. **Would you prefer to discuss this topic in small groups? With members of your own sex only? Are there topics you do not feel comfortable talking about?** Discuss students' responses.

Cooperative Learning
Respecting Others' Feelings

Have students form small groups to discuss ways to respect other classmates' feelings and privacy during the discussions of STDs. Have them draw

Check Up

Have students anonymously turn in their answers to the Check Up questions. Tally the results on the chalkboard. Identify the number of responses to each question. Discuss the correct answers to questions often missed. You might want to have students retake the Check Up at the end of the chapter and compare the class results with those obtained earlier.

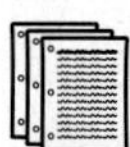

Personal Health Inventory

Have students complete the Personal Health Inventory for this chapter. The inventory helps them assess whether they are at risk for or have been infected with an STD.

Check Up

How Much Do You Already Know About STDs?

1. Can someone have an STD and not know it?
2. Are STDs common among sexually active teenagers?
3. Do birth-control pills prevent STDs?
4. Can STDs be prevented by washing carefully after sex?
5. Can the use of latex condoms greatly reduce the risk of getting an STD?
6. Can a person get an STD from oral sex?
7. Is it easy to tell if someone has an STD?

1. yes 2. yes 3. no 4. no 5. yes 6. yes 7. no

Gonorrhea

gonorrhea: *an STD transmitted by bacteria, which can infect the mucous membranes of the penis, vagina, throat, or rectum.*

One of the most common STDs is **gonorrhea** (gahn-uh-REE-uh). Gonorrhea is an infection caused by a bacterium. The gonorrhea bacterium attacks mucous membranes. It can infect the mucous membranes of the penis, vagina, throat, or the rectum.

About one million cases of gonorrhea are reported each year. Because many cases are not reported, however, the actual number is probably closer to three million cases each year.

REMINDER

Antibiotics are drugs that kill or limit the growth of bacteria.

What Are the Signs and Symptoms of Gonorrhea? As you learned in Chapter 21, a sign of a disease is something another person can see or detect. A symptom of a disease is any feeling of pain or discomfort you may experience. As many as 80 percent of women who have gonorrhea have no signs and symptoms or have signs and symptoms that are so mild that they aren't noticed. Because of this, most women with gonorrhea do not even realize that they have the disease.

One sign of gonorrhea in females is irritation of the vagina that is accompanied by a discharge. Since a female may have a vaginal discharge for other reasons, this is not a sure sign of gonorrhea. Females with gonorrhea may also have pain in the lower abdomen. But since this pain is usually mild, it is a symptom that is often ignored.

Unlike women who have gonorrhea, men infected with gonorrhea usually have signs and symptoms. One sign of gonorrhea is a heavy, yellow discharge of pus from the penis. Symptoms of gonorrhea include frequent, painful urination, tenderness in the groin or testicles, and swelling of the lymph nodes in the groin. These signs and symptoms usually appear about 2 to 10 days after infection. Sometimes the signs and symptoms go away, but that doesn't mean that the infection is gone.

One reason why gonorrhea is such a common disease is that a large number of people who are infected do not have signs or symptoms. These people may not realize that they have gonorrhea, but they can still pass the bacteria to their sex partners.

How Can a Person Become Infected with Gonorrhea? Gonorrhea is spread only by sexual contact. The gonorrhea bacteria can be passed from one person to another only by moving directly from one warm, moist body surface to another. It is not true that gonorrhea can be caught from dirty toilet seats, cups, or towels. This is because these bacteria must have the right combination of temperature, humidity, atmosphere, and nutrients to grow. A gonorrhea bacterium on a toilet seat would live for only a few seconds, because it dies when it is exposed to the air.

What Happens if Gonorrhea Is Not Treated? Gonorrhea can be completely cured by the appropriate antibiotics.

• • • TEACH continued

up a list of ways they could do this. Ask them to share their lists with the class. Have them discuss whether they were surprised by the fact that 2.5 million teenagers contract sexually transmitted diseases every year.

Journal 22B
Views on Sexual Behavior

Have students write in the Student Journal how they feel about the way sex is treated on television and in movies. Ask them to write whether they agree with their classmates about sexual behavior. Have them discuss how they would protect themselves from an STD and how they would protect someone they loved from becoming infected by them.

Class Discussion
Myths and Facts

Discuss the "Myths and Facts About STDs" table. Ask students to cover the fact column as you present each myth for discussion. Ask them to comment on each myth and provide a response that they believe is true. Have them check their responses with the fact column. One myth not on the list is that sexual activity in itself causes STDs. Students should be aware that sexual activity does not cause STDs. Sex provides the method of invasion, and sex organs provide a moist, warm location for the microbes to flourish.

Myths and Facts About STDs

Myth	Fact
Birth-control pills prevent STDs.	*Birth-control pills provide no protection against STDs.*
Washing the genitals after sex prevents STDs.	*Washing is not an effective way to prevent STDs.*
It is best to see if an STD goes away on its own before going to a doctor.	*STDs do not go away on their own. Even if the symptoms go away, it does not mean the STD is cured.*
The medicine prescribed for one kind of STD will cure any STD.	*Each STD requires different treatment. A doctor must be consulted for proper treatment.*
As soon as a person feels better, he or she can stop taking the medicine prescribed for an STD.	*All of the medicine prescribed by the doctor must be taken, even if a person starts feeling better before the medicine is all gone.*
If one sexual partner is treated for an STD, it isn't necessary for the other partner to be treated.	*Both sexual partners must be treated so they will not continue to reinfect each other.*
It is easy to tell when a person has an STD.	*Some people show no signs of illness even though they have an STD.*

(FIGURE 22-1) **A national survey, *The National Adolescent Student Health Survey*, showed that many teenagers have misconceptions about STDs that could endanger their health.**

However, without proper treatment, untreated gonorrhea in females may spread, causing an infection in the reproductive organs inside the pelvic cavity. Infection of the uterus and Fallopian tubes is called **pelvic inflammatory disease (PID).** PID can be caused by several different kinds of microorganisms, including the bacterium that causes gonorrhea. The signs and symptoms of PID may include painful sexual intercourse, uterine bleeding, vaginal discharge, abdominal pain, and fever. PID can be a very serious disease. It must be treated with powerful antibiotics and may even require hospitalization. PID can cause scarring of the Fallopian tubes, resulting in infertility.

A woman with untreated gonorrhea can also pass the gonorrhea bacterium to her baby at birth. This can cause blindness in the infant. To prevent this, it is standard procedure to treat the eyes of babies with medicated eyedrops immediately after birth.

pelvic inflammatory disease (PID):

an infection of the uterus and Fallopian tubes often caused by STDs; if untreated, may result in infertility.

Life Skills Worksheet 22A

Living With Genital Herpes

Assign the Living With Genital Herpes Life Skills Worksheet, which requires students to develop a plan of action that leads to stress reduction in a person afflicted with genital herpes.

Journal 22C
Surprising Myths

Have students write in the Student Journal the myth and fact about STDs that surprised them most.

Game
Myths and Facts About STDs

Have students play a short game using the table "Myths and Facts About STDs." A member of one team makes a statement from the table without mentioning whether the statement is from the myth or fact column. A player from the other team must identify the statement as a myth or a fact. Have students tally correct answers.

Journal 22D
Avoiding Gonorrhea

Have students write in the Student Journal what they would do to avoid contracting gonorrhea.

Writing
Dangers of Infertility

Have students write an article for the school newspaper stressing the dangers of infertility caused by STDs such as gonorrhea and chlamydia.

Journal 22E
If You Had an STD

Have students write in the Student Journal how they would feel if they found out they had an STD.

Class Discussion
Fears and Treatment for Herpes

What do people fear most about both herpes simplex I and II? *[There*

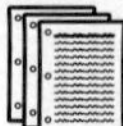

Section Review Worksheet 22.1

Assign Section Review Worksheet 22.1, which requires students to compare the characteristics of sexually transmitted diseases.

Section Quiz 22.1

Have students take Section Quiz 22.1.

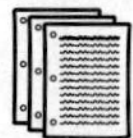

Reteaching Worksheet 22.1

Students who have difficulty with the material may complete Reteaching Worksheet 22.1, which requires students to complete descriptions of the progressive stages of syphilis and statements concerning its treatment.

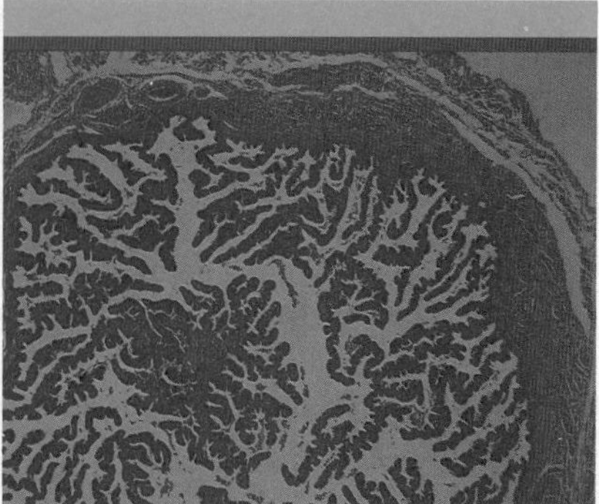

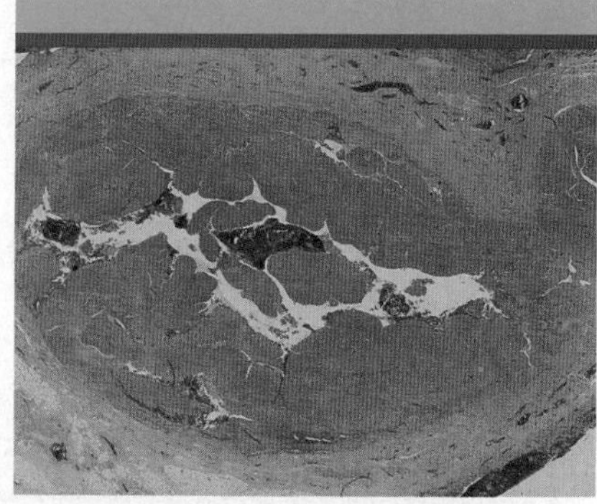

(FIGURE 22-2) **The photograph on the left shows normal tissue from a woman's Fallopian tube. The photograph on the right shows the effects of pelvic inflammatory disease (PID). Some sexually transmitted diseases can cause PID and result in infertility.**

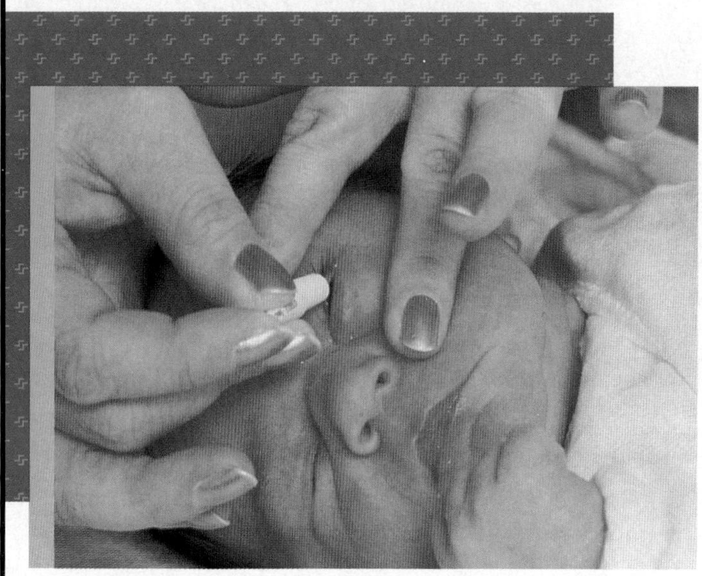

(FIGURE 22-3) **A newborn baby's eyes are treated with medicated eyedrops. This is standard procedure to prevent possible STD infections that could cause blindness.**

chlamydia: *the most common STD in the United States; caused by bacteria.*

A male who has been infected with gonorrhea may suffer serious complications in a short period of time, sometimes in just two to three weeks. Infection can spread quickly throughout the male reproductive system and cause pain, fever, and urinary problems. Eventually, the man may become infertile as a result of scarring of the sex organs.

Chlamydia

Chlamydia (klam-ID-ee-uh) is the most common STD in the United States. There are from 3 to 10 million new cases each year. Chlamydia is caused by a small bacterium. It is not a new disease, although it has become more common in recent years.

What Are the Signs and Symptoms of Chlamydia? Like gonorrhea, chlamydia does not cause signs and symptoms in the majority of women who are infected. Also, about one-fourth of infected men do not get signs and symptoms. In people who get them, the signs and symptoms of chlamydia will usually appear one to three weeks after exposure.

In males, the signs and symptoms of chlamydia infection include painful and difficult urination and a white or yellow watery discharge from the penis. In females, signs and symptoms may include painful urination, vaginal discharge, pain in the lower abdomen, and bleeding between menstrual periods.

• • • TEACH continued

is no cure for either of these viruses. Once infected you are infected for the rest of your life.] **If there is no cure for herpes, why are people treated for it?** *[Treatment reduces the pain and causes the symptoms to go away sooner.]* Mention to students that many people who have cold sores on their lips have herpes simplex type I. Remind them that the virus can be reactivated by various conditions such as irritation, stress, hormonal changes, or eating certain foods.

Role-Playing

Herpes During Childbirth

Have students role-play with a partner what a doctor might advise a pregnant woman with genital herpes to do if she has an outbreak close to childbirth. Tell them to make certain the woman is made aware of the danger to the newborn child.

Teaching Transparency 22A

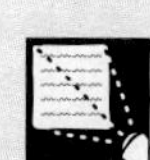

Sexually Transmitted Diseases

Show the table "Sexually Transmitted Diseases" (Figure 22-5). Ask students to group the diseases, based on similarities and differences in the causes, methods of spreading, symptoms, and cures of the disease. For example, they may group all those caused by bacteria together and all those caused by viruses together.

How Can a Person Become Infected With Chlamydia? Chlamydia is transmitted from one person to another through sexual contact. One reason chlamydia is such a common STD is that it is often spread by people who don't know that they have the disease.

What Happens if Chlamydia Is Not Treated? In women, the bacterium that causes chlamydia is another microorganism that can cause PID. Like PID caused by gonorrhea, PID caused by chlamydia can damage a woman's reproductive system, making her unable to have children. In men, an untreated chlamydia infection can also result in infertility.

Women with chlamydia are more likely to have problems during pregnancy, and babies born to women with chlamydia may get eye infections or pneumonia. Because of this, pregnant women should be screened for chlamydia even if they have no signs and symptoms.

Genital Herpes Infection with the herpes simplex virus in the genital region is called **genital herpes** (HUR-peez). Two types of the herpes simplex virus exist—type I and type II. Usually, type I is found above the waist, appearing as a cold sore or fever blister on the mouth. Type II is usually found below the waist. There are more than 30 million Americans with genital herpes. About 500,000 more become infected each year.

What Are the Signs and Symptoms of Genital Herpes? Only about 25 percent of people infected with genital herpes have signs and symptoms. The other 75 percent still have the disease and can give it to someone else.

If there are signs and symptoms, they usually take from 2 to 10 days to develop. In females, painful blisters may appear on the cervix, vagina, or vulva. In males, blisters and ulcers may appear on the penis. Pain may also be experienced when urinating. In both sexes, there are sometimes blisters on the thighs and buttocks. The infected areas may also become reddened.

In addition, some people experience itching, tingling, or burning sensations just before the sores appear. Other symptoms of herpes may include a sluggish feeling, fever, and flu-like symptoms.

There is no cure for herpes. Once you are infected with the virus that causes herpes, you are infected for the rest of your life. If you do not have signs and symptoms, or when they go away, the herpes-causing virus stays inactive in the nerves. The virus may be reactivated by various changes—irritation, stress, hormonal changes, or even certain foods.

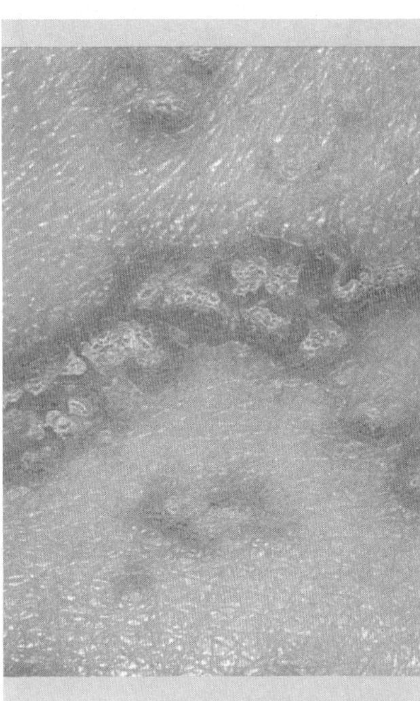

(FIGURE 22-4) **Painful blisters like these are the result of genital herpes. However, most people infected with genital herpes have no symptoms.**

genital herpes:

an STD, caused by a virus, which often causes painful blisters or ulcers; cannot be cured.

Background
On Genital Herpes

Primary symptoms of genital herpes usually last two or three weeks, but symptoms may appear as many as eight times a year. Some people have only one outbreak in a lifetime. The incidence of herpes infections has risen almost 300 percent in the last 30 years. Nonsexual transmission of herpes is possible if a person touches the genital sores of an actively infected person. The virus may then be passed by hand to the person's own genitals.

Game
What Do You Know About STDs?

Prepare two sets of cards or have students prepare them. Each card of the first set will bear one of the following terms: Cause, Method of Spreading, Symptoms, Treatment. Each card of the second set will have one of the following: gonorrhea, chlamydia, genital herpes, syphilis, nongonococcal urethritis, genital warts, vaginitis, hepatitis B, pubic lice, scabies. (You will probably want to include only those cards in the second set that have STDs covered thus far. The other cards will be added when all the diseases have been discussed.) Each player will select a card from each pile and must provide the information requested by the card of the first set about the disease mentioned on the card in the second set.

Teaching Transparency 22B

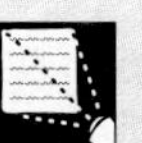

Pathogens That Cause STDs

Use the transparency *Pathogens That Cause STDs* in order to review the different cause of STDs.

Class Discussion
Treatment Is Important

Discuss syphilis as a potentially life-threatening disease. **Why is it important to seek treatment for syphilis,**

Sexually Transmitted Diseases

STD	What Causes It?	How Is It Spread?
Gonorrhea	*Neisseria gonorrhoese bacterium*	*Sexual contact; mother to infant at birth*
Chlamydia	*Chlamydia trachomatis*	*Sexual contact; mother to infant at birth*
Genital herpes	*Herpes simplex virus*	*Sexual contact; contact between sores and mucous membranes or break in skin; mother to infant at birth*
Syphilis	*Treponema pallidum bacterium*	*Sexual contact; contact between chancre or rash and mucous membranes or break in skin; mother to infant before birth*
Nongonococcal urethritis (NGU)	*Several causes, such as chlamydia, ureaplasma, mycoplasma, trichomonas, herpes*	*Most often spread by sexual contact, but some microorganisms can be spread by other means*
Genital warts	*Virus*	*Sexual contact*
Vaginitis	*Several causes, such as monilia, gardnerella, herpes, trichomonas, mycoplasma*	*Often spread by sexual contact, but some microorganisms can be spread by other means*
Hepatitis B	*Hepatitis B virus*	*Sexual contact; sharing needles; sharing items like razors, toothbrushes, eating utensils; mother to infant at birth*
Pubic lice	*Insect*	*Sexual contact, nonsexual contact*
Scabies	*Mite*	*Sexual contact, nonsexual contact*

(FIGURE 22-5) **A sexually transmitted disease (STD) is a disease that is passed from one person to another during sexual contact. AIDS is another STD, and is discussed in Chapter 23.**

• • • TEACH continued

even if the chancre disappears? *[When the chancre disappears, the disease has not been cured; instead the second stage is just beginning.]*

Role-Playing
Talking to the Doctor

Have students role-play with a partner a discussion between a doctor and a teenager who has just been diagnosed with syphilis. Have the doctor ask the teenager about common symptoms of syphilis and what has to be done to treat the disease.

Writing
Informing Partners

Ask students to write a letter to a girlfriend or boyfriend telling the friend they are being treated for syphilis. Encourage them to ask the friend to understand why they now have to change their sexual activity.

Journal 22F
On STDs and Friends

Have students write in the Student Journal how they would feel if they found out that a friend had one of the STDs. Tell them to write whether it would change their feelings for this friend. Also have them write how they would want their friend to feel if they had contracted an STD.

What Are the Signs and Symptoms?	How Is It Treated?
Females: often no signs or symptoms; vaginal irritation and discharge; pain in lower abdomen **Males:** frequent, painful urination; heavy yellow discharge of pus from penis; tenderness in groin or testicles; swollen lymph nodes on groin	Antibiotic
Females: usually no signs or symptoms; painful urination; vaginal discharge; pain in lower abdomen; bleeding between menstrual periods **Males:** often no signs or symptoms; painful, difficult urination; white or yellow discharge from penis	Antibiotic
Females: usually no signs or symptoms; painful blisters on cervix, vagina, vulva, thighs, or buttocks; sluggish feeling; fever; flu-like symptoms; lymph node enlargement **Males:** usually no signs or symptoms; blisters on penis, thighs, or buttocks; painful urination; sluggish feeling; fever; flu-like symptoms; lymph node enlargement	No cure but acyclovir can ease symptoms
First sign: small, red bumps at the point of infection, which becomes an open sore oozing fluid (called a chancre) **Later signs and symptoms:** a rash; a dull, depressed feeling; fever, joint pain; hair loss; large moist sores around the sex organs or mouth **Final stage:** Blindness; brain damage; paralysis; can cause death	Antibiotic
Painful urination; discharge	Antibiotics or other drugs depending on cause
Warts in the genital or anal area	Podophyllin, laser, liquid nitrogen, surgery
Itching or pain in vaginal area; vaginal discharge that is yellowish or has an unpleasant odor	Antibiotics or other drugs depending on cause
Flu-like symptoms; dark urine; yellowing of skin	No cure
Intense itching in groin and occasional swelling of lymph nodes in the groin	Medicated lotions and shampoos
Intense itching in genital area, under the breast, in the armpits, between the fingers, or elsewhere	Medicated lotions and shampoos

Extension

Old and New STDs

Students may want to know if people in the past had problems with STDs. Have them visit the library to find out which STDs are old and which are new diseases. They may want to read a book by Allen Chase, *The Truth About STD: The Old Ones—Herpes and Other New Ones—The Primary Causes—The Available Cures.* New York, Quill, 1983. Have students report their findings in a news article or a classroom skit.

Background

History of Syphilis

Some historians have tried to trace the terrible outbreak of syphilis in Europe in 1494 to Christopher Columbus's sailors returning from the New World. Supposedly, some bones of pre-Columbian natives resemble syphilitic bones. However, it has not been established whether the natives had syphilis. The ruins of Pompeii, A.D. 79, contain some writing about a disease that could have been syphilis. If that is the case, the disease was present in Europe long before Columbus.

syphilis:

an STD caused by bacteria, which can spread through the bloodstream to any organ of the body.

How Can a Person Become Infected With Genital Herpes? Herpes is almost always transmitted by sexual contact. However, any direct contact with a herpes sore can cause infection with herpes. The tiny blisters that form during a herpes outbreak are filled with a clear fluid that contains the virus. When blisters appear, the disease is in its most infectious state. That is the time when genital herpes can most easily be transmitted to another person. The open lesions will eventually crust over as the healing begins.

This does not mean that you cannot get herpes if you do not see herpes blisters on your partner's genitals. For one thing, although herpes is most contagious when blisters are present, it can also be transmitted when there are no blisters—for example, right before an outbreak of blisters. Also, blisters may be present but not seen. For example, if the infection were on a female's cervix, it would not be seen. Still, it could infect her sex partner.

What Happens if Genital Herpes Is Not Treated? Some people who have genital herpes will never experience signs and symptoms. Some may have signs and symptoms when they are first infected and never have them again. Still others may have herpes signs and symptoms that come and go. The signs and symptoms may appear once every few years or as often as every few weeks.

Although there is no cure, there is a drug that can be helpful to people with herpes. For people whose signs and symptoms return again and again, the drug acyclovir is used. Although acyclovir does not cure herpes, it can reduce the pain of the signs and symptoms and cause them to go away sooner than they would have without treatment. Acyclovir is available in capsules or as a cream.

The most important serious effects of genital herpes are the long-term problems. First, living with an incurable condition that can flare up at any moment can cause much stress and worry. Second, if a pregnant woman has an outbreak of herpes during childbirth, a Caesarean section may be necessary to prevent the baby from being born infected. Herpes infections in newborn babies are very serious. Fifty percent of newborns infected with herpes die, and half of the surviving babies will have severe brain or eye damage.

Syphilis

Syphilis (SIF-uh-lis) is caused by a bacterium. Syphilis is a very serious disease because it can spread through the bloodstream to any organ of the body. About 90,000 new cases of syphilis are reported each year.

What Are the Signs and Symptoms of Syphilis? The first sign of syphilis is a painless sore called a chancre (SHANG-ker). The chancre starts out as a small red bump that later becomes an open sore that oozes fluid filled with syphilis bacteria. The chancre forms at the part of the body where the infection occurred.

A chancre on the penis or on the lips of the vagina is most likely to be noticed. However, the chancre may also form on the cervix, inside the vagina, in the mouth, in the throat, or in the rectum. Since the chancre is small and painless, it is usually not noticed if it forms in these areas. A chancre on the lips may be mistaken for a cold sore. While the chancre is present, the infected person has primary syphilis.

It usually takes about three weeks for the chancre to appear after infection, although it may appear as soon as 10 days after infection. In some people it may not appear for as long as three months. Before

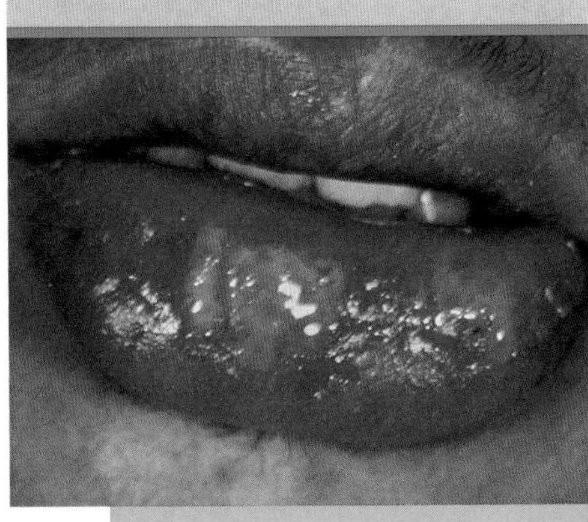

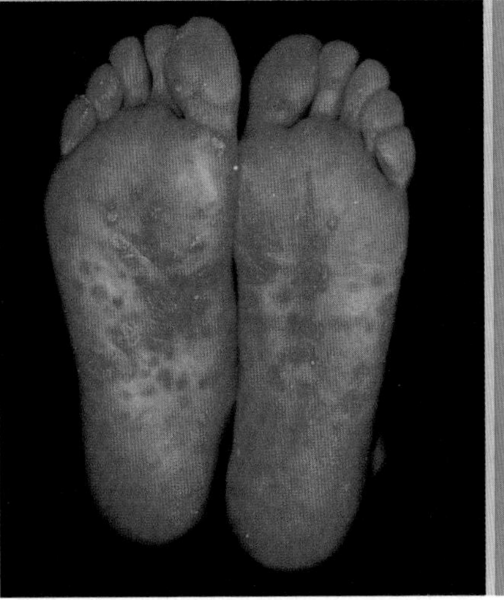

(FIGURE 22-6) **The first sign of syphilis is a painless sore called a chancre [left]. A later sign of the disease is a rash, which sometimes appears on the soles of the feet [right].**

the chancre forms, a blood test for syphilis may be negative even though the bacterium is present in the body and the disease is progressing.

The chancre disappears with or without treatment within one to five weeks. However, disappearance of the chancre does not mean the disease is cured. It is just progressing to the next stage.

The next stage of the disease is called secondary syphilis. The signs and symptoms of secondary syphilis appear about two to six months after exposure. The most common sign of secondary syphilis is a rash that appears on the body. Sometimes the rash appears on the palms of the hands and the soles of the feet. The rash does not itch, and it goes away without treatment after a few weeks, although it may come back and go away again several times.

A person with secondary syphilis may also have a dull depressed feeling, fever, joint pain, or hair loss. Large, moist sores sometimes develop around the sex organs or in the mouth. Like the chancre that is characteristic of primary syphilis, the signs and symptoms of secondary syphilis disappear without treatment. Syphilis then enters the latent stage.

Latent syphilis has no signs and symptoms. This stage may last for a few years or for an entire lifetime. However, latent syphilis may progress to tertiary syphilis. Tertiary syphilis is the stage of the disease in which the syphilis bacteria cause severe damage to parts of the body such as the skin, blood vessels, heart, bones, spinal cord, and brain. Tertiary syphilis can cause blindness, brain damage, paralysis, and, in some cases, even death.

How Can a Person Become Infected With Syphilis? The bacterium that causes syphilis is very frail and cannot survive drying or chilling. It dies within a few seconds after exposure to air. Therefore, as with gonorrhea, you cannot get syphilis from toilet seats or dirty towels. Syphilis is usually transmitted during sexual contact. The bacterium is passed from the chancre or rash of

The Spread of STDs

STD	Approximate New Cases Each Year
Gonorrhea	*1–3 million*
Chlamydia	*3–10 million*
Genital herpes	*500,000*
Syphilis	*90,000*
Genital warts	*1 million*

(FIGURE 22-7) **Sexually transmitted diseases are spreading at an alarming rate. One reason for the rapid spread is that many people do not have signs and symptoms of disease and unknowingly infect others.**

genital warts:
a viral STD in which warts appear on the genital and anal areas.

an infected person to the mucous membrane of the vagina, penis, mouth, or rectum of the other person. It is also possible for syphilis to be transmitted from a chancre or rash to an open wound or sore. An infected woman can also pass syphilis to her unborn child during pregnancy.

What Happens if Syphilis Is Not Treated? Syphilis can be cured at any stage by using the right antibiotics. Treatment for the disease is easiest during the first year of infection.

After a year, syphilis can still be successfully treated, but the medication must be taken for a longer period of time.

If syphilis progresses to the final tertiary stage, treatment can stop the progression of the disease but cannot reverse the damage that has already occurred. As you already read, tertiary syphilis can cause blindness, paralysis, and even death.

Other STDs

The most common STDs are the ones already discussed. However, there are other STDs as well.

Nongonococcal Urethritis (NGU) Any infection of the urethra—the tube that carries urine from the bladder to the outside of the body—that is not caused by gonorrhea is called nongonococcal urethritis. Several different organisms cause NGU, but most cases are caused by chlamydia. The proper antibiotic must be prescribed to cure NGU.

Genital Warts **Genital warts** may be the fastest growing STD in the United States. There are more than one million new cases each year. Warts may appear in the genital and anal areas.

Genital warts are caused by viruses. The warts may be treated with drugs, lasers, liquid nitrogen, or surgery. The viruses that cause genital warts are also associated with cervical cancer. Therefore, Pap tests at least once a year are particularly important for females who have had genital warts.

Vaginitis Vaginitis is any inflammation of the vagina. Signs and symptoms may include itching or pain in the vaginal area or any unusual vaginal discharge. It is normal for the vagina to secrete a small amount of clear liquid. It is also normal for the amount and thickness of the secretion to vary somewhat during the monthly cycle. However, if the discharge is yellowish, if it has an unpleasant odor, or if there is much more than usual, it is a sign of vaginitis.

Vaginitis can be caused by the gonorrhea or chlamydia bacteria, as well as by other microorganisms. Trichomoniasis (also called "trick") is caused by a one-celled organism that burrows under the mucus in the vagina. It is often transmitted through sexual intercourse. It can also be contracted by exposure to moist objects containing the organism. For example, this could happen if you used someone else's wet towel, bathing suit, or other clothing.

Vaginitis can also be caused by a fungus called monilia. This kind of infection, moniliasis, is commonly known as a yeast infection. A yeast infection is not necessarily sexually transmitted. Any imbalance in the normal environment inside the vagina can give monilia a chance to grow and to cause problems.

Hepatitis Hepatitis (hep-uh-TY-tis) is an inflammation of the liver that can be caused by several different viruses. The type of hepatitis that is called hepatitis A is not usually transmitted sexually, but it can be passed from one person to another by oral-anal contact.

The hepatitis B virus, on the other hand, is easily transmitted through sexual contact. It may be present in the body fluids—saliva, urine, blood, semen, and vaginal secretions—of an infected person. But sexual contact is not the only way hepatitis B is spread. Practices such as sharing toothbrushes, razors, eating utensils, or needles with an infected person can also transmit the disease.

Hepatitis B is a serious disease. It can cause damage to the liver and result in serious health problems. Early signs and symptoms may be similar to those of the flu, and may also include dark urine and yellowing of the skin. If you are exposed to hepatitis B, it is important for you to see a doctor right away.

A vaccine is now available that prevents hepatitis B. If you are concerned about this type of hepatitis, talk to a doctor or another health professional about receiving the vaccine.

Parasitic Infections Pubic lice (''crabs'') and scabies can be spread by either casual or sexual contact. Pubic lice are small insects that live in the pubic hair and attach their eggs to hair shafts. Pubic lice grip the pubic

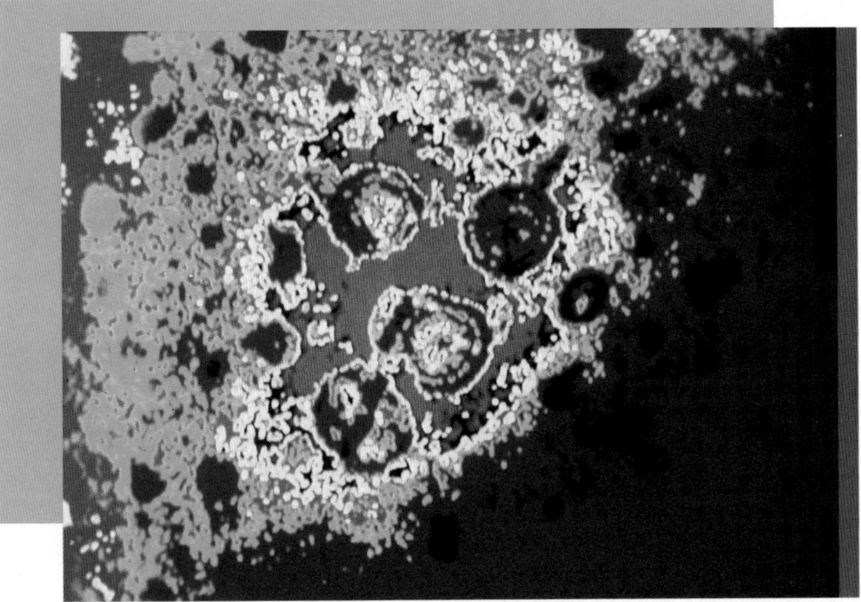

(FIGURE 22-8) **One of the early signs of hepatitis B is yellowing of the skin.**

Review Answers

1. A disease that is passed between people during sexual contact

2. The most common STDs include gonorrhea, chlamydia, genital herpes, and syphilis.

3. sexual contact; mother to infant during birth

4. In both males and females there may be no symptoms or there may be painful blisters on the sex organs and the thighs and buttocks. There may be a sluggish feeling, fever, flu-like symptoms, and enlarged lymph nodes.

5. Yes. A person with an STD but no symptoms may unknowingly infect another person. Also, some people may not recognize or may ignore the symptoms of an STD and fail to get treatment.

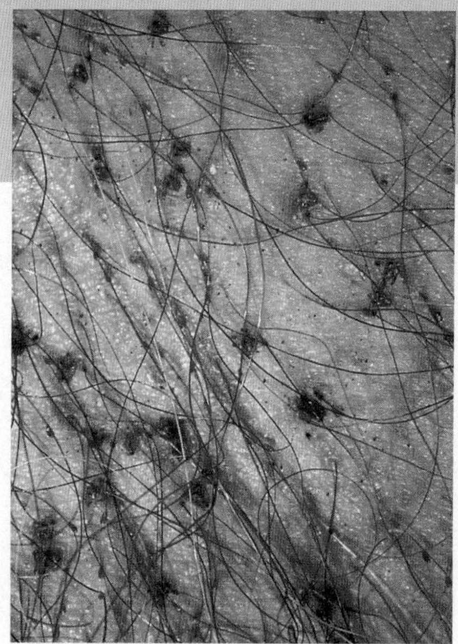

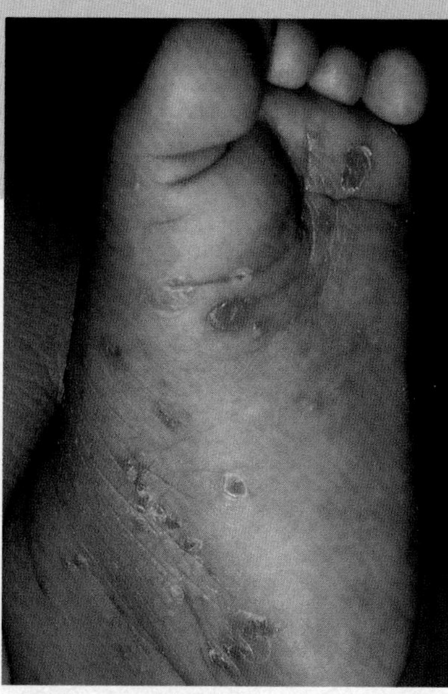

(FIGURE 22-9) **Pubic lice [left] live in the pubic hair, causing irritation and itching. Scabies is caused by a tiny mite that burrows under the skin.**

hair and feed on tiny blood vessels of the skin. The lice irritate the skin and cause itching and occasional swelling of the glands in the groin.

Scabies (SCAY-beez) is caused by a tiny mite that can barely be seen. The mite burrows under the skin and causes intense itching and the formation of pus. In addition to the genital area, scabies may appear under the breasts, in the armpits, between the fingers, and elsewhere.

Special medicated shampoo is used to treat pubic lice, and medicated lotion is used to treat scabies. However, pubic lice and scabies can be found in clothes and bed linen. Therefore, all clothing and bed linen must be washed in hot water and dried in a hot clothes dryer in order to eliminate these parasites.

Review

1. *What is a sexually transmitted disease?*
2. *Name four common sexually transmitted diseases.*
3. *Name two ways that chlamydia can be transmitted.*
4. *What are the signs and symptoms of genital herpes?*
5. ***Critical Thinking*** *Is it possible for someone to transmit an STD to another person without realizing it? Explain.*

ASSESS

Section Review

Have students answer the Section Review questions.

Alternative Assessment

The Spread of STDs

Ask students to summarize in a paragraph what the STDs discussed in this section have in common. Have them speculate about why these diseases are easily spread by sexual contact.

Closure

Remaining Questions

Ask students to list for themselves three questions they still have about STDs. Use the Question Box or initiate open discussion to encourage students to express these questions and get answers. Follow up on any questions to which you don't know the answer.

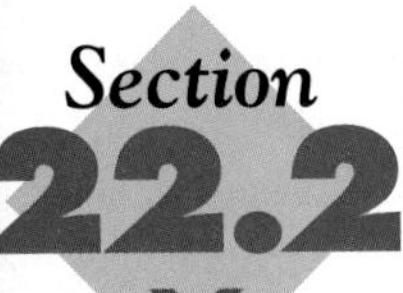

Section 22.2 Preventing Sexually Transmitted Diseases

Objectives

- *Know what you can do to decrease your chances of getting an STD.*
- *Name 10 ways you can show love for someone without sexual intimacy.*
  - **LIFE SKILLS: Communicating Effectively**
- *Know where to go for testing and treatment for STDs.*
  - **LIFE SKILLS: Using Community Resources**

Vanessa said that she thought these diseases must be pretty rare. After all, she had heard a lot of people talking about sex, but she had never known anyone personally who had gotten one of these diseases. But her mother pointed out that most people who get an STD are embarrassed about it. They aren't likely to go around telling everybody that they have one of these diseases.

Han said that she thought the people who got STDs were probably very promiscuous, with many sex partners. Vanessa's mom said that it's true that the more sex partners you have, the more likely you are to get one of these diseases. However, you can get an STD by having sexual contact just once, if your partner is infected.

Staying Healthy

STDs can be prevented by making responsible decisions. You can stay healthy by refusing to take part in behaviors that put you at risk for STDs.

Delaying Sexual Intimacy Many of these diseases are transmitted only by sexual contact or mainly by sexual contact. If you are not sexually active, you will probably never have to worry about getting gonorrhea, syphilis, or chlamydia.

Although it is theoretically possible to get genital herpes, trichomoniasis, pubic lice, or scabies in other ways besides sexual contact, it is very unlikely. You can reduce your risk of these diseases to practically zero if you avoid sexual contact and also practice good hygiene. That means not sharing towels, clothing, or bed linen with anyone else unless those items have been thoroughly washed. In addition, you must avoid direct contact with any open sores another person might have.

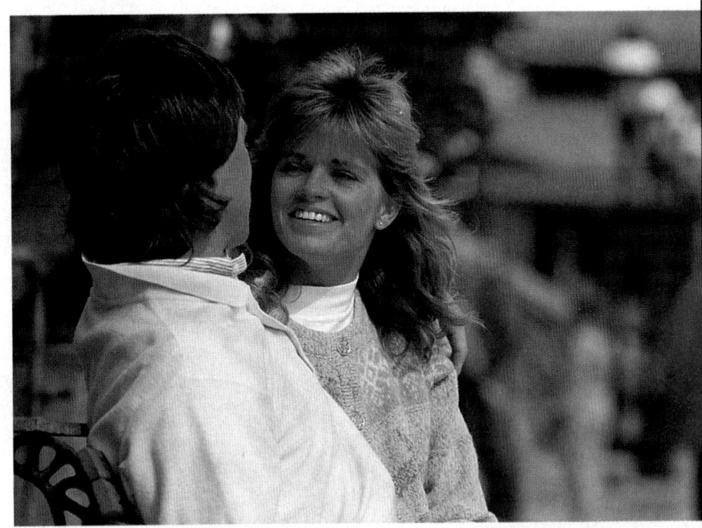

(FIGURE 22-10) **If two healthy, disease-free people marry and remain faithful to each other, they will not have to worry about most STDs.**

Background
The STD Epidemic

According to the Centers for Disease Control, the United States is in the grip of an STD epidemic that infects an average of 33,000 people a day. At this rate, one in four Americans between ages 15 and 55 eventually will acquire an STD. For those at the younger end of the scale, the risk of infertility and ectopic, or tubal, pregnancies is serious. This epidemic is having an effect on the behavior of young adults. Unfortunately, the message is taking longer to reach teenagers.

Background
It's OK to Talk About It

When a teenager is casual about having sex with someone, the chances are that the sex partner is equally casual. The odds of spreading STDs under these circumstances is enormous. Individuals should know that it's all right to ask a partner beforehand if he or she has ever had an STD or has ever had sex with someone who had an STD. Since a partner may not be completely honest on a first encounter, it's all the more reason not to have sex until much later in a relationship.

Section 22.2 Lesson Plan

MOTIVATE

Journal 22G
Prevention of STDs

This may be done as a warm-up activity. Ask students to write in the Student Journal ways to prevent sexually transmitted diseases.

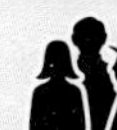

Cooperative Learning
Contracting STDs

Have the class work in small groups to prepare a bulletin board that will help teenagers understand the ways of contracting STDs and the steps they may take to avoid them.

TEACH

Class Discussion
The Spread of STDs

Discuss Vanessa's idea that STDs must be rare. You may want to remind students of Figure 22-7, which showed "The Spread of STDs." **Which of those diseases in the figure can be cured?** *[Gonorrhea, chlamydia, syphilis, and genital warts]* What do you think

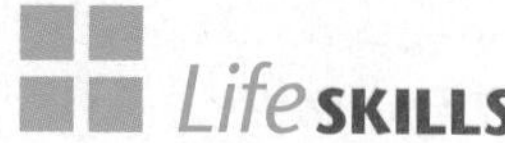

Life SKILLS

Showing Love Nonsexually

Ask students if they think the couple in the photograph love each other. Ask them how they can tell. Have them suggest other ways to show love nonsexually.

Making a Choice 22A

Public Health Campaign

Assign the Public Health Campaign card. The card asks students to design a campaign to publicize the causes and treatments of sexually transmitted diseases.

Making a Choice 22B

Designing a Game

Assign the Designing a Game card. The card requires students to design a game that teaches behaviors that prevent infection with a sexually transmitted disease.

As you already learned, delaying or abstaining from sexual intimacy is called sexual abstinence. If you decide to practice abstinence until you are older, that doesn't mean that you will not have sexual feelings for someone in the meantime. There are many safe ways to express sexual affection for someone. Talking, hugging, and holding hands, for example, are the safest possible expressions of feelings.

In spite of the messages you may be getting from advertising, movies, TV, or even your friends, the truth is that many teenagers are not sexually active. These teenagers choose to delay sexual intimacy because it makes them feel better about themselves. In addition to the peace of mind that comes from not having to worry about STDs, people are happier when they know they have set high standards for themselves and are living up to the values of their families and their communities.

Remember, if two healthy, disease-free people marry and remain faithful to each other, they will not have to worry about most STDs.

LifeSKILLS: Communicating Effectively

Showing Love Nonsexually

The teenage years are a time of strong sexual feelings. Even though you know that choosing abstinence is the best way to avoid STDs, you may want to show your affection for someone by becoming sexually intimate.

When you are in love and really care for someone, it's natural to want to show it. But sexual intercourse is not the only way to show affection. For example, one of the nicest things you can do for a person is to listen to what he or she has to say with genuine interest. This shows that you take the person seriously and that his or her thoughts and feelings are important to you.

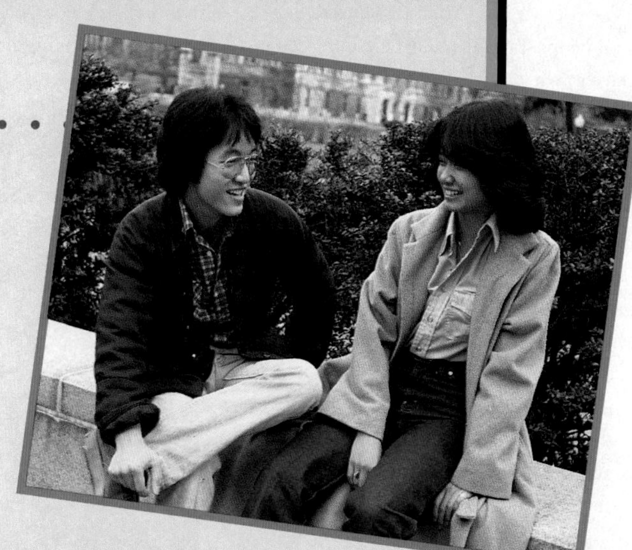

On a separate sheet of paper, write down at least 10 other ways besides sex that you can show you love your girlfriend or boyfriend.

• • • TEACH continued

of Han's conclusion that only promiscuous people contract STDs? Discuss the possibility of contracting an STD if you have just one sex partner.

Class Discussion
Sexual Abstinence

Discuss the zero risk of STDs if a person practices sexual abstinence. Ask students to name other advantages of sexual abstinence. Have them discuss whether they think it is possible to convince someone who thinks differently about sexual abstinence to change his or her ideas.

Role-Playing
Showing Love

Have students role-play these or other situations: A caring couple, both of whom have decided to abstain from sexual intercourse until later; they show their love in other ways. A caring couple, one of whom wants to show love nonsexually while the other wishes to show love sexually; they try to resolve their differences.

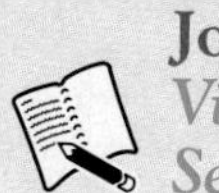

Journal 22H
Views on Sexual Abstinence

Have students write in the Student Journal what they think about sexual abstinence. Ask them to put in writing whether they think abstinence is possible for them. Ask them to think of who might help them make the right decisions about sexual activity.

Staying in Control Using alcohol and other drugs can be harmful to your health in more ways than their direct effects on your body. Drinking or doing drugs can also increase your risk of getting an STD. How? Drugs and alcohol interfere with your judgment and decision-making abilities. With drugs or alcohol clouding your thinking, it is much easier to convince yourself that it's okay ''just this once.''

Besides avoiding drugs and alcohol, it can also help to avoid situations where you might be pressured to participate in sexual activity. For example, group dating with friends who share your values can make it easier to avoid temptation. Also, getting involved in sports, after-school clubs, hobbies, or volunteer work can reduce your need to alleviate boredom or find satisfaction through sex.

Reducing the Risk of STDs Some sexual practices are not guaranteed completely safe, but they put you at much lower risk of getting an STD than unprotected sexual intercourse. For example, kissing with your mouth closed is safe unless the other person has a sore on his or her mouth. Open mouth kissing, or ''French kissing,'' carries a slight risk of passing some STDs, but it is still much less risky than sexual intercourse.

Using a latex **condom** during sexual intercourse greatly reduces the risk of getting an STD during sex. A condom is a covering for the penis that helps protect both partners from sexually transmitted diseases and also helps prevent pregnancy. Using a spermicide with a condom is even better, since the spermicide will kill some of the germs that cause STDs.

To be effective in preventing STDs, however, condoms must be used properly. The condom must be put on the penis before any physical contact, and it must be worn during the entire time of intercourse. The condom must be removed while the penis is still erect so that it doesn't slip off inside the vagina. Also, oil-based lubricants like petroleum jelly or cooking oils must never be used with a condom. These kinds of lubricants can damage the condom and cause it to break. Lubricants that are safe to use with a condom are those that have the words ''water-soluble'' on the label.

Breaking the Cycle of Infection Sexually transmitted diseases have become epidemic in the United States. One reason why so many people have them is that STDs are spread from one sex partner to another in a seemingly endless chain by people who don't know that they have a disease, who do not get proper treatment for the disease, or who don't inform their partners.

As Figure 22-11 shows, if an infected person has just two sexual partners and those people have just two partners, and so on, the disease can spread from one person to many people in a relatively short time.

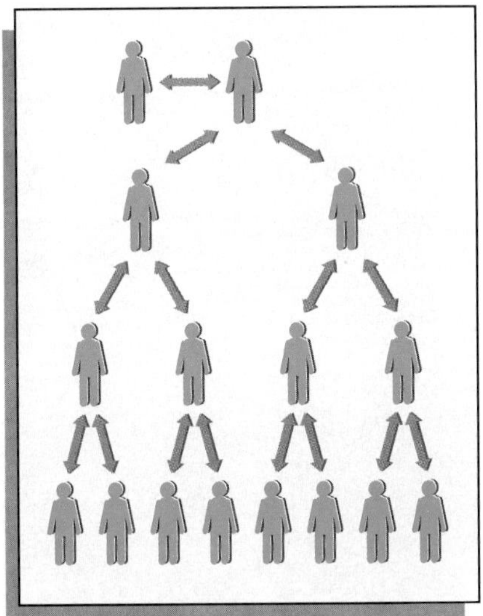

(FIGURE 22-11) **This diagram shows how rapidly an STD can spread if each infected person has two sex partners.**

condom:

a covering for the penis that helps protect both partners from sexually transmitted diseases and also helps to prevent pregnancy.

Section 22.2

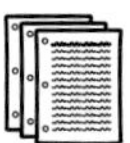

Section Review Worksheet 22.B

Assign Section Review Worksheet 22.2, which requires students to categorize practices that prevent the spread of sexually transmitted diseases.

Section Quiz 22.2

Have students take Section Quiz 22.2.

Reteaching Worksheet 22.2

Students who have difficulty with the material may complete Reteaching Worksheet 22.2, which requires students to rate various behaviors according to their effectiveness in preventing sexually transmitted diseases.

Class Discussion
Avoiding STDs

With student participation, build the following concept map on the chalkboard. Provide the title AVOIDING STDs and the two ways: Staying in Control and Reducing Risks. Ask students to state two ways to stay in control. Fill these in on the map. Ask for two ways to reduce the risks. Fill in: *Kissing* and *Using a condom.*

Ask students for one kind of kissing that is safer and one that is less safe. Fill these in. Ask for ways to use condoms that are safer and fill these in on the tree.

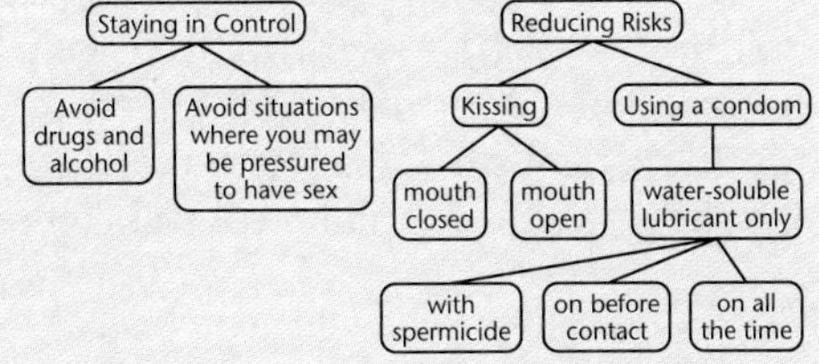

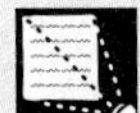

Teaching Transparency 22C
The Chain of Infection

Show the transparency that demonstrates the spread of STDs if one of the partners has two sex partners (Figure 22-11). Encourage students to express their views on how they would feel if they found out someone they had sex with was also having sex with another person. Ask them to discuss the responsibility of a person with an STD to himself or herself, to a sex partner, to all the others infected.

Background
The Law and STDs

If a case or reportable STD is made known to public officials, they will contact all recent sex partners of the infected person. When voluntary treatment is not obtained, police action may force the person to have a medical examination and to start treatment if necessary. Many states now have laws that authorize the treatment of minors for STDs without requiring parental consent.

If you think you might have an STD, it is very important that you break this chain of infection. If you do not act responsibly to stop the disease, there could be serious consequences to your own health. You could also be responsible for the infection of many other people.

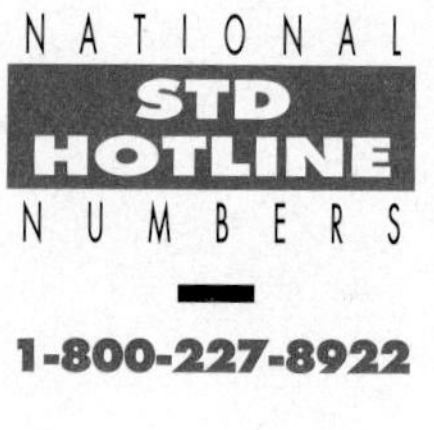

If You Think You Might Have an STD

If you have any reason to think you have been exposed to one of these diseases, you must find out for sure if you have it even if you do not have signs or symptoms. Only a doctor or a health professional at a clinic can diagnose STDs.

Where to Go for Help You have several choices about where to go for proper diagnosis and treatment. You can go to your family doctor or to another private doctor. Remember, doctors have a professional duty to keep information regarding their patients confidential.

If you don't have a private doctor, or if you cannot afford to pay for private treatment, there are public health clinics that offer free or low-cost treatment. These clinics are listed in the phone book. Depending on where you live, the clinic nearest you may be listed under "Sexually Transmitted Diseases Clinic," "Health Department," "Public Health Clinic," or "Rural Health Clinic."

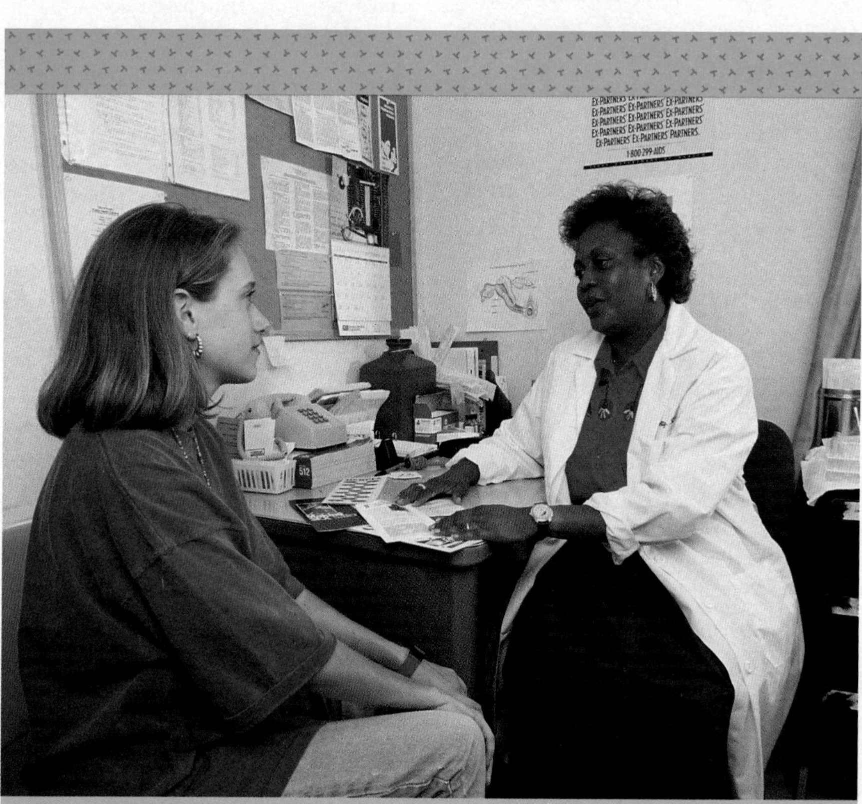

(FIGURE 22-12) **Public health clinics will keep your name, your diagnosis, your treatment, and any other information about you completely confidential.**

• • • TEACH continued

Reinforcement
Seeking Help

It is normal that someone may not want to admit that he or she has an STD. What is not right is to inflict the disease on someone else knowingly. Ask students what the consequences of not seeking help would be to themselves and to any sex partners.

Debate the Issue
Revealing Names

Tell students that a person who has been diagnosed as having an STD may be asked for the names of sex partners. Hold a class debate on whether this is an invasion of privacy. Tell them to consider this both as a matter of law and as a matter of moral responsibility.

Role-Playing
Coping With the Diagnosis

Ask students to role-play with a classmate a situation in which one player finds out he or she has an STD and the other player is the sex partner. Encourage role players to consider the correct line of action from the viewpoint of the person infected and also from the viewpoint of the person's sex partner.

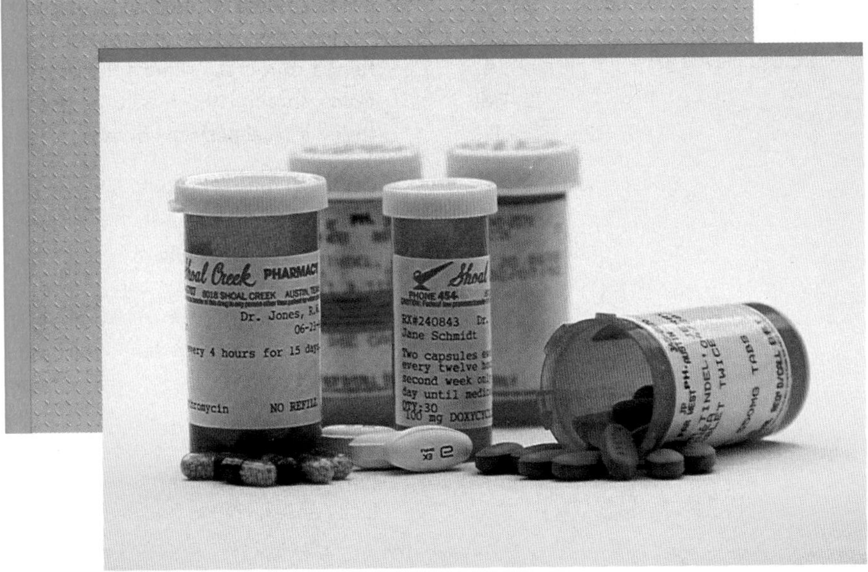

(FIGURE 22-13) **People with STDs should take all the medicine they are prescribed and follow the doctor's orders exactly.**

You can also call the National STD Hotline number shown at the left to find out where in your area you can go for STD testing and treatment. The people staffing the National STD Hotline can also answer any questions you have about STDs.

It is the law in every state that anyone can be treated for a communicable disease. You will not be required to get permission from your parents, and your parents will not be notified.

Don't worry about the health workers in the clinics being shocked or upset that you might have an STD. Remember, dealing with STDs is just part of their daily routine. Their goal is to stop the spread of these diseases. Public health workers are more likely to be upset by people who do not get treatment and who continue to spread the disease. Public health clinics will keep your name, your diagnosis, your treatment, and any information you give them completely confidential.

If you are diagnosed with certain STDs, workers at the clinic may ask for the names of your sex partners. They do this so that they can inform your partners of possible exposure to the disease. For many people, telling their partners is the hardest part of dealing with an STD. If a person with an STD wishes, a health clinic worker will contact the sex partners but not reveal the name of the person with the STD.

Treatment for STDs Different STDs require different treatments, so a visit to a health professional is necessary to receive the correct treatment.

Many people think they have to take their medicine only until they feel better. This is not true! Once a person feels better and is not so worried, it may take some effort to keep taking the medicine until it is gone. However, it is very important to do so. People with STDs should take all the medicine they are prescribed and follow the doctor's instructions exactly.

Journal 22I
Hotline Questions

Have students write in the Student Journal any questions they might want to ask on the National STD hot line.

Reinforcement
See a Doctor

Remind students that, since many of the symptoms of an STD do not show up immediately, it is important to see a doctor if they think they may have become infected with an STD. This would be especially advisable if they discovered that a sex partner had an STD or even if they found out that a sex partner was having sexual intercourse with someone else.

Class Discussion
STD Treatment

Why is it necessary that a patient take all the medicine prescribed in order to cure the STD? *[Many STDs are treated with antibiotics. Physicians prescribe a certain amount of antibiotics to be taken. A smaller amount may not kill all the harmful bacteria. It may kill only the weaker ones, leaving the stronger ones to develop a resistance to the antibiotic.]* Discuss why it is necessary for both partners to be treated at the same time for certain STDs.

Extension
STDs and Teens

Encourage students to do library research about the prevention of STDs among teenagers.

Review Answers

1. Answers will vary. Students may answer: avoid sexual intercourse; do not share towels, clothing, or bed linens; do not use alcohol or other drugs; try group dating; become involved in sports, clubs, hobbies, or volunteer work.
2. Answers will vary. Some answers may include hugging, holding hands, doing something nice for the person, listening to the person, respecting the opinions and feelings of the person, and talking.
3. Look up phone numbers in the telephone book under headings such as "Sexually Transmitted Diseases Clinic," "Health Department," "Public Health Clinic," or "Rural Health Clinic"; or call the National STD Hotline, 1-800-227-8922.
4. Antibiotics are only effective against bacterial infections. Antibiotics cannot cure viral infections, such as genital herpes.

Medicine must not be shared with anyone else. For one thing, it might be the wrong medicine to cure someone else's disease. And if two people are taking medicine prescribed for one person, there may not be enough medicine to completely cure both people.

Though they shouldn't share the same medicine, sex partners should be treated at the same time for certain STDs. A person with an STD should ask a health professional if his or her partner should also be treated. If both sex partners are not treated at the same time, they could continue to reinfect each other.

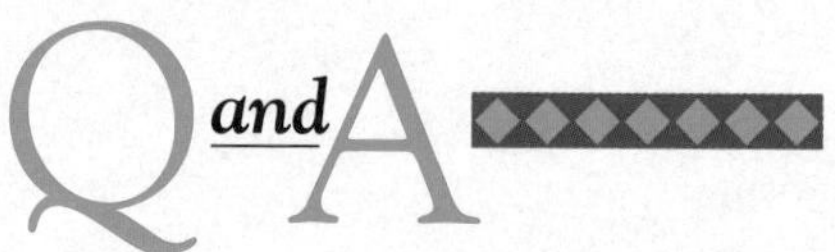

Q. A friend told me that the best way to avoid STDs is to take a shower right after having sex. He said that if you can't take a shower right away, you should at least wash off the best you can. Is this true?

A. No. Washing after sexual contact will not prevent STDs. If you have unprotected sexual contact with an infected partner, disease-causing microorganisms can cross mucous membranes and enter your body before you can wash them off.

Q. Is it true that taking birth-control pills can prevent STDs?

A. No, definitely not. Birth-control pills prevent pregnancy but do nothing to prevent STDs.

Q. My boyfriend told me that he has gonorrhea. I feel fine, though. I don't think I caught it. What's the point of going through the hassle of getting tested if I feel perfectly okay?

A. Not everyone who gets an STD has signs or symptoms of the disease. And almost everyone who finds out that he or she has or might have an STD is upset or embarrassed about it. These two things together make it very tempting for people to convince themselves that they can ignore the situation. They tell themselves that even though they were exposed, they were lucky enough not to be infected.

This is a very dangerous attitude. If you have any reason to think you may have been exposed to an STD, get tested immediately.

Review

1. *Name five actions you can take that will eliminate or reduce your risk of getting an STD.*
2. ***LIFE SKILLS: Communicating Effectively*** *Name 10 ways you can show love for someone without becoming sexually intimate.*
3. ***LIFE SKILLS: Using Community Resources*** *If a friend told you that he thought he might have an STD but didn't know where to go to find out for sure, how could you help him?*
4. ***Critical Thinking*** *Antibiotics are ineffective against the herpes simplex virus. Explain why this is true.*

ASSESS

Section Review

Have students answer the Section Review questions.

Alternative Assessment

Stopping the Spread

Have students explain in a paragraph how STDs are spread and how they can be contained.

Closure

Letter to a Friend

Have students write a letter to a friend who has told them that he or she has an STD but can't bring himself or herself to get treatment or to tell any sex partners of the infection. The letter should try to convince the friend why someone infected with an STD is obliged to receive treatment and to report his or her sex partners.

Chapter 22 Highlights

Summary

- The most dangerous STD (sexually transmitted disease) is AIDS. It cannot be cured and is eventually fatal.
- Some other serious STDs include gonorrhea, chlamydia, genital herpes, and syphilis.
- Gonorrhea is an infection caused by a bacterium. Many people with gonorrhea do not have symptoms but can pass the bacteria to their sex partners.
- Genital herpes is caused by a virus; there is no known cure. Fifty percent of newborns infected with herpes die, and half of the surviving babies will have severe brain or eye damage.
- Syphilis is caused by a bacterium and progresses in stages. It can be cured at any stage with the right antibiotic, but if it progresses to the final stage, the damage that has occurred cannot be reversed.
- Other common STDs include genital warts, hepatitis, and pubic lice.
- Using a spermicide with a condom greatly reduces the risk of getting an STD. Safe lubricants for a condom are "water-soluble" ones.
- Confidential diagnosis and treatment for STDs can be obtained from a private doctor or a public health clinic.
- Sexual partners should be treated at the same time for STDs, though they shouldn't share the same medicine.

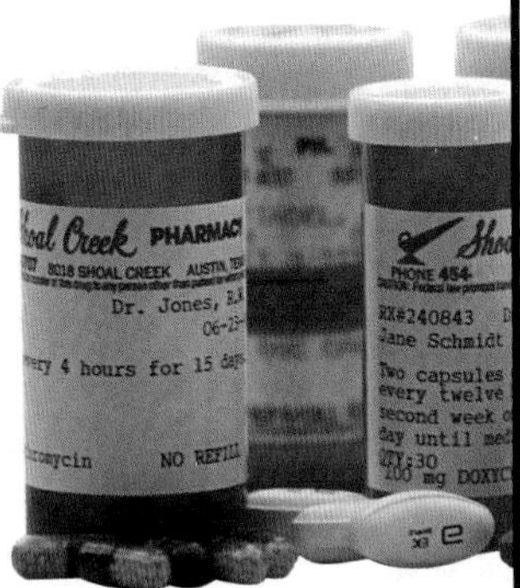

Vocabulary

sexually transmitted disease (STD) a disease that is passed from one person to another during sexual contact.

gonorrhea an STD transmitted by bacteria that can infect the mucous membranes of the penis, vagina, throat, or rectum.

pelvic inflammatory disease (PID) an infection of the uterus and Fallopian tubes often caused by STDs; if untreated, may result in infertility.

chlamydia the most common STD in the United States; caused by bacteria.

genital herpes an STD caused by a virus that often causes painful blisters or ulcers; cannot be cured.

syphilis an STD caused by bacteria that can spread through the bloodstream to any organ of the body.

genital warts an STD caused by viruses that cause warts to appear on the genital and anal areas.

Chapter 22 Highlights Strategies

Summary
Have students read the summary to reinforce the concepts they learned in Chapter 22.

Vocabulary
Have students write questions that use the vocabulary words. Have them work in pairs, asking questions of their partner and answering their partner's questions.

Extension
Have students write an article for a teen magazine discussing what they think every teenager should know about STDs. Tell them to keep the article upbeat but serious.

Chapter 22 Assessment

Chapter Review

Concept Review

1. b
2. d
3. a
4. d
5. d
6. c
7. d
8. b

Expressing Your Views

Sample responses:

1. Genital herpes can also be transmitted when there are not blisters, for example right before an outbreak of blisters. Therefore, condoms should be used all the time.

2. Sexual intercourse needs to take place only once with an infected person in order for the other partner to become infected. His partners need to be told so that they can seek treatment. Both partners need to be treated to prevent passing the disease back and forth and to other people.

3. People do not use protection, such as condoms, during sexual intercourse; people do not recognize symptoms and/or are reluctant to seek treatment; people do not inform their sexual partners that they have been exposed to an STD.

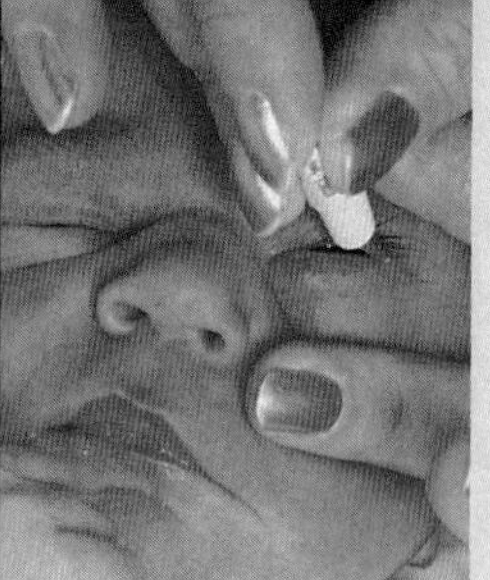

Chapter Review

Concept Review

1. An incurable STD is
a. gonorrhea.
b. herpes.
c. syphilis.
d. hepatitis.

2. An STD that can cause sterility and pelvic inflammatory disease is
a. syphilis.
b. genital warts.
c. vaginitis.
d. chlamydia.

3. How are some sexually transmitted diseases commonly spread?
a. from mother to fetus
b. by kissing
c. by using dirty toilet seats
d. all of these

4. An STD associated with cervical cancer is
a. vaginitis.
b. NGU.
c. scabies.
d. genital warts.

5. Hepatitis B can be spread by
a. sharing toothbrushes.
b. sexual contact.
c. sharing eating utensils.
d. all of these.

6. Special medicated shampoos or medicated lotions are used to treat
a. genital warts.
b. PID.
c. parasitic infections.
d. genital herpes.

7. Which of the following behaviors provides the best protection against STDs?
a. using a condom
b. using a condom with spermicide
c. postponing sexual intercourse
d. all of the above

8. To find out if you have an STD, you should
a. talk to a counselor.
b. visit a doctor or clinic.
c. talk to your sexual partner.
d. get an "over-the-counter" drug from the pharmacist.

Expressing Your Views

1. Your friend has confided to you that she has genital herpes. Her boyfriend does not use a condom during sexual intercourse. She says she will not infect her boyfriend as long as she doesn't have an outbreak of blisters. How would you respond to this statement?

2. You have a friend who has been diagnosed as having a sexually transmitted disease. He has received treatment but is too embarrassed to tell his sexual partners about his problem. He keeps telling himself that he didn't have sexual intercourse with them often enough for them to be infected. Why is it important for him to tell his partners?

3. Why do you think sexually transmitted diseases continue to spread?

Life Skills Check

Sample responses:

1. Carmen could do something nice for Ben and respect his opinions and feelings. Carmen and Ben could spend more time holding hands, hugging, and talking.

2. Visit your doctor or a clinic to have the sore properly diagnosed.

Projects

Have students plan and carry out the projects on STDs.

Personal Pledge

Have students read and sign the personal pledge for Chapter 22.

Life Skills Check

1. **Communicating Effectively**
Carmen has been dating Ben for almost a year. She likes him very much, but lately they have been arguing about the same old issue. He thinks she doesn't really care about him because she won't have sexual intercourse. She feels, for many reasons, that it would be better to wait. What could Carmen do nonsexually to convince Ben she cares about him?

2. **Communicating Effectively**
You have noticed a small, painless sore in your mouth. Ordinarily you would dismiss it as a cold sore. But you realize that lately you have been behaving in a way that would put you at risk for a sexually transmitted disease, and you wonder if that is what it could be. How could you find out for sure in a confidential manner?

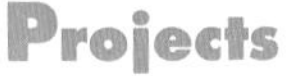

Projects

1. Use telephone books and library research to compile a list of telephone numbers and addresses of local agencies that could provide information, counseling, and testing for sexually transmitted diseases. Display the lists in the classroom and around the school.
2. Work with a group to create a bulletin board describing the STDs covered in this chapter. Include symptoms, dangers, and treatments of each disease.
3. Design a cartoon illustrating a way for people to cope with a risky situation or peer pressure.

Plan for Action

STDs are a major health concern because of their increase among teens and young adults. Make a plan to protect yourself and to help control the spread of these diseases.

Plan for Action

Have students work in pairs. Give students folded pieces of paper with the name of an STD they have been diagnosed as having, the name of their sex partner, something about their relationship, and the person to whom they are talking. Have each student work with a partner to act out a responsible way to discuss the situation. Students may add to the situations as they like. An example might include the following:

genital herpes
boyfriend of six months, Chris
doctor

Assessment Options

Chapter Test
Have students take the Chapter 22 Test.

Alternative Assessment
Have students do the Alternative Assessment activity for Chapter 22.

Test Generator
The Test Generator (Macintosh® or IBM® format) contains an additional 50 assessment items for this chapter.

HIV INFECTION AND AIDS

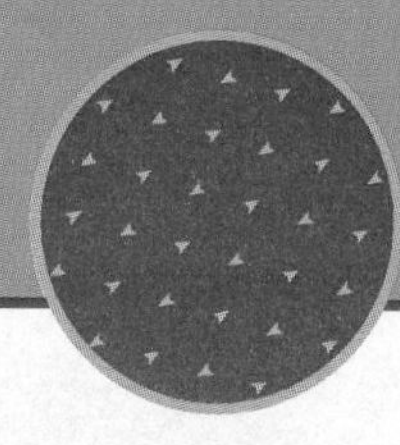

PLANNING GUIDE

TEXT SECTIONS	OBJECTIVES	TEXT FEATURES	OUTSIDE RESOURCES	NOTES
23.1 What Is HIV Infection? pp. 485-491 2 periods	• Define AIDS. • Describe how HIV works in the body. • Describe the three phases of HIV infection. ■ Find out where to get an HIV-antibody test.	• Check Up, p. 487 **ASSESSMENT** • Section Review, p. 491	**TEACHER'S RESOURCE BINDER** • Lesson Plan 23.1 • Personal Health Inventory • Journal Entries 23A, 23B • Life Skills 23A • Section Review Worksheet 23.1 • Section Quiz 23.1 • Reteaching Worksheet 23.1 **OTHER RESOURCES** • Transparencies 23A, 23B, 23C • Parent Discussion Guide • English/Spanish Audiocassette 6	
23.2 Transmission of HIV pp. 492-497 1 period	• Name the three body fluids that may contain enough HIV to infect another person. • List the four behaviors that put you at risk for HIV infection. • Name at least five behaviors that don't put you at risk for HIV infection. ■ Find out where you can get answers to any questions that are not covered in this chapter.	■ LIFE SKILLS: Using Community Resources, p. 495 **ASSESSMENT** • Section Review, p. 497	**TEACHER'S RESOURCE BINDER** • Lesson Plan 23.2 • Journal Entries 23C, 23D • Section Review Worksheet 23.2 • Section Quiz 23.2 • Reteaching Worksheet 23.2 **OTHER RESOURCES** • Transparency 23D	
23.3 How to Protect Yourself From HIV pp. 498-501 1 period	• Discuss abstinence as the most effective way to prevent the sexual transmission of HIV infection. ■ Practice resisting pressure to be sexually intimate. ■ Know how to reduce your risk of HIV infection if you are sexually active.	■ LIFE SKILLS: Resisting Pressure, p. 499 **ASSESSMENT** • Section Review, p. 501	**TEACHER'S RESOURCE BINDER** • Lesson Plan 23.3 • Journal Entry 23E • Life Skills 23B • Section Review Worksheet 23.3 • Section Quiz 23.3 • Reteaching Worksheet 23.3 **OTHER RESOURCES** • Making a Choice 23A, 23B	
23.4 HIV Infection and Society pp. 502-504 1 period	• Describe medical treatments available for HIV infection. • Name at least two actions you can take to help people with HIV infection.	**ASSESSMENT** • Section Review, p. 504	**TEACHER'S RESOURCE BINDER** • Lesson Plan 23.4 • Journal Entry 23F • Life Skills 23C • Ethics Worksheet • Section Review Worksheet 23.4 • Section Quiz 23.4 • Reteaching Worksheet 23.4	

■ Denotes LIFE SKILLS objectives

• Items in blue are also part of the *Holt Health Activity Book*.

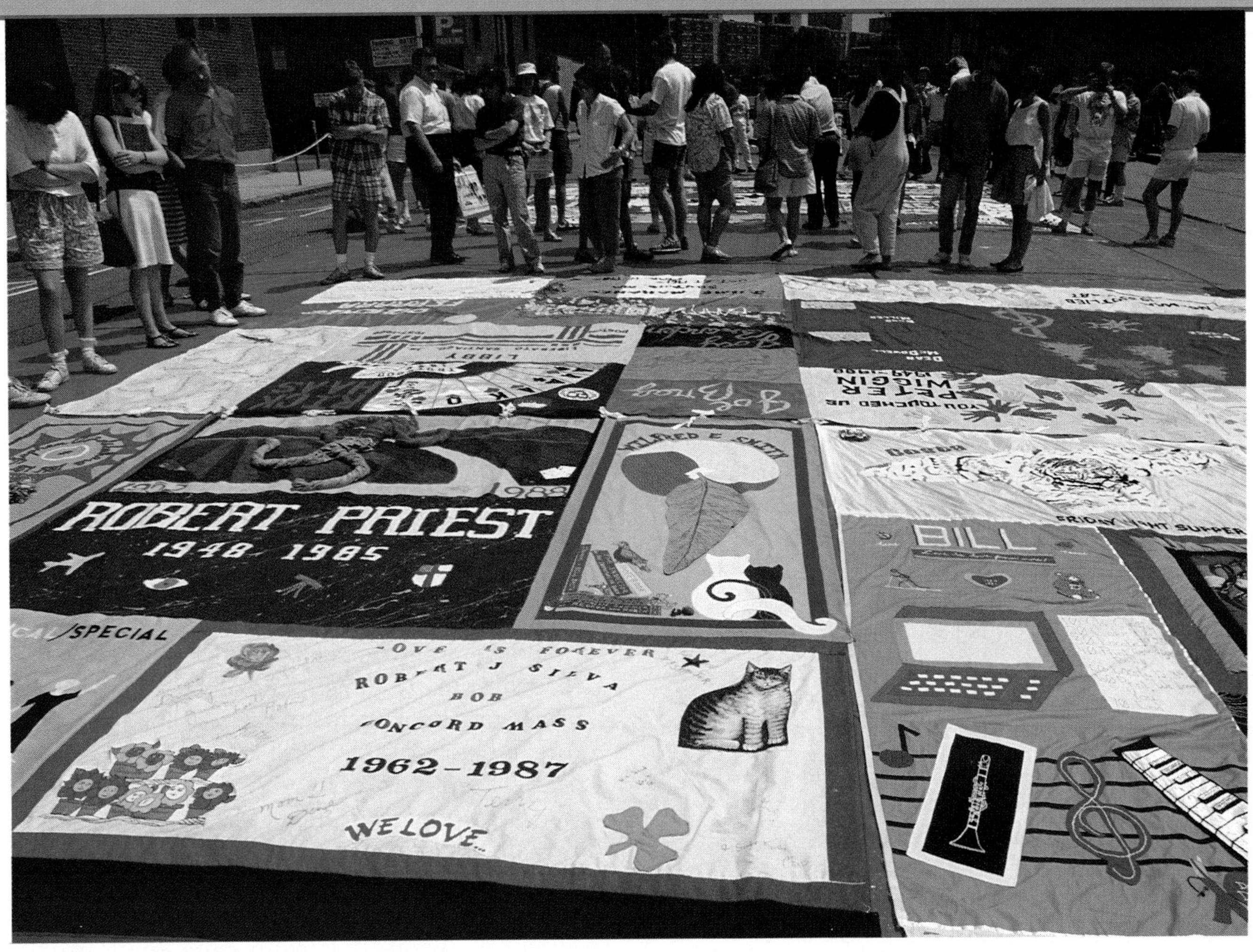

CONTENT BACKGROUND

AIDS and Teenagers

FOR ALL THE PUBLICITY THAT HIV INFECTION and AIDS receive, most people do not view AIDS as significant to their lives: it happens to other people. This view permeates our approach to educating adolescents about AIDS—especially our prevention education. But look at the facts: of the more than 206,000 cases of AIDS reported to the federal Centers for Disease Control and Prevention (CDC) by the end of 1991, 20 percent were people 20 to 29 years old. HIV infection can remain silent and symptomless for 10 years; this means that many of the 20- to 29-year-olds who have AIDS today became infected as teenagers. Between 1989 and 1991, there was a 70 percent increase in the number of AIDS cases in teens (from 401 to 789). Among people aged 15 to 24, AIDS is the sixth leading cause of death nationally.

We have no nationwide statistics on the rate of HIV infection among teens for several reasons: (1) unlike having AIDS, being HIV-positive is not a condition that must be reported to the CDC; (2) testing is not as readily available to teens as it is to adults; and (3) our cultural attitude that adolescents are at low risk makes teens think they don't need to be tested or makes them fearful of being tested. But we do have some clues about what is happening. One is a CDC study of students in selected colleges across the nation who had blood drawn for non-HIV-related medical reasons. A small sample of blood from each student was tested: 1 in 500 was HIV-positive. Another clue is a study done in New York state. Each baby born there since December 1987 has been tested for HIV antibodies. (The HIV-antibody test on a newborn gives the status of the mother, not of the baby.) Of 106,812 newborns of mothers ages ten to seventeen, 370 were HIV-positive.

Other facts tell us that we must acknowledge the adolescent risk for HIV infection:

- **Sexual maturation is occurring earlier than it did a generation ago.**
- **By age twenty, 68 percent of all females and 86 percent of all males are sexually active.**
- **By their senior year, 25 percent of high school students have had at least four sexual partners; of these, 6.2 percent of the males and 2.6 percent of the females have used intravenous drugs.**
- **Fewer than 50 percent of teens report having used a condom the last time they had sex.**
- **One in four sexually active adolescents contracts a sexually transmitted disease each year.**
- **More than one million adolescent pregnancies occur each year; at least 50 percent of these are thought to begin when one or both partners are high from alcohol or drugs.**

Clearly, adolescents—and large numbers of them—are engaging in behaviors that put them at risk for HIV infection.

Abstinence from sex is the best way to avoid HIV infection, sexually transmitted diseases, and unintended pregnancy. Avoiding drugs, including alcohol, reduces the likelihood of making bad decisions that lead to infection, pregnancy, automobile accidents, and accidents of other kinds. Many adults feel that promoting abstinence is the *only* acceptable message. But the facts show that many adolescents choose not to heed this advice, at least initially. That does not mean that the messages cannot be heard. Early sexual experiences are often hurried, awkward, and unsatisfactory. They may be cries for affection, expressing "a need to be needed." For young women especially, sex may even be painful, but they may engage in it to keep a boyfriend, or continue because "it is expected." By acknowledging that adolescents are making choices about sex, by teaching them about prevention using condoms and responsible decision making, and by helping them improve their self-esteem, we can create a trust that allows us to discuss options. We can then tell teens that just because they have had sex does not mean that they have to have it again; that if they had sex with a previous partner, they do not "owe it" to a new partner. We can teach adolescents—male or female—that it is all right to say no to sex until they feel ready. We can teach them that there are many ways to express one's sexuality without intercourse.

When discussing sex with teens, it is necessary to be clear and explicit. Adults typically interpret the phrase "having sex" as meaning sexual, usually vaginal, intercourse. As anyone who has talked with many adolescents on an AIDS hotline can tell you, adolescents may not think this way. Some adolescents think that kissing or other nonrisky behaviors can lead to STDs, HIV infection, and even pregnancy. Others equate having sex only with vaginal intercourse, and they may practice oral or anal sex as a "safe" alternative.

Another difficult topic that may arise is same-gender sex. Many adolescents experiment sexually with members of the same sex. Some students are in fact homosexual, but they must live in a society that is predominately heterosexual. Sometimes this leads to sexual confusion. If you are successful in creating a trusting environment for discussion of HIV and AIDS, students experiencing confusion may seek advice. Steering them toward caring, nonjudgmental counseling could save their lives. Many homosexual adolescents, and those who think they may be homosexual, attempt suicide or become addicted to drugs to deal with their pain and confusion.

Because of our unwillingness to do large-scale surveys of adolescent sexuality, we have only limited data on what adolescents actually do. But the statistics cited above clearly indicate that many teens are placing themselves at risk for HIV infection. Their survival may well depend on their receiving complete, accurate information and support in making healthful decisions.

PLANNING FOR INSTRUCTION

KEY FACTS

- **HIV attacks and weakens the body's immune system, causing AIDS.**
- **There is no cure for, or vaccine against, AIDS.**
- **The transmission of HIV can be prevented.**
- **The riskiest behaviors include sexual intercourse and the sharing of equipment to pierce ears, tattoo, or inject drugs.**
- **Abstinence or a monogamous relationship with someone who is not infected are the only sure methods of avoiding sexual transmission of the virus.**
- **Using condoms and spermicides makes sexual intercourse less dangerous.**

MYTHS AND MISCONCEPTIONS

MYTH: It is possible to get AIDS from casual contact.

Behaviors such as touching, breathing the same air, sharing utensils, and so on, do not transmit HIV. There hasn't been a single documented case of anyone getting HIV from casual contact with an HIV-positive person.

MYTH: People with HIV look very sick.

People in the final stages of AIDS look wasted and very weak. For a period that may last years, however, a person who has tested positive for HIV may show no symptoms at all.

MYTH: It is dangerous to donate blood.

It was never unsafe to give blood. Sterile, new needles are used to draw blood. Furthermore, since 1985 all donated blood has been tested, so it is extremely unlikely that a blood transfusion will cause infection.

MYTH: If you use a condom, you won't get AIDS.

Condoms can leak, break, or come off during sex. And to be effective against HIV transmission, a condom must be made of latex, must be used with a water-based, spermicidal lubricant, must be used from beginning to end of every sexual encounter, and must be replaced by a new one each time.

VOCABULARY

Essential: The following vocabulary terms appear in boldface type:

AIDS	**HIV-positive**
HIV	**mucous membranes**
HIV-antibody test	**monogamy**

Secondary: Be aware that the following terms may come up during class discussion:

homosexual	hemophiliac
heterosexual	spermicide
antibody	chronic condition

FOR STUDENTS WITH SPECIAL NEEDS

LEP Students: Have students read the book *AIDS: You Can't Get It by Holding Hands* (Lapis, 1987), by Niki de Saint Phalle, and share their findings with the class.

Visual Learners: Collect images that reinforce key points of the chapter. Display them on a bulletin board or on posters. Images might include young people enjoying each other's company in a nonsexual way, the action of a virus in a cell, people who are ill with AIDS, and young people with tattoos or pierced ears. Have students make collages showing positive ways of expressing affection nonsexually.

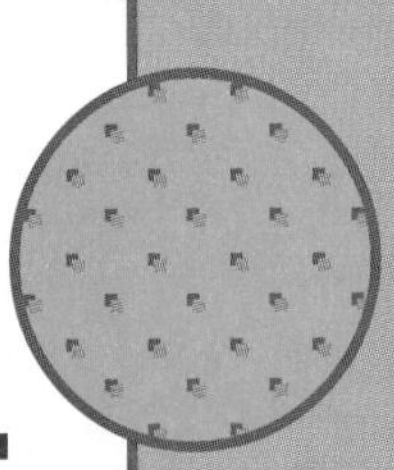

ENRICHMENT

- Create an AIDS Update newsletter. Assign students investigative stories, features, cartoons, and editorials. Students can interview teachers, administrators, parents, or classmates about common myths and misconceptions surrounding AIDS and HIV. Library research and telephone interviews are good ways to get information. Then ask them to type up their articles and publish the paper within the school.
- Arrange for someone from an agency that helps people with AIDS and HIV to speak to the class. Ask the person to tell stories about the people the agency serves and to describe ways in which students can help.

CHAPTER 23
CHAPTER OPENER

GETTING STARTED

Using the Chapter Photograph

Ask students how the person in the picture is taking action against AIDS. Discuss how this action might increase public awareness of the disease and why increased awareness is important.

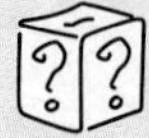

Question Box

Have students anonymously write out any questions they have about HIV and AIDS and put them in the Question Box. To ensure that students with questions are not embarrassed to be seen writing, have students who do not have questions write a fact they already know about HIV on the paper instead.

Preview the questions and then answer them at appropriate points in the chapter. You may wish to allow students to write additional questions as they go through the chapter.

Personal Issues *ALERT*

The discussion of AIDS may make students uncomfortable. To explain the spread of the disease, it is necessary to discuss sexual activities explicitly, including some practices students may know little about. In addition, a student may know someone who has the disease, or may be HIV-positive himself or herself. Students who have had homosexual feelings or experiences are particularly vulnerable; they may have already faced angry or violent responses to homosexuality. This chapter presents an opportunity to clear up the myth that homosexuals are responsible for the AIDS epidemic. Prepare the class to be respectful of privacy, tolerant of differences, and receptive to new information.

CHAPTER 23

HIV Infection and AIDS

◆ ◆ ◆ ◆

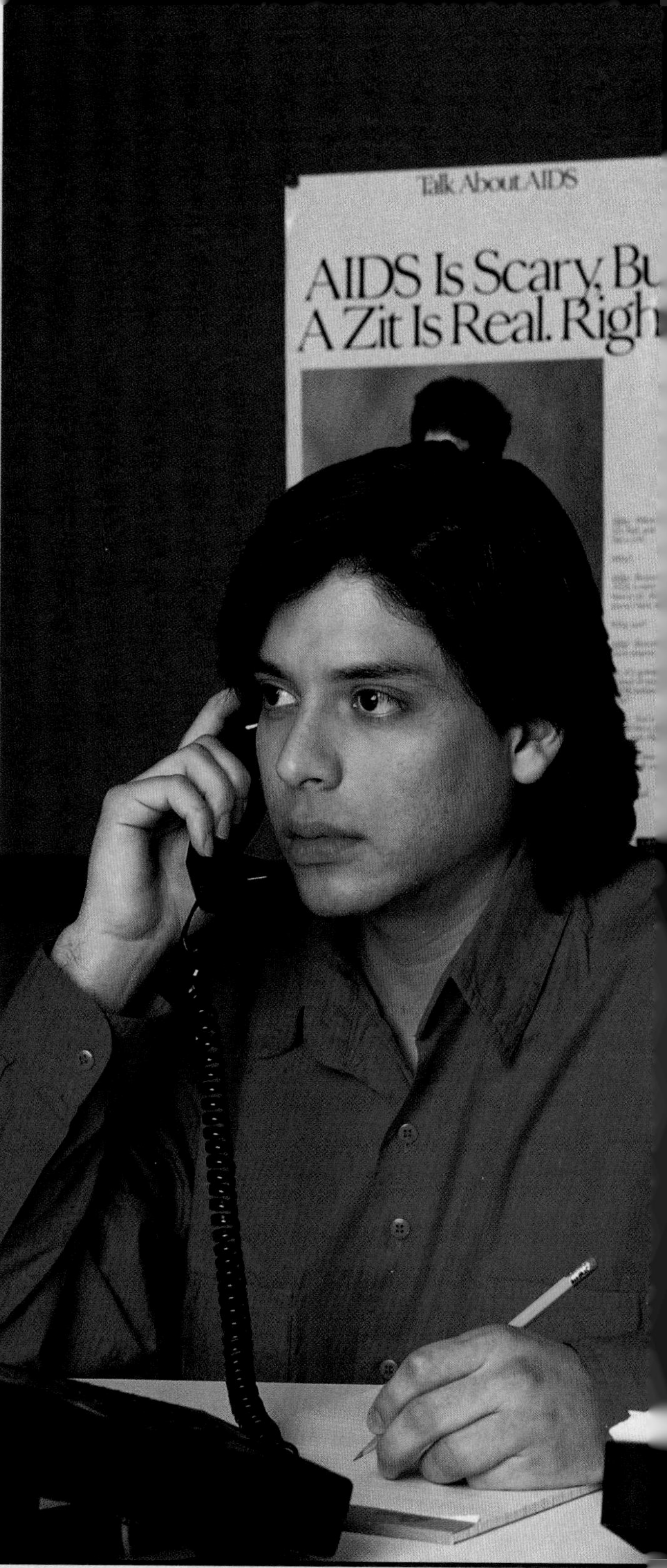

A young man takes positive action against AIDS by staffing an AIDS information hotline.

Michael and Bryan met when they both got jobs at a fast-food hamburger restaurant. After a few months, they were pretty good friends. Michael felt that he could tell Bryan just about anything. But he got the feeling that Bryan wasn't as open with him; Bryan got quiet and sad-looking sometimes, and he refused to tell Michael what was wrong.

Finally Michael lost his patience and told Bryan that he'd better tell him what was bothering him. Bryan said he'd think about it, which made Michael really nervous about what the problem could be. A couple of days later, Bryan told Michael that he had tested positive for the AIDS virus. Michael felt like he had just been punched in the stomach. He had no idea what to say. "Does that mean you have AIDS?" he blurted out, and then wanted to kick himself for asking that question. But Bryan didn't seem surprised. He told Michael that so far he hadn't gotten any of the illnesses that people with AIDS get. Then Bryan said that he trusted Michael not to tell the other people at work, because he could lose his job if they found out.

Michael was in a daze the rest of the day. Was his friend going to die? How could he help him? Was there any possibility that Bryan had infected him with the AIDS virus? Michael decided to call the AIDS hotline number to get some answers.

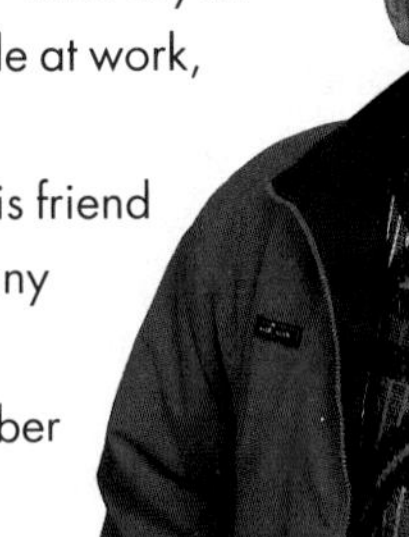

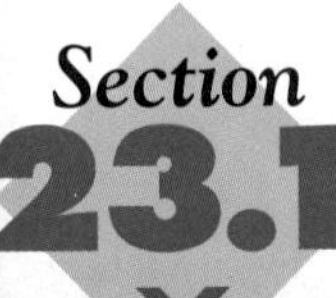

Section 23.1 What Is HIV Infection?

Objectives

- *Define AIDS.*
- *Describe how HIV works in the body.*
- *Describe the three phases of HIV infection.*
- *Find out where to get an HIV-antibody test.*

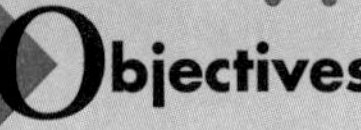

LIFE SKILLS: Using Community Resources

The person who answered the hotline number helped Michael cope with the news of his friend's situation and sent him a packet of information about HIV infection. In this chapter, you'll learn what Michael learned as he read the information he received.

The most important thing to know about HIV infection is that it is preventable. You can keep from getting it by learning about how it is spread and then avoiding behaviors that might allow you to be infected. In other words, you can choose responsible behaviors to protect yourself. And you can relax about behaviors that don't put you at risk.

Background

Origins of AIDS

Some scientists believe that AIDS originally developed in central Africa, where certain monkeys are known to carry a similar virus that is harmless to them. Humans may have become infected with the virus through monkey bites or by eating monkey meat. After being introduced to humans, the virus may have changed into the deadly AIDS virus.

Background

History

Scientists think AIDS may have existed as early as 1959. A sample of stored blood taken from an African in 1959 was tested in the 1980s and shown to be HIV-positive.

Section 23.1 Lesson Plan

MOTIVATE

Journal 23A
Concerns About AIDS

This may be done as a warm-up activity. Encourage students to record the concerns about AIDS in their Student Journal in the Student Activity Book. They could also write down their feelings about the above story of Michael and Bryan.

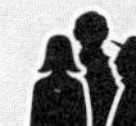

Cooperative Learning
Michael's Response

Have students form small groups to discuss Michael's reaction to the news that his friend has AIDS. How would they have reacted?

TEACH

Class Discussion
AIDS Can Be Prevented

Write on the chalkboard "AIDS is a preventable disease." **What does this mean?** *[Actions people take can affect whether they get the disease.]* **What are some other diseases that are influenced by a person's actions?** *[In some cases, lung cancer, heart disease, diabetes]* **What are some diseases that a person cannot prevent?** *[Hereditary diseases, including hemophilia, sickle cell anemia, and muscular dystrophy]* **If a person gets a disease that could have been prevented, is that person responsible? Why or why not?** *[It would depend on how well informed the*

Background
On the Virus

A virus is like a living organism in that it contains hereditary material. But, unlike a living organism, it is not a cell and cannot, in the usual sense, reproduce itself. In order to reproduce, it must enter a living host cell. When HIV enters the T4 cells, it gives instructions to have itself reproduced; this process results in the destruction of the host cell. The AIDS virus does not survive long outside the human body, but it moves easily in blood.

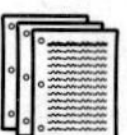

Personal Health Inventory

Have students complete the Personal Health Inventory for this chapter. The inventory helps students assess whether they are at risk for HIV infection.

AIDS: *a disease, caused by a virus, that cripples a person's immune system; AIDS is classified as a sexually transmitted disease, but it can also be spread in other ways, such as through sharing infected equipment for injecting drugs, tattoing, or ear piercing. AIDS is the last phase of HIV infection.*

REMINDER

A virus is a microscopic agent that can cause disease.

HIV: *(human immunodeficiency virus) the virus that causes AIDS; also called the "AIDS virus."*

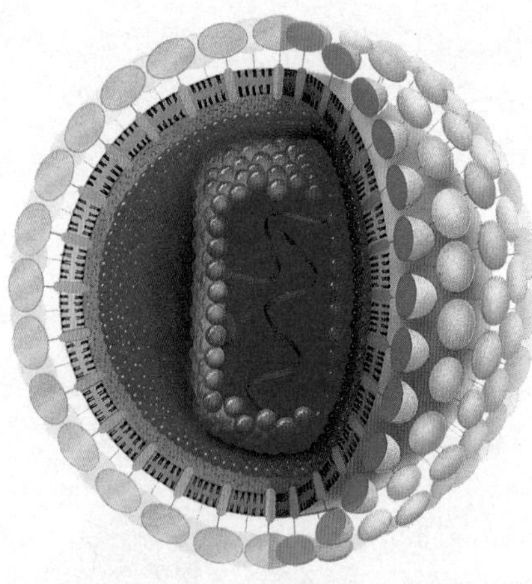

(FIGURE 23-1) **The virus that causes AIDS is called HIV (human immunodeficiency virus).**

AIDS, the last phase of HIV infection, is considered to be a sexually transmitted disease because it is most often spread through sexual contact. The name **AIDS** stands for Acquired Immune Deficiency Syndrome. When you break the name of the disease down into its parts, the name makes sense.

Acquired means that a person gets AIDS during his or her lifetime, rather than inheriting it from parents (although a pregnant woman with HIV infection can pass the virus on to her baby).

Immune Deficiency means that the body's immune system, the system that defends the body against infection and disease, is no longer able to do its job. In other words, the immune system becomes deficient.

Syndrome refers to the many diseases and conditions that result from having AIDS.

AIDS is caused by a kind of virus called **HIV** (human immunodeficiency virus). HIV is often referred to as the "AIDS virus." You can see a diagram of one of these viruses in Figure 23-1.

HIV actually attacks the body's immune system, making it difficult for the immune system to defend the body against infection. What this means is that infections that normally wouldn't be very dangerous can kill a person with AIDS.

As this book is being written, there is no cure for HIV infection. Once the virus is in a person's body, there is no way to get it out. Neither is there any kind of vaccination that can keep you from getting infected with HIV. That's why it's important to read this chapter carefully and take precautions to protect yourself from HIV infection.

The Spread of HIV Infection

The first cases of AIDS were diagnosed in the United States in 1981. Since that time, the number of people with AIDS has grown tremendously, as you can see in Figure 23-2. At the end of 1981, there were 379 cases of AIDS in the United States. Ten years later, the number had increased to more than 200,000.

These numbers don't even include people who are infected with HIV but haven't yet become ill. That number is estimated to be around one million in the United States alone.

The World Health Organization estimates that by the year 2000 there will be six million people in the world sick with AIDS and 30 million infected with HIV.

Many of the people who first had AIDS were homosexual men. As a result, some people thought that only homosexuals could get AIDS. That is now known to be a myth. Anyone who does certain things can get HIV, whether that person is homosexual or heterosexual. Heterosexual contact is becoming an increasingly common method

• • • TEACH continued

person was about the risks and whether he or she had an opportunity to prevent the disease.]

Class Discussion
AIDS on the Increase

Have students look at Figure 23-2 and speculate about how many more people in this country will have AIDS by the year 2001. Will the incidence of the disease increase sharply? Will it fall? Have students support their conclusions with data from the graph.

Demonstration
Statistics in the Classroom

Have students stand up where they are in the classroom. Hand each an index card with an HIV status on it. There should be two AIDS cards, ten HIV-positive cards, and the rest negative. Have students with AIDS cards stand at the front of the class. Have those with HIV-positive cards walk toward the front of the class, one long step for each year you call out: first year, second year, and so on. After ten years, those with HIV-positive cards should be at the front of the room. **Is this a fair representation of the epidemic's progress?** *[It is in the sense that all HIV-positive people eventually develop the disease, and there are about five times as many people infected with the virus as have the disease.]* **What would have to be added to make it more accurate?** *[More people would have to become HIV-positive and begin the "trip" toward AIDS over the ten years.]*

of transmission. In fact, in some parts of the world, heterosexuals make up the largest group of people with AIDS.

Something that is particularly disturbing about the spread of HIV is the large number of people in their twenties who have it. It often takes years from the time of infection until a person actually gets sick.

What this means is that many people were in their teens when they were originally infected with HIV. Among people 15 to 24 years of age, AIDS is now the sixth leading cause of death.

How HIV Works

In Section 23.2, you'll learn exactly which behaviors put you at risk of getting infected with HIV. Now you are going to learn how the virus works. If you know the way in which HIV works in the body, you'll understand why certain behaviors increase your chances of being infected with the virus.

Check Up

How Much Do You Already Know About HIV Infection?

1. Can you get HIV by drinking from a glass that someone with HIV has just used?
2. Can you get HIV by holding hands with a person with HIV?
3. Can you get HIV by having sexual intercourse with a person with HIV?
4. If a restaurant cook with HIV sneezes on your food, could you get HIV?
5. Can a woman with HIV infect her baby during delivery?
6. Can you get HIV by donating blood?
7. Can you tell by looking at someone whether he or she has been infected with HIV?
8. Is there a blood test that shows whether a person has been infected with HIV?

(The correct answers are shown below.)

1. no 2. no 3. yes 4. no 5. yes 6. no 7. no 8. yes

Check Up

Have students anonymously turn in their answers to the Check Up questions. Tally the results on the chalkboard. Identify the number of correct responses to each question. Discuss the correct answers to questions often missed. You might want to have students retake the Check Up at the end of the chapter and compare the class results obtained earlier.

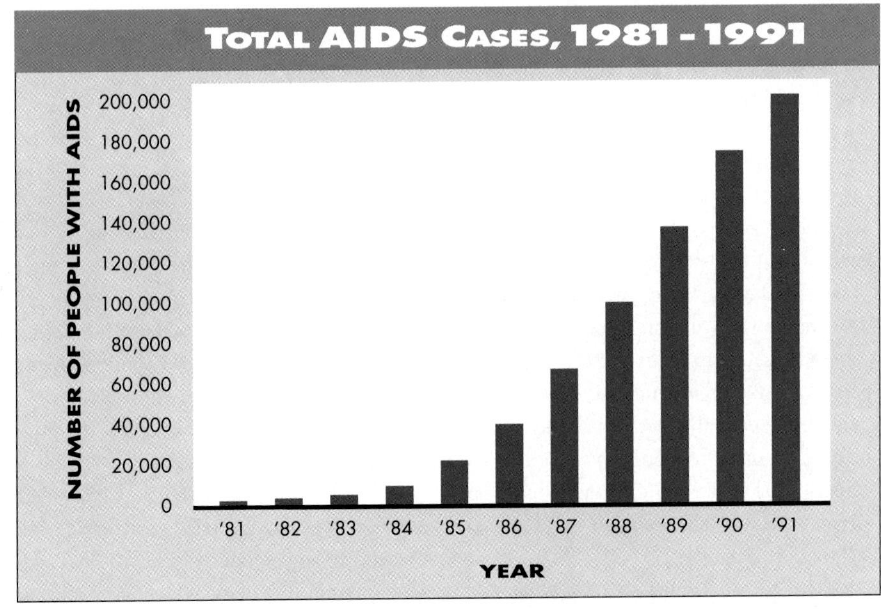

(FIGURE 23-2) **The total number of people diagnosed with AIDS has grown tremendously since 1981.** (Source: U.S. Centers for Disease Control, Atlanta, Georgia.)

Reinforcement
About the Epidemic

Tell students that the AIDS epidemic in the United States first took hold in the homosexual community. This led to early speculation that the disease might be related to homosexuality and would be confined to that group. That turned out not to be the case. The disease began among heterosexuals in other countries and is spreading among them in the United States as well. At the same time, it has slowed down among homosexuals, who not only have lobbied for funds to support research and care but also have become highly organized to prevent the spread of AIDS and attend to those who already have the disease.

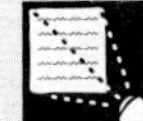

Teaching Transparency 23A
HIV

Show the illustration of the human immunodeficiency virus (Figure 23-1). Ask students to describe the process by which HIV enters and eventually destroys blood cells.

Journal 23B
"AIDS Among Youth"

Have students write the thoughts that occur to them while looking at Figure 23-3. What do the figures mean to them? Are the numbers reassuring or alarming? What would they answer to a friend who argues, "A few thousand cases is nothing. There's hardly any chance you'll come into contact with someone who has AIDS if you're not in the main risk groups."

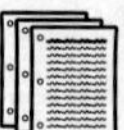

Life Skills Worksheet 23A

Local Antibody Testing

Assign Life Skills Worksheet 23A, which asks students to find out about local antibody testing.

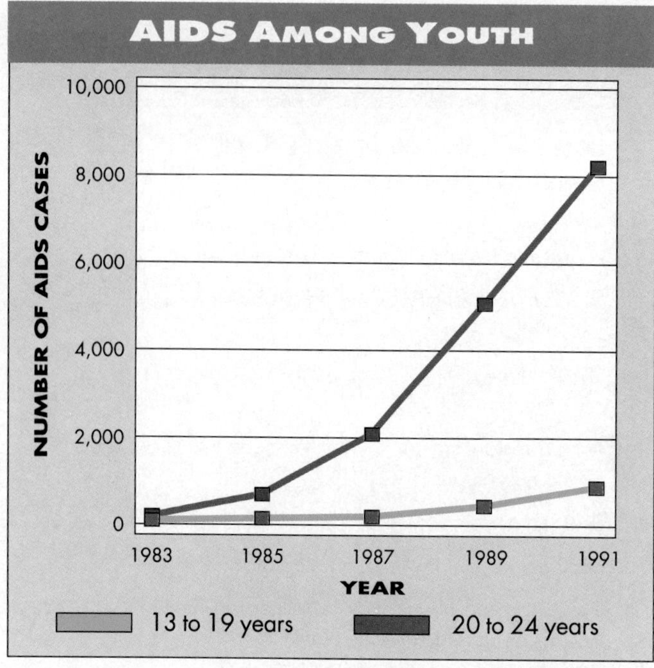

(FIGURE 23-3) **The graph shows the alarming increase in the number of teens and young adults with AIDS.**

First, HIV must get into a person's bloodstream. The virus can get into the bloodstream directly, when an infected person's blood goes directly into another person's blood (by sharing needles or syringes while using drugs, for example). Or the virus can first enter the body another way (when a person has sexual intercourse with an infected person, for example) and then get into the bloodstream.

In the body, HIV targets a special kind of blood cell—white blood cells called T4 cells. T4 cells are an extremely important part of a person's immune system, because they are the cells that coordinate the body's defense against infection. The attack on T4 cells is what makes HIV so dangerous—it targets the cells that are most important in fighting off infection.

HIV-antibody test:

a test used to determine whether a person has been infected with HIV.

The viruses enter the T4 cells and slowly begin destroying them. They force the T4 cells to start making thousands of copies of HIV. The T4 cells become tiny factories, making nothing but HIV, and the cells die in the process.

The newly made viruses then go on to target and attack other T4 cells. As more and more cells are destroyed, the person's immune system gets weaker and weaker. Without a working immune system, a person's body is defenseless against other viruses, bacteria, fungi, and cancer cells. These other infections and cancers are what kill a person with AIDS, not HIV itself.

There are two main points to remember about how HIV works. First, the virus has to get into a person's bloodstream before it can cause trouble. What this means to you is that you have to avoid doing things that might let HIV into your bloodstream.

Second, HIV can be in a person's body for years before it causes illness. The destruction of T4 cells may take place slowly; sometimes more than 10 years pass before an infected person shows any outward signs of disease. That means you can't tell by looking at people whether they have been infected with HIV. But people infected with HIV can pass the virus along to others, even if they don't look or feel sick.

HIV-Antibody Tests

A person can find out if he or she is infected with HIV by going to a health clinic, hospital, or doctor's office and asking for an **HIV-antibody test.** The HIV-antibody test checks a person's blood for antibodies to HIV. Antibodies are substances the body makes to fight infectious agents.

The test is usually free at public health clinics but may be fairly expensive elsewhere. Many clinics offer what is called "anonymous" testing, which means that no

• • • TEACH continued

Reinforcement

How HIV Strikes

Reassure students that the AIDS virus cannot affect a person unless it enters his or her body. It must reach the bloodstream to have an effect. Stress the fact that symptoms of HIV infection do not show up immediately. A person who appears healthy may be infected with HIV and can pass the disease to others.

Reinforcement

Myths and Consequences

After students read the myths and facts in Figure 23-4, ask if they can think of any additional myths or misconceptions. For each myth, ask students to explain what the consequences would be of believing it. Do they believe that misconceptions about HIV and AIDS are contributing to the spread of infection?

Role-Playing

HIV With No Symptoms?

Have students role-play a situation in which one member of a couple is trying to convince the other that he or she is not infected with HIV because he or she has no symptoms. The other person should use facts about the virus to counteract the arguments. In a variation, the first person says he or she has had an antibody test and the other asks questions to determine whether the results would be reliable.

one at the clinic knows your name. (You don't give your name at the clinic. Instead, you are assigned a number.) You can call your community AIDS hotline number or the national AIDS hotline number shown on **page 497** to get the location of the nearest anonymous testing clinic. The call is free, and you don't have to give your name.

Myths and Facts About HIV Infection

Myth	Fact
HIV and AIDS are the same thing.	*HIV (human immunodeficiency virus) is the name of the virus that causes AIDS. AIDS is the last phase of HIV infection.*
People who are infected with HIV look very sick.	*Although people with advanced AIDS may look very sick, many people with HIV look perfectly healthy. You can't tell by looking at people whether they have the virus. Even HIV-positive people who look healthy can infect others.*
A person who is young and healthy cannot be infected with HIV.	*Anyone who takes part in risky behavior can be infected with HIV. Unfortunately, many teenagers see themselves as "immune" to misfortunes such as HIV infection.*
Birth-control pills can prevent the transmission of HIV.	*Birth-control pills have no effect whatsoever on the spread of HIV.*
A person who uses a new latex condom each time he or she has intercourse runs no risk of getting HIV.	*Although latex condoms provide good protection, they are not 100% effective in preventing HIV transmission. Condoms sometimes tear or are used incorrectly.*
Sharing needles to inject medicines such as insulin or antibiotics is not risky for HIV transmission.	*Sharing needles for any purpose is risky, even if the injected drugs are legal.*
It is possible to get HIV by donating your blood.	*Donating your blood does not put you at risk for HIV. Blood donation centers use a new, sterile needle with each donor.*
If a mosquito bit someone with HIV and then bit you, you could get HIV.	*There have been no cases of HIV transmission by an insect or any other animal. If mosquitoes could transmit HIV, there would already be many reported cases of that happening by now.*
It is possible to get HIV by eating food that a person with HIV has handled.	*There have been no cases of HIV transmission through food or beverages.*

(FIGURE 23-4)

Class Discussion
Anonymous Testing

Ask students for possible reasons why many clinics offer anonymous testing for HIV. List the reasons on the chalkboard. Then lead a discussion about the need for anonymous testing. Who should have access to the results of an HIV-antibody test?

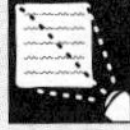

Teaching Transparency 23B
"AIDS Among Youth"

Have students study the graph "AIDS Among Youth" (Figure 23-3). Ask a volunteer to interpret the information it gives. To help the student out, you might ask: **What is the pattern for teenagers from 1983 to 1991? How does the pattern for young adults differ? What might account for the difference? Are teenagers therefore less at risk than young adults?** *[Many of the AIDS sufferers between 20 and 24 became HIV-positive as teenagers.]*

Class Discussion
HIV Testing

Why might an HIV infected person get a negative result from an HIV-antibody test? *[It can take up to 18 months after infection for antibodies to form.]* Stress the importance of retesting if a person has engaged in any high-risk behaviors during the six months prior to the previous test.

Have students give reasons why at-risk individuals should be tested. *(In*

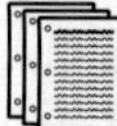

Section Review Worksheet 23.1

Assign Section Review Worksheet 23.1, which requires students to complete a chain of events to describe the effects of HIV.

Section Quiz 23.1

Have students take Section Quiz 23.1.

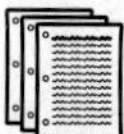

Reteaching Worksheet 23.1

Students who have difficulty with the material may complete Reteaching Worksheet 23.1, which requires them to characterize the three phases of AIDS.

The HIV-antibody test has one major drawback. It takes a while for an infected person's body to make enough antibodies to show up on the test—usually from 6 to 12 weeks, and sometimes up to 18 months. If a person went in for testing immediately after being infected, the results would be negative. So even when the test results are negative, there is still some chance that a person may be infected with HIV.

Some people say they wouldn't want to find out if they were infected with HIV because it would be too frightening. But there are two very compelling reasons to have the test if you think you might be infected. First, it may be possible to slow down the progress of the disease with early treatment. You may be able to prolong your life by beginning medication before you get sick. The earlier you know, the better. And second, you could protect others from HIV infection. You wouldn't want to be responsible for infecting other people.

Phases of HIV Infection

There isn't a timetable for the progression of HIV infection, but people tend to go through the following three phases.

Phase 1: Infection With No Signs or Symptoms of Illness Some people—infants, people who already have chronic diseases, and older people, for example—show signs and symptoms of infection very quickly. Others can be infected with HIV for years, sometimes 10 years or longer, without any noticeable illness. They seem perfectly healthy and wouldn't even know they were infected if they hadn't tested positive on the HIV-antibody test.

HIV-positive: *the condition of being infected with HIV.*

People who have been infected with HIV are said to be **HIV-positive**. It's important to remember that people can be HIV-positive and not have AIDS. People who are HIV-positive probably will get sick eventually, however, unless researchers find a way to prevent the disease from progressing. The main thing to remember now is that people who are infected with HIV but don't show any signs or symptoms of illness can still transmit the virus to other people.

Phase 2: Infection With Signs and Symptoms of Illness During the second phase of HIV infection, a person's immune system will begin to fail. A person in this phase may have one or more of the following signs and symptoms:

- swollen lymph glands in the neck and armpits
- extreme tiredness
- fever
- diarrhea
- severe weight loss
- excessive sweating during the night
- white patches on the inside of the mouth

You might be thinking to yourself, "I've had some of those signs. Does that mean I might be infected with HIV?" Remember that these signs and symptoms can also be caused by other infections, such as a cold or the flu. If you have these signs and symptoms, it doesn't necessarily mean that you're infected with HIV. One difference between the signs and symptoms of an HIV infection and a cold or flu is that the signs and symptoms of HIV infection tend to last a lot longer. If you have any of the signs or symptoms for more than two weeks, it's a good idea to see a doctor just to be on the safe side.

In addition to these infections, females can develop problems of the reproductive system. Often the first symptom of a weakened immune system in women is a series of severe vaginal infections.

Phase 3: AIDS According to the Centers for Disease Control and Prevention, there are two ways in which an HIV-infected per-

• • • TEACH continued

addition to getting treatment to delay the onset of disease and prevent the infection of others, students may mention putting worries to rest and being motivated to stop risk behaviors.)

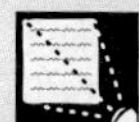

Teaching Transparency 23C
Phases of HIV Infection

Use this transparency to complement the three phases described in the text.

Extension

Information on the HIV-Antibody Test

Encourage students to visit a local health clinic to get pamphlets about the HIV-antibody test. Display the literature on a bulletin board.

The Research Frontier

Interested students may find recent articles describing promising medical research, medicines, and techniques for fighting HIV and AIDS. Have them report to the class on their findings.

son is considered to have AIDS. One way is for tests to indicate that the number of T4 cells in the blood is fewer than 200 cells per microliter of blood, or less than 14 percent of the white blood cells in the blood. This statistic would indicate that the person's immune system has been severely damaged.

The second way in which a person is considered to have AIDS is if he or she develops serious conditions that result from long-term damage to his or her immune system.

Among these serious conditions are what are called opportunistic infections. They are called opportunistic infections because they take the "opportunity" provided by a weakened immune system to attack the person's body.

One of the most common opportunistic infections people with AIDS get is a kind of pneumonia called Pneumocystis carinii, which causes difficulty in breathing, chest pain, and coughing. Kaposi's sarcoma, a rare cancer that causes purple patches or bumps on the skin and on the internal organs, is another serious disease that people with AIDS get. It is very unusual for people who don't have AIDS to get Pneumocystis carinii or Kaposi's sarcoma, because their immune systems can successfully defend against them. And HIV-infected women are also more likely than other women to get infections or cancers of the uterus and ovaries.

People with AIDS who have a relatively high amount of functioning T4 cells often appear healthy. They are energetic for long periods of time and can work or go to school. Those with fewer T4 cells are more likely to become ill and to develop opportunistic infections and cancers.

There is now no cure for AIDS. But you'll learn later in the chapter about new treatments that can help people with AIDS lead longer, healthier lives.

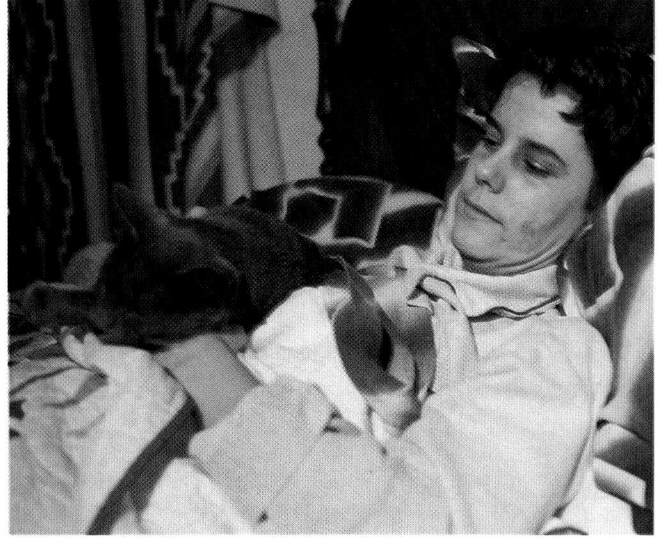

(FIGURE 23-5) **People with AIDS are more susceptible to infections and cancers than people who have fully functioning immune systems.**

Review

1. *Define AIDS.*
2. *Define HIV.*
3. *Can a person infected with HIV who shows no outward signs of illness infect another person? Explain your answer.*
4. ***LIFE SKILLS: Using Community Resources*** *Write down a hotline number you could call to find out the location of the nearest anonymous HIV-testing clinic.*
5. ***Critical Thinking*** *Is it possible for a person who was infected with HIV at the age of 14 to have no outward signs of illness at the age of 19? Explain your answer.*

Section 23.1

Review Answers

1. AIDS (Acquired Immune Deficiency Syndrome) is a disease caused by a virus that harms a person's immune system; AIDS is the last stage of HIV infection.
2. HIV (human immunodeficiency virus) is a virus that attacks the body's immune system, so that it can't defend the body against infection.
3. Yes, if an HIV-positive person's blood or body fluid comes into contact with another person's blood. Also, some people can be infected with HIV for years without knowing it or showing symptoms.
4. The national AIDS hotline number is 1-800-342-2437.
5. Yes. It can take ten years for symptoms to show.

ASSESS

Section Review

Have students answer the Section Review questions.

Alternative Assessment

The Price of Showing No Symptoms

Have students explain what the delay between HIV infection and the appearance of symptoms means for individuals and for society.

Closure

HIV and AIDS

Have students write a brief paragraph that explains the difference between being infected with HIV and having AIDS.

Background
Other Bodily Fluids
HIV has been found in small amounts in tears, saliva, and urine. However, the amounts present in these fluids are considered insufficient to infect someone, and there are no documented cases of HIV having been transmitted by them.

Section 23.2 Transmission of HIV

Objectives

- *Name the three body fluids that may contain enough HIV to infect another person.*
- *List the four behaviors that put you at risk for HIV infection.*
- *Name at least five behaviors that don't put you at risk for HIV infection.*
- *Find out where you can get answers to any questions about HIV that are not covered in this chapter.*
  LIFE SKILLS: Using Community Resources

HIV isn't transmitted like the viruses that cause the common cold or flu. Cold and flu viruses are transmitted pretty easily. If you shake hands with a person who has a cold or flu, for example, and then you touch your mouth, you are pretty likely to catch the virus from that person. HIV is much harder to catch, because it is not transmitted through the air. By far the most common way that HIV is transmitted from one person to another is through bodily fluids. And only some of these fluids may contain enough of the virus to infect someone else. These are the body fluids that may contain enough HIV to infect another person:

- blood
- semen
- vaginal secretions

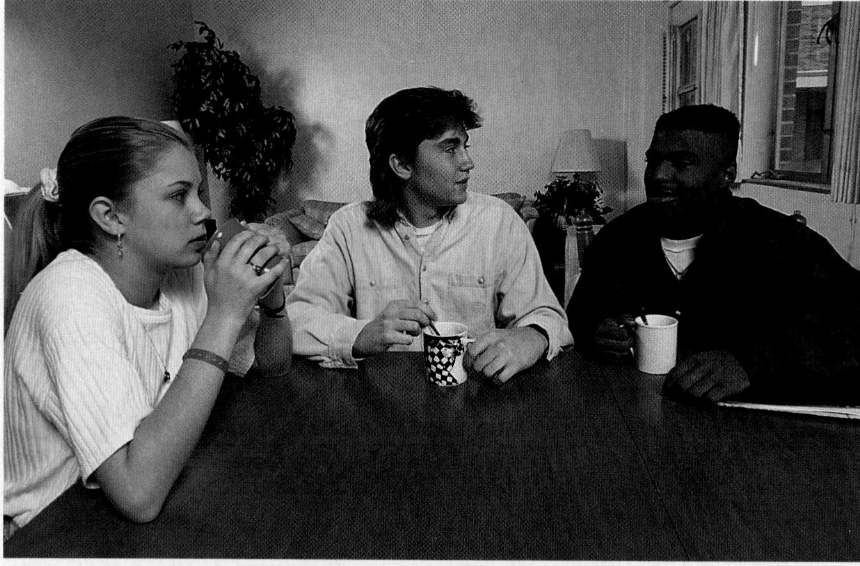

(FIGURE 23-6) **You can't get AIDS from being around a person in an ordinary, everyday kind of way.**

Section 23.2 Lesson Plan

MOTIVATE

Journal 23C
How a Person Gets AIDS

This may be done as a warm-up activity. Have students complete this sentence in their Student Journal: "A person can get AIDS by . . ."

TEACH

Class Discussion
Transmission of HIV

Ask: **What conditions are necessary for one person to pass the HIV virus to another?** *[It must be conveyed in one of three body fluids without being exposed to air, and it must enter the person's bloodstream.]*

Draw a fishbone diagram on the chalkboard and use it to organize the answers students supply:

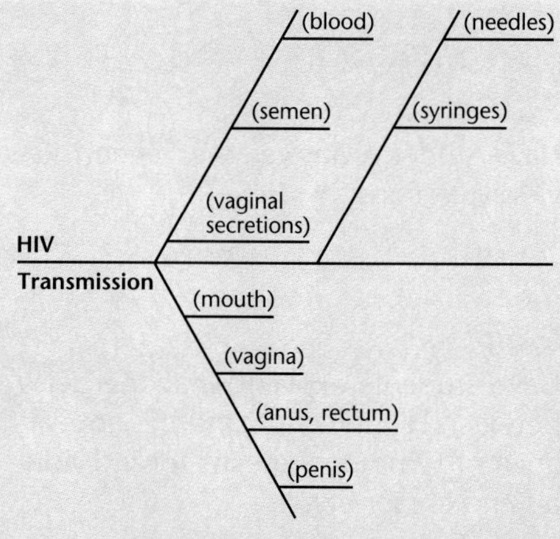

Transmission of HIV

Risky Behaviors	Safe Behaviors ("Casual Contact")
1. Sharing equipment for injecting drugs, tattooing, or piercing	*1. Working at the same place or going to the same school*
2. Vaginal intercourse with an infected person	*2. Living in the same home*
3. Oral intercourse with an infected person	*3. Sharing food, eating from the same plate, or using the same knives, forks or spoons*
4. Anal intercourse with an infected person	*4. Shaking hands, holding hands, or hugging*
	5. Sharing a toilet or using a public toilet
	6. Using the same locker room
	7. Using the same telephone
	8. Using the same water fountain
	9. Swimming in the same pool
	10. Being breathed on, coughed on, or sneezed on
	...and any other ordinary, everyday kind of contact with people

(FIGURE 23-7) **Risky behaviors involve blood, semen, or vaginal secretions. Safe behaviors don't involve those body fluids.**

Remember that HIV must get into a person's bloodstream before it can cause any trouble. It must go from the blood, semen, or vaginal secretions of an infected person into the bloodstream of another person. But how can HIV get into a person's bloodstream?

First, HIV can go directly from an infected person's blood into another person's bloodstream. The most common way this happens is when needles and syringes are used to inject drugs.

Second, HIV can enter the bloodstream through the **mucous membranes** of the body. Mucous membranes are moist, pink tissues that line the openings to the body—the mouth, the vagina, the anus and rectum, and the opening at the tip of the penis. Sores or tiny breaks in the mucous membranes make it easier for HIV to enter the body. But even if a person has no breaks in the mucous membranes, HIV can still enter the body through the mucous membranes.

mucous membranes:

moist, pink tissues of the body; HIV can enter the body through the mucous membranes of the mouth, vagina, anus and rectum, and the opening at the tip of the penis.

Be alert for misconceptions students have about the way HIV is spread. *(They may think it is spread in urine, tears, saliva, by sneezing, by sharing a toilet, by kissing, and so on.)*

Game
Stump the Guest

Have students form teams to play Stump the Guest. Each team prepares 10 questions. They should try to word the questions so as to make them challenging for opponents. (Can you get AIDS from sharing a soft drink? Can you get AIDS from having anal intercourse with someone who is not infected?) Teams take turns sending a representative to the other side. The other team poses one of its questions to this guest. The guest gets one point for a correct answer. The asking team gets a point if they stump the guest.

Reinforcement
Two Ways Into the Bloodstream

Remind students that HIV has two ways to get into the bloodstream: directly (through shared needles, breaks in the skin, or contaminated blood products) or indirectly (through mucous membranes). HIV can pass through these membranes even if they are not torn.

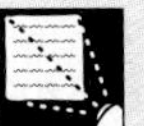

Teaching Transparency 23D
Transmission of HIV

Show the transparency called "Transmission of HIV" (Figure 23-7). Have students think of other risky behaviors that might be added to the left half of

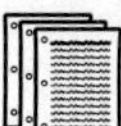

Section Review Worksheet 23.2

Assign Section Review Worksheet 23.2, which requires students to complete a concept map showing methods of HIV transmission.

Section Quiz 23.2

Have students take Section Quiz 23.2.

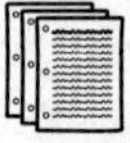

Reteaching Worksheet 23.2

Students who have difficulty with the material may complete Reteaching Worksheet 23.2, which requires them to choose among safe and unsafe behaviors.

How You Can Get HIV

People used to talk about HIV "risk groups"—certain groups of people who were more likely than others to get HIV. Now we know that anyone who takes part in certain risky behaviors can be infected with HIV.

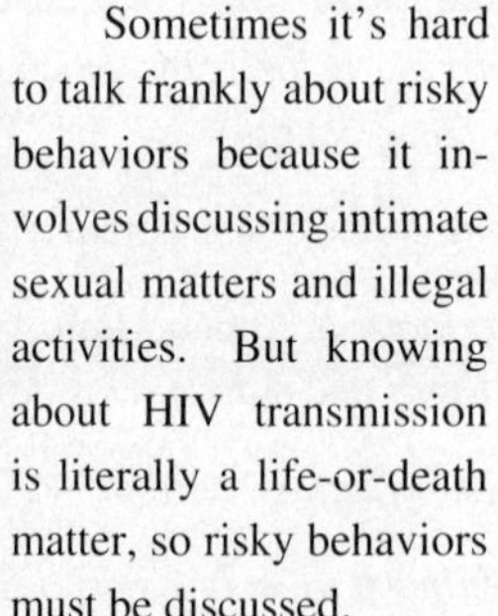

"I was really scared about AIDS until I took this health class. I'd heard all kinds of wild stories about how you could get it."

Mei

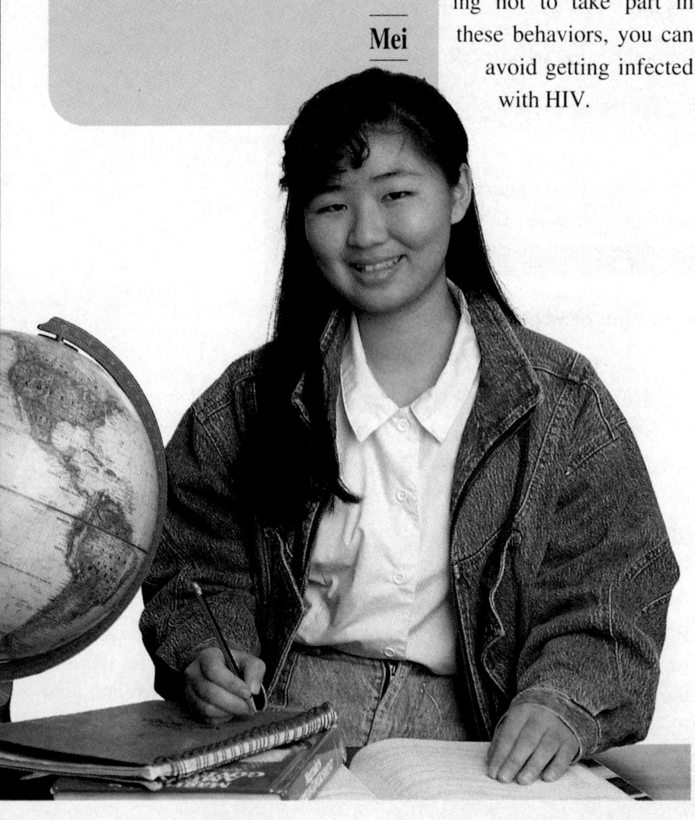

Sometimes it's hard to talk frankly about risky behaviors because it involves discussing intimate sexual matters and illegal activities. But knowing about HIV transmission is literally a life-or-death matter, so risky behaviors must be discussed.

There are four behaviors that put you at risk for getting HIV. By choosing not to take part in these behaviors, you can avoid getting infected with HIV.

Sharing Equipment for Injecting Drugs, Tattooing, or Piercing Any sharing of needles or other equipment for injecting drugs, tattooing, or piercing is risky behavior. When people share a needle to inject drugs, the blood from the first person may go directly into the second person's body. If the blood contains HIV, the viruses will be injected along with the blood. It doesn't matter what substance is being injected; it might be heroin, cocaine, or steroids. Even injecting vitamins, insulin, or antibiotics can expose a person to HIV if needles or syringes are shared.

If you share needles with an infected person to tattoo or pierce any part of your body, you are risking HIV infection. You won't get HIV if you go to a professional tattoo artist or ear-piercing salon where the equipment is sterilized after each use. Make very sure, however, that they do sterilize their equipment.

Vaginal Intercourse With an Infected Person Vaginal intercourse is usually just called "sexual intercourse," and it's the most common kind of intercourse between men and women. It's when a man puts his penis into a woman's vagina.

During vaginal intercourse a man can pass HIV to a woman, and a woman can pass it to a man. If the man is infected with HIV, viruses in his semen can get into the woman's bloodstream through the mucous membranes of her vagina.

If the woman is infected with HIV, the viruses can be passed from her vagina to the man. They may get into the man's bloodstream through the mucous membranes that are in the opening at the tip of his penis.

Although either partner can transmit the virus to the other, it is easier for a woman to become infected. A woman has a much larger area of mucous membranes exposed to fluids than a man does. Also,

• • • TEACH continued

the chart; discuss their suggestions. Ask for additional safe behaviors for the right half.

Journal 23D
Considering Risk Activities

Have students use the Student Journal to write down their feelings and thoughts about the four main risk activities. Do they feel that any of these activities, aside from being dangerous, are wrong under some circumstances? Are they uncomfortable discussing them? Do they agree with Dr. C. Everett Koop, the former U.S. surgeon general, that it is necessary to discuss these risk behaviors?

Cooperative Learning
The Path of Transmission

Have students form groups to analyze the path of transmission of HIV for each of the four main risk activities. What fluids and tissues are involved? How does the virus reach the bloodstream? Have each group make a list of questions that have not been answered by the discussion so far. Answer any questions you can; write the others on the chalkboard and keep them there until answers are found. (Sample questions: When transmission is possible, does it always occur? How many times must you be exposed to contract HIV? Can HIV live in dried blood? Can you prevent the transmission of HIV by early withdrawal during sexual intercourse? Can you become pregnant at the same time you contract the disease?)

semen may remain in the woman's vagina for quite a while after intercourse. Therefore, more women than men become infected with HIV from vaginal intercourse.

Oral Intercourse With an Infected Person Oral intercourse, also called oral sex, is contact between one person's mouth and another person's genitals. The viruses can be passed to either partner through tiny cuts or through the mucous membranes of the mouth and genitals.

Anal Intercourse With an Infected Person Anal intercourse is when a man puts his penis into the anus of another person. It is possible for either partner to transmit the virus to the other. HIV can get through the mucous membranes of the anus, the rectum, or the opening in the penis.

LifeSKILLS: Using Community Resources

Getting HIV Information

You may have questions about HIV infection that haven't been answered in this chapter. Don't worry; you can get answers to your questions. You may be comfortable talking to a parent or teacher, or you may prefer to call someone who doesn't know you. After you do the following exercise, you'll be able to get the information you need.

1. Look in the phone book under "AIDS" and write down the name of every organization you see.
2. Write down the phone number of the local AIDS hotline.
3. Write down the phone number of the national AIDS hotline, which is given in this chapter.
4. Where could you call to talk to someone about whether you are at risk of being infected with HIV?
5. Write down the name and phone number of a place where you can get an HIV-antibody test. (You may have to call one of the phone numbers you've already looked up to get this information.)

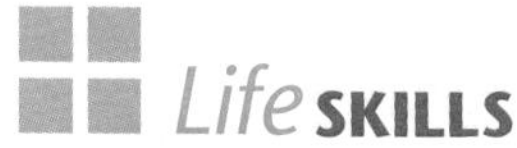

Getting HIV Information

Have students gather the information requested in steps 1-5 in the text. Each student should do this exercise independently in order to benefit from the experience. Give each student an index card on which to record and retain the information gathered.

Students may wish to do research and report to the class on questions you cannot immediately answer.

Reinforcement

Other Methods of Transmission

Draw a simple network on the chalkboard, with four lines extending from a central circle labeled "Other Methods of Transmission." Ask students to name methods of transmitting HIV other than the four main risk behaviors, and write them on the spokes leading to the center. Remind students that although these are not common sources of infection, they are important to know about.

Class Discussion

Thoughts on HIV Transmission

Ask questions like the following to extend students' thinking about other methods of transmission: Is it a good idea for an HIV-positive woman to become pregnant? If a woman who is HIV-positive bears a child who is not infected, should she breast-feed the baby? What kinds of precautions should be taken with hypodermic needles? Is it reasonable to be afraid of going to the dentist because of the possibility of AIDS infection? Is it reasonable to be afraid of receiving a blood transfusion?

Debate the Issue

Testing of Health Personnel

Hold a class debate on the topic, "Should doctors and other health-care professionals undergo mandatory HIV

Background
HIV and Pregnancy

According to one estimate, pregnant women who are infected with HIV have a 25 to 30 percent chance of infecting their babies with the virus. Generally, the baby is infected through an exchange of blood before or during birth, or, more rarely, by nursing on breast milk after birth. Some children with AIDS develop severe symptoms and die before they are two years old. The disease progresses more slowly for other children, who may suffer from frequent bacterial infections but can live for a number of years.

An Especially Risky Behavior It is especially risky to have intercourse with many people. The more people a person has intercourse with, the more likely that person is to have intercourse with someone who has HIV—it's just a matter of probability.

Other Methods of Transmission Some people have gotten HIV even though they didn't take part in risky behaviors. Infants have gotten HIV from their mothers while still in the womb or during birth. And there is evidence that an HIV-infected woman can infect her baby through breast-feeding. Therefore, any woman who is thinking about becoming pregnant should consider getting an HIV-antibody test.

A few doctors, nurses, and other health-care workers have gotten HIV from their patients. Some of the health-care workers had cuts or other breaks in their skin and were exposed to infected blood. Others accidentally stuck themselves with needles they had used to draw blood from people with HIV infection.

A few people have gotten HIV as a result of dental procedures done in the office of an HIV-infected dentist. Therefore, new federal guidelines were established in 1991 to protect patients.

Before 1985, some people got HIV from receiving blood transfusions or other blood products that contained HIV. Hemophiliacs (people whose blood does not clot properly) were particularly at risk because they used a product made of blood from many different donors. Since 1985, all blood donated in the United States has been tested for HIV, and any HIV-infected blood is discarded. So now there is very little chance of getting the virus from blood products.

(FIGURE 23-8) **All blood that is donated in the United States is tested for HIV, and all blood that is infected is discarded.**

How You Can't Get HIV

You could fill a book with a list of all the ways that you can't get HIV. You can't get HIV by having what's called ''casual'' contact with an HIV-infected person. In other words, you can't get HIV by being around a person in an ordinary, everyday kind of way. Scientists who do HIV research are almost 100-percent sure of this because there hasn't been one single case of anyone getting HIV from casual contact with an infected person. Even family members or friends who live with people with AIDS and help care for them have not been infected with HIV from casual contact.

• • • TEACH continued

tests?" Have students do some research, then allow presentations, counterarguments, and questions from the audience. Remind students that in a debate you are not always arguing the side you believe in, but are trying to put forth the best possible arguments for an assigned position.

Class Discussion
Jobs and HIV

Ask students their opinions about the way health-care workers with AIDS are treated. Should HIV-positive workers continue in their jobs?

Writing
Health-Care Workers

Ask students to write a persuasive essay or letter to the editor about how we should provide for health-care workers who have contracted HIV infection on the job.

Extension
Health-Care Precautions

Suggest that students visit a dental or medical office to find out what precautions its personnel take against transmission of HIV.

Q and A

Q: Is it possible to get HIV from kissing?

A: You can't get HIV from a "simple" kiss, the kind in which people just put their lips together. If you could, a lot of people would already have been infected this way. There have been no reported cases of this happening. But it is theoretically possible for the virus to be transmitted through "French" kissing—deep, open-mouth kissing—since HIV has been found in the saliva of infected people. HIV researchers think it usually takes many viruses to cause infection, however, and saliva contains very few viruses. And here again, there have been no reported cases of HIV being transmitted in this way.

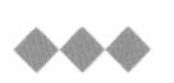

Q: Isn't it true that you can get AIDS if you donate your blood?

A: No, absolutely not. This is something that many people are confused about. Blood-donation centers use a new, sterile needle with each donor. Don't let a myth like this keep you from donating blood to those who need it.

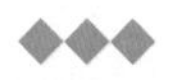

Q: I've heard people say that you could get HIV if a mosquito bites a person with HIV and then bites you. Is that true?

A: No. If mosquitoes could transmit HIV, there would already be many cases of that happening by now. In fact, there are no reported cases of HIV being transmitted by any kind of insect or other animal.

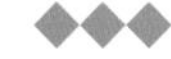

Q: What should I do if I think I might be infected with HIV?

A: Talk to someone you trust about getting an HIV-antibody test—a parent, teacher, coach, school nurse, counselor, doctor, or someone at a health clinic. You can also call one of the AIDS hotline numbers shown at the right, to find out where you can go for HIV testing and counseling.

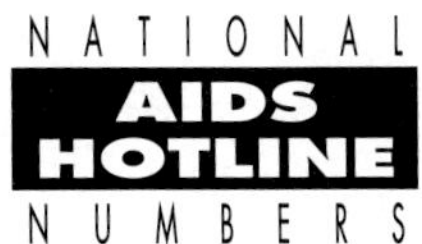
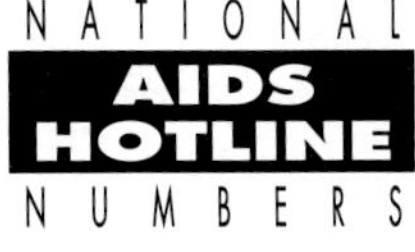

1-800-342-2437

1-800-344-7432
(SPANISH)

1-800-243-7889
(HEARING IMPAIRED)

Review

1. *Name the three body fluids that may contain enough HIV to infect another person.*
2. *Name the four behaviors that put you at risk for HIV infection.*
3. *Name at least five behaviors that don't put you at risk for HIV infection.*
4. ***LIFE SKILLS: Using Community Resources*** *Name two people you could talk to about whether a certain behavior could put you at risk for getting HIV.*
5. ***Critical Thinking*** *Could you get infected with HIV by wiping away the tears of a baby with HIV? Explain your answer.*

Review Answers

1. Blood, semen, and vaginal secretions
2. Sharing equipment for injecting drugs, for tattooing, or for ear piercing; vaginal, oral, or anal intercourse with an infected person
3. Students should list five of the safe behaviors listed in the table shown in Figure 23-7.
4. You could talk with someone you trust, or you could call an AIDS hotline.
5. Extremely unlikely. Tears can contain HIV, but wiping tears does not allow for direct contact between the virus and the bloodstream or the mucous membranes.

ASSESS

Section Review

Have students answer the Section Review questions.

Alternative Assessment

The Nature of HIV and Infection

Have students write a brief narrative about how the AIDS epidemic would differ if HIV could be transmitted through casual contact.

Closure

Risk of Infection

Ask students to speculate about how a person who has never injected drugs and has only one sexual partner might become infected with HIV.

Section 23.3 How to Protect Yourself From HIV

Background

Students and Monogamy

Studies have shown that many sexually active teenagers have serial monogamous relationships. This practice is not truly monogamous and does increase risk of becoming infected with HIV.

Making a Choice 23A

Couple's Discussion

Assign the Couple's Discussion card. The card asks students to answer questions about a couple who is contemplating sexual intimacy and to role-play the situation.

Making a Choice 23B

Advertising

Assign the Advertising card, which asks students to discover some of the methods advertisers use to sell products.

Skills for delaying sexual intimacy are discussed in Chapter 17.

Objectives

- *Discuss abstinence as the most effective way to prevent the sexual transmission of HIV infection.*
- *Practice resisting pressure to be sexually intimate.*
  LIFE SKILLS: Resisting Pressure
- *Know how to reduce your risk of HIV infection if you are sexually active.*
  LIFE SKILLS: Solving Problems

In this section you'll learn exactly how to reduce your risk of becoming infected with HIV. Protecting yourself requires knowledge about HIV and the skills to put your knowledge to use.

Abstinence

The only way to be 100 percent safe from getting HIV sexually is to avoid the three kinds of sexual intercourse that were discussed in Section 23.2. When a person decides against taking part in sexual intercourse, that person is said to be choosing abstinence.

Abstinence doesn't mean that a person has no sexual feelings. Everyone has sexual feelings—they are a perfectly natural and pleasurable part of being human. It's just that people who choose abstinence decide not to act on their sexual feelings in ways that could endanger them. There are many ways to show affection for other

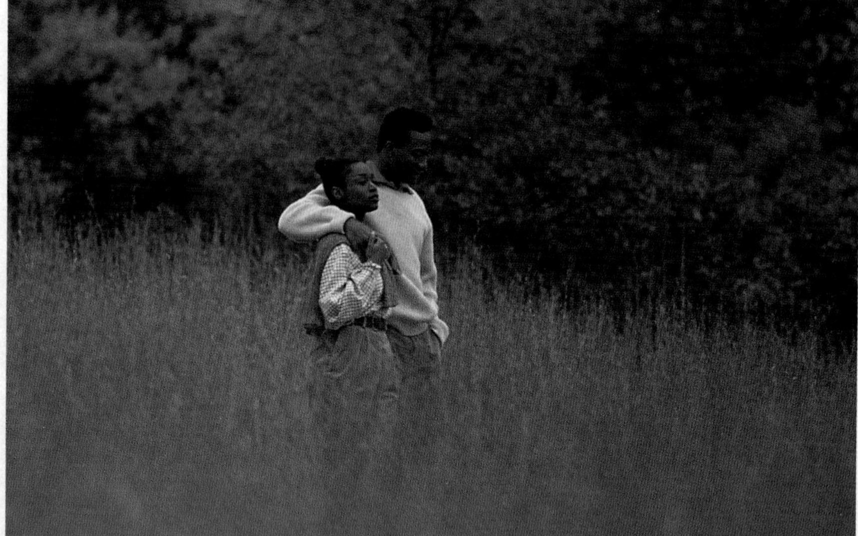

(FIGURE 23-10) **People who are sexually abstinent can show affection for each other in ways that don't put them at risk for getting HIV.**

Section 23.3 Lesson Plan

MOTIVATE

Journal 23E
On Sexual Abstinence

This may be done as a warm-up activity. Have students write down the pros and cons of sexual abstinence. Are there more reasons not to have sex than to have sex? Do the reasons for having sexual intercourse make the risk of getting AIDS worthwhile?

TEACH

Class Discussion
Social Pressures

Most HIV is transmitted sexually; abstaining from sex is the surest way to avoid this transmission. Ask students to comment on social pressures for or against delaying sexual activity. If there is peer pressure to have sex, is there a good way to cope with it? Stress the value of anticipating and avoiding situations in which there is pressure to have sex, and remind students that no one has the right to force them to have sex. They can refuse verbally or simply leave the situation.

Reinforcement
Understanding the Dangers of Serial Monogamy

Many teens are serially monogamous. Have students differentiate clearly between lifelong monogamy and serial monogamy. Stress to students that

people that don't put you at risk for getting HIV. The Life Skills activity on page 499 will help you to prepare to resist the pressure to do the things that you don't really want to do.

One final note about abstinence: You'll have a harder time sticking to your decision to remain abstinent if you drink or use drugs. The best of resolutions can be forgotten when a person is drunk or high.

Safer Sex

The only sexual intercourse that is completely safe from HIV infection is between two people who are emotionally mature enough to be faithful to each other for their

Life SKILLS: Resisting Pressure

Saying No

One of the ways to keep from doing things that put you at risk for HIV is to become resistant to pressure. See if you can think of a resistant response to each of the statements below.

1. "We'll just play around some. We can stop whenever you want."
2. "If you really loved me, you would make love to me."
3. "You must not have any sexual feelings at all."
4. "But I hate using condoms. It takes all the fun out of it."
5. "I'll pierce your ears and then you can pierce mine."

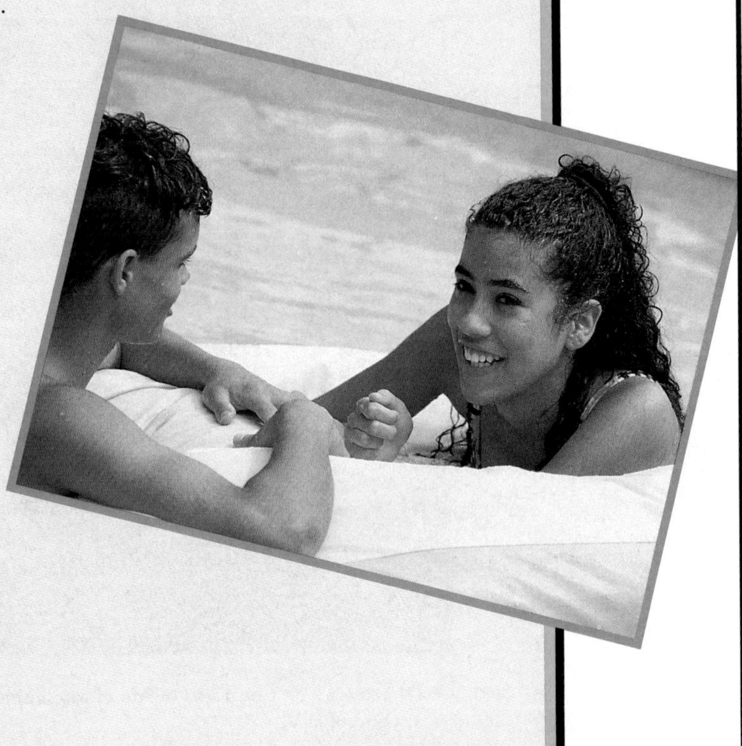

Although it helps to think of responses to certain statements, remember that you aren't required to have a reason. If you don't want to explain, all you have to say is "I don't want to." You don't have to debate what to do with your own body.

Life SKILLS

Saying No

Have students do the Life Skills exercise in this section, answering the five questions on paper. After they have done the exercise, have students role-play the five situations. For each situation, give several pairs of students a chance to use their resistant responses. If students are comfortable with the exercise, ask those in the audience to critique the resistant responses of the role players.

serial monogamy is *not* an effective preventive strategy. **Can you believe that a partner is telling the truth about their previous sexual encounters?** *[Not necessarily]*

Demonstration
Latex Condoms

Bring a package of latex condoms to class. Have students read the package label to verify that the condoms are made of latex. Unwrap a condom to show students what it looks like and how it is used. Demonstrate how the condom is put on by pulling one over two fingers or an object such as a banana. You might also wish to bring other protective devices, such as vaginal foams and jellies that contain nonoxynol-9.

Debate the Issue
Condoms on Campus?

Despite the risks involved, some young people will choose to be sexually active. Have students debate the question, Should condoms be distributed on high school campuses? Divide the class into two teams: one pro and one con. Each team should prepare for the debate by listing arguments the other side is likely to make and by composing their counterarguments.

Reinforcement
Drugs and Alcohol and Judgment

Aside from the direct danger of infection from injecting drugs, there is an-

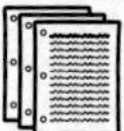

Life Skills Worksheet 23B

Magazine Advertisements

Assign the Magazine Advertisements Life Skills Worksheet, which asks students to analyze magazine advertisements in terms of the sexual messages.

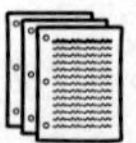

Section Review Worksheet 23.3

Assign Section Review Worksheet 23.3, which requires students to note safe and unsafe behaviors.

Section Quiz 23.3

Have students take Section Quiz 23.3.

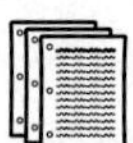

Reteaching Worksheet 23.3

Students who have difficulty with the material may complete Reteaching Worksheet 23.3, which asks them to respond to statements about sexual intimacy.

monogamy: *when two people have intercourse with only each other for their entire lives.*

entire lives. When two people have sexual relations with only each other over a lifetime, they are said to be practicing **monogamy**.

What if someone says that he or she has never had sexual relations before? That person wouldn't pose a risk of HIV infection, right? Unfortunately, people don't always tell the truth when it comes to sexual matters. In a recent study of college students, 34 percent of the men and 10 percent of the women surveyed admitted lying to a partner in order to have sexual relations.

Sometimes a person has intercourse out of fear of losing a boyfriend or girlfriend. It is difficult to resist this kind of pressure, especially when it comes from someone you love. A young woman named Amy Dolph has something to say about this problem. She says you shouldn't allow another person, even someone you love, to determine when you will die. ''Do you want to put your life in that other person's hands?'' she asks. ''Is that boy or girl worth dying for? I doubt it.'' Amy Dolph contracted HIV during high school from her second sexual partner.

Those who do not practice abstinence or monogamy must take precautions to reduce their risk of getting HIV. The following two steps must be taken to practice ''safer'' sex:

1. **Limit the Number of Partners** The fewer sexual partners a person has, the less likely he or she is to have intercourse with someone who is HIV-positive. But remember that it takes only one HIV-infected partner to infect a person with the virus.
2. **Use Latex Condoms During Intercourse** Sexual partners must use latex condoms

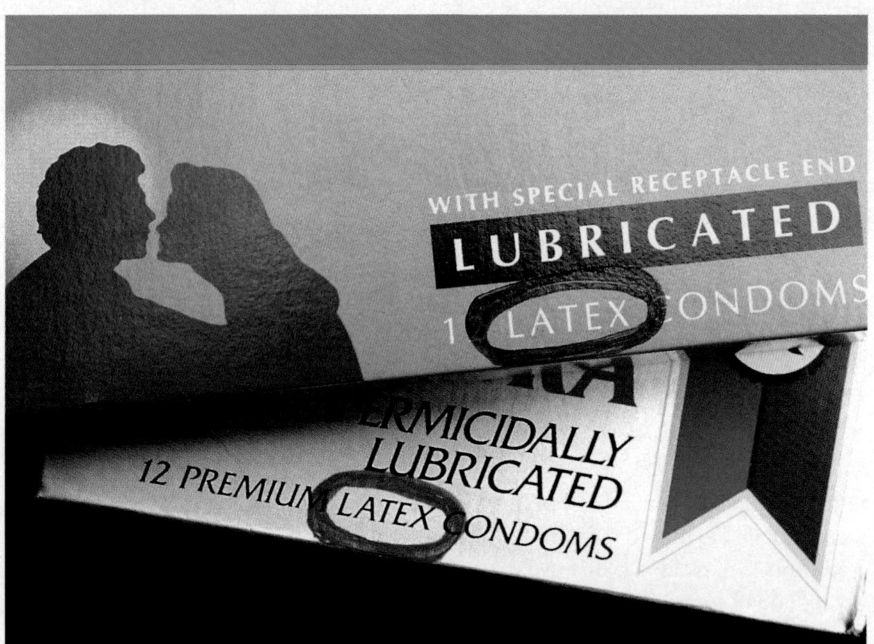

(FIGURE 23-10) **Condoms made of latex are the most effective in preventing the spread of HIV.**

• • • TEACH continued

other danger. Remind students that drugs and alcohol impair body functions and cloud judgment. Research shows that when people are on drugs and alcohol they are much less likely to use condoms.

Cooperative Learning

Protection From HIV

Have the class prepare a bulletin board describing the ways people can protect themselves from HIV. They might divide the bulletin board in half—one half showing decisions they personally can make to protect themselves, and the other half showing steps society can take.

Extension

HIV in Your Community

Have students visit or telephone the local health department to find out its approach to AIDS prevention, education, and treatment.

to reduce their risk of HIV infection. Condoms aren't 100-percent effective in preventing the spread of HIV, but they make sexual relations much less risky for both partners. To be effective against HIV, a condom must be made of latex (a kind of rubber). Condoms made of natural lambskin aren't as good as latex condoms at keeping HIV from spreading from one partner to another; the viruses might be able to pass through a lambskin condom. If a condom is made of latex, the label on the package will say so.

It's important to remember that a condom must be used the whole time—from start to finish—during vaginal, anal, or oral intercourse. A new condom should be used each time a person has intercourse.

Some brands of condoms are made with a spermicide on them. The product label on these condoms will say they have nonoxynol-9, a kind of spermicide. Some studies have shown that nonoxynol-9 offers additional protection against HIV, although recent evidence suggests that this may not be true. Still, using condoms with spermicides is a good idea because they do help prevent pregnancy and may help prevent the transmission of some other STDs.

Don't Use Injected Drugs

If you haven't used injected drugs, don't start. If you do use them, seek treatment to help you quit. See Chapter 15 for information about drug-treatment programs.

For those who use injected drugs and share equipment, doctors recommend that they clean their equipment with a solution of 1 part household bleach to 100 parts water before and after each use. This precaution reduces the risk of HIV infection.

What if You've Already Engaged in Risky Behavior?

What if you haven't followed these guidelines? Should you just forget about it because it's already too late? No, absolutely not. You haven't necessarily been infected, even if you know you've engaged in risky behavior with an HIV-infected person.

If you think there is a chance you've been infected, get an HIV-antibody test immediately. Protect yourself and protect other people.

Review

1. *What is the best way to prevent the sexual transmission of HIV?*
2. *Why is a latex condom more effective against HIV than a lambskin condom?*
3. **LIFE SKILLS: Resisting Pressure** *If your friend wanted the two of you to give each other tattoos, what would you do or say to protect yourself against the possibility of HIV infection?*
4. **LIFE SKILLS: Solving Problems** *If you have decided to have intercourse, how could you reduce your risk of becoming infected with HIV?*
5. **Critical Thinking** *Explain the reasoning behind this statement about the transmission of HIV: "When you have intercourse with someone, you're also having intercourse with everyone that person has ever had intercourse with."*

Review Answers

1. Abstinence or sexual activity only within a lifelong monogamous relationship with an uninfected person are means of avoiding sexual transmission of HIV.
2. Viruses may pass through a lambskin condom but not through a latex condom.
3. Get a tattoo only at a place you know uses sterilized equipment.
4. (a) Practice monogamy with a person who is not infected, (b) Use latex condoms treated with nonoxynol-9, (c) Avoid drugs and alcohol.
5. Because the virus is transmitted sexually, every previous partner of a person may have given him or her the virus. You can become infected, too.

ASSESS

Section Review

Have students answer the Section Review questions.

Alternative Assessment

HIV Among Teens

Ask students whether they think education about HIV and AIDS will make a great difference in HIV transmission in teens. Have them specify what they think the effect will be (for example, HIV transmission among teens will level off in the next five years). Have students then support their conclusion with references to the protective measures they have learned about.

Closure

Feelings on Delayed Sexual Intercourse

Ask students how they would feel toward a student who has made the decision not to be sexually active.

Section 23.4 HIV Infection and Society

Background
Treatments for HIV

AZT and DDI inhibit the function of an enzyme necessary for viral replication. This enzyme is encoded by the virus's own genetic material. These drugs cannot cure the disease, but they may delay the onset of debilitating symptoms, keeping a person healthier longer.

Background
Tips for Helping AIDS Patients

Some positive, helpful actions a friend can take for someone with AIDS:

- Don't stay away.
- Keep touching—hugs and hand holding.
- Call and ask if it is okay to visit; the person may not feel well enough every day.
- Respond to the person's feelings.
- Bring a favorite dish and share the meal.
- Go for a walk or outing, if possible.
- Help answer their correspondence.
- Ask for a shopping list of needed items and deliver them.
- Bring books, periodicals, music tapes, posters, and so on.

Objectives

- *Describe medical treatments available for HIV infection.*
- *Name at least two actions you can take to help people with HIV infection.*

HIV doesn't just affect individuals. It affects society. Millions of dollars are being spent searching for new treatments for HIV infection, even as discrimination against people with HIV continues.

But a society is made up of individuals. Each individual can do his or her part to eliminate the disease and care for the people affected by it.

Medical Advances

Recent medical advances have made it possible to ease the symptoms of HIV infection and perhaps delay the onset of illness. Researchers discovered that the drugs AZT (zidovudine) and DDI (dideoxyinosine) show promise in postponing symptoms in people who have tested HIV-positive but are not yet sick. AZT and DDI slow down the rate at which the viruses reproduce inside a person's body. Another drug, aerosol pentamidine, is a spray breathed into the lungs that helps prevent Pneumocystis carinii pneumonia.

Because of the development of drugs and other treatments, HIV infection is now considered to be a chronic condition that can be managed for many years. Researchers continue to search for a cure for HIV infection and for a vaccine to prevent infection in the first place. Still, it may take many years before these attempts are successful. In the meantime, your first line of defense against HIV is you.

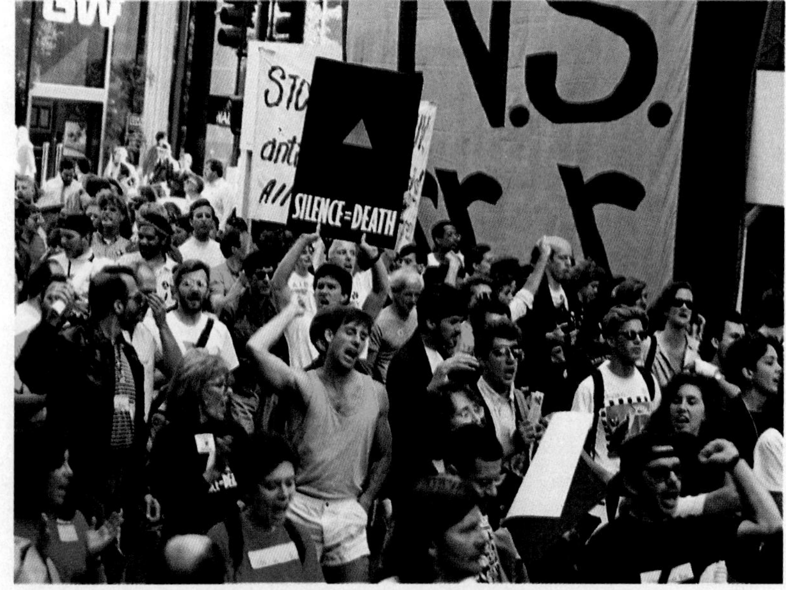

(FIGURE 23-11) **AIDS activists put pressure on governmental agencies to increase spending on HIV programs. AIDS activists were also responsible for raising public awareness about HIV infection.**

Section 23.4 Lesson Plan

MOTIVATE

Journal 23F
A Roommate With HIV

Pose the following situation to students and have them write their response in the Student Journal: You are attending a convention or athletic event away from home. As soon as you meet your assigned roommate, he or she tells you, "I am infected with HIV." How would you feel about the revelation? Would it change your expectations about the person? about sharing a room? Would it matter to you how the person contracted HIV? What questions would you want to ask?

TEACH

Writing
Asking a Person With AIDS

Have students make a list of questions they might wish to ask a person who has AIDS. Questions might include: How do you feel? What are your needs? What kind of help are you getting? How are you being treated by old friends? by acquaintances? by family? Suggest that students write the questions into a letter. It may be possible to send one or more letters to real AIDS patients by contacting a local AIDS organization.

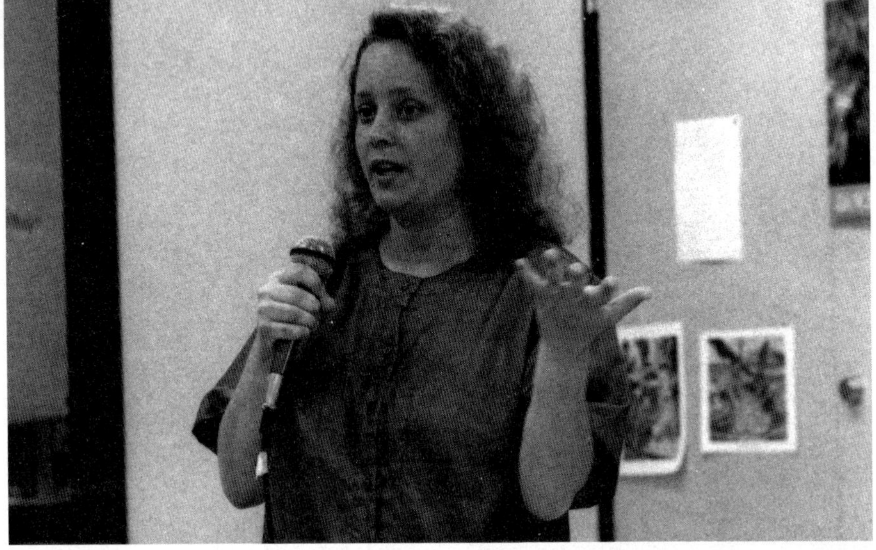

(FIGURE 23-12) **Dawn Marcel was infected with HIV when she was a senior in high school. She is now a speaker for an AIDS-education program in San Francisco. "I've been on AZT for three years," Dawn said. "I take it for one month, then go off it for one month because it destroys my liver. I don't look sick. I'm chubby, or I think I'm chubby. People don't imagine that I could be sick, but you can't tell by looking at someone."**

Teenagers' Special Needs

Teenagers have some special needs when it comes to HIV prevention. They tend to be experimental and eager to try new things and new styles of living. Much of this experimentation is healthy and valuable, but some of it, as you've found out, can be dangerous. When it comes to HIV, teenagers who have intercourse or experiment with injected drugs may be risking their lives and the lives of their friends.

There is also a special set of ethical and legal issues regarding testing teenagers for HIV infection. Some people argue, for example, that teenagers' parents or guardians should be told about the results of HIV-antibody tests, especially if the results are positive. Others argue that to do so would make teenagers reluctant to be tested and keep them from getting the medical treatment they might need. What do you think about this dilemma?

Living With HIV Infection

People often avoid and isolate people who have HIV infection. When the people in Ryan White's town found out he had AIDS,

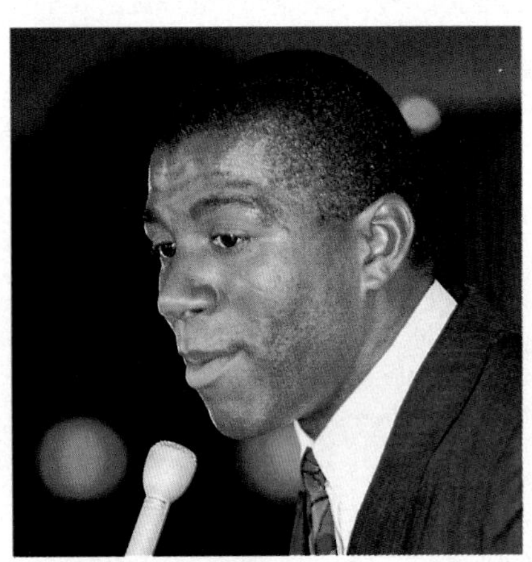

(FIGURE 23-13) **Earvin "Magic" Johnson, former Los Angeles Lakers basketball star, discovered in 1991 that he was HIV-positive.**

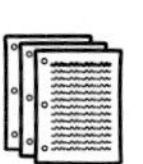

Life Skills Worksheet 23C

Decision Making

Assign the Decision Making Life Skills Worksheet, which has students consider feelings and attitudes about sexual activity.

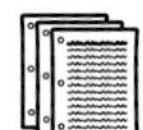

Ethics Worksheet

Have students complete the Ethics Worksheet for Unit 6.

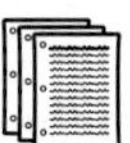

Section Review Worksheet 23.4

Assign the Section Review Worksheet 23.4, which requires students to tell about AIDS medications and respond to various AIDS-related situations.

Section Quiz 23.4

Have students take Section Quiz 23.4.

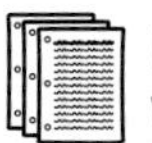

Reteaching Worksheet 23.4

Students who have difficulty with the material may complete Reteaching Worksheet 23.4, which requires them to suggest ways they could help in the AIDS epidemic.

Class Discussion

Ryan White's Situation

Ask students how they feel about the way Ryan White was treated. Would a student today be treated differently at school? Tell students what the AIDS policy is in your school system.

Role-Playing

An Acquaintance With HIV

Have students act out a situation in which they meet a person who has AIDS. After students act out their parts, lead a discussion about the feelings and reactions of each person.

Debate the Issue

Athletes With HIV

Divide the class into two teams to debate the question: Should athletes with HIV have to retire? Students on both sides of the argument should support their positions with information about AIDS and HIV.

Writing

AIDS and Discrimination

Ask students to write a poem or short story about the types of discrimination and hardship people with AIDS face. Collect the writings in a book to remain in the classroom.

Review Answers

1. AZT (zidovudine) and DDI (dideoxyinosine) help delay the onset of symptoms. Aerosol pentamidine, breathed into the lungs, helps prevent Pneumocystis carinii pneumonia.
2. Raise money for AIDS programs, volunteer for organizations that help people with AIDS, educate others about HIV infection and AIDS, and treat people who have AIDS with respect, compassion, and acceptance.
3. HIV-positive people fear discrimination and the loss of their jobs.

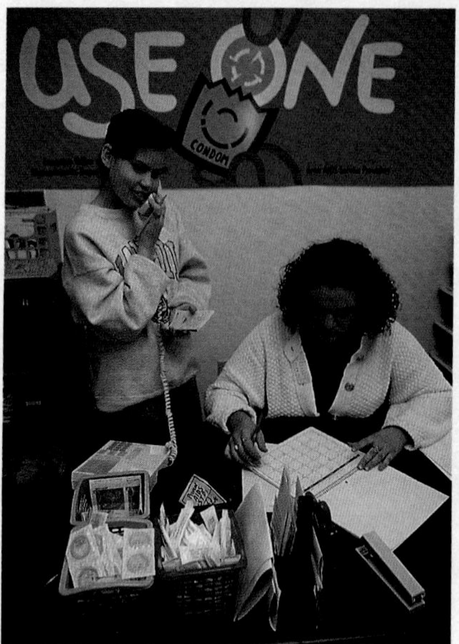

(FIGURE 23-14) **You can help people with HIV infection by doing volunteer work for AIDS organizations. These teens are working at an AIDS education center in Massachusetts.**

for example, they made life rough for him. "Lots of kids in school flattened themselves against walls when I walked by," Ryan said. "When I went to restaurants, people would get up and leave. Even in church, no one would shake my hand."

Michael's friend Bryan was afraid that he would lose his job if people found out he had HIV. Bryan knew only too well that some people think they can become infected with HIV just by being around someone with HIV.

People with HIV infection may face discrimination at work, at school, and in their personal relationships. They must face all this at the same time they are fighting a deadly disease. People with AIDS are sometimes called "AIDS victims." But when you think about their struggle, it is no surprise that they do not want to be thought of as passive "victims."

Take Positive Action Against HIV

You've already learned what you can do to protect yourself against HIV infection. But what can you do to help people who are already infected with HIV?

First, you can help raise money for AIDS programs. Your school or a community organization can sponsor a fundraiser for an agency that gives support to children, adults, and families affected by HIV.

Second, you can do volunteer work for organizations that help people with AIDS. Volunteers may run errands for homebound people with AIDS, deliver food, answer telephones for a hotline, or perform clerical work.

Third, you can educate others. If someone says something that is not true about how HIV is spread, for instance, give him or her the correct information. You can help people with HIV infection by helping others overcome prejudices based on misinformation.

Fourth, and most important, you can treat people with HIV infection as you would any person who has a life-threatening illness—or anyone else, for that matter: with respect, compassion, and acceptance.

Review

1. *Describe medical treatments that may delay the onset of HIV symptoms.*
2. *Name two actions you could take to help people with HIV.*
3. ***Critical Thinking*** *Why do many people with HIV infection choose not to tell their fellow students or co-workers about their HIV test results?*

• • • TEACH continued

Extension

Volunteering

Have students volunteer once a week in some capacity—fundraising, working in a hospice, and so on.

ASSESS

Section Review

Have students answer the Section Review questions.

Alternative Assessment

Have students write a public service announcement that they think will persuade teenagers to treat people with HIV as they would want to be treated if they contracted HIV.

Closure

Ask students to explain why teens have special needs when it comes to HIV prevention.

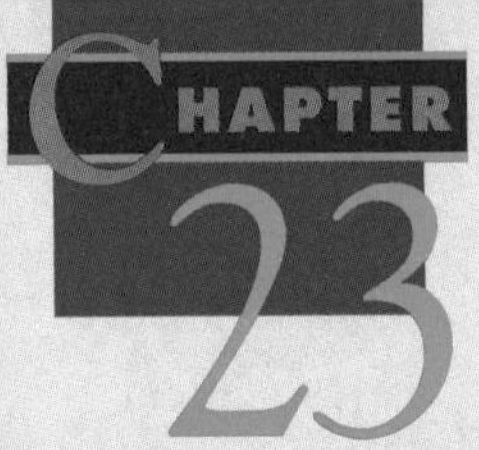

Highlights

Summary

- AIDS is a sexually transmitted disease that is caused by a virus.
- The virus that causes AIDS is called HIV (human immunodeficiency virus).
- AIDS is the last phase of HIV infection.
- Even though an HIV-infected person appears healthy, he or she can still transmit the virus to another person.
- The four behaviors that put a person at risk for getting HIV are: 1) sharing equipment for injecting drugs, tattooing, or ear piercing with an infected person; 2) having vaginal intercourse with an infected person; 3) having oral intercourse with an infected person; and 4) having anal intercourse with an infected person.
- You can find out more about HIV infection by calling the free AIDS hotline number, 1-800-342-2437.
- The behaviors that are most effective in preventing HIV infection are abstinence from sexual intercourse and abstaining from drugs.
- Using latex condoms reduces the risk of sexual transmission of HIV.
- People with HIV infection must struggle with discrimination at the same time they are fighting a deadly disease. They do not want to be thought of as passive "victims."

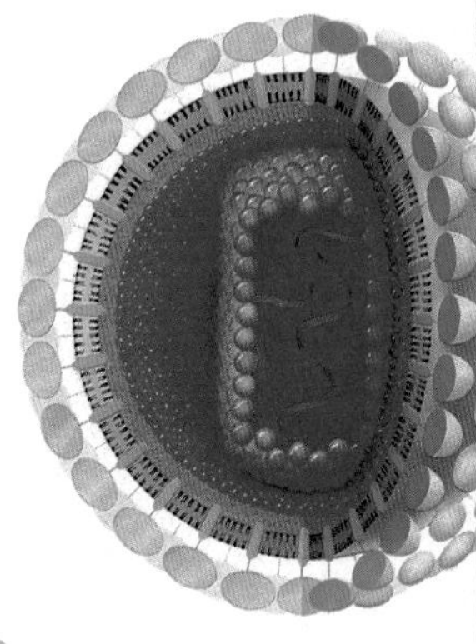

Vocabulary

AIDS a disease, caused by a virus, that harms a person's immune system; AIDS is classified as a sexually transmitted disease, but it can also be spread in other ways, such as through sharing infected equipment for injecting drugs, tattoing, or ear piercing. AIDS is the last stage of HIV infection.

HIV (human immunodeficiency virus) the virus that causes AIDS; also called the "AIDS virus."

mucous membranes moist, pink tissues of the body; HIV can enter the body through the mucous membranes of the mouth, vagina, anus and rectum, and the opening at the tip of the penis.

monogamy when two people have sex with only each other for their entire lives.

condom a covering for the penis that helps protect both partners from sexually transmitted diseases and also helps to prevent pregnancy.

Chapter 23 Highlights Strategies

Summary
Have students read the summary to reinforce the concepts they learned in Chapter 23.

Vocabulary
Have students write a paragraph about AIDS that uses the vocabulary words correctly.

Extension
Have students make AIDS awareness posters to be displayed in the school. The posters could concern myths about AIDS, steps that can be taken to prevent HIV infection, or volunteer opportunities for students to help people with AIDS.

CHAPTER 23 ASSESSMENT

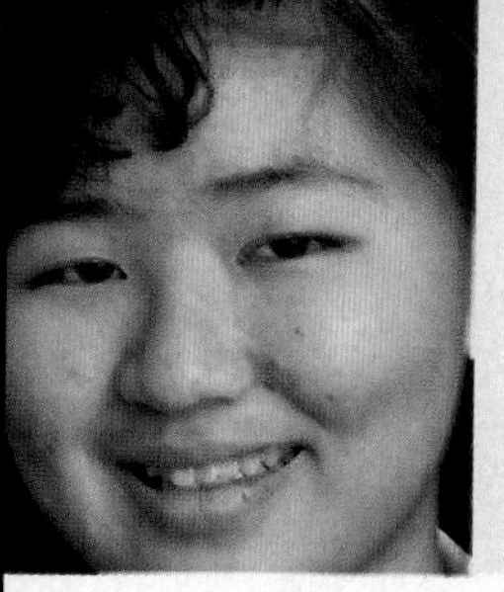

Chapter Review

CHAPTER REVIEW

Concept Review

1. b
2. a
3. a
4. d
5. a
6. c

Expressing Your Views

Sample responses:

1. If an unsterilized needle used to pierce ears was previously used on a person who was HIV-positive, the next person who used it could become infected.

2. Discourage your friend from having sexual intercourse because of the risk of HIV infection, among other reasons. Practicing safer sex does not eliminate the risk of HIV infection. A person who is under the influence of drugs is less likely to practice safe sex.

3. Some people are prejudiced against people who are HIV-positive because they do not fully understand how HIV can be transmitted. They may believe that they could become infected by touching or working near the infected person.

Life Skills Check

Sample student responses:

1. Look in the phone book under AIDS and call an organization that deals with AIDS. Call the local or national AIDS hotline.

2. Condoms can help prevent HIV infection, but they are not 100 percent effective. Abstinence from sexual intercourse, or sexual intercourse only with one other, uninfected partner, is the most effective way to prevent HIV infection.

Concept Review

1. When a person has HIV infection, it means that he or she
   a. has AIDS.
   b. can infect other people with HIV.
   c. has Kaposi's sarcoma.
   d. has used injected drugs.
2. A person can find out if he or she has been infected with HIV by
   a. getting an HIV-antibody test.
   b. calling the AIDS hotline.
   c. asking all previous sexual partners if they are HIV-positive.
   d. talking with a school counselor.
3. Which of the following behaviors can put a person at risk for HIV infection?
   a. sharing needles to inject steroids with an HIV-infected person
   b. sharing a glass of water with an HIV-infected person
   c. sharing an elevator with an HIV infected person
   d. all of the above
4. Which of the following types of sexual intercourse with an HIV-infected person is risky for HIV infection?
   a. vaginal intercourse
   b. oral intercourse
   c. anal intercourse
   d. all of the above
5. Which of the following behaviors provides the best protection against HIV infection?
   a. practicing abstinence from sexual intercourse
   b. using condoms
   c. showering every day
   d. practicing French kissing
6. Which of the following actions would help people with HIV infection?
   a. raising money for agencies that help people with HIV infection
   b. treating people with HIV infection no differently from anyone else who had a life-threatening illness
   c. all of the above

Expressing Your Views

1. You are planning to get your ears pierced. One of your friends offers to pierce your ears for free. What problems could develop in accepting your friend's offer?
2. At a party your best friend gets drunk and confides to you that he or she is going to "do it" tonight. What do you think you should do?
3. Why do you think some people are prejudiced against people who have HIV infection?

Skills Check

1. **Using Community Resources**
   You need to find out if something you are doing is risky behavior for HIV. You feel that you cannot talk to your parents or any of your teachers or counselors. In fact, you feel that you cannot talk about this to anyone you know. How could you get the information you need?

2. **Resisting Pressure**
   You are being pressured by your boyfriend or girlfriend to have sexual intercourse. In talking about this situation with a friend, she tells you that you have nothing to worry about if you use a condom. How would you respond to this statement?

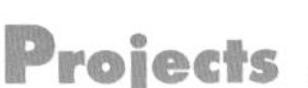

Projects

1. Design a survey to find out how much other students in your school know about HIV infection. Think of five questions to ask in your survey, and work in a group of 3-4 students to collect responses from the whole student body. Tabulate your results and present your data and conclusions to your class.
2. Work with a group of students to come up with a plan to inform the students in your school about HIV prevention. Present your group plan to the principal.
3. Have a health fair at your school in which a variety of health topics are introduced, including HIV infection.

Plan for Action

HIV infection is a communicable disease that can be prevented. Devise a plan to protect yourself from getting infected with HIV.

Projects

Have students plan and carry out the projects for HIV infection and AIDS.

Plan for Action

Hold a class discussion to brainstorm suggestions that could help teenagers

- resist peer pressure to engage in risk behaviors
- avoid situations in which risk behaviors are likely
- promote healthy sexuality without promoting pre-marital sex

ASSESSMENT OPTIONS

Chapter Test

Have students take the Chapter 23 Test.

Alternative Assessment

Have students do the Alternative Assessment activity for Chapter 23.

Test Generator

The Test Generator (Macintosh® or IBM® format) contains an additional 50 assessment items for this chapter.

NONINFECTIOUS DISEASES AND DISORDERS

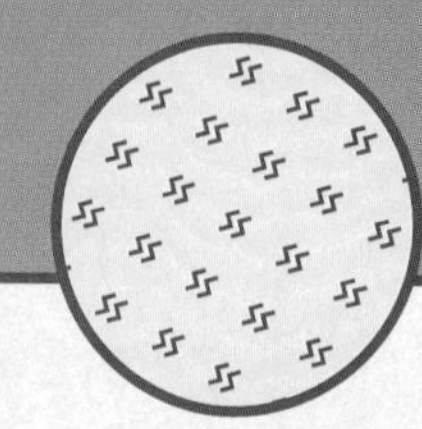

PLANNING GUIDE

TEXT SECTIONS	OBJECTIVES	TEXT FEATURES	OUTSIDE RESOURCES	NOTES
24.1 Hereditary and Congenital Diseases pp. 509-517 2 periods	• Define noninfectious disease. • Distinguish between hereditary and congenital diseases. • List three factors that may cause congenital disease.	**ASSESSMENT** • Section Review, p. 517	**TEACHER'S RESOURCE BINDER** • Lesson Plan 24.1 • Personal Health Inventory • Journal Entry 24A • Section Review Worksheet 24.1 • Section Quiz 24.1 • Reteaching Worksheet 24.1 **OTHER RESOURCES** • Transparency 24A	
24.2 Autoimmune Diseases pp. 518-520 1 period	• List three common autoimmune diseases. • Explain the difference between autoimmune disease and AIDS.	**ASSESSMENT** • Section Review, p. 520	**TEACHER'S RESOURCE BINDER** • Lesson Plan 24.2 • Journal Entry 24B • Section Review Worksheet 24.2 • Section Quiz 24.2 • Reteaching Worksheet 24.2	
24.3 Degenerative Diseases pp. 521-530 3 periods	• Describe what happens to arteries during the development of atherosclerosis. • Explain the relationship between atherosclerosis and high blood pressure. • List five kinds of cancer to which tobacco use contributes. ■ Name four things you can do to reduce your risk of cardiovascular disease. ■ Name two things you can do to reduce your risk of getting cancer.	■ LIFE SKILLS: Practicing Self-Care, pp. 528-529 **ASSESSMENT** • Section Review, p. 530	**TEACHER'S RESOURCE BINDER** • Lesson Plan 24.3 • Journal Entries 24C, 24D • Life Skills 24A, 24B, 24C, 24D • Section Review Worksheet 24.3 • Section Quiz 24.3 • Reteaching Worksheet 24.3 **OTHER RESOURCES** • Transparency 24B, 24C • Making a Choice 24A, 24B	
End of Chapter pp. 531-533		**ASSESSMENT** • Chapter Review, pp. 532-533	**TEACHER'S RESOURCE BINDER** • Chapter Test • Alternative Assessment **OTHER RESOURCES** • Test Generator	

■ Denotes LIFE SKILLS objectives

• Items in blue are also part of the *Holt Health Activity Book.*

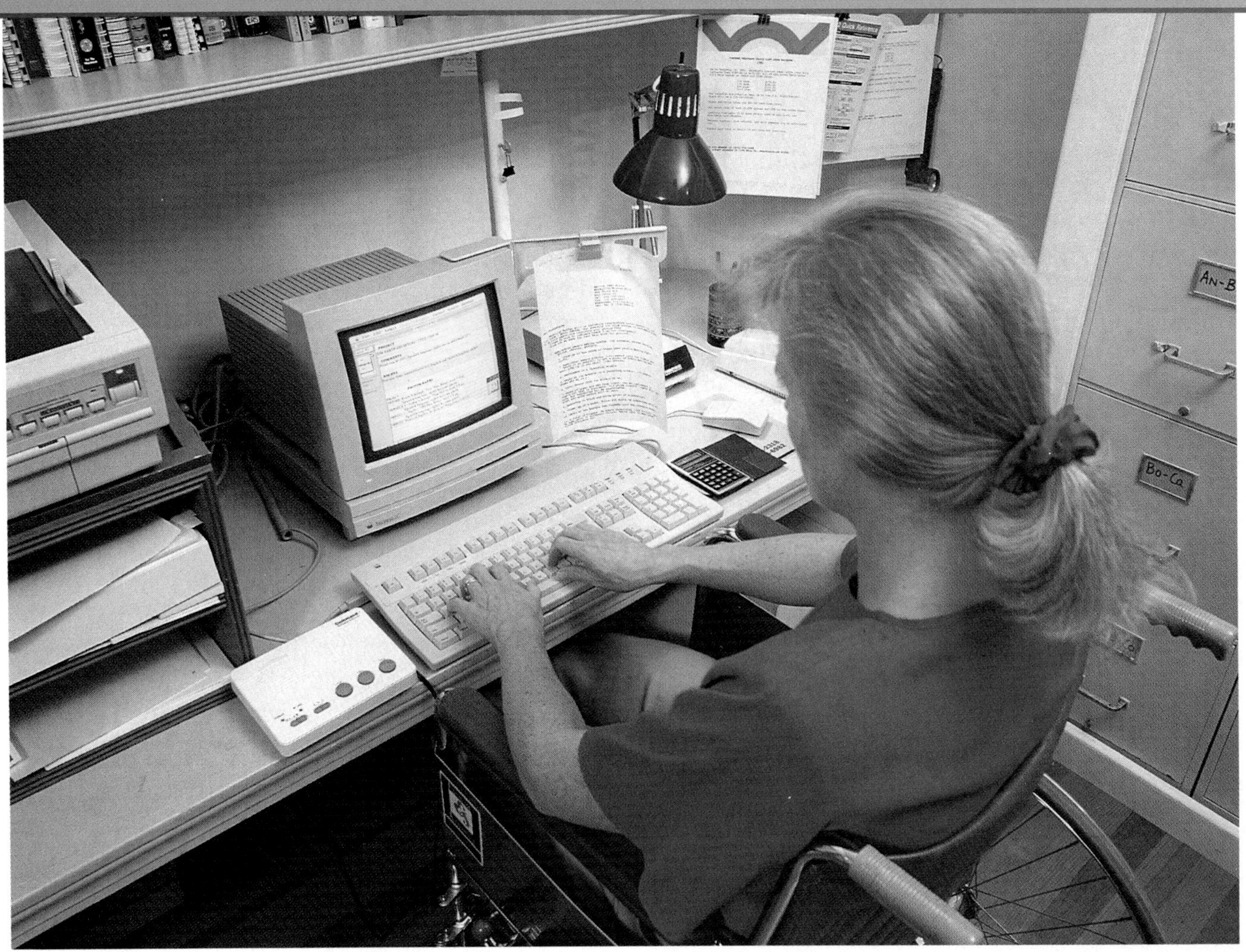

Content Background
Living With Multiple Sclerosis

ONE OF THE FIRST SIGNS MOIRA GRIFFIN had of her multiple sclerosis (MS) was a fall from a horse. As a young woman, she had a job cleaning out a stable and caring for the horses; she thought she was just overtired from the demands of physical labor. To build herself up, she ran and swam every day, and then went into training for a triathlon. But the tiredness persisted, and sometimes the ground would seem to wobble beneath her, or her body would delay in its response to her mental commands to move or stop. She became depressed.

The diagnosis of MS was one of elimination. Tests showed Moira did not have a brain tumor and had not had a stroke. Other tests showed abnormalities with her vision and hearing and her body's sense of position. After her diagnosis, Moira gradually became accustomed to the rhythms of her disease: sometimes she had strength and coordination to ride again (the disease was in remission), sometimes not (a period called exacerbation). The underlying physical cause of the disease was the gradual destruction of areas of the brain or spinal cord called myelin. Small, hard areas called plaques form in the myelin—which is the fatty sheath surrounding nerves—preventing the nerve pathways from functioning normally. As Moira learned, the disease is rarely fatal, but it can eventually cause serious disabilities, including paralysis.

Most people who have MS first experience symptoms between the ages of 20 and 45. In young adults, it is the most common neurological disease of the central nervous system. For some, the disease will appear suddenly, go through one or two attacks, and then move into long-lasting remission. For others, there are less complete remissions or none at all. For about 15 percent, the disease is chronic-progressive, never letting up and resulting in chronic disability. A patient doesn't know at the outset what course the disease will follow with her or him, but most will live a nearly normal life span.

Moira continued to exercise to her limits. She joined a group called Achilles, for disabled people who want to run. Through that experience, she learned that her own disability was not as bad as that of others, and she began to put her disability in perspective. There were still many things she could do: walk to the store, write, paint, and exercise. She did feel angry and defensive in many social situations, however. Sometimes she wondered whether she was somehow to blame for having the disease, though she knew that was not true. The causes of MS are not fully understood; it strikes more women than men and is most common among populations from the colder regions of the world. It does not seem to be hereditary.

People with MS experience various symptoms. For Moira, the most alarming were the breaks into sudden weakness or spasticity, a kind of walking she describes as galumphing. These episodes were embarrassing to her. Other symptoms include tingling, blurred vision, trembling, numbness, bladder problems, and lack of coordination. The disease can be aggravated by emotional upset, infections, overexertion, fatigue, injuries, surgery, and pregnancy. Specific drugs can be used to treat individual symptoms; research is underway to find treatments that will stop MS from progressing once it begins.

Moira worked on maintaining a positive attitude because she knew emotions play a key role in handling the disease. She focused on the abilities she did have. She recalled that when she had been able to do more, she was often critical of herself for not doing better. Now she took pleasure in things just because they were possible. People with chronic conditions often find they can lead full lives focused on activities they like with people they enjoy. They may join support groups for their own diseases, participate in group therapy, or seek individual counseling. One of the greatest problems young people with MS face is maintaining their self-esteem and the feeling of being attractive. Sometimes anger they feel at having the disease makes relations with friends difficult. People with MS must struggle with self-esteem problems and overcome them in much the same way anyone else does. As Moira Griffin explains in her book, *Going the Distance: Living a Full Life with Multiple Sclerosis and Other Debilitating Diseases,* "disabled people are full-fledged individuals with hopes and hates and loves."

PLANNING FOR INSTRUCTION

KEY FACTS

- **A noninfectious disease cannot be passed from person to person either by viruses or other microorganisms.**
- **A hereditary disease, such as sickle cell anemia, cystic fibrosis, or Tay-Sachs disease, is passed from both parents to the child.**
- **A congenital disease is present from birth but is not hereditary. Cerebral palsy and epilepsy are caused by brain damage during pregnancy or birth.**
- **An autoimmune disease occurs when a person's immune system attacks and damages an organ of his or her own body.**
- **Common autoimmune diseases are multiple sclerosis, Type I diabetes, rheumatoid arthritis, Hashimoto's thyroiditis, and Graves' disease.**
- **Degenerative diseases, such as osteoarthritis, cardiovascular diseases, and cancer, result from gradual damage to organs over time.**
- **Cardiovascular disease results in progressive damage to the heart and blood vessels.**

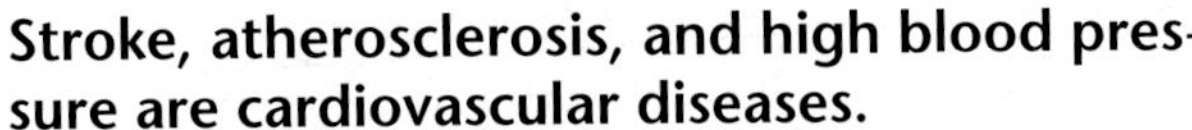

Stroke, atherosclerosis, and high blood pressure are cardiovascular diseases.

- A heart attack occurs when one of the coronary arteries that supply blood to the heart tissue is blocked. A stroke occurs when the blood supply to a part of the brain is cut off.
- Cardiovascular disease and cancer can be prevented or delayed by eating a healthy diet, exercising regularly, and avoiding alcohol and tobacco.

MYTHS AND MISCONCEPTIONS

MYTH: Diseases such as cancer and arthritis can be caught from someone who has the disease.

These diseases are noninfectious and cannot be passed from one person to another by viruses or microorganisms.

MYTH: Both parents must have a disease like sickle cell anemia, cystic fibrosis, or Tay-Sachs disease in order for their children to inherit it.

Each parent may have only one gene for the trait and be a carrier without having the disease. If both parents are carriers, the child may inherit the disease.

MYTH: If someone in your family has cancer, there's nothing you can do to prevent your contracting the disease.

Cancer can be prevented by eating a healthy diet with less fat and avoiding alcohol, tobacco, and overexposure to the sun.

VOCABULARY

Essential: The following vocabulary terms appear in boldface type:

noninfectious disease	**cardiovascular disease**
hereditary disease	**atherosclerosis**
chromosomes	**arteriosclerosis**
gene	**high blood pressure**
congenital disease	**coronary arteries**
autoimmune disease	**stroke**
degenerative disease	**cancer**

Secondary: Be aware that the following terms may come up during class discussion:

sickle cell anemia	cerebral palsy
cystic fibrosis	epilepsy
Down's syndrome	multiple sclerosis
muscular dystrophy	rheumatoid arthritis
diabetes	malignant tumor
asthma	benign tumor

FOR STUDENTS WITH SPECIAL NEEDS

At-Risk Students: Provide students with the name of a young person who has one of the noninfectious diseases, such as multiple sclerosis or Type I diabetes. Encourage students to correspond with the young person. Mutual encourage-ment may help both the at-risk students and the person with the disease to achieve their goals in life.

Less-Advanced Students: Some students may have difficulty in remembering the different hereditary, congenital, autoimmune, and degenerative diseases. Write these titles each on a separate piece of paper. Give students self-stick note sheets on which to write the names of the diseases discussed in the chapter. Have them stick each name under the proper category of disease.

ENRICHMENT

- Have students write a story about someone who has a noninfectious disease, showing how the disease changes the person's life and how he or she has learned to cope with it.
- Arrange for a speaker from one of the foundations established to assist those with a noninfectious disease to address the class. Ask the speaker to tell stories about some of the people they have helped. Have students prepare questions about the disease being discussed.

Chapter 24 Chapter Opener

GETTING STARTED

Using the Chapter Photograph
Ask students how the person in the picture is dealing with his or her illness in a way that will help him or her to achieve the same goals that others achieve in the class. Discuss how mainstreaming helps both the student with a health problem and the others in the class.

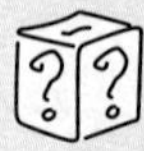

Question Box
Have students write out anonymously any questions they have about noninfectious diseases and put them in the Question Box. To ensure that students with questions are not embarrassed to be seen writing, have those who do not have questions write a fact they already know about noninfectious diseases on the paper instead.

Preview the questions and then answer them at appropriate points in the chapter. You may wish to allow students to write additional questions as they go through the chapter.

Personal Issues *ALERT*
Discussion of diseases may make students uncomfortable. Some students or someone close to them may have one of the noninfectious diseases. They might be interested in finding out more about the disease, or they might be embarrassed and want to avoid the subject. Prepare the class to be respectful of privacy, and receptive and sensitive to other people's feelings.

Chapter 24

Noninfectious Diseases and Disorders

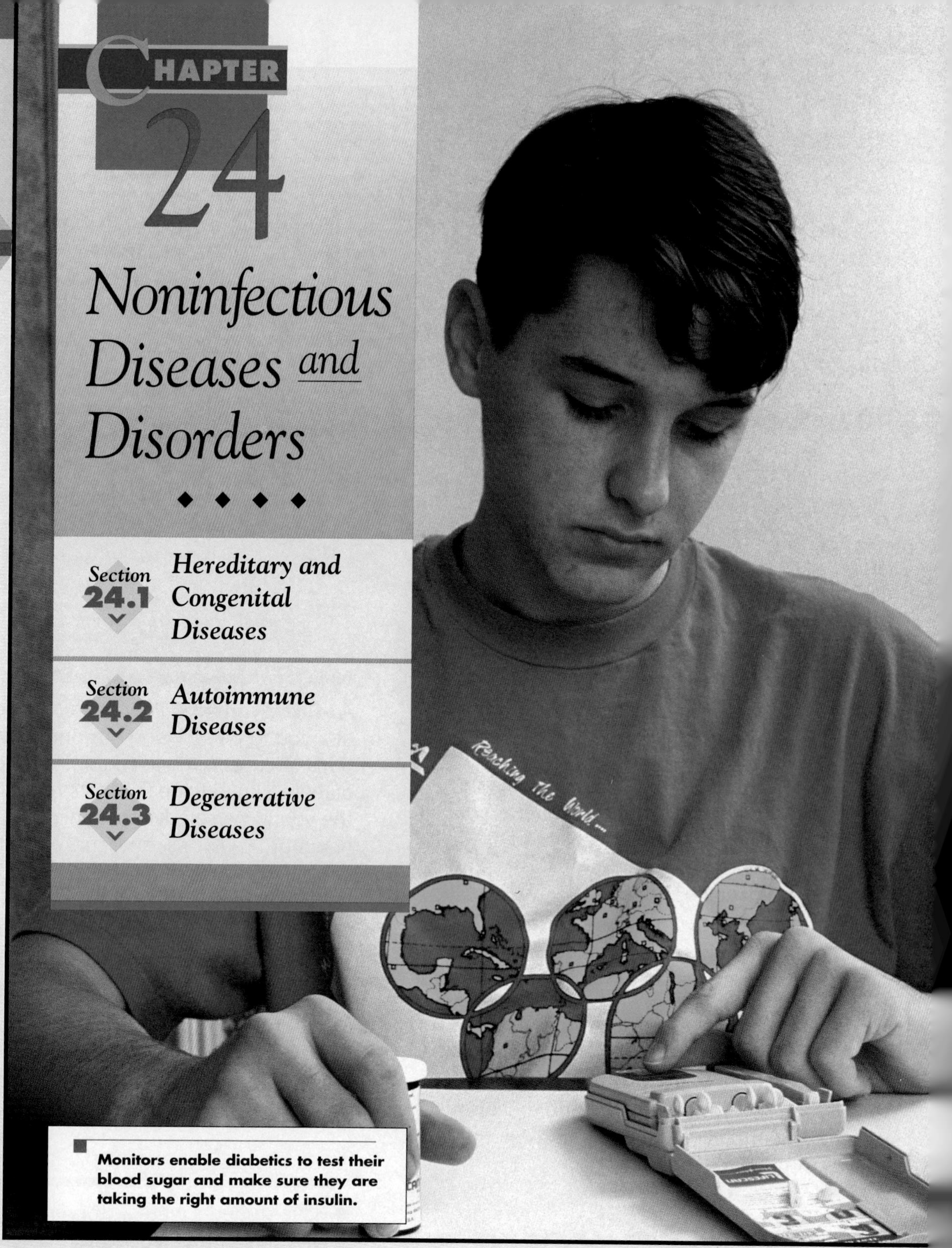

Monitors enable diabetics to test their blood sugar and make sure they are taking the right amount of insulin.

Shawn's pretty lucky; he had ear infections and a case of the chickenpox when he was very young, but during the last few years the only disease he's had to worry about has been an occasional cold. Some of the people he knows, and even some people in his own family, have had much more serious illnesses. His mother has high blood pressure. His cousin has sickle cell anemia. And two years ago, his grandfather died of lung cancer. Shawn has some questions about these diseases.

For example, is there any need to worry about being around people who have these diseases? Are any of them "catching"? Could he inherit high blood pressure from his mother, or lung cancer from his grandfather? Is there anything he can do to avoid getting these diseases?

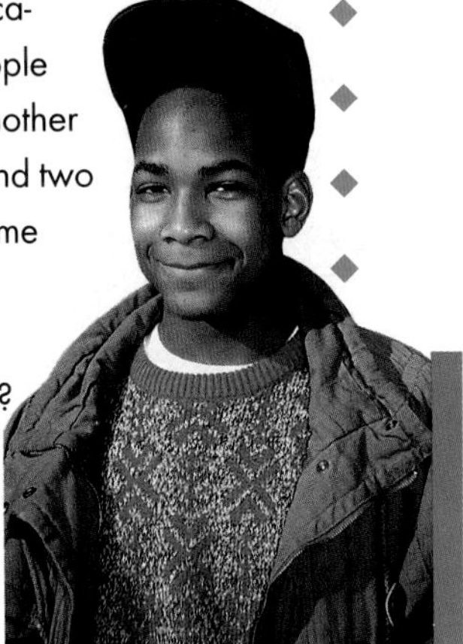

Personal Health Inventory

Have students complete the Personal Health Inventory for this chapter. The inventory helps them assess their experience of noninfectious diseases.

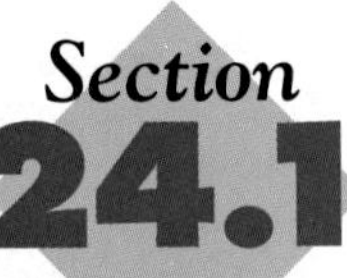

Section 24.1 Hereditary and Congenital Diseases

Objectives

- *Define noninfectious disease.*
- *Distinguish between hereditary and congenital diseases.*
- *List three factors that may cause congenital disease.*

High blood pressure, sickle cell anemia, and cancer are all examples of **noninfectious diseases**. A disease is a condition that prevents your body from functioning normally. When a disease is noninfectious, it means that you can't catch it from viruses or microorganisms that pass from another person, or other organism. You can "catch" a cold from your sniffling, sneezing best friend, because some of the viruses that are attacking your friend's nose and throat leave your friend's body and attack your nose and throat. You can't catch cancer or sickle cell anemia, though, because they are not caused by viruses or microorganisms.

There are many different noninfectious diseases. Some people are born with a disease such as sickle cell anemia or cystic fibrosis and are affected by the disease throughout their lives. Other noninfectious diseases, like cancer and heart disease, usually show up later in life. When you say that a person was "born with" a certain disease, you are referring to either a hereditary or a congenital disease.

Hereditary Diseases

A **hereditary disease** is a disease caused by defective genetic information passed from one or both parents to a child. In order to understand how this happens, it is important

REMINDER

A microorganism is a living thing that can be seen only under a microscope.

noninfectious disease: *a disease that a person cannot catch from another person or any other organism.*

hereditary disease: *a disease caused by defective genes passed from one or both parents to a child.*

Section 24.1 Lesson Plan

MOTIVATE

Journal 24A
Finding Out About Diseases

This may be done as a warm-up activity. Encourage students to record in the Student Journal in the Student Activity Book their concerns about diseases they have heard about. They could also write their reactions to Shawn's concerns about the diseases of those around him and include similar concerns of their own.

Cooperative Learning
Infectious vs. Noninfectious Diseases

Have students form small groups to discuss the difference between infectious and noninfectious diseases. Have them list ways to avoid getting both kinds of diseases.

TEACH

Class Discussion
Inheriting a Disease

Write on the chalkboard: Some diseases can be inherited from parents. **How can a disease be inherited?** *[If a gene inherited from one parent has incorrect information, it can cause a hereditary disease.]* **What is a gene?** *[A gene is a short segment of the DNA molecule that serves as a code for a particular bit*

Background

Adaptive Value of the Sickle Cell Gene

People who carry one gene for sickle cell anemia are much less susceptible to malaria, a disease that is a leading cause of death in certain parts of Africa. This explains why, although people who have both genes for sickle cell anemia die from the disease before they are old enough to reproduce the gene, it is still passed on by parents who have just one gene for the condition.

chromosomes: *cell structures that carry hereditary information.*

gene: *a short segment of the DNA molecule that serves as a code for a particular bit of genetic information.*

to know something about heredity. Many of your characteristics, such as the way you look and certain talents you have, were passed on to you from your parents. This kind of information is carried from your parents to you in the form of tiny structures within the body's cells known as **chromosomes**. Chromosomes contain the hereditary material deoxyribonucleic acid, better known as DNA.

Each chromosome is made up of thousands of genes. A **gene**, which serves as a code for a particular bit of inherited information, is a short segment of the DNA in a chromosome. The genes that you inherited from your parents determined many of your characteristics; for example, whether you have blue, green, or brown eyes. Tens of thousands of genes determine the inherited characteristics of an individual. Genes don't always carry correct information, however. If one single gene does have incorrect information, it can cause a hereditary disease.

Sickle Cell Anemia One hereditary disease that occurs when genes carry incorrect instructions is sickle cell anemia, the illness Shawn's cousin Nelson has. The genes that carry incorrect information in Nelson's body affect the construction of a protein called hemoglobin. This protein, which is found inside the body's red blood cells, carries oxygen from the lungs to the other tissues in the body.

Because the hemoglobin inside Nelson's red blood cells isn't constructed correctly, the hemoglobin forms long, stiff chains. This causes the red blood cells—normally smooth, round disks—to sickle, or become spiky, such as those that are shown in Figure 24-2.

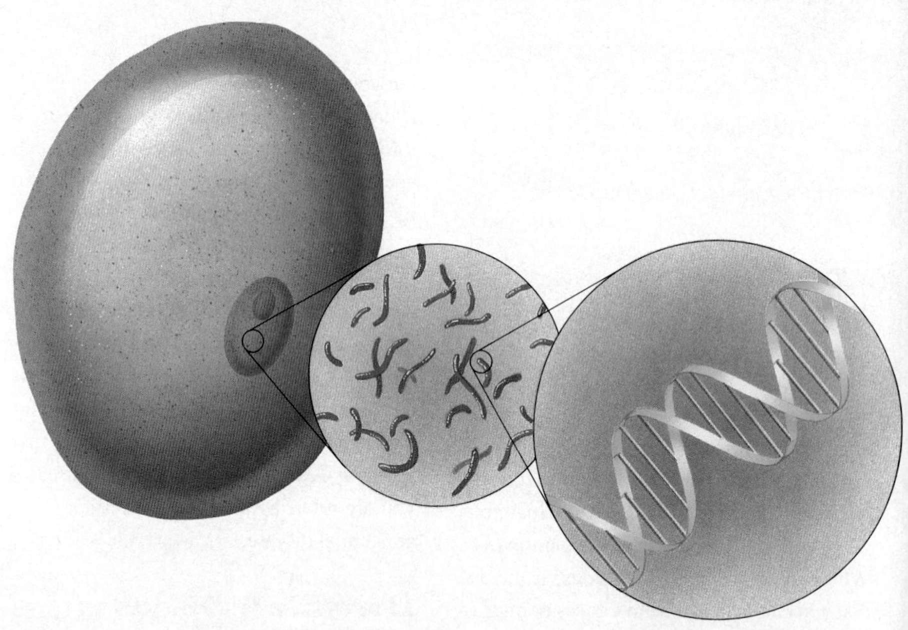

(FIGURE 24-1) **Each chromosome in the cell nucleus contains a DNA molecule. The genes that determine all your inherited characteristics are segments of a DNA molecule.**

• • • TEACH continued

of genetic information that provides a person with a characteristic he or she receives from a parent.] **What is sickle cell anemia?** *[Sickle cell anemia is a hereditary disease that causes the hemoglobin in the red blood cells to have a different shape. This causes the red blood cells to become stuck inside the smallest blood vessels. This in turn causes intense pain and damage to the vital organs.]* **From which parent does a child inherit sickle cell anemia?** *[For a child to inherit sickle cell anemia, he or she has to inherit a gene for the disease from each parent.]*

Teaching Transparency 24A
Cell Nucleus, Chromosomes, and DNA

Show the illustration of a chromosome with the DNA blowup (Figure 24-1). Ask students to describe how the chromosomes separate during meiosis.

Reinforcement
Genes Specific to Geographic Locations

Remind students that one in ten African-Americans carries one gene for sickle cell anemia. One in twenty white Americans carries one gene for cystic fibrosis. People of eastern European extraction are more likely to have a gene for Tay-Sachs disease. At one time, these genes may have had a useful function, due to climate or other environmental factors.

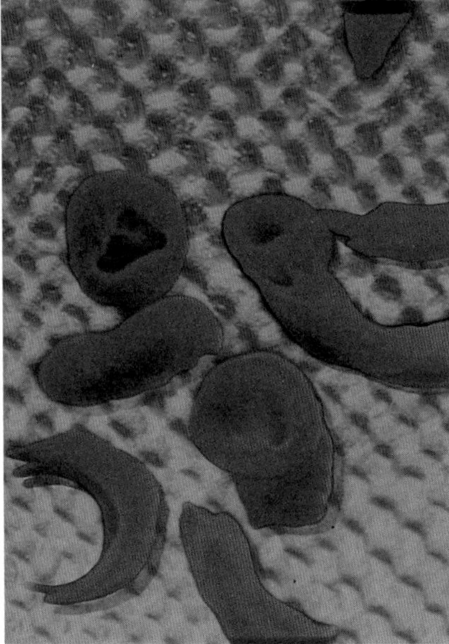

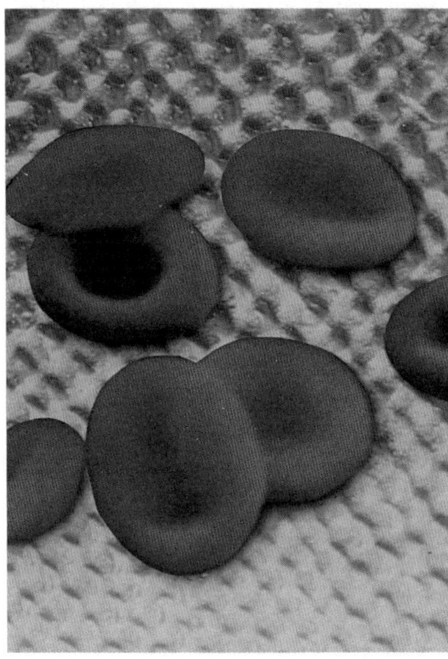

(FIGURE 24-2) **The red blood cells of a person who has sickle cell anemia (left) become long, spiky, and sickled. Note how different they look from normal red blood cells (right).**

Anything that reduces oxygen in Nelson's body, such as stress, respiratory disease, or strenuous exercise, can cause a sickle cell crisis. During the crisis, a high percentage of red blood cells sickle. Spiky, sickled red blood cells rupture easily and tend to become stuck inside the smallest blood vessels, the tiny capillaries. Intense pain and damage to vital organs may result.

For a person to have sickle cell anemia, he or she must inherit two copies of the sickle cell gene, one from each parent. People who have inherited only one sickle cell gene from one parent are usually quite healthy. Almost 10 percent of African-American people carry the gene for sickle cell anemia.

Cystic Fibrosis The most common serious inherited disease among white Americans is cystic fibrosis. Cystic fibrosis is a hereditary disease that results in the secretion of very thick mucus in the lungs and digestive tract.

Unlike normal mucus, which is regularly cleared from the lungs, the thick mucus produced by people with cystic fibrosis builds up and blocks small air passages inside the lungs. This makes breathing difficult and increases the likelihood of lung infections. Mucus in the digestive tract interferes with the action of digestive enzymes. Because of this, people with cystic fibrosis have difficulty getting adequate nourishment from their food.

The symptoms of cystic fibrosis can be treated with physical therapy and drugs that loosen mucus in the lungs. These drugs may be delivered to the lungs by using a vaporizer, like the one shown in Figure 24-3. Unfortunately, this treatment provides only temporary relief. Cystic fibrosis is a very serious, and eventually fatal, disease.

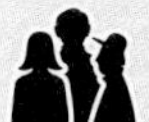

Cooperative Learning
Disease Symptoms

Have students work in groups to make a chart that shows the symptoms of the hereditary diseases studied so far.

Class Discussion
Genetic Counseling

Discuss with students that when couples plan to marry, they often seek genetic counseling to find out if there is a possibility that they would have children with one of these diseases: sickle cell anemia, cystic fibrosis, or Tay-Sachs disease. Someone with one gene for one of these diseases would take a serious risk for their future children by marrying someone who also has the gene. Have students offer their opinions on what a couple could do if they found out they both carried the gene. Mention that with each birth there would be one chance in four that the child would have a serious disease and would die before growing up. In addition, there would only be one chance in four that they would have a child without any gene for the disease in question. There would be a 50 percent chance that every child born to this couple would have one gene for the disease.

Reinforcement
Cystic Fibrosis

Remind students that in cystic fibrosis an unusually thick and sticky mucus interferes with the normal functioning of the lungs and the digestive system. It also blocks sweat glands, making peo-

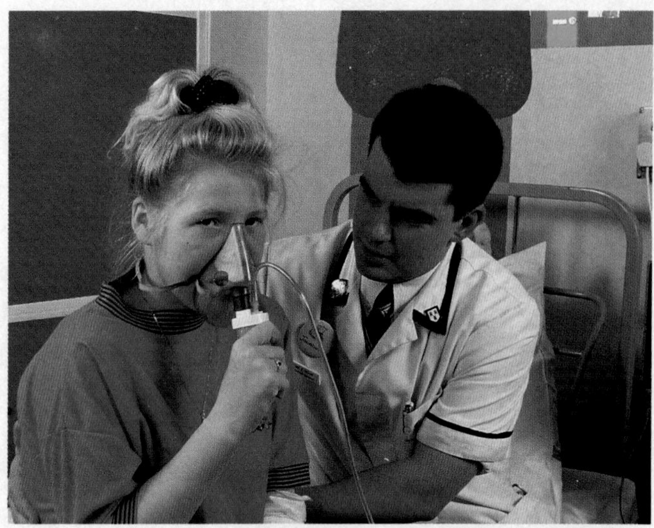

(FIGURE 24-3) **Cystic fibrosis causes mucus to build up and block air passages in the lungs. Vaporizers that deliver special medications to clear these air passages can help people with this disease breathe more easily.**

Like sickle cell anemia, cystic fibrosis strikes only those who have inherited two cystic fibrosis genes—one from each parent. About one in twenty white Americans carries one gene for cystic fibrosis.

Tay-Sachs Disease Tay-Sachs disease is a condition caused by a defective gene that causes fat to accumulate in the brain, destroying normal brain tissue. Although babies born with Tay-Sachs seem normal at first, by the time they are a few months old, symptoms begin to appear. These symptoms include seizures, mental retardation, and blindness. Death generally occurs by the age of three or four.

The gene that causes Tay-Sachs disease is most common in families of eastern European origin.

Muscular Dystrophy Muscular dystrophy refers to several genetic diseases that cause muscles to weaken and degenerate. One of the more common forms, Duchenne muscular dystrophy, affects only boys.

Children with this form of muscular dystrophy develop normally at first, but between the ages of two and ten, they become clumsy and uncoordinated as their muscles begin to weaken. As the disease progresses, they have difficulty standing and they fall frequently. By their teens, people with muscular dystrophy must use a wheelchair. The disease is fatal when it progresses to the point that the muscles that control breathing fail. This usually occurs in the sufferer's early twenties.

There is currently no cure for muscular dystrophy. However, the gene that is responsible for Duchenne muscular dystrophy has been identified and the protein for which it codes is being studied. Researchers hope that better understanding will lead to an effective treatment for this disease.

Diabetes Mellitus Diabetes is a disease that results when a substance called insulin is lacking in, or is not used properly by, the body. Insulin is a natural chemical that helps blood sugar enter the body's cells. Blood sugar is the body's major source of energy, even for people who don't eat many sweets. Starchy foods like potatoes and rice contain sugars that are broken down and used for energy. But when insulin is lacking or cannot be used properly, as is the case in people with diabetes, the body's cells are unable to use the blood sugar that enters them.

When a person's cells cannot use sugars for energy, the cells begin to use fats and proteins for energy. Breaking down large amounts of fats and proteins produces dangerous levels of toxic waste products. For this reason, diabetes that is not treated is often fatal.

The most common form of diabetes, called Type II diabetes, usually appears in middle age. People with Type II diabetes do produce insulin; however, their bodies cannot use it properly. There is evidence

• • • TEACH continued

ple with the disease unusually sensitive to heat. The recent discovery of the gene locus for the disease may permit the detection of the disease before it shows itself in families.

Class Discussion
Coping With Diabetes

Discuss with students the symptoms of diabetes and the necessary lifestyle changes that a person who is diagnosed with the disease must make. **What lifestyle changes do people diagnosed with diabetes have to make?** *[Those with Type II diabetes have to adhere to a strict, balanced diet and exercise. People with Type I must take daily injections of insulin.]*

Case Study
Allergies

Have students put together a case study of a person with allergies. They should describe the difficulties the person has in pinpointing the substances causing the allergies.

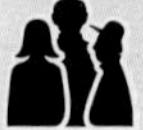

Cooperative Learning
Asthma

Have students prepare a skit in which an asthma patient discusses his or her problem with a doctor. The doctor should explain what happens when a person has an asthma attack. Have the doctor discuss the treatment needed. The patient should ask meaningful questions specific to asthma.

that Type II diabetes is hereditary. Studies have shown that if one identical twin has Type II diabetes, there is a 100-percent chance that the other twin will have the disease. Other factors that may contribute to the onset of Type II diabetes include age and obesity. Type II diabetes can usually be controlled by a strict, healthy diet (most Type II diabetics are obese) and exercise. Drug therapy may also be recommended for those whose diabetes cannot be controlled by diet alone.

Type I diabetes is a more serious form of the disease that usually begins during childhood. Only about 10 percent of diabetics have Type I diabetes. Unlike Type II diabetes, Type I diabetes does not appear to be an inherited illness. People with Type I diabetes must take daily injections of insulin to replace this substance, which is missing from their body. You'll learn more about Type I diabetes in the next section.

Allergies Allergies affect about one of every seven people in the United States—more than 35 million Americans. An allergy is the overreaction of a person's immune system to a common substance—such as dust, pollen, certain foods, mold spores, or animals—that has no effect on nonallergic people. Allergies are usually inherited.

Allergic reactions take many forms. When an inhaled substance triggers an allergic attack, the person may experience a stuffy nose, red itchy eyes, and sinus pain. Allergies to foods or certain drugs sometimes cause hives, itchy welts, or bumps to develop on the skin.

Although allergies are generally not life-threatening, they do make life miserable. If you have an allergy, the best way to treat it is to avoid the thing that you're allergic to. For example, if you are allergic to cat dander and saliva, as many people are, you'd be wise to choose another kind of pet.

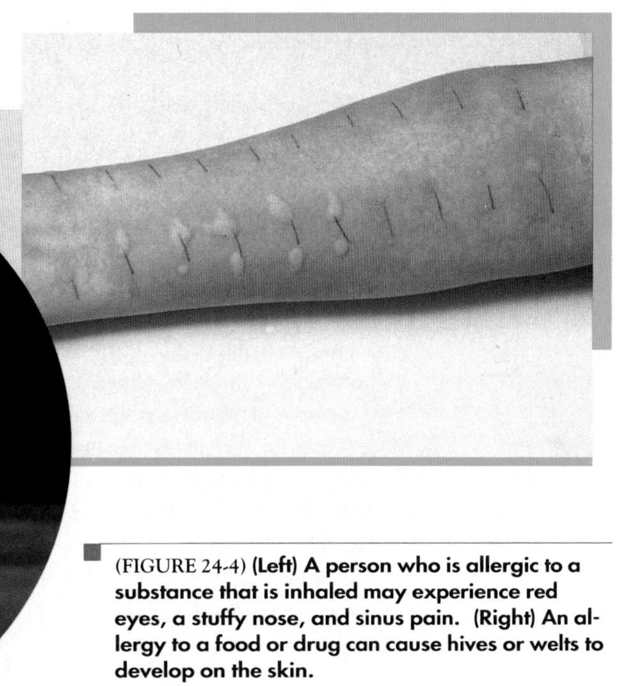

(FIGURE 24-4) **(Left) A person who is allergic to a substance that is inhaled may experience red eyes, a stuffy nose, and sinus pain. (Right) An allergy to a food or drug can cause hives or welts to develop on the skin.**

SECTION 24.1

Background
Epilepsy
Living tissue from the brain of a person with epilepsy has been placed in a chamber with circulating fluids at body temperature, to be studied in the laboratory. A microelectrode records the electrical activity of individual cells. Drugs can be tested on this tissue to control the excessive electrical activity of the cells. This unusual experiment has yielded useful information for treating the disease.

Class Discussion
Congenital vs. Hereditary Disease

How does a congenital disease differ from a hereditary disease? *[A congenital disease is caused by an incident that occurred during pregnancy or at birth, whereas a hereditary disease is caused by an abnormal gene.]* **What is an example of an incident occurring during pregnancy that could cause a disease in the child?** *[If a woman has German measles during pregnancy, her child may be born with cataracts or heart defects. Exposure to drugs, radiation, or pollutants in the environment could also cause congenital diseases.]*

Class Discussion
Cerebral Palsy

What causes cerebral palsy? *[Brain damage resulting from lack of oxygen during a difficult birth as well as exposure during pregnancy to radiation, certain drugs, and some diseases.]* **What are the symptoms of cerebral palsy?** *[A person with severe cerebral palsy cannot control his or her muscles. The person may not be able to walk or talk because both of these functions require the use of muscles. Some people with cerebral palsy are retarded, but others have normal intelligence.]*

Class Discussion
Epilepsy

What does an electroencephalograph measure? *[It measures the electrical im-*

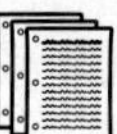

Section Review Worksheet 24.1

Assign Section Review Worksheet 24.1, which requires students to complete a network and sentences to demonstrate understanding of heredity and congenital diseases.

Section Quiz 24.1

Have students take Section Quiz 24.1.

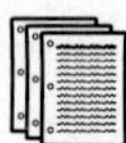

Reteaching Worksheet 24.1

Students who have difficulty with the material may complete Reteaching Worksheet 24.1, which requires them to recognize hereditary diseases and their causes.

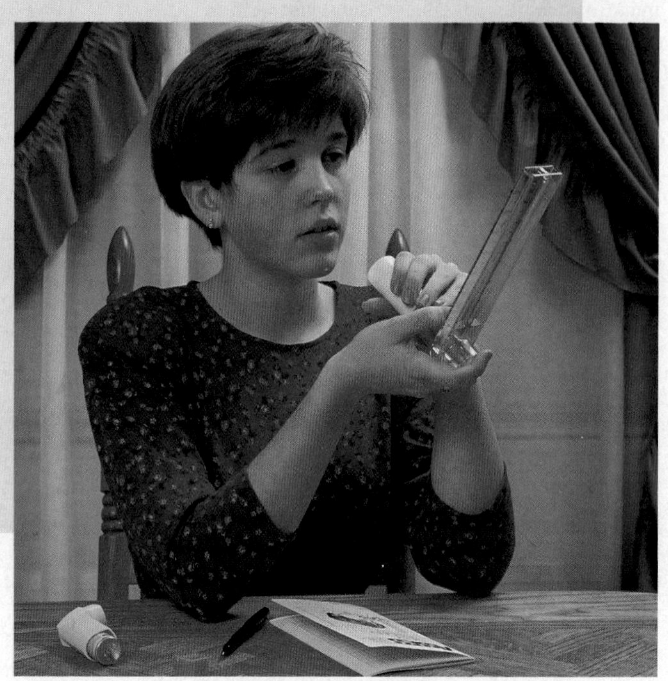

(FIGURE 24-5) **Specially prescribed inhalers can prevent asthma attacks or lessen their severity.**

If you're allergic to house dust, on the other hand, you will suffer much less if you live in a house that has wood or tile floors rather than carpeting.

Sometimes it is simply impossible to avoid the substance causing the allergic reaction. In that case, medicines called antihistamines can help relieve the allergic symptoms. Histamine is the substance released by the immune system that causes the unpleasant effects of an allergy. Antihistamines work by interfering with the action of histamine. Some allergies can also be treated by a series of injections that reduce the sensitivity of the allergic person to a particular substance.

Asthma Even though hay fever or hives can make a person very uncomfortable, these types of allergic reactions are not really serious. However, about 15 million people suffer from asthma, which is a very serious disease that is often a form of allergic reaction.

Take a deep breath. The air you just inhaled travels through a series of air passages that branch into smaller and smaller tubes inside your lungs. These tubes are encircled by small muscles that adjust the width of the tubes.

Changing the diameter of the tubes is one of the ways in which your body adapts to allow you to take in more air when you are exercising, and less air when you are sitting quietly.

During an asthmatic attack, these muscles overreact, causing the air passages to become constricted. Taking in enough air becomes very difficult. To make matters worse, the linings of the air passages may swell and become filled with mucus. Sometimes the small tubes collapse and make it even more difficult to exhale than it is to inhale.

An asthmatic attack can be life-threatening. More than 4,000 people a year die from asthma, and the number is increasing. Fortunately, there are effective treatments for asthma. Most deaths from asthma occur because the person had not been diagnosed or was not getting proper treatment.

Once they understand that asthma must never be taken lightly, asthmatics can usually lead normal, healthy lives, provided they faithfully follow the treatment prescribed by a doctor. Drugs breathed into the lungs from an inhaler, like the one shown in Figure 24-5, can often prevent asthmatic attacks or reduce their severity.

Such treatments have made it much safer for people with asthma to participate in athletic activities. In fact, not only is exercise beneficial for most people with

• • • TEACH continued

pulses generated by the nerve cells of the brain.] **If it is normal to have electrical impulses in the brain, what is epilepsy?** *[Epilepsy is abnormal electrical activity in the brain.]*

Role-Playing

Helping Someone With a Seizure

Have students role-play a family who is expecting a visit from a cousin with epilepsy. They should discuss what everyone should do if the cousin has an epileptic seizure. They should also discuss how to handle the time after the seizure, so that the relative feels support and understanding from the family.

Extension

Research on Noninfectious Diseases

Have students investigate the organizations that sponsor research on such diseases as muscular dystrophy, cystic fibrosis, sickle cell anemia, and Tay-Sachs disease. Encourage students to find out how they can help the organization of their choice. Have them collect brochures telling of the research being done on one of the diseases and post them on the bulletin board, to be followed by a discussion.

asthma, but many people with this condition excel at sports.

A person with asthma who does perform strenuous exercise, however, must follow certain precautions. For some people, this may mean avoiding exercising in cold, dry air or where air pollution levels are high. To prevent attacks, most asthmatics must take medication before engaging in strenuous exercise.

Down's Syndrome: An Inherited Disorder

One in 600 babies is born in the United States each year with a disorder called Down's syndrome. Down's syndrome is caused by the presence of an extra chromosome in body cells.

Normally, cells in the human body contain 46 chromosomes. The exceptions are the sperm and egg cells, which each contain 23 chromosomes. When the sperm and egg unite at fertilization, the fertilized egg has the normal complete set of 46. Sometimes, however, a sperm or egg with 24 chromosomes is produced. Sperm with extra chromosomes are usually so abnormal that they are unable to fertilize an egg. For this reason, sperm with extra chromosomes are unlikely to contribute to the formation of an abnormal embryo. However, an egg with an extra chromosome can be fertilized.

Having an extra chromosome always causes serious problems in the development of an embryo. In most cases, the deformities caused by the extra chromosome are so severe that the embryo dies before birth. Survival is possible, however, if the extra chromosome is one of the smaller ones. Down's syndrome results when there is an extra copy of chromosome 21, one of the smallest chromosomes.

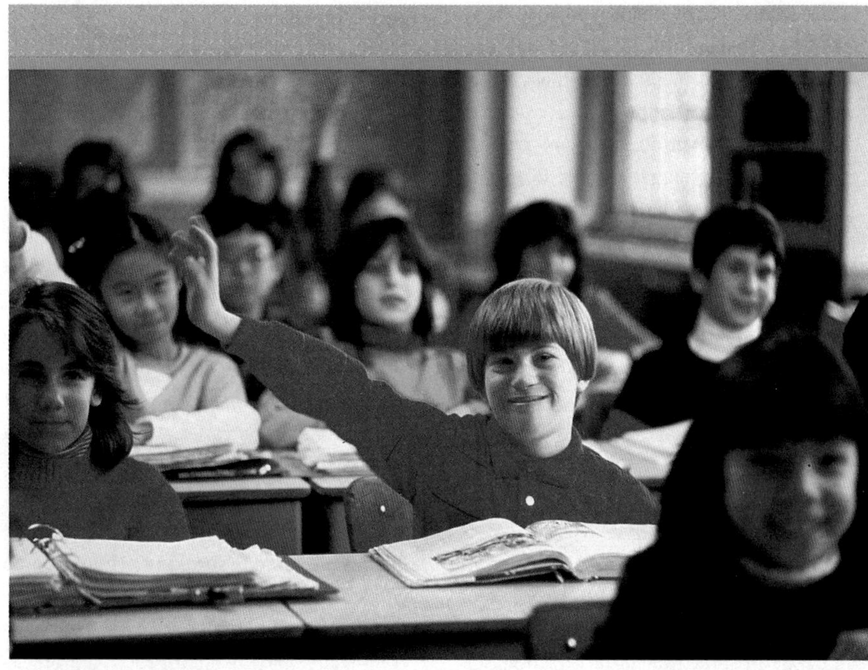

(FIGURE 24-6) **Down's syndrome results from an extra copy of chromosome 21 in body cells.**

Background

Cause of Down's Syndrome

The extra copy of chromosome 21 present in persons with Down's syndrome occurs more often in eggs of women over age 30. For women in their twenties, the possibility of giving birth to a Down's child is 1 in 1,400 births. In those between the ages of 30 and 35, the risk increases to 1 in 750, while for those over 45, it rises to 1 in 16 births. The overall incidence is about 1 in 700 live births. It is possible to tell, on the basis of tests comparing the parents' and child's chromosomes, whether the egg or the sperm carried an extra chromosome 21. It has been found that about 20 percent of Down's syndrome cases are attributable to an extra paternal chromosome.

Every person who is born with Down's syndrome suffers from mental retardation, although the degree of retardation varies from person to person. Some people with Down's syndrome also suffer a defective thyroid gland or other health problems. The severity of the symptoms of Down's syndrome varies greatly. People born with Down's syndrome who have the less severe symptoms often live long and healthy lives. On the other hand, heart defects, which are fairly common in babies with Down's syndrome, may be so serious that they are fatal in infancy.

Genetic Screening Owing to sophisticated genetic testing and prenatal screening, couples who are planning to have babies can find out whether they are at risk of passing defective genes on to their unborn children. Tests can determine the presence of genes that may carry Tay-Sachs disease, cystic fibrosis, and sickle cell anemia.

In addition, a woman who may be at risk of having a child with a hereditary disorder can undergo specific tests that can detect some genetic defects. For example, women who are over the age of 35 are at a higher risk than younger women of giving birth to a child with Down's syndrome. Many doctors recommend that pregnant women over the age of 35 undergo a test called amniocentesis, given at the end of a woman's first trimester of pregnancy. Amniocentesis can detect the presence of Down's syndrome, as well as other chromosomal defects.

Fetal alcohol syndrome is also discussed in Chapter 13.

Congenital Diseases

A **congenital disease** is a disease that is present from birth but is not hereditary. In other words, a congenital disease is not caused by an abnormal gene present in the egg or sperm at the time of fertilization, but by an accident or incident that happened during the pregnancy or birth. For example, if a woman has rubella (German measles) during pregnancy, her baby may be born with cataracts or heart defects. Besides certain diseases, exposure during pregnancy to certain drugs or to environmental dangers such as radiation or pollutants can cause congenital disease.

congenital disease:

a disease that is present from birth, but is not hereditary.

Fetal Alcohol Syndrome One drug that can cause a serious congenital disease is alcohol. A woman who drinks alcohol during pregnancy is at risk of having a baby with fetal alcohol syndrome. The symptoms of this congenital disease include small size, mental retardation, facial deformities, and heart defects.

Many doctors believe that a milder form of fetal alcohol syndrome, which may result in mental retardation with less obvious physical deformities, can be caused by drinking smaller amounts of alcohol during pregnancy. For this reason, pregnant women are often advised to drink no alcohol during pregnancy.

Cerebral Palsy Cerebral palsy is caused by brain damage that results in a form of paralysis that makes it impossible for a person to control his or her muscles. The muscles may be limp and unresponsive, or they may contract in a random and uncontrolled way. The type of paralysis that causes muscles to contract randomly is known as spastic paralysis.

The inability to control muscles may result in the inability to walk and in facial expressions that don't seem appropriate to the situation. People with cerebral palsy sometimes find it difficult or impossible to talk, because of the difficulty of controlling the muscles used in speaking. Some people with cerebral palsy have mental retardation. But many people with cerebral palsy are of completely normal intelligence and are as capable of achievement as those born without the disease.

Review Answers

1. A noninfectious disease is one that a person cannot catch from another person, animal, or other organism. An infectious disease is one that a person can catch in any of these ways.

2. A hereditary disease is caused by a defective gene or genes passed from one or both parents to a child. A congenital disease is present from birth but is not hereditary. A hereditary disease involved a defective gene that was present in the egg or the sperm, or both, at the time of fertilization. A congenital disease is not caused by an accident or incident that happened during the pregnancy or birth.

The brain damage that causes cerebral palsy can result from several factors. Lack of oxygen during a difficult birth is one possible cause of the disease, but it can also be caused by exposure during pregnancy to radiation, certain drugs, and some diseases.

Epilepsy Another type of brain damage may result in epilepsy. Epilepsy is a disease in which electrical activity in the brain becomes abnormal for short periods. Epilepsy is not mental retardation. People with this disorder have the same mental abilities as people who are not epileptic.

Epilepsy takes different forms, depending on which type of abnormal brain activity occurs. The periods of abnormal brain activity are called epileptic seizures.

The most serious form of epilepsy is grand mal epilepsy. During a grand mal seizure, the person loses consciousness, falls to the floor, and begins to flail and thrash about uncontrollably. The movements are so forceful that epileptics may injure themselves when they hit objects such as desks or other furniture.

A grand mal seizure is often very frightening to witness. If someone around you should have a grand mal seizure, the best thing you can do to help the person is to move furniture out of the way to reduce the risk of injury. Do not try to touch or move the person while he or she is having a seizure. Grand mal seizures usually last only a few minutes. After the seizure, the person will probably sleep for a short time.

Grand mal seizures are also frightening for the person who experiences them. The person may feel disoriented and confused after a seizure. Many epileptics are embarrassed by their seizures or feel guilty because of the disruption and worry they have caused. It is very important that people who witness a seizure be understanding and supportive.

Fortunately, medication helps most people with grand mal epilepsy avoid having seizures. Once the proper drug therapy is prescribed, an epileptic may go for many years, or for the rest of his or her life, without a seizure.

There are two other forms of epilepsy. Petit mal epilepsy causes a person to simply "go blank" for a minute or two. Convulsions do not occur. This form of epilepsy usually occurs during childhood and disappears by adolescence. Psychomotor epilepsy causes seizures in which the person does not fall or have convulsions but may repeat simple movements over and over. Epilepsy may be a hereditary or congenital disease, or it may be caused by a head injury or a tumor later in life.

People with epilepsy, or with any type of congenital or hereditary disease, should be treated the same way as anyone else: with compassion and respect.

Review

1. *What is a noninfectious disease? How does it differ from an infectious disease?*
2. *Define hereditary disease and congenital disease. How do they differ?*
3. *List three factors that can cause a congenital disease.*
4. ***Critical Thinking*** *Should a person born with fetal alcohol syndrome be able to sue his or her mother for damages if it can be proven that the mother used alcohol during pregnancy, knowing of its risks? Why or why not?*

SECTION 24.1

Answers to Questions 1 and 2 are on p. 516.

3. Answers may include radiation, pollution, drugs, diseases, or lack of oxygen during birth.

4. Answers will vary. Students may say yes, because the mother knew she was potentially damaging the child and anyone who inflicted such damage on another person could be prosecuted in other circumstances. Others may say that even if she knew the consequences, the mother may have been unable to refrain from drinking, or that a lawsuit for such a reason within a family is inappropriate.

ASSESS

Section Review

Have students answer the Section Review questions.

Alternative Assessment

Symptoms of a Disease

Have students explain in their own words the cause and symptoms of one of the diseases studied in this chapter.

Closure

Preventing Noninfectious Diseases

Ask students to write a brief paragraph about how some diseases, such as fetal alcohol syndrome, can be prevented.

Background
Type I Diabetes
Young people with juvenile-type or insulin-dependent diabetes must be even more careful than other teens to develop a healthy lifestyle. They must exercise to keep their weight and body composition within the healthy range, and to keep their body using insulin efficiently. And they must eat well-selected foods. Eating too much sugar or eating irregularly can throw off the carefully regulated insulin levels. If there is too much insulin in the body, a condition called insulin reaction or insulin shock may occur. The condition can be handled by eating a sugar-rich food immediately; for that reason, diabetics often carry candy with them. The young person with Type I diabetes has to take responsibility early in life for exercising, eating well, and following a healthy lifestyle.

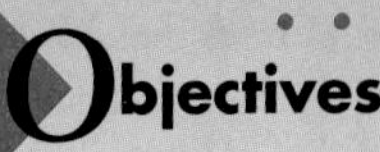

Section 24.2 Autoimmune Diseases

Objectives

- *List three common autoimmune diseases.*
- *Explain the difference between autoimmune disease and AIDS.*

Your immune system consists of an amazing set of specialized cells that destroy potentially dangerous viruses, microorganisms, and poisons that enter your body. Cells of the immune system constantly patrol your blood and tissues, checking out every cell and substance they meet. When an immune system cell recognizes a cell or molecule, it leaves it alone. But an immune system cell will attack and destroy anything that it does not recognize.

You could not survive without this patrol system. However, in some people, the immune system mistakes a cell type or a certain kind of body tissue for a foreign invader and attacks it. When a person's immune system attacks and damages an organ of his or her own body, the person has an **autoimmune disease.**

autoimmune disease: *a disease in which a person's own immune system attacks and damages an organ of his or her own body.*

What Causes Autoimmune Disease?

There seem to be several factors that trigger the immune attack. Some tissues in the body are not normally patrolled by, or exposed to, the immune system. An example is the thyroid gland. If an injury or infection brings immune cells into contact with thyroid cells, the immune system behaves as if this "new" tissue is foreign.

Sometimes a virus or bacterium contains molecules that are very similar to molecules found in the human body. If a person is infected by one of these viruses or bacteria, the immune system fights the infection in the normal way. However, after the infection is over, the immune system then goes on to attack the similar molecules in the body. For example, molecules on heart valves are similar to molecules found in the streptococcus bacterium that causes strep throat. After a strep throat infection, the immune system may attack the heart valves and damage them. This autoimmune disease is called rheumatic fever.

Even though autoimmune diseases are disorders of the immune system, it is important not to confuse them with HIV infection or AIDS. Infection with HIV leads to the gradual destruction of the immune system until it is unable to defend the body against invaders. With autoimmune disease, the immune system is strong and effective against foreign invaders, but it also attacks some part of the "self."

The most important distinction between AIDS and autoimmune diseases is that AIDS is a communicable disease. That is, it is passed from one person to another. Autoimmune diseases are noncommunicable diseases. You do not have to worry about "catching" them from someone else.

Multiple Sclerosis Multiple sclerosis (MS) is the result of an immune system attack on the fatty coverings of nerves. The resulting nerve damage affects different

Section 24.2 Lesson Plan

MOTIVATE

Journal 24B
What Is an Autoimmune Disease?

This may be done as a warm-up activity. Ask students to write in the Student Journal in the Student Activity Book what they think their immune system does. Then they should write what they think an autoimmune disease is. Tell them to reread what they have written after they have studied this section.

TEACH

Class Discussion
Why AIDS Is Not an Autoimmune Disease

How does your immune system protect your body? *[Cells of the immune system constantly patrol your blood and tissues, attacking and destroying anything that it does not recognize.]* **What is an autoimmune disease?** *[This is a disease that occurs when a person's immune system attacks and damages an organ of his or her own body.]* **Why is AIDS not an autoimmune disease?** *[AIDS is an infection caused by the HIV virus that leads to the gradual destruction of the immune system, until it is unable to defend the body against invaders. A person with an autoimmune disease has a strong immune system*

parts of the nervous system in each patient. Early symptoms include vision disturbances, stiffness and fatigue in limbs, dizziness, and emotional disturbances. Complete paralysis, numbness, double vision, speech problems, general weakness, difficulty in swallowing, and other problems may occur in the advanced stages.

The exact trigger for the autoimmune attack is unknown. The disease usually shows up in early adulthood. One characteristic of multiple sclerosis is the cycle of temporary recovery from symptoms followed by periods when the disease gets worse. There is no cure for the disease, and the periods during which the symptoms are less severe make it very difficult to judge the value of any particular treatment.

Type I Diabetes You have already learned how important it is for the body's cells to be able to use sugars for energy, and that in order to use the sugars, the body must have insulin. Insulin is a hormone that is made by the pancreas.

Type I diabetes, which is sometimes called juvenile diabetes, is believed to be caused by an autoimmune attack on the insulin-producing cells of the pancreas. Once their insulin-producing cells are destroyed, people with Type I diabetes must receive insulin every day. There is no "insulin pill" that works, because the insulin would be destroyed by acids and enzymes in the digestive tract. The insulin must be delivered directly to the bloodstream, either by injections ("shots") or by an insulin pump. Diabetics must carefully monitor the level of sugars in their blood to make sure that they are taking the right amount of insulin. Some diabetics use a device like the one shown at the beginning of this chapter.

Some symptoms of diabetes are excessive thirst, excessive hunger, excessive urination, unexplained weight loss, slow healing of cuts and bruises, low energy, intense itching, vision changes, and pain in the extremities. If these symptoms appear, a doctor can perform a urine or blood test to determine whether the person has diabetes.

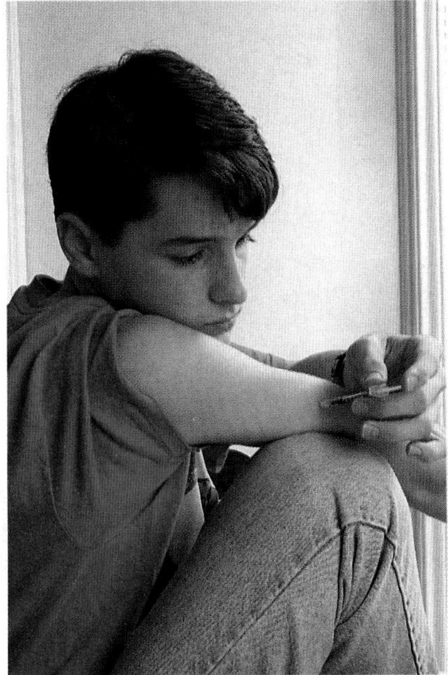

(FIGURE 24-7) **People with Type I diabetes must take insulin every day.**

When a diabetic does not get enough insulin, a diabetic coma may occur. A person about to enter a diabetic coma may develop a fever, appear quite ill, complain of thirst, and vomit. A diabetic who receives too much insulin may suffer from insulin shock. Weakness, moist pale skin, and tremors or convulsions are all symptoms of insulin shock. Sugar (orange juice, soft drinks, granulated sugar on the tongue) may be given if the person is conscious.

Although diabetes is a serious disease, treatment is very effective. Diabetics who monitor and control their intake of insulin carefully, maintain a healthy, specially designed diet, get regular exercise, and avoid tobacco can lead healthy lives.

SECTION 24.2

Background

Hypoglycemia

Hypoglycemia, the condition of having too little glucose or sugar in the blood, most commonly occurs among diabetics who take insulin. If the dosage of insulin is too large or overcorrects the condition, low blood sugar results. Symptoms can include hunger, headache, nervousness, sweating, and accelerated heartbeat. In extreme cases, convulsions, unconsciousness, even death can result. In nondiabetics, the condition can be either organic or functional. The more severe organic form can result from physical abnormalities, such as those caused by liver diseases. Functional hypoglycemia is usually an overreaction to high blood sugar following a meal, especially one including a lot of carbohydrates. Symptoms of hypoglycemia can be treated by eating something containing sugar. A balanced diet of foods containing proteins and carbohydrates is recommended for the management of hypoglycemia.

that is still effective against foreign invaders. The immune system of a person with an autoimmune disease attacks the cells and organs of its own body. An autoimmune disease cannot be contracted from someone else.]

Cooperative Learning

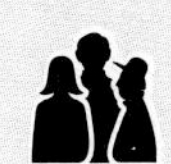

Symptoms of Some Autoimmune Diseases

Have students work together in groups to produce a chart of autoimmune diseases, showing the symptoms of each disease and its effect on the body.

Extension

Research on Autoimmune Diseases

Have students obtain brochures from local chapters of the Multiple Sclerosis Society, the Diabetes Research Foundation, and the Rheumatic Diseases Research Foundation. Ask them to display the brochures with posters soliciting support for research on these three diseases.

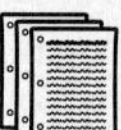

Section Review Worksheet 24.2

Assign Section Review Worksheet 24.2, which requires students to supply information about autoimmune diseases and to match diseases with their symptoms and the body parts they affect.

Section Quiz 24.2

Have students take Section Quiz 24.2.

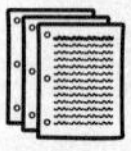

Reteaching Worksheet 24.2

Students who have difficulty with the material may complete Reteaching Worksheet 24.2, which requires them to recognize autoimmune diseases and their characteristics.

Review Answers

1. Answers may include rheumatic fever, multiple sclerosis, Type I diabetes, rheumatoid arthritis, Hashimoto's thyroiditis, and Graves' disease.
2. AIDS is a communicable disease; an autoimmune disease is not communicable.
3. Too much insulin can cause insulin shock. Not enough can cause a diabetic coma.

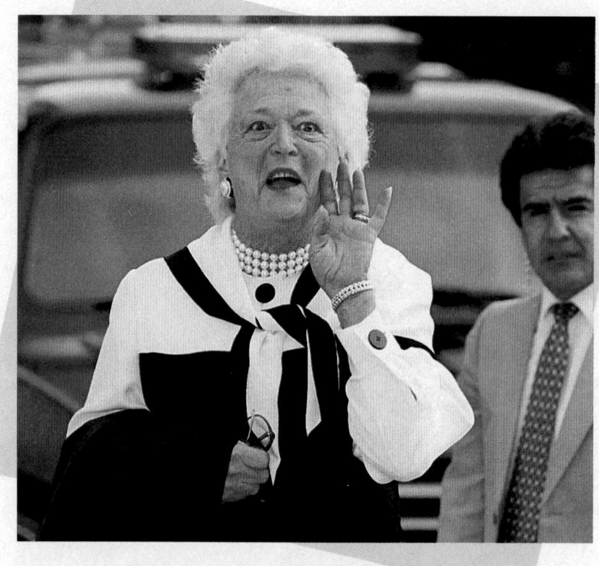

(FIGURE 24-8) **Former First Lady Barbara Bush suffers from Graves' Disease, a disorder that causes irregular heartbeat and a protruding of the eyeballs.**

Rheumatoid Arthritis Rheumatoid arthritis occurs when the immune system attacks the membranes that line the spaces between joints. Eventually, the joints may be destroyed and the bones may even fuse together. Unlike osteoarthritis, which is very common in older people, rheumatoid arthritis usually shows up at a younger age. It is more common in women and often first appears between the ages of 30 and 40.

Rheumatoid arthritis may also cause other problems, like anemia and heart disease. It is treated with anti-inflammatory drugs and gentle exercise.

Hashimoto's Thyroiditis and Graves' Disease Hashimoto's thyroiditis and Graves' disease are both caused by an immune attack on the thyroid gland, but oddly, they have opposite effects. In the case of Hashimoto's thyroiditis, the immune system destroys tissues of the thyroid gland and not enough thyroid hormone is produced. People with this disease must take thyroid hormone pills every day to replace the missing hormone.

In Graves' disease, the immune system attacks the thyroid, and the thyroid gland is tricked into making too *much* thyroid hormone. The usual treatment for this disease is to remove the thyroid or destroy it with radioactive iodine. Then the person takes thyroid pills to restore and maintain a normal level of the hormone.

Review

1. *Name three common autoimmune diseases.*
2. *What is an important distinction between AIDS and autoimmune diseases?*
3. ***Critical Thinking*** *Why is it so important for a person to monitor the amount of insulin he or she takes?*

ASSESS

Section Review

Have students answer the Section Review questions.

Alternative Assessment

Autoimmune Diseases

Have students work together to make up a game about the autoimmune diseases. On separate index cards, they should list each of the diseases described in this section. On other cards, they should list what each disease causes in the body. On a third set of cards, they should write the symptoms. To play the game, a player selects a card. If the card has the name of a disease, the player must tell what causes the disease or give one of its symptoms. If the card has a symptom or what causes the disease, the player must give the name of the disease. When a player misses, the other team begins its turns and plays until someone misses.

Closure

Graves' Disease in the White House

Have students consider the diagnosis of physicians that former President Bush, his wife Barbara, and their dog all suffer from Graves' disease. Ask them to write whether this could be coincidental or could the disease have spread from one to the others? *(It must be coincidental, because Graves' disease is a noninfectious disease.)*

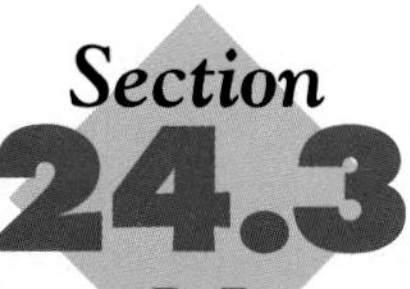

Section 24.3 Degenerative Diseases

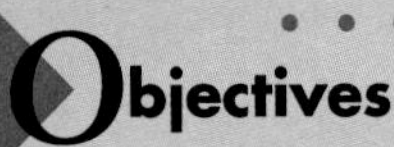

Objectives

- *Describe what happens to arteries during the development of atherosclerosis.*
- *Explain the relationship between atherosclerosis and high blood pressure.*
- *List three kinds of cancer to which tobacco use contributes.*
- *Name four things you can do to reduce your risk of cardiovascular disease.*
  LIFE SKILLS: Practicing Self-Care
- *Name two things you can do to reduce your risk of getting cancer.*
  LIFE SKILLS: Practicing Self-Care

Degenerative diseases are diseases that result from gradual damage to organs over time, and that are more likely to occur as a person gets older. In this section, you will learn about three degenerative diseases: osteoarthritis, cardiovascular disease (disease of the heart and blood vessels), and cancer.

Osteoarthritis

Osteoarthritis is very different from rheumatoid arthritis, the autoimmune disease. Osteoarthritis seems to be caused by wear and tear on joints over time. Osteoarthritis is very common among the elderly, although the age at which it appears varies from person to person. Some people begin to feel its effects in middle age or even earlier, while other people in their seventies or eighties are free of it. Some researchers think that the age at which osteoarthritis appears is determined by your genes, but that everyone who lives long enough would eventually get it.

Osteoarthritis is usually treated with aspirin or ibuprofen. Gentle exercise, which is often prescribed by a doctor or therapist, can slow the progression of the disease, relieve stiffness and pain, and prolong freedom of movement.

Cardiovascular Disease

Progressive damage to the heart and blood vessels is called **cardiovascular disease.** Damage to blood vessels usually occurs slowly, over many years. It may even begin in childhood. In the early years of the disease, it causes no pain or other symptoms, which means that some people in their teens and early twenties are suffering from cardiovascular disease and don't know it.

Although the early stages of cardiovascular disease don't have symptoms, the effects of the illness can be deadly. Heart disease is the leading cause of death in the United States. Stroke, which is also caused by cardiovascular disease, is the nation's third leading killer.

Atherosclerosis **Atherosclerosis**, the most common cause of cardiovascular disease, is a narrowing of the arteries caused by a buildup of fatty material. Arteries are blood vessels that carry blood away from the heart. Atherosclerosis begins with a small injury to the inner wall of an artery.

cardiovascular disease: *progressive damage to the heart and blood vessels.*

degenerative diseases: *diseases that result from gradual damage to organs over time.*

Background

Causes of Osteoarthritis

Running and other forms of vigorous exercise do not appear to advance osteoarthritis. Investigators have found that obesity, rather than exercise, creates the highest risk. Runners actually strengthen their bones: they accumulate 40 percent more mineral in their bones than do nonrunners, and their ligaments, tendons, and cartilage become thicker and stronger with exercise. Although most people will develop osteoarthritis as they grow older, severe or repeated joint injuries may cause degeneration earlier. Other causes include trauma, infection, and anatomical abnormality in a joint. Exercise by itself does not appear to harm healthy joints and it does strengthen bones.

Section 24.3 Lesson Plan

MOTIVATE

Journal 24C

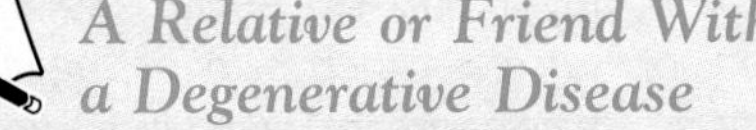

A Relative or Friend With a Degenerative Disease

This may be done as a warm-up activity. Have students write in the Student Journal what they would like to know about the degenerative diseases—osteoarthritis, cardiovascular diseases, and cancer—and why. Mention that perhaps someone they know, or someone in a friend's family, has one of these diseases. Ask them to write whether they ever worry about having one of these diseases someday.

TEACH

Class Discussion

Osteoarthritis

What seems to cause osteoarthritis? *[Wear and tear on the joints over time]* **At what age do people develop osteoarthritis?** *[It can begin in middle age or even earlier, but is more common in older people.]* **Why does the age at which it develops vary?** *[Researchers believe genes determine the age at which it begins.]*

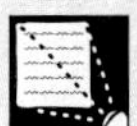

Teaching Transparency 24B

Artery Blockage

Show the transparency of the blocked artery (Figure 24-9). Ask students to describe the process by which the fatty material accumulates in the arteries and to describe its effects.

Background

Avoiding High Blood Pressure

Excessive salt is one cause of high blood pressure. Americans consume from two to six times the recommended daily allowance of sodium, which is 1.1 to 3.3 g. Since salt is the main source of sodium for most people, the daily allowance of salt is ½ to 1½ teaspoons of salt. Abstaining from salty foods and not adding salt to food at the table are two ways to lower your blood pressure.

This triggers cells lining the artery to multiply and take in certain substances circulating in the bloodstream. One of these substances is cholesterol.

Cholesterol is made only in animal cells. A certain amount of cholesterol is absolutely essential. Cholesterol makes up part of your cell membranes and provides the raw material for certain essential hormones. Your body can make all the cholesterol it needs. Even strict vegetarians who eat no animal products do not suffer from cholesterol deficiency. If you eat a small amount of cholesterol, your body will make less and use some of the cholesterol from your food for its needs. However, the average American eats far more cholesterol than the body is able to use.

A diet high in fats can also increase a person's cholesterol numbers to an unhealthy level. When this occurs, the amount of cholesterol floating through the bloodstream rises to unhealthy levels, and more fat is deposited inside the artery walls. For more information on fats and cholesterol, see Chapter 4.

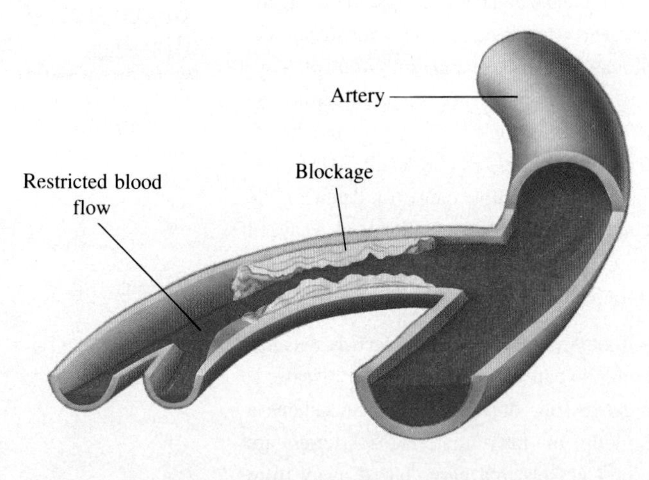

(FIGURE 24-9) **Fatty material that accumulates in the arteries can interfere with or block blood flow.**

The regions where fat is deposited tend to thicken over time, narrowing the artery, as shown in Figure 24-9. Eventually, the arteries stiffen, making blood flow difficult. When the disease becomes this severe, it is called **arteriosclerosis,** or "hardening of the arteries."

People who have high cholesterol levels can develop atherosclerosis at an early age. In addition to eating too much cholesterol-rich food, high levels of cholesterol in the blood can be caused by a diet high in other fats, smoking, lack of exercise, and heredity—or in most cases, several of these factors combined.

High Blood Pressure Another major cause of cardiovascular disease is **high blood pressure**. As you now know, your blood circulates from your heart to the rest of your body through tubular blood vessels called arteries. Your blood travels through your arteries in much the same way that water travels through a garden hose. Just like water in a garden hose, the blood in your arteries is under pressure. To picture what is happening inside your arteries, imagine that you turn the water faucet connected to your garden hose on and off repeatedly. The pressure rises when water squirts out of the faucet and then falls when you turn the water off.

A person with a strong, healthy heart and flexible, healthy arteries should have a blood pressure reading of about 120/80 or less. A blood pressure measurement higher than 140/90 is considered to be high blood pressure. These numbers measure the highest and lowest pressure inside your arteries.

While your heart contracts, squeezing blood into your arteries, the pressure inside your arteries is at its highest. This pressure is your systolic blood pressure, which is what the first number represents. When the heart muscle relaxes, the pressure in your arteries falls. The lowest pressure—the

• • • TEACH continued

Demonstration

Change in Blood Flow

Use a rubber tube to demonstrate how blood flows through a normal artery. Pour water into one end of the tube and call attention to the diameter of the water flow from the other end. Insert a plastic tube that fits snugly into the far end of the rubber tube. When you pour water into the other end of the rubber tube, ask students what they notice about the water flowing from the tube this time. Have them relate the demonstration to the flow of blood through an artery damaged by atherosclerosis. Discuss with students how high blood pressure can cause the damage to the inner walls of arteries that begins the process of atherosclerosis.

Class Discussion

Heart Attack and Stroke

To help students understand the cause of a heart attack, call their attention to a diagram of a heart showing the coronary arteries. **What causes a heart attack?** *[If the coronary arteries are narrowed by atherosclerosis, a spasm in the muscle layer of the artery —or a tiny blood clot—can block the coronary artery. When part of the heart muscle receives no oxygen, it begins to die in a few minutes.]* **Why do some people survive a heart attack?** *[When the damaged region is not too large and the person receives medical treatment quickly, a heart attack victim may survive, but the damaged tissue will be re-*

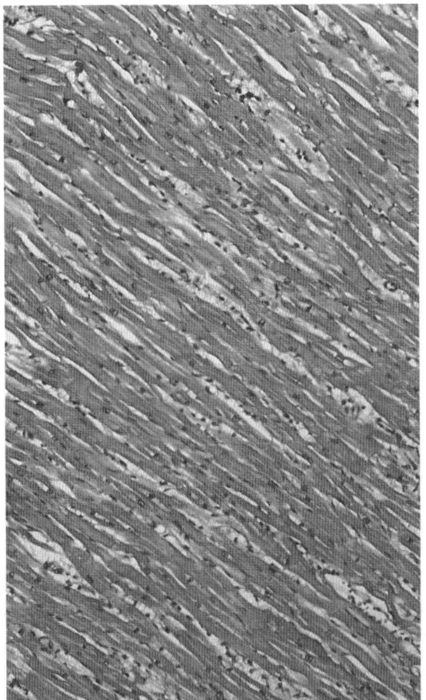

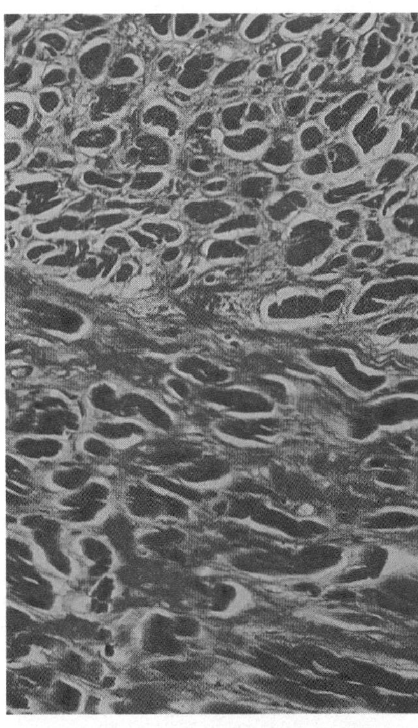

(FIGURE 24-10) **A heart attack does permanent damage to the heart by replacing healthy muscle (left) with scar tissue (right).**

pressure of the blood in between contractions of the heart—is the second number. This is called your diastolic blood pressure.

High blood pressure can cause the damage to the inner walls of arteries that begins the process of atherosclerosis. As fat is deposited and arteries narrow, the heart must pump harder in order to push blood through the body. Blood pressure rises even higher, causing even more damage to blood vessel walls.

Heart Attack The heart is the hardest working muscle in your body. It contracts continually throughout your life, never resting, not even when you sleep. A plentiful, oxygen-rich supply of blood is essential to the health of your heart.

Since the heart is filled with blood, you might think that the blood inside the heart supplies the heart muscle with all of the oxygen and nutrients that it needs. However, this is not the case. In fact, the inner lining of the heart actually acts as a barrier to the transfer of oxygen and nutrients.

When blood leaves the heart, it is pumped out through the largest artery in the body, the aorta. However, before blood is carried to any other part of the body, some of the blood detours into small blood vessels leading off from the aorta where it connects to the heart.

These vessels, on the outside of the heart, are the **coronary arteries.** They have one of the most important jobs in the entire blood vessel system—that is, to supply blood to the heart muscle itself.

If the coronary arteries have been narrowed by atherosclerosis, a spasm in the muscle layer of the artery—or a tiny blood

The circulatory system is discussed in greater detail in the Body Systems Handbook on pages 662–63.

The symptoms of a heart attack are discussed in Chapter 28.

Making a Choice 24A

Smoking

Assign the Smoking card. The card asks students to summarize their knowledge about the health consequences of smoking cigarettes.

Making a Choice 24B

Avoiding Arterial Damage

Assign the Avoiding Arterial Damage card. The card asks students to analyze foods in terms of their consequences for heart disease.

placed by scar tissue.] **How are a stroke and a heart attack similar and how are they different?** *[Both a stroke and a heart attack involve loss of the blood supply to a vital organ. A stroke occurs when a part of the brain is deprived of its blood supply, while a heart attack happens when a part of the heart does not receive blood.]*

Game

Cardiovascular Concentration

Ask students to work in pairs to make five cards, each with the name of one of the cardiovascular diseases mentioned in this section. Have these pairs of students also make five cards with a definition of the disorder. Have students play concentration by matching the name with the definition.

Class Discussion

Learning About Cancer

Discuss with students what cancer is and what it does to the body. **Why is cancer a noninfectious disease?** *[Cancer is not caused by an organism outside the body and it cannot be passed on to someone else.]* **What is the difference between a benign tumor and a malignant tumor?** *[A benign tumor is harmless and can often be ignored. A malignant tumor invades and destroys tissues of the body.]*

Cooperative Learning

Treatment for Cancer

Have students form groups to research and report on cancer treatments. They should find out about surgery, radia-

Background
Diet and Cancer Prevention

Many foods contain nutrients that help reduce one's chances of getting cancer. Cabbage-type vegetables, such as broccoli, cauliflower, kale, and brussels sprouts, protect against cancers of the colon, rectum, stomach, and lungs. High-fiber foods, such as bran cereals, whole wheat bread, rice, popcorn, and potatoes protect against cancer of the colon. Foods with vitamin A, such as carrots, peaches, squash, and broccoli protect against cancer of the esophagus, larynx, and lungs. Foods with vitamin C, such as grapefruit, oranges, strawberries, and red peppers guard against cancer of the esophagus and stomach.

clot—can block the coronary artery. Part of the heart muscle receives no oxygen and begins to die within a few minutes. When this happens, a heart attack has occurred. If the damaged region of the heart is not too large, and the person receives medical treatment quickly, there is a good chance that the heart attack victim will survive. After recovery, however, the damaged heart muscle will be replaced by scar tissue.

The symptoms of stroke are discussed in Chapter 28.

Stroke Like the heart, the brain needs blood and the nutrients it carries in order to survive. When a region of the brain is cut off from its blood supply, a **stroke** occurs. Some strokes result when blood traveling through blood vessels damaged by cardiovascular disease can't reach the brain. A stroke can also occur when a blood clot that can't pass through an artery narrowed by atherosclerosis cuts off the brain's blood supply, when a blood vessel breaks, or when a blood vessel swells and puts pressure on the brain.

Nearly 150,000 people die each year of stroke. If you think someone you're with is having a stroke, call a doctor immediately and describe the symptoms. If a physician is unavailable, call an ambulance or take the person to the hospital immediately.

cancer:

a disease caused by cells that have lost normal growth controls and that invade and destroy other tissues.

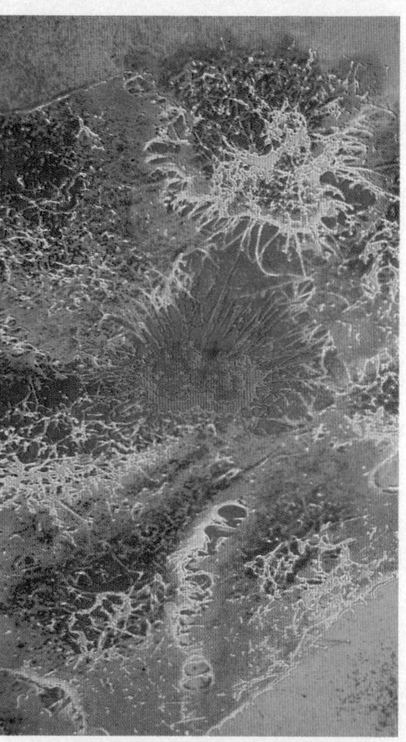

(FIGURE 24-11) **Cancer results when cells that have undergone a rapid and uncontrolled growth invade other cells and body tissue.**

Cancer

Your body makes millions of new cells every day. Normally, this is a tightly controlled process, and cells divide to provide replacement cells for the ones that are worn out. Sometimes, though, cells will begin to divide and multiply in an uncontrolled way. These cells may form a solid mass called a tumor. A tumor is not necessarily cancerous. A noncancerous tumor is called a benign tumor. Most benign tumors are essentially harmless. Some may be safely ignored, whereas others will need to be removed through surgery.

Cancer is a disease caused by cells that have lost normal growth controls and that invade and destroy other tissues. Eventually, damage to vital organs caused by a cancer may be fatal. A cancerous tumor is called a malignant tumor.

Cells in almost any part of the body can become cancerous. When a cancer arises, it usually grows for a while in the part of the body where it began—sometimes for years. Eventually, however, some of the cancer cells may metastasize, or move to other parts of the body. The cancer cells often travel through the blood or lymph fluid and give rise to new malignant tumors.

Cancer Treatments At one time, the vast majority of cancers were incurable. Today,

• • • TEACH continued

tion, chemotherapy, and alternative therapies such as visualization and meditation. For what kinds of cancer are they each used? For what stages of a cancer's development? Are they sometimes used together, or in sequence?

Class Discussion
Early Detection of Cancer

Discuss the chart "Seven Warning Signals for Cancer" (Figure 24-13). Emphasize that early detection may mean the difference between life and death. At an early stage, cancer does not move to other parts of the body. It can more easily be controlled at this stage. Have students read the information about breast self-examination and testicular self-examination. Ask them to outline the steps appropriate to them.

Journal 24D
Promise of Monthly Self-Examination

Have students write in the Student Journal their promise to carry out the monthly self-examination and their personal reasons for doing so.

Class Discussion
Your Risks of Getting a Cardiovascular Disease

Discuss the factors that can't be controlled in contracting a degenerative disease. **How can heredity place one**

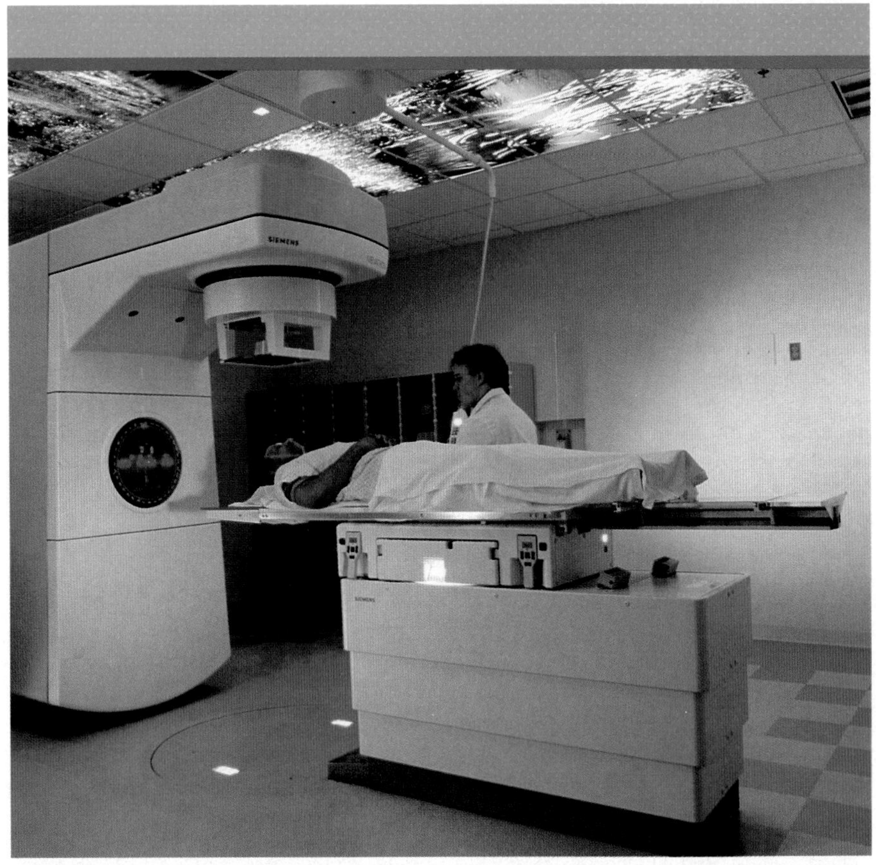

(FIGURE 24-12) **Cancer patients sometimes require radiation therapy after surgery to kill any cancerous cells that may remain in the body.**

Cancer Treatments At one time, the vast majority of cancers were incurable. Today, many cancers can be controlled, and often cured. Even so, cancer remains a very serious disease. It is the second leading cause of death in the United States.

The first step in treating cancer is usually to surgically remove the cancerous growth. Cancer surgery is often performed with lasers, which can cut through the cancerous tissue without causing damage to the surrounding tissue. Surgery is most effective in the early stages of cancer. A small cancer that has not spread to other parts of the body can be completely removed in this way.

After surgery, some patients also receive radiation treatments or chemotherapy. Some patients receive both. The purpose of radiation therapy is to kill any cancer cells near the original tumor that were not removed by surgery. The goal of chemotherapy, which is treatment with special anticancer drugs, is to destroy cancer cells that have traveled to other parts of the body.

When cancer is not diagnosed until after it has grown and spread into vital organs such as the lungs, the pancreas, or the brain, surgery is often useless. Radiation or chemotherapy may be used to treat advanced cases of cancer. In these cases, a cure is very unlikely. However, treatment

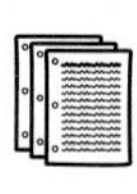

Life Skills Worksheet 24A

Giving Good Health-Care Advice

Assign the Giving Good Health-Care Advice Life Skills Worksheet, which requires students to provide informed advice in several situations.

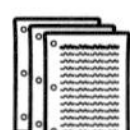

Life Skills Worksheet 24B

Knowing When to See a Doctor

Assign the Knowing When to See a Doctor Life Skills Worksheet, which requires students to recognize serious symptoms.

person more at risk than another to contract a cardiovascular disease? *[If several members of a person's family have cardiovascular problems, that person may have inherited a tendency toward these problems.]* **What could you do to reduce the risk of your contracting one of the cardiovascular diseases?** *[You could avoid the factors that you can control, such as poor dietary habits, high blood pressure, lack of exercise, smoking, and drinking alcohol.]*

Role-Playing
Preventing Cancer

Have students role-play a situation where a teen is trying to convince his or her father or mother to quit smoking. Have them mention the five kinds of cancer caused by cigarette smoking and any ideas they have learned about reducing the risk of cancer.

Debate the Issue
Avoiding the Risk Factors

Hold a class debate on the topic: People should not deprive themselves of so many things they want to do all their life, just to add a few years to their life at the end. Divide the class into two teams, one pro and one con. Each team should prepare for the debate by listing arguments the other side is likely to make and composing their counterarguments.

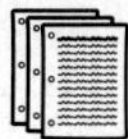

Life Skills Worksheet 24C

National and Local Organizations

Assign the National and Local Organizations Life Skills Worksheet, which has students look into organizations that provide support groups and research for specific diseases.

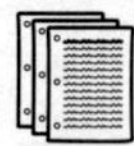

Life Skills Worksheet 24D

Making Healthy Lifestyle Decisions

Assign the Making Healthy Lifestyle Decisions Life Skills Worksheet, which asks students to respond to pressure to participate in activities that undermine health.

Seven Warning Signals for Cancer

- ***C**hange in bowel or bladder habits.*
- ***A** sore that does not heal.*
- ***U**nusual bleeding or discharge.*
- ***T**hickening or lump in breast or elsewhere.*
- ***I**ndigestion or difficulty in swallowing.*
- ***O**bvious change in wart or mole.*
- ***N**agging cough or hoarseness.*

(FIGURE 24-13) **Having one or more of the above signs and signals does not mean that you have cancer. But to be on the safe side, see a doctor.**

sometimes reduces the size of tumors, reduces pain, and prolongs life.

Complete information on breast and testicular self-examinations is provided in Chapter 16.

Early Detection of Cancer It is important that everyone know the early warning signs of cancer. Remember, cancer caught early is very often completely curable. You can begin protecting yourself by learning the seven warning signals for cancer that have been developed by the American Cancer Society, listed in Figure 24-13. If you have one of these warning signals, see your doctor immediately.

Some cancers do not have symptoms that you can feel or see in their early stages, yet they can be detected by certain diagnostic tests. This is one reason why regular checkups are so important. Regular self-examination of breasts or testicles is the most effective way to detect cancer in these regions at an early stage. See Chapter 16 for more information regarding these important self-exams.

Preventing Cardiovascular Disease and Cancer

It's not always easy to determine the exact reason why a particular person gets cardiovascular disease or cancer. There is evidence that a person can inherit a tendency to suffer a certain degenerative disease from his or her parents, and it is also known that older people are more likely to get degenerative diseases than are younger people.

Risk Factors for Degenerative Disease

Factors You Can't Control	Factors You Can Control
Gender	*Poor Dietary Habits*
Heredity	*High Blood Pressure*
Age	*Lack of Exercise*
	Smoking
	Drinking Alcohol

(FIGURE 24-14) **Most of the risk factors for degenerative disease are within your control.**

• • • TEACH continued

Cooperative Learning
Environmental Cancer Risks

Have students work together to chart the risks of cancer that may be present in the environment and plan how to counteract them. Suggest they make a simple chart with four categories down the left side (radiation, toxic chemicals, tobacco, sun) and two wide columns across the top (times you may be exposed to these dangers, and ways to minimize exposure). When each group has finished, combine all the ideas on a single chart on the chalkboard.

Teaching Transparency 24C
Factors That Increase the Risk of Heart Disease or Cancer

Use the transparency to reinforce the connections between diet, exercise, smoking, and other habits and the development of heart disease and/or cancer.

Extension
Visiting a Hospital

Encourage students to visit a hospital to find out about volunteer work. What kinds of work are available for high school students? What are the demands of the job, and what are the requirements of applicants? Have students talk with volunteers, if possible, to learn about what they do.

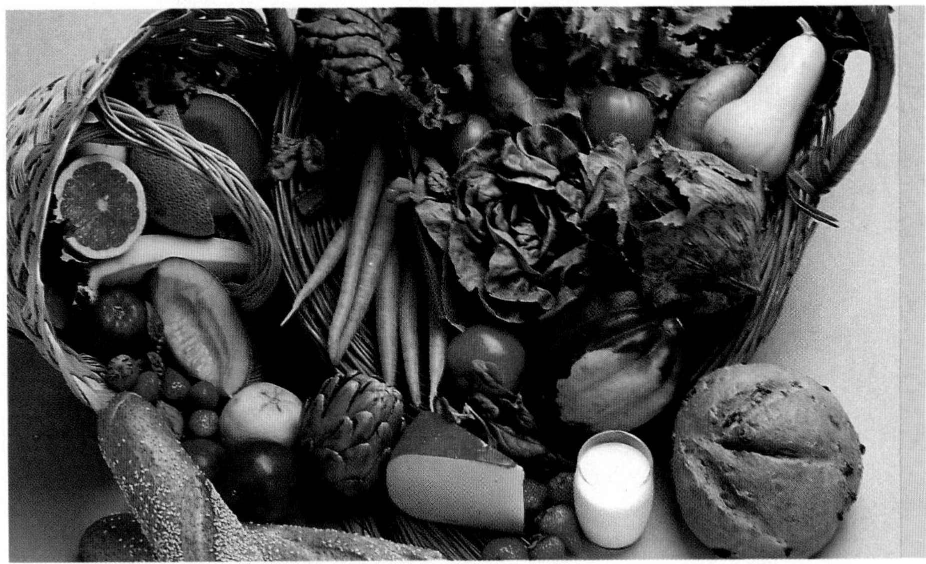

(FIGURE 24-15) **Some studies have shown that certain foods contain nutrients that may reduce a person's chances of suffering cancer.**

Age and heredity are two disease-causing factors a person can't do anything about. But there are things you *can* do to decrease your chances of getting certain diseases. The decisions you make concerning the care of your body—starting now—can have a very strong influence on your health as you grow older.

By making healthy choices, you may be able to avoid getting a certain degenerative disease. Even if you don't avoid the disease entirely, you may be able to postpone the age at which a disease shows up, or reduce its severity.

Cardiovascular Disease It may not seem especially important to think about preventing cardiovascular disease while you're still a teenager. But in fact, the choices you make now about diet, exercise, tobacco, and alcohol are already affecting your heart and blood vessels. For some measures you can take to reduce your risk of getting cardiovascular disease, read the Life Skills feature on pages 528–29.

Preventing Cancer In order for cells to become cancerous, a series of changes must occur in cells in a particular sequence. These changes cause the cells to lose their normal growth controls. Scientists have discovered several factors that cause some of these changes in cells. Regular exposure to these factors increases your risk that some of the cells in your body will undergo the unlucky combination of changes that results in cancer.

High doses of radiation and certain very toxic chemicals are known to cause cancer. Fortunately, you are unlikely to be exposed to these factors. However, many people are concerned that low doses of less toxic chemicals common in the environment may also be causing cancer in some people. Research continues to explore the relationship between environmental factors and cancer.

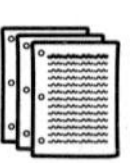

Section Review Worksheet 24.3

Assign Section Review Worksheet 24.3, which requires students to answer questions and complete sentences about degenerative diseases.

Section Quiz 24.3

Have students take Section Quiz 24.3.

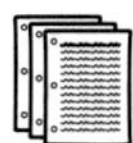

Reteaching Worksheet 24.3

Students who have difficulty with the material may complete Reteaching Worksheet 24.3, which requires them to recognize the chain of events leading to arteriosclerosis.

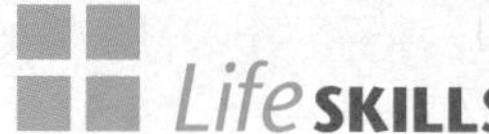

Reducing Your Risk of Cardiovascular Disease

Have students read the Life Skills feature in the text. Ask them whether they feel the steps suggested are practical. Are there any that would be difficult for them to take? Are some easy, requiring only a minimal adjustment? What are the rewards of following these steps?

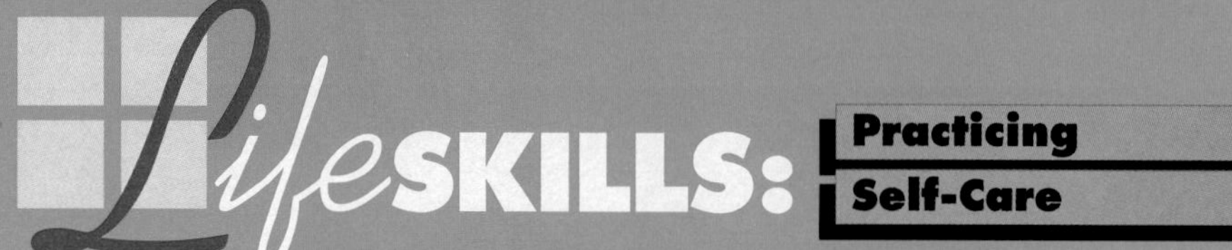

Reducing Your Risk of Cardiovascular Disease

Here are some steps you can take—starting now—to reduce your chances of getting cardiovascular disease.

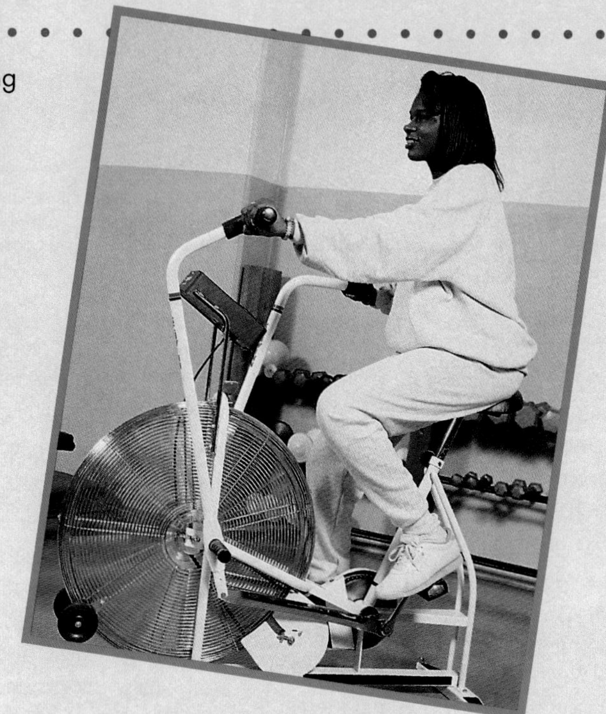

1. *Don't smoke.* Smoking cigarettes or using any other form of tobacco increases your risk of heart attack and stroke more than any other factor that you can control. Smokers are two to six times more likely to have a heart attack than are nonsmokers. Smokers who have heart attacks are more likely to die from them. The best thing that you can do to maintain good health is to never start smoking. If you have started, quit. For some suggestions on ways to stop smoking, see Chapter 14.
2. *Have your blood pressure checked regularly.* Most people with high blood pressure can bring their blood pressure down to normal levels and greatly reduce their risk of heart attack and stroke. Many people return to normal blood pressure readings simply by quitting smoking, not drinking alcohol, maintaining a normal weight, and getting regular exercise. Some people also need to take medication to lower their blood pressure.

3. *If you are diabetic, be sure you follow medical advice to control it.* Diabetics develop more severe atherosclerosis earlier in life. If you have diabetes, be sure that you see a doctor regularly, and follow his or her instructions regarding insulin shots and general self-care. In addition, a healthy lifestyle is even more important for you than for nondiabetics.
4. *Eat healthy foods.* Eating a healthy variety of foods in moderate amounts reduces your risk of obesity, which in turn reduces your risk of suffering cardiovascular disease. You should make a special effort to avoid foods that are high in fat. Chapter 4 offers specific information on choosing a nutritious diet.
5. *Exercise regularly.* Regular aerobic activity can strengthen the heart and has been shown to increase the internal diameter of arteries, allowing more blood to pass through. Exercise can also lower blood cholesterol. If you don't exercise, not only will you lose these protective effects, but you will find it much more difficult to maintain normal weight.
6. *Learn how to manage stress.* Everyone suffers from stress now and then. But having a continuous amount of high stress can contribute to heart disease. Learning how to manage the stress in your life can make you not only happier, but healthier too. Some specific approaches for stress management are discussed in detail in Chapter 9.
7. *Schedule regular medical checkups.* An examination by a doctor can let you know if you are developing risk factors such as high blood pressure, diabetes, or high blood cholesterol levels. You can then treat these conditions before they cause serious damage to your heart and blood vessels.

Review Answers

1. Atherosclerosis is a condition in which the arteries become narrow because of a build-up of fatty material. Eventually the arteries stiffen, making blood flow difficult.
2. High blood pressure can cause damage to the inside walls of the arteries, damage that begins the process of atherosclerosis.
3. Answers may include lung, bladder, kidney, and pancreas cancers.
4. Answers may include don't smoke; have your blood pressure checked regularly; eat healthy foods; exercise regularly; manage stress; control your diabetes if you are a diabetic; get regular medical checkups.
5. Answers may include don't smoke or use tobacco products; avoid exposure to radiation, toxic chemicals, and pollutants; avoid overexposure to the sun; and use a sunscreen with a high sun protection factor.
6. What you do now can affect you later in life. Cardiovascular disease can begin in childhood. The accumulative effects of years of smoking greatly increase your chance of developing cancer and cardiovascular disease later in life.

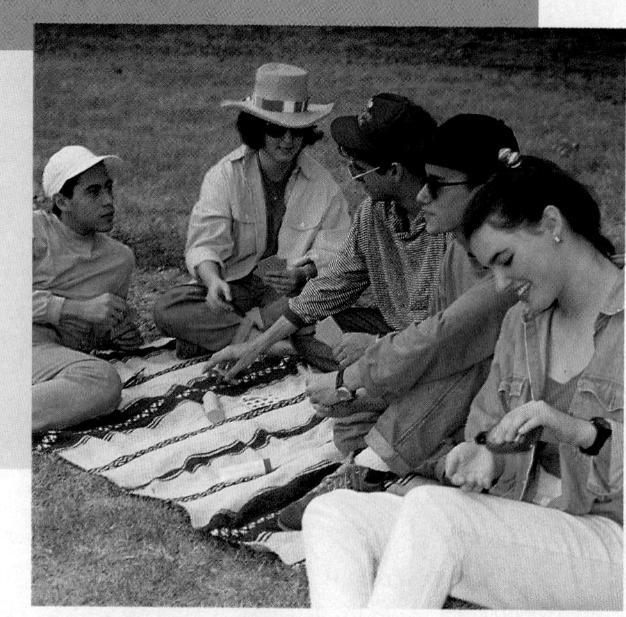

(FIGURE 24-16) **Too much sun can cause skin cancer. If you do spend time in the sun, be sure to cover up as much as possible and to use proper protection.**

There are several proven measures you can take to decrease your risk of getting cancer. First, don't use tobacco or alcohol. Smoking cigarettes is the number-one cause of lung cancer in this country. Chewing tobacco and snuff can cause cancers of the bladder, pancreas, and kidney. Long-term tobacco use is associated with a higher risk of liver, esophagus, larynx, and pharynx cancers. By avoiding tobacco, you can significantly lessen your chances of getting any of these diseases.

It is also important to follow a healthy diet and exercise plan. Eating low-fat foods and getting plenty of exercise can help you maintain a healthy body weight and reduce your chances of getting many diseases—including cancer. In addition, some evidence indicates that certain nutrients are anticarcinogens, which are substances that can prevent cancer.

Another thing you can do to help protect yourself from cancer is to avoid overexposure to the sun. Ultraviolet rays from the sun are known to cause skin cancer.

Some forms of skin cancer are easily treated and rarely fatal. However, one form of skin cancer that is on the rise, melanoma, can be incurable unless detected early. A single case of sunburn in childhood serious enough to cause blisters can dramatically increase the risk of melanoma.

If you do spend time in the sun, be sure to use a sunscreen with a high sun protection factor number. For more information on selecting a proper sunscreen, see Chapter 6.

Review

1. *Explain the ways in which the arteries are affected by atherosclerosis.*
2. *Describe the relationship between atherosclerosis and high blood pressure.*
3. ***LIFE SKILLS: Practicing Self-Care*** *List three kinds of cancer that tobacco use can cause.*
4. ***LIFE SKILLS: Practicing Self-Care*** *Name four things you can do to reduce your risk of cardiovascular disease.*
5. *Name two things you can do to reduce your risk of getting cancer.*
6. ***Critical Thinking*** *A friend of yours who smokes cigarettes and eats a diet high in fats tells you it's stupid to worry about cardiovascular disease while you're still a teenager. What could you say in response?*

ASSESS

Section Review

Have students answer the Section Review questions.

Alternative Assessment

Looking Back

Have students write the resolutions they would make after suffering a heart attack. Do they think they would keep the resolutions after they felt better again?

Closure

Choosing to Live Longer

Ask students to suggest steps they could take to avoid one of the degenerative diseases later in life.

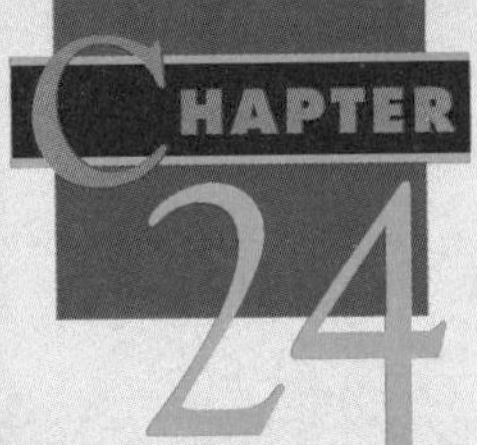

Highlights

Summary

- Diseases that are not transmitted from one organism to another are called noninfectious diseases. Hereditary, congenital, autoimmune, and degenerative diseases are all types of noninfectious diseases.
- Hereditary and congenital diseases are diseases people are "born with."
- Genes are responsible for transmitting hereditary characteristics. Some hereditary conditions are sickle cell anemia, cystic fibrosis, Tay-Sachs disease, Down's syndrome, muscular dystrophy, Type II diabetes, allergies, and asthma.
- Exposure during pregnancy to some drugs, environmental factors, and certain diseases can cause congenital diseases. Some congenital diseases are fetal alcohol syndrome, cerebral palsy, and epilepsy.
- Autoimmune diseases are disorders of the immune system. The most important distinction between AIDS and autoimmune diseases is that AIDS is an infectious disease, and autoimmune diseases are not.
- Three types of degenerative disease are osteoarthritis, cardiovascular disease, and cancer.
- Many types of cancer and heart disease can be prevented by avoiding certain environmental and lifestyle risks. Early detection and treatment can cure some types of cancer and control cardiovascular disease.

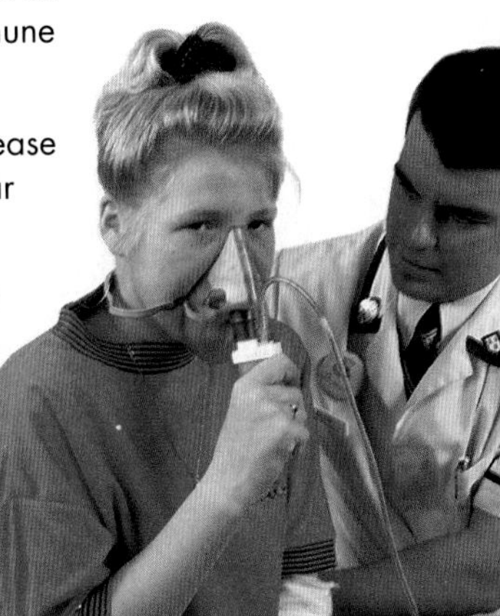

Vocabulary

noninfectious disease a disease that a person cannot catch from another person, animal, or other organism.

hereditary disease a disease caused by defective genes passed from one or both parents to a child.

congenital disease a disease that is present from birth but is not hereditary.

autoimmune disease a disease in which a person's own immune system attacks and damages an organ of his or her own body.

degenerative diseases diseases that cause gradual damage to organs over time.

cardiovascular disease progressive damage to the heart and blood vessels.

cancer a disease caused by cells that have lost normal growth controls and invade and destroy other tissues.

Chapter 24 Highlights Strategies

Summary

Have students read the summary to reinforce the concepts they learned in Chapter 24.

Vocabulary

Have students write a paragraph about noninfectious diseases that uses the vocabulary words for this chapter correctly.

Extension

Encourage students to find out how responsible adults whose opinions they respect are attempting to prevent degenerative diseases in their own lives and the lives of their children. Have them interview at least three such adults to find how the new information about these diseases is affecting their lives. Have students report on their interviews and compare findings.

Chapter 24 Assessment

Chapter Review

Concept Review

1. noninfectious
2. chromosomes or genes
3. cystic fibrosis
4. Down's syndrome
5. autoimmune
6. atherosclerosis
7. noncancerous
8. melanoma
9. diet, exercise

Expressing Your Views

Sample responses:

1. He might be experiencing a heart attack. I should call 911 for emergency help.
2. Yes. I would move furniture out of the way to reduce the risk of injury to Wendy. I would also not try to touch or move her while she is having a seizure. I would be understanding and supportive.
3. I would suggest he eat a low cholesterol diet and begin an exercise program. If he smoked, I would suggest that he quit.
4. Some people may want to know if they have inherited a fatal disease so they can make plans for things they might like to do and make plans for their deaths.

Life Skills Check

Sample responses:

1. I would use a waterproof sunscreen of SPF 15. I would also wear sunglasses that block UV radiation.
2. No. I would follow my doctor's advice on how to control my asthma when I participate in athletic activities or exercise. The advice is usually to avoid activities or exercise in cold, dry air or when air pollution levels are high, and to premedicate before the activity or exercise.
3. I might be experiencing an allergic reaction. I might see an allergist for testing to find out what I am allergic to. Then I would try to find that source in the house and eliminate or minimize it. I might also need to take medication, called antihistamines, if I can not avoid the substance causing the allergic reaction.

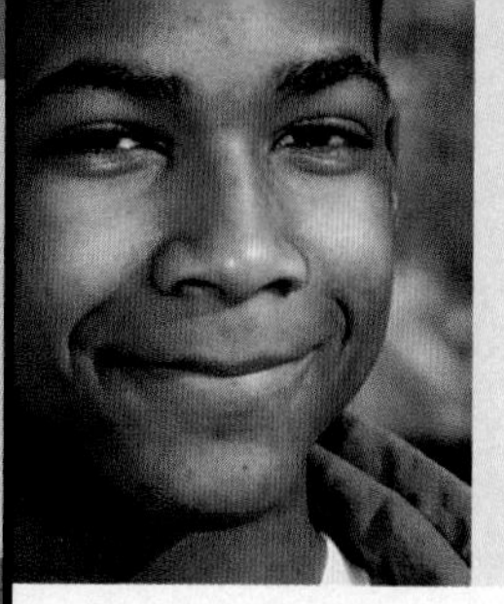

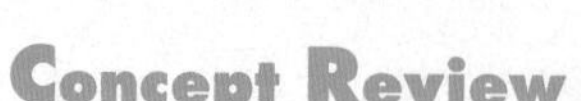

Chapter 24 Chapter Review

Concept Review

1. High blood pressure, sickle cell anemia, and cancer are all examples of ________ diseases.
2. The characteristics that were passed from your parents to you are carried on tiny structures within the body's cells known as ________.
3. ________ is a hereditary disease that results in breathing and digestive difficulties caused by the secretion of thick mucus in the lungs and digestive tract.
4. ________ is caused by the presence of an extra chromosome in the body cells.
5. When a person's immune system attacks and damages an organ of his or her own body, the person has an ________ disease.
6. The most common cause of cardiovascular disease is ________, a narrowing of the arteries caused by a buildup of fatty materials.
7. A ________ tumor is called a benign tumor.
8. ________ is one form of skin cancer that is on the rise and can be fatal unless detected early.
9. The choices you are making now concerning ________, ________, alcohol, and tobacco are already affecting your heart and blood vessels.

Expressing Your Views

1. Your uncle, who has just returned from jogging, says he has an uncomfortable feeling of pressure in the middle of his chest and then becomes short of breath and dizzy. What might he be experiencing, and what should he do?
2. Your new friend, Wendy, has just told you that she suffers from epilepsy. Would you ask her any questions about her disease? What would you do if she had a seizure when you were alone with her?
3. Your father just found out that his cholesterol level is dangerously high. What things would you suggest he do to bring his cholesterol level down?
4. Do you think most people would want to know if they had possibly inherited a fatal disease? Explain.

Life Skills Check

1. **Practicing Self-Care**
   On a hot summer day, you and your friends plan to go to the beach. You are sure you will spend all day there and you are worried about sunburn. What could you do to protect yourself?

2. **Practicing Self-Care**
   You have recently been diagnosed as having asthma. Does this mean you can no longer participate in athletic activities? What can you do to minimize your attacks?

3. **Practicing Self-Care**
   Since your family moved to a new house, you have had a stuffy nose, itchy eyes, and frequent sneezing. What might you be experiencing? What could you do to relieve your misery?

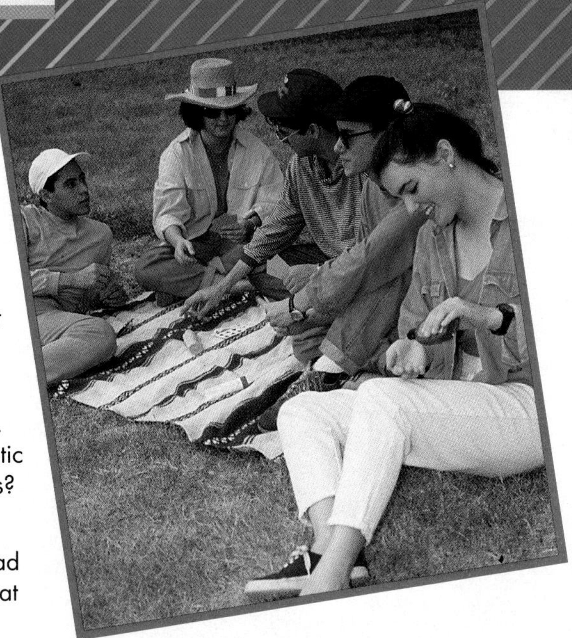

Projects

1. Research the cause and nature of a given noninfectious disease. Then prepare an oral report that describes the disease, its prevention, and its treatment, and that identifies any behaviors that could minimize the risk of getting the disease.
2. Work with a group to write public service announcements that inform the public of ways to prevent cancer. Deliver your announcements to the class.
3. Work with a group to create a bulletin board that illustrates ways to lower your chances of developing cardiovascular disease.
4. Several cultures around the world have low rates of heart disease. Work with a partner to research the diet of one of these cultures. Prepare a meal that is representative of the foods they eat.

Plan for Action

Early habits and attitudes play an important role in the prevention of cardiovascular disease and cancer. Create a plan to reduce your chances of getting one of these diseases.

Projects
Have students plan and carry out the projects for noninfectious diseases.

Plan for Action
Have students work in cooperative groups to plan how they can avoid contracting any of the degenerative diseases. Tell them to draw up strategies to improve their lifestyle with regard to diet, exercise, and avoiding carcinogens. Ask students to communicate their plans by means of a skit or a newsletter to present to the class.

ASSESSMENT OPTIONS

Chapter Test
Have students take the Chapter 24 Test.

Alternative Assessment
Have students do the Alternative Assessment for Chapter 24.

Test Generator
The Test Generator (Macintosh® or IBM® format) contains an additional 50 assessment items for this chapter.

Issues in Health

ETHICAL ISSUES IN HEALTH

ISSUE: *Should clean needles be distributed to intravenous drug users in order to slow the spread of AIDS?*

Have students read the Ethical Issues in Health feature. Ask them which side of the controversy they are on. If the class divides over the issue of needle exchange programs, hold a debate. Allow students to do library research to support their arguments. If the class agrees—either pro or con—have them do research to counteract the arguments that might be raised against their positions. Finally, ask for ideas about how to prevent HIV infection of infants.

Ethical Issues in Health

ISSUE: Should clean needles be distributed to intravenous drug users in order to slow the spread of AIDS?

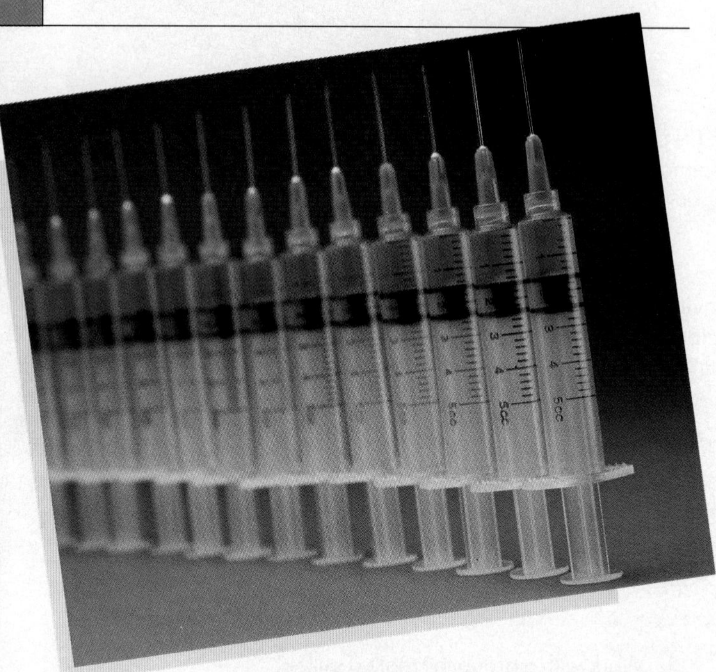

Intravenous drug use has become a major factor in the spread of AIDS because of a very dangerous practice—sharing needles. According to the Centers for Disease Control and Prevention, 23 percent of AIDS cases reported in the United States in 1992 resulted from intravenous drug users sharing needles contaminated with HIV.

Public-health authorities have proposed a method to slow the spread of HIV infection by intravenous drug users. The method involves distributing clean needles and supplies such as bottles of bleach and water for cleaning needles and syringes. These items are included in a ''survival kit.'' The popular name for such an effort is ''needle exchange program.'' Reactions to this method have sparked national and international debate.

Those who oppose needle exchange programs argue that the programs will increase intravenous drug use and encourage youngsters to use drugs. Some opponents also argue that intravenous drug users will not take advantage of programs to protect their health. They believe that by using drugs, users show a lack of concern for themselves.

Advocates of needle exchange programs contend that most persons addicted to drugs are concerned about AIDS and will take steps to prevent HIV infection, if they are assisted in doing so. Supporters also argue that making clean needles available will not increase the use of drugs but will improve the relationship between public-health workers and people addicted to drugs. This improved relationship, they believe, will increase the likelihood that people with addictions will get into treatment programs.

During a two-year experiment in New Haven, Connecticut, researchers at Yale University collected information about the effects of a needle exchange program. Their data showed that the program had several positive effects. First, the needles returned for exchange were in circulation for a shorter length of time than needles in circulation before the program began. This indicates that fewer people used each of the needles. Second, the percentage of needles infected with HIV dropped by one-third. Third, referrals to drug treatment centers increased.

The Yale study showed that in New Haven, drug use did not increase when a needle exchange program was begun, as many had feared. In fact, it may have decreased somewhat. In addition, the chief of police in New Haven reported a 20-percent decrease in the area's crime rate. He speculated that the reason for the drop may have been an improved relationship between public-health workers and the drug-using community. Since the average participant in the program was 35 years old and had been shooting drugs for an average of seven years, the Yale study also suggests that the New Haven program did not encourage more adolescents to use drugs.

Currently, there are many legal barriers to conducting needle exchange programs. In some states, it is just as illegal to carry needles and syringes as it is to use or possess drugs. Public-health workers who distribute ''survival kits'' in these states often risk being arrested.

State and federal lawmakers who support needle exchange programs have begun to address the legal barriers. On the local level, several city governments have authorized needle exchange programs despite unanswered legal questions. These cities have obtained police cooperation to prevent the arrest of health workers and needle recipients.

One group that could benefit from needle exchange programs is children. Seventy percent of all AIDS cases among children are linked to intravenous drug use by a parent. These children were infected with HIV before birth. One mayor who had opposed a needle exchange program in his city changed his mind and became an advocate after seeing HIV-infected newborns in a hospital.

Situation for Discussion

Ben is a 28-year-old married man who has used intravenous drugs for more than 10 years. He frequents a "shooting gallery" where needles are shared. Ben is aware of the danger of HIV infection and the possibility of infecting his wife and future children, but his wife is unaware of his addiction and wants to start a family. Ben wants to get treatment for his addiction but worries that he will be fired if he uses the insurance his employer provides. He has heard about a needle exchange program near the shooting gallery but fears he will be arrested for carrying needles if he participates.

a. What course of action is open to Ben? What keeps him from getting help? What are some positive and negative aspects of participating in the needle exchange program?

b. If you were a public official, would you support or oppose a needle exchange program? What data would you gather to support your position? What steps would you take to start or stop such a program?

UNIT 7

HEALTH AND SOCIETY

CHAPTER OVERVIEWS

CHAPTER 25

ENVIRONMENTAL AND PUBLIC HEALTH

Students learn that a healthy environment is important to personal and public health. The chapter defines *ecosystem* and discusses interactions within an ecosystem. It describes the elements of a healthy environment and explains how overpopulation and pollution threaten the health of the environment. The major types of pollution, their causes, and their health effects are discussed. Students learn the benefits of conservation, recycling, and reuse in fighting pollution and explore specific ways they can help. The chapter defines public health and describes public health activities. The public health concerns of developed and developing countries are compared. The chapter ends with a description of the functions of local, state, national, and international public and private health organizations.

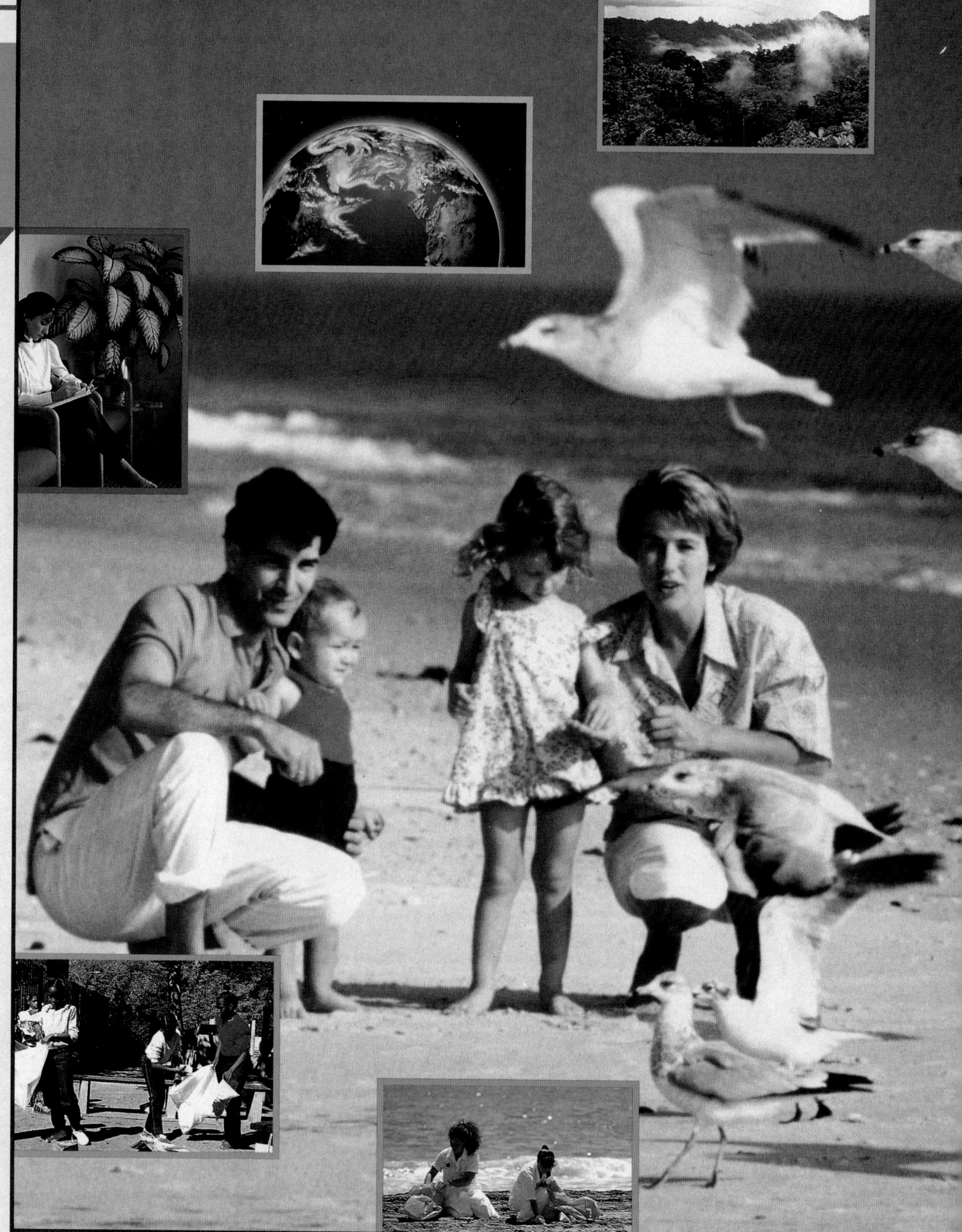

CHAPTER 26

BEING A WISE CONSUMER

The chapter describes the process of selecting a doctor and explains the Patient's Bill of Rights. Students learn why health care costs in the United States are rising. They learn about the advantages and disadvantages of traditional health insurance policies and HMOs. They learn how to find and use free health services and how to protect themselves against quackery.

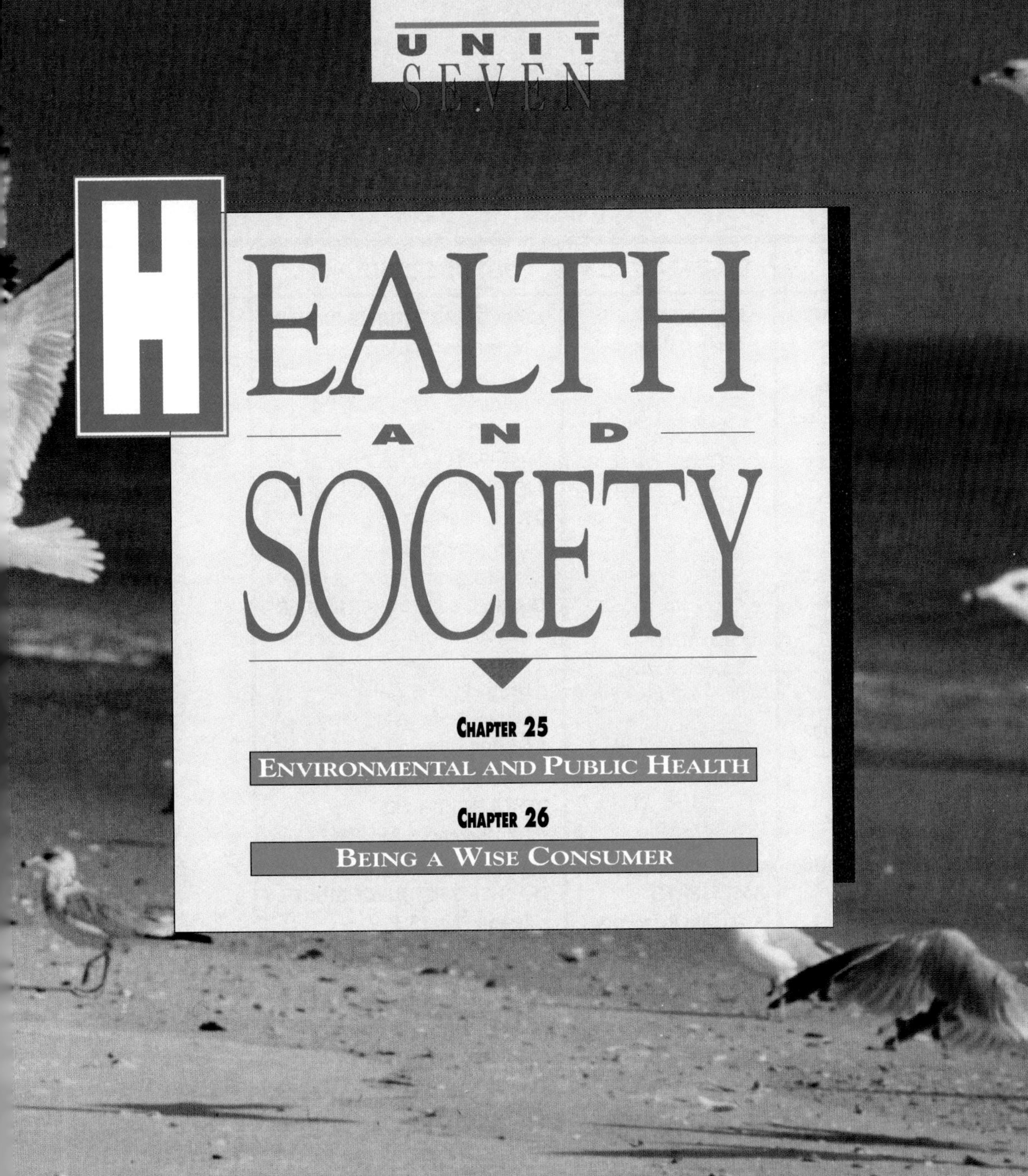

UNIT PREVIEW

This unit provides information that helps students understand how a healthy environment is essential to personal and public health. This in turn helps them make responsible decisions about environmental issues. Students learn the roles of various agencies and organizations in maintaining public health. To prepare them to be informed consumers of health care, the unit describes how to select and communicate with a doctor. It explains the rights of patients as well as some of the plans that are available to pay for health care costs. The five major health themes are emphasized throughout the unit, as indicated in the chart below.

THEMES TRACE

	WELLNESS	BUILDING SELF-ESTEEM	DECISION MAKING	DEVELOPING LIFE-MANAGEMENT SKILLS	ACCEPTANCE OF DIVERSITY AMONG PEOPLE
Chapter 25	pp. 539, 560		p. 558	pp. 547, 555–556, 563–566	
Chapter 26			pp. 572–573	pp. 571–574, 578, 580	pp. 578–579

ENVIRONMENTAL AND PUBLIC HEALTH

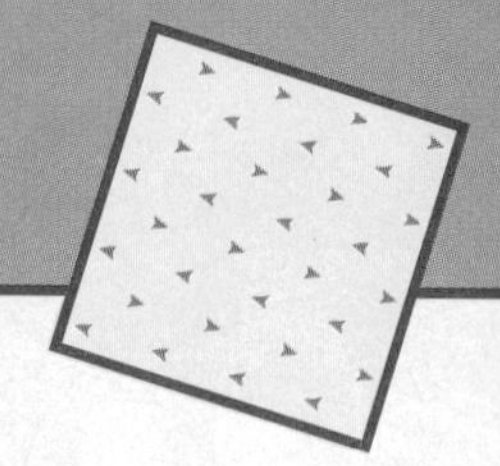

PLANNING GUIDE

TEXT SECTIONS	OBJECTIVES	TEXT FEATURES	OUTSIDE RESOURCES	NOTES
25.1 The Environment and Health pp. 539-544 4 periods	• Identify the characteristics of an ecosystem. • Describe the components of a healthy environment. • Identify the consequences of overpopulation and pollution.	**ASSESSMENT** • Section Review, p. 544	**TEACHER'S RESOURCE BINDER** • Lesson Plan 25.1 • Personal Health Inventory • Journal Entries 25A, 25B • Section Review Worksheet 25.1 • Section Quiz 25.1 • Reteaching Worksheet 25.1 **OTHER RESOURCES** • Transparency 25A	
25.2 Environmental Pollution pp. 545-552 4 periods	• Identify the main cause of environmental pollution. • Describe the environmental consequences of air pollution. • Identify health problems caused by various types of pollution.	• Check Up, p. 552 **ASSESSMENT** • Section Review, p. 552	**TEACHER'S RESOURCE BINDER** • Lesson Plan 25.2 • Journal Entries 25C, 25D • Life Skills 25A, 25B • Section Review Worksheet 25.2 • Section Quiz 25.2 • Reteaching Worksheet 25.2 **OTHER RESOURCES** • Transparencies 25B, 25C	
25.3 What Can You Do? pp. 553-556 2 periods	• Describe the benefits of responsible waste management, recycling, and conservation. • List specific ways each individual can help reduce pollution. ■ Make a recycling and reuse plan for your household.	**ASSESSMENT** • Section Review, p. 556	**TEACHER'S RESOURCE BINDER** • Lesson Plan 25.3 • Journal Entries 25E, 25F • Life Skills 25C • Section Review Worksheet 25.3 • Section Quiz 25.3 • Reteaching Worksheet 25.3 **OTHER RESOURCES** • Making a Choice 25A, 25B	
25.4 Public Health pp. 557-566 3 periods	• Define public health. • Describe four public-health activities. • Compare the public-health concerns of developed and developing countries. ■ Discover what the major public-health issues are in your community and find out where to get help for a public-health problem.	• What Would You Do?, p. 558 • LIFE SKILLS: Using Community Resources, p. 565 **ASSESSMENT** • Section Review, p. 566	**TEACHER'S RESOURCE BINDER** • Lesson Plan 25.4 • Journal Entries 25G, 25H, 25I • Life Skills 25D • Section Review Worksheet 25.4 • Section Quiz 25.4 • Reteaching Worksheet 25.4	
End of Chapter pp. 567-569		**ASSESSMENT** • Chapter Review, pp. 568-569	**TEACHER'S RESOURCE BINDER** • Chapter Test • Alternative Assessment • Personal Pledge **OTHER RESOURCES** • Test Generator	

■ Denotes LIFE SKILLS objectives

• Items in blue are also part of the *Holt Health Activity Book*.

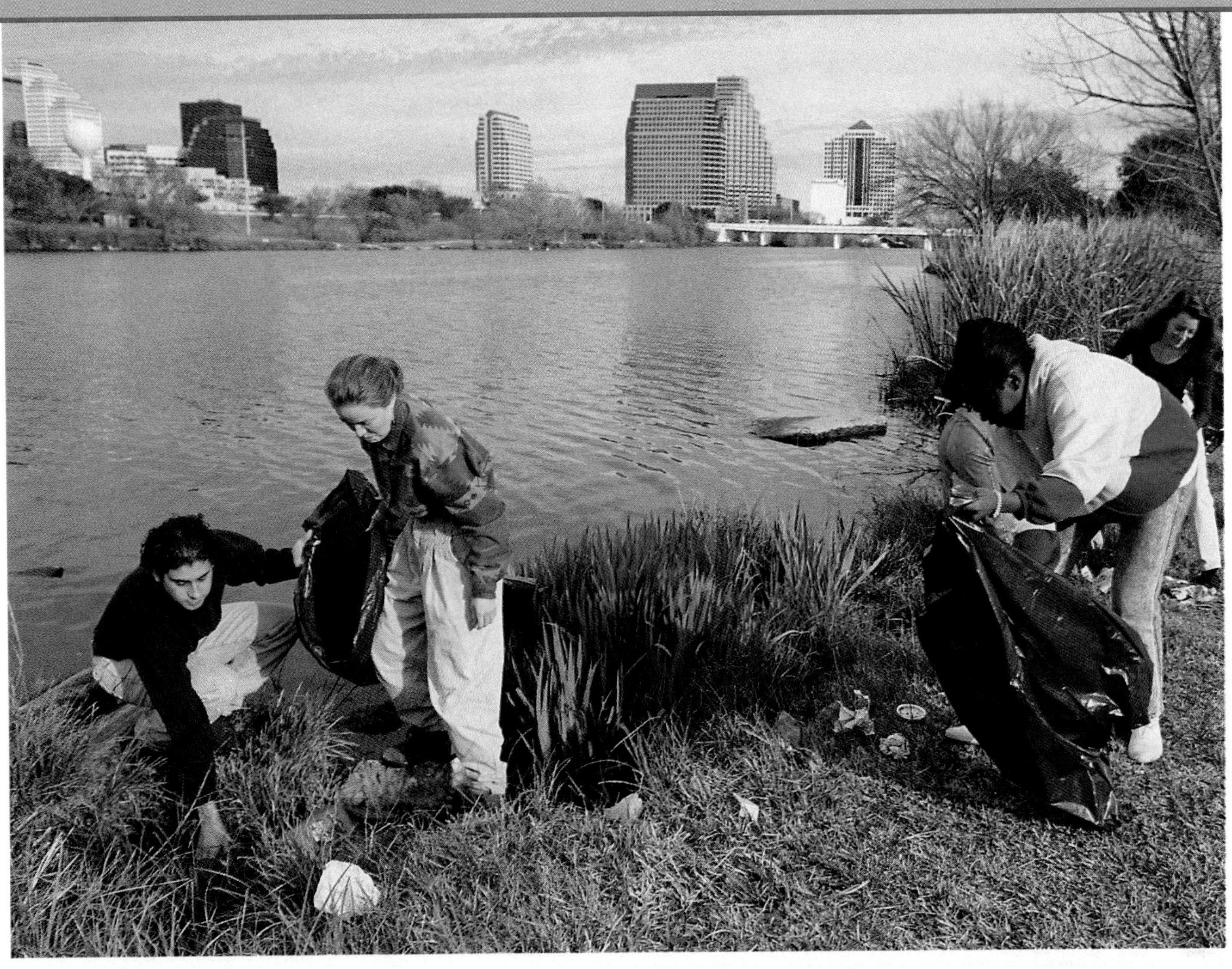

CONTENT BACKGROUND Environmental Action

MANY PEOPLE BELIEVE THAT THE PLANET'S environmental health is the most important public-health issue today. If the planet cannot support life, all other issues will be moot. More subtly, environmental degradation contributes to the deterioration of health; people in a sick environment cannot experience complete wellness.

Students are aware of the numerous environmental challenges we face: from oil spills and smog to DDT in breast milk and pesticides in groundwater; from global warming to deforestation to acid rain. They may be aware that many of these problems are interrelated. Population growth, for instance, underlies the loss of forests and the creation of air pollution. They will be asking what they can do to help.

Students are organizing themselves on college campuses, and colleges themselves are capitalizing on student interest in the environment. For example, at Kalamazoo College in Michigan, a course on managing the Earth is stimulating attention from students with a wide variety of majors and divergent political orientations. More students are choosing careers that meet environmental concerns. Colleges are encouraging activities that reflect environmental concerns. Some colleges require participation in community activities, some of which are environmentally oriented. New student-designed multidisciplinary majors combine business, sociology, foreign language, and international and environmental law. Another program offers a major in English with a minor in environmental studies, leading to a career in environmental journalism. Extracurricular activities that reflect environmental concerns sometimes turn into vocational opportunities for college students after graduation.

An educational computer network now available for environmental information provides students with up-to-date information. Global Action Network (GAN), based at Tufts University, is accessed through an electronic network called EcoNet. Technology and education are now working cooperatively and powerfully to address the environmental crisis.

National governments, industries, and research institutions traditionally involved in environmental politics are now sharing the arena with participants from the media, nongovernmental and international organizations, and political parties. Established institutions must adapt to new situations and cooperate with new groups that arise out of environmental concern. Policy coordination is needed so that interrelated ecosystems are not treated separately and therefore ineffectively. One vital role for government is to provide information and coordination—while decision making is done at the local level.

Individuals, rather than large groups, are gaining in importance and are becoming the catalyst of environmental policy formation. Leaders are needed who learn and who willingly admit mistakes and the limited scope of their knowledge. Leaders are needed who will act on new information when it arises. Young people like those in your classroom may very well assume these leadership roles someday.

PLANNING FOR INSTRUCTION

KEY FACTS

- **Living things and their physical surroundings (environment) make up ecosystems. The living things and nonliving parts of an ecosystem are interdependent.**
- **The environment provides water, air, food, and living space for living things.**
- **Overpopulation, overuse of resources, and pollution can disturb the environment and disrupt ecosystems.**
- **Water pollution, including water contaminated with hazardous materials, and air pollution, which results from toxic gases and particles in the air, can damage health.**
- **Destruction of the ozone layer and global warming both affect the health of people on a worldwide scale.**
- **Conservation, the wise use of natural resources, helps protect the environment. Recycling reduces land pollution and helps preserve the environment.**
- **Individual actions can do much to help preserve the environment.**
- **Public-health concerns are those that deal with the health of people in a community. Public-health practices include providing good sanitation and using quarantine and immunization to control disease.**
- **Public-health problems and priorities in developed countries may differ from those in developing countries.**
- **Public-health agencies provide services at local and state, national, and international levels. Many private organizations provide support for public-health efforts around the world.**

MYTHS AND MISCONCEPTIONS

MYTH: The world is so huge that there is nothing that I can do to change it — for better or for worse.

The actions of every individual count. It is only through the collective action of individuals that changes needed to preserve the environment will take place.

MYTH: Lower levels of pollutants in the atmosphere are safe.

Even minute quantities of toxic materials in the environment can have devastating effects on ecosystems. For some toxins, there is no safe level of exposure.

MYTH: Except for AIDS, infectious disease is not a problem in the United States.

Infectious diseases, such as pneumonia, kill many people in the United States, particularly the young and the elderly. In August 1992 a man in Tucson, Arizona, died of pneumonic plague, a particularly virulent form of bubonic plague. Tuberculosis is becoming a threat again, as strains that resist antibiotics develop.

VOCABULARY

Essential: The following vocabulary terms appear in boldface type.

ecosystem
homeostasis
food chain
overpopulation
nonrenewable resources
renewable resources
greenhouse effect
global warming
hazardous wastes
conservation
epidemic
public health

Secondary: Be aware that the following terms may come up during class discussion.

environment
interdependency
CFCs
life expectancy
ozone layer
recycling
solid waste
nuclear wastes
infectious diseases
immunization

FOR STUDENTS WITH SPECIAL NEEDS

Visual Learners: Have students collect pictures from magazines and newspapers showing a variety of unspoiled ecosystems, the effects of pollution in different settings, and the causes of pollution. Use these pictures as you discuss ecosystems and pollution.

At-Risk Students: Organize a project to improve the environment in and around the school. Allow students to select tasks that they wish to participate in, and provide recognition for students' accomplishments.

LEP Students: Many terms from this chapter are drawn from the fields of science and medicine. Have pairs of students write these terms on a set of index cards and have them write the definitions on a second set of cards. Have these pairs of students work together, matching terms and definitions.

ENRICHMENT

- Suggest students read *Silent Spring,* by Rachel Carson, published by Houghton Mifflin in 1962. The book alerted the public to how activities of humans were destroying the environment.
- Invite an official of the local public-health department to speak to the class about important public-health issues. If possible, ask the official to distribute printed information about physical and mental health services available to the community.

CHAPTER 25 CHAPTER OPENER

GETTING STARTED

Using the Chapter Photograph

Ask students what they find appealing about the photograph showing people enjoying a ride down white-water rapids. Elicit from students the relationship between a clean, healthy environment and an individual's feeling of personal health and well-being.

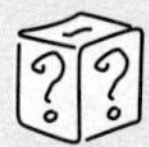

Question Box

This chapter analyzes the relationship between environment and health. The Question Box provides students with an opportunity to ask questions anonymously. To ensure that students with questions are not embarrassed to be seen writing, have those who do not have questions write something else—such as three things in the environment that affect their health—instead.

Preview the questions and then answer them at appropriate points in the chapter. You may wish to allow students to write additional anonymous questions as they go through the chapter.

Personal Issues *ALERT*

It is not likely that all students come from comparable environments. The environmental quality in some areas may be poorer than in others, due to various types of pollution, including pollution from nearby industries. Students should not be made to feel that their surroundings reflect their personal worth, or that a better environment means a better individual. Nor should they be made to feel responsible for environmental problems. Instead, emphasize that they take responsibility for improving the environment.

Access to health care, including use of public-health facilities, is a private matter. Be cautious about discussions that might cause students to be uncomfortable about their health care and how it is obtained.

CHAPTER 25

Environmental and Public Health

For many people, enjoying the outdoors is part of a healthy lifestyle. But even if you don't enjoy outdoor activities, a healthy environment is essential to your health and to the health of all people.

The trouble started when Teresa's sister wound up in the hospital with pains in her abdomen. Before long, several other people in the neighborhood began to have the same symptoms. People were upset because the doctors at the local clinic hadn't been able to figure out what was making everyone sick. Eventually, officials from the health department were called in to help solve the mystery.

Within a few weeks, health officials announced that Teresa's sister and her neighbors were suffering from gasoline poisoning. Small amounts of gasoline in the neighborhood's drinking water had caused liver and neurological damage. In other words, the environment in the neighborhood was unhealthy. To inform as many people as possible of the danger, a neighborhood meeting was arranged. Teresa decided to go to find out what was going on.

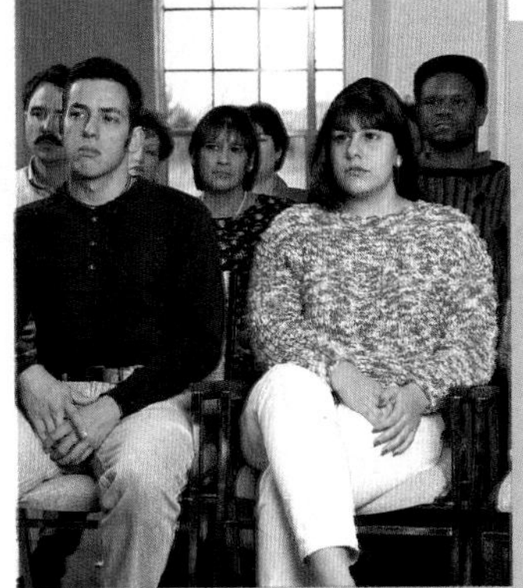

Section 25.1 The Environment and Health

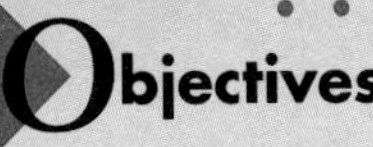

Objectives

- *Identify the characteristics of an ecosystem.*
- *Describe the components of a healthy environment.*
- *Identify the consequences of overpopulation and pollution.*

Talking about the environment in a health class may seem strange, but a healthy environment is an important element in both personal and public health. Every year thousands of people—like the people in Teresa's neighborhood—find out how important the environment is to their health. In this chapter, you will discover how the environment is important to your health.

At the meeting, several environmental and health specialists spoke to people from Teresa's neighborhood. As she listened to the speakers, Teresa began to get a better idea of how all living things are related to their environment. Teresa learned that a healthy environment promotes good health, and that when the environment is damaged, the health effects can be enormous.

Ecosystems

Every living thing is part of an **ecosystem**, which consists of many groups of living things and their physical surroundings (environment). For example, a lake and all the organisms that live in it make up an ecosystem. All the living things on Earth and the places where they live make up a worldwide ecosystem. From the smallest to the largest, all ecosystems have several things in common.

ecosystem:
a system made of living things and their physical surroundings.

Background
The Gaia Hypothesis
The idea that the Earth itself is a living being is found among the mythologies of ancient peoples. However, in 1979 a scientist named James Lovelock proposed the Gaia hypothesis, stating that the Earth is a giant organism. The Gaia hypothesis (*Gaia* is from the ancient Greek name for Mother Earth) envisions all of Earth's creatures, as well as Earth's physical components, as parts of the organism called Earth. The complex interactions between organisms and between organisms and physical systems, such as the ocean and atmosphere, maintain conditions suitable for life. Thus, according to the Gaia hypothesis, Earth actively maintains its homeostasis. Although discounted by many scientists, Lovelock's hypothesis has generated considerable discussion and debate.

Section 25.1 Lesson Plan

MOTIVATE

Journal 25A
Your Environment
This may be done as a warm-up activity. Ask students to record in the Student Journal in the Student Activity Book some things about their environment that affect their health in positive ways. Then ask them to record some things that affect their health in negative ways. Suggest that they review their lists as they read the chapter and modify the lists if necessary.

TEACH

Class Discussion
Teresa's Environment
Discuss with students how they might react to the situation in Teresa's neighborhood if they lived there. Ask them to consider whether they would become involved and in what ways. Have them identify questions they might ask at a neighborhood meeting and the kind of action they would want the community to take.

Demonstration
Ecosystems
Display a small ecosystem, such as an aquarium or a terrarium, to the class. (You may be able to borrow such an ecosystem from the biology department.) Have students identify the living things in the ecosystem. Have

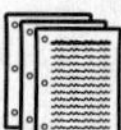

Personal Health Inventory

Have students complete the Personal Health Inventory for this chapter. The inventory helps them assess their own behavior with respect to the environment and their health.

Interactions One characteristic of an ecosystem is that its living and nonliving parts interact with one another. Some living things feed on others. Living things also take the water and nutrients they need from the environment. They return materials that are needed by other living things. For example, you inhale oxygen and exhale carbon dioxide. Plants take in carbon dioxide and give off oxygen. In other words, each living thing provides something that other living things need.

Nonliving materials interact as well. For example, oxygen reacts chemically with elements such as iron to form new compounds. The rusting of iron and steel is such a reaction. Such processes help turn rocks into soil. Another example of interaction between nonliving parts of the environment is the effect of the carbon dioxide in the atmosphere. Carbon dioxide helps maintain the temperature of our surroundings by trapping heat from the sun.

Interdependency Now, consider what could happen if most of Earth's plants died. For one thing, there would be less oxygen and more carbon dioxide. Both you and the environment would be affected. Your body would have to adjust to having less oxygen. The extra carbon dioxide might make the climate warmer. Just think how it would be if summertime temperatures were 10 to 20 degrees warmer than they are now. This could happen if certain human activities (releasing large amounts of carbon dioxide by burning oil and gas and clearing large areas of the world's forests) are not reduced.

You can see that whatever happens to one part of an ecosystem affects other parts. In other words, the parts of an ecosystem are interdependent. The water, air, land, and climate, plus the kinds of organisms and the size of their communities, are all important to the health of an ecosystem. If one part of an ecosystem is damaged, the environment in the ecosystem could become unhealthy.

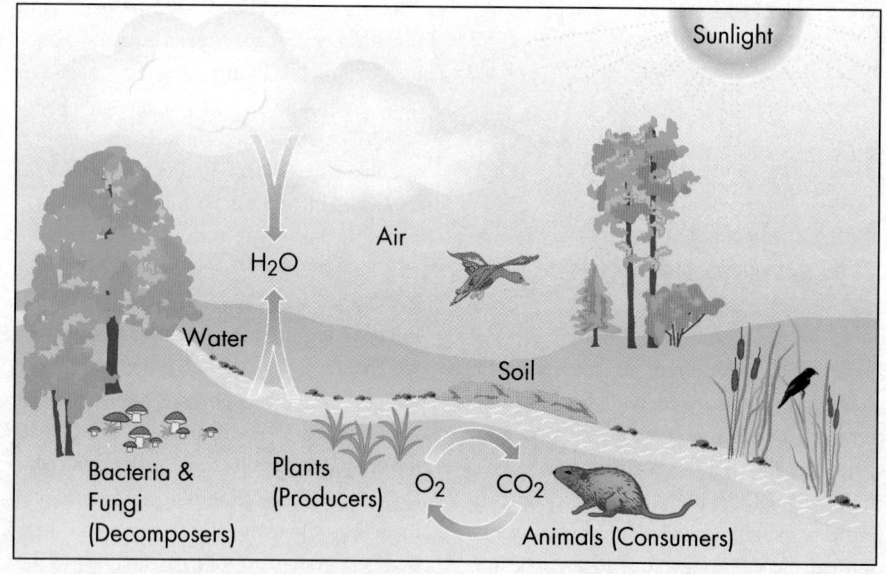

(FIGURE 25-1) **The parts of an ecosystem interact and are interdependent. Constant change is another feature of an ecosystem.**

• • • TEACH continued

them identify the nonliving parts, or physical factors, in the ecosystem. If you cannot display a small ecosystem, try to take students outdoors to observe a local ecosystem and have them identify the living and nonliving parts.

Class Discussion
People and the Environment

Emphasize the interaction between people and the environment. **What are some things the environment supplies that are necessary for life?** *[Air, water, food, and a proper temperature are examples.]* Point out that animals depend on plants for oxygen. Plants are also a source of food, both directly and indirectly. Ask students to explain how eating meat is, indirectly, dependent on a supply of plant life. Finally, remind students that animals breathe out carbon dioxide, which plants need to make food.

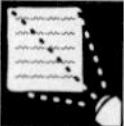

Teaching Transparency 25A
Parts of an Ecosystem

Show the diagram of the parts of an ecosystem (Figure 25-1). Have students distinguish the ecosystem's living and nonliving parts.

Journal 25B
Personal Water Use

Have students record in the Student Journal in the Student Activity Book the ways in which they use water each day. Then have them decide if they are

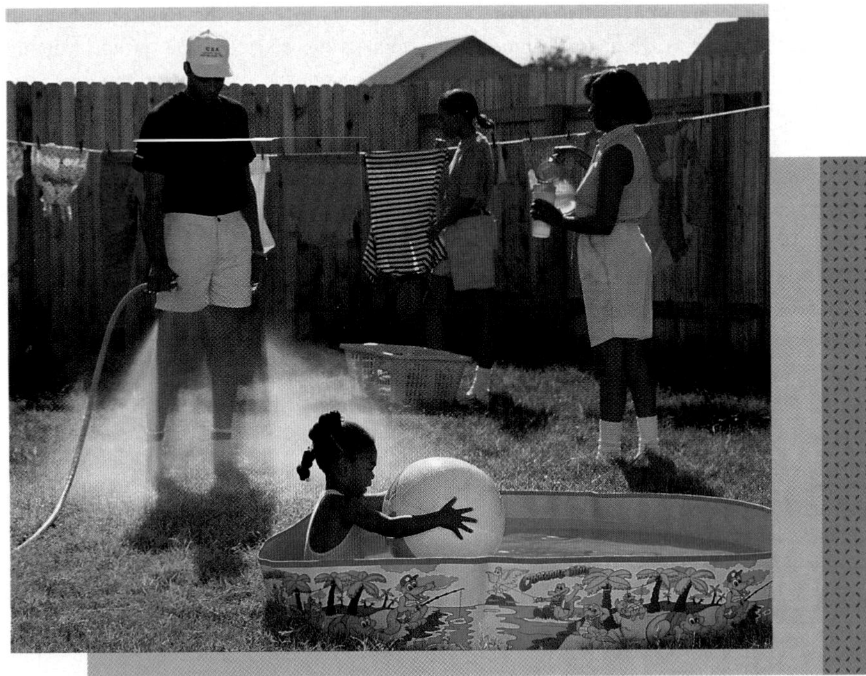

(FIGURE 25-2) **In addition to the many everyday activities for which we use water, each of us uses about 40 gallons of water per day just for personal washing and toilet flushing.**

Change and Homeostasis Fortunately, living things are able to adjust to changes in their environment. When it's cold, for instance, you shiver and get goose bumps. This is an automatic change your body makes to warm you up. Organisms rely on such changes to maintain a balance inside their bodies. Maintaining this balance is called **homeostasis**.

Ecosystems also change constantly. For example, the temperature changes from day to night and from season to season. Materials such as water and air, as well as the living things, constantly come and go. In healthy ecosystems, there is a balance between the materials that are entering and leaving. The internal balance that exists in an ecosystem can also be thought of as homeostasis.

Elements of a Healthy Environment

Even though living things can adjust to many of the changes in their surroundings, there are limits to this ability. The environment provides certain materials and conditions that are essential for the healthy existence of living things. Among these essentials are water, air, and adequate food and living space.

Water Water is one substance that is vital to all living things. It is home to many organisms (living things). But more important, all of the body processes that sustain life require water. In fact, most of an organism's body is water. For instance, water makes up as much as 65 to 70 percent of your body as a whole, and 80 percent

homeostasis:

the tendency of any living thing to maintain a balance in its inner systems.

wasting water in any of these uses. Students can also record ways to reduce their water usage.

Demonstration
A Food Chain

Divide the class into groups of three or four. In each group, students should assume the identity of an organism that could be part of a food chain. Students must adhere to the following rules: one person in each group must be a plant; at least one person in each group must be a plant-eater; at least one person in each group must be a meat-eater. (grass, cow, person) Have each group demonstrate how the organisms might form a food chain. To extend the activity, allow groups to exchange members to construct different food chains.

Debate the Issue
Overpopulation

Select two teams of students to debate the question: Should national governments limit family size in their countries? Give students time to research factors involved in the issue, including the relationship between birth rate and population growth, and attitudes toward an individual's right to privacy. Allow each team to present its arguments. Then allow other members of the class to question team members about their stand on the question.

Background
Population Growth

Population growth is often expressed in terms of doubling time, that is, the time required for a population to double in size. Earth's population in 1600 was approximately 500 million. It was not until 1850, 250 years later, that the population had doubled, reaching 1 billion. However, as population size increases, doubling time declines, if the birth rate is constant. Thus, Earth's population reached 2 billion in the first part of the twentieth century and about 3 billion by 1960. Even though the birth rate is declining, Earth's population will likely reach 6 billion early in the twenty-first century.

of your brain. Human activities require a great deal of water as well. In addition to the water we must drink daily to maintain good health, we also use water for personal and household cleanliness, food preparation, and recreation. Agriculture and industry use huge amounts of water to grow food, process food and raw materials, and manufacture other necessities.

food chain: *a sequence of organisms that begins with a food producer and continues with one or more organisms, each of which eats the one before it.*

Unfortunately, less water is available for our use than most people realize. About 97 percent of Earth's vast water supply is salt water. Most of the remaining 3 percent is frozen in the polar icecaps and glaciers. This means that only about 0.5 percent of Earth's water supply is fresh water that is suitable for human use. However, we must share that water with the other organisms that live in and require fresh water.

Air Air is another substance that is vital to all living things. Without it, you could survive for only a few minutes. Oxygen is the important gas you get from air. It allows you to obtain energy from your food. Other gases, such as carbon dioxide and ozone, are also important to you. In addition to trapping the sun's heat, carbon dioxide is used by plants to make the food on which all animals depend. Ozone protects living things from the damaging ultraviolet rays in sunlight.

Other Essentials Nutrients (food and minerals) are another requirement for living that comes from the environment. All living things are part of a **food chain**. In a food chain, an organism, such as a frog, eats another organism, such as a dragonfly. The frog may then be eaten by a fish, and the fish may be eaten by a human. As you can see in Figure 25-3, all food chains begin with a life form, such as a plant, that makes its own food out of nonliving materials from the environment.

If something affects one of the life forms in a food chain, the others are usually affected as well. For example, if all of the frogs disappeared, there would be more dragonflies. And because the fish would have less food, there would be fewer fish, which would mean there would also be less food for the humans.

Living things also require a certain amount of room in which to live. The amount of space needed by a particular type

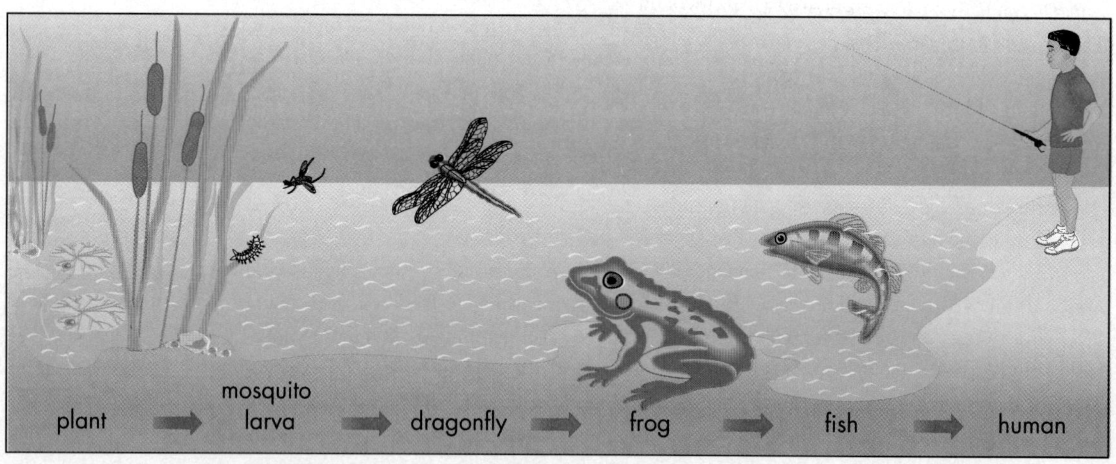

(FIGURE 25-3) **A typical food chain.**

• • • TEACH continued

Extension
Looking at the Problems

Have students check newspapers and weekly newsmagazines for stories about human hardships that are in some way connected to problems in the environment. Such stories might range from local environmental problems, similar to the problem in Teresa's neighborhood, to more extensive tragedies, such as famine. Have students bring the stories to class. Select stories to discuss and emphasize the relationship between environmental degradation and human hardship.

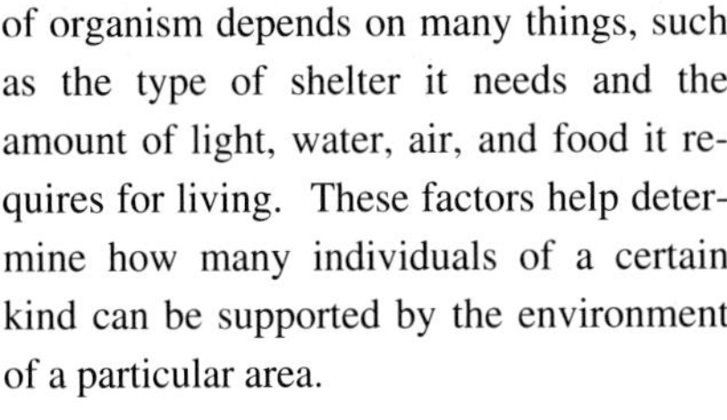

of organism depends on many things, such as the type of shelter it needs and the amount of light, water, air, and food it requires for living. These factors help determine how many individuals of a certain kind can be supported by the environment of a particular area.

Upsetting the Balance

If you have ever had food poisoning from eating contaminated food or become dehydrated from perspiring too much, you know how bad you can feel when your homeostasis is disrupted. Your health suffers when your internal balance is upset. Likewise, the health of the environment is threatened when the homeostasis of an ecosystem is disturbed. **Overpopulation** and pollution are two factors that disturb the healthy balance in an ecosystem.

Overpopulation If you had been born in 1900, you could have expected to live about 47 years. Babies born in the United States in the 1990s are expected to live about 76 years. Better health care and cleaner living conditions are primary reasons for this dramatic increase in *life expectancy* (the average length of time a person is expected to live). However, as life expectancy has increased, the number of people living on Earth has also increased.

The world's population is currently growing at a rate of about 255,000 people per day, or 90 million people per year. About 90 percent of this growth is occurring in the developing countries. Such a rapidly growing human population places a burden on the natural resources of some regions. When the population of a region becomes too large to be supported by the available resources, overpopulation has occurred.

The effects of increasing population are serious. At its worst, overpopulation results in poverty and starvation when food production cannot keep up with population growth. In addition, there are severe shortages of usable land and other natural resources. Currently, Earth's **nonrenewable resources** such as petroleum and mineral ores are being used at an alarming rate. Even **renewable resources** such as timber and seafood are being consumed at a much faster rate than they are currently being replaced.

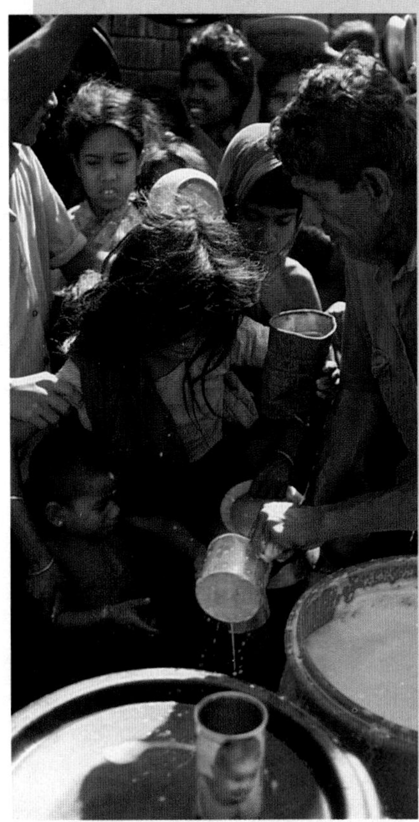

(FIGURE 25-4) **Overpopulation has resulted in a shortage of food in Dacca, Bangladesh. These conditions have made it necessary for the people there to wait in long lines just to get a small ration of milk for their children.**

overpopulation: *the point at which the population of an area is so large that it can no longer be supported by the available resources.*

nonrenewable resources: *natural resources such as coal and oil that cannot be replaced once they are used.*

renewable resources: *natural resources such as trees that can be replaced continually.*

Section 25.1

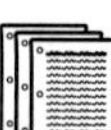

Section Review Worksheet 25.1

Assign Section Review Worksheet 25.1, which requires students to demonstrate an understanding of interactions in ecosystems.

Section Quiz 25.1

Have students take Section Quiz 25.1.

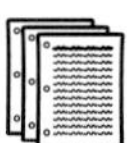

Reteaching Worksheet 25.1

Students who have difficulty with the material may complete Reteaching Worksheet 25.1, which requires them to complete and interpret a graphic showing interactions in an ecosystem.

Review Answers

1. The parts of an ecosystem interact, are interdependent, and are able to adjust to changes.
2. Water, air, nutrients, and space
3. Overpopulation can lead to poverty, starvation, and shortages of usable land and natural resources. Pollution can lead to the extinction of life forms, climate changes, and shortages of food and clean water.
4. Yes. Humans should make sure that the environment remains balanced and healthy. They can do so by not polluting the environment and by using natural resources wisely.

Consequences of Pollution and Removal of Resources

Extinction of life forms, such as the dinosaurs.

Destruction of ecosystems, such as the tropical rain forests of Central and South America.

Climate changes, such as global warming due to the greenhouse effect.

Shortages of food and clean water, which lead to famine and disease.

(FIGURE 25-5) **Since the parts of the environment are interrelated, any one of these events could trigger the others.**

Pollution The balance in an ecosystem is also disturbed when one or more of its parts is damaged by pollution. Pollution occurs when substances that are harmful to living things contaminate the air, water, or soil. Such substances include poisonous chemicals, garbage, and radioactive wastes. Even excess amounts of otherwise beneficial materials such as carbon dioxide can also be considered as pollutants (substances that cause pollution). It is difficult to predict how pollution will ultimately affect Earth and its inhabitants, but it has already greatly affected human and environmental health. In Figure 25-5, you will find some of the many possible consequences of pollution.

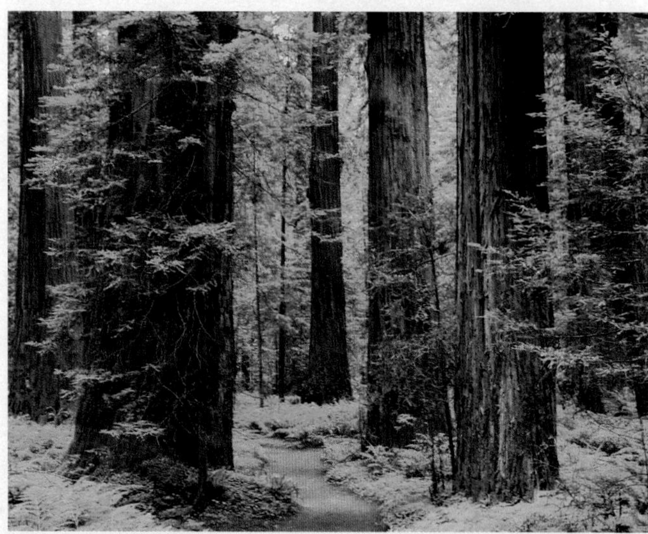

(FIGURE 25-6) **When properly managed, forests like this one, and many other natural resources as well, can be renewable resources.**

Review

1. *List the characteristics of an ecosystem.*
2. *What do living things need from their environment for a healthy existence?*
3. *How do overpopulation and pollution affect an ecosystem?*
4. ***Critical Thinking*** *Do you think that humans are a part of the natural ecosystems on Earth? If so, what responsibility, if any, do you think humans should take for the other parts of ecosystems?*

ASSESS

Section Review

Have students answer the Section Review questions.

Alternative Assessment

Parts of an Ecosystem

Have students give an example of an ecosystem. Then have them name some living and nonliving things in that ecosystem. Finally, have students identify one or more ways in which the homeostasis of that ecosystem might be upset.

Closure

Overpopulated Ecosystems

Have students explain how overpopulation in a natural ecosystem, such as a pond or a forest, places a burden on the resources of that ecosystem. *[The rapid reproduction of algae in a pond is an example. Decomposing algae cause an oxygen shortage in the water; the algae on the surface block sunlight from reaching lower levels, killing plants that depend on photosynthesis and animals that depend on those plants.]*

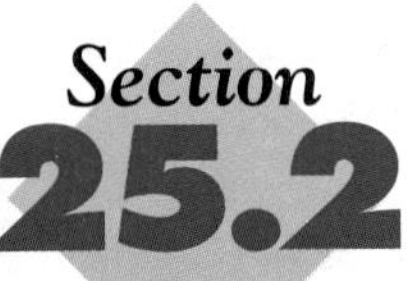

Section 25.2 Environmental Pollution

Objectives

- *Identify the main cause of environmental pollution.*
- *Describe the environmental consequences of air pollution.*
- *Identify health problems caused by various types of pollution.*

The situation in Teresa's neighborhood is just one example of how pollution can damage the environment and affect human health. You have probably heard or read about many other incidents that are similar, or even more serious. In this section, you will learn about several forms of environmental pollution and discover how they may affect your health.

Although Teresa had learned a lot at the neighborhood meeting, she was still upset. "Did you hear?" Teresa asked her boyfriend, Jaime. "The health department found out there's gasoline in our drinking water! That's what made my sister and our neighbors sick. They say the gasoline's coming from some gasoline storage tanks in our neighborhood."

"I heard," Jaime said. "My dad works for a company that owns some of those tanks. That's all he talked about last

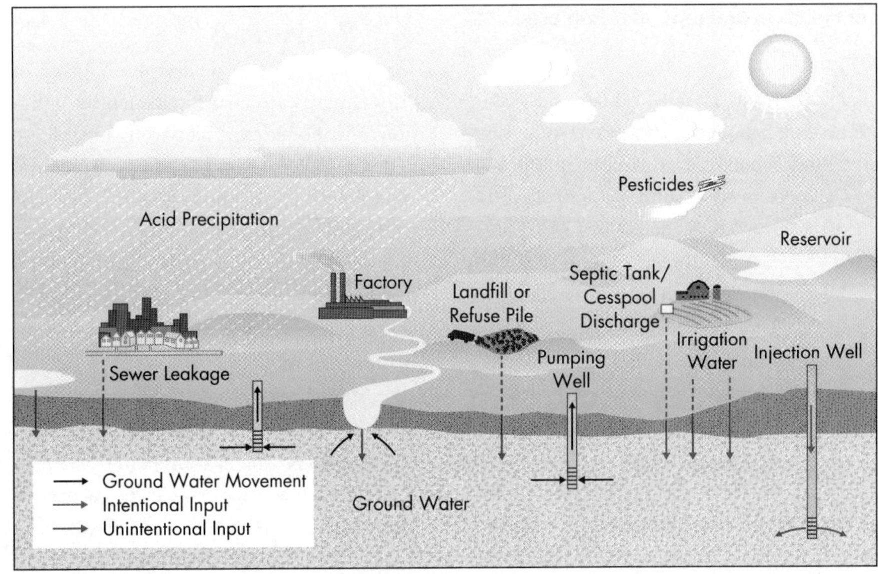

(FIGURE 25-7) **Sources of water pollution. Public drinking water comes from two main sources: surface waters (precipitation that collects in rivers, lakes, and reservoirs) and ground water (precipitation that seeps into the ground). The quality of drinking water varies, depending on its source and its exposure to pollutants.**

Background

Magnifying Pollutants

Dumping even small amounts of pollutants into bodies of water can result in serious damage to the environment. Organisms that live in the water may take in the pollutants, concentrating them in their tissues. The pollutants are further concentrated as they are passed along the food chain. Thus, an animal, such as an eagle, that consumes fish, may be affected by pollutants that were initially absorbed by aquatic plants. The increasing concentration of pollutants through the food chain is called biomagnification.

Section 25.2 Lesson Plan

MOTIVATE

Journal 25C

Pollution Around You

This may be done as a warm-up activity. Encourage students to record in the Student Journal examples of pollution in their environment. Suggest that they look for pollution both in their neighborhoods and around the school. Have them identify the sources of the pollution, if possible.

Role-Playing

Community Concerns

Have two or three students play the roles of officials from companies that own the underground tanks in Teresa's neighborhood. Have five or six students play the roles of community representatives. The company officials should try to convince the community representatives that they are serving the needs of the community and that the tanks should be repaired but not removed. Allow the community representatives to respond as they believe they should.

TEACH

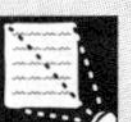

Teaching Transparency 25B

Sources of Water Pollution

Show the transparency of the diagram that illustrates possible sources of water pollution (Figure 25-7). Have students identify the sources in the diagram and then indicate if any of

Background
Acid Rain
Acid rain is another harmful outcome of air pollution. It damages soil and surface waters, destroys forests and agricultural crops, and endangers human health. The main causes of acid rain are the sulfur dioxide and nitrogen oxides given off by coal-burning power plants and motor vehicles. These gases interact with sunlight and water vapor in the air, forming acid compounds. When ordinary precipitation (rain or snow) passes through air containing acid compounds, it picks them up and falls to the ground as acid rain, snow, or sleet.

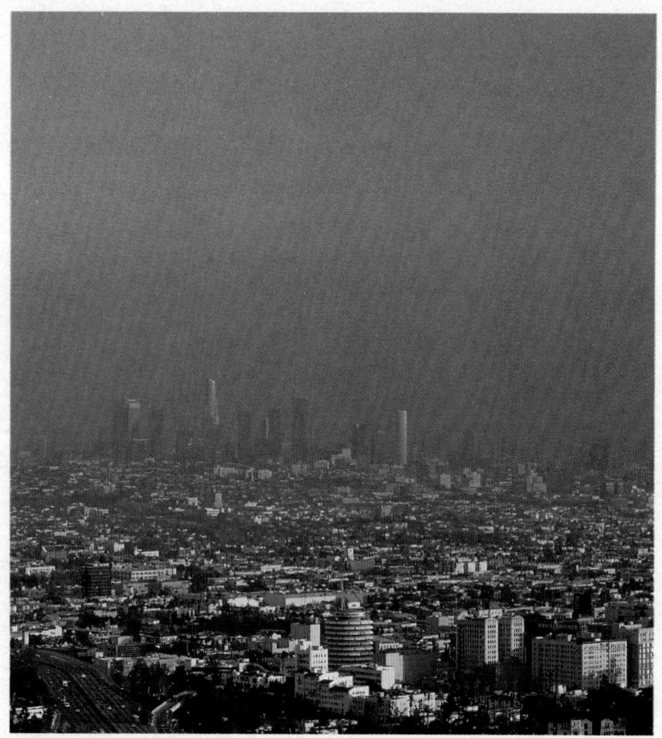

(FIGURE 25-8) **Smog is a visible form of air pollution that causes the hazy appearance of the air in and around urban areas.**

night. The way he tells it those tanks can't be leaking gasoline. They have some kind of pollution controls. But, come to think of it, I always smell gasoline when I drive by the tank farm."

"Me too," Teresa agreed. "Well, we're going to demand that all the tanks be removed from our neighborhood! Those companies don't have the right to make everybody in our neighborhood sick by polluting the water!"

Water Pollution

Our increasing need for water and the pollution of our water supply are moving us steadily toward a health disaster. Already, part of our limited supply of fresh water is too polluted for human use. As a result, many communities in this country, like Teresa's, have more health problems than normal due to polluted drinking water. Entire populations of some countries suffer from many life-threatening health problems caused by severe shortages of clean, fresh water. Imagine what it would be like if you did not have enough water for drinking, bathing, cooking, or washing clothes.

Industry, agriculture, and our everyday activities create a vast amount of waste water, which contains many dangerous chemicals and disease-causing organisms. Although cholera and typhoid (two diseases spread by polluted water) have been eliminated in the United States, chemicals such as lead, gasoline, oil, and disinfection by-products impose many health risks. These and other hazardous chemicals increase the risk of cancer and birth defects as well as neurological, gastrointestinal, kidney, and liver disorders.

Air Pollution

The quality of our air and the balance of critical gases are also threatened by pollution. Air pollution is caused by the release of toxic gases and particles into the atmosphere by automobiles, factories, power-generating plants, and burning trash. These pollutants can be carried long distances by the wind or can rise into the upper levels of the atmosphere, where they cause major worldwide problems.

Many health problems are linked to air pollution. The Environmental Protection Agency (EPA) blames air pollution for at least 2,000 new cases of cancer each year. There is also evidence that polluted air is a factor in birth defects and many other health problems. Young children, the elderly, and people who suffer from allergies or respiratory diseases such as asthma, bronchitis, and emphysema are especially at risk.

• • • TEACH continued

these sources could affect the drinking water in their communities.

Class Discussion
Your Drinking Water
Determine if students know where their household water comes from—a reservoir or other surface water, such as a river, or underground water obtained from wells. Tell them that water from reservoirs and rivers is treated to remove bacteria and is tested periodically for toxic materials. If some students obtain water from underground sources, ask them how the water is tested to ensure that it is free of contaminants. If the community has experienced problems with its water supply, discuss this situation with the class.

Cooperative Learning
How's the Air?
Have students form groups to discuss the air quality in their area. Students should note whether smog or atmospheric haze is common. Ask them to check local newspapers to see if air quality data are given. Have each group suggest what they think is the most important factor contributing to air pollution in the area.

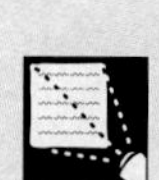

Teaching Transparency 25C
Friend in the Sky, Foe on the Ground
Use this transparency to help students understand how ozone can be both helpful and harmful.

Destruction of the Ozone Layer Ozone is an unstable form of oxygen. In the lower atmosphere, ozone is an undesirable gas that contributes to air pollution and is often a major component of smog. But the ozone found in the region of the upper atmosphere called the ozone layer is vital to living things.

The ozone layer completely surrounds the planet and protects living things from the ultraviolet (UV) light rays of the sun. UV light is dangerous to living things because it damages cells. In the early 1970s, scientists discovered a hole in the ozone layer over Antarctica. In the early 1990s, another hole was detected over the Northern Hemisphere. These holes in the ozone layer allow more of the damaging UV light to reach the Earth's surface.

Chemicals called chlorofluorocarbons (CFCs) have been linked to the destruction of the ozone layer. Sunlight causes these chemicals to break down. When they do, chlorine released from CFCs breaks apart ozone molecules. Aerosol sprays (such as hairspray and deodorant) and chemicals used for cooling in air-conditioning systems and refrigerators are the main sources of ozone-damaging CFCs.

Increased exposure to UV rays has been linked to an increase in several health problems, including skin cancer. Each year, approximately 8,000 people die from skin cancer, and over 500,000 new cases are discovered. Jaime was wondering if all this bad news meant that he would have to give up having fun in the sun. Then he read that he could still enjoy the outdoors by taking a few precautions.

Precautions you can take to avoid overexposure to the sun are discussed in Chapter 6.

Global Warming and the Greenhouse Effect A greenhouse is a great place to be when it's cold outside, but not such a great place to be in the summer when it's hot.

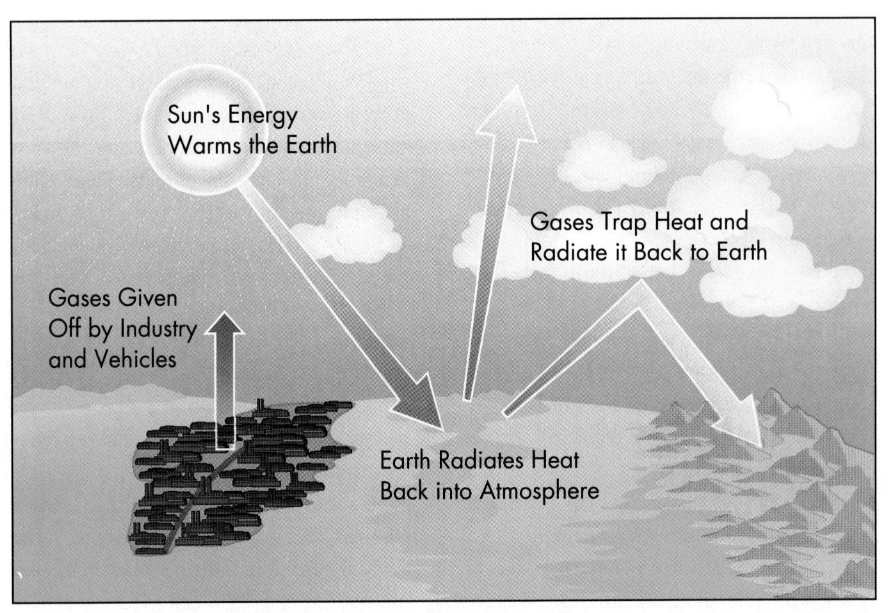

(FIGURE 25-9) **The greenhouse effect causes warming of the atmosphere. As the concentration of greenhouse gases in the atmosphere increases, an overall rise in the temperature of the air, called global warming, is expected.**

SECTION 25.2

Background
Ozone: Increase and Decrease

The thinning of the ozone layer in the stratosphere, caused by CFCs, leads to an increase in ultraviolet radiation reaching the earth's surface. According to one EPA study, a decrease of 1 percent in stratospheric ozone could lead to a 5 percent rise in skin cancer in the United States. Increased UV radiation also damages plants and animals, including the microscopic plankton that form the base of the food chains in the sea.

Additionally, human activities—such as driving gas-powered vehicles, manufacturing, and power production—indirectly add ozone to the lower atmosphere, where it is neither needed nor wanted. Ozone in the lower atmosphere is a pollutant that damages plants and causes respiratory problems in humans. Thus, our activities are destroying ozone where we need it and adding it where it is harmful.

Debate the Issue
No More CFCs

Although aerosols containing CFCs are banned in the United States, most air-conditioning and refrigeration systems still use CFCs. Research is underway to find alternatives to these gases but such products may be years away. Have students debate the issue: Should the manufacture and sale of all CFCs be banned immediately? Have students consider the environmental consequences, as well as the effects on the economy and personal comfort.

Demonstration
Global Warming in a Car

On a sunny day, heat trapped within a car that has the windows closed can raise the inside air temperature considerably. Even on a cool day, the effect is noticeable. Demonstrate this effect by having students measure the temperature inside and outside the car, using thermometers. Have students report any difference in warmth between the inside air and the outside air. Use the car as an analogy to help students understand how such a greenhouse effect could lead to global warming.

Class Discussion
A Warmer Future

Point out that global warming not only means a rise in sea level but a wide range of other consequences as well. For example, dramatic changes in climate, including patterns of rainfall

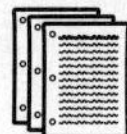

Life Skills Worksheet 25A

Avoiding Tobacco Smoke

Assign the Avoiding Tobacco Smoke Life Skills Worksheet, which requires students to examine strategies nonsmokers can use to avoid secondhand smoke.

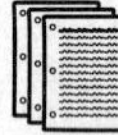

Life Skills Worksheet 25B

Protection from Noise Pollution

Assign the Protection from Noise Pollution Life Skills Worksheet, which requires students to explore strategies for avoiding noise pollution.

Indoor Air Pollutants

Formaldehyde—*chemical used in making furniture, foam insulation,and pressed wood; can cause dizziness, headaches, nausea, and burning eyes and lungs.*

Asbestos—*fibrous mineral once used in insulation; linked to lung cancer and other respiratory diseases.*

Radon—*radioactive gas that occurs naturally in certain kinds of rocks; linked to lung cancer.*

Carbon monoxide—*invisible, odorless gas that escapes from faulty furnaces; causes drowsiness and death.*

(FIGURE 25-10) **Your home, school, or workplace could contain one or more of these indoor air pollutants. Your local health department can help you find out how to determine if any of these pollutants are present in your home.**

greenhouse effect: *the trapping of heat from the sun by certain gases in the atmosphere called greenhouse gases.*

The glass or plastic that covers a greenhouse traps heat from the sun's rays, warming the inside. The **greenhouse effect** is the name given to this warming. The term is also used to describe the warming effect of certain gases in the atmosphere that trap heat from the sun's rays. These gases, called greenhouse gases, include carbon dioxide, water vapor, methane, ozone, nitrous oxide, and CFCs. In the right amounts, the greenhouse gases keep Earth's surface warm enough for life.

global warming: *long-term change in temperature (warming) of Earth's climate that is related to air pollution and the greenhouse effect.*

Today, certain agricultural, industrial, and consumer practices are increasing the amount of greenhouse gases—such as carbon dioxide—in the atmosphere. At the same time, vast numbers of trees, which consume carbon dioxide, are cut down each year. Water pollution also threatens to kill algae and small water plants that take up carbon dioxide and give off oxygen. The overall effect of these changes may be a gradual increase in the temperature of the planet—**global warming**.

Already, global warming has resulted in a rising sea level and the erosion of many coastal areas. Experts believe that by the year 2100, increasing temperatures could melt many glaciers and raise the sea level another two to seven feet. A seven-foot rise of sea level would flood 50 to 80 percent of our coastal wetlands (bays and swamps) and cause extensive destruction of coastal property, wildlife, and beaches.

Indoor Air Pollution Most of us are exposed daily to air pollution in our homes, schools, and workplaces. In tightly sealed buildings, indoor air pollutants may be more concentrated than outdoor air pollutants. In general, indoor air pollution tends to aggravate health problems such as asthma, bronchitis, heart disease, and emphysema. But certain pollutants can cause cancer and other serious illnesses

Tobacco smoke is a common indoor air polluter. You learned in Chapter 14 that if you smoke you are more likely to develop cancer, cardiovascular disease, or respiratory diseases than someone who does not smoke. Recent studies have shown that nonsmokers who are exposed to secondhand and sidestream smoke also have an increased risk of developing these same health problems. Other indoor pollutants and their effects are listed in Figure 25-10.

Land Pollution

Overpopulation and modern technology are creating another pollution problem. Land pollution is the spoiling of the land so that it is unfit to be inhabited by living things. As population grows, more land area will be required to house the human race. This land will become unfit for other purposes, such as growing food and supporting wildlife. But an even greater land-pollution problem is the accumulation of wastes that are produced and discarded by humans.

• • • TEACH continued

and average annual temperatures, would likely occur in most regions. Ask students to consider how such changes might affect agricultural production, recreational activities, fuel consumption, and other human activities.

Debate the Issue

Diapers: Cloth or Disposable?

Have students find out about the differences between disposable and cloth diapers, in terms of their environmental impact. They should look at the amount and kinds of material used in manufacture, the energy consumed in manufacture, the energy used in washing, the landfill space used in disposal, and so on. Have them debate the question: Which is better, cloth or disposable? Then discuss whether there is a clear preference between the two kinds of diapers in terms of the environmental impact.

Journal 25D

My Garbage

Have students refer to Figure 25-11 to identify the types of garbage that humans produce. Then ask them to record in the Student Journal the types of garbage they throw away each day for a week. Have them classify the materials based on the categories shown in Figure 25-11. Then ask them to outline steps they could take to help reduce the problem of garbage disposal.

Solid Wastes Solid wastes include all of the materials that humans discard. In the United States, human activities—agriculture, manufacturing, mining, health care, and just everyday living—produce more than 150 million tons of solid wastes each year. In fact, each one of us generates about four pounds of trash per day. Figure 25-11 shows the types and relative amounts of the materials that the average American throws away.

The most common way of dealing with solid wastes has been to dump them "as far away as possible" so that they could be forgotten. But open dumps (where wastes are left on the ground) are breeding grounds for disease-carrying insects and rodents (rats and mice). Today the amount of solid wastes has grown to the point that finding a safe place to put them (where they will not affect health) is a serious problem.

Most solid wastes are now placed in sanitary landfills. At these sites, the wastes are covered with a layer of soil to prevent the spread of disease. However, materials often escape from landfills to pollute the air and water. Some wastes are burned in incinerators, which reduces the amount of the solid waste but may pollute the air. Sanitary landfills and incinerators (plants where solid wastes are burned) are healthier alternatives to open dumps. Unfortunately, all of these methods take up land that could be used for other purposes, and none are completely safe for human and environmental health.

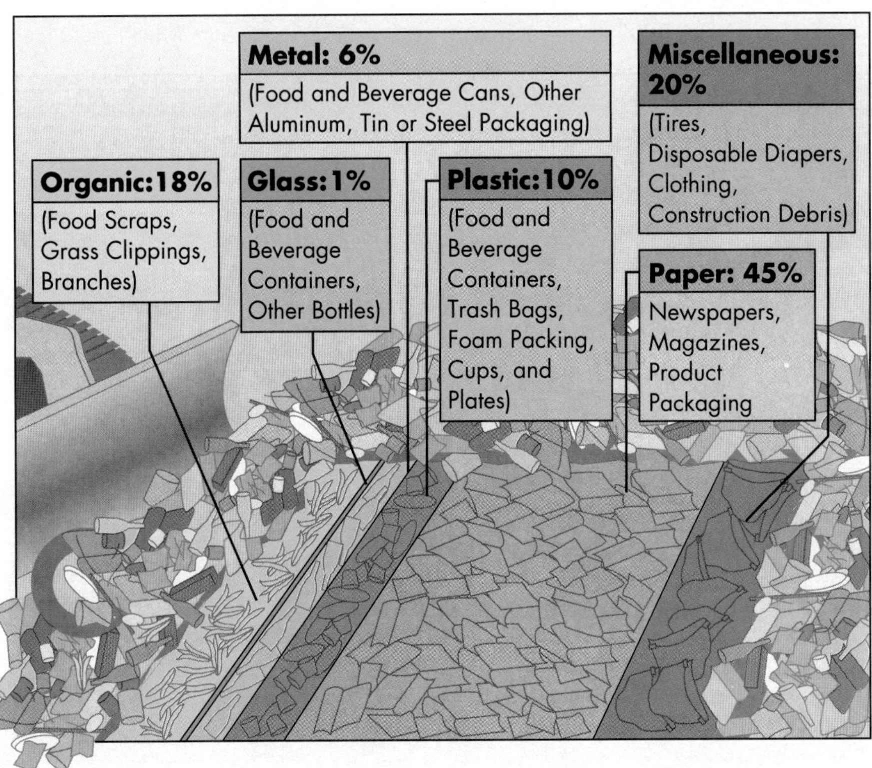

(FIGURE 25-11) **Do you know what's in your trash? Some of these figures may surprise you.**

SECTION 25.2

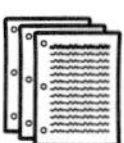

Section Review Worksheet 25.2

Assign Section Review Worksheet 25.2, which requires students to classify factors that contribute to pollution, and to relate health problems to specific types of pollution.

Section Quiz 25.2

Have students take Section Quiz 25.2.

Reteaching Worksheet 25.2

Students who have difficulty with the material may complete Reteaching Worksheet 25.2, which requires them to identify pollutants and their related health risks.

Cooperative Learning
Hazardous Chemicals in Common Use

Obtain Material Safety Data Sheets (MSDSs) for hazardous chemicals that are commonly used in a school or home. They may include cleaning materials, paint thinners, herbicides, and pesticides. (Schools are required to have such sheets on file for the products they use.) Have students form small groups and give each one an MSDS. Have them review the sheet to identify the hazardous chemicals, the kinds of hazards they present, and the recommendations for handling and disposing of the chemicals. Have each group report its findings to the class.

Reinforcement
The Problem of Solid Wastes

Have students distinguish the three categories of wastes that can pollute the land:

- Solid wastes—garbage, or refuse, that is disposed of in open dumps or in sanitary landfills
- Hazardous wastes—toxic materials that can cause serious health problems for all living things
- Nuclear wastes—hazardous wastes that are radioactive and that cause health problems even in small doses

Ask students to suggest ways in which the three types of waste must be disposed of, so that they do not pollute the environment and endanger health.

Background

Nuclear Wastes—Where to Put Them

Nuclear power plants, nuclear weapons plants, research facilities, and medical facilities all generate radioactive wastes. The radiation released by such wastes varies, and it decreases slowly over time. At present, there are no permanent nuclear waste storage facilities in the United States. Such wastes are stored in temporary facilities, often in large pools of water located at the sites where they are produced. A plan for a permanent storage facility envisions burying the radioactive wastes in underground salt domes. Such salt domes are thought to be geologically stable—that is, they are unlikely to change over thousands of years. However, opponents of this plan argue that there is no guarantee that geologic events, such as earthquakes, would not damage the storage areas, releasing radioactive materials into the environment. At present, no plan for permanent storage has been approved.

hazardous wastes:

wastes that are dangerous to the health of living things or that are harmful to the environment.

Hazardous Wastes Certain types of wastes are classified as **hazardous wastes** because they may cause injury, illness, or death. Heavy metals, such as lead and mercury, and many chemical wastes, such as pesticides and herbicides, are examples of hazardous wastes. These substances are toxic (poisonous) to living things and are responsible for many human health problems, including birth defects and cancer. Even plastic bags are considered hazardous wastes. When swallowed by wildlife, they block the digestive system, causing starvation or disease.

Nuclear wastes are another type of hazardous waste. These highly dangerous radioactive materials result from nuclear weapons research and production, nuclear power generation, and medical research. Nuclear wastes must be kept out of the environment for at least 10,000 years—the time it takes for dangerous radioactive elements to decay to safer substances. Exposure to a large dose of radiation from nuclear wastes can be deadly. Even small amounts of radiation have been shown to cause bone marrow damage, skeletal abnormalities, and cataracts, as well as leukemia and other types of cancer.

Noise Pollution

The average volume of sound in our environment doubles every 10 years. Each day, you are exposed to many sources of noise pollution, including cars, trucks, heavy equipment, and jet aircraft. Sounds from radios, televisions, stereos, and rock concerts are also major noise pollutants.

Loud or constant noise not only can damage your hearing but also can cause stress, fatigue, irritability, anger, tension, and anxiety. Prolonged exposure to loud sounds can even rupture your eardrum and may cause permanent hearing loss. Figure 25-13 shows some sources of noise pollution, their volume, and the type of damage they may cause to your hearing.

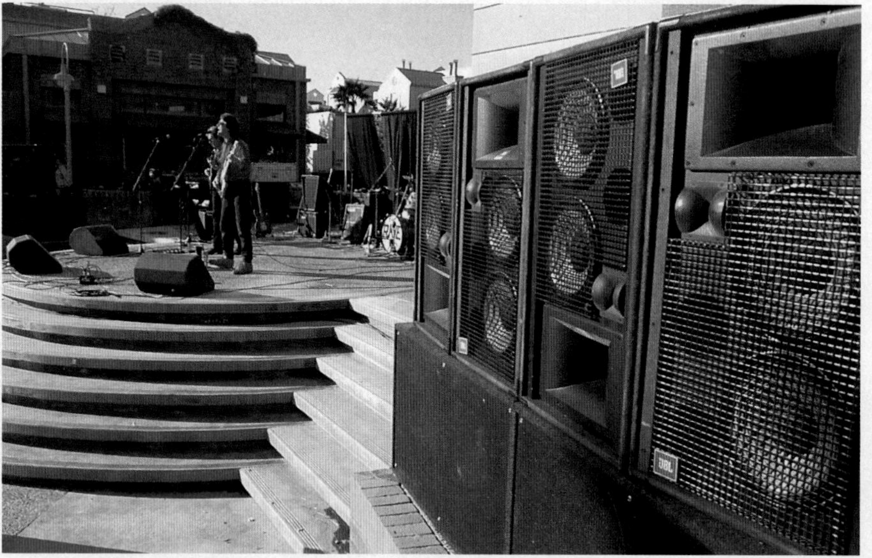

(FIGURE 25-12) **Live rock concerts often produce sound levels that can cause some people pain and may even result in hearing loss.**

• • • TEACH continued

Class Discussion

Noise Around Me

Have students identify sources of noise in and around their homes. The stereo, vacuum cleaner, and lawn mower are some examples. Suggest they discuss with family members ways of reducing noise around the home or ways of reducing exposure to noise.

Extension

Your Community's Garbage

Have a speaker from the local sanitation department speak to the class about the ways in which the community's solid wastes are disposed of. Also have the speaker discuss any plans for changing the way that solid wastes will be disposed of in the future.

LOUDNESS OF COMMON SOUNDS

THE DECIBEL SCALE. The decibel (dB) is the unit of sound loudness. It was arbitrarily based on the faintest sound people can hear. The decibel scale is logarithmic, which means that an increase of 10 dB produces a sound that is ten times louder. Therefore, an increase from 20 dB to 40 dB does not double the loudness of sound—it increases it by 100 times. The graph below compares the loudness of some common sounds.

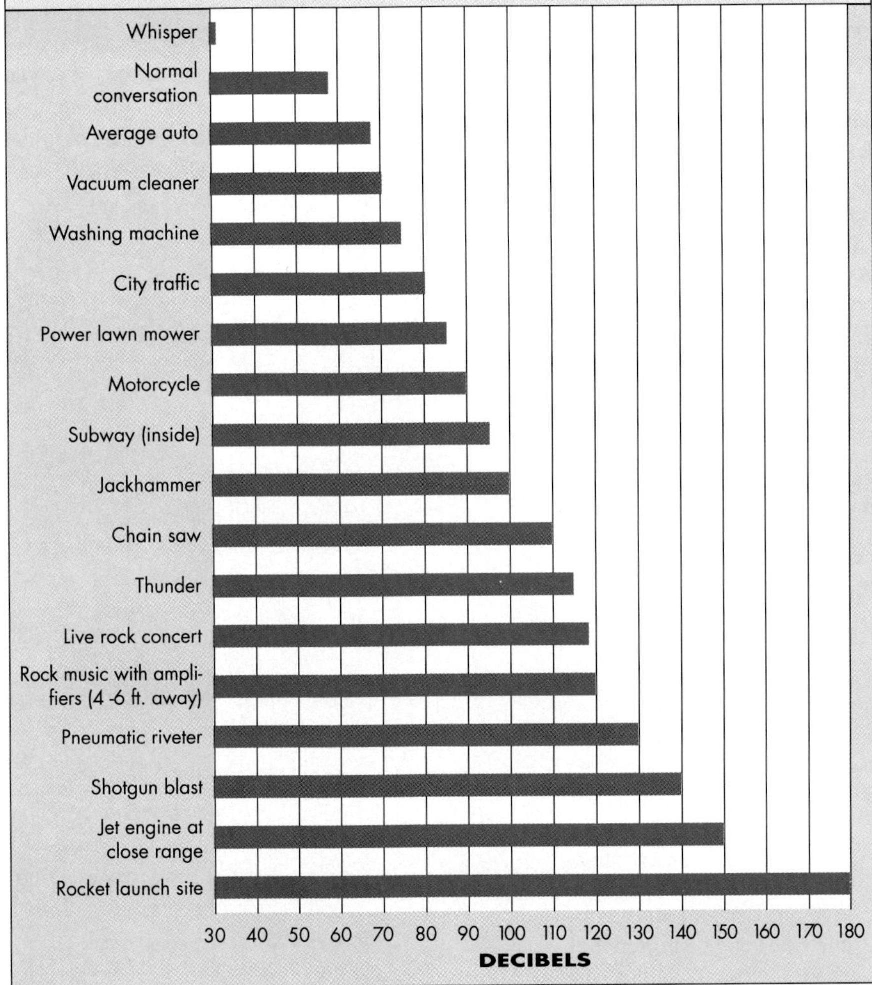

(FIGURE 25-13) **The slightest sound that the human ear can detect has a loudness of 0 decibels (dB). Sounds in the 40- to 60-dB range are considered comfortable. Constant exposure to sounds above 70 dB (10 million times louder than the slightest sound) can be annoying and may begin to damage your hearing. Serious damage to hearing occurs with exposure to sounds of 120 dB. Sounds of 140 dB or more can cause pain, and at 180 dB, immediate and irreversible hearing loss occurs.**

Review Answers

1. Human activities are the main cause of environmental pollution.

2. Agricultural, industrial, and consumer practices are increasing the amount of gases that trap heat from the sun's rays and increase Earth's temperatures. This global warming has resulted in a rising sea level and erosion of many coastal areas. If global warming continues, many coastal wetlands will be flooded, causing destruction of more coastal property, wildlife, and beaches. Chlorofluorocarbons (CFCs) from aerosol spray cans and coolants are broken down by sunlight, releasing chlorine. The chlorine destroys the ozone layer. As the ozone layer is destroyed, more UV rays reach Earth's surface, causing an increase in health problems such as skin cancer.

Check Up

Are You Protecting Your Hearing?

Have students complete the Check Up, using Figure 25-13 as a guide to the decibel levels of noises in the environment. After completing the Check Up, have students record their conclusions concerning personal hearing loss. Students should also record any action they think they should take to protect their hearing.

Answers to Questions 1 and 2 are on p. 551.

3. These wastes may cause illness, injury, death, birth defects, and starvation.

4. Answers will vary depending on the individual opinions of students.

Check Up

Are You Protecting Your Hearing?

There are a number of ways noise can increase your anxiety level or permanently damage your hearing: Prolonged exposure to sounds above 70 dB (annoying), 8 hours of exposure to 90 dB or more (hearing damage), short-term exposure to 120 dB or more (serious hearing damage), or exposure to 150 dB or more for any length of time (eardrums may rupture). Unfortunately, damage may occur with or without apparent symptoms.

Use Figure 25–13, Loudness of Common Sounds, as a guide, and evaluate your potential for hearing loss by responding "yes" or "no" to the following questions. Write your answers on a separate sheet of paper.

1. Do you attend rock concerts?
2. Do you frequently go to places that play loud music?
3. Do you listen to your stereo with the volume turned very high?
4. Do you use earphones when you listen to music or watch television?
5. Do you live or work around sources of loud noises, such as construction, airports, or major industry?
6. Do you sit up front when you go to:
   Movies?
   Concerts?
   Other places that play loud music?
7. Do you hunt with a rifle or a shotgun or practice using firearms at a shooting range?
8. Have you ever been exposed to extremely loud noises (above 120 dB)?

If you responded yes to any of the questions above or if you frequently have trouble hearing certain sounds, you may have suffered some hearing loss. You also need to consider changing your behavior so you do not further damage your hearing.

Many teenagers have already damaged their hearing. Studies indicate that over 50 percent of college freshmen have some type of hearing loss. Much of this damage occurs during the middle school and high school years, in spite of the fact that hearing can easily be protected. Turning down the volume of radios and televisions and using protective earplugs when operating loud machinery and firing guns are ways that you can protect your hearing. To determine whether you may have impaired hearing, complete the "Check Up: Are You Protecting Your Hearing?" box to the left.

Review

1. *What is the main cause of environmental pollution?*
2. *How does air pollution cause the greenhouse effect? destruction of the ozone layer? What are the potential dangers of each?*
3. *List five ways in which solid and hazardous wastes are harmful to the health of living things.*
4. ***Critical Thinking** Recently, smoking has been banned or restricted in most public places—schools, transportation systems, the workplace, and restaurants. This poses a difficult ethical question. Smokers often feel unfairly treated and resentful when they are not allowed to smoke. Nonsmokers usually find the smell of cigarette smoke very unpleasant. It is also hazardous to their health. How do you think this problem should be handled?*

ASSESS

Section Review

Have students answer the Section Review questions.

Alternative Assessment

Pollution and Health

Have students make up charts that show health risks associated with each type of pollution. The chart should have the heads WATER POLLUTION, AIR POLLUTION, LAND POLLUTION, and NOISE POLLUTION. Students can then fill in the charts.

Closure

Pollution Around Me

Have students give examples of pollution they have observed or experienced. In each case, have the student classify the pollution as water pollution, air pollution, land pollution, or noise pollution.

Section 25.3 What Can You Do?

Objectives

- *Describe the benefits of responsible waste management, recycling, and conservation.*
- *List specific ways each individual can help reduce pollution.*
- *Make a recycling and reuse plan for your household.*
  LIFE SKILLS: Setting Goals

After what they had learned about the effects of environmental pollution on health, both Teresa and Jaime wanted to know what they could do to protect their health. By collecting brochures and reading books and articles on the subject, they found that there are many ways to protect environmental and personal health.

Protecting Natural Resources and the Environment

As you learned in Section 25.1, the environment provides the materials that living things need for survival. This includes the many materials that people use for manufacturing the growing number of products and appliances they depend on. Currently, many natural resources are being used at an

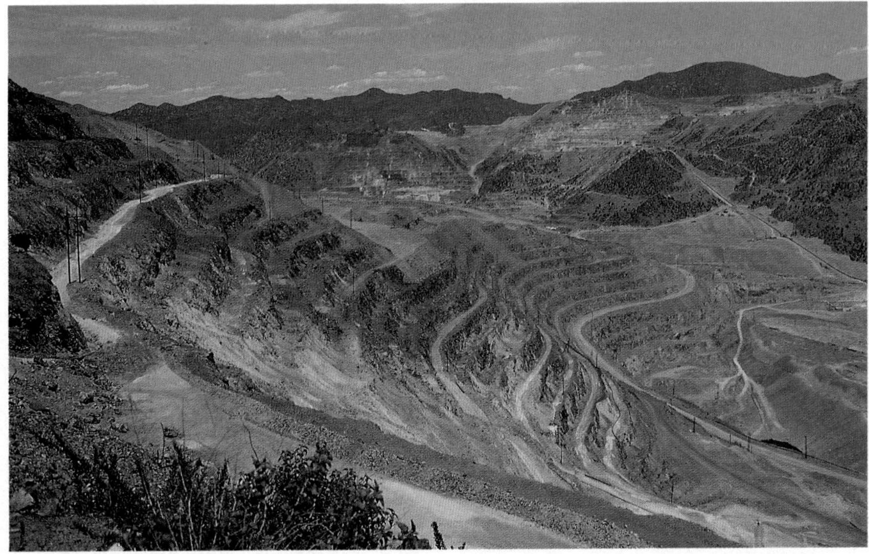

(FIGURE 25-14) **Strip mining is one way that natural resources such as copper and coal are gathered. Frequently, these methods are very harmful to the environment.**

Background

Alternative Energy Sources—Wind

In past centuries, wind was a source of mechanical energy. Windmills were used to pump water and to grind grain into flour. As electric motors came into use, windmills became rare. Now, windmills are making a comeback—to generate electricity. Large windmills are efficient generators of electricity. Windmills have certain advantages—the wind is free and windmills produce no pollutants. Of course, wind does not blow steadily and some areas experience more wind than others. However, some experts think that wind-generated electricity could supply most electrical needs in many parts of the United States, particularly in the Midwest.

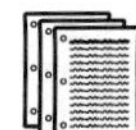

Life Skills Worksheet 25C

Caring for the Environment

Assign the Caring for the Environment Life Skills Worksheet, which requires students to react to behaviors that can have an adverse impact on the environment or on health.

Section 25.3 Lesson Plan

MOTIVATE

Journal 25E

Environmental Awareness

This may be done as a warm-up activity. Have students record in the Student Journal the things they are currently doing to help preserve and protect the environment. Point out that they will learn more ways of protecting the environment as they read this section.

TEACH

Cooperative Learning

Resources From the Environment

Have students meet in small groups to brainstorm ways in which they are dependent on resources from the environment. Suggest that they consider materials that they use every day, materials needed for a comfortable home, materials needed for transportation, and materials that help them remain healthy. Each group should compile a list of resources from the environment that supply these needs.

Writing

Conservation Ads

Have students compose advertisements or slogans that commend the benefits of conservation. Students might want to include artwork with their advertisements and construct posters. They could display their posters in the school or community.

Background

Radon

Another important indoor pollutant is *radon,* a naturally occurring radioactive gas found in many types of rocks and soils. Outdoors, it is relatively harmless. Indoors, however, radon can build to unhealthy levels, especially in basements. High levels of radon can damage lung tissue and eventually cause lung cancer. The EPA recommends that all homes be tested for radon. Test kits are available at most hardware stores. In most homes, the radon level is safe. However, if the radon level is found to be above a safe level, a ventilation system should be installed and any cracks in the building's foundation should be sealed.

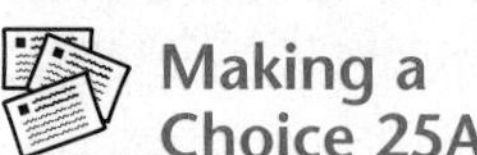

Making a Choice 25A

Producing Less Waste

Assign the Producing Less Waste card. The card requires students to examine ways to reduce their use of disposable products.

alarming rate, while the manner in which they are used pollutes the environment. If we don't reverse this trend, we will be left with an environment that can no longer support life as we know it. Fortunately, there are healthier and more responsible alternatives to the activities that are endangering the health of our environment.

conservation: *the wise use and protection of natural resources.*

Conservation **Conservation** is the protection and wise use of natural resources. By using less of the materials we take from the environment, particularly those resources that are nonrenewable, we can help ensure that those materials will still be available in the future. One example of a pressing need for conservation efforts is in the way we produce energy. Much of our electricity is generated by burning coal and oil. The burning of gasoline is used to power most motor vehicles. Burning fuels such as coal, oil, and gasoline is highly damaging to the environment. In addition, supplies of these fuels are limited. Using less electricity and driving less will help to extend the supplies of burnable fuels and slow down the rate of pollution. It will also help each of us save money.

Conservation also means protecting the environment from pollutants by using products that are less toxic (safer). Safer alternatives to many toxic products are available. For example, pump sprays do not contain CFCs and do not damage the ozone layer. Low-phosphate and no-phosphate laundry detergents are less polluting to the water than high-phosphate detergents. Safer alternatives to burning fuels for energy include solar power, wind power, and water power. These energy sources are also renewable.

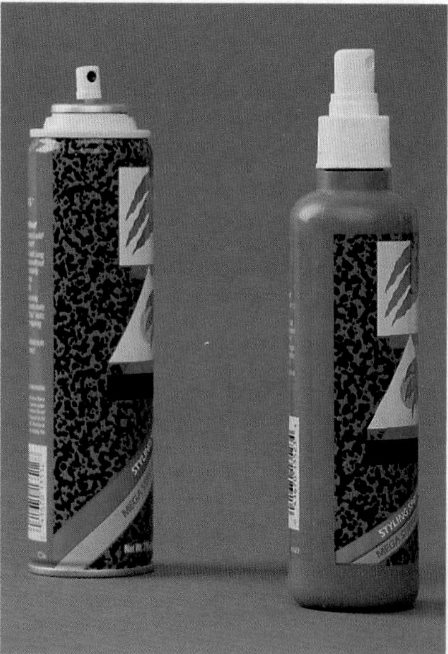

(FIGURE 25-15) **Many products that are sold in aerosol cans are available in pump sprays, which do not contain CFCs or damage the ozone layer.**

Recycling and Reusing Many of the materials that we discard can be reused. Ways of reusing materials include:

- recycling—the reusing of materials either directly or indirectly by making them into another product (For example, glass bottles can be used again or ground up and remelted to make a new item.)
- composting—the converting of organic matter into fertilizer by allowing it to be broken down by the action of bacteria
- pulverizing and compacting—the pounding of solid wastes into bricks that can be used in constructing landfills, roads, or other structures

About 80 percent of the solid waste produced is reusable. The advantages of reusing these materials include reducing the volume of solid waste and slowing down the rate at which resources are removed from the environment. Unfortunately, it costs more in many instances to recycle items than to produce them from scratch. As a

• • • TEACH continued

Class Discussion

Conserving Health

Point out that conserving resources will make those resources last longer. Ask students why conservation is a good choice for a healthier life. (*Decreased use of fuels and toxic materials that pollute the environment means a more healthful existence for all of us.*)

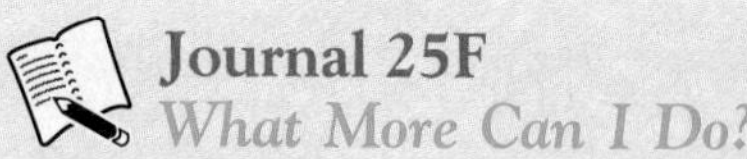

Journal 25F

What More Can I Do?

Tell students to review the list of things that Teresa and Jaime have identified as personal goals to help make the environment cleaner and safer. Have them record in the Student Journal things listed under Preserving the Air, Preserving the Water, and Reducing Solid and Chemical Waste that they are willing to do to have a better environment. Suggest that they review their activities periodically to see if they are meeting their goals.

Role-Playing

Everyone Must Pitch In

Select two students to role-play a disagreement between two people on environmental action. One student will play a person who feels that his or her personal actions have such limited impact that inconveniencing oneself to preserve the environment in not worth it. The second student will play a person who thinks that everyone must

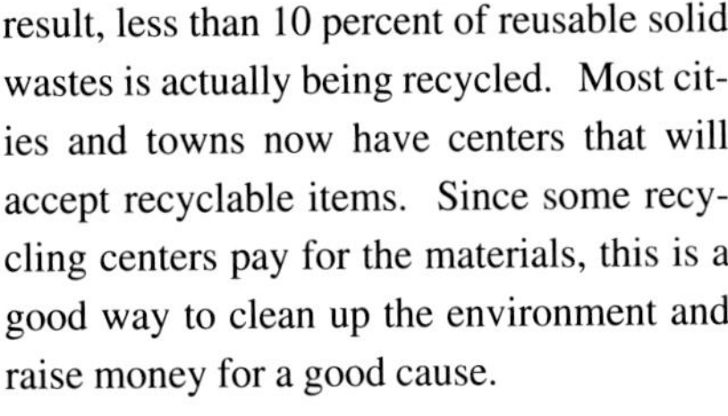

result, less than 10 percent of reusable solid wastes is actually being recycled. Most cities and towns now have centers that will accept recyclable items. Since some recycling centers pay for the materials, this is a good way to clean up the environment and raise money for a good cause.

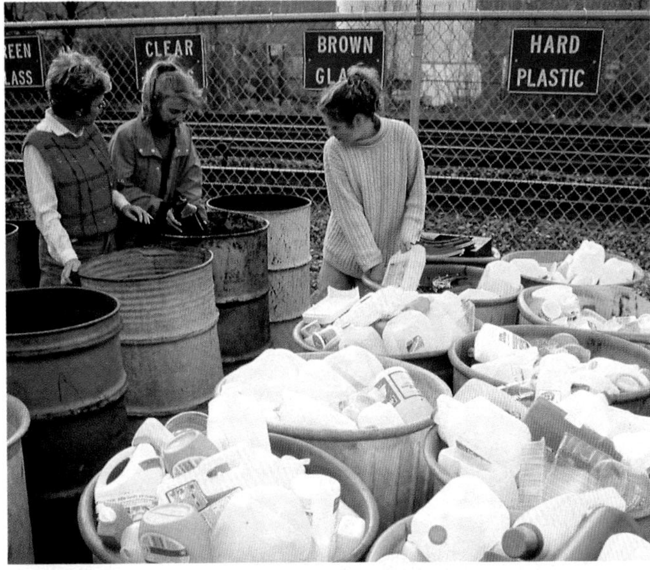

(FIGURE 25-16) **Community recycling centers accept a variety of recyclable materials. These materials must be separated according to their type. It's a good idea to do this ahead of time if you plan to recycle.**

Reducing Personal Pollution

There is much that each individual could do to limit the amount of pollution that enters the environment. Teresa and Jaime decided to list ways that they could begin to make their environment cleaner and safer. Even though they knew carrying out these activities would require making a major change in their lifestyles, Teresa and Jaime realized that their reward would be a cleaner, healthier environment. The following are some of the things they listed as personal goals.

Preserving the Air To help keep the air as clean as possible, we will:

- Walk, bicycle, or carpool whenever possible.
- Purchase safer alternatives to products sold in aerosol cans.
- Choose not to smoke or spend time with those who do.
- Keep the car well tuned, and have the exhaust system checked frequently.
- Avoid purchasing products that contain formaldehyde or CFCs.
- Use less electricity.
- Plant trees by participating in a community Releaf program. (Information about the Global Releaf campaign can be obtained by calling 1-800-368-5748.)

Preserving the Water To conserve water and help keep it cleaner, we will:

- Use only biodegradable, low-phosphate detergents.
- Fix leaky faucets and toilets quickly.
- Put displacement devices in all toilet tanks.
- Take shorter showers, use less water in the tub for baths, and replace shower heads with water-conserving models.
- Fertilize and water lawns sparingly.
- Avoid using pesticides, and use the least-toxic products available when they are necessary.
- Dispose of all household chemicals safely. (Contact the local EPA office or city sanitation department for instructions and disposal sites in your community.)

Reducing Solid and Chemical Waste To help reduce pollution and preserve nonrenewable resources, we will:

- Recycle and reuse whenever possible.
- Reduce household trash by purchasing reusable items and products with minimal packaging.

Making a Choice 25B

Assessing Threats to Health

Assign the Assessing Threats to Health card. The card requires students to consider environmental threats to health in their local community.

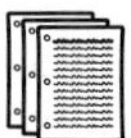

Section Review Worksheet 25.3

Assign Section Review Worksheet 25.3, which requires students to identify and give reasons for strategies that help reduce pollution.

Section Quiz 25.3

Have students take Section Quiz 25.3.

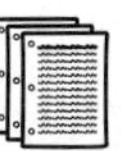

Reteaching Worksheet 25.3

Students who have difficulty with the material may complete Reteaching Worksheet 25.3, which requires them to identify sound environmental strategies.

help, if environmental health is to be ensured. After the discussion, have other members of the class evaluate the effectiveness of the arguments.

Class Discussion
Local Issues

Have students check the local newspaper for several days to find out about environmental issues that concern the local community. Engage the class in a discussion of those issues. Students should decide how the issues affect them, what they think should be done, and what actions, if any, they want to take.

Extension
Time to Recycle

Have students find out if their community has a recycling program. If so, have students report on the types of materials recycled and how the community handles such materials. If recycling is voluntary, have students organize a campaign to increase participation among community residents. Students can help distribute information about what to recycle and how. If no recycling program exists, have students organize a campaign to start a recycling program in the community. Students can write letters to local officials and put up posters in the school and around the community urging that the local government start a recycling program.

Review Answers

1. Recycling reduces the volume of solid waste and slows the rate at which resources are removed from the environment. Conservation helps ensure we will have natural resources in the future and helps protect the environment from pollutants.

2. Water pollution: Answers may include to fertilize and water lawns sparingly, to avoid using pesticides, and to dispose of all household chemicals safely. Air pollution: Answers may include to walk, cycle, or carpool whenever possible, to use less electricity, and to not smoke. Land pollution: Answers may include to recycle and reuse, to start a compost pile, and to purchase environmentally safe cleaning products.

3. Students might use the Yellow Pages, their city government, or the local library to find the locations of recycling centers. Students' plans will vary depending on the type of materials students plan to recycle and reuse.

4. Students might use symbols that convey the dangers of hazardous and nuclear wastes.

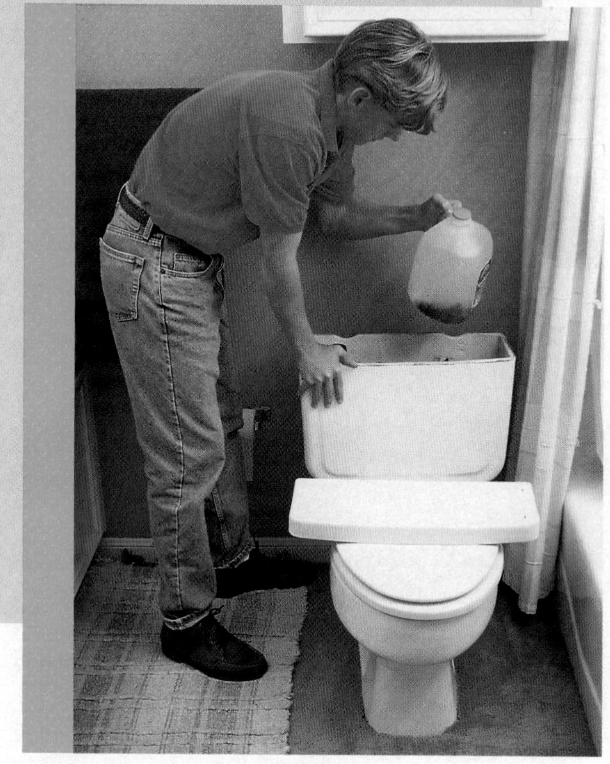

(FIGURE 25-17) **You can reduce the amount of water used in flushing the toilet by placing a displacement device into the tank. A plastic milk or juice bottle filled with water and a few rocks to weight it down is ideal for this purpose. Your city water board should be able to give you more information on how to conserve water.**

- Start a compost pile for biodegradable garbage.
- Limit the use of chemical fertilizers and pesticides.
- Purchase environmentally safe cleaning products.

Other Ways to Make a Difference

In addition to adopting personal behaviors that reduce pollution, there are many ways people can work together to promote a cleaner, safer environment. Some of the ways you could help are listed here.

- Join or support the efforts of environmental groups such as the Sierra Club, Friends of the Earth, the Wilderness Society, and the Nature Conservancy.
- Call problems to the attention of those who can help, such as conservation groups, newspapers, and city hall.
- Help attorneys prosecute violators by identifying sites of pollution and providing evidence such as photos.
- Participate in the law-making process by voting and by writing or talking to elected officials about your concerns.
- Encourage the school to obtain and use programs that build environmental awareness: Project WILD, Project Learning Tree, and the National Wildlife Federation CLASS PROJECT.

Review

1. *What are the benefits of recycling and conservation?*
2. *List three ways individuals can help reduce each of the following: water pollution, air pollution, and land pollution.*
3. ***LIFE SKILLS: Setting Goals** Find out where the recycling centers are in your community and what materials they accept. Then outline a recycling and reuse plan for your household and plan to carry it out.*
4. ***Critical Thinking** How would you label hazardous and nuclear wastes so that someone living 10,000 years in the future would be able to understand their danger even though they may not speak your language?*

ASSESS

Section Review

Have students answer the Section Review questions.

Alternative Assessment

For My Own Good

Have students write a brief paragraph showing the connection between helping protect the environment and protecting their own health.

Closure

Protecting the Environment

Have each student suggest three things that he or she thinks are most important in protecting the environment. List these on the chalkboard as they are suggested. Keep a tally of the number of students mentioning each one. Then reorder or number the steps in the order of importance to the class.

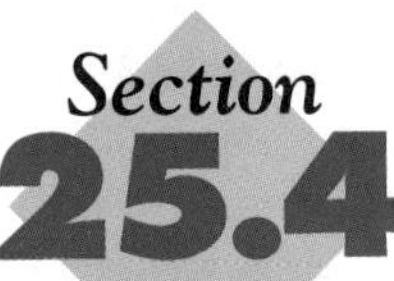

Section 25.4 Public Health

Objectives

- *Define public health.*
- *Describe four public-health activities.*
- *Compare the public-health concerns of developed and developing countries.*
- *Discover what the major public-health issues are in your community, and find out where to get help for a public-health problem.*

LIFE SKILLS: Using Community Resources

In most of the chapters in this book, your attention is focused on your personal health. However, your health and well-being is affected by the health and well-being of other people, and vice versa. For example, communicable diseases (infectious diseases that are passed from person to person) spread when people who are sick come in contact with healthy people. Infectious diseases (diseases caused by bacteria, viruses, or other parasites) cause many people to suffer poor health. Certain infectious diseases are among the leading causes of death. And as Teresa and Jaime learned, environmental problems can also affect the health of large numbers of people.

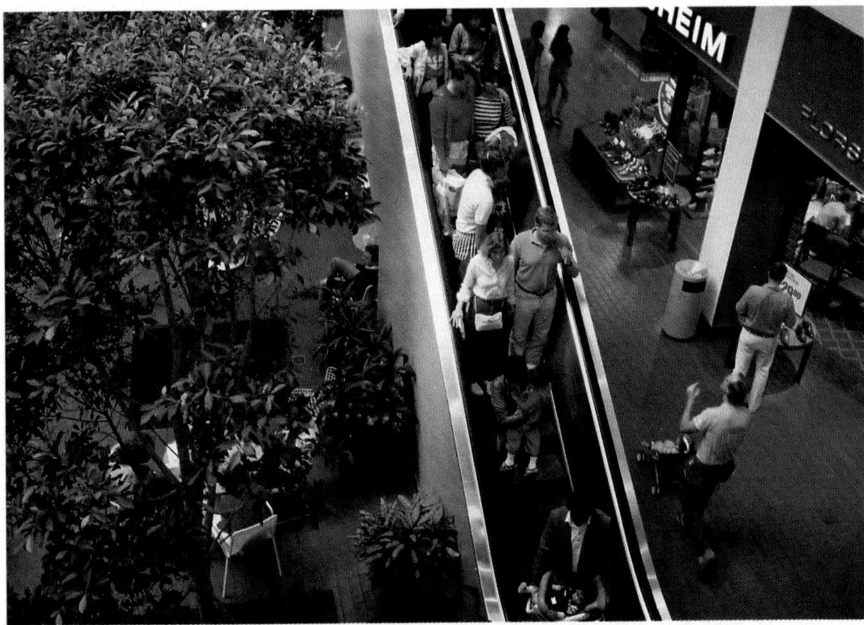

(FIGURE 25-18) **Because the people living together in a community interact with one another, they affect each other's health and well-being.**

Background
History and Disease

The history of the human race is marked by episodes of epidemic disease. Perhaps the most famous is that of the bubonic plague, which killed as much as one-third of the population of Europe in the 14th century and reoccurred several times in succeeding centuries. The arrival of Europeans in the Americas also meant the arrival of new diseases, against which the native people had no immunity. As Cortés besieged the Aztec capital of Tenochtitlan, smallpox, a disease introduced by the Europeans, was ravaging the city. The Aztec defeat may have resulted primarily from disease, rather than Spanish arms. An epidemic of flu that traveled around the world in 1918 and 1919 killed more people than did the fighting in World War I.

Section 25.4 Lesson Plan

MOTIVATE

Journal 25G
Public-Health Awareness

This may be done as a warm-up activity. Have students write in the Student Journal any public-health announcements or notices that they recall having seen or heard. Such announcements may be broadcast on television or radio, printed in newspapers, or even displayed on products or outdoor advertisements. Have students record whether any of these announcements affected their health practices or attitudes toward health.

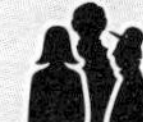

Cooperative Learning
Living in Crowds

Have students design a public-health campaign consisting of radio messages and posters to warn people of the dangers of spreading infectious diseases, such as colds and flu. They should recall from Chapter 21 what measures are recommended to prevent the spread of these diseases.

TEACH

Class Discussion
AIDS and Public Health

Point out that, although many people think of epidemics as catastrophes of the past, the worldwide AIDS epidemic is a present-day catastrophe. Have students recall how AIDS is caused and

What Would You Do ?

Review the seven steps of the decision-making model with students or refer them to Chapter 2, Section 2, to read over the steps of the model.

What Would You Do ?

You're Sick but You're Needed at Work

Making Responsible Decisions

Imagine that you work at a popular fast-food restaurant near a high school. Lots of kids go there every day for lunch. One day you get really sick with a stomach flu and call as soon as possible to report why you cannot make it to work. Your supervisor insists that they can't handle the lunch crowd without you and tells you that you have to come in, sick or not! What would you do?

Remember to use the decision-making steps:

1. State the Problem.
2. List the Options.
3. Imagine the Benefits and Consequences.
4. Consider Your Values.
5. Weigh the Options and Decide.
6. Act.
7. Evaluate the Results.

epidemic:
an outbreak of disease that affects many people in a particular area.

public health:
the health of a community as a whole; the organized efforts of a community to promote the health and well-being of all its members.

Controlling the spread of infectious disease and problems like the one in Teresa's neighborhood are public-health concerns. **Public health** is the health of the people in a community. The term is also used to refer to the actions a society takes to protect and promote the health of its people.

Public-health problems cannot be solved by individual efforts alone. Cooperation is key. Through government and privately sponsored activities, individuals work together to create a healthier environment for all the people living on Earth. In this section, you will learn about public-health activities and some of the agencies that deal with public-health problems.

Public-Health Activities

For most of human history, public health was endangered because of a lack of healthy, clean living conditions and because people did not understand how they got diseases. As the human population grew, large numbers of people died during repeated **epidemics** (widespread outbreaks) of infectious disease. A variety of public-health activities developed out of a desire to control the spread of disease.

Sanitation Sanitation is the practice of providing pure drinking water, sewage disposal and treatment systems, waste disposal sites, and clean living and working conditions. It was the first community-wide method of controlling the spread of infectious disease. From collecting garbage to inspecting the food preparation and storage areas in restaurants for sanitary conditions, modern sanitation efforts play an important role in protecting public health.

Hygiene Practicing personal hygiene (cleanliness) is one way you can play an important part in protecting public health. For instance, washing your hands can eliminate many disease-causing agents. This protects not only your own health but helps keep you from passing certain communicable diseases to others. Chapters 22 and 23 contain other examples of personal behaviors that prevent the spread of sexually transmitted diseases such as AIDS.

Quarantine The practice of quarantine (separating the sick from the healthy to stop the spread of disease) is another public-health activity that was begun to combat massive epidemics. People, as well as animals, plants, and agricultural crops, may be placed in quarantine if they are suspected of carrying an easily transmitted infectious disease. The period of separation lasts until the disease-causing agents are no longer

• • • TEACH continued

how it can be spread. Ask them how public-health officials in the United States are attempting to reduce the spread of the disease. Finally, have the class consider all of the reasons why AIDS is a public-health problem.

Journal 25H
Quarantined!

Have students record in the Student Journal instances when they had infectious diseases and, as a result, had limited physical contact with others, including family and friends. Ask students to record how they felt about being kept separated from others or told they could not attend a family gathering. Then ask them to describe the benefits of such isolation.

Debate the Issue
Get Your Shots

Have two teams of students debate the question: Is mandatory immunization an invasion of privacy? One team should advance the position that public-health concerns override an individual's right to refuse shots. The other team should argue the position that an individual's health is his or her concern and society has no right to demand that a person submit to medical practices that are either not wanted or that violate religious beliefs.

infectious or until they can be destroyed by antibiotic or chemical treatments.

Immunization and Antibiotic Treatments Two of the most important public-health activities are immunization and antibiotic treatments. Before you entered school, for instance, you were required to have immunizations against several infectious diseases. Such requirements have eliminated the deadly diseases of smallpox and polio in the United States and greatly reduced the occurrence of other serious diseases such as whooping cough and measles.

Although immunization programs have completely or nearly eliminated several serious diseases, such programs must be continued to prevent the return of these diseases. Recently, the number of measles cases has been on the rise in the United States. This rise has been blamed on poor immunization rates and the high cost of health care. More information about antibiotic drugs and the process of immunization is found in Chapter 21.

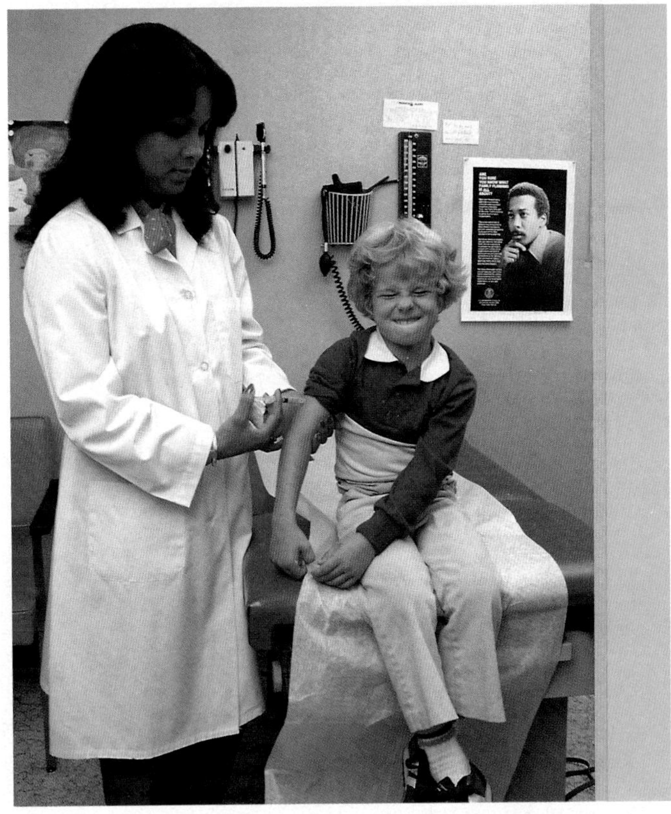

(FIGURE 25-19) **Immunizations given in doctors' offices and public-health clinics like this one protect the health of the individuals in a community. Although some serious diseases have almost been eliminated, they could return if people do not take advantage of the immunizations that are available.**

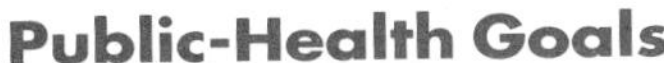

Public-Health Goals

Even though great progress has been made in protecting public health, modern methods are not available in all parts of the world. As a result, public-health problems and priorities are very different in different parts of the world.

Developed Countries In the developed countries such as the United States, modern health care (including immunization programs and antibiotic treatments) and modern sanitation systems have greatly reduced the number of deaths from infectious diseases. Chronic (long-lasting or recurring) noninfectious diseases and the problems of homelessness have become greater public-health concerns. Heart disease, for instance, is the number-one cause of death in developed countries. Also among the leading causes of death in the United States today are homicide, suicide, and accidental injury.

A list of some of today's major public-health priorities is found in Figure 25-20. Although disease prevention is still a priority in developed countries, effective public-health efforts must address all of these issues. The ultimate goal of public-health programs in developed countries is to create an environment in which each member of a community can enjoy a healthy and productive life.

SECTION 25.4

Life Skills Worksheet 25D

Community Organizations

Assign the Community Organizations Life Skills Worksheet, which requires students to gather information about private organizations in the community that focus on protecting the environment.

Cooperative Learning
Health Objectives 2000

Have students meet in groups to discuss the selected health objectives for the year 2000 listed in Figure 25-21. Ask students to rank the objectives in the order of importance, based on the group's assessment. Also, have students comment on the feasibility of the objectives. Finally, ask them if they can suggest objectives they feel should have a higher priority than those listed.

Class Discussion
Public Health Beyond the U.S.

Have students bring in articles from newspapers and newsmagazines that deal with public-health problems in developing countries. As part of a class discussion, have students compare these problems with those that occur in the United States. Ask them to note similarities and differences and to explain why some problems common elsewhere are not common in the United States.

Class Discussion
Local Health Facilities

Use Figure 25-22 to initiate a discussion of the services provided by local and state public-health agencies. Find out where local facilities are located and what services and information they provide. Ask students whether the public is adequately aware of available services and, if not, how to increase public awareness.

Background
WHO's Success

Smallpox is caused by a virus and infects only humans. Thus, no animal reservoir for the disease exists. Therefore, it has been possible, through the coordinated efforts of the World Health Organization, to eliminate the disease entirely. Vaccination against smallpox dates back to the late eighteenth century in Great Britain. By the 1940s, smallpox had been eliminated in Europe and North America. In 1967, the World Health Organization began a final campaign of vaccinations and quarantine to eliminate smallpox in regions—including Africa, Asia, and South America—where it remained. Vaccination teams traveled throughout infected countries. The last naturally occurring cases were found in 1977; by May 1980, WHO was able to announce that smallpox, one of the most deadly diseases to afflict the human race, had been wiped out.

Major Public Health Priorities and Selected Examples

Maternal, Infant, and Child Health
prenatal care
nutrition
detection of birth defects and risks
infant mortality
immunization programs

Adolescent and Adult Health
teen sex and pregnancy
sexually transmitted diseases and AIDS
teenage smoking and other drug and alcohol abuse
accidental injury
violence and homicide
suicide

Aging and the Elderly
physical activity and fitness
mental health and mental disorders
diseases of aging

Environmental Health
community injury control
community water and waste management
housing
community disease vector control
air and noise pollution

Access to Health Care and Rehabilitation Resources

Community Mental Health, Stress, and Violence

Communicable Disease Control

Lifestyle and Health Promotion

(FIGURE 25-20) **Public-health programs today are aimed at solving a variety of problems in an attempt to provide a healthier, more productive life for all. Some of the public-health problem areas that are currently being targeted by public-health agencies in the United States are listed here.**

Our nation's goals for public health are stated in a lengthy report that was prepared through a joint effort sponsored by the U. S. Public Health Service. The report, which is titled *Healthy People 2000*, lists several hundred specific health objectives. But the major goals of this report can be summarized as follows.

- Increase the healthy life span of all Americans.
- Reduce the health disparities among different ethnic groups in America.
- Provide access to preventive services and care to all Americans.

The objectives listed in *Healthy People 2000* are being used by various agencies to plan public-health activities that will improve the overall health of Americans. A sample of these objectives appears in Figure 25-21.

Developing Countries Adequate health care and sanitation are not facts of life for many people in the world. As a result, infectious disease remains a leading cause of illness and death in many of the world's developing (unindustrialized) countries. Achieving effective disease control in developing countries depends on:

- financial resources—to provide the necessary health-care supplies, facilities, and professionals.
- political stability—so that public-health efforts can be carried through.

Unfortunately, these factors are not present in many developing countries. Instead, they are often characterized by poverty, unstable governments, and a lack of resources, which along with growing populations, have led to famine (a severe lack of food) in many of these countries. Thus, in addition to infectious disease, starvation and malnutrition are major public-health problems in developing countries.

• • • TEACH continued

Debate the Issue
Rejoin UNESCO

The United States and several other Western nations have recently withdrawn their support for UNESCO. Allow students some time to research the issues involved in this dispute. Then hold a class debate on the proposal that the United States rejoin UNESCO and provide financial support for this organization.

Role-Playing
International Health

Select one student to play the role of a WHO official who is seeking financial support for health concerns in several foreign countries. Allow several other students to play the role of American citizens who need to be convinced that it is in their own interests to contribute to the health of people throughout the world.

Writing
The Peace Corps

Suggest that students write to the Peace Corps to request information about requirements for joining, the types of work that Peace Corps volunteers do, and countries that are currently being served. Have several students report to the class on what they found out about this international agency.

Selected Health Objectives From *Healthy People 2000*

Reduce coronary heart disease deaths to no more than 100 per 100,000 people. (In 1987, it was 135 per 100,000.)

Reduce the proportion of overweight persons to no more than 20% among people aged 20 and older and no more than 15% among adolescents aged 12 to 19. (From 1976 to 1980, it was 26% for people aged 20 to 74, 24% for men and 27% for women; and 15% for adolescents aged 12 to 19.)

Increase to at least 30% the proportion of people aged 6 or older who engage regularly, preferably daily, in light to moderate physical activity for at least 30 minutes per day. (In 1985, 22% of people aged 18 or older were active for at least 30 minutes, 5 or more times per week.)

Increase to at least 20% the proportion of people aged 18 or older, and to at least 75% the proportion of children and adolescents aged 6 to 17, who engage in vigorous maintenance of cardiorespiratory fitness 3 or more days per week for 20 or more minutes per occasion. (In 1985, it was 12% for people 18 and older; and in 1984, it was 66% for youth aged 10 to 17.)

Reduce to no more than 15% the proportion of people aged 6 or older who engage in no leisure-time physical activity. (In 1985, it was 24% for people aged 18 or older.)

Increase to at least 40% the proportion of people aged 6 or over who regularly perform physical activities that enhance and maintain muscular strength, muscular endurance, and flexibility. (Baseline data available in 1991.)

Increase to at least 50% the proportion of overweight people aged 12 or older who have adopted sound dietary practices combined with regular physical activity to attain an appropriate body weight. (In 1985 for people aged 18 or older, it was 30% of overweight women and 25% of overweight men.)

Increase to at least 50% the proportion of children and adolescents in 1st through 12th grade who participate in daily school physical education. (From 1984–1986 it was 36%.)

(FIGURE 25-21) **These are some of the several hundred specific health objectives proposed in *Healthy People 2000*. This report was prepared through the cooperative efforts of agencies of the U. S. Department of Health and Human Services and the U. S. Public Health Service.**

Reinforcement
Public-Health Agencies

To facilitate student knowledge of the various public-health organizations and their levels of service, put the following chart on the chalkboard:

- State and Local Public-Health Agencies: Regulate public-health activities of hospitals, clinics, local health departments; provide health services to community residents.
- National Public-Health Agencies: Support research concerning medical and health issues; provide support for disease control and health matters of national scope; monitor the quality and effectiveness of drugs and food products.
- International Public-Health Agencies: Conduct activities to raise the level of health care in countries with inadequate care; provide support to help prevent the spread of diseases from country to country.
- Private Health Organizations: Provide relief and health services in disaster areas and in poor areas; fund research for a variety of health problems.

Journal 25I
Personal Support

Have students review the list of private health organizations in Figure 25-25. Encourage each student to write in the Student Journal the organization that he or she would most like to support and why. Suggest that students also record what they are willing to do to provide support for their organization.

Background
Health Statistics

An important, if seemingly mundane, task of public-health agencies is the gathering of statistical data relating to health. Data on births, deaths, and causes of deaths, stillbirths, and diseases and their incidence are examples of the kinds of data gathered by these agencies. The organization and study of such data are part of the science of biometrics. Courses in biometrics are required in all schools that offer studies in public health. Biometric data are used to identify public-health concerns and to gauge the effectiveness of public-health measures.

Public-Health Agencies

Promoting and protecting public health require the coordinated efforts of government agencies and private organizations. Public-health agencies work at local, state, national, and international levels.

Local and State Agencies Public-health activities are usually carried out by state and local agencies. Each state has a board of health, which is made up of several elected officials. The board establishes laws and regulations that direct the public-health activities of local health departments, public-health clinics, and state hospitals throughout the state. When Teresa called the local health department to find out what services it provides for the community, she was given a long list. Figure 25-22 contains some of the major public-health activities occurring in most communities.

Public Health Activities in a Community

Regulation of community food, water, and milk supplies; medication; and toys and recreational equipment.
Prevention of communicable and chronic diseases.
Planning the development, availability, and quality of health facilities, personnel, and services.
Maintaining and analyzing vital records systems.
Educating and motivating the public in personal and community health.
Scientific, technical, and administrative research.
Control of environmental pollution.

(FIGURE 25-22) **Local public-health agencies protect the health of the people in a community in a variety of ways.**

National Agencies The primary public-health agency of the United States is the Department of Health and Human Services. The Department of Health and Human Services itself is divided into five separate public-health agencies.

Four of these agencies, the Social Security Administration (SSA), the Health Care Financing Administration (HCFA), the Office of Human Development Services (OHDS), and the Family Support Administration (FSA), oversee entitlement programs. These programs provide support to people who are "entitled" to services because they belong to a specific group or because they can demonstrate a certain level of need. Examples of entitlement programs include Medicare, Medicaid, and Aid to Families With Dependent Children.

Most of the federal government's public-health activity is handled by the Public Health Service (PHS). The agencies that make up the Public Health Service and the primary responsibilities of these agencies are listed in Figure 25-23. The surgeon general of the United States, who serves as our country's chief health adviser, is an appointed official of the PHS.

International Public Health

Because similar health problems can affect many nations at the same time, an organized system that conducts public-health activities across many nations is necessary. AIDS, tropical diseases such as malaria, diarrheal diseases, and environmental pollution are international health problems that require international efforts. Other critical issues affecting international health are poverty, natural disaster, war, and famine. Several government and private organizations are attempting to deal with the massive health problems that exist internationally.

• • • TEACH continued

Extension
National Health Issues

Have students bring in articles from newspapers and newsmagazines that concern national health issues. In particular, suggest that they look for stories about the role of the Food and Drug Administration in product labeling. This agency is responsible for ensuring that medical and health claims made for drugs and food are true. Have the class discuss cases in which the FDA has required manufacturers or producers to substantiate claims or to stop making claims.

Public Health Service Agencies

The Alcohol, Drug Abuse and Mental Health Administration *(ADAMHA)—focuses on problems related to alcohol and drug abuse, and mental health issues.*

The National Institutes of Health *(NIH)—directs and conducts basic research on the prevention, diagnosis, and treatment of diseases.*

The Centers for Disease Control and Prevention *(CDC)—works directly with state health departments to monitor health status, detect health problems, and control epidemics.*

The Health Resources and Services Administration *(HRSA)—concerned with such issues as access to, equity, quality, and cost of health care.*

The Food and Drug Administration *(FDA)—responsible for assuring that food is safe and wholesome; drugs, biologicals, and medical devices are safe and effective; and that radiological equipment is used appropriately and safely.*

The Indian Health Service *(IHS)—provides hospitals, health centers, and health stations for American Indians and Alaska Natives.*

The Agency for Health Care Policy and Research *(AHCPR)—administers several research programs designed to identify problems and solutions to encourage adequate access to health care for all Americans.*

The Agency for Toxic Substances and Disease Registry *(ATSDR)—monitors and provides information to the public regarding exposure to hazardous substances in the environment.*

(FIGURE 25-23) **The Public Health Service, a division of the Department of Health and Human Services, conducts most of the public-health activities of the United States government. The PHS is divided into eight smaller agencies. Each of these agencies concentrates on a separate area of public health.**

The United Nations The United Nations (UN) plays a major role in international public health. The UN is an alliance of over 170 nations dedicated to working together for the purpose of preserving world peace and human dignity. Several agencies established by the UN have had an impact on the health of the world's inhabitants. Among these agencies are:

- The United Nations Children's Fund (UNICEF)
- The United Nations Educational, Scientific and Cultural Organization (UNESCO)
- The Food and Agricultural Organization (FAO)
- The World Food Council (WFC)
- The World Health Organization (WHO)

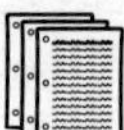

Section Review Worksheet 25.4

Assign Section Review Worksheet 25.4, which asks students to categorize public-health activities and answer questions about public-health agencies.

Section Quiz 25.4

Have students take Section Quiz 25.4.

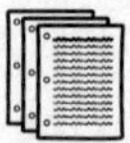

Reteaching Worksheet 25.4

Students who have difficulty with the material may complete Reteaching Worksheet 25.4, which requires them to compare public-health concerns in developing countries and to classify public-health agencies.

The World Health Organization The primary health organization of the United Nations is the World Health Organization. It was created after World War II to deal with the devastation and disease that the war brought to Europe. Today, the goals of the WHO are worldwide prevention of disease and attaining a level of health that will permit all people of the world to lead socially and economically productive lives.

The main targets of WHO programs are developing countries. WHO programs provide the citizens of these countries with access to health care by training health-care professionals, building hospitals and clinics, and sponsoring a variety of preventive health-care services.

The WHO is also involved in fighting the AIDS pandemic (an epidemic that affects many countries at the same time). In 1987, WHO formally began its Global Strategy for the Prevention and Control of AIDS. Other WHO activities include working toward universal childhood immunization and organizing effective family-planning programs.

Other International Agencies The United States government sponsors several international health efforts, especially in developing countries. The Peace Corps, for example, sends volunteers to these countries to provide education and assistance with agriculture, construction, sanitation, and health services. The Agency for International Development (AID) has provided billions of dollars in emergency assistance to regions such as Africa that have serious problems with famine. With UNESCO and other international organizations, AID also sponsors programs for immunization and oral rehydration therapy (the giving of fluids to a person who is dehydrated from excessive diarrhea or vomiting).

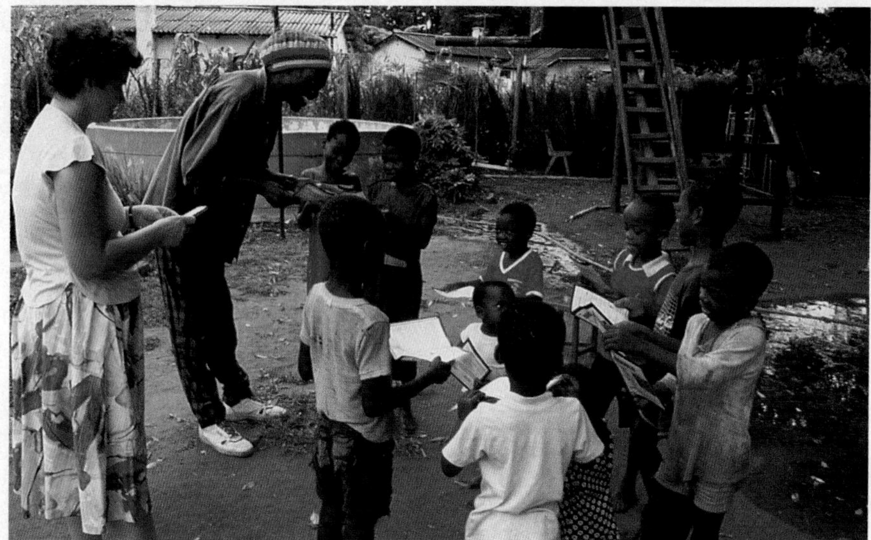

(FIGURE 25-24) **The WHO coordinates many activities that are designed to combat the spread of AIDS. Here, Dr. Kristina Baker and her assistant are distributing information about AIDS to a group of Zambian school children and helping them start an anti-AIDS club. The activities of more than 260 such clubs are teaching the children of Zambia how to avoid getting AIDS.**

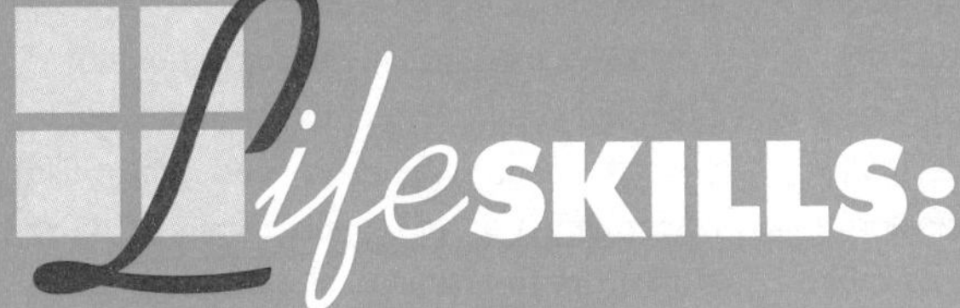

Using Community Resources

Being Aware of Public-Health Issues in Your Community

Teresa and Jaime became aware of public-health issues in their community through personal experience. You may or may not have had a similar experience. The public-health problems in your community are probably very different, but problems do exist. There are also places in your community where you can get help for problems related to public health.

To make yourself better aware of the public-health problems and resources in your community, follow your local newspaper for two weeks. Look for any articles that have to do with health issues, especially in your community. On a piece of paper, complete the following activity.

1. List five public-health problems that exist in your community. How have these problems affected the quality of life in your community? How have these problems affected your friends and relatives?
2. Choose one of these problems and write down your thoughts about the problem. What is the reason for the problem? How do you think it could, or should, be solved? What may happen in the future concerning the problem?
3. Find out which public-health agencies or organizations in your community can help with the problem you choose. Call or write to one of these groups for more information about the problem and the group's public-health programs.

Life SKILLS

Being Aware of Public-Health Issues in Your Community

You might wish to have students bring the newspaper articles to class to share with others. Suggest that interested students carry out their strategy for finding more information about the problem they selected. Have them report their findings to the class.

Review Answers

1. The health of the community as a whole; the organized efforts of a community to promote the health and well-being of all its members

2. Sanitation provides pure drinking water, sewage disposal and treatment systems, waste disposal sites, and clean living and working conditions. Hygiene promotes personal cleanliness. Quarantine separates the sick from the healthy. Immunizations protect people from certain infectious diseases.

Answers to Questions 1 and 2 are on p. 565.

3. Developed countries: answers may include chronic noninfectious diseases, homelessness, homicide, and accidental injury. Developing countries: answers may include infectious diseases, starvation, malnutrition, and adequate health care.

4. Answers may include city, county, and state public-health departments, as well as the Agency for Toxic Substances and Disease Registry.

5. Yes. Since it is easy to travel from country to country today, people from developed countries could visit and contract an infectious disease in a developing country. They could return home and spread the disease to others in their country.

Private Organizations Private organizations also provide important public-health support around the world. One such organization is the International Red Cross, which was originally created in 1859 to provide assistance to soldiers and others during war. Since then, it has expanded its relief efforts to include natural disasters such as floods and earthquakes.

Goodwill Industries of America is another privately funded public-health and assistance organization. This international nonprofit organization collects and distributes reusable materials to the poor and provides job training and rehabilitation services to the disabled.

The Salvation Army is yet another international organization that performs a valuable public-health service. Salvation Army volunteers help provide shelter and health services to the homeless and the poor worldwide. Figure 25-25 lists several other private health organizations.

Private organizations depend on donations and volunteers to fund health research, education, and support services. They also offer many types of support groups for those who suffer from a particular health problem or have friends or family who do. These support groups provide an opportunity for people to meet, discuss the frustrations they feel, and share positive skills and experiences. Private volunteer health agencies also provide excellent opportunities for young people to become actively involved in the health of their communities.

Private Health Organizations
The American Cancer Society
The American Diabetes Association
The American Foundation for the Blind
The American Heart Association
The American Lung Association
The American Red Cross
The Arthritis Foundation
The Cystic Fibrosis Foundation
The Epilepsy Foundation of America
The March of Dimes
The Multiple Sclerosis Foundation
The Muscular Dystrophy Association
The National Council on Alcoholism
The National Hemophilia Foundation
The United Cerebral Palsy Association

(FIGURE 25-25) **Private and voluntary health agencies such as these play a vital role in solving many public-health problems.**

Review

1. *Define public health.*
2. *Describe three types of public-health activities that control the spread of communicable disease.*
3. *What are four of the major public-health problems in developed countries today? in developing countries?*
4. ***LIFE SKILLS: Using Community Resources*** *What public-health agencies would play an active role in resolving problems like the one in Teresa's neighborhood? Write to one of these agencies to get more information on the public-health programs they provide.*
5. ***Critical Thinking*** *Could the massive public-health problems of developing countries affect public health in developed countries? Explain.*

ASSESS

Section Review

Have students answer the Section Review questions.

Alternative Assessment

Public-Health Services

Have students identify three public-health problems or issues: one that would be addressed by a local or state public-health department, one that would be addressed by a national public-health agency, and one that would be addressed by an international public-health agency.

Closure

Levels of Service

With students suggesting what should be included, make a diagram on the chalkboard that shows the various levels of public-health service available in the world today.

Highlights

Summary

- All living things are part of a worldwide ecosystem. If overpopulation or pollution damages that ecosystem, all forms of life are threatened.
- Human activities are the primary cause of environmental pollution.
- Pollution can be controlled or prevented by conserving resources, choosing safer alternatives to toxic chemicals, and recycling materials.
- The ultimate goal of public-health programs is to create an environment in which each member of a community can enjoy a healthy, productive life.
- Modern health care and sanitation systems have greatly reduced the number of deaths from infectious diseases.
- Government and private public-health agencies work at local, state, national, and international levels.

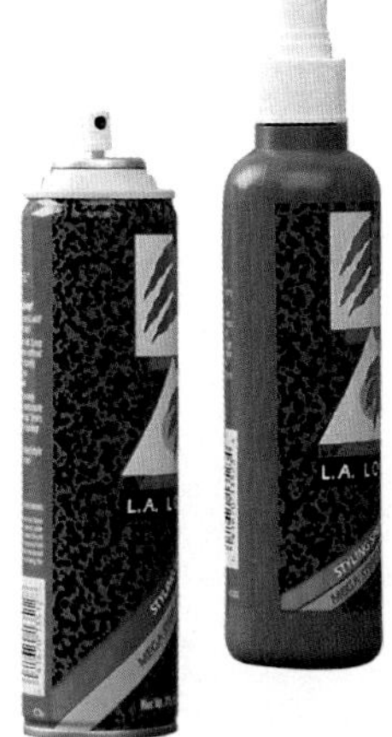

Vocabulary

ecosystem a system made up of living things and their physical surroundings.

homeostasis the tendency of any living thing to maintain a balance in its inner systems.

food chain a sequence of organisms that begins with a food producer and continues with one or more organisms, each of which eats the one before it.

overpopulation the point at which the population of an area is so large that it can no longer be supported by the available resources.

nonrenewable resources natural resources such as coal and oil that cannot be replaced once they are used.

renewable resources natural resources such as trees that can be replaced continually.

greenhouse effect the trapping of heat from the sun by certain gases in the atmosphere called greenhouse gases.

global warming long-term change in temperature (warming) of Earth's climate that is related to air pollution and the greenhouse effect.

hazardous wastes wastes that are dangerous to the health of living things or that are harmful to the environment.

conservation the wise use and protection of natural resources.

public health the health of a community as a whole; the organized efforts of a community to promote the health and well-being of all its members.

epidemic an outbreak of disease that affects many people in a particular area.

Chapter 25 Highlights Strategies

Summary

Have students read the summary to reinforce the concepts they learned in Chapter 25.

Vocabulary

Have students write a paragraph that expresses their concerns about the environment and uses at least five of the vocabulary words correctly.

Extension

Have students create an Environmental Action bulletin board. The bulletin board can be used to continuously highlight news about the local environment and display suggestions for improving the environment.

Chapter 25 Assessment

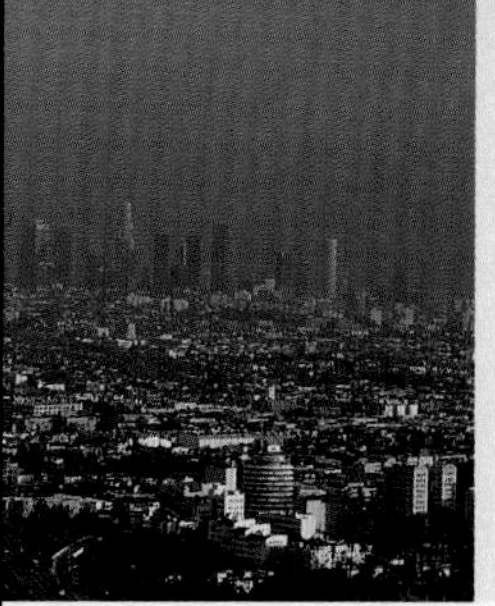

Chapter Review

Concept Review

1. What is an ecosystem?
2. Name two factors that disturb the healthy balance in an ecosystem.
3. What are the major causes of water pollution? What are some important health problems caused by water pollution?
4. How is destruction of the ozone layer linked to skin cancer?
5. How can a landfill cause water pollution and air pollution?
6. What are three sources of nuclear wastes? Why are they so dangerous?
7. Identify three alternatives to burning fuels for energy. Why are these alternatives safer?
8. List three ways to reuse materials. What are the advantages to reusing materials?
9. What are three ways in which individuals can help make a difference in protecting the environment?
10. In the past, why was public health endangered? What was the first community-wide method of controlling the spread of infectious diseases?
11. What is famine, and how does it affect public health? What causes famine in developing countries?
12. Four federal government agencies oversee entitlement programs. What do these programs provide? What are three examples of entitlement programs?

Expressing Your Views

1. Why is pollution an international problem?
2. Who do you think should be responsible for protecting the environment: individuals, industry, local governments, or the federal government?
3. Do you think quarantine is a violation of personal freedom? Why or why not?

Chapter Review

Concept Review

1. A system made up of living things and their physical surroundings

2. Overpopulation and pollution

3. Industry, agriculture, and everyday activities. Diseases such as cholera and typhoid, as well as increased risk of cancer, birth defects, and neurological, gastrointestinal, kidney, and liver disorders

4. As the ozone layer is destroyed, more UV rays reach the earth. Increased exposure to UV rays is directly related to skin cancer.

5. Rainwater trickles through landfills, carrying substances from the landfills with it as it seeps into the ground to become groundwater. Burning solid wastes in landfills causes air pollution.

6. Nuclear weapons research and production, nuclear power generation, and medical research. Exposure to radiation can be deadly—or cause various types of cancer, skeletal abnormalities, and cataracts.

7. Solar power, wind power, and water power. These do not cause pollution and help conserve natural resources.

8. Recycling, composting, and pulverizing and compacting. Reusing materials reduces the volume of solid waste and slows down the rate at which natural resources are removed.

9. Preserving the air by car pooling and purchasing safer alternatives to aerosol cans; preserving the water by using biodegradable detergents and taking shorter showers; reducing solid and chemical wastes by recycling and reusing; joining or supporting the efforts of environmental groups

10. There was a lack of healthy, clean, living conditions; sanitation.

11. A severe lack of food. Poverty, unstable governments, a lack of resources, and growing populations

12. Entitlement programs provide support to people who are "entitled" to services because they belong to specific groups or because they can demonstrate a certain level of need. Medicare, Medicaid, and Aid to Families with Dependent Children

Expressing Your Views

1. The air pollution created in one country can be carried by global wind currents to

Chapter 25 Assessment

Life Skills Check

1. **Communicating Effectively**
   Write a letter to one of your local legislative representatives describing an environmental concern and what you would like him or her to do about it.
2. **Setting Goals**
   Someday you will move into a place of your own. Suppose you were to design your house or apartment. What are some things you would put in your plans that would be energy efficient and foster environmental protection? Include plans for landscaping, materials for building the house, and plumbing fixtures.
3. **Using Community Resources**
   You would like to provide public-health support by doing volunteer work. You don't really want to work with a government agency. Who else might need your help? What could you do for them?

Projects

1. Write a brief report about your community's trash disposal system. Does your community have a sanitary landfill? If not, how does your community dispose of trash? Is the system environmentally safe? If your community has a landfill, does the landfill prevent environmental pollution? How? If possible, include pictures with your report.
2. With a group, create bumper sticker designs and slogans about the dangers of pollution. Display your finished projects in the classroom.
3. Interview a person who works for a public-health agency. Ask about the work the organization does and the services and job training it offers. Report your findings to the class.

Plan for Action

The responsibility for your community's environment ultimately rests with the individuals of the community. Devise a plan to adapt your behaviors in order to promote a healthy environment in your community.

other countries. Pollution of ocean water can affect living things in the ocean, and upset the balance of this ecosystem, as well as contaminate fish and other food sources.

2. Students may suggest that all parties are responsible.

3. Students might answer no because they feel the quarantine prevents the spread of infectious diseases and in this way saves many lives.

Life Skills Check

1. Letters will vary according to students' concerns.

2. Answers may include skylights, solar panels, computer-controlled thermostat, composting areas, gardening area, landscaping with trees and shrubs, water-conserving faucet heads.

3. Answers will include a variety of volunteer agencies that deal with problems such as AIDS, drug abuse, homelessness, and teen pregnancies.

Projects

Have students complete the projects on environmental and public health.

Plan for Action

Have the class vote on a single environmental or health issue that they would like to support or promote as a group. Have students brainstorm a list of actions they can take to help achieve their goal.

Personal Pledge

Have students read and sign the personal pledge for Chapter 25.

Assessment Options

Chapter Test

Have students take the Chapter 25 Test.

Alternative Assessment

Have students do the Alternative Assessment activity for Chapter 25.

Test Generator

The Test Generator (IBM® or Macintosh® format) contains an additional 50 assessment items for this chapter.

Being a Wise Consumer

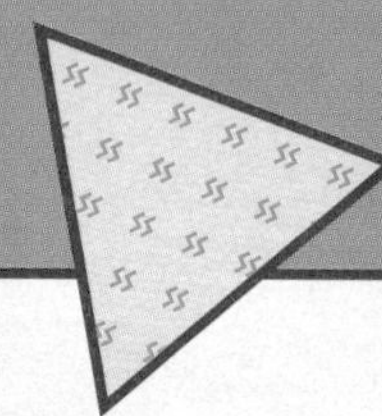

PLANNING GUIDE

TEXT SECTIONS	OBJECTIVES	TEXT FEATURES	OTHER RESOURCES	NOTES
26.1 What You Can Expect in Health Care pp. 571-573 1 period	■ Develop a plan to select a physician. ■ Learn how to communicate with medical personnel. • Understand your rights as a patient.	**ASSESSMENT** • Section Review, p. 573	**TEACHER'S RESOURCE BINDER** • Lesson Plan 26.1 • Personal Health Inventory • Journal Entries 26A, 26B • Life Skills 26A • Section Review Worksheet 26.1 • Section Quiz 26.1 • Reteaching Worksheet 26.1 **OTHER RESOURCES** • Making a Choice 26A	
26.2 Financing Your Medical Costs pp. 574-580 2 periods	• Understand why health-care costs in the United States are rising. ■ Know the advantages and disadvantages of traditional private health-care insurance and HMOs. ■ Learn how to locate free health care in your community. ■ Learn how to recognize quackery.	■ LIFE SKILLS: Being a Wise Consumer, p. 577 **ASSESSMENT** • Section Review, p. 580	**TEACHER'S RESOURCE BINDER** • Lesson Plan 26.2 • Journal Entries 26C, 26D • Life Skills 26B, 26C • Ethics Worksheet • Section Review Worksheet 26.2 • Section Quiz 26.2 • Reteaching Worksheet 26.2 **OTHER RESOURCES** • Making a Choice 26B • Transparency 26A	
End of Chapter pp. 581-583		**ASSESSMENT** • Chapter Review, pp. 582-583	**TEACHER'S RESOURCE BINDER** • Chapter Test • Alternative Assessment **OTHER RESOURCES** • Test Generator	

■ Denotes LIFE SKILLS objectives

• Items in blue are also part of the *Holt Health Activity Book.*

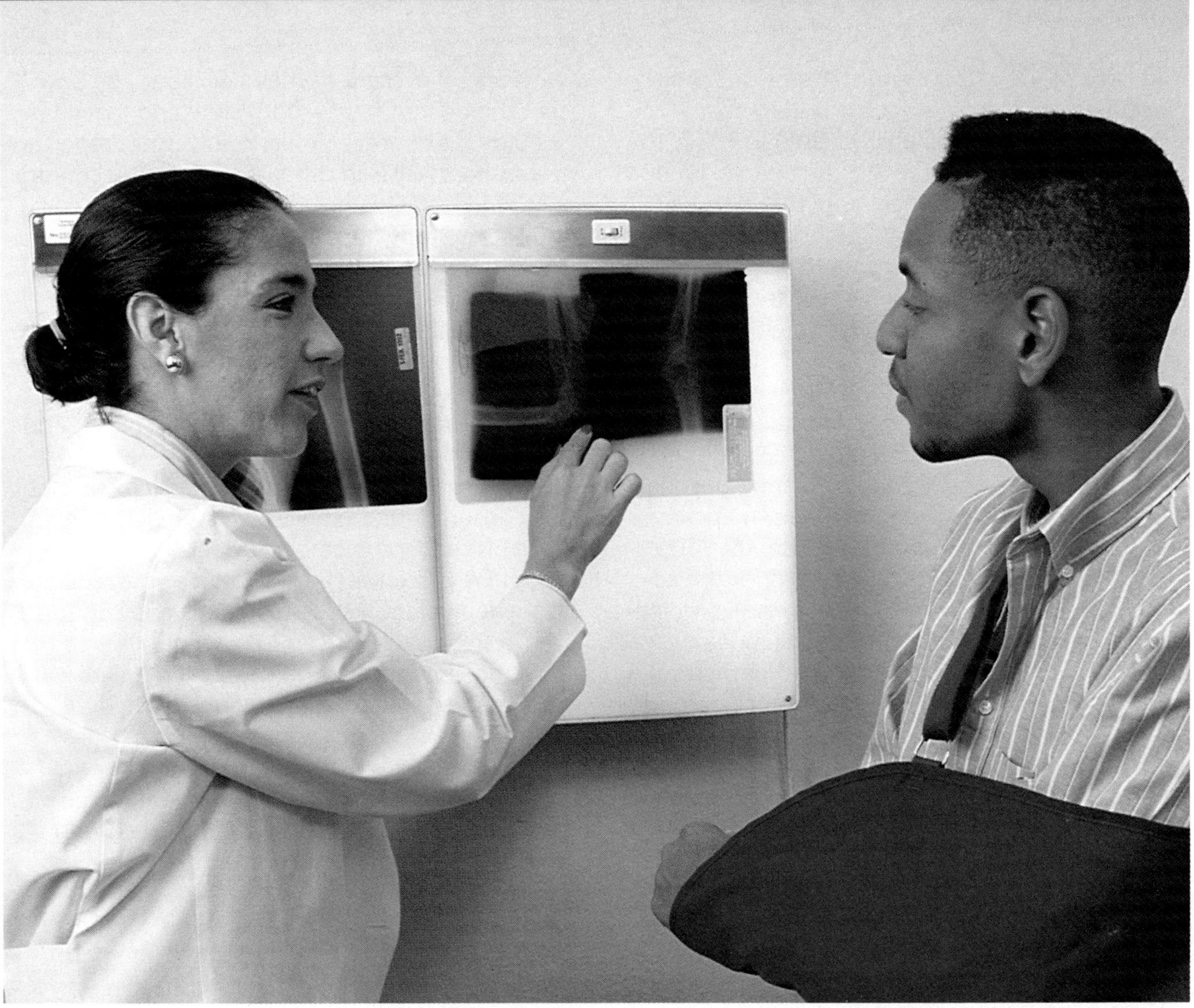

CONTENT BACKGROUND

The Current Health-Care System in the United States

HEALTH-CARE COSTS HAVE RISEN dramatically in the United States during the last 10 years. It is estimated that they are doubling every five years and that by 1996 the annual cost of health care could reach $1.4 trillion.

According to data from the Office of National Health Statistics, about one-third of the 1990 "health dollar" came from private health insurance; 42 cents from Medicare, Medicaid, and other government programs; 20 cents from out-of-pocket payments; and the remaining nickel from industrial in-plant health services, nonpatient revenues, and privately financed construction. Thirty-eight percent of the health dollar went toward hospital care; 23 percent toward dental and other professional services, home health care, drugs and other medical products; 19 percent toward services provided by medical personnel; and 12 percent to administration and the net cost of private health insurance, government public health, research in the medical fields, and construction of medical facilities. The remaining 8 percent of the nation's health dollar was spent on nursing-home care.

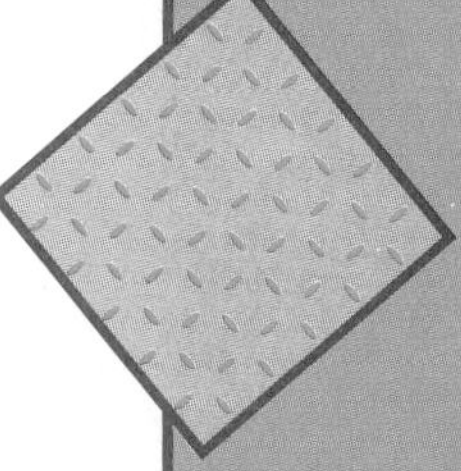

In light of such staggering statistics, the pharmaceutical journal *Drug Topics* conducted a survey of its readers (all pharmacists) in 1992, to determine the state of the health-care system in the United States and what, if anything, should be done to change it. Eighty-eight percent of the 408 pharmacists sampled agree that some kind of reform is necessary. Two percent of the respondents were neutral and 10 percent felt that changes in the present health-care system aren't necessary. Most respondents (85 percent) attributed the failing health-care system to insurance administration, government-regulated programs such as Medicare and Medicaid, soaring hospital costs, a growing population of older Americans, and societal woes such as drug abuse, the AIDS epidemic, and violence. Other causes for the ailing health-care system include malpractice/defensive medicine, antitrust status for insurance companies, the cost of drugs and other medical devices, and people having no insurance or inadequate insurance.

All of the respondents agreed that every American should be provided with basic health-care coverage. About one-quarter felt that legal aliens whose permanent place of residence is the United States should also be provided basic health-care coverage. Those polled were split, however, as to who should administer this basic health-care system. Forty percent of pharmacists in the western part of the country believe that the private sector should be in charge of health-care reform, whereas 60 percent of their colleagues believe that the government—both state and federal—should take charge. Similar results were reported from pharmacists in other regions of the country.

What is a "basic health-care system"? According to the study, inpatient hospital services, emergency services, and surgery were the minimum services that should be provided under a reformed health-care program. Other services considered important by the pharmacists included doctor visits, prenatal care, care in case of catastrophic illness, outpatient hospital services, and prescription drugs.

Well over half the pharmacists polled felt that the consumer of the health-care services should have his or her choice of providers and services. About 20 percent believed that a single regulator at the federal level should administer a centralized system. A little over 20 percent believed that a balance between a single federal regulator and a consumer choice system would be the most workable plan for health-care reform in the United States.

To pay for reform, the pharmacists favored higher taxes and employer mandated contributions to the program.

The responses of the pharmacists seem to echo the feelings of most individuals in this country regarding health services and the need for reform. With annual national health-care costs currently exceeding $738 billion, however, just how and when this much-needed reform will occur is unclear.

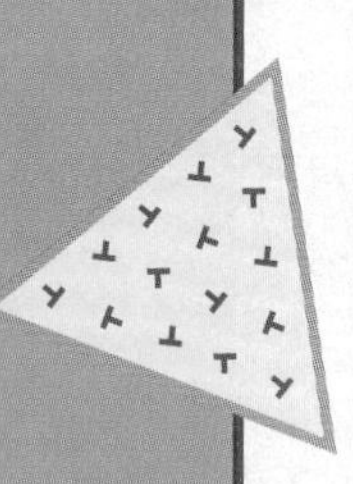

PLANNING FOR INSTRUCTION

KEY FACTS

- **A primary-care physician is critically important to maintaining good health.**
- **Your doctor must learn all about you by checking you and learning your medical history. You must tell the doctor your symptoms and any other important information.**
- **You have the right to obtain a second opinion from another doctor.**
- **If you are hospitalized, you should be given a Patient's Bill of Rights.**
- **Health-care costs are increasing every year because of the use of high-tech equipment, organ transplants, the AIDS epidemic, malpractice insurance, and defensive medicine.**
- **Everyone needs insurance to help pay for health care.**
- **Health-care options include traditional health insurance, health maintenance organizations, and free or low-cost health care provided by government.**
- **Quackery is the promotion of worthless or unproven medical services or products.**

MYTHS AND MISCONCEPTIONS

MYTH: Malpractice is a major cause of rising medical costs.

The U.S. Department of Health and Human Services says malpractice accounts for less than 1 percent of the national health-care cost. Hospital expenses are the biggest single factor in rising medical costs; they account for 38 percent.

MYTH: Health-care advertising must be true, because government agencies check it.

Several government agencies try to limit fraudulent services and products, and most broadcasters and publishers try to check ads to some extent, but no thorough controls over health-care advertising exist. Quack ads are common. All health-care advertising should be viewed skeptically.

VOCABULARY

Essential: The following vocabulary terms appear in boldface type.

- **primary care physician (family doctor)**
- **defensive medicine**
- **premium**
- **quackery**
- **deductible**
- **HMO (health maintenance organization)**

Secondary: Be aware that the following terms may come up during class discussion.

- medical history
- health insurance
- second opinion
- socialized medicine
- group insurance policy
- dependents
- grace period
- Medicaid
- disability or lost-income protection
- previously existing illness
- preventive medicine
- chronic disease
- copayment

FOR STUDENTS WITH SPECIAL NEEDS

LEP Students: Provide students with one index card for each vocabulary term for this chapter. Ask them to write the term on one side of the card and the definition on the other and practice saying the terms and defining them.

Less-Advanced Students: To help students identify quackery, have them find examples of quack advertising in magazines, using Figure 26-7 for guidance.

ENRICHMENT

- Ask the school nurse to visit the class to talk about finding a doctor, hospitals, health insurance, clinics, pharmacies, and to answer students' questions concerning health care.
- Have students who are interested in business conduct library research on the cost of health care, the growth of the health-care industry, and the profitability of the industry.

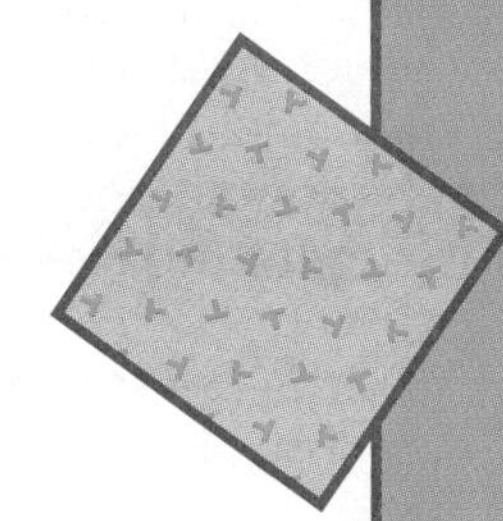

Chapter 26 Chapter Opener

GETTING STARTED

Using the Chapter Photograph

Ask students: **How is the boy in the picture taking responsibility for maintaining his health?** *[By visiting a doctor]* Ask how they think the boy went about choosing the doctor and how he or his family might be paying for the visit.

Question Box

Have students write out any questions they have about choosing a doctor and paying for medical services and put them in the Question Box. The Question Box provides students with an opportunity to ask questions anonymously. To ensure that students with questions are not embarrassed to be seen writing, have those who do not have questions write something else on the paper instead, such as something they already know about choosing a doctor and paying for medical services.

Preview the questions and then answer them at appropriate points in the chapter. You may wish to allow students to write additional anonymous questions as they go through the chapter.

Chapter 26

Being a Wise Consumer

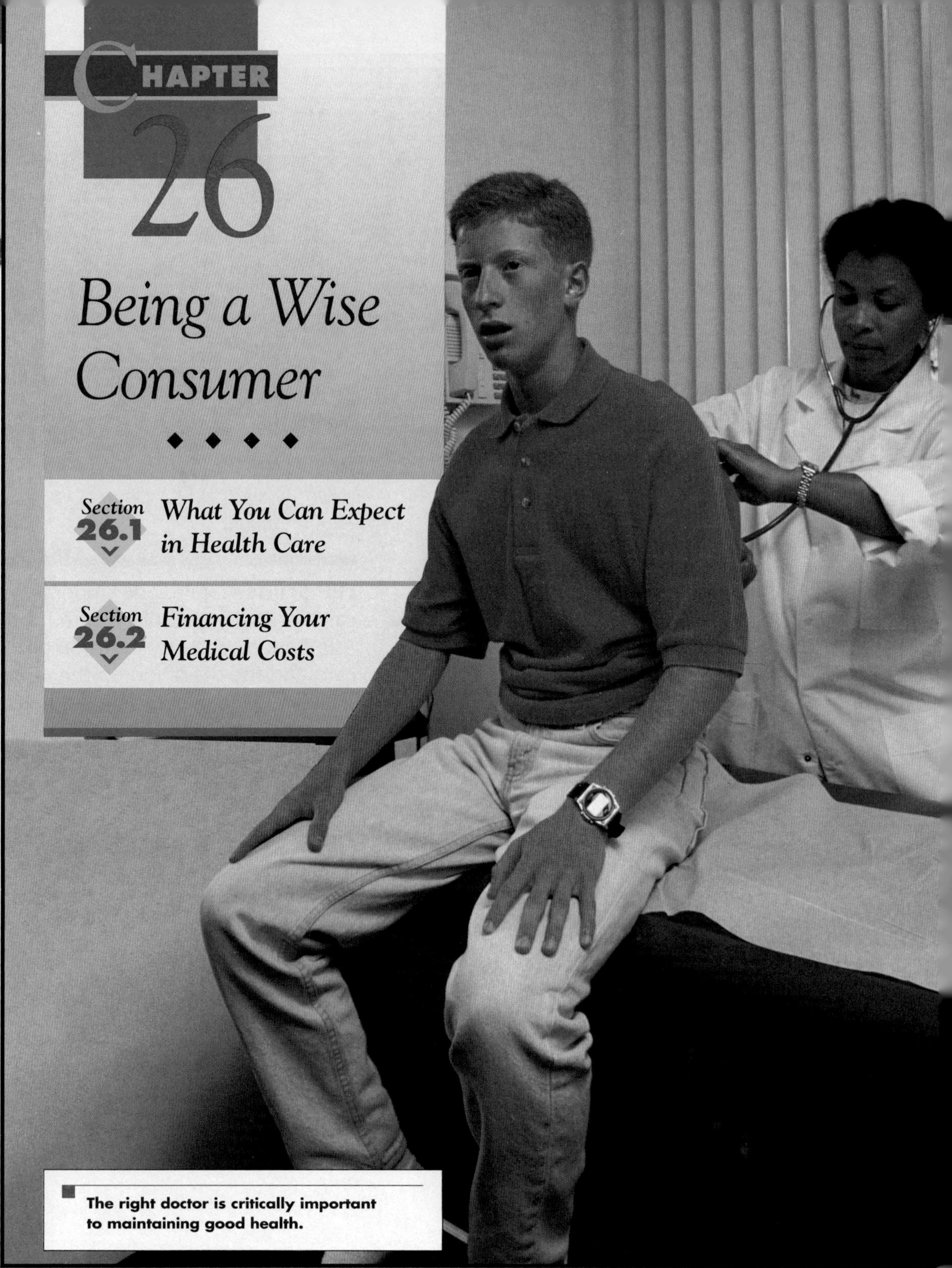

The right doctor is critically important to maintaining good health.

Personal Issues *ALERT*

At one time, only the poor lacked health care and a choice of doctor. Today, many middle-class and self-employed people have no health insurance, family doctor, or dentist, and have difficulty paying for health care. Because one student's routine health care may be unavailable to another—an orthodontist for one, Medicaid for another—be sensitive to these varying economic levels in your class. Don't assume that everyone has or can afford regular health care. Also, a student undergoing treatment for a personal problem, such as a psychological disorder or drug abuse, may become uncomfortable discussing medical services, so be alert to discomfort levels in students.

Cam sat in the middle of the living room looking at all the boxes that surrounded her. Books were strewn across the floor, and her cat was having a great time running through the maze. Cam could hear her parents in the next room hanging pictures. It seemed they had been here longer than just two days.

All of a sudden, Cam began to wheeze from all the dust in the room. "Oh, no," she thought. "I hope I don't get an asthma attack *now*. Not when we just moved to this town. We don't even have a doctor yet."

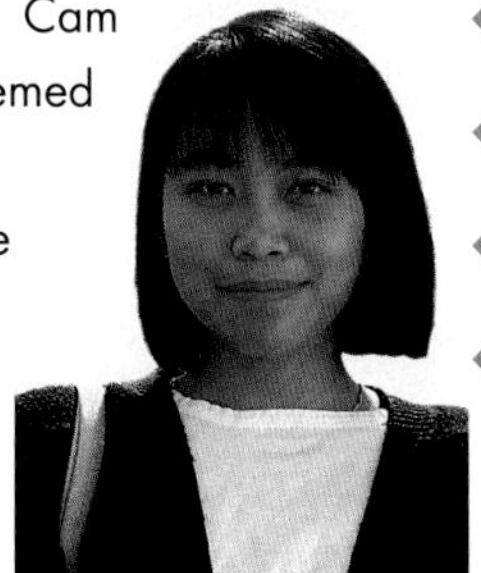

Section 26.1 What You Can Expect in Health Care

Objectives

- *Develop a plan to select a physician.*
  - **LIFE SKILLS: Being a Wise Consumer**
- *Learn how to communicate with medical personnel.*
  - **LIFE SKILLS: Communicating Effectively**
- *Understand your rights as a patient.*

Like Cam and her family, practically everyone needs a **primary care physician** (family medicine physician). Although the right doctor is critically important to maintaining good health, many people don't know how to find a good doctor. People often seem unconcerned with how they choose their physician. In fact, some studies indicate that the average American spends more time selecting a mechanic than in selecting a doctor. In this chapter, you'll learn how to select a doctor and how to communicate with doctors. You'll find out what your rights are in dealing with them. And you'll learn about some of the plans that are available to pay for the costs of health care.

primary care physician:

a family medicine physician, a pediatrician, or a general internal medicine physician.

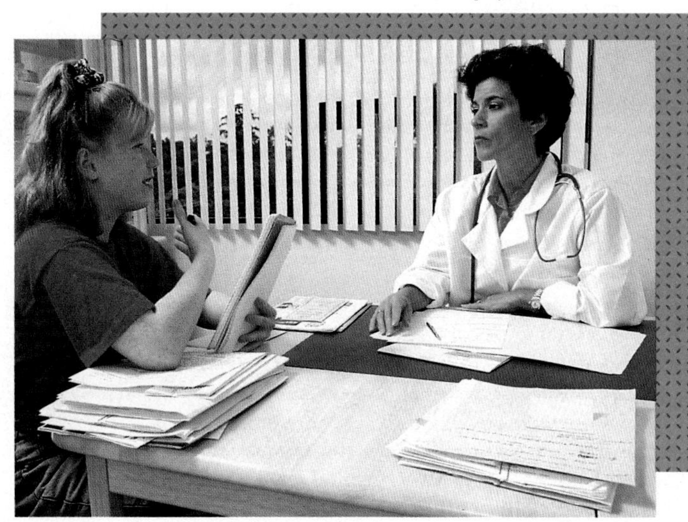

(FIGURE 26-1) **It is important that you feel free to be direct and assertive with your doctor and to ask any questions that concern you.**

SECTION 26.1

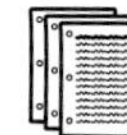

Personal Health Inventory

Have students complete the Personal Health Inventory for this chapter. The inventory helps them rate the health care they receive.

Life Skills Worksheet 26A

Making Responsible Decisions

Assign the Making Responsible Decisions Life Skills Worksheet, which requires students to get recommendations for a primary care physician, interview one of the doctors recommended, and decide whether they would want to be a patient of that doctor.

Making a Choice 26A

Doctor-Patient Interactions

Assign the Role-Playing Doctor-Patient Interactions card, which requires students to role-play an interview between a doctor and prospective patient and between a doctor and first-time patient.

Section 26.1 Lesson Plan

MOTIVATE

Journal 26A
Your Medical Services

This may be done as a warm-up activity. In the Student Journal in the Student Activity Book, ask students to list all the medical services they use, such as doctors, specialists, dentists, eye doctors, clinics, hospitals, pharmacies, and so on.

TEACH

Class Discussion
Why You Need a Doctor

On the chalkboard, write *Why You Need a Doctor.* Write the reasons as students volunteer them. *[To maintain good health; for physicals and immunizations; for care if there is illness; someone to call in emergencies; someone you trust to help with personal problems]* Have students discuss the role of the family doctor and why their family chose that particular doctor, or have them discuss where they go when they need medical attention. **If you don't have a family doctor, or if you can't get your doctor during an emergency, where can you go for medical help?** *[A public hospital emergency department is the best place to go.]*

Journal 26B
Your Medical History

Have students write their own medical histories in the Student Journal. Tell

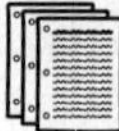

Section Review Worksheet 26.1

Assign Section Review Worksheet 26.1, which encourages students to recognize ways to select a doctor, ways to communicate with a doctor, and their rights as patients.

Section Quiz 26.1

Have students take Section Quiz 26.1.

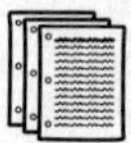

Reteaching Worksheet 26.1

Students who have difficulty with the material may complete Reteaching Worksheet 26.1, which requires them to decide if their rights as patients are being violated in particular situations.

The Selection Process

Soon you will be on your own and will need to decide who your doctor will be. You may decide to keep the same physician you have always had. If you decide to change doctors, there are several ways you can do so. One way is to ask your relatives and friends about their physicians. Another method is to locate a medical school in your area. The school will be affiliated with a nearby hospital, where some of its professors will serve on the staff. Call the school and ask for a list of its staff physicians. The county medical society can also provide you with a list of physicians.

After making your choice, call the doctor's office to make sure new patients are welcome and to check on hours, fees, and other information. Avoid making a final decision until after a few visits. If you sense a communication problem, questionable practices, or do not feel comfortable, continue your search for a doctor.

Your doctor will want to know why you scheduled your first visit. He or she will record your reason for coming in, specific signs and symptoms (temperature, blood pressure, heart rate, type of pain, etc.), medication taken, and your exercise habits. Information about previous illnesses, surgery, treatment, allergies, and reactions to medications will also be needed to begin your medical history. During the examination, you can help by pointing out pains, lumps, growths, and previous injuries that cause pain or concern. Keep in mind that your doctor is trying to learn and record as much about you as possible to aid diagnosis and treatment.

It is important for you to feel comfortable being direct and assertive with your doctor, and to ask any questions that concern you. You might ask, How long will it take to heal? Will the medicine produce any side effects? Should I take the medicine with food or on an empty stomach? When should I come back? Can I go to school? Can I exercise and go to soccer practice? You should expect an answer to all of your questions, no matter how trivial they may seem. Some people like to write down their questions and bring the list with them. You may also want to write down any special instructions the doctor gives you during the office visit. It is important that you not allow the doctor to rush you or brush you off to get to the next patient. If

(FIGURE 26-2)

Patient's Bill of Rights

- *Considerate and respectful care*
- *The right to obtain complete information concerning your diagnosis, treatment, and prognosis in terms you can understand*
- *The right to all information you need to give informed consent (risks, benefits, alternative treatments) before treatment*
- *The right to refuse treatment, once you are aware of the facts, to the extent permitted by law*
- *Privacy and confidentiality (refusal to be examined in front of people not involved in your case, confidentiality of records)*
- *A reasonable response when you ask for help*
- *Information about any possible conflicts of interest (hospital ownership of labs, professional relationships among doctors who are treating you)*
- *The right to be told if the hospital plans to make your treatment part of a research project or experiment*
- *The right to an explanation of your hospital bill*
- *The right to know what hospital rules apply to your conduct as a patient*
- *The right to expect good follow-up care*

• • • TEACH continued

them to list significant past illnesses, surgeries, injuries, allergies, reactions to medicines, therapies, regular exercise and sports, and risky personal behaviors. Also, have them list any serious illnesses in relatives (explain that certain diseases are inherited).

Students' privacy should be respected since this information is considered very confidential.

Role-Playing
Visiting the Doctor

Assign roles: nurse (obtains brief statement of symptoms, takes temperature and blood pressure), doctor (examines, recommends treatment, and prescribes medications and therapy), receptionist (receives payment for the visit), and patients. Have each patient prepare a brief list of symptoms for an actual illness and questions to ask the doctor during the visit. Upon leaving, each patient must request an itemized bill and tell the receptionist how they will pay it.

Reinforcement
Caring for Yourself

Emphasize that each student is responsible for his or her own health care. Point out that students also should apply the Patient's Bill of Rights any time they see a doctor or dentist. They should always communicate clearly with medical people, be assertive, ask questions, and feel free to find a second opinion or another doctor.

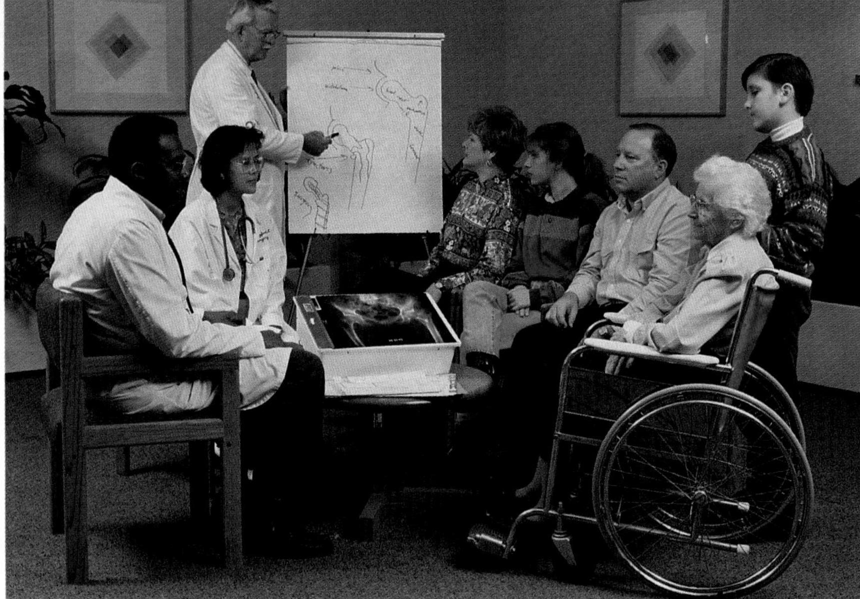

(FIGURE 26-3) **You and your family may have to consult a team of doctors if someone close to you has a major illness and requires long-term medical care.**

you are hurried, treated like a child, or cannot get direct answers, change doctors.

Remember that you have a right to get the opinion of another doctor at any time. This can be especially important when surgery or another major procedure has been recommended. The recommendation of the second doctor is called a "second opinion."

Patient's Bill of Rights

The basic rights of human beings include freedom of expression, the right to make one's own decisions and to act upon them, and the right to maintain one's personal dignity. These rights should be preserved for you when you are a patient. If you are hospitalized for any reason, you should receive your copy of the Patient's Bill of Rights, shown in Figure 26-2. Although it is not a legal document, it does set forth standards that hospitals are expected to follow. Becoming aware of your rights as a patient is your first step toward getting quality health care. It is your own personal responsibility to look out for yourself, insisting on good care and freely expressing your needs and concerns.

Review

1. ***LIFE SKILLS: Being a Wise Consumer*** *List three ways to select a physician.*
2. ***LIFE SKILLS: Communicating Effectively*** *This is your third visit to your doctor about the headaches you have been having. Your doctor hasn't told you what is causing the headaches or whether they will go away. Write down four questions you can ask your doctor to get clear information on your condition.*
3. ***Critical Thinking*** *Why should a hospital tell you if it plans to make your treatment part of an experiment it is conducting?*

Review Answers

1. Ask relatives and friends about their physicians, locate a medical school in your area and call its affiliated hospital for a list of its staff, contact your county medical society.
2. Answers will vary. Some questions might be: What do you think is causing the headaches? Can I expect the headaches to go away? What tests might be done to find the cause of the headaches? What can I do to prevent the headaches? What can I do to treat the headaches once they start?
3. You have a right to know whether the treatment received is experimental or approved, and if the treatment is experimental, you have a right to know the risks involved and how your medical information will be used.

Extension

Choosing a Hospital

Have students visit a hospital admissions department to obtain literature on services and facilities available through the hospital, a copy of the Patient's Bill of Rights, and a list of affiliated doctors.

ASSESS

Section Review

Have students answer the Section Review questions.

Alternative Assessment

A Dangerous Mistake

Suppose you don't tell a doctor all of your symptoms or don't ask all of your important questions. Why is this a dangerous mistake?

Closure

Health Care Is Your Responsibility

Ask students to think about what they will do after high school, such as go to college, get a job, or start a family. Discuss whose responsibility it will be to find a family doctor.

Background
History
In colonial America medical care was rare and doctors were few. Most people lived with diseases they could not cure, such as strep throat. Hospitals began to appear in the 1700s. Modern health-care innovations include health insurance, HMOs, and Medicare for the elderly and Medicaid for the poor. Today, many people think our massive health-care system needs overhauling, but people can't agree on how to change it.

Background
Wasteful Spending
Studies estimate that $130 billion is spent on unnecessary surgery, tests, and hospitalization days, and that $70 billion is wasted through administrative inefficiency. Various studies indicate that many Caesarean births, hysterectomies, back surgeries, and MRI scans (Magnetic Resonance Imaging, which displays computer-generated images of the body) are unnecessary.

Section 26.2 *Financing Your Medical Costs*

Objectives

- *Understand why health-care costs in the United States are rising.*
- *Know the advantages and disadvantages of traditional private health-care insurance and HMOs.*
  LIFE SKILLS: Being a Wise Consumer
- *Learn how to locate free health care in your community.*
  LIFE SKILLS: Using Community Resources
- *Learn how to recognize quackery.*
  LIFE SKILLS: Being a Wise Consumer

defensive medicine: *use of numerous diagnostic tests to avoid a lawsuit.*

premium: *payment a person makes to an insurance company in exchange for coverage.*

We are spending more and more each year for personal health care, as physician costs, dental costs, and hospital-care costs rise rapidly. You can see this trend in Figure 26-4. High-tech equipment, organ transplants, the AIDS epidemic, malpractice insurance, and **defensive medicine** (use of numerous diagnostic tests to avoid a lawsuit) are some of the causes, and they will increase costs even more in the future. Unless something is done to reduce costs, the number of Americans unable to afford medical or dental care will continue to grow.

The U.S. government and businesses are exploring ways to make medical care affordable for everyone, by examining proposals on socialized medicine (free health care paid from tax dollars), shared-cost programs, and other approaches.

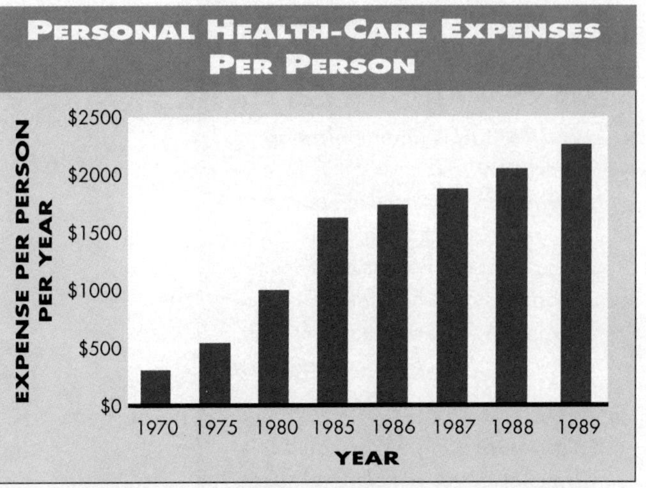

(FIGURE 26-4) **The cost of health care in the United States has been rising rapidly, making it difficult for many people to obtain quality health care. (Source: U.S. Bureau of the Census.)**

Your Family Health Insurance Plan

A good health insurance plan is an absolute necessity in the United States today. Employees of major industries, the government, and other companies often receive free health insurance or pay a small fee, called a **premium,** for their insurance coverage. For an additional fee, they may add family members. Unfortunately, many small businesses and other employers have no such plans, and their employees cannot afford the high health insurance premiums of individual policies. High medical costs have also forced many companies to reduce their benefits and to increase the premiums of employees. The monthly insurance premium is taking a bigger and bigger portion

Section 26.2 Lesson Plan

MOTIVATE

Writing
How Are Medical Costs Paid For?
This may be done as a warm-up activity. Tell students to suppose that someone in their family needs a $15,000 operation but has only $500. Ask them to write down all the ways they can think of for paying this large bill.

TEACH

Class Discussion
Why Are Health-Care Costs Rising?
Call attention to the graph in Figure 26-4. Discuss why health-care costs have gone up so much. Solicit personal anecdotes about the high cost of doctors, hospital bills, tests, and prescriptions. Ask students to multiply 1989's health-care cost per person ($2,274) by the U.S. population (250 million) to discover how much we spent on health care that year. *($568,500,000,000, or $568.5 billion)* Ask them to speculate about where this enormous amount of money comes from. *(From health insurance that people and companies pay for; from government programs for the elderly (Medicare) and the poor (Medicaid))*

Debate the Issue
Can We Cut Health-Care Costs?
Have students select one of the reasons for rising health-care costs, for-

Check Your Insurance Coverage

(FIGURE 26-5)

Is there "first dollar" coverage? That is, do you have to pay anything before the insurance company begins paying?

How does the deductible affect premiums? What amount is suited to your family income?

Is disability or lost-income protection provided? Is there a lump-sum payment to dependents in case of death?

Is full coverage provided for hospital, medical, and surgical cost?

Is major medical insurance available for serious illness and accidents?

Are expenses for care during pregnancy and delivery covered?

Is this a "commercial policy" (one that can be canceled if the holder becomes a bad risk after the claim for a current illness is paid)?

Is a group policy available? These are less expensive.

Is coverage provided for mental and emotional disorders?

Is coverage provided for dental care?

Are dependents covered?

What is the grace period for late premiums before cancellation?

Do any restrictive clauses eliminate payment for previously existing illnesses or require a waiting period before such illnesses are covered?

What happens if I am covered by a group policy at work and I get fired or resign? Could I keep my insurance, or would the policy be canceled?

of the employee's take-home pay. In addition, health insurance pays only part of the bill. For those who are stricken with a serious illness, family savings are often quickly drained.

Traditional Policies Traditional private health insurance policies have advantages and drawbacks. One big advantage is that the insurance company will pay for treatment by any doctor or hospital the insured person chooses. This can be very important if a person has had the same physician for a long time and does not want to change.

One drawback is that the insured person must first pay for many medical expenses and then fill out a claim form in order to be reimbursed.

Another disadvantage is that the insured person must pay a yearly **deductible,**

deductible: *the amount of medical costs an insured person must pay before the insurance company begins paying.*

Background
What Health Insurance Covers

Coverage usually includes hospital expense (shared room, meals, tests, medications, nursing, operating room), surgical expense (doctor's fee), outpatient expense (nonsurgical), and major medical (cost from a serious illness or accident, office visits, therapy, medications). Some policies include dental, vision, and disability income.

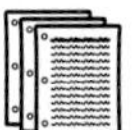

Ethics Worksheet

Assign the Ethics Worksheet for Unit 7.

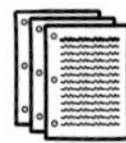

Life Skills Worksheet 26B
Using Community Resources

Assign the Using Community Resources Life Skills Worksheet, which requires students to call and find out about local health clinics that offer free or low-cost services.

mulate a question, and debate the pros and cons. Some sample questions to debate are: Should doctors stop performing organ transplants to save money? Should laws be passed to exempt doctors from malpractice lawsuits so they will stop practicing defensive medicine?

Demonstration
Teacher's Health Insurance

As an example, explain to students your school district's health-care plan for teachers. Describe where the money comes from, the types of coverage provided, any additional fees for family coverage, deductibles, any premium you must pay, and so on. Show the arithmetic for a specific claim on the chalkboard to illustrate how the system works.

Journal 26C
Your Family's Health Insurance

Have students ask the adults at home questions about their health insurance and explain in the Student Journal what services the insurance pays for.

Case Study
How Health Insurance Works

Present the following information to students: Anna has health insurance at work with $500 deductible, 80 percent payment, and no dental or eye coverage. Last year she had hospital bills ($1,100), doctor bills ($300), prescriptions for drugs ($100), dental care ($75), and new glasses ($125). **How**

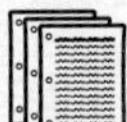

Life Skills Worksheet 26C

Resisting Pressure

Assign the Resisting Pressure Life Skills Worksheet, which helps students frame responses to people selling quack health-care products.

Making a Choice 26B

Choosing a Health Insurance Plan

Assign the Choosing a Health Insurance Plan card. This card directs students to make up a list of questions to help them decide whether to enroll in a traditional health insurance plan or in an HMO.

HMOs (health maintenance organizations): *organizations that offer subscribers complete medical care in return for a fixed monthly fee.*

or set fee, before the insurance company begins paying for any of the costs. In addition, routine checkups at a doctor's office are usually not reimbursed—only office visits for illness or injury. Insurance companies will reimburse only a percentage of office visit costs (often 80 percent). The remaining amount is paid by the insured person. Insurance companies will also pay only a percentage of hospital costs, usually 80 percent.

If your family is searching for a traditional health insurance policy, it would be helpful to find out the answers to the questions in Figure 26-5 before purchasing a policy. Also, you might find it helpful to call your state insurance department for assistance. A representative can help analyze any policy, explain its terms, and provide information on how easy it is to get reimbursed for claims.

HMOs (Health Maintenance Organizations) A more recent type of health-care plan is provided by **HMOs (health maintenance organizations)**. An HMO is a group of doctors and other health-care workers who offer complete medical care in return for a fixed monthly fee. In addition, some HMOs charge a small fee for office visits and prescriptions.

HMOs have several advantages. First, patients do not have to submit claim forms for reimbursement.

Another advantage is that HMOs practice preventive medicine. Because HMOs receive almost the same amount of money from members no matter how many times members use their services, it is financially advantageous for HMOs to have healthy members who don't constantly need their services. Therefore, HMOs emphasize checkups, immunizations, and other ways of staying healthy.

(FIGURE 26-6)

Traditional Insurance Policies Versus HMOs

Traditional Insurance Policies	HMOs
Regular checkups usually not covered; only a percentage (often 80 percent) of hospital cost and office visits reimbursed; reimbursement doesn't begin until cost exceeds the deductible	*Most health-care cost paid, except for a small fee (copayment) charged by some HMOs for office visits or prescriptions*
Can see any primary care physician you choose	*Must use one of the HMO's participating primary care physicians*
Can see any specialist you choose	*Must have the HMO's consent to see specialist or the HMO will not pay costs*
Often must submit claim forms in order to be reimbursed	*No need to submit claim forms*

• • • TEACH continued

much did Anna pay? How much did her insurance pay? *[Anna paid $200 for dental and eye care. Her insurance covers the $1,500 for hospital, doctor, and prescriptions, but she had to pay the first $500 (the deductible). That left $1,000, of which the insurance company paid 80 percent or $800; Anna paid the remaining $200. Altogether, the insurance company paid $800, and Anna paid $900.]*

Cooperative Learning
Finding Free Health Care

Divide the class into three groups to use telephone directories to find free health-care sources. The sources should include city, county, state, and U.S. government health and human services, public welfare and assistance, and so on. Have each group call appropriate organizations and explain that they are doing a school project. Have the groups each describe a family of four (children aged 2 and 4; the woman is pregnant; $12,000 family income) and ask where they can get doctors, immunizations, dental care, and glasses. Then have them ask what it will cost. (A referral service such as Community Action or United Way may be able to identify all needed services.) Have each group keep a log of calls showing the agency, the telephone number, the name of the person they spoke to, and the information received.

In addition, some HMOs have all their services in one building, including special testing with high-tech machinery. This means that patients can see their doctor and get their tests in one location.

A big drawback of HMOs is that you can't freely see any doctor of your choice. If you see a specialist outside the HMO without the consent of the HMO, you must pay for the services yourself.

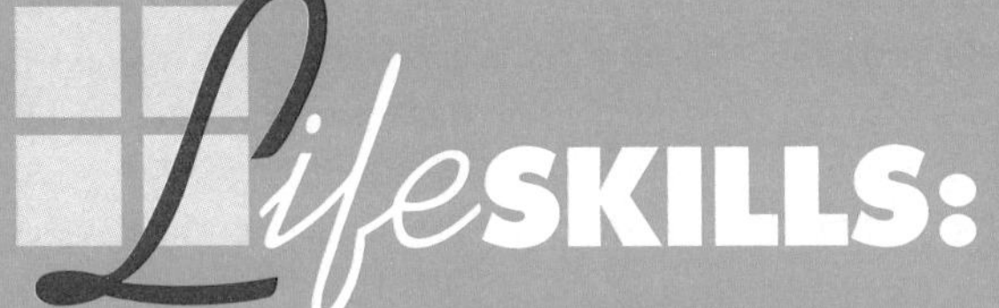

Being a Wise Consumer

Traditional Policy or HMO?

You may need to select a health insurance policy in a few years. Get some practice now by evaluating the following situation.

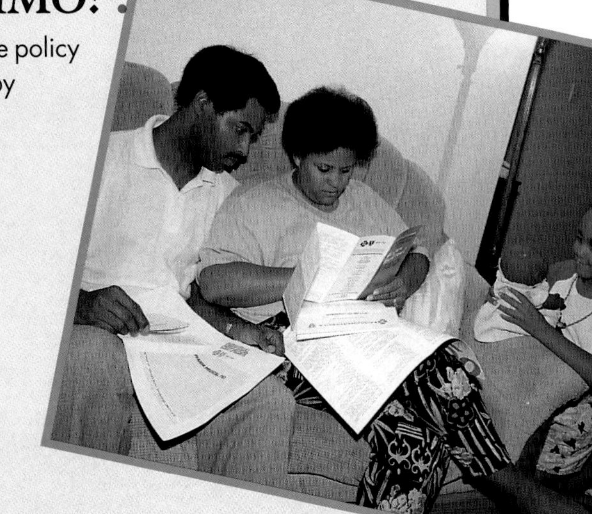

At your new job, your take-home pay is $1,100 a month. You're married and have a small child. Your spouse does not have health insurance at work, but you can get either a traditional policy or join an HMO where you work.

The traditional policy would cost you $71 per month. It would cost you $22 per month to add your spouse and child. The traditional policy has a $250-a-year deductible for you, or $500 for you and your dependents (spouse and child), and it pays 80 percent of hospital costs.

You would pay $56 per month for the HMO. It would cost $22 per month to add your spouse and child. In addition, each time you or a member of your family visited the doctor or bought a prescription medicine, you would pay a $5 copayment. There would be no copayment required of you if you or a member of your family entered the hospital.

Everyone in your family is enjoying good health right now. Your child will need a checkup at least once a year. You are happy with the pediatrician who cares for your child. You and your spouse, however, have not yet chosen a primary care physician.

Which family members would you insure? Would you choose the HMO or the traditional policy? Why?

Life SKILLS
Traditional Policy or HMO?

Have students consider the facts presented in the text and decide on their own whether the traditional health insurance policy or the HMO is more advantageous in this case.

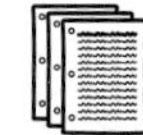

Section Review Worksheet 26.2

Assign Section Review Worksheet 26.2, which encourages students to compare traditional insurance plans, HMOs, and free clinics by listing advantages and disadvantages of each.

Section Quiz 26.2

Have students take Section Quiz 26.2.

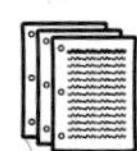

Reteaching Worksheet 26.2

Students who have difficulty with the material may complete Reteaching Worksheet 26.2, which requires them to compare traditional insurance plans with HMOs.

Debate the Issue
Traditional Insurance or HMO?

Have student teams debate whether traditional insurance or an HMO is the better deal for a family. Ask students to prepare for the debate by studying the text, Figure 26-6, and magazine articles. Close by having the leader of each team summarize on the chalkboard why his or her team's method is better.

Journal 26D
Your Health-Care Sources

In the Student Journal, have students list agency names and phone numbers that are useful to them. Tell them to use the following column headings: Type of Care, Agency Name, Phone, and Address, and have them title the list "Sources of Free or Low-Cost Health Care."

Class Discussion
Spotting Quackery

Obtain a supermarket tabloid and have the class study and discuss the ads for quack products, using the guidelines in Figure 26-7. Likely candidates include weight-control products; intelligence enhancers; cures for cancer, arthritis, and migraine; breast enlargers; baldness cures; sex enhancers; and 900-line health advisers. For 900 numbers, have students calculate the charge for a 10-minute call.

Background

Health Care for the Poor and Uninsured

People who are poor and lack insurance have difficulty getting health care. Medicaid patients sometimes are refused service by doctors and hospitals because Medicaid pays too little to cover the total cost. Private hospitals make money from well-insured patients, often leaving public and nonprofit hospitals to serve the poor and uninsured, limiting the care they can provide.

How to Find and Use Free Health Services

Most states and communities have some form of free health care. Medicaid provides federal aid to the elderly, blind, disabled, and families with dependent children. It also assists those who live at or below the federally designated poverty level.

Community health resources are also available to everyone. State health departments and county or city health units exist to help residents with specific health problems. Immunization centers for disease control, special clinics for sexually transmitted diseases, and maternal and child health services are generally available. Some fees may be charged, but they are generally small.

"Free clinics" have also been established in most cities to treat or counsel people for undesired pregnancies, sexually transmitted diseases, and drug abuse. Many of these clinics also treat other types of ailments for those people who are unable to afford medical care.

However, the funding for their clinics

Cultural DIVERSITY

Native Americans and Health Care

The United States health-care system is enormous. It includes a large number and variety of hospitals, health-care centers, doctors, nurses, and other health professionals. Some people find that the options available within this system meet their health needs quite effectively. Others, however, have customs and beliefs that lead them to seek different sources of treatment, called "alternative" health-care systems. Native American cultures are examples of cultures that provide alternative health systems for their people.

According to the philosophy of these cultures, all elements of the world—inanimate objects as well as living things—have life, spirit, power, and specific roles to play. Each element is related to the others, and each affects the entire universe. When there is harmony among these elements, a state of well-being results. But an imbalance among the elements can cause illness.

When such an imbalance occurs, a Native American may seek the help of a traditional healer. Healers are trained men and women who perform ceremonies to right the imbalance and in so doing heal the illness. Such healing ceremonies may include prayers, rituals, special medicines, and the use of visual symbols.

Though the practices of Native American healers may seem quite differ-

• • • TEACH continued

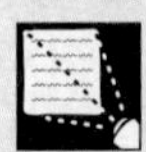

Teaching Transparency 26A

Quack Health-Care Products

Use this transparency to give students extra practice in identifying quack health-care products and claims.

Extension

Another Viewpoint

Ask the school nurse, or a doctor, dentist, or representative from a hospital or HMO, to visit the class, discuss the problem of providing affordable health care for everyone, and answer students' questions.

is usually low, so they must restrict the medical services they offer to a small number of patients and limit the services provided. Check the yellow pages for a list of health-care clinics that are in your area, or call your state or county health department.

Quackery

Quackery—the promotion of medical services or products that are worthless or unproven—can endanger your health.

Worthless so-called miracle remedies for arthritis, cancer, epilepsy, and other serious disorders flood the market and confuse the public. Fake treatments and worthless medication may delay accurate diagnosis and appropriate treatment until the problem is very serious.

And even when worthless treatments don't actually endanger your health, such as creams that are advertised as breast enlargers, they waste your money.

It is often very difficult to know which health products and services to purchase for special problems and which ones to avoid. Television, radio, magazine, and mail advertising is designed to get you to buy vari-

quackery: *the promotion of medical services or products that are worthless or unproven.*

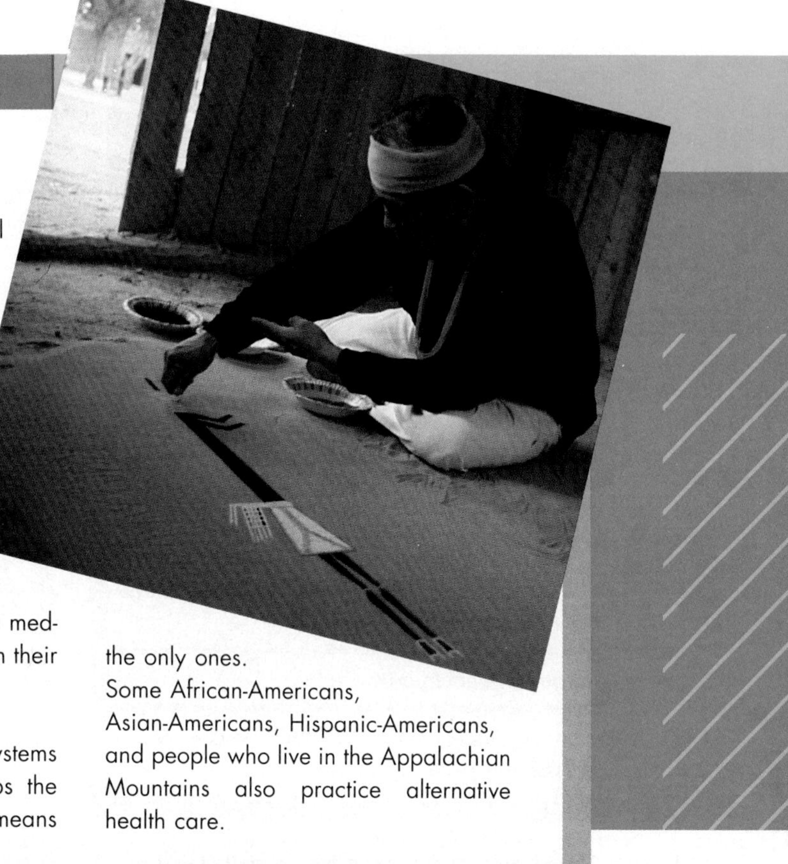

ent from those of medical doctors, there are similarities. Like medical doctors, Native American healers must undergo years of special training. They must learn the right ceremonies and rituals to perform for the different types of imbalance. Also like medical doctors, Native American healers sometimes specialize in certain kinds of health problems. The healers may refer a patient to another healer or to a medical doctor if an illness is not within their area of expertise.

The alternative health-care systems of Native Americans are perhaps the best known, but they are by no means the only ones. Some African-Americans, Asian-Americans, Hispanic-Americans, and people who live in the Appalachian Mountains also practice alternative health care.

Review Answers

1. Answers may include high-tech equipment, organ transplants, the AIDS epidemic, malpractice insurance, and defensive medicine.
2. Answers may vary. Students might say that they would choose a traditional insurance policy so that they could continue to see the same doctor, otherwise they would have to change to a doctor who participates in the HMO.

Answers to Questions 1 and 2 are on p. 579.

3. Answers may include the elderly, blind, disabled, families with dependent children, and those who live at or below the poverty level.

4. Answers may include National Health Council, World Health Organization, Food and Drug Administration, Department of Health and Human Services, American Heart Association, and American Lung Association.

5. Answers may include those who are unemployed, those who cannot afford high health-care costs or individual insurance policy premiums and whose employers don't provide health-care plans, those who work part-time jobs, and those who are poor, elderly, or disabled.

ous products. Each media message does its best to convince you that its product is the absolute best way to eliminate a particular health concern.

Quackery is not always practiced by dishonest people. Some people who sell worthless products or services truly believe in what they are selling.

Your best protection is to analyze carefully every product or treatment method you are considering. You may have to contact your physician or a reputable agency or nonprofit organization for advice. One good resource for information on drugs and cosmetics is a book called *The Medicine Show,* an unbiased report on numerous products by the editors of *Consumer Reports* magazine. Other sources of health-related consumer information are the National Health Council, the World Health Organization, the Food and Drug Administration, the Department of Health and Human Services, and various nonprofit associations such as the local offices of the American Heart Association and the American Lung Association. Any time you are in doubt, check the product out before you purchase it. Figure 26-7 gives you some tips to help identify a quack or an unsound product.

Are You Dealing with a Quack?

If you encounter the following, you may be dealing with a quack:

- *The promise or guarantee of a quick cure*
- *The use of a "secret remedy" or an unorthodox treatment*
- *The use of advertising to gain patients*
- *Testimonials by patients who have been cured*
- *Claims that a product will cure a wide variety of ailments*
- *Claims that sound too good to be true*
- *Request for a large payment in advance*
- *Claims by the manufacturers or sponsors of the product that the medical profession is persecuting them*

(FIGURE 26-7) **Spectacular claims are often a sign that you're dealing with a quack.**

Review

1. *List three reasons why health costs are rising in the United States.*
2. **LIFE SKILLS: Being a Wise Consumer** *You have a chronic condition for which you've been seeing the same doctor for years. You have a great deal of confidence in your doctor and don't want to change. Would you choose a traditional insurance policy or an HMO? Explain your answer.*
3. **LIFE SKILLS: Using Community Resources** *List three groups of people who can receive health care through Medicaid.*
4. **LIFE SKILLS: Being a Wise Consumer** *You are considering buying a health product that guarantees a quick cure for your condition. Name two groups you could consult to determine whether you are dealing with a quack.*
5. ***Critical Thinking*** *Which people in the United States are least likely to have access to good health care?*

ASSESS

Section Review

Have students answer the Section Review questions.

Alternative Assessment

Health-Care Systems Improvements

Have students write a paragraph on improvements they would like to see made in the health-care system.

Closure

Being a Wise Consumer

Ask students: **What things can you do to get the best health care at the lowest cost?** *[The many possibilities include avoiding unnecessary treatment; comparison-shopping for doctors, hospitals, dentists, eye care, pharmacies, therapists, and health-care plans; using free clinics if you qualify to do so; being alert to quackery, and never spending money for suspicious services or products.]*

Highlights

Summary

- When choosing a doctor, ask friends and relatives about their physicians, or obtain a list of the staff physicians at a nearby hospital from the hospital, from a medical school, or from the county medical society.
- It is important to feel comfortable and communicate well with your doctor.
- A medical examination includes a medical history, physical examination, and a talk with the doctor. Patients should ask any questions that concern them and insist that the doctor explain special instructions clearly.
- As a patient, you have the right to get another doctor's opinion at any time.
- An advantage of traditional private health insurance policies is that the insured person can choose any doctor. Disadvantages of traditional policies are that the insured person must pay a yearly deductible and also must pay medical fees before being reimbursed. In addition, traditional health insurance does not reimburse the cost of routine checkups.
- Advantages of HMOs are that their practitioners stress preventive medicine, and patients do not have to submit claim forms for reimbursement. One drawback of HMOs is that patients can't always see a doctor of their choice.
- There are public-health resources that are available to everyone. Some services are free, while others are provided for small fees.
- To avoid fake treatments and worthless medications, carefully analyze every product or treatment method you are considering.

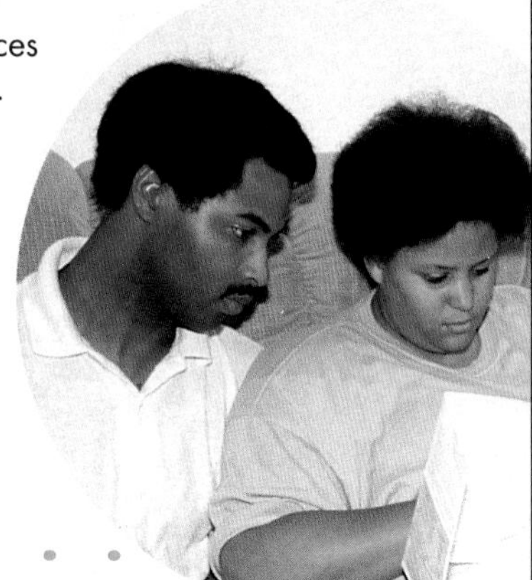

Vocabulary

primary care physician a family medicine physician, a pediatrician, or a general internal medicine physician.

defensive medicine the use of numerous diagnostic tests to avoid a lawsuit.

premium the payment a person makes to an insurance company in exchange for coverage.

deductible the amount of medical costs an insured person must pay before the insurance company begins paying.

HMOs (health maintenance organizations) organizations that offer subscribers complete medical care in return for a fixed monthly fee.

quackery the promotion of medical services or products that are worthless or unproven.

Chapter 26 Highlights Strategies

Summary

Have students read the summary to reinforce the concepts they learned in Chapter 26.

Vocabulary

Review the vocabulary list and ask students if they have questions about any of the terms.

Extension

Have students prepare a poster for display in the community showing major health-related hotlines such as those related to alcohol and drugs, pregnancy, AIDS, and so on.

Chapter 26 Assessment

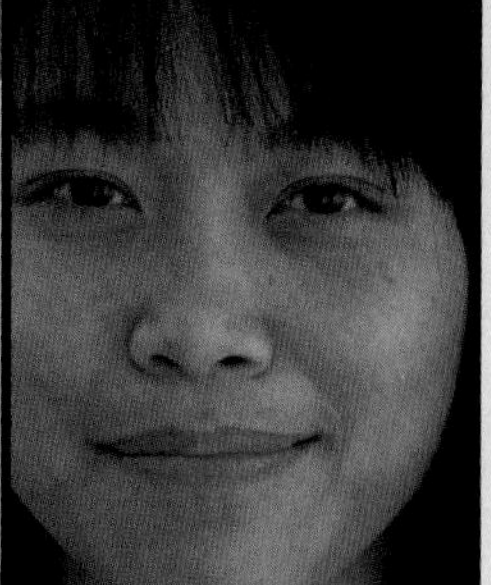

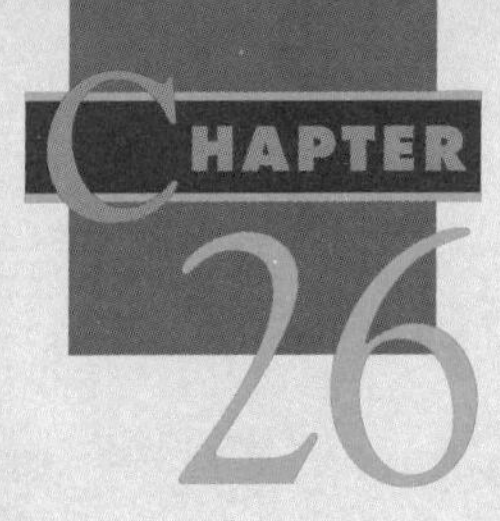

Chapter Review

Concept Review

1. What types of information make up a medical history?
2. What is included in a routine physical examination?
3. What is a "second opinion"? When might a patient need one?
4. When would an individual receive a copy of the Patient's Bill of Rights? What does it do?
5. Are health-care costs rising or falling? Why? What is the outlook for health-care costs in the future?
6. What are two approaches being considered by the U.S. government and businesses to make medical care affordable for everyone?
7. Why have many companies had to reduce the health insurance benefits they provide for employees?
8. Name one advantage and one disadvantage of traditional private health insurance policies.
9. Who can you contact to help you choose a traditional health insurance policy? How can they help you?
10. What is an HMO? Describe its service.
11. Name three types of health services that are available through state health departments and county or city health units.
12. What kind of treatment or counseling do "free clinics" provide? Who do they treat?
13. Name four instances in which a health consumer should suspect quackery.

Expressing Your Views

1. You need to select a primary care physician. What professional and personal characteristics of a doctor are important to you? What would you do if, after you found a doctor, you were not satisfied with him or her?
2. Your primary care physician has recommended that you have surgery. You are wondering if you should see another doctor for a second opinion. What advantages are there to getting an opinion from another doctor?
3. Why do you think some people continue to buy worthless products?

Chapter Review

Concept Review

Sample responses:

1. Reason for visit; specific signs and symptoms; medication taken; exercise habits; information about previous illnesses, surgery, allergies, and reactions to medications

2. The doctor will record your specific signs and symptoms, such as temperature, blood pressure, heart rate, and weight.

3. The recommendation of a second doctor. When surgery or any other major procedure is recommended by the first doctor

4. When a person is hospitalized for any reason; it sets forth standards that hospitals are expected to follow.

5. Health-care costs are rising because of high-tech equipment, organ transplants, the AIDS epidemic, malpractice insurance, and defensive medicine. Health-care costs in the future are likely to be higher still.

6. Socialized medicine and shared-cost programs

7. High medical costs

8. An advantage of a traditional private health insurance policy is that the insured person can choose any doctor. Disadvantages of traditional policies are that the insured person must pay a yearly deductible and also must pay medical fees before being reimbursed. Traditional health insurance does not reimburse the cost of routine checkups.

9. The state insurance department. They will help a person analyze any policy, explain its terms, and provide information on how easy it is to get reimbursed for claims.

10. HMOs, or health maintenance organizations, offer subscribers complete medical care and preventive medicine in return for a fixed monthly fee. HMOs offer services such as special testing with high-tech machinery.

11. Medicaid, immunization centers, clinics for STDs, maternal and child health services.

12. Treatment and counseling for undesired pregnancies, sexually transmitted diseases, and drug abuse. They treat people who cannot afford medical care.

13. Students should list four of the instances listed in Figure 26-7.

Chapter 26 Assessment

Life Skills Check . . . .

1. Communicating Effectively
You have your first appointment with your new primary care physician concerning a recent health problem. What information should you take to the doctor with you? What are three questions you could prepare to ask the doctor?

2. Being a Wise Consumer
Your family has been offered a fantastic deal on a traditional health insurance policy. What questions should you ask the insurance agent before purchasing the policy? Where else could you check to be sure the company is sound and that the policy is a good one for your family?

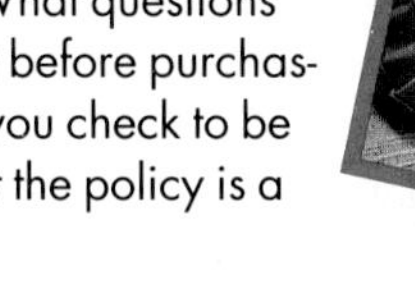

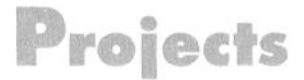

Projects . . . .

1. Some countries have a national health insurance program. Many people think we should have such a program in the United States. Work with a group to research the national health insurance program of another country and compare that program with the health services available in our country. Organize a class debate on whether our federal government should institute national health insurance.

2. Work with a partner to create a short skit about quackery. The skit can be humorous or outrageous. One partner should pretend to be a quack using some of the common practices listed in Figure 26-7. The other partner should pretend to be a consumer. Lead the audience to see the possible negative consequences of being misled by quackery.

Plan for Action . . . .

A health-care system cannot be expected to care for your health if you are not willing to do your part in caring for yourself. Make a plan to find a doctor if you do not have one and list three local health-care facilities you could use if necessary.

Expressing Your Views

1. Answers concerning personal characteristics will vary. Students should find another doctor if they are not satisfied with their current one.

2. Surgery may not be necessary. You would be saved the cost, time, and pain of surgery.

3. They are hoping for a fast or easy cure to their medical problems.

Life Skills Check

1. The results of any tests you had and any medication you are taking or have taken for the health problem; How long will my condition take to heal? Should I take medicine with food? Can I go back to school? Can I exercise?

2. What is the deductible? Is full coverage provided for hospital, medical, and surgical costs? What is the monthly premium? State insurance department

Projects

Have students plan and carry out the projects for health care.

Plan for Action

Ask students how they think they will pay for their health care five years from now? Have them discuss the responses. Do they believe the health-care system will be improved by then? If so, in what ways? If not, how will that affect them?

Assessment Options

Chapter Test

Have students take the Chapter 26 Test.

Alternative Assessment

Have students do the Alternative Assessment activity for Chapter 26.

Test Generator

The Test Generator (Macintosh® or IBM® format) contains an additional 50 assessment items for this chapter.

Issues in Health

ETHICAL ISSUES IN HEALTH

ISSUE: *Should family leave be an employment benefit in the same way as sick leave?*

Have students read the Ethical Issues in Health feature. Ask students to speculate—or report—about how families without family leave handle the needs described in the article. Sometimes parents use their own sick days to care for children, sometimes parents or other caretakers work part time, or sometimes people lose their jobs or have to quit. In what way are the needs of a family the responsibility of the society as a whole? Have each student write a paragraph, story, or poem about a family crisis that would be affected by family leave.

Ethical Issues in Health

ISSUE: Should family leave be an employment benefit in the same way as sick leave?

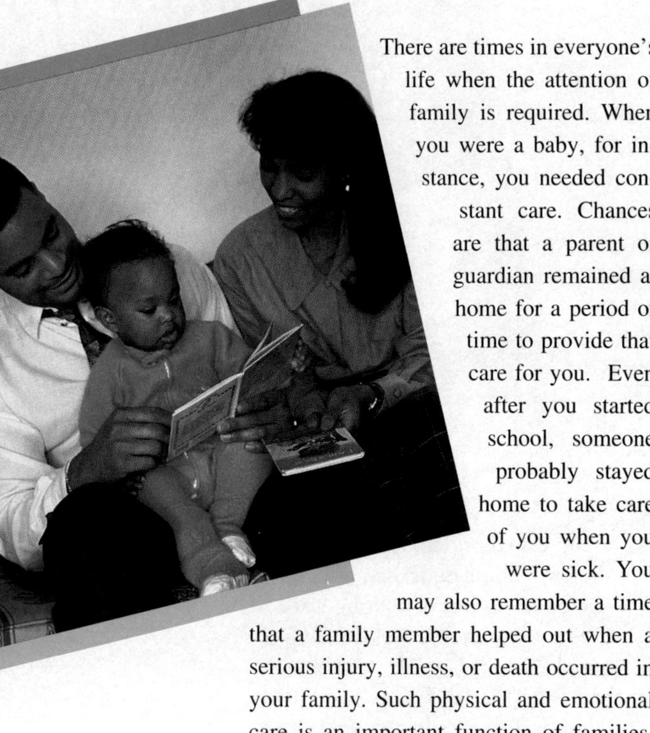

There are times in everyone's life when the attention of family is required. When you were a baby, for instance, you needed constant care. Chances are that a parent or guardian remained at home for a period of time to provide that care for you. Even after you started school, someone probably stayed home to take care of you when you were sick. You may also remember a time that a family member helped out when a serious injury, illness, or death occurred in your family. Such physical and emotional care is an important function of families.

For many families, caring for each other is also a financial necessity. Today's soaring medical costs make hospital care unaffordable for many people, especially when they require continuous care for a long period of time. For example, someone who has been seriously hurt in an accident may require 24-hour care for weeks, months, or even years. People who have Parkinson's or Alzheimer's disease also require constant care. Since the number of older persons in our society is rapidly increasing, family members will be called on more and more in the future to care for older adults suffering from cancer, heart disease, arthritis, loss of memory, or muscle disease. Unfortunately, people with full-time jobs often find it impossible to work and still provide regular care for a family member in need.

Employers can make such situations easier to manage by allowing employees to take a leave of absence from their jobs—as they would if they were sick—to take care of family members. This type of leave is usually called family leave. Some companies continue paying an employee's salary and insurance premiums while he or she is on family leave. Others simply provide assurance that the same job, or a similar one, will be available when the employee is able to return to work. Child-care leave is a specific type of family leave that many companies provide for women who have just had babies. In some companies, child-care leave is available to new fathers as well.

Many people believe family and child-care leave should automatically be part of the benefits and rights for all employees. These advocates contend that government and the business community have a responsibility to help families cope with the consequences of birth, death, illness, and disability. They stress that home care is better and much less expensive than the care given in a hospital, day-care center, or nursing home. Since health-care costs are often paid for by the insurance plans provided by employers or by tax dollars (as with Medicare and Medicaid), some experts predict that family leave would reduce the overall cost of health care.

In one of the first acts of his administration, President Clinton signed into law the Family and Medical Leave Act. This legislation requires all businesses with more than 50 employees to provide up to 12 weeks of unpaid family leave to all employees who have worked at the company at least one year and who work at least 25 hours per week. Employers must also offer the same job or a comparable job to employees returning from leave and must pay employees' health insurance costs while they are on leave. Several states have laws that require smaller companies to provide family-leave benefits as well.

Opponents of family-leave laws argue that a company should be responsible only for providing its employees fair salaries and reasonable benefits. They argue that a company should not have to take responsibility for the well-being of an employee's entire family. They predict that if employers are required to provide family-leave benefits, some private businesses could be driven out of existence as a result.

Those who oppose family-leave laws also point out that such policies would increase taxes as well as the price of products and services. Taxes would increase because the large number of government employees would receive family-leave benefits. The price of products and services would increase because the cost of temporarily replacing an employee is high. In order to survive, many companies will have to add this cost to the prices customers pay.

Situation for Discussion

In the Garcia family, both parents work at a small company in order to support their four children, who range in age from 8 to 16. Mrs. Garcia's 78-year-old father, Mr. Pena, lives alone in an apartment near the family's home. Several years ago, Mr. Pena began to have trouble walking, his hands started shaking, and he fell several times. The doctor diagnosed Mr. Pena as having Parkinson's disease and prescribed medication to manage the disease. But now, even with the medication, Mr. Pena is no longer able to care for himself and live alone safely.

a. How can the Garcia family manage this situation? What choices do they have?

b. If Mr. Garcia or Mrs. Garcia could take family leave, should the company hold a job until he or she returns, or hire a person who is equally qualified for the job? Should the company pay full salary during the leave? What would the company have to do to continue normal operations during the leave?

c. Should the government reimburse a company for the cost of family leave?

UNIT 8

SAFETY AND EMERGENCY CARE

CHAPTER OVERVIEWS

CHAPTER 27

SAFETY AND RISK REDUCTION

This chapter examines ways in which personal behaviors can be modified to reduce accidents. Students learn to recognize the factors that contribute to motor vehicle and bicycle accidents. They also learn behaviors that reduce their risks of being injured in such accidents. The most common accidents around the home and how to avoid them are discussed. Students learn how to reduce their risk of injury in the workplace and in the event of disasters. A discussion of safety in sports, swimming and diving, and camping, hiking, and hunting ends the chapter.

CHAPTER 28

FIRST AID AND CPR

Students learn that first aid often makes the difference between life and death when an accident or other emergency occurs. The chapter describes the first steps that should be taken during an emergency. The ABC procedure for assessing and treating medical priorities is explained. The CPR procedure is described, and students are encouraged to attend a training class in CPR. First aid for injuries, choking, and heart attack is covered thoroughly. Students also learn how to deal with emergencies caused by extreme heat and cold, bites, stings, and poisoning.

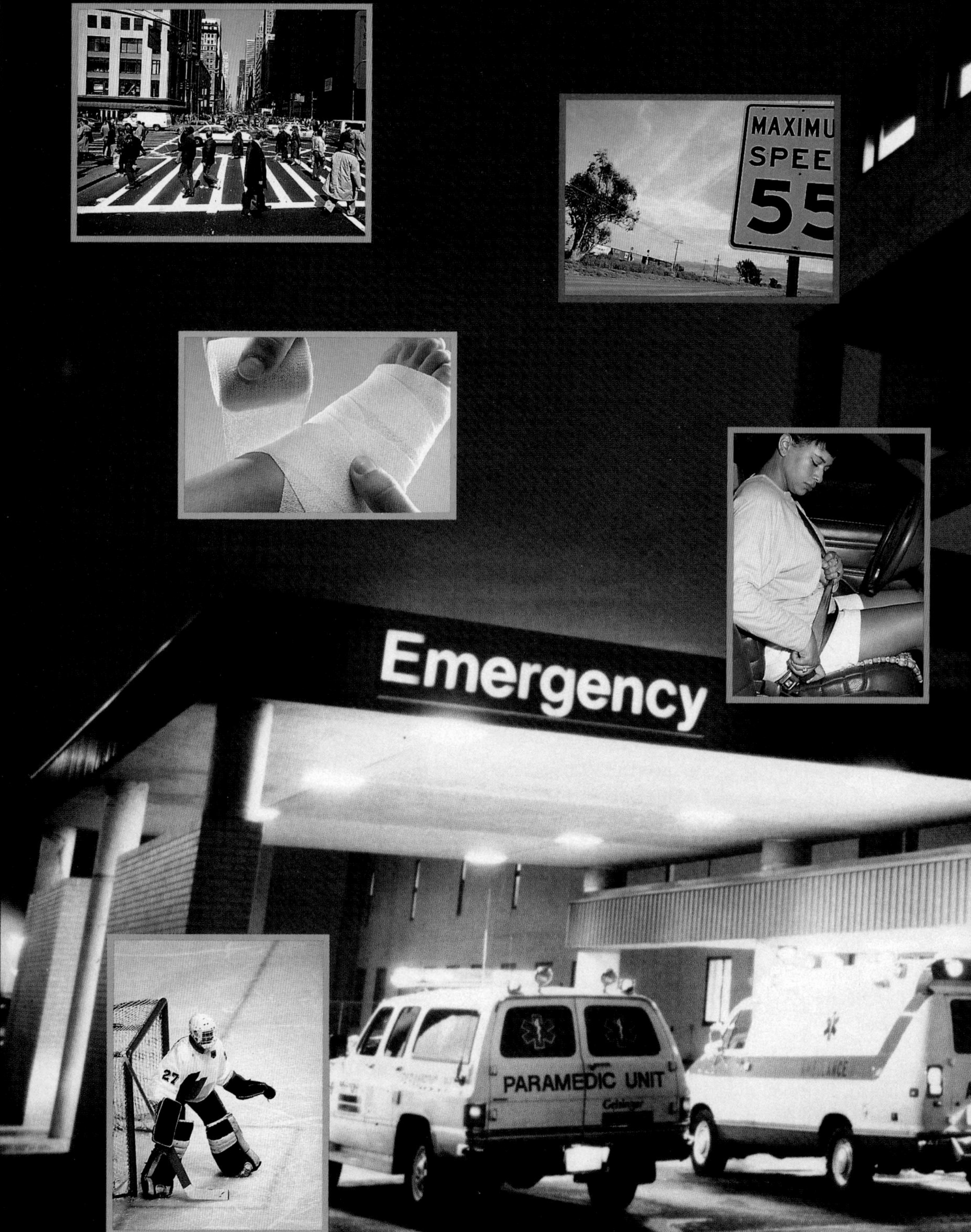

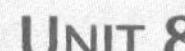

UNIT EIGHT

SAFETY AND EMERGENCY CARE

CHAPTER 27

SAFETY AND RISK REDUCTION

CHAPTER 28

FIRST AID AND CPR

UNIT PREVIEW

Accidents are the leading cause of death for people between the ages of 15 and 24. In this unit, students learn that carelessness and taking unnecessary risks are factors in most accidents. Students' safety awareness—knowledge about risks and how to reduce them—is raised by thorough coverage of vehicle safety; home, workplace, and community safety; and recreational safety. Students' readiness to deal with accidents and other emergencies is enhanced through the unit's presentation of first aid procedures.

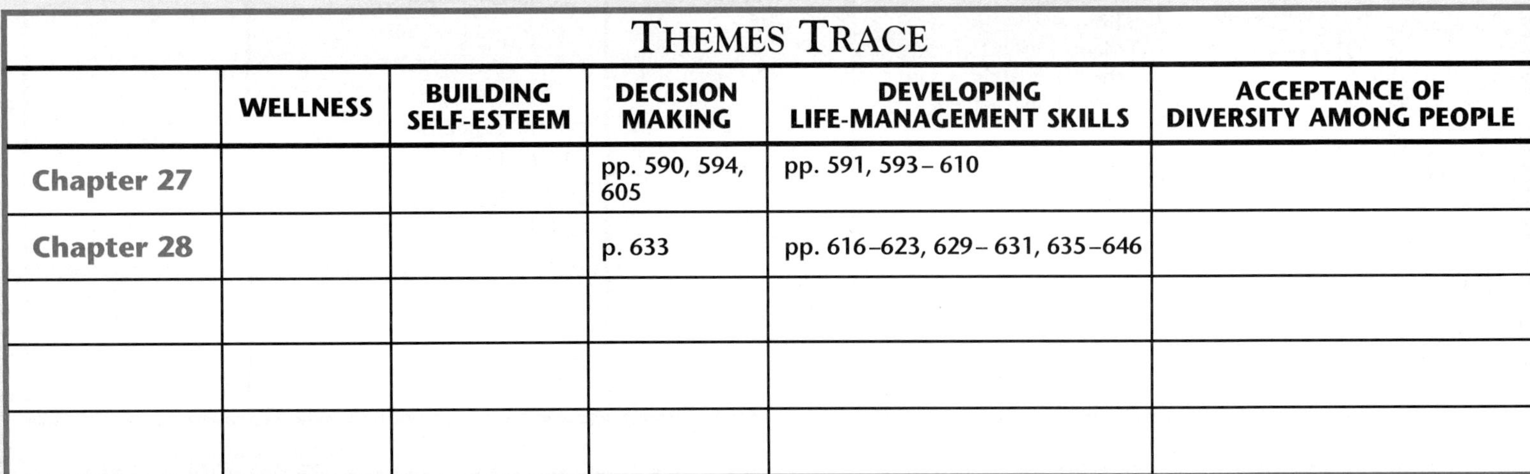

THEMES TRACE

	WELLNESS	BUILDING SELF-ESTEEM	DECISION MAKING	DEVELOPING LIFE-MANAGEMENT SKILLS	ACCEPTANCE OF DIVERSITY AMONG PEOPLE
Chapter 27			pp. 590, 594, 605	pp. 591, 593–610	
Chapter 28			p. 633	pp. 616–623, 629–631, 635–646	

CHAPTER 27

SAFETY AND RISK REDUCTION

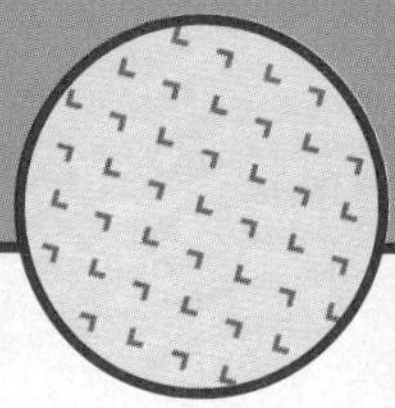

PLANNING GUIDE

TEXT SECTIONS	OBJECTIVES	TEXT FEATURES	OUTSIDE RESOURCES	NOTES
27.1 **Accidents and Risks** pp. 589-592 1 period	• Recognize that accidents are the leading cause of death for people between the ages of 15 and 24. • Recognize that risky or careless behaviors are factors in most accidents. ■ Identify ways in which your personal behavior can be modified to reduce your risk of accidents.	• LIFE SKILLS: Practicing Self-Care, p. 591 **ASSESSMENT** • Section Review, p. 592	**TEACHER'S RESOURCE BINDER** • Lesson Plan 27.1 • Personal Health Inventory • Journal Entry 27A • Section Review Worksheet 27.1 • Section Quiz 27.1 • Reteaching Worksheet 27.1 **OTHER RESOURCES** • Making a Choice 27A	
27.2 **Vehicle Safety** pp. 593-597 1 period	• Recognize factors that contribute to motor-vehicle accidents. • Identify behaviors that reduce the risk of being injured in a motor-vehicle accident. • List some ways to maintain a bicycle for safety. ■ Identify behaviors that reduce the risk of being injured in a bicycle accident.	**ASSESSMENT** • Section Review, p. 597	**TEACHER'S RESOURCE BINDER** • Lesson Plan 27.2 • Journal Entry 27B • Section Review Worksheet 27.2 • Section Quiz 27.2 • Reteaching Worksheet 27.2 **OTHER RESOURCES** • Transparency 27A	
27.3 **Safety at Home and at Work** pp. 598-606 2 periods	• Recognize the relationship between accidents that frequently occur in the home and personal behavior. • Identify potential accident hazards in the home and in the community. ■ Recommend steps to reduce the potential for accidents in the home and in the community. • Identify ways to maintain safety in the workplace.	• What Would You Do? p. 605 **ASSESSMENT** • Section Review, p. 606	**TEACHER'S RESOURCE BINDER** • Lesson Plan 27.3 • Journal Entry 27C • Life Skills 27A • Section Review Worksheet 27.3 • Section Quiz 27.3 • Reteaching Worksheet 27.3	
27.4 **Recreational Safety** pp. 607-610 1 period	• Recognize potential hazards in recreational activities. ■ Identify ways to reduce the risk of accidents in recreational activities.	**ASSESSMENT** • Section Review, p. 610	**TEACHER'S RESOURCE BINDER** • Lesson Plan 27.4 • Journal Entries 27D, 27E • Ethics Worksheet • Section Review Worksheet 27.4 • Section Quiz 27.4 • Reteaching Worksheet 27.4 **OTHER RESOURCES** • Making a Choice 27B	

■ Denotes LIFE SKILLS objectives

• Items in blue are also part of the *Holt Health Activity Book.*

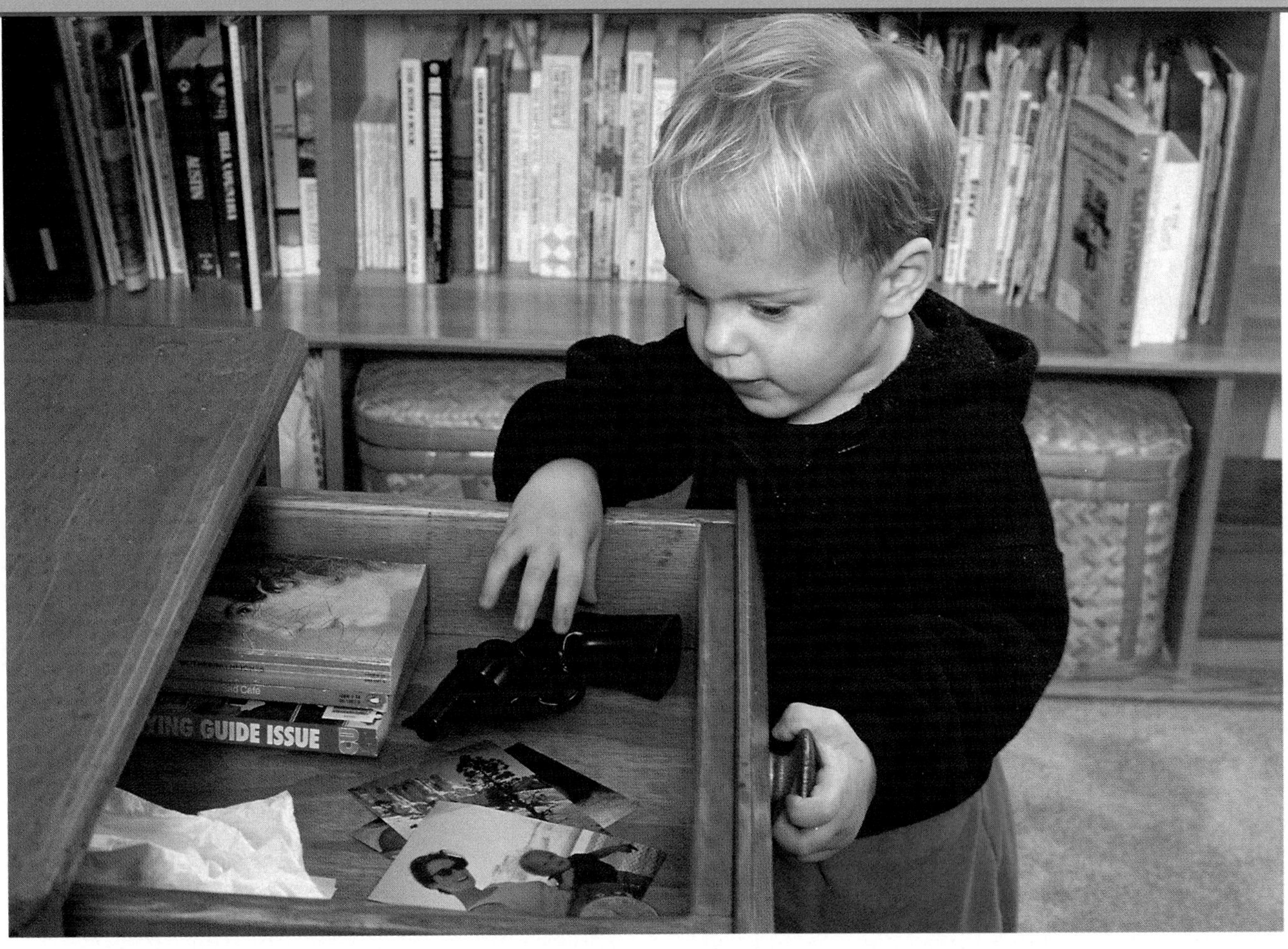

Content Background
Gun Safety

American children are accidentally killed with handguns at the rate of one every day—mostly by themselves or by other children. Ten times as many are injured. Sometimes these accidents occur in school, sometimes at home, sometimes at the homes of relatives or friends. One youngster in a highchair picked up a pistol from the counter top in his grandmother's kitchen and fatally shot himself; a 10-year-old boy fatally shot his friend while playing with a shotgun they found in a closet; a two-year-old dropped or fired a handgun found on a closet shelf, seriously injuring his four-year-old sister. In all these cases, guns were stored irresponsibly, and those children who were old enough to learn about gun safety had not been taught.

A major study by the Center to Prevent Handgun Violence, in Washington, D.C., analyzed 266 accidental shootings of children—140 of which ended in death, 126 in injury. They found that 50 percent took place in the victim's home, 30 percent occurred in a friend's home, 17 percent happened outdoors, and 14 percent occurred in a car. Accidents at home tended to be self-inflicted (42 percent) or committed by a sibling (42 percent), while those at a friend's house were more often committed by the friend (61 percent).

Typically, the handguns were found by the children where the shootings took place; they did not carry them far. The guns were kept in easily accessible places where children play. Forty-five percent were found in bedrooms—in dressers, closets, and night stands; between mattresses; or under pillows and beds. The next largest number were found in living rooms—on coffee tables, between couch cushions, or in end tables. Handguns in cars were found under the seats, on the seats, or in the glove compartments.

The owners of these guns were not practicing even elementary gun safety. Guns should never be put away loaded. They should be kept in locked containers or secured with trigger guards. Children should not be left alone where guns are stored. But even if parents practice gun safety at home and do their best to ensure that friends and relatives do the same, children may still encounter guns. For this reason, the other half of gun safety for children is education.

Education programs must reach boys especially, must cover unintentional encounters with guns when adults are not present, and must begin early. Eighty percent of the victims of accidental shootings are boys, and 60 percent are older children (9 to 16), according to the Center to Prevent Handgun Violence study. Those who fire the guns are even more likely to be male (92 percent) and older children (67 percent). The youngest victims in the study, ages 0 to 4 years, were most often involved in self-inflicted shootings; those 5 to 8 were most often shot by siblings; and those 13 to 16 by friends. About 60 percent of the time, no adults were at home when shootings took place; about 40 percent of the shootings took place while adults were home but not supervising the children.

One place children may encounter guns unexpectedly is in school. Despite metal detectors and security guards at some schools, weapons still get in. According to one high school student, weapons are brought to school for protection, for revenge, to show off, or to have available in case a fight begins. Guns are commonly brought to school by students who deal in drugs, even if they are not dealing in school.

One approach to education about guns, taken by the Gun Safety Institute in Cleveland, Ohio, is to challenge assumptions about firearms and their purposes. Children learn that possessing a handgun can be more dangerous for the owner than for potential intruders. Another education program, developed by the Youth Crime Watch of Dade County, Inc. and the Center to Prevent Handgun Violence, was introduced in the Dade County, Florida, schools. It is called KIDS + GUNS: A Deadly Equation. Children are taught through a multi-activity approach, and asked to sign a pledge that expresses their knowledgeable respect for guns: "If I ever see a gun or anything that looks like a gun or a part of a gun, I won't touch it. I'll go and tell an adult because guns can hurt me." For older children, emphasis is placed on resolving conflicts without violence, understanding and handling anger, and countering peer pressure.

Guns must be kept away from children and adolescents, as far as that is possible, through good gun safety measures. No child should encounter a gun accidentally in a home, and no gun a child might find should be loaded. But children need to know how to handle themselves if they do encounter guns, because the possibility is too real and too dangerous to dismiss.

PLANNING FOR INSTRUCTION

KEY FACTS

- **Accidents are the leading cause of death for those between the ages of 15 and 24.**
- **Risky behavior and carelessness are factors in most accidents. Accidents can be reduced by changing behavior.**
- **The highest number of motor vehicle fatalities occur in the 15 to 24 age group.**
- **Drugs and alcohol, speeding, and reckless driving are responsible for most car accidents.**
- **The risk of being injured in a motor vehicle accident can be reduced by not using drugs or alcohol, by driving within the speed limit, and by avoiding reckless driving.**
- **Bicycle accidents can be avoided by not engaging in risky behavior and carelessness.**
- **Careless behavior is strongly related to accidents that frequently occur in the home.**
- **Plans should be drawn up beforehand to determine what to do during a disaster.**

- **Accidents in the workplace are due to carelessness and a disregard for safety requirements.**
- **Recreational activities have potential hazards. The activity that results in the greatest number of accidental deaths is swimming.**

MYTHS AND MISCONCEPTIONS

MYTH: Most people aren't responsible for accidents that happen to them.

In many cases—because they allow themselves to be distracted or they take risks—people are at least partly responsible for the accidents that happen to them.

MYTH: Defensive driving means demanding that others respect your rights when you are driving.

Defensive driving involves expecting other drivers to do the unexpected—like change lanes suddenly—and being able to deal with what happens quickly and safely.

MYTH: Home is where you are safe from accidents.

Most falls occur in the home or just outside the home; fires and poisonings are most likely to occur at home.

VOCABULARY

Essential: The following vocabulary terms appear in boldface type:

accident	**drown proofing**
assault	**electrocution**
defensive driving	**risk**
disaster	**safety awareness**

Secondary: Be aware that the following terms may come up during class discussion:

fatalities	amperage	circuit breakers	tornado
hazards	smoke detector	fuses	hurricane
		fire extinguisher	earthquake
		appliances	asbestos
		pesticides	firearms

FOR STUDENTS WITH SPECIAL NEEDS

Visual Learners: Have students draw, sketch, paint, or use other means to illustrate a scene in which an accident is bound to happen. Ask them to imagine dangerous circumstances around the home, at school, or in another familiar place. Display their pictures in the classroom.

At-Risk Students: Have students interview family members, neighbors, or fellow students to compile statistics on one category of accident each. They could choose recreational, home repair, automobile, and so on. They should ask for information about the victim, time of day, state of health, and so on. Then have them get together to make a complete set of statistics. What seem to be the most common causes among the accidents they covered? Are some people more accident-prone than others? Have them present their statistical conclusions to the class.

ENRICHMENT

- Invite a paramedic or police officer to speak to the class about his or her experiences with accident injuries and fatalities. Ask the speaker to tell stories, particularly of teens who are injured in motor vehicle or bicycle accidents. Have students prepare questions to ask the speaker.
- Have students work in groups to prepare a handbook for avoiding accidents. Each group may handle one of the following categories: motor accidents, falls, fires, poisonings, disasters, sports accidents, and other recreation accidents. Each group can prepare a page or two, illustrated if they wish, to provide guidelines to be followed in each situation.

Chapter 27 Chapter Opener

Getting Started

Using the Chapter Photograph

Ask students how the person in the picture could have taken action to foster safety and reduce risks while riding a bicycle. Discuss how using a helmet not only protects a person's life but also helps reduce insurance costs.

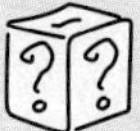

Question Box

Have students anonymously write out any questions they have about safety and risk reduction and put them in the Question Box. To ensure that students with questions are not embarrassed to be seen writing, have those who do not have questions write a fact they already know about safety and risk reduction on the paper instead.

Preview the questions and then answer them at appropriate points in the chapter. You may wish to allow students to write additional questions as they go through the chapter.

Personal Issues *ALERT*

Students who have been injured in an accident or who have a close friend or relative who has been injured may feel self-conscious. They may feel regretful, guilty, or defensive; it may make them unhappy to read that caution might have prevented the accident. Others may be from families who believe their freedom is unfairly limited by state laws requiring helmet or seat belt use. Students should be alerted to the need to be sensitive to other people's feelings.

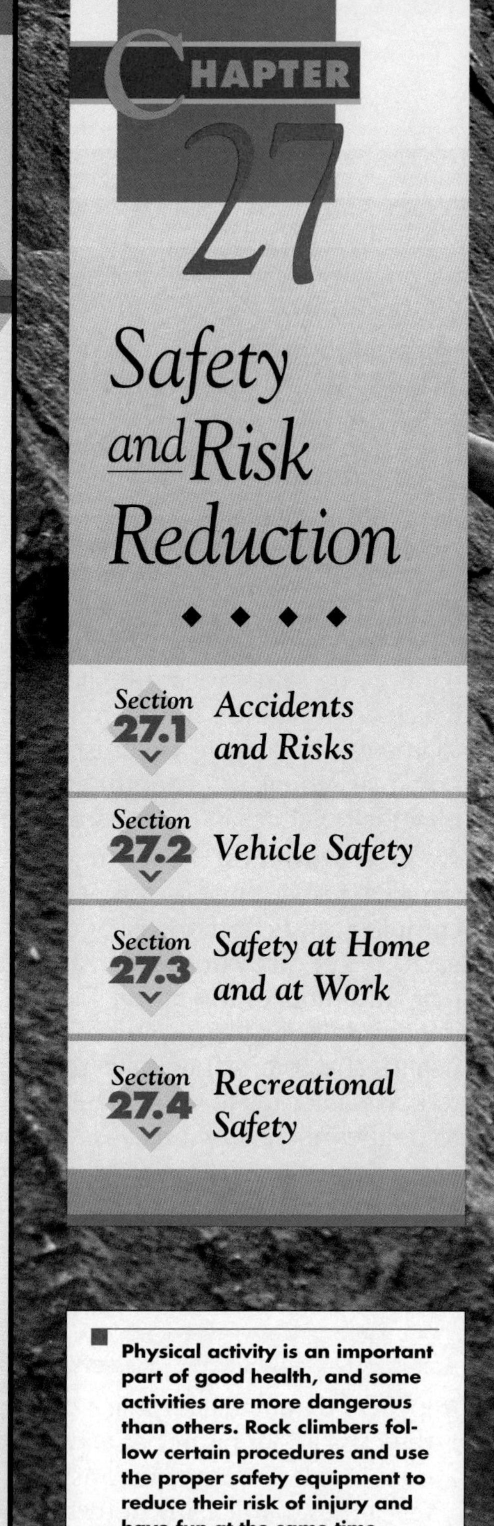

Chapter 27

Safety and Risk Reduction

Physical activity is an important part of good health, and some activities are more dangerous than others. Rock climbers follow certain procedures and use the proper safety equipment to reduce their risk of injury and have fun at the same time.

Sarah hung up the telephone and turned toward her mother. "That was Jan, Mom. Her little brother, Billy, just got back from the emergency room. He flipped off his bike today and broke his wrist. The lace of his sneaker jammed the bike chain and he was thrown over the handlebars."

"Poor Billy, he won't have much of a summer vacation this year," said Sarah's mother.

"It could've been a lot worse," said Sarah. "He hit his head on the curb, but his bicycle helmet cushioned the blow. The doctor told his mother that if he hadn't been wearing a helmet, Billy's injuries would've been more serious."

Sarah thought of her younger sister, Lynette. "Mom, I think it's time we bought a bike helmet for Lynette."

"And what about you, Sarah? Can you be sure that you'll never take a fall from your bike?"

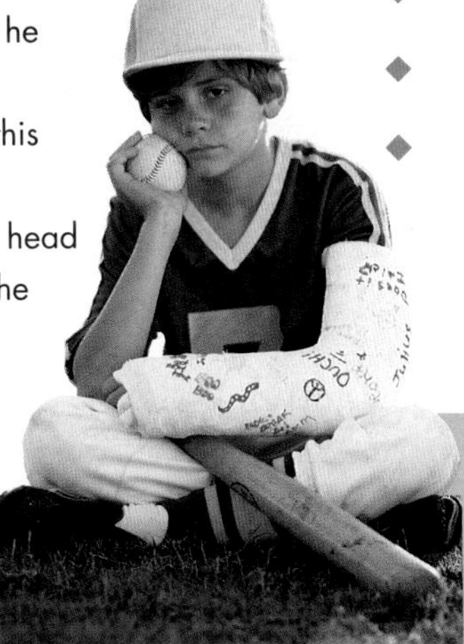

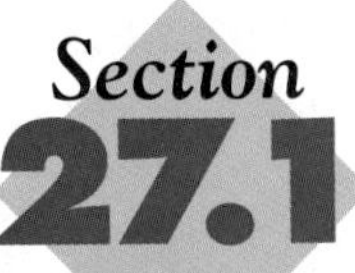

Section 27.1 Accidents and Risks

Objectives

- *Recognize that accidents are the leading cause of death for people between the ages of 15 and 24.*
- *Recognize that risky or careless behaviors are factors in most accidents.*
- *Identify ways in which your personal behavior can be modified to reduce your risk of accidents.*
  LIFE SKILLS: Practicing Self-Care

Billy's broken wrist was the result of an **accident**. In this chapter, you will learn that even though they are unexpected, many accidents can be prevented.

Accidental Deaths

Accidents are the number-one cause of death in the United States among people 15 to 24. Overall, accidents are the fourth leading cause of death. Figure 27-1 on the next page shows the number of deaths that occurred because of some specific types of accidents in the United States in 1990. Notice that motor-vehicle accidents were responsible for the greatest number of accidental deaths—approximately the same number as all other categories combined.

Different age groups tend to have different types of accidents. Among 15- to 24-year-olds, for example, most fatal accidents involve motor vehicles or alcohol, or both. Very young children and elderly people are more likely to be injured or killed in falls. Children under five account for many cases of accidental poisoning.

accident: *any unexpected event that causes damage, injury, or death.*

SECTION 27.1

Background
Lowering Risks

A safe life is not necessarily a dull, inactive one. The dangerous regions of the world—such as deserts, mountains, and the polar regions—have been explored by successful risk takers who knew how to anticipate and prepare for emergencies. Mountain climbers condition themselves slowly to the higher altitudes so as to avoid sickness and disorientation; explorers in the cold regions carefully store food and supplies at intervals along their way to supply their return trip. Anyone planning to engage in a risky activity should first master the related safety rules. It's important to be aware of one's own physical capabilities, reactions, and emotional state before beginning.

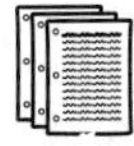

Personal Health Inventory

Have students complete the Personal Health Inventory for this chapter. The inventory helps them assess their own behavior with respect to safety and avoiding assault.

Section 27.1 Lesson Plan

MOTIVATE

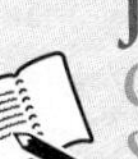

Journal 27A
Critiquing One's Own Safety Awareness

This may be done as a warm-up activity. Encourage students to judge themselves on a scale of one to five as someone who makes an effort to practice safety and avoid risks. Have them record in the Student Journal in the Student Activity Book a critique of their own safety-related behavior.

Cooperative Learning
Accidents as News

Have students form small groups to read newspapers for stories about accidents. Have them draw up a list of the accidents they find. (They might also add to the list accidents that happened to people they know.) Have them note how each of these accidents might have been avoided.

TEACH

Class Discussion
Statistics on Accidental Deaths

Before students look at Figure 27-1, have them write down what they think are the three most frequent causes of accidental death in the United States. Tally their choices on the chalkboard. Have them compare their class list with the table. Ask them why they think motor vehicles cause the most deaths.

SECTION 27.1

Making a Choice 27A

Accident Survey

Assign the Accident Survey card. The card asks students to list accidents in which group members have been involved and discuss possible ways each accident could have been prevented.

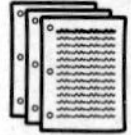

Section Review Worksheet 27.1

Assign Section Review Worksheet 27.1, which requires students to correct false statements about accidents and risks.

Section Quiz 27.1

Have students take Section Quiz 27.1.

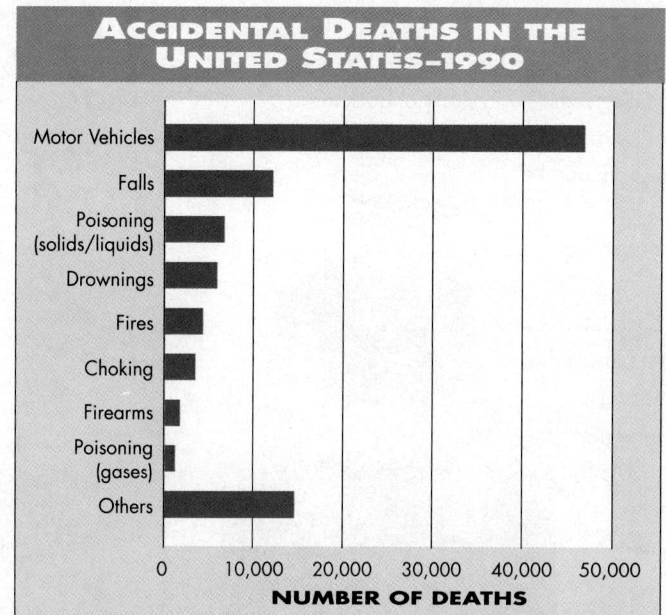

(FIGURE 27-1) **Accidents are currently the fourth leading cause of death in the United States. For young adults 15 to 24, they are the leading cause of death.**

risk: *an action that is potentially dangerous; the chance of injury.*

Risks and Carelessness

Sometimes a person has no control over the things that lead to an accident. For example, when an earthquake causes bricks to fall from a building, someone may be injured. Such events, however, make up a minority of accidents.

Most accidents result from the actions, or inactions, of people. Have you noticed that certain people seem to have more accidents than others? You've probably also heard or used phrases such as "He is an accident waiting to happen" and "She's accident prone" many times. Such phrases suggest that the person may be at least partly responsible for many of the accidents that happen to him or her. A person's behavior may greatly affect his or her chances of being involved in an accident. Understanding why accidents occur can help you avoid most accidents.

safety awareness: *knowledge about risks and how to reduce them.*

Taking Risks One type of behavior that increases the likelihood of having an accident is taking risks. A **risk** is an action that involves danger of some kind. Many everyday activities involve risk. Every time you cross a busy street, for example, you are taking a risk. But your chances of being injured are fairly low if you pay attention and obey traffic signals.

Many people, however, take unnecessary risks. Dodging traffic to cross the street in the middle of the block is far more likely to lead to an accident than crossing at the corner. Drinking alcohol and taking drugs increase the risk of having accidents because these substances impair a person's ability to make good judgments.

The high number of accidents among teenagers is related to the fact that they take more risks than older people. You can minimize risk by making responsible decisions. For example, you can choose to cross a street at the corner or not to use drugs.

Being Careless Putting dishes away, as the boy in Figure 27-2 is doing, is not, by nature, dangerous. But notice that by not paying attention to his task, the boy has managed to push a bowl off the shelf—and possibly onto his head! His behavior is not risky—it is careless. Carelessness is a lack of concern about the possible effects of one's actions, or not paying attention while performing a task. As with taking unnecessary risks, carelessness can lead to accidents that could have been avoided.

Safety and Behavior

Avoiding unnecessary risks and being attentive are important to your safety. **Safety awareness** is knowing about risks and how to reduce them. Assuming that they don't wish to be injured, why do so many people lack safety awareness? There are several answers to this question.

• • • TEACH continued

Discuss why they think the insurance for drivers between the ages of 15 and 24 is so high.

Role-Playing

Who's Responsible?

Have students role-play a situation in which several teens are urging another to do something dangerous. Examples might include climbing a water tower, climbing under a suspension bridge, jumping into a river from a rock, eating food that may be spoiled—anything that involves risk. The lone person should assess the situation and decide whether to resist the pressure or to go along.

Class Discussion

Necessary vs. Unnecessary Risks

Write on the chalkboard the headings: *Necessary Risks* and *Unnecessary Risks.* Have students suggest some necessary risks they take often, such as crossing the street or riding a bike. List these on the chalkboard. Have students discuss whether the risks mentioned are truly necessary or simply a more convenient or easier way of completing a task. Ask students to suggest unnecessary risks that they might be tempted to take, such as crossing the street in the middle of the block or riding a bike without a helmet. List these on the board and have students discuss why these risks should be avoided.

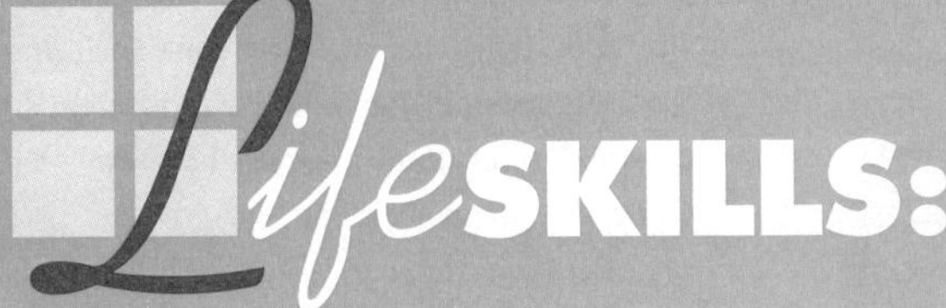

Practicing Self-Care

Analyze Your Safety Awareness

The teens in this photo are demonstrating their safety awareness by buckling their seat belts. You can protect yourself from many accidental injuries by being safety-conscious and practicing behaviors that promote safety as well.

To analyze your safety awareness and behavior, answer the following questions on a separate sheet of paper. Thousands of 10th-graders answered similar questions when they took the *National Adolescent Student Health Survey*, a project developed by health educators and funded by agencies of the U.S. Department of Health and Human Services. Later in this chapter, you will discover how your behavior and safety awareness compares to that of these 10th-graders.

1. How many times in the past month did you ride with a driver who had used alcohol or drugs?
0 times 7–10 times
1–3 times 11–20 times
4–6 times Over 20 times

2. Did you wear a seat belt the last time you rode in an automobile?
Yes No Don't remember

3. How often do you wear a helmet when riding a bicycle?
Never Usually
Rarely Always
Sometimes

4. How often do you warm up before exercising?
Never Usually
Rarely Always
Sometimes

5. How often do you swim alone or in a restricted or unsupervised area?
Never Sometimes

Once you have identified behaviors that place you at risk of being injured in an accident, work on modifying these risky behaviors to protect yourself.

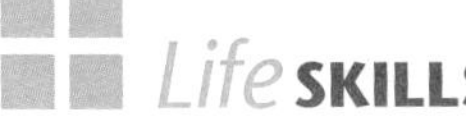

Analyze Your Safety Awareness

Have students review their daily activities and analyze them for risky behavior. Ask them to determine their role in accidents that affect others. Give each student an index card on which to record and retain the results of their review and analysis.

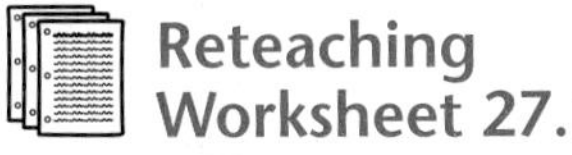

Reteaching Worksheet 27.1

Students who have difficulty with the material may complete Reteach Worksheet 27.1, which requires them to evaluate behaviors and to identify risk taking, carelessness, and safety awareness.

Extension

Interviews on Risk Taking and Accidents

Encourage students to interview family members, neighbors, or adult friends about risks they took as teens or young adults. Do the adults now regret the risks they took? Have students share their findings.

Review Answers

1. Accidents
2. Risks and carelessness. A risk is an action that involves danger of some kind. Carelessness is inattentive behavior while one is performing a task.
3. Answers will vary based on students' behaviors.
4. Yes. Infants and toddlers can put small objects into their mouths and choke. They can chew on electrical cords and reach for hot items on a stove. They can also easily fall from high objects such as a chair, bed, or the top of the stairs. Since infants and toddlers do not yet understand risk behavior, they need constant adult supervision in order to minimize risks.

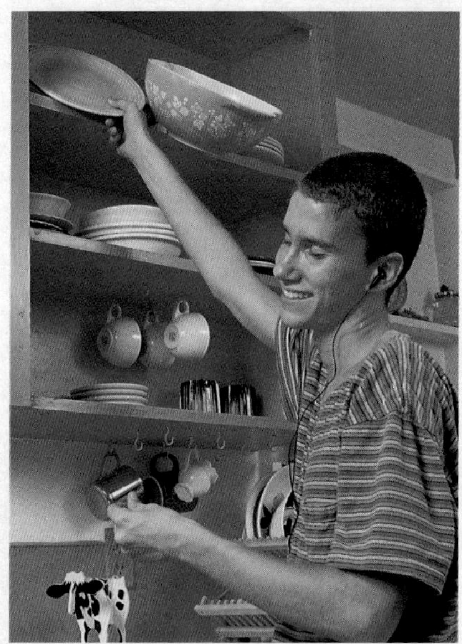

(FIGURE 27-2) **Not paying attention to what you are doing is a factor in many accidents.**

Ignorance and lack of caution can lead to dangerous situations. For example, Rob is on the school swimming team. While out with friends, he decided to swim across a small river to show his ability. Rob assumed the current was not very strong. However, he was swept downstream and had to be rescued by people fishing from a small boat. Rob did not know the strength of the current. He exercised poor judgment and was not cautious. Among young people, such lack of caution can stem from the feeling that "it can't happen to me."

The use of drugs and alcohol increases risky behavior and carelessness as well. A person is far more likely to attempt a foolish—even dangerous—act if he or she is under the influence of drugs or alcohol.

A person's emotional state can also contribute to risky behavior. For example, someone who is angry is likely to act on impulse and with little or no regard for what might happen. Such a person may drive over the speed limit, putting himself or herself and others at risk. Someone suffering from depression may also be indifferent to personal safety and may act in a way that could lead to an accident.

Peer pressure can influence individuals to take unnecessary risks. For example, Meda was with a group of friends when they found a fallen tree that made a bridge over a deep gorge. Her friends took turns walking on the tree to cross the gorge. Meda could see the tree wasn't steady, but her friends dared her to cross and she did. Everyone, at some point, has been dared to do something dangerous. Taking a dare, even though the results could be fatal, becomes a test of one's courage, but it is neither mature nor responsible behavior.

Personal responsibility is the key to avoiding accidents. To discover whether your behavior demonstrates safety awareness, complete the Life Skills activity on page 591.

Review

1. *What is the leading cause of death among young people 15 to 24?*
2. *Name and describe the two factors that contribute to avoidable accidents.*
3. ***LIFE SKILLS: Practicing Self-Care*** *This week, eliminate or modify at least one behavior that contributes to your likelihood of having an accident.*
4. ***Critical Thinking*** *Can infants and toddlers engage in risky behaviors that lead to accidents? Support your answer with examples.*

ASSESS

Section Review

Have students answer the Section Review questions.

Alternative Assessment

Learning to Be Cautious

Have students write a fable about a foolish person who ignores prudent advice and takes an unnecessary risk. The story should include a moral.

Closure

Proper Procedures When in a Motor Vehicle

Have students suggest factors that contribute to motor vehicle accidents (emotions, inexperience, inattention, showing off). List them on the chalkboard. For each one, have another student suggest an accident it could cause. What are ways of handling these factors so that they do not cause an accident?

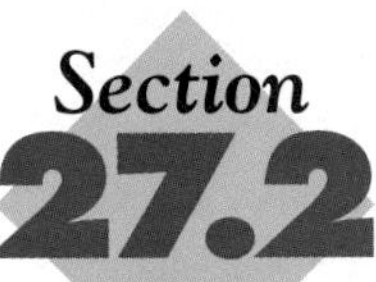

Section 27.2 Vehicle Safety

Objectives

- *Recognize factors that contribute to motor-vehicle accidents.*
- *Identify behaviors that reduce the risk of being injured in a motor-vehicle accident.*
- *List some ways to maintain a bicycle for safety.*
- *Identify behaviors that reduce the risk of being injured in a bicycle accident.*

Riding in or on any vehicle involves risk. And because of their size, weight, and the speed at which they travel, motor vehicles have great potential for doing damage. Now look again at Figure 27-1 and recall that motor-vehicle accidents account for more deaths than any other kind of accident. For these reasons alone, vehicle safety should be a priority for you.

As a teenager, you may already have a license and be driving. You probably also ride with friends. Unfortunately, drivers under the age of 24 have more accidents than drivers in other age groups. There are also more deaths from motor-vehicle accidents among 15- to 24-year-olds than in any other age group. In fact, three-fourths of all accidental deaths in this age group are related to motor vehicles. Half of these deaths also involve alcohol. By learning to avoid certain risky behaviors, you could avoid having an accident that could result in injury or death.

Behavior and Auto Accidents

As with accidents in general, motor-vehicle accidents are usually linked to human behavior. The automobile in Figure 27-3 was demolished in an accident, and the driver and passengers were injured. Quite possibly, the driver's behavior was at fault.

Using alcohol or drugs is a behavior that is a factor in most motor-vehicle accidents. In Chapters 13 and 15, you studied some of the effects of these substances: reaction time is slowed, judgment is impaired, and general awareness is lowered. Thus, a person driving under the influence of drugs or alcohol is not in full control of a vehicle that can be a deadly weapon.

The effects of alcohol and drugs on the body are discussed in Chapters 13 and 15.

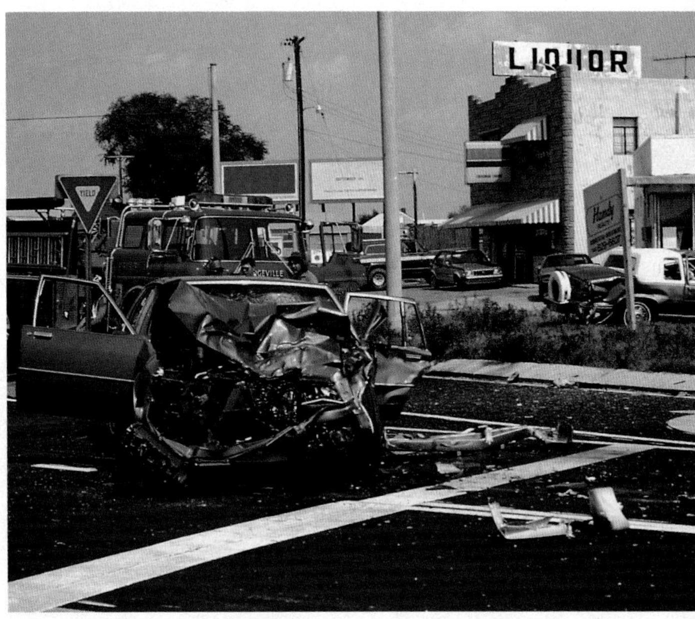

(FIGURE 27-3) **Alcohol is a factor in at least half of all automobile accidents.**

Background

Effect of Drugs and Alcohol on Driving

Fifty percent of traffic fatalities occur when the driver is on drugs or alcohol. When a person drinks alcohol faster than it can be oxidized by the liver, the blood alcohol level (BAL) rises, and judgment and critical thinking are somewhat impaired. When the BAL reaches 0.10 percent (one part alcohol to 1,000 parts blood), every state considers a drinker legally intoxicated and incapable of operating a vehicle safely. Maine, Oregon, Utah, and California have established a lower limit —0.08 percent—for the BAL. Since mandatory drug testing of transportation workers began in the 1980s, personal injuries on railroads have fallen dramatically.

Section 27.2 Lesson Plan

MOTIVATE

Journal 27B

Reducing Risks in Motor Vehicles

This may be done as a warm-up activity. Encourage students to record in the Student Journal in the Student Activity book any risky behavior they engage in when in a motor vehicle, such as clowning around, racing other cars, or making threatening signals at the driver of another car. Have them mention the possible outcome of any of these behaviors.

TEACH

Reinforcement

Behavior and Auto Accidents

Ask students why they think teens are more prone to motor vehicle accidents than any other group. Have them suggest unnecessary risks that teens may take when driving a motor vehicle. Ask them to suggest ways to avoid accidents in motor vehicles. If they do not mention being careful and paying attention to what they are doing, bring this up for discussion. Lead students to the conclusion that thinking about what might result from their actions is good common sense.

Background
Rescuing Accident Victims
Technology has helped in rescuing accident victims trapped inside a car or pinned underneath wreckage. Air bags have been developed that are less than 2.5 cm wide, making it possible to insert them into tight places where a person is trapped. Air is then pumped into the bag, forcing apart whatever is trapping the victim. Air bags have the power to move objects weighing over 50,000 kg.

Other behaviors that increase the risk of having an accident are speeding and reckless driving. Mark is a high school senior who enjoys driving his own car. But in three months he has received three speeding tickets. His response is, ''What's the big deal? I like to drive fast.'' This attitude is dangerous to Mark and to others.

For several reasons, speeding increases the risk of accidents and injuries. One reason is a driver's reaction time (the time between deciding to apply the brakes and applying them). Although reaction time is usually less than one second, a car moves some distance in that second. And a car traveling at 45 mph goes much farther in that time than a car traveling at 25 mph. Furthermore, a car traveling at a faster speed has a longer braking distance and takes more time to stop. Finally, the faster a car is traveling upon impact, the more likely it is that people will be seriously injured. So speeding increases both the likelihood that an accident will occur and the risk of serious injury or death.

Reckless driving is careless behavior. Being distracted from driving for just a moment—tuning the radio, talking to a passenger, reading signs or a road map, or trying to get a wasp out the window—can get you into trouble. Even more serious are deliberate actions, such as not obeying traffic rules and signs, trying to turn or pass with too little time, or running a light.

Reducing Auto Injuries

Avoiding automobile accidents is the best way to reduce your risk of injury. The first step is never drink and drive or ride in a car with a driver who is under the influence of alcohol or drugs. If you know someone is under such influence, try to keep him or her from driving.

Obeying traffic laws, including posted speed limits, will also reduce your risk of being involved in an auto accident. If you know someone who disregards safe driving practices, is careless, or takes chances behind the wheel, don't ride with that person.

10th Graders Who Rode With Drivers Who Had Used Alcohol or Drugs

Number of Times	Male	Female	Total
0 times	57.0%	54.0%	55.6%
1—3 times	23.4%	30.8%	27.0%
4—6 times	7.6%	7.1%	7.4%
7—10 times	4.5%	4.5%	4.5%
11—20 times	3.1%	1.8%	2.5%
over 20 times	4.4%	1.8%	3.2%

(FIGURE 27-4) **This is how the 10th-graders who participated in the *National Adolescent Student Health Survey* responded to the question: "How many times in the past month did you ride with a driver who had used alcohol or drugs?"**

• • • TEACH continued

Class Discussion
Braking Time

How does the speed at which you are driving affect your braking time? *[The faster you are going, the longer it takes to stop.]* **What other factor might affect your braking time?** *[The condition of the road—whether it is wet, icy, or dry; and the condition of the brakes—good, fair, or poor.]* **How should these conditions affect your driving?** *[Under unfavorable conditions, you should always drive more slowly and more cautiously.]*

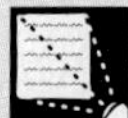

Teaching Transparency 27A
Crash Speeds

Use this transparency to discuss how speed influences motor vehicle accidents. It shows a comparison of crash speeds to a car being dropped from different heights.

Role-Playing
Responsible Driving

Have students role-play situations in which someone who has been drinking or using drugs wants to drive a car. The others should provide alternatives, such as offering to drive the car.

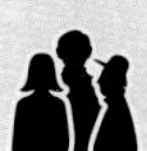

Cooperative Learning
Reducing Injuries From Motor Vehicle Accidents

Have students work in groups to produce a bulletin board to convince

Seatbelt Use Among 10th Graders

Wore Seat Belts	Female	Male	Total
Yes	39.9%	40.3%	40.1%
No	58.3%	57.6%	57.9%
Don't Remember	1.8%	2.1%	1.9%

(FIGURE 27-5) **This is how the 10th-graders who participated in the *National Adolescent Student Health Survey* responded to the question: "Did you use a seat belt the last time you rode in a vehicle?"**

When you drive, practice **defensive driving** to avoid accidents. Defensive driving involves expecting other drivers to drive recklessly, like changing lanes suddenly or turning from the wrong lane. You will be better able to handle such situations if you assume they might happen.

Wearing a seat belt is a way to reduce your risk of injury if you should be involved in an auto accident. But as Figure 27-5 indicates, most 10th-graders do not wear a seat belt. This is a risky behavior.

defensive driving:

driving as though you expect other drivers to drive recklessly.

Safety and Other Motor Vehicles

Motorcycles, minibikes, snowmobiles, and all-terrain vehicles (ATVs) are other types of motor vehicles. They are fun to ride, but they can also be dangerous. In accidents involving these vehicles, the risk of serious head injury is very high. Approximately 60 percent of 10th-graders surveyed recently reported having ridden on a motorcycle or minibike, but less than 30 percent reported that they always wore a helmet.

To protect yourself from injury, take the following safety measures when riding on one of these vehicles. Always wear a helmet to reduce your risk of suffering a serious head injury. Wear goggles to protect your eyes, especially if the vehicle has no windshield. Sturdy clothing can also help prevent an injury in the event of an accident. Obey all traffic laws as you would when driving a car. Don't use alcohol or drugs or ride with someone who does.

Bicycle Safety

As with any vehicle, there are hazards involved in bicycle riding. And once again, risky behavior and carelessness—the human factors—contribute to many bicycle accidents.

When Billy's shoelace got caught in his bicycle chain, it resulted in an accident. Clothing catching in the chain or wheels is a leading cause of bicycle accidents. The sudden jamming of the chain or wheel can cause the rider to be thrown from the bike. When riding a bicycle, make sure your laces are tucked into your shoes or tied so that they hang toward the outer side of your shoes. It is also best to wear clothing that is closefitting.

Losing control of a bicycle can also result in an accident. Hitting a hole or turning suddenly to avoid a person walking can cause a rider to lose control. As with motor

teens to drive carefully and avoid unnecessary risks. They should include messages about not speeding, avoiding drugs and alcohol, driving defensively, obeying all traffic laws, using seat belts, and wearing helmets and goggles when on motorcycles.

Class Discussion

Causes of Bicycle Accidents

Discuss with students the causes of bicycle accidents. List the causes on the chalkboard as they mention them. Have them state a way to avoid accidents from each cause.

Role-Playing

Good Advice

Have students role-play a parent and adolescent in conflict over the use of a bicycle helmet. One student should play a young person who is reluctant to wear the helmet and gives his or her reasons; another student should play the parent or guardian who explains why the helmet is important. In a variation, the young person could be insisting on getting a helmet and the parent is reluctant to go along.

Extension

Safety in the Community

Have students visit a bicycle shop to inquire about safety devices on bicycles. Encourage them to contact a cycling club to find out how safety rules are promoted by the club.

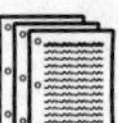

Section Review Worksheet 27.2

Assign Section Review Worksheet 27.2, which requires students to complete statements related to vehicle safety.

Section Quiz 27.2

Have students take Section Quiz 27.2.

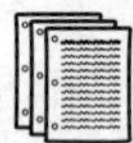

Reteaching Worksheet 27.2

Students who have difficulty with the material may complete Reteaching Worksheet 27.2, which requires them to identify which safety statements apply to different vehicles and pedestrians.

Review Answers

1. Answers may include driving under the influence of drugs or alcohol, speeding, and reckless driving.

2. Answers may include do not speed, do not drive recklessly, do not drive while under the influence of drugs or alcohol, do not ride with a driver who is under the influence of drugs or alcohol or who drives recklessly, obey traffic laws, drive defensively, and always wear a seat belt.

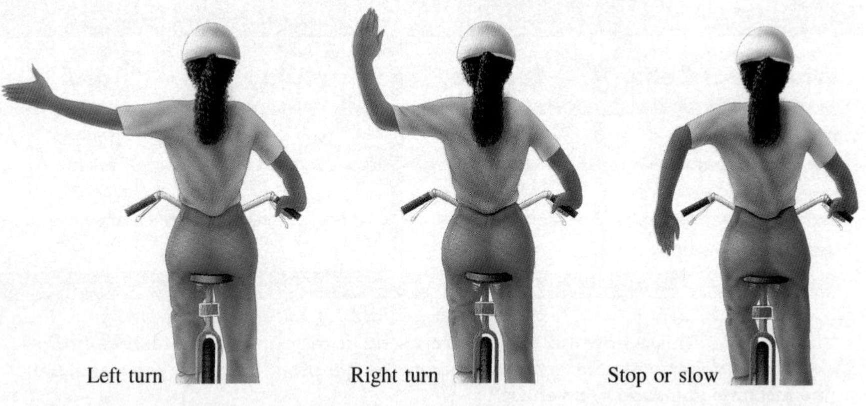

(FIGURE 27-6) **By warning the traffic behind you that you intend to change direction or speed, you can help to protect yourself from being injured in an accident while riding a bicycle.**

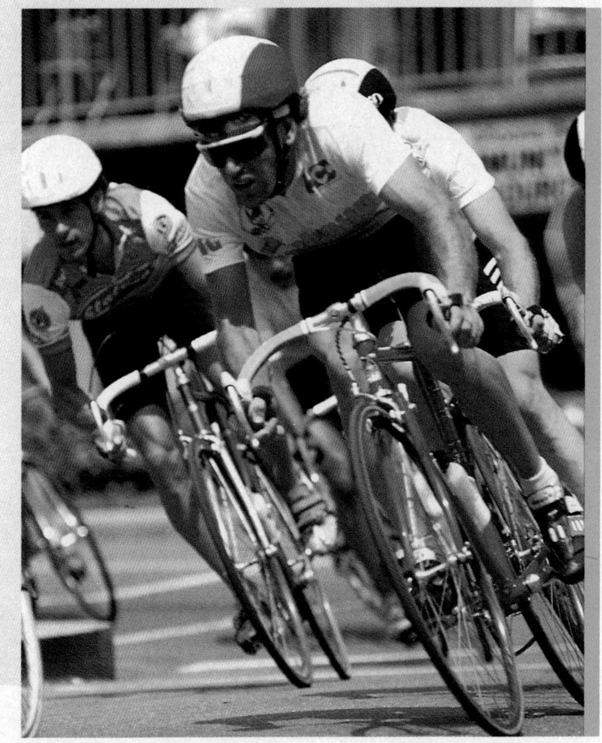

(FIGURE 27-7) **Serious cyclists wear specialized equipment to reduce their risk of having an accident or being seriously injured in an accident.**

vehicles, maintain control by not speeding and ride defensively.

Bicyclists must generally obey the same traffic laws as other vehicles. A bicycle, for example, should be ridden in the direction that traffic flows. Hand signals, as shown in Figure 27-6, should be used to signal a change in direction or speed. If you ride at night, your bicycle should be equipped with lights and reflectors.

Sometimes bicycle accidents are caused by mechanical problems with the bicycle. Maintaining the bicycle in a safe condition is important. Keep the fenders, spokes, pedals, and handlebars undamaged and tightly attached. Adjust the saddle height and handlebars for comfortable fit. Keep the chain lubricated, and be sure it is in good condition. The bell or horn, lights, and reflectors should be working perfectly. Keep the tires filled with air, and check them for wear, leaks, or embedded pebbles and nails.

The cyclists in Figure 27-7 are skilled riders—they race bicycles. Notice that they are wearing helmets. But as Figure 27-8 indicates, 10th-grade bicycle riders

Bicycle Helmet Use Among 10th Graders

Helmet Is Used	Female	Male	Total
Never	94.3%	89.2%	91.6%
Rarely	2.9%	5.2%	4.1%
Sometimes	1.4%	3.4%	2.5%
Usually	0.7%	1.7%	1.3%
Always	0.7%	0.4%	0.6%

(FIGURE 27-8) **This is how the 10th-graders who participated in the *National Adolescent Student Health Survey* answered the question: "How often do you wear a bicycle helmet when riding a bicycle?"**

almost never wear helmets. Head injuries account for the majority of fatal injuries in bicycle accidents. Deciding to wear a helmet will reduce your risk of being seriously injured or killed in a bicycle accident.

Pedestrian Safety

People riding in motor vehicles are not the only victims of motor-vehicle accidents. Pedestrians are often struck and killed by motor vehicles, in many cases, while crossing streets. Some accidents involve young children running into streets from between parked cars. In other cases, improperly crossing a busy street leads to an accident. In New York City, five times as many people are struck and killed by moving vehicles as die in fires!

Only about one-third of 10th-graders questioned said that they always or usually cross busy streets at the corner. At busy intersections, pedestrian walk signs may be provided, and there is usually at least a painted crosswalk. Once again, the behavior you choose affects the probability that you will be involved in an accident.

Review

1. *Describe two factors that contribute to motor-vehicle accidents.*
2. *What are some ways that a person can reduce his or her chances of being injured in a motor-vehicle accident?*
3. *List some ways to maintain a bicycle for safety.*
4. *What are some ways that a person can reduce his or her chances of being injured in an accident while riding a bicycle?*
5. ***Critical Thinking*** *Some drugs, such as stimulants, increase awareness and may cause a person to react more quickly. Why, then, would a person who is under the influence of such a drug still be a hazard when driving a motor vehicle?*

SECTION 27.2

Answers to Questions 1 and 2 are on p. 596.

3. Keep the fenders, spokes, pedals, and handlebars undamaged and tightly attached. Adjust the saddle height and handlebars for comfortable fit. Keep the chain lubricated and in good condition. The bell or horn, lights, and reflectors should be working well. Keep the tires filled with air and check them for defects.

4. Answers may include wear close-fitting pants; do not wear scarves, long coats, or other items that can get caught in the spokes or chain; don't ride over objects or holes; don't speed; ride defensively; ride with traffic; use hand signals; ride with lights and reflectors at night; keep the bicycle in a safe condition; and always wear a helmet.

5. That person may respond too quickly or too much. An overreaction can be as dangerous as a sluggish response in driving.

ASSESS

Section Review

Have students answer the Section Review questions.

Alternative Assessment

Appeal for Safer Roads

Ask students to write an article for the school newspaper on vehicle safety, especially as it relates to teens.

Closure

Personal Vehicle Safety

Have students write a brief paragraph in which they evaluate their own compliance with the rules of safety when driving or riding in vehicles.

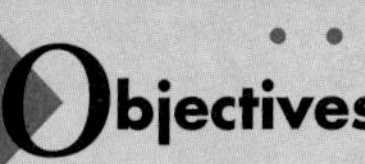

Section 27.3 Safety at Home and at Work

Objectives

- *Recognize the relationship between accidents that frequently occur in the home and personal behavior.*
- *Identify potential accident hazards in the home and in the community.*
- *Recommend steps to reduce the potential for accidents in the home and in the community.*
  LIFE SKILLS: Problem Solving
- *Identify ways to maintain safety in the workplace.*

People spend much of their time at home. Most adults and some teenagers also spend part of their day at the place where they work. Unfortunately, accidents are common in both places. This section contains tips that will help you reduce your risk of accidental injury at home and at work.

Safety Around the Home

Look again at Figure 27-1. Many of the types of accidents listed are likely to occur at home. Most falls, which are the cause of the second greatest number of accidental deaths, do not occur outdoors while hiking or climbing but in the home. Accidents involving fires and poisons are also most likely to occur at home. So making sure that your home is a safe place to be is extremely important.

Falls About 50 percent of fatal accidents that occur in the home are due to falls. The chances of dying in a fall increase with age. In fact, for people over 65, falls make up from one-third to one-half of all accidental deaths! Young children are also more likely to be injured or killed in falls, often as a result of climbing onto or off of furniture and other items.

Many falls occur on staircases. Surprisingly, however, falls on level surfaces are more numerous and cause more fatalities. Examine the photos in Figure 27-9 for hazards that could lead to falls. Notice the objects on the floor at the top of the staircase. Anyone could stumble over one of these objects and fall down the stairs. The curled rug is another hazard that could lead to a fall. Finally, that highly polished floor may look very nice, but it could easily cause someone to slip and fall. Check your home for such hazards when you go home today.

The following are some measures that can be taken to help reduce the risk of falls:

- If you have staircases, the handrails should be sturdy and the steps should have nonslip treads or flat carpeting.
- Floors should be kept free of clutter—toys, electrical cords, or books—that could cause someone to trip.
- Frayed rugs and broken floor tiles should be repaired.
- The bottom of the bathtub should have a nonskid texture. If elderly people live in the house, there should be handrails on the walls beside the bathtub as well.
- Floor mats in the bathroom should also be nonskid to prevent slipping when stepping into and out of the tub or shower.

Section 27.3 Lesson Plan

MOTIVATE

Journal 27C
Accidents at Home

This may be done as a warm-up activity. Encourage students to record in the Student Journal in the Student Activity Book the more serious accidents that occurred at home as they were growing up — fractures of limbs, cuts, falls, or other injuries.

TEACH

Class Discussion
Danger of Falling

Have students discuss the photographs on page 599. **How could each of these potential dangers be avoided?** *[The toys should be stored in a safe place when not in use; the carpet should be held down by a metal strip that is tacked down; the floor might receive other care, such as a vinegar rinse that maintains the shine without slippery waxes.]* **How should the danger from a slippery sidewalk be lessened?** *[By covering it with salt, sand, or other material that will cause friction]*

Class Discussion
Fire Hazards

Call attention to the photograph of the smoker dozing in a chair. **What is likely to happen to the cigarette?** *[It will fall and could start a fire.]* **Why do many fires start in the kitchen?** *[The*

(FIGURE 27-9) **Any of these situations could cause someone to fall and be injured.**

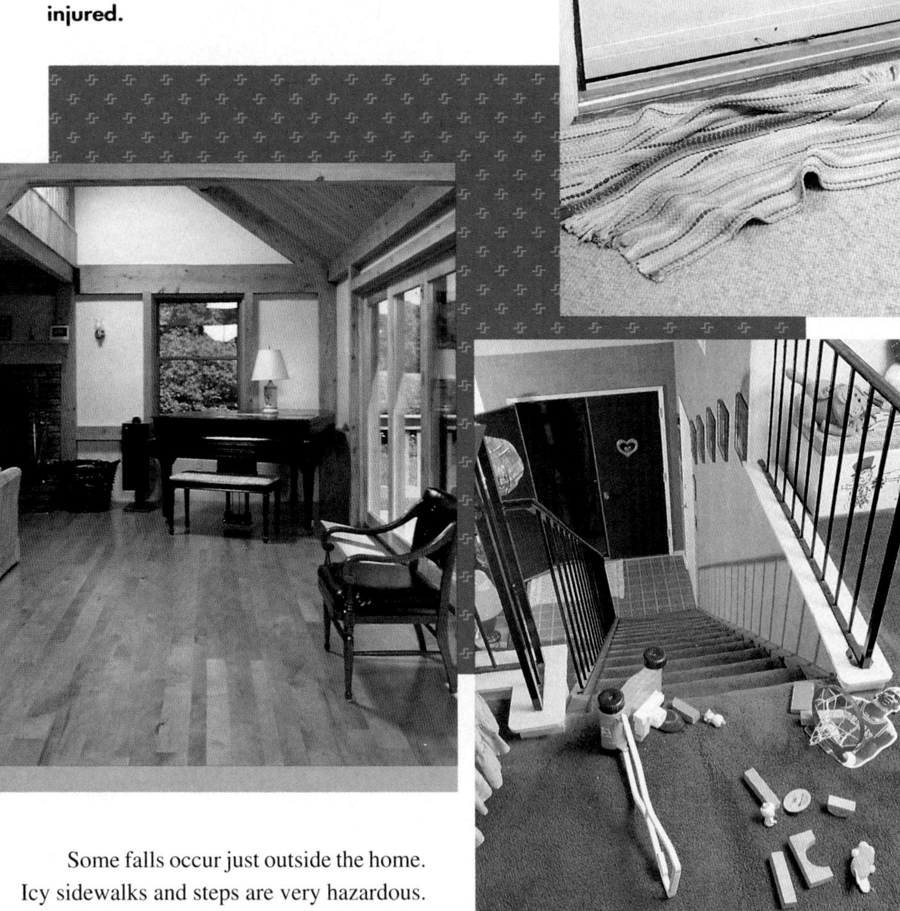

Some falls occur just outside the home. Icy sidewalks and steps are very hazardous. Broken sections of pavement, exposed tree roots, and objects left on the ground should be fixed, covered, or cleared away.

Fires Fires are the third most common cause of accidental death in the home. Careless smoking is a leading cause of home fires. Other causes include faulty electrical wiring and faulty heating units, cooking accidents, children playing with matches, and improper use of fireplaces.

Carelessness, whether while cooking, smoking, or using electricity, contributes to many household fires. The following list can be used to check your home for potential fire hazards:

- Do not overload electrical outlets.
- If you have fuses, use only fuses of the specified amperage. If you have circuit breakers, keep them in good working order.
- Have the heating system inspected regularly by a professional.
- If you have a fireplace, use a protective metal screen and have the chimney cleaned regularly.
- Keep the kitchen stove free of grease.

SECTION 27.3

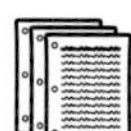

Life Skills Worksheet 27A

Looking at Fire Extinguishers

Assign the Looking at Fire Extinguishers Life Skills Worksheet, which requires students to evaluate different brands and types of extinguishers.

burners get too hot and the food or cooking oil catches fire.] **How would a smoke detector and a fire extinguisher help in both these cases?** *[The person who started the fire would be alerted to the fire by the smoke detector and so would others in the home. The fire extinguisher would put out the fire before it spread.]*

Role-Playing

Rules to Be Observed During a Fire

Have students role-play a situation in which a family discovers that a fire has broken out in the house. They should illustrate the appropriate behaviors outlined in the text. Ask students to evaluate the behaviors demonstrated in the skits and point out any adjustments that should be made.

Cooperative Learning

Preventing Fires at Home

Have students write a one-paragraph summary of information they would convey to a youngster about fire prevention in the home. *(The summaries should be clear and complete, and they should include signs of danger that a younger child could perceive.)*

Background
Electrical Accidents

If a person comes into contact with a "hot" wire, the current can flow through parts of the body. If the circuit is completed through the hand, a shock or a burn would result. But if the circuit is completed through the body from one hand to the other or from hand to foot, the person may lose muscle control and not be able to let go. Large amounts of current can cause breathing difficulties and uncontrolled contractions of the heart.

To rescue a person who has had an electrical accident, the rescuer should first disconnect the equipment, touching only the plug. Then the rescuer should pull the victim away from the contact with a long, dry pole, a rope, or cloth. The rescuer must have dry hands and be standing on a dry surface.

(FIGURE 27-10) **Smoke detectors should be checked at regular intervals to be sure they are working properly. Place fire extinguishers where they will be visible and easily accessible in case of an emergency.**

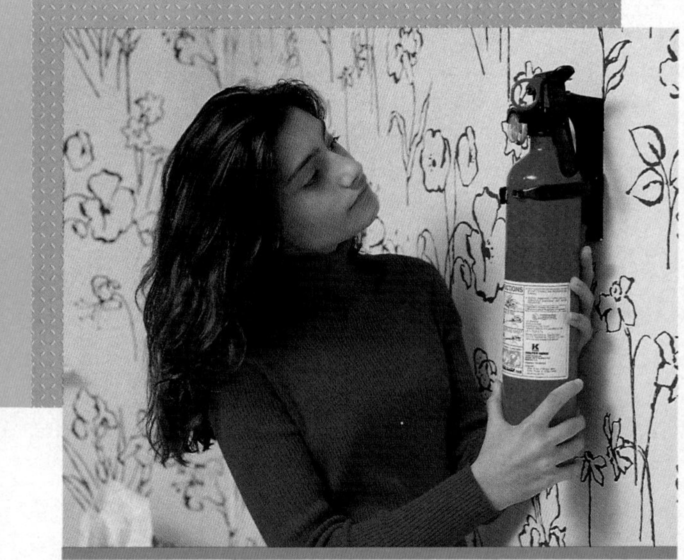

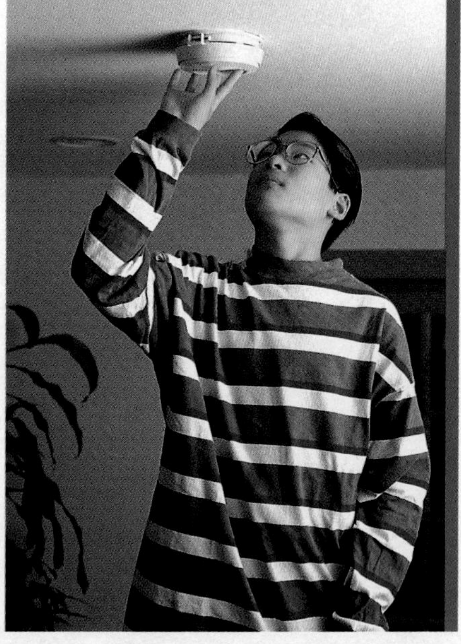

All homes should have smoke detectors and fire extinguishers. But in a recent study, about 20 percent of students questioned reported not having smoke detectors in their homes. Smoke detectors should be located on every floor and should be tested regularly to make sure they are working. It's a good idea to make a chart showing the dates smoke detectors have been checked. Fire extinguishers should be placed in kitchens, basements, and storage areas to deal with small fires.

electrocution: *death resulting from the flow of electrical current through the body.*

Finally, you should have a plan for escape in case of fire. The plan should be practiced, and all family members should take part in fire drills. If a fire does break out in your home, observe the following safety precautions:

- If possible, alert the other members of your household, and leave by one of the exits established in your escape plan.
- If there is smoke, cover your nose and mouth with a wet cloth, drop to the floor, and crawl toward the prearranged exit.
- If a closed door is warm to the touch, do not open it. There could be fire on the other side of the door.
- Close doors behind you, if possible.
- Once outside, call the fire department from the nearest phone.
- Meet other family members at the place designated by your escape plan. Do not go back into a burning building for any reason!

Electrical Safety Faulty electrical wiring and improper use of fuses can result in fires. Electricity also presents an additional danger. **Electrocution** is death resulting from the passage of electric current through the body. About 1,000 people are accidentally electrocuted each year.

Many electrical accidents involve appliances that are not installed or used properly. Any electrical appliance that is not working properly should be unplugged right away. It should be repaired by a qualified

• • • TEACH continued

Class Discussion
Accidents Caused by Electricity

What is the purpose of a fuse? *[A fuse melts when the circuit is overloaded and prevents an electrical fire.]* **When might a person be in danger of electrocution in or near the home?** *[After a severe storm, an electrical wire may fall to the ground. Anyone touching the wire could be electrocuted. Using an appliance when standing in water can do the same. Touching a worn wire of a plugged-in appliance can also cause electrocution.]* **How can young children be protected from the dangers of electricity?** *[By not letting them play with electrical wires or plugs; by placing outlet caps over electrical outlets so they cannot stick objects into the holes.]*

Reinforcement
Accidental Poisonings at Home

Discuss ways in which young children become victims of accidental poisoning. Ask where medicine should be stored if there is a young child in the house. Also discuss the danger of chemicals, such as cleaning fluids and pesticides, and the proper places where they should be stored. Discuss ways in which other family members may also be poisoned accidentally when poisonous substances are not properly labeled or stored.

technician, or it should be replaced. Never attempt to fix an appliance that is plugged into an outlet!

Careless use of electrical appliances around water is very dangerous. Because water is a good conductor of electricity, someone who is wet or has wet hands can become a pathway for electric current. Avoid using hair dryers and other appliances in the bathroom. Never place a radio or other electrical device near a tub or sink. Bathroom outlets should have built-in circuit breakers.

A worn electrical cord is both a fire hazard and an electrocution hazard. Inspect the electrical cords in your home. Tell a parent or guardian about any defective wiring that you find.

Electricity is especially dangerous to young children. They should not be allowed to play with electrical cords or appliances nor permitted to plug in or unplug such appliances. Outlet caps should be placed over electrical outlets to keep young children from sticking objects into the holes.

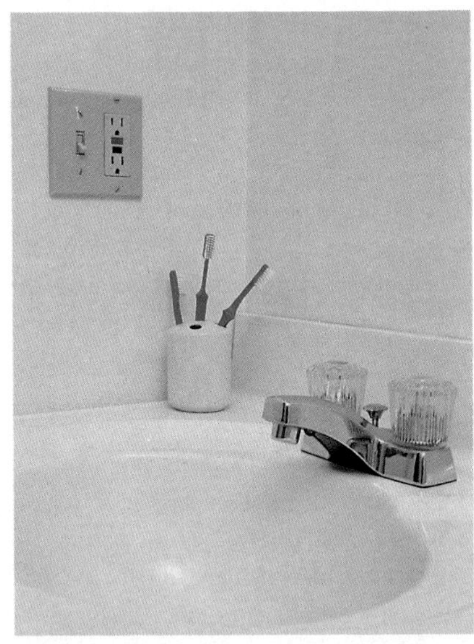

(FIGURE 27-11) **This outlet has a built-in ground fault protector to break the circuit automatically in case an electrical appliance comes in contact with water.**

Poisoning Most cases of accidental poisoning involve children under five. These children may swallow medicines, cleaning chemicals, pesticides, or other poisons. Improper storage of poisonous substances or failure to put them away after use are the most common ways that poisons get into the hands of youngsters.

To make your home safer for children, all medicines should be placed in cabinets that are out of a child's reach. Cleaning fluids and other poisonous materials should not be stored under sinks or in closets where children can reach them. A locked cabinet is the best storage location. Since basements are often collection places for a variety of dangerous chemicals, they should be inspected carefully and childproofed.

Older children and adults can also be victims of accidental poisoning. Storing liquids in plastic soda bottles, as shown in Figure 27-12, is a practice that can lead to someone accidentally drinking a poisonous material. Always store materials in their original containers, and make sure they are clearly marked.

Sometimes people are accidentally poisoned when handling pesticides and weedkillers. Before using any of these chemicals, read the label carefully and follow the instructions given. When using such products, you should wear gloves. If you spray pesticides indoors, the windows should be open, and it is a good idea to go outside afterward. If you need to spray outdoors, do not do so on a windy day.

Accidental poisoning can also result from taking medicine that was prescribed for someone else. Since your present health condition can affect how you react to a drug, you should take only medicines that were

Cooperative Learning
Unsafe Materials in the Home

Have students work in groups to prepare posters that show how dangerous household products should be stored, labeled, and kept from the hands of young children. Some posters should point out that older members of the family are also in danger from mislabeled bottles.

Reinforcement
Natural Disasters

Discuss with students the kinds of natural disasters that strike from time to time. Certain disasters are more likely to threaten one part of the country than another. For example, the West Coast has concerns about earthquakes, the Atlantic and Gulf Coasts about hurricanes, the Midwest about tornadoes. Many parts of the country have severe thunderstorms. Any low-lying region near a river may be flooded. Ask students how injuries can occur during each of these disasters.

Cooperative Learning
Preparing for a Disaster

Have students work in cooperative groups to draw up plans of action for when a severe thunderstorm or tornado occurs in their area. Their plans should include meetings with family members to review the proper procedures to protect themselves and their

Background

Preparing for an Emergency

After a major earthquake or other disaster, electricity, water, and gas may be out of service. Emergency aid may not reach victims for several days. Homes, offices, and cars should be equipped with the following items: fire extinguisher, first aid kit, wrench for turning off gas and water valves, flashlight and extra batteries, water and disinfectant, radio and extra batteries, dry or canned food that does not require cooking, blankets, clothing, and shoes for walking through the debris. Everyone in an at-risk area should have these items located in a place where they can easily be reached.

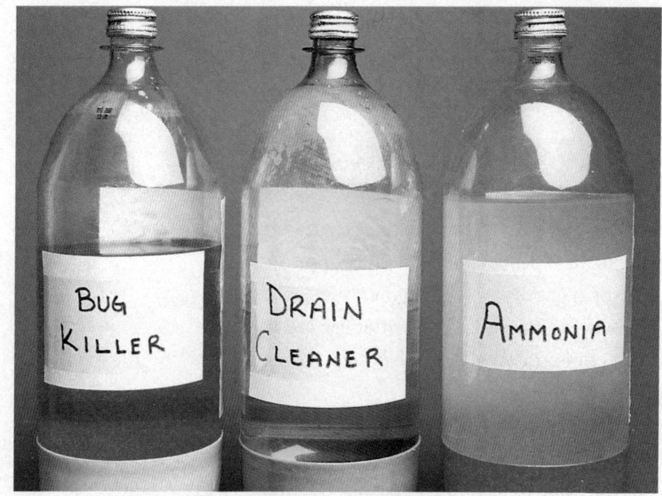

(FIGURE 27-12) **This photo shows a very unsafe practice. Poisons should be stored in their original containers, with their original labels intact.**

prescribed for you. Combining drugs is another risky behavior. It can result in a drug interaction that is dangerous to health. Such a situation is also a case of accidental poisoning.

Everyone should inspect his or her home for poison hazards and take steps to poison-proof it. One step that is a must is to have the telephone number of the nearest Poison Control Center next to your phone. By calling that number, you can get instructions for helping someone who has been poisoned.

Safety in a Disaster

disaster:

an event that affects the lives and health of people in one or more communities.

An event that seriously affects the lives and health of the people living in one or more communities is called a **disaster**. Many disasters, such as storms and earthquakes, are acts of nature. People have no control over such events. However, it is possible to reduce your risk of injury from these events.

Thunderstorms Thunderstorms are powerful but short-lived events that are most common in spring and summer. Although most thunderstorms would not be considered disasters, strong winds that sometimes accompany thunderstorms can blow objects around and cause widespread damage as well as injuries.

The most dangerous aspect of any thunderstorm is the lightning. Lightning is a gigantic discharge of electricity. It often strikes the tallest object in the area. However, the electricity can move from an object to your body if you are nearby. More people are killed each year by lightning than by other weather-related events.

To reduce your risk of being injured during a thunderstorm, observe the following precautions:

- If you are outdoors, try to find shelter in a building or car.
- If you are on or in water, such as a lake or swimming pool, leave the water immediately. High winds, waves, and lightning are dangerous to boaters and swimmers.
- Never stand under a tall, isolated tree or other tall object.
- If you are in an open area, discard anything that might attract lightning, such as a large metal belt buckle, metal-frame backpack, or golf club. Crouch down to avoid being the tallest object in the area.
- If you are indoors, close the windows and stay away from them. Do not use the telephone or other electrical appliances. If lightning strikes a nearby electrical transmission line, the electricity can be transferred to you.

Tornadoes Like thunderstorms, tornadoes are most common in the spring and summer. Although they are fairly brief, the winds in tornadoes can be as high as 300 mph. Thus, tornadoes are able to destroy homes and send objects, including cars, flying through the air. The following are some safety tips to follow if a tornado is sighted or a warning is issued in your area:

• • • TEACH continued

property when a watch has been put into effect or in case the disaster occurs without warning.

Class Discussion

Hurricanes and Tornadoes

What are some dangers during a hurricane? *[People can be struck by flying objects, including broken glass, bricks, boards, and debris. Vehicles and mobile homes can be overturned.]* **What precautions should be taken during a tornado?** *[If you are outdoors, try to go indoors. Go to the lowest part of the building, such as a basement or cellar. Stay away from windows or doors. Get out of a car or mobile home. If you cannot go indoors, lie in a ditch or on the lowest ground you can find.]*

Class Discussion

How to Avoid Assault

Discuss the reasons why people are assaulted. **What should you do to reduce the possibility of being assaulted?** *[Keep the doors locked both day and night. Have a service person show identification through a window before you open the door. Never let a stranger know you are home alone. Do not walk alone outside, especially at night. When in a car, keep the doors locked. At night, keep the windows partially rolled up.]*

Debate the Issue

To Fight, or Not to Fight

Have students debate the question of whether it is best to resist an attacker

- Try to get indoors, then go to the lowest part of the building. Basements and interior bathrooms, closets, and hallways on the ground floor will provide the most protection.
- Stay away from windows and doors. Windows may be shattered by the winds. Doors can be ripped from their hinges and thrown about.
- If you are in a vehicle or mobile home as a tornado approaches, get out of it and go to a safer place. A tornado can overturn most vehicles and mobile homes. If you cannot get indoors, lie in a ditch or the lowest place you can find.

Hurricanes Hurricanes are strong tropical storms that occur most often in late summer and fall. Hurricane winds range from 75 to more than 150 mph, and the rain from a hurricane is usually very heavy. Hurricanes are very large storms that may travel great distances. Fortunately, there is usually some time to prepare for a hurricane. Observe the following precautions if a hurricane is forecast for your area:

- If you live along the coast, be prepared to leave if local officials advise it. The huge ocean waves and flooding produced by a hurricane do great damage to coastal areas and are a major cause of injuries and deaths from these storms.
- Have a supply of canned food, drinking water, flashlights, fresh batteries, candles, and first-aid materials in your home.
- If possible, board up windows or tape the inside of each pane. Place indoors all objects that might be blown away if left outside, such as lawn chairs or bicycles.
- Remain indoors until authorities advise that the storm is over. Once outside, avoid downed electrical wires and flooded areas.

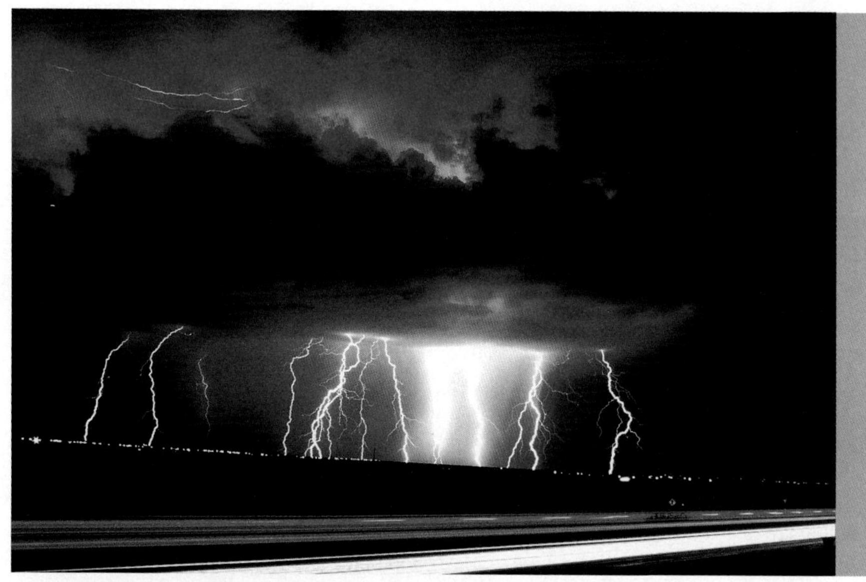

(FIGURE 27-13) **Severe thunderstorms, like the one shown here, can produce dangerous lightning, damaging winds, hail, heavy rain, flash flooding, and even tornadoes. If you live in a part of the country that is prone to these types of storms, learn to recognize the signs of an approaching storm, and know what to do to protect yourself from storm-related injuries.**

or to give in. After each side has presented its case, have students arrive at a list of conditions, if any, under which they agree resistance is advisable.

Class Discussion
Occupational Safety

Ask students what they think are the most dangerous occupations. Then have them look at the graph that shows the death rates among workers in various industries. **Why do you think you hear more about accidents that occur in manufacturing plants than in farming?** *[More people are usually involved in a single manufacturing accident, but many more farm accidents may occur every day.]* Discuss the kinds of accidents that occur in the mining industry.

Cooperative Learning
Possibility of a Disaster in Your Area

Have students research newspapers and magazines to find information on the kinds of disasters that have struck your part of the country in the past. Some students may have experienced these disasters. Encourage them to share their experiences with the class. Ask students to discuss how they will respond to similar problems in the future.

Extension
Safety in the Workplace

Have students interview the managers of local manufacturing plants or businesses to find out how they handle occupational safety.

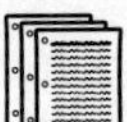

Section Review Worksheet 27.3

Assign Section Review Worksheet 27.3, which requires students to select the path through a puzzle that describes only safe behaviors and to identify why those actions should be undertaken.

Section Quiz 27.3

Have students take Section Quiz 27.3.

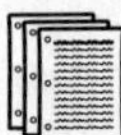

Reteaching Worksheet 27.3

Students who have difficulty with the material may complete Reteaching Worksheet 27.3, which requires them to place statements about home accidents in correct categories.

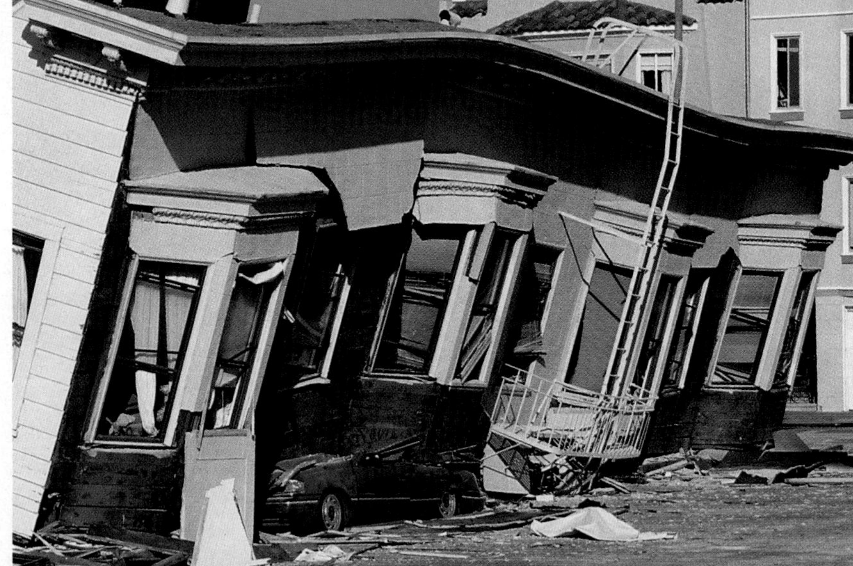

(FIGURE 27-14) **This building collapsed during an earthquake in San Francisco, CA. In earthquake-prone areas, building codes now specify earthquake-resistant designs.**

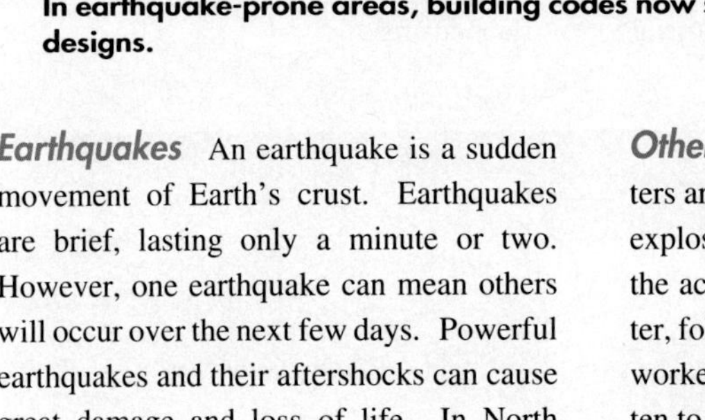

Earthquakes An earthquake is a sudden movement of Earth's crust. Earthquakes are brief, lasting only a minute or two. However, one earthquake can mean others will occur over the next few days. Powerful earthquakes and their aftershocks can cause great damage and loss of life. In North America, most serious earthquakes occur near the West Coast. Safety during an earthquake is often a matter of thinking quickly. The following are suggestions that could save your life:

- If you are outdoors, get away from buildings and other tall objects. Material falling from them could injure or kill you.
- If you are in a car, pull over but remain in the car.
- If you are indoors, stand in a doorway between rooms or get under a heavy table. Stay away from windows, doors with glass panes, and objects that might shake loose from walls.

Other Disasters Although many disasters are caused by nature, some, such as gas explosions and forest fires, often result from the activities of people. During any disaster, follow the instructions of the emergency workers in charge. It is a good idea to listen to the emergency information on a local radio station so that you know what to do.

assault:

a personal attack in which you are threatened or harmed.

Assaults

A personal attack in which you are threatened or harmed is called an **assault**. Many assaults occur in connection with robberies. Some assaults involve bias on the part of the attacker, often based on the victim's race or ethnic background. Sexual assault includes rape and any other type of sexual contact with a person without his or her consent. Chapter 20 contains more information about sexual assault and how to prevent it.

Ways to avoid being a victim of violence are discussed in Chapter 20.

To reduce your risk of being assaulted, observe the following safety precautions:

- When at home, keep doors locked both day and night. Never unlock the door for a stranger. If a service person comes to the door, have the person show identification at a window.
- Never let a stranger know that you are home alone, even if the stranger is on the telephone. If you receive a threatening or obscene phone call, hang up and then call the police.
- Do not walk outside alone, particularly at night. Even when you are with friends, avoid deserted areas, alleys, and poorly lighted parks.
- When in a car, keep the doors locked. At night, keep the windows partially rolled up. If a stranger approaches your car, drive away.

If you are attacked, let good judgment determine your actions. Escape if you can. If your attacker has a weapon, do not try to resist unless you think that your life is in immediate danger. Afterward, report the attack to the police.

Occupational Safety

Many people are injured or killed each year in job-related accidents. According to a study by the National Safety Council, personal behavior—such as being careless and disregarding safety requirements—is a factor in 82 percent of these accidents. Close to 20 percent of work-related accidents are caused wholly by such behavior. Faulty machinery and unsafe working conditions also contribute to many injuries and deaths.

As a student, you are preparing for your future occupation. Some occupations, such as mining and the manufacturing of chemicals and explosives, are obviously risky. But as the graph in Figure 27-15 indicates, agriculture, construction, and transportation can also be considered risky occupations.

What Would You Do?

Making Responsible Decisions

Your On-the-Job Safety Is Threatened

Suppose that you work for a company that uses hazardous materials in its everyday operation. You like the job and the people you are working with. Then one day, one of your co-workers shows you a copy of the *Material Safety and Data Sheet* for a chemical that you use frequently, saying that you should read it carefully.

Material Safety and Data Sheets are government publications that contain information about the hazards of chemicals and the types of protective clothing and equipment that are needed for handling them safely. After reading the data sheet, you realize that you have not been provided with the proper protective equipment. What would you do?

Remember to use the

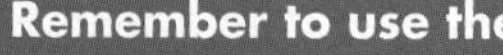

decision-making steps:

1. **State the Problem.**
2. **List the Options.**
3. **Imagine the Benefits and Consequences.**
4. **Consider Your Values.**
5. **Weigh the Options and Decide.**
6. **Act.**
7. **Evaluate the Results.**

What Would You Do?

Your On-the-Job Safety Is Threatened

Have students do the exercise, using the decision-making model to decide what to do as a worker who has to handle hazardous chemicals but who has not been provided with the proper protective equipment.

Review Answers

1. Answers will vary but might include being careless while cooking, or not repairing frayed rugs or broken tiles.
2. Answers will vary but might include not using bath mats or overloading electrical outlets.
3. Plans for fire safety will vary with each student and home. Fire safety plans should enable fires to be detected as early as possible, and escape routes should be as direct an exit from the house as possible.
4. Occupational Safety and Health Administration, or OSHA. OSHA helps protect workers by setting safety standards such as requirements for storing large amounts of chemicals, types of safety equipment workers must wear, and allowable amounts of exposure to dangerous materials.
5. Answers will vary according to occupation. Accept any answer that demonstrates the ability to recognize potential hazards and ways to eliminate or reduce those hazards.

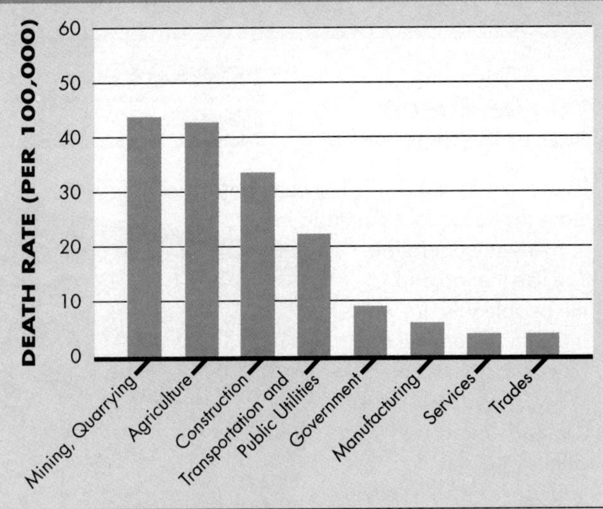

(FIGURE 27-15) **This data from 1990, supplied by the National Safety Council, indicates the most hazardous occupations. If you work in one of these industries, remember that *both* you and your employer are responsible for your safety.**

The Occupational Safety and Health Administration (OSHA) is a federal agency that sets safety standards in the workplace. State and local governments may also set standards for safety in various occupations. Fire safety, requirements for storing large amounts of chemicals, and the types of safety equipment that workers must wear are examples of factors the government regulates. In industries that expose workers to dangerous materials such as poisonous vapors and radiation, the government sets limits on how much exposure a worker is permitted to have.

Work-related illnesses and injuries affect close to two million Americans each year. Many workers once employed in the asbestos industry developed serious lung diseases as a result of contact with asbestos. Illnesses caused by contact with irritating or toxic materials continue to affect the health of many workers each year. To practice protecting yourself at work, complete the "What Would You Do?" activity on page 605.

Although the accident rate in the workplace has, in general, been declining, such accidents are still an important factor in the total number of accidental injuries and deaths. The same principles that apply to accidents in general also apply in the workplace. Both employers and employees are responsible for ensuring safe working conditions and preventing accidents.

Review

1. *Cite some examples of how careless behavior can contribute to accidents in the home.*
2. *What unsafe conditions can you identify in your home that might lead to accidental falls? to electrical accidents?*
3. ***LIFE SKILLS: Problem Solving*** *Review the fire safety of your home. Then develop a plan to improve it. Discuss your plan with a parent or guardian. With his or her assistance, put your plan into action.*
4. *What federal agency oversees the safety of workers? List three ways this agency helps protect workers from injury on the job.*
5. ***Critical Thinking*** *Choose one of the occupations shown on the graph in Figure 27-15. What potential hazards associated with that occupation might be regulated by government agencies to help ensure the safety of the workers?*

ASSESS

Section Review

Have students answer the Section Review questions.

Alternative Assessment

Government Help During Disasters

Ask students to speculate about what it would be like if the government did not help restore things to normal after a disaster strikes an area.

Closure

Student Responsibility to Safety at School

Ask students to suggest ways students sometimes endanger themselves and others when at school (for instance, by not being careful when riding their bicycles or skateboards, or by leaving articles in places where others may trip over them).

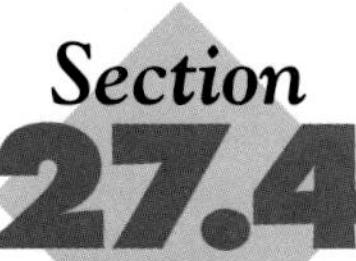

Section 27.4 Recreational Safety

Objectives

- *Recognize potential hazards in recreational activities.*
- *Identify ways to reduce the risk of accidents in recreational activities.*
  LIFE SKILLS: Problem Solving

Activities such as swimming, hiking, and playing baseball provide fun and exercise, and can reduce stress. Recreation also involves risk, but there are things you can do to reduce the risk of accidents and injury.

Sports and Safety

The student in Figure 27-16 is on a high school track team. But right now he is not running; he is warming up. Figure 27-17 gives information about warm-up practices among 10th-graders who exercise or play sports outside of school.

Warming up stretches ligaments and tendons—tissues that hold bones to muscles and muscles to other muscles, respectively.

(FIGURE 27-16) **Warming up protects against sports injuries.**

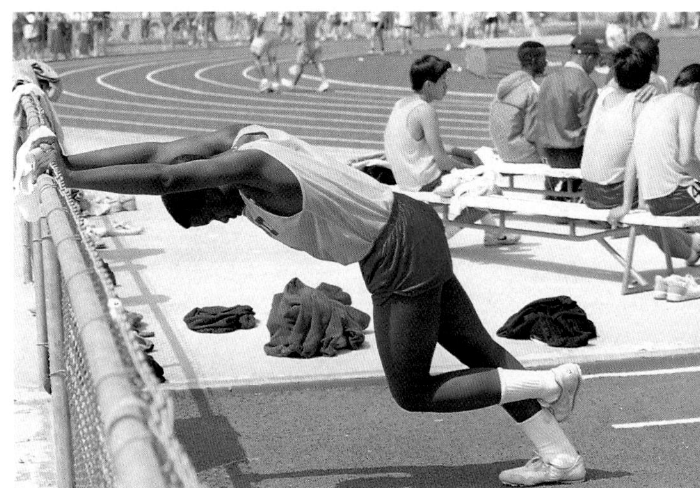

Background
Warming Up the Joint Fluid
Warming up before sports activities helps prevent injury during playing time. Warming up causes an increase in the amount of synovial fluid that lubricates the joints. Without a sufficient amount of this fluid, the bones that meet at the joints are stressed and are more easily injured.

Warm-up Practices of 10th Graders

Warm Up Before Exercises	Female	Male	Total
Never	*9.8%*	*14.9%*	*12.5%*
Rarely	*11.1%*	*14.1%*	*12.7%*
Sometimes	*20.7%*	*18.1%*	*19.3%*
Usually	*22.7%*	*20.7%*	*21.6%*
Always	*35.7%*	*32.1%*	*33.8%*

(FIGURE 27-17) **This is how the 10th-graders who participated in the *National Adolescent Student Health Survey* answered the question: "How often do you warm up before exercising?"**

Section 27.4 Lesson Plan

MOTIVATE

Journal 27D
Sports and Safety

This may be done as a warm-up activity. Encourage students to record in the Student Journal ways in which they could participate in sports activities while following safety guidelines.

Cooperative Learning
Warm-up Activities

Have students form groups. Have them discuss the importance of warm-ups, then tally how many in the group always warm up before exercising, usually warm up, sometimes do, rarely do, and never do. Copy the categories on the chalkboard and find the class profile by combining the totals for each category for all the groups. Compare the results with the national averages.

TEACH

Class Discussion
Proper Equipment for Sports and Exercise

Ask students to name the sports and other forms of exercise they participate in. Write them on the chalkboard. Then ask what kinds of equipment are needed to make these activities safe, and write these next to the activity. Have students mention accidents they

Background

Swimmers Who Drown

Many people who drown are accomplished swimmers. They may swim out too far, then become too tired to return to shore. Strong currents may carry them into deep water. Sometimes cramped muscles cause a swimmer to lose the ability to continue swimming. Some swimmers take unnecessary risks; others swim while under the influence of alcohol. Swimming is usually safe for those who follow the rules and are aware of the risks.

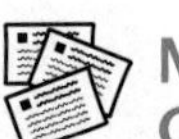

Making a Choice 27B

Planning for Safety

Assign the Planning for Safety card. The card requires students to analyze safety hazards of their activities, and to plan how to avoid potential accidents.

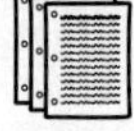

Ethics Worksheet

Assign the Ethics Worksheet for Unit 8.

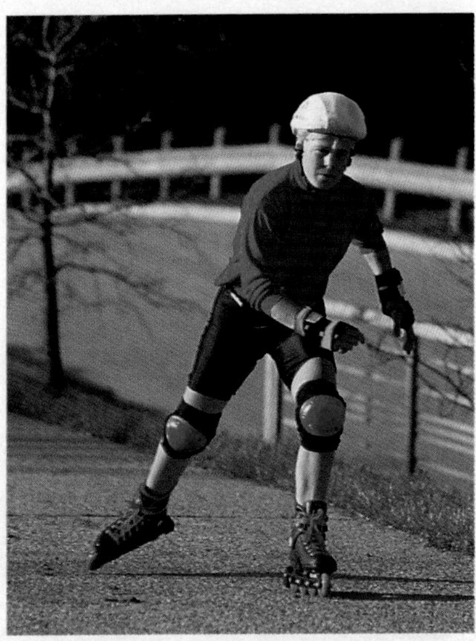

(FIGURE 27-18) **In-line skaters wear protective gear to reduce their risk of injury.**

The importance of warming up properly is discussed in greater detail in Chapter 3.

Warming up also slowly increases the flow of blood, and thus oxygen, to muscles. Beginning physical activity without first warming up can result in pulled ligaments and muscles, and in muscle strains. Such injuries are common among people who participate in sports.

Water Safety Among 10th Graders

Behavior	Never Do	Sometimes Do
Swim alone	*62.0%*	*38.0%*
Swim in restricted/ unsupervised area	*70.7%*	*29.3%*

(FIGURE 27-19) **This is how the 10th-graders who participated in the *National Adolescent Student Health Survey* answered the question: "How often do you swim alone or in restricted or unsupervised areas?"**

The most serious injuries in sports often occur because of the misuse—or no use—of protective equipment. As with bicycles and motorcycles, helmets are an important piece of safety equipment in many sports. Batting helmets are required in Major League Baseball. No player in the National Football League would head onto the field without his helmet. Professional athletes reduce their risk of injury by using helmets. Unfortunately, amateurs don't always take the same precautions.

In-line skating, which has become very popular, is a sport that causes many broken bones and other injuries. Notice the types of protective equipment being worn by the skater in Figure 27-18. If you participate in this activity or a similar activity, such as roller-skating or skateboarding, be sure you are protected against accidental injury—wear protective equipment.

Water Safety

As you might suspect, the recreational activity that results in the greatest number of accidental deaths is swimming. Figure 27-1 shows that drowning is the fourth leading cause of accidental death. This is partly because a great number of people head for the water on hot summer days.

Swimming and Diving Many drownings occur in home swimming pools. Because of carelessness, young children are frequently the victims. Children should never be left unattended in or near a pool. Many communities require pools to be fenced so that youngsters cannot wander into them.

Older children and adults, including those who can swim, are also victims of drowning. In many cases, risky behavior contributes to an accidental drowning. Swimming alone and swimming in an unprotected area are two such behaviors.

• • • TEACH continued

know of that occur during these activities, and the effect of proper equipment on reducing injuries.

Demonstration

Drown Proofing

Have students act out a situation where they are in deep water and are in danger of drowning. Ask them to go through the steps to demonstrate drownproofing to the class. When they have finished, ask the class to suggest improvements, if necessary.

Journal 27E

Water Safety

Have students look at the table in Figure 27-19. Ask them to write in the Student Journal their opinion of students who neglect water safety.

Class Discussion

Safe Procedures in Boats

Ask students to mention some unsafe boating practices to be avoided. Discuss the consequences of these risky behaviors.

Role-Playing

Safe Hiking

Have students role-play a situation in which teens are planning a hike. Ask some groups to demonstrate plans that include safeguards to avoid getting lost. Other groups can illustrate what not to do. When the skits are completed, let the class mention improvements that should be made to the plans to make them safer.

Figure 27-19 shows that approximately one-third of 10th-graders surveyed engage in such risky behavior at least some of the time. To reduce the risk of drowning, you should always swim with a friend and swim where there are lifeguards.

Learning how to swim will reduce your risk of drowning. But if you are in trouble in deep water and no immediate help is available, a technique called **drown proofing** can help keep you afloat. The steps in drown proofing are as follows:

- First, take a deep breath and relax, allowing your face to enter the water. Let your legs hang down in the water and your arms float forward.
- Next, slowly exhale underwater. Then move your arms downward as you kick with your feet to raise your head above the surface.
- Finally, take a breath and begin the process again.

Diving into water can be thrilling but requires caution. Learn to dive from someone who knows how. Diving into an unknown area or into water of unknown depth is a very risky behavior. Hitting bottom can cause serious head, neck, and spinal injuries. Paralysis or death often results from such accidents.

Boating Safety Some drownings occur as a result of boating accidents. The girls in Figure 27-20 are reducing their risk of drowning by wearing life jackets. All boaters, regardless of their swimming ability, should wear a life jacket or have some type of flotation device close at hand.

Boating accidents usually result from carelessness or risky behavior. As with a car, speeding in a boat can result in loss of control. Alcohol is another factor in many boating accidents. Ignoring warning buoys and other markers and weaving unnecessarily can also result in accidents. Sudden

drown proofing: *a technique to stay afloat that can be used even by those who cannot swim.*

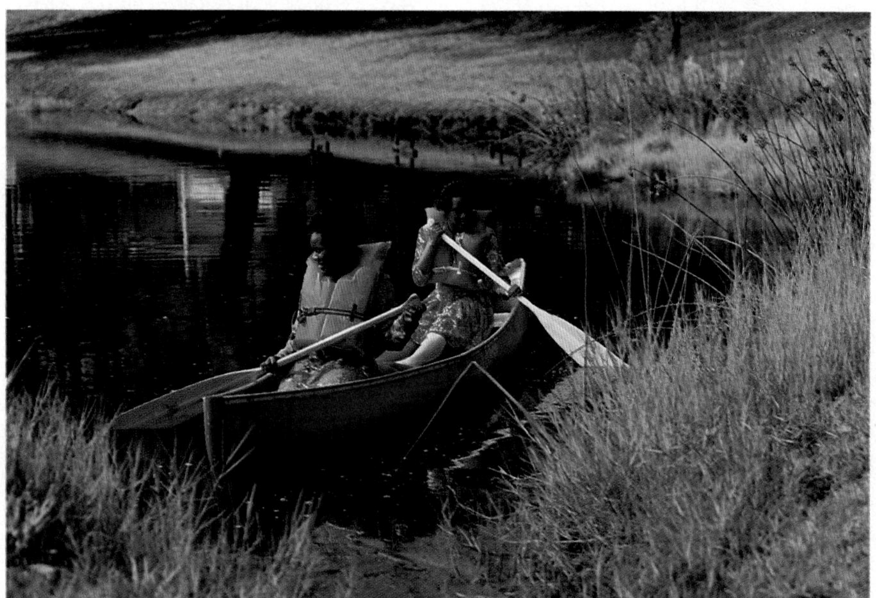

(FIGURE 27-20) **As these girls are demonstrating, every person in a boat should have his or her own life jacket.**

SECTION 27.4

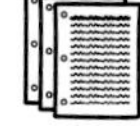

Section Review Worksheet 27.4

Assign Section Review Worksheet 27.4, which requires students to answer questions related to recreational safety.

Section Quiz 27.4

Have students take Section Quiz 27.4.

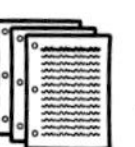

Reteaching Worksheet 27.4

Students who have difficulty with the material may complete Reteaching Worksheet 27.4, which requires them to identify unsafe behaviors in recreational activities.

Extension

Safe Camping

Have students visit or contact a forest preserve or park near them to find out the rules by which campers must abide. Ask them if they can think of any other restrictions that might make camping safer.

Review Answers

1. Some people are careless and do not watch children near pools or at beaches. As a result, the children can fall into the pool and drown. Risky behaviors that can result in drowning include: swimming alone; swimming in an unprotected area; not wearing a life jacket when in a boat or when participating in water sports, such as water skiing; swimming while under the influence of alcohol or drugs; and diving in water of unknown depth.

2. Stretching, doing warm-up exercises, and using protective equipment can reduce sports-related injuries.

3. Answers will vary depending on students' recreational activities.

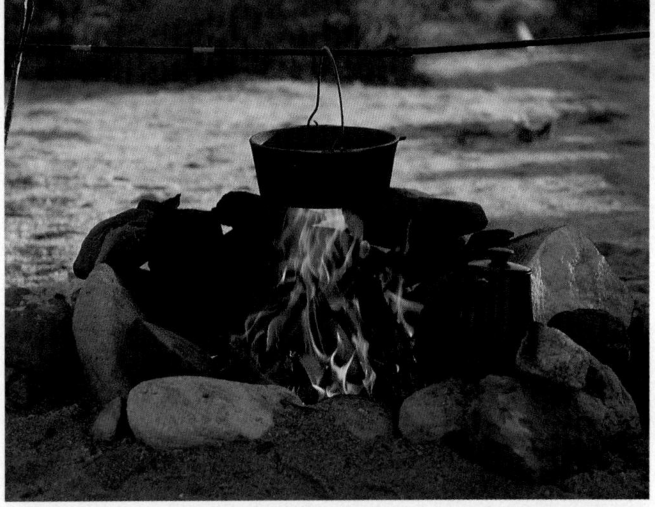

(FIGURE 27-21) **This is one safe way to manage a campfire. Campfires should not be left unattended and should be extinguished completely before the last person leaves the area.**

storms and overloading a small boat with people and equipment can result in capsizing, or turning the boat over. If you use a boat, learn how to handle it. Also learn the rules of boating safety.

Wilderness Safety

Hiking, camping, and hunting are outdoor activities enjoyed by millions of people. Although some people are injured by animals such as bears and snakes, such incidents are rare. Hazards such as getting lost, losing control of a fire, and being injured with firearms are far more common.

Hiking in the woods involves thinking ahead. For example, when Gary and Lien planned to hike for a day, they bought a trail map of the area, studied it, then let their parents know where they were going and when they expected to return. As they hiked, Gary and Lien followed the marked trail. They did not try to cut across the forest to reach their destination. Carrying a map and staying on the trail helped Gary and Lien avoid getting lost. Letting people know where they were going hiking was another good precaution to take in case something went wrong.

Careless handling of campfires and other fires results in many forest fires each year. Damage runs into the millions of dollars, and loss of life can result. Like the campfire in Figure 27-21, a campfire should be built only in a fire ring of metal or stone, or in a stone fireplace. Using inflammable liquids to start a fire or get it burning better is a risky behavior that can result in injuries. A fire of any kind must never be left unattended. If the fire danger in the area is high, it is unlikely that campfires will be permitted.

Hunting accidents often result from carelessness. If you hunt, wear bright red or orange clothing so that you are visible to other hunters. When preparing to shoot, be sure that your target is the intended animal. If you are not certain about what you are shooting at, don't shoot. Firearms should always be stored and transported unloaded. But when you are handling a firearm, always assume that it is loaded until you have checked it!

Review

1. *In what ways do careless and risky behaviors contribute to accidental drowning?*
2. ***LIFE SKILLS: Problem Solving*** *Discuss some ways to reduce injuries resulting from participation in sports.*
3. ***Critical Thinking*** *Review your recreational activities for potential hazards. Identify actions that you can take to reduce the risk of accidents.*

ASSESS

Section Review

Have students answer the Section Review questions.

Alternative Assessment

Making Recreation Accident Free

Have students choose one form of recreation that they enjoy most. Ask them to write a radio announcement that promotes safer practices for those who participate in that activity.

Closure

Safe Camping

Have students suggest safe ways to enjoy camping. Write these suggestions on the chalkboard.

Highlights

Summary

- To reduce the risk of accident or injury in a motor vehicle, wear seat belts, obey traffic laws, drive defensively, and never drive after using alcohol or drugs or ride with a driver who is under the influence of alcohol or drugs.
- To reduce the risk of accident or injury on a bicycle or motorcycle, wear a helmet and proper clothing, avoid speeding, ride defensively, obey traffic laws, and keep bikes in good working order.
- To reduce the risk of injury from falls, keep walkways and stairways free of clutter, install nonslip surfaces, and repair carpets, tiles, sidewalks, and handrails.
- To prevent injury from fire, install fire extinguishers and smoke detectors; properly maintain heaters, stoves, fireplaces, and electrical wiring; and have a home evacuation plan.
- To reduce the risk of accidental poisoning, keep medicines and other poisonous substances out of the reach of children, store them in properly marked original containers, and follow the directions for their proper use.
- To reduce the risk of being assaulted, keep doors locked, avoid strangers and deserted areas when alone, and follow community disaster plans.
- To reduce the risk of accidental injury or death when engaging in outdoor activities, use the proper safety equipment and follow the safety rules for each activity, tell someone where you are going and when you will be back, and never go alone.

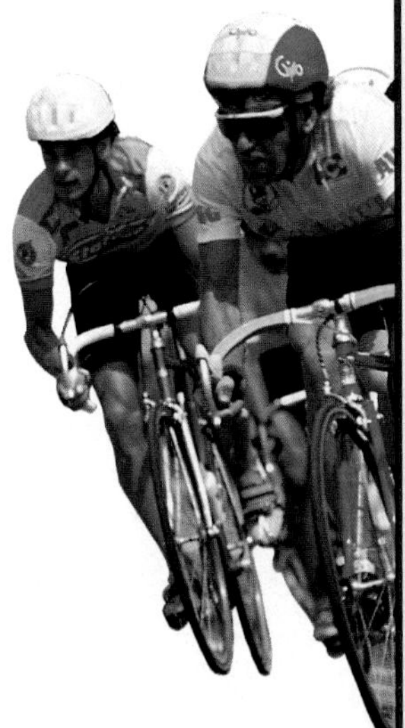

Vocabulary

accident any unexpected event that causes damage, injury, or death.

risk an action that is potentially dangerous; the chance of injury.

safety awareness knowledge about risks and how to reduce them.

defensive driving driving as though you expect other drivers to drive recklessly.

electrocution death resulting from the flow of electrical current through the body.

disaster an event that affects the lives and health of people in one or more communities.

assault a personal attack in which you are threatened or harmed.

drown proofing a technique to stay afloat that can be used even by those who cannot swim.

Chapter 27 Highlights

Summary

Have students read the summary to reinforce the concepts they learned in Chapter 27.

Vocabulary

Have students write several safety rules in which they use all the vocabulary words correctly.

Extension

Have students make posters that raise community awareness to the need for safer practices in sports activities. Have students ask that their posters be displayed in the public library, banks, and health clubs.

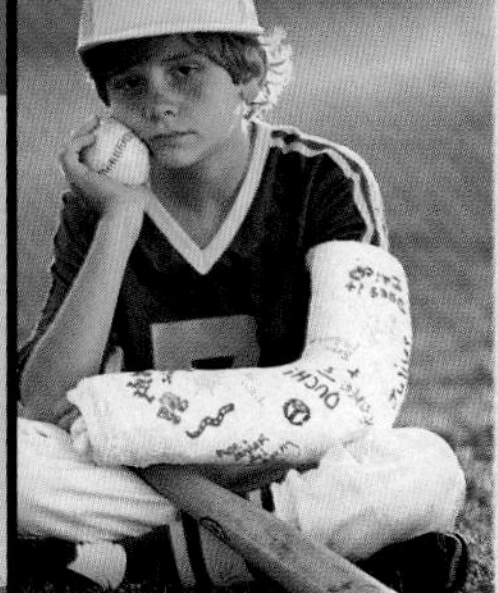

Chapter Review

Concept Review

1. Avoiding risky behavior and being attentive are part of being ________.
2. ________ accidents account for more deaths than any other kind of accident.
3. You can reduce your risk of being involved in a motor-vehicle accident by not riding with a person who ________.
4. ________ involves expecting other drivers to do the unexpected.
5. Wearing a ________ when riding a bicycle or motorcycle can reduce your chances of suffering a serious injury.
6. For people over 65, ________ cause from one-third to one-half of all accidental deaths.
7. Two types of devices that reduce the risk of injury from a fire are ________ and ________.
8. Electrical appliances should never be used around ________.
9. ________ have the highest risk of being poisoned by improperly stored medicines and poisons.
10. ________ and ________ are the most dangerous aspects of a thunderstorm.
11. The two most risky occupational fields are ________ and ________.
12. The recreational activity that results in the greatest number of accidental deaths is ________.
13. All boaters should wear a ________ or have some type of ________ nearby.
14. For safety, firearms should be stored and transported ________.

Expressing Your Views

1. Why do you think so many teenagers fail to use safety equipment such as seat belts and bicycle helmets, as indicated by the tables in Figures 27-5 and 27-8?
2. Many states have laws that require passengers in cars to wear seat belts and motorcyclists to wear helmets. Do you think people should be required by law to wear such equipment? Why or why not?
3. If your one-year-old cousin were coming to your house for a visit, what changes would you make in your home to assure his safety?

Chapter 27 Assessment

Chapter Review

Concept Review

1. safety aware
2. motor vehicle
3. is under the influence of alcohol or drugs
4. driving defensively
5. helmet
6. falls
7. smoke detectors, fire extinguishers
8. water
9. children under five
10. lightning, strong winds
11. mining, agriculture
12. swimming
13. life jacket, flotation device
14. unloaded

Expressing Your Views

Sample responses:

1. Teenagers often take more risks than other people would because they typically feel that an accident "can't happen to me." Some teenagers may feel that wearing a seat belt or a bicycle helmet doesn't look "cool." Also, some teenagers may not wear safety devices because their friends don't.

2. Answers will vary with individual opinions. However, most students will probably answer yes because wearing seat belts and helmets has been shown to save lives.

3. Lock all medicines in a cabinet that is out of reach, lock all cleaning materials in a cabinet, put away all small items that the child might put in his or her mouth and possibly swallow or choke on, put out of reach all items that are breakable or have sharp edges, put electrical outlet safety plugs in all outlets that are not in use, and close and lock doors that lead to stairs or put up a child safety gate in front of stairs.

Life Skills Check

Sample responses:

1. If I did not drive to work I would have someone pick me up directly in front of the restaurant or I would get a ride home with another employee who I knew well and could trust. If I did drive to work I would park as close to work as possible, in a well-lighted area, and lock all doors when I left the car. I would have my car keys in my hand as I walked to my car. I would make sure no one was in the back seat before I got into the car. If there were strangers near my car, I would go back into the restaurant and find someone to escort me to my car, or call the police.

Chapter 27 Assessment

2. I would not go with my friend. Swimming and diving at night is not safe, especially in an area not open to swimmers and without lifeguards. I would continue trying to convince my friend to do something else.

3. I could make a disaster plan for each of the natural disasters. One plan would tell what I would do if I were at home; the other plan would tell what I would do if I were at school. I would practice my plan so that it would be familiar to me, if and when I should need to put it into action.

Life Skills Check

1. **Practicing Self-Care**
   You just got a late-night job at a restaurant downtown, about eight blocks from your house. What safety precautions could you take to make sure you get home safely each night?
2. **Making Responsible Decisions**
   Your friend tries to talk you into going swimming and diving with him in a water-filled quarry late one night. You try to persuade your friend to do something less dangerous, but he won't listen. What should you do?
3. **Problem Solving**
   Tornadoes, hurricanes, and earthquakes are natural disasters. What could you do at home and at school to prepare for each of these disasters?

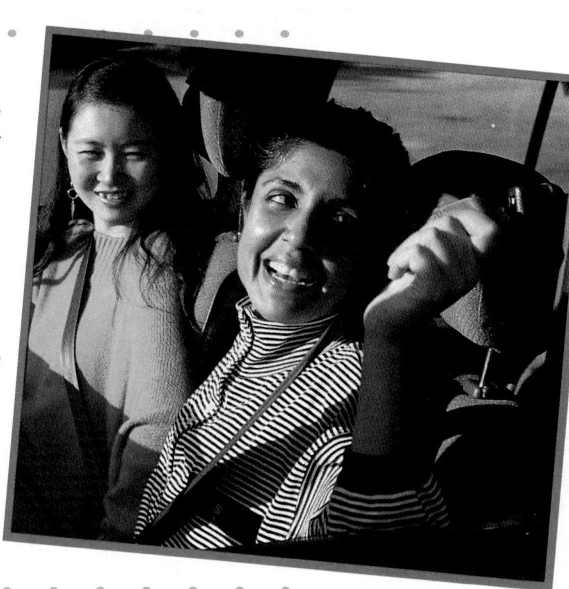

Projects

1. Divide a sheet of poster board into four parts. Create a "What Is Wrong?" picture in each part, showing an important safety rule being violated. Present these to the class and have volunteers guess what is wrong in each picture.
2. Working with a group, contact your local police department, hospital, or EMS squad to find out the numbers and types of accidents that are most common in your community. Ask if any prevention programs are being used to reduce these problems. Present your findings to the class along with your suggestions for ways to limit these accidents.
3. Develop a fire-escape plan for your home. On a floor plan of your home, diagram the escape routes for every member of your household, and make a list of the directions to share with your family.

Plan for Action

The home is a place where people spend much of their time, and unfortunately, it is a place where accidents are common. Create a plan to help reduce the risk of accidents in your home.

Projects

Have students plan and carry out the projects for safety and risk reduction.

Plan for Action

Hold a class debate on the topic: Should people be forced to follow safety rules that do not affect the safety of others but only of themselves? Have students research and present their cases followed by counter-arguments and questions from the audience.

Assessment Options

Chapter Test

Have students take the Chapter 27 Test.

Alternative Assessment

Have students do the Alternative Assessment activity for Chapter 27.

Test Generator

The Test Generator (Macintosh® or IBM® format) contains an additional 50 assessment items for this chapter.

Chapter 28

First Aid and CPR

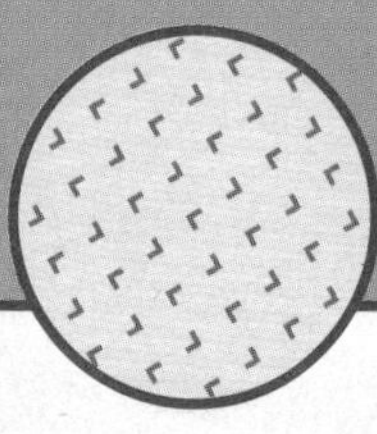

Planning Guide

TEXT SECTIONS	OBJECTIVES	TEXT FEATURES	OUTSIDE RESOURCES	NOTES
28.1 Emergency Priorities pp. 615-623 4 periods	• Name the first steps that should be taken during an emergency. ■ Describe the procedure for rescue breathing. ■ Describe the procedures for stopping or controlling bleeding. • Describe the signs of shock and its treatment. ■ List two facilities that might offer CPR training.	■ LIFE SKILLS: Using Community Resources, p. 617 **ASSESSMENT** • Section Review, p. 623	**TEACHER'S RESOURCE BINDER** • Lesson Plan 28.1 • Personal Health Inventory • Journal Entries 28A, 28B, 28C • Section Review Worksheet 28.1 • Section Quiz 28.1 • Reteaching Worksheet 28.1 **OTHER RESOURCES** • Transparencies 28A, 28B	
28.2 Injuries pp. 624-628 2 periods	• Differentiate among five types of wounds and their treatments. • Describe the first-aid steps for a fracture. • Describe the first-aid procedures for suspected injuries of the head and spine.	**ASSESSMENT** • Section Review, p. 628	**TEACHER'S RESOURCE BINDER** • Lesson Plan 28.2 • Journal Entries 28D, 28E • Section Review Worksheet 28.2 • Section Quiz 28.2 • Reteaching Worksheet 28.2	
28.3 Choking, Heart Attack, and Other Emergencies pp. 629-633 2 periods	• Describe the first aid for a heart attack victim. • Explain what to do if you find a person unconscious from an unknown cause. ■ Know how and when to perform the Heimlich maneuver.	• What Would You Do? p. 633 **ASSESSMENT** • Section Review, p. 633	**TEACHER'S RESOURCE BINDER** • Lesson Plan 28.3 • Journal Entry 28F • Life Skills 28A • Section Review Worksheet 28.3 • Section Quiz 28.3 • Reteaching Worksheet 28.3	
28.4 Common Emergencies pp. 634-646 4 periods	• Contrast two health emergencies caused by heat, and compare their treatments. ■ Know how to identify and protect your body from cold-related health emergencies. • Describe three types of burns and their treatment. • List the steps to be taken when poison is swallowed.	■ LIFE SKILLS: Practicing Self-Care, p. 637 **ASSESSMENT** • Section Review, p. 646	**TEACHER'S RESOURCE BINDER** • Lesson Plan 28.4 • Journal Entries 28G, 28H • Life Skills 28B, 28C, 28D • Section Review Worksheet 28.4 • Section Quiz 28.4 • Reteaching Worksheet 28.4 **OTHER RESOURCES** • Making a Choice 28A, 28B	
End of Chapter pp. 647-649		**ASSESSMENT** • Chapter Review, pp. 648-649	**TEACHER'S RESOURCE BINDER** • Chapter Test • Alternative Assessment **OTHER RESOURCES** • Test Generator	

■ Denotes LIFE SKILLS objectives

• Items in blue are also part of the *Holt Health Activity Book.*

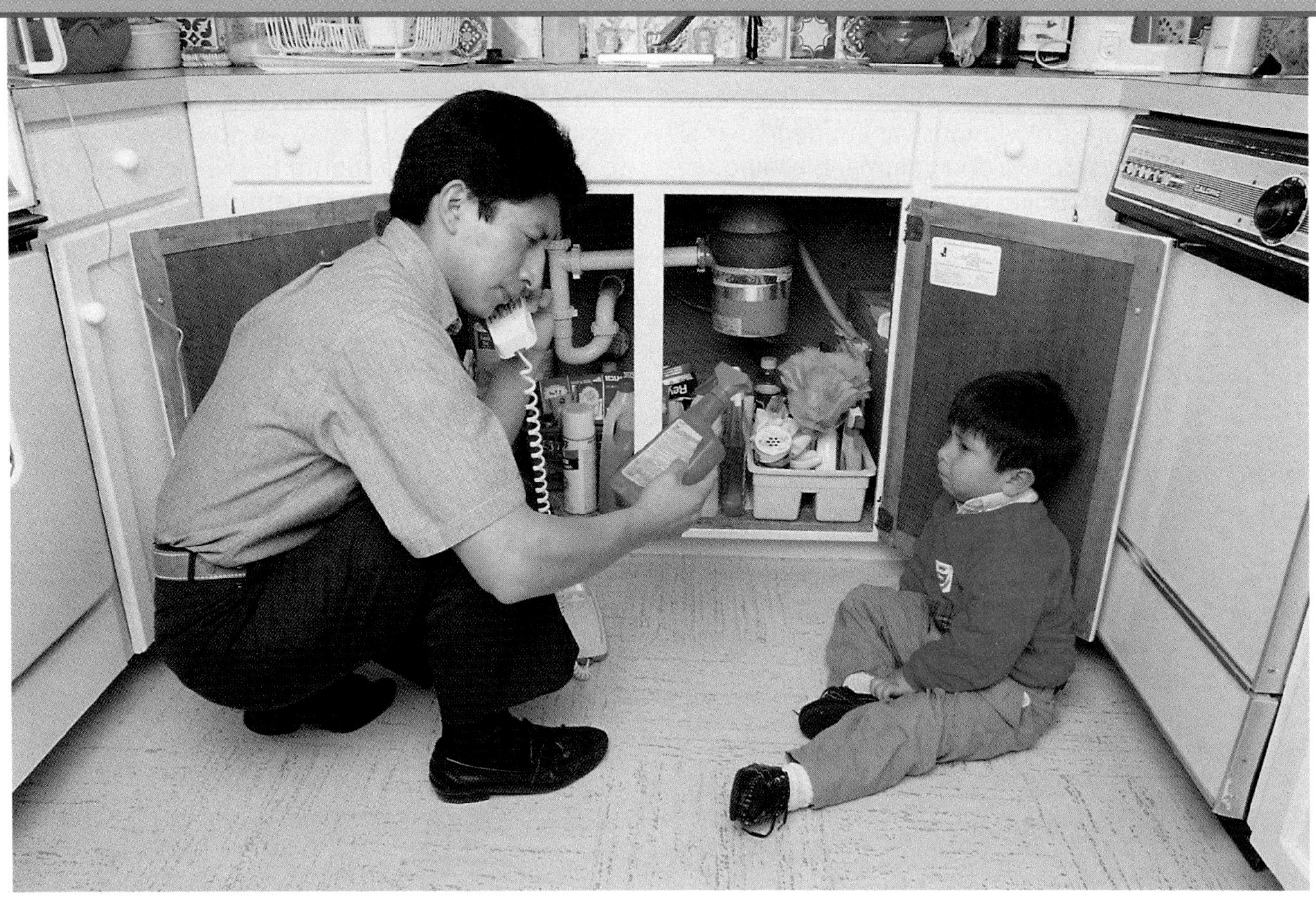

CONTENT BACKGROUND Misconceptions About First Aid

STAY CALM, USE COMMON SENSE, AND apply basic information: these are the first rules of administering first aid. In many situations, however, people are confronted with misconceptions and fears that get in their way. Preparedness is crucial. Following are some common misconceptions about medical emergencies. The person who learns about these ahead of time can avoid making poor decisions under the pressure of a real emergency.

Most frightening to any witness of an accident is the large amount of blood on and around the victim. The sight of blood is terrifying to the person offering first aid, and the natural inclination is to attend to the wounds first. This can be a fatal mistake. Head wounds are very common and bleed profusely, inordinately in proportion to their severity. In a documented incident, an individual who had received a minor head wound, which the first-aid giver attended immediately, died because no one attended to an airway obstruction. If a wound is so severe as to be immediately life threatening, it must be attended to, but not at the expense of restoring breathing. Severe brain damage occurs after four minutes without oxygen. Usually, breathing is the primary consideration for aiding the survival of the victim.

Fainting is another symptom that can frighten bystanders, but it is not a cause for panic, as people sometimes think. It is an indicator that something is wrong, and the fainting victim needs to be revived as quickly as possible. Fainting will cause an individual who is lacking blood circulation to the brain to establish a horizontal posture. The horizontal posture is best for getting the brain at or below the level of the heart and restoring oxygenation. Fainting is the body's natural defense mechanism to restore muscular relaxation and equilibrium.

Misconceptions about convulsions or seizures, are also common. Convulsions vary in degree and may be caused by low blood volume, bleeding, dehydration, heatstroke, previous head injuries, epilepsy, or diabetes. The first step in helping a person who has convulsions is to place the person in a horizontal position to increase blood flow to the brain. Lay the person on his or her side. Do not restrain the person, except when injury may be caused by thrashing. Restraining the individual can cause back and joint injuries. Never place any object into the mouth, because it can push the tongue into a position that restricts the airway. The object could potentially be aspirated. If the convulsions are clearly a result of overheating and the skin is clammy, rehydrate the person after the convulsions stop. If the skin is dry, cool the person as a first priority and then rehydrate.

Another source of confusion is poisoning. Many people panic because they do not know whether to give a universal antidote to the victim or to induce vomiting. A universal antidote does not actually exist. For unconscious victims, or those having convulsions or any difficulty breathing, call 911. If the person is not in distress, can swallow, and can breathe, call your poison control center. Do not follow the directions on the back of the bottle or container of the poison, because they are often in error. Follow the directions given to you by the poison control center only.

Misconceptions about first aid can be fatal. Learning the correct ways of responding to and dealing with emergencies can help ensure the survival of a person in need of first aid. The best way of becoming informed is to enroll in a first-aid class and receive CPR training.

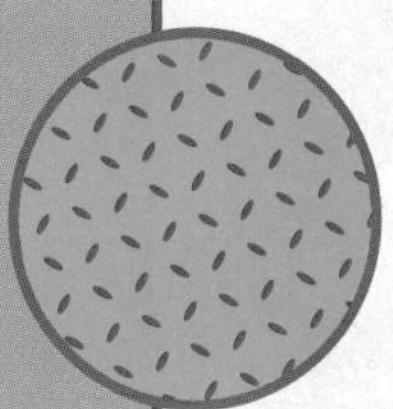

PLANNING FOR INSTRUCTION

KEY FACTS

- **First aid, immediate care given before professional medical help is available, can mean the difference between life and death.**
- **In an emergency, the recommended first steps are: evaluate the situation; rescue the victim if it is necessary and can be done safely; send for medical help.**
- **In giving first aid, check immediately to see if the victim's airway is open, if the victim is breathing, and if the victim's heart is beating.**
- **In giving first aid, treat problems in this order: restore breathing, restore heart action (if you have been trained to do so), control bleeding, treat poisoning, assess other injuries, and treat for shock.**
- **In cases where the victim has suffered an injury to the head, neck, or spine, the victim should not be moved.**
- **The Heimlich maneuver is the recommended method for dislodging an object from the throat of a person who is choking.**
- **A victim of heat exhaustion should be moved to a cool place and, if conscious and not nauseated, given fluids. A victim of heatstroke must be cooled with water or wet cloths, given fluids in small quantities if conscious, and taken to an emergency room.**
- **Frostbite should be treated by slow warming of the affected area. Hypothermia should be treated by warming the trunk of the body and obtaining medical help immediately.**
- **To prevent infection, bites—whether from a human, dog, snake, or other animal—should be treated by cleaning the wound with soap and water. Medical attention should be obtained as soon as possible for poisonous bites, allergic reactions to venom, possibility of rabies, and prevention of tetanus.**
- **Treatment of burns depends on the severity of the burn. Medical attention is required for all second-degree and third-degree burns.**
- **When poisoning is suspected, the nearest poison control center should be contacted immediately for instructions.**

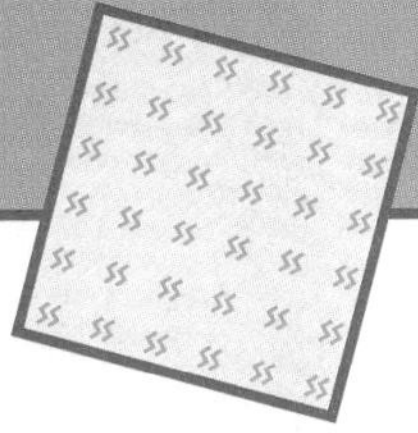

MYTHS AND MISCONCEPTIONS

MYTH: In a life-threatening emergency, the safest action is to wait for medical help to arrive.

Medical help may not arrive in time to save a person's life, and first aid administered by a lay person can mean the difference between life and death.

MYTH: Frostbite should be treated by rubbing snow on the affected area.

Frostbite is the freezing of tissues; treatment involves slowly warming the tissues, not making them colder.

MYTH: Burns should be treated by covering the affected area with butter.

Neither butter nor any over-the-counter ointment should be applied to severe burns. First-degree burns can be treated with an ointment specifically designed for the purpose and administered by a doctor.

MYTH: A person who swallows poison must be made to vomit.

Many poisons are caustic and should be diluted with fluids rather than evacuated by vomiting.

VOCABULARY

Essential: The following vocabulary terms appear in boldface type.

first aid
cardiopulmonary resuscitation (CPR)
fracture
dislocation
sprain
strain
Heimlich maneuver
cardiac arrest
stroke
hypothermia

Secondary: Be aware that the following terms may come up during class discussion.

rescue breathing
shock
Good Samaritan law
splint
epilepsy
scalds

FOR STUDENTS WITH SPECIAL NEEDS

Kinesthetic Learners: Students might be helped by practicing the first-aid skills learned in this chapter in role-playing situations.

At-Risk Students: During role-playing situations, assign these students roles that involve decision making and treatment. Such assignments will help build self-esteem.

LEP Students: Have students make a chart that lists the types of emergencies covered in this chapter. Then ask them to write in the chart any words concerning each emergency that they do not understand. Go over the charts with them to clarify definitions.

ENRICHMENT

- Encourage students to organize a first-aid information booth in the school cafeteria or in some other suitable location. Students can obtain pamphlets on first aid and health emergencies from professional organizations, such as the local fire department and hospital, and distribute them at the booth. Students could also give information on how to sign up for first-aid courses, CPR training, and other similar courses.
- Have interested students interview the nurse or health clerk at the school to find out what kinds of emergencies the school is prepared to handle. Have them list the accidents, disasters, and conditions covered, and the location and kind of equipment available.

CHAPTER 28
CHAPTER OPENER

GETTING STARTED

Using the Chapter Photograph

Ask students to describe what is taking place in the photograph. Have them speculate on what may have occurred. As students suggest possible reasons for the medical emergency, list their speculations on the chalkboard. Then have students discuss how they might respond to each emergency if medical help were not available.

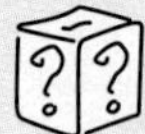 **Question Box**

In this chapter, students will study procedures for dealing with emergency situations. The Question Box provides students with an opportunity to ask questions anonymously. To ensure that students with questions are not embarrassed to be seen writing, have students who do not have questions write something else—perhaps a description of a medical emergency that they witnessed.

Preview the questions and then answer them at appropriate points in the chapter. You may wish to allow students to write additional anonymous questions as they go through the chapter.

CHAPTER 28

First Aid and CPR

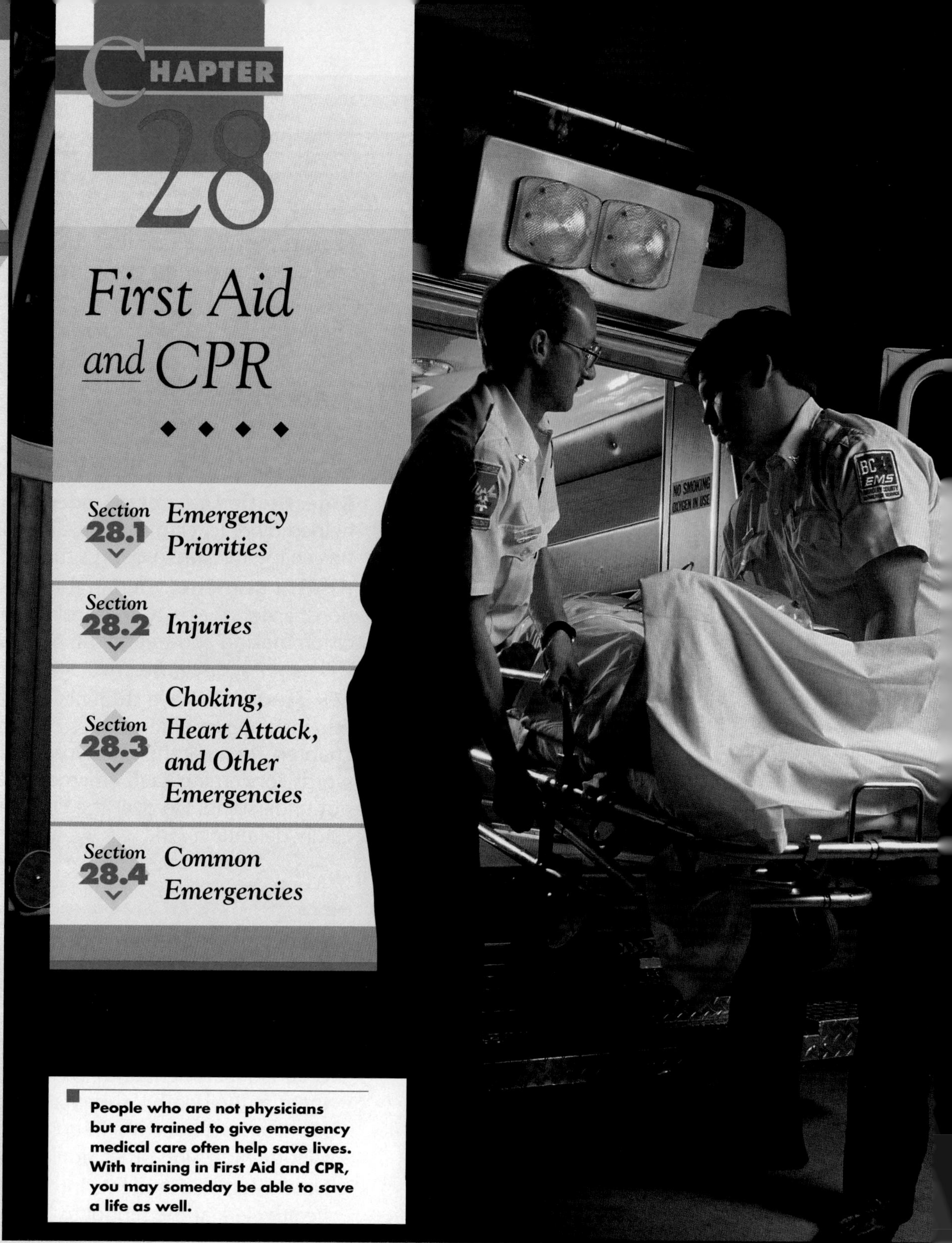

People who are not physicians but are trained to give emergency medical care often help save lives. With training in First Aid and CPR, you may someday be able to save a life as well.

Personal Issues *ALERT*

Some students may have experienced a serious medical emergency. A student who has been injured in such a situation may find that recalling his or her experience is painful and troublesome. A student who has witnessed such an emergency involving a family member or friend may also find that recalling the situation is upsetting. Care must be exercised in eliciting personal experiences concerning these situations.

Some medical emergencies are the result of violent personal attacks. Students who have experienced or witnessed such attacks are likely to be uncomfortable discussing these incidents, particularly where family violence is involved.

The late afternoon sun hung low in the sky as Sonya walked home, her jacket collar pulled up against the chill autumn air. She heard the swish of leaves behind her, and Masahiko streaked past her on his bicycle.

While Sonya watched in horror, a driver pulled out of a parking place directly in front of Masahiko. Unable to brake in time, Masahiko crashed into the side of the car and flew off his bike. His head slammed into the curb.

Looking around for help, Sonya saw no one. She was on her own. What should she do first? How could she tell whether Masahiko was injured seriously? How should she treat his injuries?

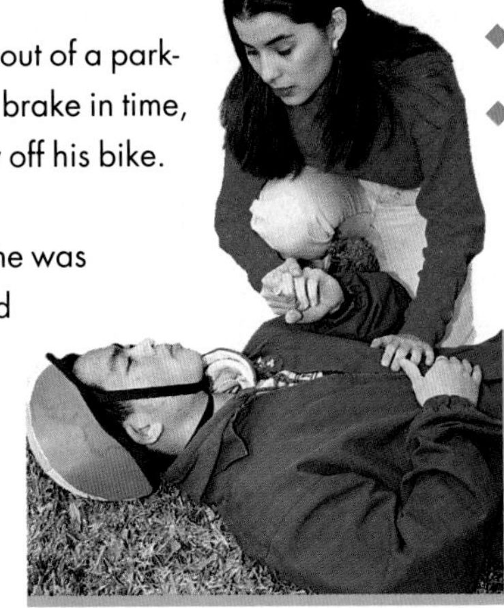

Section 28.1 Emergency Priorities

Objectives

- *Name the first steps that should be taken during an emergency.*
- *Describe the procedure for rescue breathing.*
  LIFE SKILLS: Intervention Strategies
- *Describe the procedures for stopping or controlling bleeding.*
  LIFE SKILLS: Intervention Strategies
- *Describe the signs of shock and its treatment.*
- *List two facilities that might offer CPR training.*
  LIFE SKILLS: Using Community Resources

You never know when an emergency may occur, or in what form. You could be needed to help the victims of a hurricane, earthquake, car collision, or sporting accident. A classmate could be wounded in metal shop, or a person near you at a concert could collapse from a drug overdose.

In this chapter you will learn how to respond in an emergency when lives could depend on what you do next. You will learn what to do first and about treatment priorities. After studying the chapter, you will know how to treat many medical emergencies. To find out how to get specialized training, complete the Life Skills activity on page 617.

First Aid: The Difference Between Life and Death

First aid is the immediate care given until professional medical personnel arrive at the

first aid: *emergency care given to an ill or injured person before medical attention is available.*

Background
First Aid
Standard first-aid techniques were introduced by the St. John's Ambulance Association in 1877 in London. In 1882, the State Charities Association in New York became the first American group to offer training in first aid. Other groups, including the American National Red Cross, became interested in first aid and began teaching courses. In 1907, Clara Barton was instrumental in setting up the International First Aid Committee, an organization of groups from many countries committed to instruction in first aid.

Section 28.1 Lesson Plan

MOTIVATE

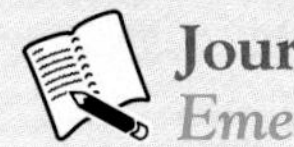

Journal 28A
Emergencies
This may be done as a warm-up activity. Encourage students to record in the Student Journal in the Student Activity Book descriptions of their involvement in emergency situations in which another person was the victim. Suggest that they write down any steps that they took to help the victim. Or have them note what others did to help the victim.

TEACH

Role-Playing
What Should Sonya Do?
Select students to play the roles of Masahiko, the driver, and Sonya. Have the students act out the situation described in the text from the point just after Masahiko is injured. Point out that it is up to Sonya to take whatever steps are necessary to assist Masahiko. Have the class jot down the actions that Sonya takes. You may wish to have several groups act out these roles.

Class Discussion
What Actions Were Needed?
Have students discuss why someone in an emergency situation might fail to take appropriate action. Point out that, in an emergency, someone with knowledge about how to proceed is

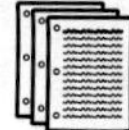

Personal Health Inventory

Have students complete the Personal Health Inventory for this chapter. The inventory helps them assess their own behavior with respect to injuries and emergency situations.

scene of an accident or sudden illness. Sonya knew that appropriate first aid could mean the difference between life and death or between recovery and permanent injury. If Masahiko was seriously injured, Sonya had only seconds to act. Prompt medical attention was essential.

Sonya made an effort to compose herself, then ran to Masahiko. He wasn't moving. The car's driver, a man of about 50, seemed unhurt but was almost hysterical. He was beating his fists on the steering wheel and crying, "What have I done?" Grabbing the man by the arm, Sonya asked him to calm down, find a telephone, dial 911, report the emergency, and then come back to tell her when the ambulance and paramedics would arrive.

Sonya then turned to Masahiko, tapped him on the shoulder, and asked in a loud voice, "Masahiko, are you all right?"

Masahiko still did not move, but he groaned and muttered "No."

Steps To Take in a Medical Emergency

1. *Survey the scene.*
2. *Rescue the person if necessary to prevent further injury.*
3. *Send for help.*
4. *Treat life-threatening conditions.*
5. *Go for help yourself if nobody has done so.*
6. *Identify other injuries, and provide first aid.*
7. *Remain with the victim until medical help arrives. Monitor breathing and heart rate, and prevent further injury.*

(FIGURE 28-1) **Follow these steps if you are the first person to arrive at the scene of a medical emergency. Do not risk your safety to rescue or give first aid to someone else.**

First Steps in a Medical Emergency

If you are the first person to arrive on the scene of a medical emergency, there are certain steps you should take. Figure 28-1 summarizes these steps. Do not, however, risk your own safety in order to rescue or provide first aid to another person.

Survey the Scene First, evaluate the situation and the area for possible danger to you or to the victim. Determine what happened and how many people are injured. Look for and call out for bystanders who can help you.

Rescue If you can do so safely, your next step is to rescue anyone whose life is endangered. For example, a victim in deep water, a burning car, or a room full of poisonous fumes will need to be moved to a safer place before you can even begin to check for injuries. Otherwise, *never* move an injured person until medical help arrives. Moving someone who has a head, neck, or spine injury could cause further serious, or fatal, injury. Instead, do what you can to protect the person from further injury.

Because of the nature of Masahiko's accident, Sonya knew that he could have suffered a head or neck injury. Until she knew the full extent of Masahiko's injuries, moving him would risk making his injuries worse. Luckily, a motorist stopped to help. Sonya asked her to park her car crosswise in the street, providing a barrier to protect Masahiko from oncoming traffic. This was Sonya's rescue step.

Send for Medical Help If others are available, send them for medical help. If not, shout "Help!" Do not leave the injured person, even to go for help, until you have checked for and treated life-threatening conditions. People who call for help in an emergency should use the procedure given at the top of page 619.

• • • TEACH continued

better prepared to deal with the situation than someone who has never thought about what he or she might do. How do students judge Sonya's actions as described in the text?

Reinforcement
Dealing With an Emergency

Review with students Figure 28-1, which outlines the steps that a person should take in dealing with an emergency. Have students describe Sonya's action for each step.

Case Study
When to Rescue

Rescue is the second step to be taken in an emergency—if it can be done safely. Read a news story to the class about a rescue that involved serious risk to the rescuer. Pose the question, "Do people who risk their lives to save others violate recommended steps for dealing with an emergency?"

Role-Playing
Getting Help

Have one student play the victim of an accident. Allow this student to describe the kind of accident that occurred, where the accident took place, and the nature of the injuries. Have a second student role-play a citizen who is using the telephone to call for assistance. Repeat the role-playing procedure with other students, changing the circumstances of the accident.

Life SKILLS: Using Community Resources

First Aid and CPR Training

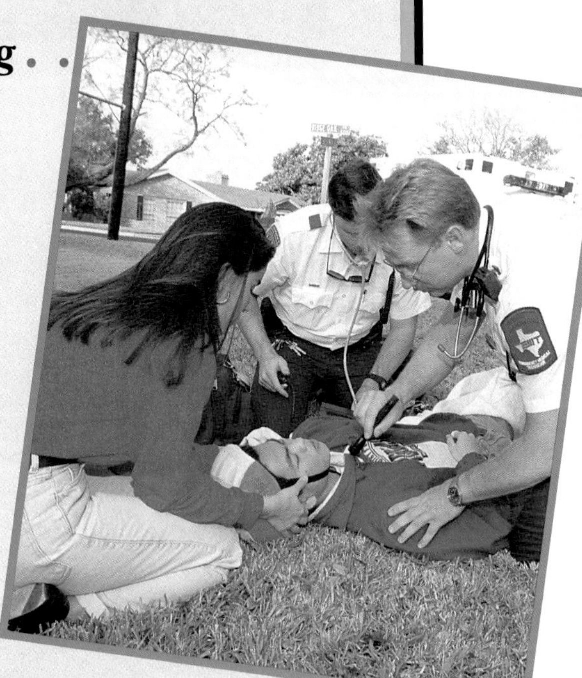

You never know when you may be called upon to give emergency care to help save a life, prevent further injury, or simply lessen discomfort. People in certain professions are required to study emergency care. For example, boat captains, flight attendants, police officers, and firefighters all need to be certified in first aid and cardiopulmonary resuscitation (CPR). Knowledge of emergency care can also be extremely important for anyone who spends time in the wilderness. On a hunting or backpacking trip, for instance, people may be miles from the nearest vehicle or medical facility. First aid may be the only care an injured person receives for hours, days, or even weeks.

First-Aid Training If you have not already taken a first-aid course, you may wish to do so. The course will give you hands-on experience that will help you remember the techniques described in this book. First-aid courses are given by the American Red Cross, local community colleges, and hospitals.

CPR Training Someday you may be able to save a life if you are trained in CPR. A local chapter of the American Red Cross or the American Heart Association will be able to tell you where training is available.

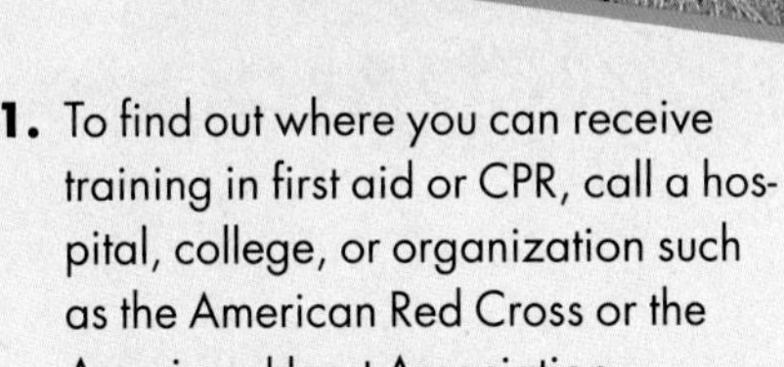

1. To find out where you can receive training in first aid or CPR, call a hospital, college, or organization such as the American Red Cross or the American Heart Association.
2. Find out when the courses are given.
3. Ask if there is a charge for the course.
4. Find the number of the nearest poison control center, and post it near a telephone you use.

Life SKILLS
First Aid and CPR Training

Have students read the Life Skills feature. Then have them investigate where they can obtain first-aid training and training in CPR. Encourage students to consider enrolling in such courses with friends.

Demonstration
Opening the Airway

Have a volunteer play the role of an unconscious accident victim. Demonstrate for the class the proper method of opening the victim's airway. Have several students rehearse the method under your supervision.

Demonstration
Rescue Breathing

Bring in a doll to use in demonstrating how to perform rescue breathing. Ask for a volunteer to act as a rescuer who must save a young child who has stopped breathing. Allow the student to refer to Figure 28-2 as he or she administers rescue breathing. Have the class critique the procedure.

Demonstration
Finding the Carotid Artery

Show students how to locate their carotid artery. They can refer to Figure 28-3 for assistance. Have selected students find the artery on each other, demonstrating the proper technique for the class.

Role-Playing
Controlling Bleeding

Select one student to play the role of an accident victim with severe bleeding from the upper arm. Select another student to play the role of a person who is administering first aid. The rescuer must control the bleeding with whatever materials he or she can obtain in the class. Allow the student to refer to Figure 28-5 as he or she proceeds.

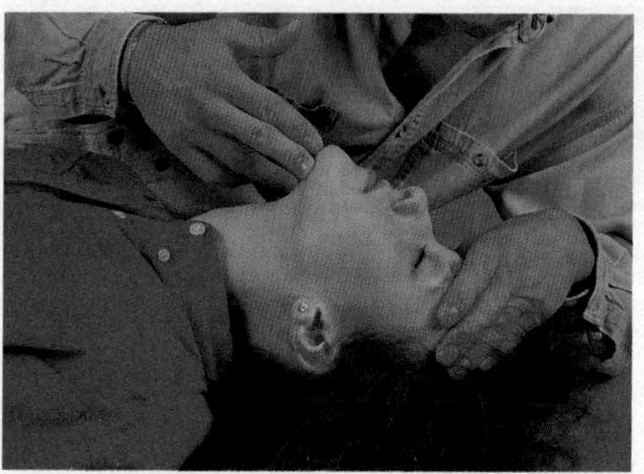

1. Open the airway by tipping the head back and lifting the chin.

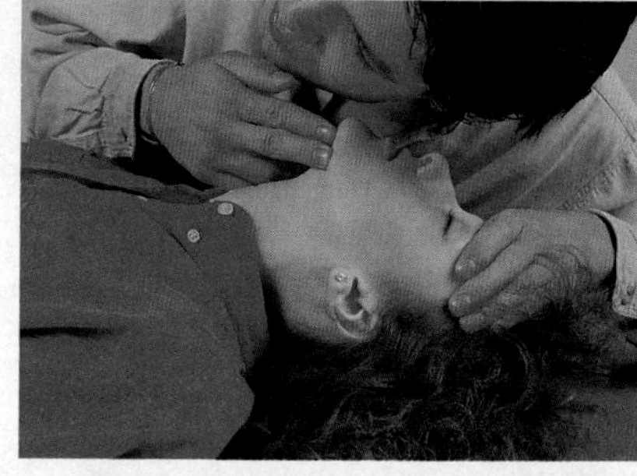

2. Check for breathing by placing your cheek next to the person's nose, then listening and feeling for breath.

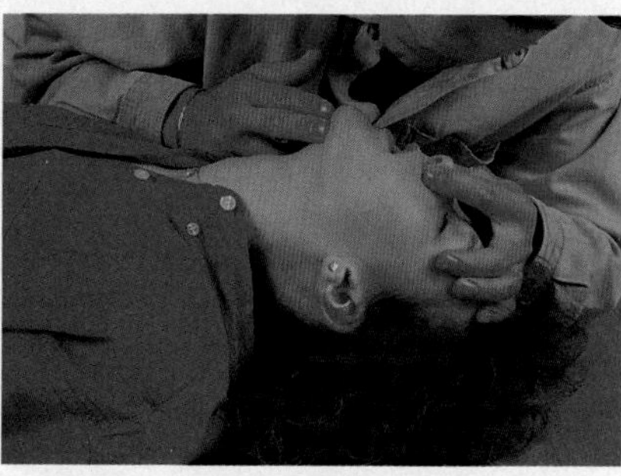

3. Pinch the nose closed with one hand while keeping the airway open by holding the chin up with the other hand.

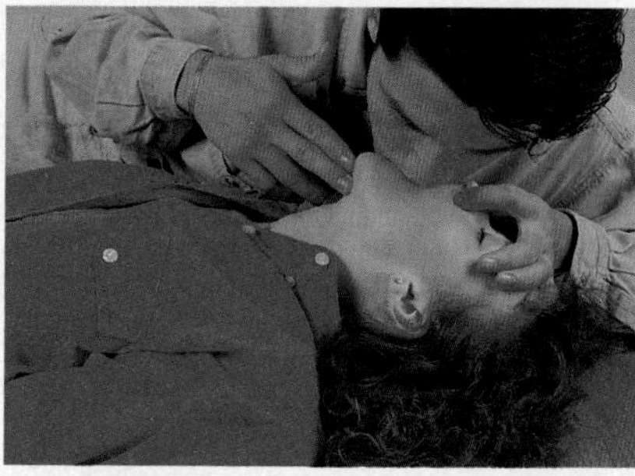

4. Tightly seal your mouth over the victim's mouth and blow air into the victim's lungs, or hold the mouth closed and blow into the nose.

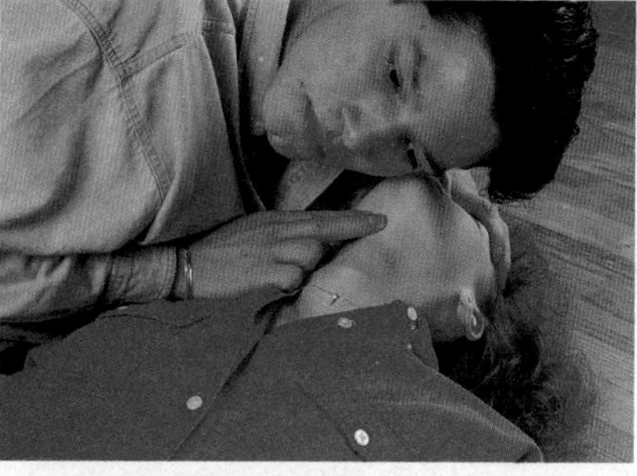

5. After two breaths, check for a pulse and signs of breathing.

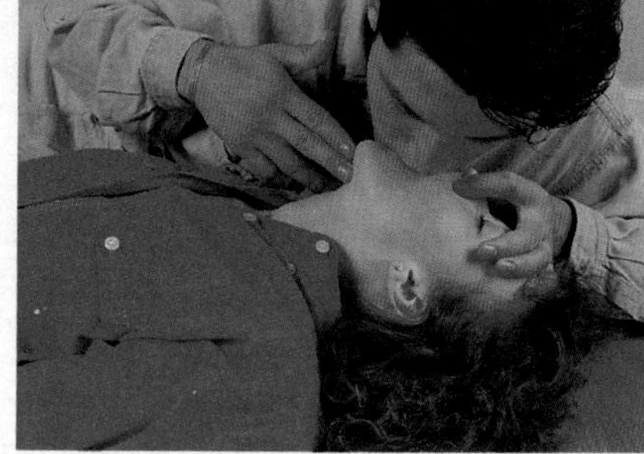

6. Continue to give one breath every 5 seconds until medical help arrives or you are too exhausted to continue.

For young children and babies:
1. Blow into the mouth and nose at the same time.
2. Give one breath every 3 seconds.
3. Use smaller puffs of breath, since the lungs are smaller.

(FIGURE 28-2) **Procedure for opening the airway and giving rescue breathing. Note the differences in the procedure for young children and babies.**

• • • TEACH continued

Journal 28B
AIDS and Accidents

Have students record in the Student Journal in the Student Activity Book any concerns they may have about administering first aid to a person who is HIV-positive or has AIDS. Then encourage them to review what they know about how AIDS is transmitted. Finally, ask them to write how to minimize the risks involved in giving first aid to a person with AIDS.

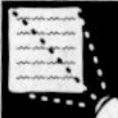

Teaching Transparency 28A
Rescue Breathing

Use the transparency and discuss the procedure for opening the airway and giving rescue breathing.

Class Discussion
What Is Shock?

Although the victim of a serious accident is likely to experience shock, many students may misunderstand the nature of shock. Point out the difference between electric shock (the passage of electric current through the body) and shock (a general collapse of the circulatory system). Although electric shock may produce shock, so may any serious injury. Have students note the signs of shock. **What indications are there that shock involves the circulatory system?** *[Rapid breathing, rapid heart beat, weak pulse, blue color around lips and fingernails]* Some students may have experienced mild or severe shock as a result of injury. Ask

When calling for help:

- Speak slowly and clearly.
- Tell exactly where the victim is, including town, address, description of the location, and any landmarks.
- Describe the accident, number of people injured, and nature of the injuries.
- Ask what you should do while waiting for medical help to arrive, and listen carefully to the instructions.
- Let the other person hang up first, to be sure they have no more questions or advice for you.

Initial Assessment Priorities

When giving first aid, treat life-threatening conditions first by following the procedure described below.

Determine Whether the Victim Is Conscious Tap the person on the shoulder, and ask loudly, "Are you all right?" Even though Masahiko answered "No," his answer told Sonya that he was conscious.

Check ABCs If the person is unconscious, check the ABCs: *A*irway, *B*reathing, and *C*irculation of blood. Check in this order, because a person whose airway is closed will stop breathing, and when breathing stops, the heart will soon stop circulating blood. Sonya checked all ABCs at once by asking if Masahiko was all right. Anyone who can talk, however poorly, has an open airway, can breathe, and has a beating heart.

Airway To open the airway, turn the person gently onto his or her back after checking for head, neck, and spinal injuries. If the person has such injuries, do not move him or her until the head and neck have been stabilized. With one hand under the chin and one on the forehead, lift the chin and tip the head back as shown in Figure 28-2.

Breathing Check for breathing by putting your cheek next to the person's nose and mouth and listening and feeling for breath. Also watch the chest to see if it is rising and falling. If the victim is not breathing, start rescue breathing at once, using the procedure shown in Figure 28-2. If the person's airway is open, your breath should easily enter his or her lungs and the chest will rise. The person should exhale automatically when you remove your mouth to take a breath. If your breath will not enter the victim's lungs, repeat the procedure for opening the airway.

Circulation of Blood Look for a pulse to determine whether the heart is working. The easiest pulse to find is usually at the carotid artery in the neck. You can find it in the groove on either side of the windpipe, beside the Adam's apple, as shown in Figure 28-3.

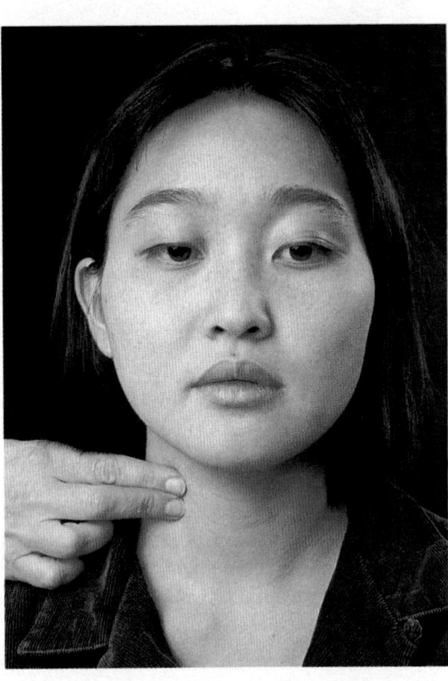

(FIGURE 28-3) **Check circulation by feeling for a pulse at the carotid artery on the side of the neck.**

those students to describe what being in shock was like.

Role-Playing
Treating Shock

Have a student role-play an accident victim who is going into shock. Have another student play the role of a person who is administering first aid. Have this person demonstrate the proper procedure for preventing and treating shock. Have the class critique the effort. Repeat the role-playing with two more students.

Debate the Issue
Being a Good Samaritan

Select two small teams of students to debate whether it is okay to refuse to give first aid to an injured person because of the risk of being sued for incompetent treatment. Point out to the debaters that, although most states have laws protecting individuals who try to help victims, laws vary and final interpretation may be in the hands of a judge or jury. After the debate, poll the class about their attitudes on the proposition.

Journal 28C
Reviewing First Aid

Have students read over their journal entries describing emergencies they witnessed. Have them compare how the emergencies were handled with what they now know about dealing with emergencies. Ask them to write in the Student Journal whether they would have acted any differently, in view of the knowledge they now have about handling emergencies.

CPR for Adults:

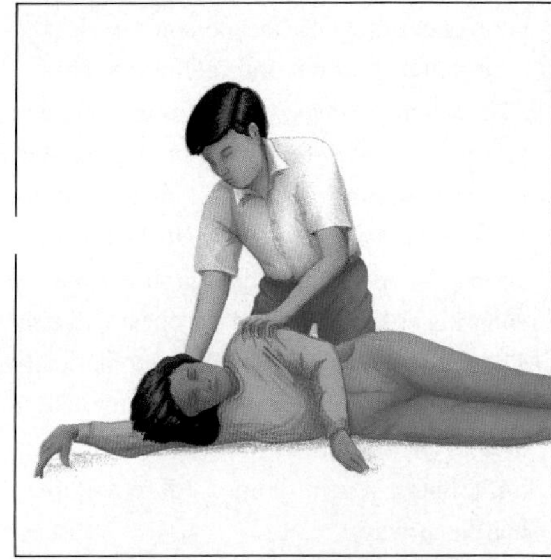

1. Lay the person on his or her back.

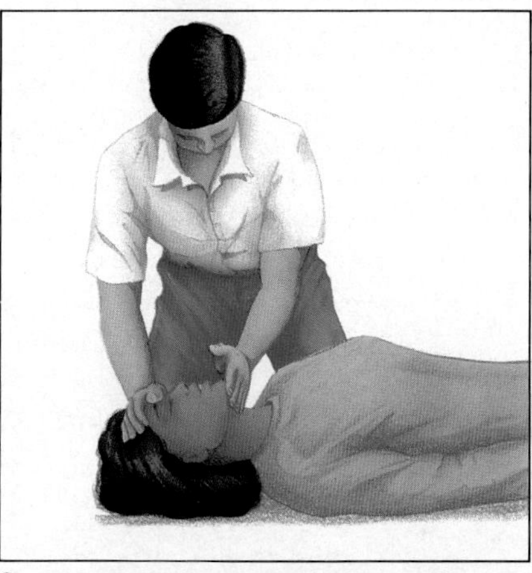

2. Open the airway as previously described, and give two quick but full breaths.

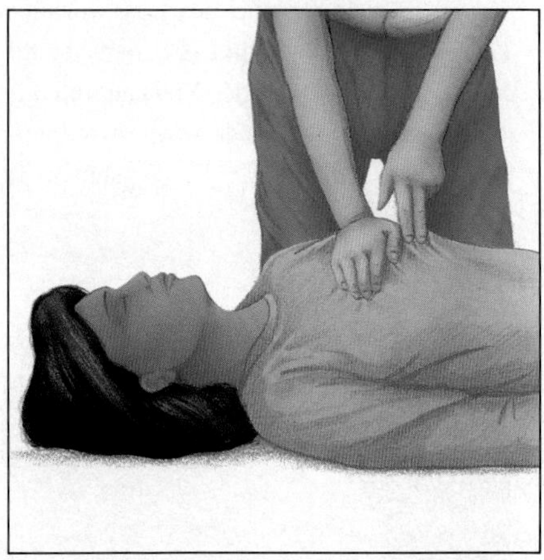

3. Place the heel of the hand nearest the victim's head on the breastbone, starting two finger-widths up from the bottom of the victim's breastbone, and your other hand directly on top of your first hand.

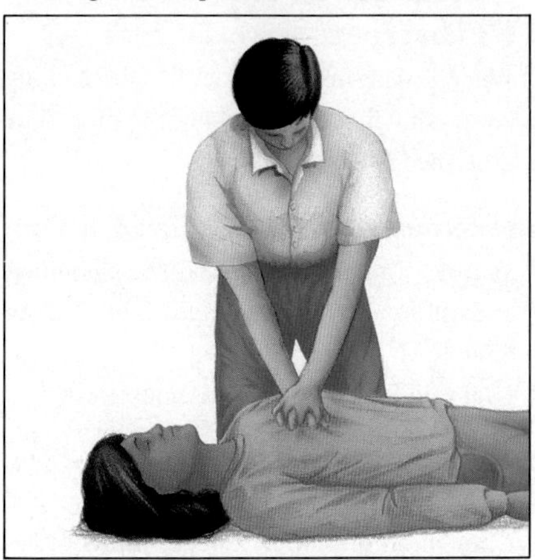

4. With your arms straight, put your weight on your hands and press down on the sternum, then release the pressure so the chest can expand. Give compressions at a rate of 80-100 thrusts per minute. After 15 compressions, give two rescue breaths. After 4 sets of 15 compresssions and two breaths, stop and check for a pulse. If the victim has a pulse, stop giving compressions. If not, repeat this step.

CPR for Young Children and Babies:
Follow the same basic procedure as above, with the following exceptions.

1. An infant should be held, with one hand supporting the head.
2. Use two or three fingers instead of your hands.
3. Depress the sternum only 1/2 to 1 inch.
4. Give compressions at a rate of 2 per second, about as fast as you can do it.

(FIGURE 28-4) **Procedure for performing CPR. Note the differences for young children and babies. If two rescuers know CPR, one does the chest compressions and the other gives a rescue breath after every five compressions.**

• • • TEACH continued

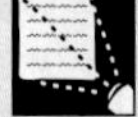

Teaching Transparency 28B
Unconscious Victim

Use the transparency and discuss emergency priorities. Discuss how a rescuer checks items in order and provides treatment at every step before moving on to the next.

Extension
Obtaining Expert Advice

Have students write a class letter to a paramedic team that works in your area, describing the accident used as an example at the beginning of this section (Masahiko's bicycle accident). Have students describe what Sonya did and ask the paramedics whether she acted correctly and what else, if anything, she should have done.

CPR Procedures If you cannot find the victim's pulse and you are trained in the procedure, you may be able to save his or her life with **cardiopulmonary resuscitation (CPR)**. Figure 28-4 describes CPR. *Do not attempt CPR with the instructions from this or any other book unless you've had CPR training.* Improperly administered, CPR can cause further injury. Study these directions for understanding of CPR, or use them for review if you are trained or for study if you plan to receive training.

CPR is hard work. It's all right not to start CPR if you don't feel up to it or aren't sure you know how. If you do start CPR, be prepared to keep on without pause until (1) you are relieved by another trained CPR provider, (2) a professional medical person pronounces the victim dead, or (3) you are simply too exhausted to continue. If, after CPR, the victim's heart starts beating on its own, check for breathing and continue rescue breathing if needed.

CPR is given *only* when a person is not breathing and has no pulse (heartbeat). Such a person is technically dead. If CPR is successful in reviving the person, he or she will most likely require additional medical treatment to remain alive. For this reason, you should always call 911 for emergency medical assistance, or send someone to call for you, before beginning CPR.

Control Bleeding If an injured person's breathing and circulation are adequate, the next priority is to stop severe bleeding that is life threatening. Use direct pressure, as described in Figure 28-5.

If you do not have sterile gauze, you will have to make do with whatever clean materials you have. Sanitary napkins make ideal dressings, and sometimes they are available when other materials are not. They are sold in restroom vending machines, and female bystanders may be carrying them in their purses.

cardiopulmonary resuscitation (CPR): *a lifesaving procedure designed to revive a person who is not breathing and has no heartbeat.*

Procedure to Stop Bleeding

1. *If possible, cover the wound with a clean dressing, such as several layers of sterile gauze.*
2. *If possible, raise the bleeding wound above the heart.*
3. *Use your palm to apply pressure directly over the dressing on the bleeding wound. Keep applying pressure for at least 10–12 minutes, to give blood clots time to form.*
4. *If bleeding starts again, resume pressure until it stops.*
5. *Wrap a pressure bandage tightly over the dressing. Do not remove blood-soaked bandages or dressings. If blood soaks through, place another dressing on top.*

(FIGURE 28-5) **Follow these steps to stop or control severe bleeding. If it is not stopped, the victim might bleed to death before medical help arrives. Take steps to avoid direct contact with someone else's blood.**

SECTION 28.1

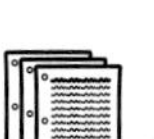

Section Review Worksheet 28.1

Assign Section Review Worksheet 28.1, which requires students to supply information about first-aid priorities and evaluate statements about shock.

Section Quiz 28.1

Have students take Section Quiz 28.1.

Reteaching Worksheet 28.1

Students who have difficulty with the material may complete Reteaching Worksheet 28.1, which requires them to supply and sequence the first steps in an emergency health-care crisis.

Background

Shock

Shock can be thought of as severe circulatory distress. Shock can result from fluid loss, most commonly blood loss. But shock can accompany injuries in which there is no noticeable loss of blood. During shock, blood supply to the extremities, including skeletal muscles and skin, is reduced. Heart action is weak. Breathing is shallow. The victim may become lightheaded and weak. Shock may be immediate, or it may develop several hours after an injury. In treating a victim during an emergency, the rescuer must always be alert for signs of shock. Untreated, shock can be fatal.

Review Answers

1. Survey the scene; rescue the person if necessary to prevent further injury; send for help.

2. Answers should agree with information shown in Figure 28-2.

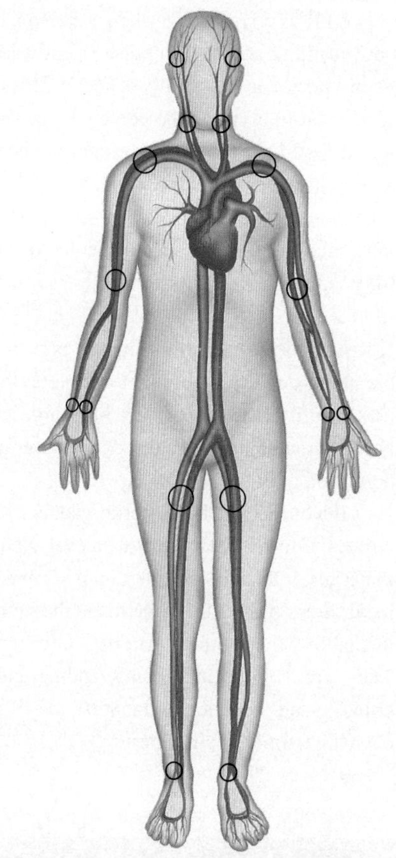

(FIGURE 28-6) **The body's pressure points are the locations of main arteries and veins. To stop bleeding, apply pressure with your fingers or the heel of your hand to the pressure point *nearest* the bleeding wound that is *between* the heart and the wound. Except for the head, this point would be just above the wound.**

If direct pressure and elevation do not stop bleeding on the head or a limb, apply pressure to the main artery supplying blood to the affected part. The places on the body where these arteries are located are called pressure points. Figure 28-6 shows the body's pressure points.

Try to avoid direct contact with someone else's blood, because it can carry an organism or a virus that causes a very serious disease such as hepatitis or AIDS. If your first-aid kit has rubber gloves, wear them. Otherwise, put something between your hand and the wound. You can, for example, place the victim's hand between yours and the wound. After providing first aid to a bleeding victim, wash your hands immediately. Meanwhile, do not eat or drink, and keep your hands away from your eyes, nose, and mouth.

Treat Poisoning As soon as the victim's ABCs are in order and bleeding is stopped, you must treat poisoning if it has occurred. (You'll learn how to treat poisoning later in the chapter.)

Assess Other Injuries The next step in handling an emergency is to look carefully for other injuries. If the person is conscious, ask him or her what hurts. Very gently, inspect the person's body for anything that looks broken or not quite right.

Look for Signs of Shock You must watch for signs of shock when helping an injured person or a victim of a serious accident. Shock is a condition in which the body's vital processes are severely depressed—circulation and breathing slow way down. If the shock process is not stopped, the person will die. Shock can result from major injuries, loss of blood, burns, poisoning, electric shock, allergic reactions, and sudden temperature changes. Even when the victim of a serious accident appears uninjured, he or she can have hidden injuries that could cause shock. Shock can kill a person even when the injury that triggered it is not life threatening.

The signs of shock include rapid, shallow breathing; rapid heartbeat; a weak pulse; pale, clammy skin; blue color around lips and fingernails; nausea; apathy; agitation; and weakness. Any time you start to see signs of shock, call immediately for an ambulance equipped with oxygen.

Treatment for Shock To treat shock, keep the victim calm, lying face up with feet elevated 10 to 12 in. This helps supply more blood to the brain. Victims who are unconscious or who may vomit should have their head turned to the side so they will not choke on their vomit. Do not elevate the feet if you suspect a head injury.

A shock victim's normal body temperature needs to be maintained. In some cases, you may need to cool an overheated shock victim, but usually you need to keep the victim warm. Cover or wrap the victim just enough to maintain body temperature.

Sonya treated Masahiko for shock immediately after checking his ABCs and determining that he was not bleeding severely. She knew that treatment is much more likely to be successful, and to save a life, if it is begun *before* signs of shock have started to appear. This means that any time you are treating an injury that might cause shock, you should begin treating for shock right away.

Because it was a chilly afternoon and getting colder, Sonya sent the motorist who had stopped to help to get blankets from a nearby home. She covered Masahiko with them and watched him closely. Knowing that a shock victim's breathing or heartbeat can fail, Sonya was ready to provide rescue breathing and, because she was trained, start CPR if necessary.

Attitude

It is important to approach an emergency situation with a calm and reassuring attitude. If you are upset or panicky, the victim will sense it and possibly become more panicked. That's why Sonya took control of herself after Masahiko's accident. Try to reassure injured persons that you will help them and that they will be all right. Since fear can bring on shock, calm reassurance can help save a victim's life. The power of fear is so great that people have died after being bitten by nonpoisonous snakes!

Good Samaritan Laws

Most states have a Good Samaritan law that will protect you from legal liability if you help someone in an emergency. As long as you do your best, use common sense, and are careful not to cause unnecessary harm to the injured person, the law should shield you from any legal problems. However, do not attempt procedures in which you have had no training.

Review

1. *What are the first three steps that should be taken in an emergency?*
2. ***LIFE SKILLS: Intervention Strategies*** *Explain how to provide rescue breathing.*
3. ***LIFE SKILLS: Intervention Strategies*** *How would you stop severe bleeding?*
4. *When and how would you treat a person for shock?*
5. ***LIFE SKILLS: Using Community Resources*** *Find out where you can get CPR and first-aid training in your community. Write or call two of these places and obtain a schedule of their classes.*
6. ***Critical Thinking*** *You are the first to arrive on the scene of an auto accident where there are two victims. How will you decide which victim to treat first?*

Section 28.1

Answers to Questions 1 and 2 are on p. 622.

3. Answers should agree with information given in Figure 28-5.

4. When the person has suffered major injuries or shows one of the following signs of shock: rapid, shallow breathing; rapid heart beat; a weak pulse; pale, clammy skin; blue color around lips and fingernails; nausea; apathy; agitation; and weakness. Treatment involves keeping the victim calm, lying face up with feet elevated. Unconscious victims should have their head turned to the side. Cover the victim to maintain body temperature.

5. Answers may include the local chapter of the American Red Cross or the American Heart Association, the fire department, continuing education classes at a high school or college, the community education department of the local hospital, or the YWCA or YMCA.

6. Answers will vary, but students should indicate that they first need to assess each victim and treat the victim whose life is in the greatest danger.

ASSESS

Section Review

Have students answer the Section Review questions.

Alternative Assessment

Responsible Action

Tell students to imagine that they have witnessed an accident in which a person has fallen down a flight of stairs and is not moving. Have students write down the steps that they would take if they were the first or only person on the scene.

Closure

The Danger of Shock

Have students describe shock and how to treat it. Then have them explain why an accident victim must always be checked for signs of shock. Ask each student, in turn, to suggest an incident in which a victim might go into shock.

Background
Tourniquets
A tourniquet is a constricting device that is used as a last resort to control severe bleeding. A tourniquet is applied only when a large artery in a limb is severed and cannot be closed or when a section of a limb has been partially or totally severed.

A tourniquet is made by wrapping a length of cloth twice around the limb, just above the wound. The cloth is then tied once, and a stick, piece of metal, or other sturdy, elongated object is centered on the tied cloth. The cloth is then knotted over the stick and the stick is twisted in a circle until the bleeding stops. Once applied, a tourniquet should be released only by a doctor.

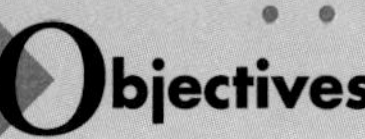

Section 28.2 Injuries

Objectives

- *Differentiate among five types of wounds and their treatment.*
- *Describe the first-aid steps for a fracture.*
- *Describe the first-aid procedures for suspected injuries of the head and spine.*

Injuries that may require first aid occur frequently in daily life. For instance, during athletic events, outdoor activities, or even common activities in the home, you or someone nearby may require first aid for an injury. The following are the recommended first-aid treatments for some common types of injuries.

Wounds

Wounds are among the most common injuries. Figure 28-7 shows the different kinds of wounds and their treatment.

Infections With any type of wound, there is danger that an infection will later develop as invading bacteria begin to multiply. Signs of infection include fever, pus, pain, swelling, and redness. Immunization helps prevent tetanus, which is a very serious, life-threatening infection. Anyone with a serious wound should have a tetanus shot if they are not up-to-date with their immunizations. Anyone who has not had a tetanus shot for more than 10 years should get one whether they have a wound or not.

Scalp Wounds The head has a large supply of blood, and much of it runs near the surface. Consequently, a relatively minor wound of the scalp or face can cause profuse bleeding that must be stopped by applying pressure.

Embedded Foreign Body When a foreign body, such as a piece of glass or even a knife, is embedded in a body part, it should be left in place. If you attempt to take it out, you could easily do more damage than good. Bandage the wound with the foreign body held in place, and get medical help for the victim.

Avoid Contact With Blood Remember that blood and some other body fluids can carry organisms and viruses that cause serious diseases. As much as possible, avoid getting blood or other body fluids on your hands whenever you are treating another person's bleeding wounds.

Blisters

Pressure or friction may cause blisters. Treat blisters as follows:

- Protect an unbroken blister and avoid further pressure or friction.
- Wash a broken blister with soap and water and cover it with a sterile dressing.
- If a blister is likely to break,
  1. wash the area with soap and water,
  2. *do not* attempt to pierce and drain the blister,
  3. cover the blister with a bandage or sterile dressing,
  4. watch for signs of infection, and seek medical attention as needed.

Section 28.2 Lesson Plan

MOTIVATE

Journal 28D
My Injury

This may be done as a warm-up activity. Have students recall an incident in which they were injured. Encourage them to write in the Student Journal a description of how they became injured, how they felt, and what type of assistance or treatment they received immediately after being injured.

TEACH

Class Discussion
Treating Wounds

Use Figure 28-7 to discuss the various types of wounds, their characteristics, and their treatment. Most students have experienced minor wounds; a few students may have had more serious wounds. Allow students to describe how they were wounded and what treatment was required. Then have them compare the recommended treatment for each type of wound. **Which types of wounds might require emergency treatment to stop bleeding?** *[Lacerations, incisions, and avulsions]* **Why should bleeding be encouraged with a puncture wound?** *[To help clean it and reduce the chance of infection]* Help students recognize that many wounds result from accidents, and have them recall that risky behavior and carelessness contribute to many accidents.

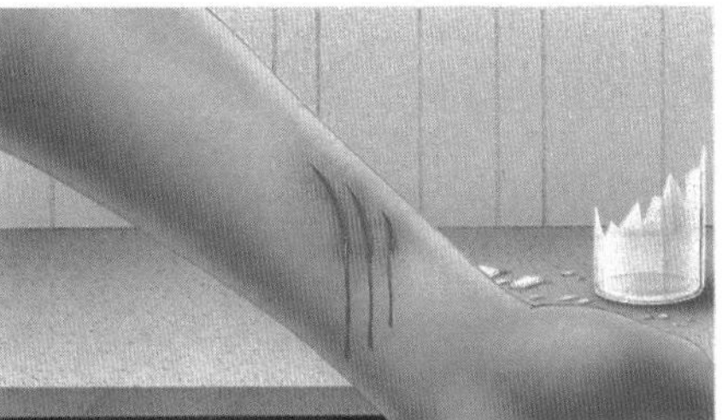

Laceration

In a laceration the skin is torn. Lacerations usually bleed freely, and risk of infection is small if the wound is kept clean. First-aid steps:

1. Stop severe bleeding.
2. Make sure the cut is clean.
3. Cover with a clean sterile dressing.
4. Take victims with serious wounds to a doctor. If you have any doubt about seeing a doctor, you should do so.

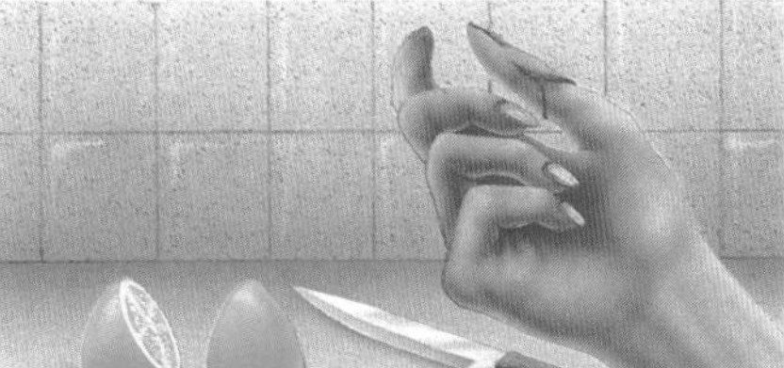

Incision

An incision is a clean cut, as made by a knife or a sharp piece of glass. Incisions usually bleed freely, and risk of infection is small if the wound is kept clean. First-aid steps:

1. Stop severe bleeding.
2. Make sure the cut is clean.
3. Cover with a clean sterile dressing.
4. Take victims with serious wounds to a doctor. If you have any doubt about seeing a doctor, you should do so.

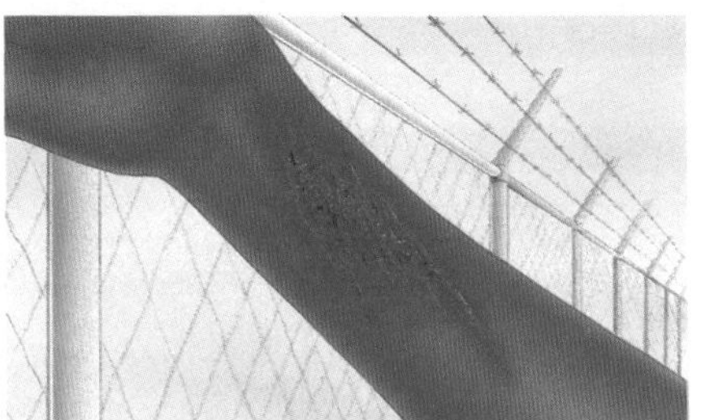

Abrasion

Skin is scraped away or worn away in an abrasion. A skinned knee from falling off a bicycle is a typical abrasion. Many abrasions do not bleed very freely and will need to be washed clean to aviod infection. First-aid steps:

1. Rinse carefully under running water.
2. If dirt or other matter is stuck in the abrasion, try to remove larger pieces by wiping very gently with a clean, damp cloth or tissue. Small bits can be left in place, if necessary, and will work their way out as the wound heals.
3. Cover with a bandage.

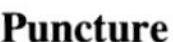

Puncture

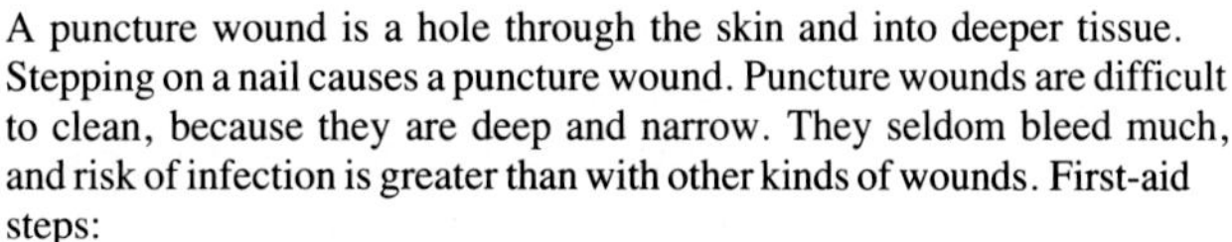

A puncture wound is a hole through the skin and into deeper tissue. Stepping on a nail causes a puncture wound. Puncture wounds are difficult to clean, because they are deep and narrow. They seldom bleed much, and risk of infection is greater than with other kinds of wounds. First-aid steps:

1. Encourage the wound to bleed, to help clean it.
2. Wash the area around the wound to help prevent infection.
3. Because tetanus germs can thrive in a puncture wound, any victim of such a wound should be up-to-date on tetanus shots or make arrangements for a booster immediately.

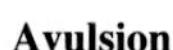

Avulsion

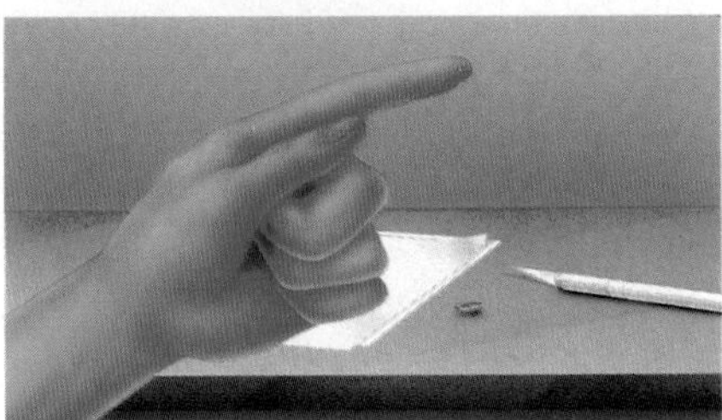

In an avulsion, skin or another part of the body is torn off, or nearly torn off and attached by a flap of skin. First-aid steps:

1. Use direct pressure on the wound to stop the bleeding.
2. If a flap of skin is cut off or hanging loose, gently lay it back in place before bandaging the wound.
3. If a body part (such as a finger) has been removed, send it to the hospital with the victim. If possible, pack the part in ice, but don't delay getting the victim to an emergency room or hospital.
4. Treat for shock.

(FIGURE 28-7) **Types of wounds and their treatment.**

Background
Tetanus

In any type of wound, including an open fracture, the danger of infection exists. Tetanus is a serious infection caused by the bacterium *Clostridium tetani.* The bacteria thrive under conditions of low oxygen, which helps explain why puncture wounds are candidates for infection with this microbe. The bacteria release a toxin that affects the nervous system, eventually causing paralysis. Death occurs when the respiratory muscles cease to function. Vaccines that give immunity are available, but periodic booster injections are required to ensure immunity. If untreated, the fatality rate exceeds 50 percent.

Role-Playing
Treating a Fracture

Obtain some wooden splints, gauze padding, adhesive tape, and a towel (to use as a sling). Select a student to play the role of a person who has suffered a closed fracture of the lower arm in a fall from a tree. Have two or three other students play the roles of passersby who must administer first aid. Have them place a splint on the injured person, securing it loosely with tape. Then have them place the arm in a sling. Allow other members of the class to inspect the splint to see how effective it is. Repeat the exercise with other students.

Reinforcement
Injuries and Shock

Have students review the procedures for treating wounds, fractures, dislocations, and injuries to the neck and spine. Have them note that in all cases, it may be necessary to treat the victim for shock. Elicit from students that shock is a possible consequence of any serious injury. A person giving first aid must always be alert for signs of shock and must always be ready to treat it.

Demonstration
Pupils of the Eye

If possible, obtain a number of penlights. Have students form pairs. Distribute penlights to as many pairs as possible. Darken the classroom and have students wait five minutes. Then have one member of each pair use the

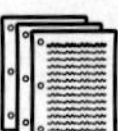

Section Review Worksheet 28.2

Assign Section Review Worksheet 28.2, which requires students to classify characteristics of wounds and to complete multiple choice items about fractures.

Section Quiz 28.2

Have students take Section Quiz 28.2.

First Aid for Fractures

1. *Avoid moving fracture victims unless you need to move them out of danger or transport them to a medical facility. If medical help is on the way, keep the injured person still.*
2. *Build a splint to hold the broken bone in whatever position you find it. Trying to straighten out a fractured bone could cause further damage.*
3. *Place the splint so it immobilizes both the broken bone and the joints immediately above and below the fracture.*
4. *Provide padding between the splint and the skin. For example, for a broken forearm, you can splint the break so the wrist is supported as well as the bone, and then support the forearm in a sling so the elbow doesn't move.*
5. *Don't make the splint too tight. Fractures often cause swelling. Check to make sure the victim has a pulse on the side of the splint away from the heart; that tells you that the splint is not too tight.*
6. *Treat fracture victims for shock.*

(FIGURE 28-8) **A splint prevents further injury by immobilizing a bone. Splints can be made from pieces of wood; from rolled-up magazines, newspapers, or pillows; or from pieces of stiff cardboard.**

fracture:

a broken bone.

Fractures

A broken bone is called a **fracture**. Fractures can be either open or closed. With a closed fracture, also called a simple fracture, the skin is unbroken. If the skin is broken at the site of the fracture, it is called an open fracture, or a compound fracture. Open fractures are more serious because germs and contamination that cause infection can reach the bone, making the fracture more difficult to treat.

Sometimes a fracture is obvious, because the bone is exposed or a limb is lying at a strange angle that would be possible only with a broken bone. Sometimes the victim cannot move toes or fingers without pain. You may even hear a snap as the bone breaks. Swelling, discoloration, or loss of movement are often present with fractures.

A fracture must be immobilized so that the bone can't move and further injure the victim. To immobilize a bone, use a splint as described in Figure 28-8. A splint is a rigid strip of wood, metal, or some other material that will not easily bend. Other parts of the body can also be used as a splint. For example, a broken leg may be bound to the other leg to immobilize the broken bone. If the fracture is open, cover the wound with a clean dressing before applying a splint. You may need to stop bleeding as well.

You won't always know whether an injury is a fracture or something else. Sometimes all you know is that the victim is in pain. To administer first aid, you need not be certain that the injury is a fracture. If you suspect a fracture, treat it as such and splint it.

• • • TEACH continued

penlight to examine the eyes of the other member. Have them note how the pupil of each eye responds as the penlight is shone on the eye. Then have the remaining pairs of students do the demonstration.

Class Discussion
Head Injuries

Discuss whether head injuries tend to be more serious than injuries to other parts of the body. Have students consider why protective headgear is required or recommended in so many diverse activities (baseball, football, bicycle riding, motorcycle riding). In addition, ask students to consider nonfatal consequences of head injuries as opposed to nonfatal consequences of other types of injuries.

Demonstration
Treating a Sprain

Obtain an elastic bandage. Demonstrate for students the proper method for wrapping a sprained ankle or wrist with the bandage. Allow students to examine the secured bandage. If possible, have students practice placing the bandage on their own wrists.

Journal 28E
My Injury—Evaluated

Have students review in the Student Journal their description of an injury they experienced and its treatment. Encourage students to evaluate the treatment they received, in light of what they have learned about proper treatment

Dislocations

In a **dislocation**, the end of a bone comes out of its joint. The dislocated joint will be swollen and deformed, and the person will feel severe pain. Dislocations should be splinted in the same way as fractures. For a dislocated shoulder, splint the upper arm with the elbow supported in a sling and the upper arm strapped to the side of the chest. This gives the dislocated joint the greatest possible support. Treat the victim for shock.

Neck and Spine

An accident victim who complains of pain in the neck or back may have a fractured neck or spine. Moving someone with a broken spinal column could paralyze or kill the person. If the slightest chance of a broken neck or back exists, do not move the person. Treat for shock, send for medical help, and stay until help arrives. Place your hands or a rolled-up blanket or coat on either side of the person's head to keep it from moving.

Head Injury

Any bump on the head that causes a victim to lose consciousness, even if only for a second or two, is potentially serious. Blood vessels sometimes break inside the skull, and then pressure may build and squeeze the brain. This can happen quickly or take place slowly over hours or days. Nausea, slurred speech, slowed breathing, convulsions, and loss of memory can be signs of a head injury, as can blood or body fluid leaking from the ears or nose.

You can sometimes find clues to internal head injuries by examining the pupils of the victim's eyes. Pupils are normally the same size on both sides, or nearly so, and they react to light, becoming smaller in bright light and bigger in dim light. If one pupil is significantly bigger than the other, or if the pupils do not react to light and dark, assume the individual has a serious head injury. You can check for reaction to light by shining a flashlight into one eye then the other, or by shading first one eye then the other from a strong light.

When you suspect a head injury, do the following:

- Treat for shock, but *do not* elevate the victim's feet.
- Stay with the victim, watching carefully for signs of deterioration.
- Monitor breathing. Be ready to give rescue breathing if needed, or CPR if you are trained. If you do so, however, do not tilt the head back. Keeping the head and neck still, pull the jaw forward. Use this procedure also when you suspect an injury to the neck or spine.

dislocation:
an injury in which the end of a bone comes out of its joint.

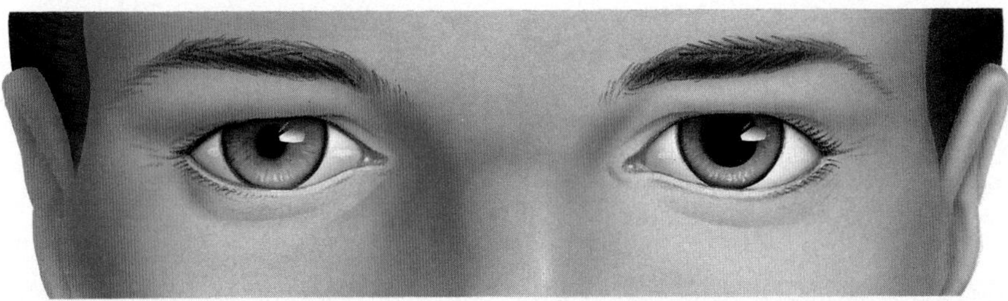

(FIGURE 28-9) **Examine the eyes if you suspect a head injury. If the pupils are not the same size or do not react to light, it may indicate a serious head injury.**

SECTION 28.2

Background
Concussion

Any head injury that results in unconsciousness, and even injuries that do not result in such, may include concussion. *Concussion* can be defined as a brain bruise. It results in a temporary state of confusion or in unconsciousness that can be fleeting, or it may last for hours or even days. A concussion is produced by the slamming of the brain tissue into the bones that form the skull. Any type of blow to the head can toss the head rapidly, causing the brain tissue to be compressed against the skull. Concussions can involve damage to the blood vessels and the nerve tissue in the brain. In all cases of concussion, medical treatment is required.

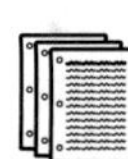

Reteaching Worksheet 28.2

Students who have difficulty with the material may complete Reteaching Worksheet 28.2, which requires them to complete a chart about treatment of types of wounds.

of injuries. Have them include any thoughts on how the treatment could have been improved.

Extension
Paramedics

Have a member of a local emergency squad speak to the class about how to treat wounds. Ask the person to demonstrate the proper techniques for treating wounds, using students as simulated victims. In many communities, emergency squads are composed of trained volunteers. Some students may be interested in finding out how to become members of such squads.

Review Answers

1. Laceration—torn skin; incision—clean cut; abrasion—skin scraped or worn away; puncture—hole through the skin and into deeper tissue; avulsion—skin or other part of the body torn off, or nearly torn off
2. Avoid moving fracture victim; build a splint to hold the broken bone in the position it is in; place the splint so it immobilizes both the broken bone and the joints above and below; provide padding between the splint and the skin; don't make the splint too tight; check for swelling; treat for shock.
3. Do not move the victim because this could paralyze or kill the person.
4. A puncture wound, because it is harder to clean and thus the risk of infection is greater. Also, at the time of treatment for a puncture wound, the victim can receive a tetanus shot or a booster, because tetanus germs can thrive in a puncture wound.

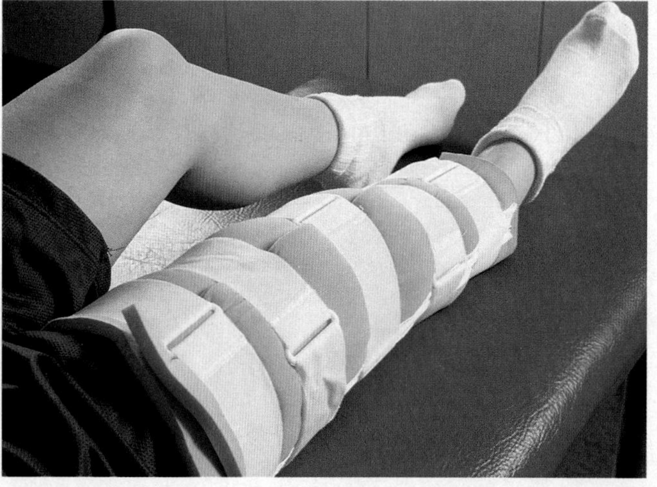

(FIGURE 28-10) **A splint can be used to immobilize a limb that has suffered a sprain or a strain, as well as to immobilize a fracture.**

sprain: *a torn or stretched ligament or tendon.*

strain: *a torn or stretched muscle.*

Sprains and Strains

When a ligament or tendon that joins a muscle to a bone is torn or stretched, the resulting injury is called a **sprain**. In a **strain**, the muscle itself is torn or stretched. Sharply twisting a joint, for example, may cause a sprain, while strains often occur when a person is lifting a heavy weight. With either a sprain or a strain, the victim will experience pain and swelling.

It can be difficult to tell a sprain or strain from a fracture. If you think the injury might be a fracture, you should treat it as a fracture instead of as a sprain. Leave off the elastic bandage and apply a splint instead. It never does any harm to treat a sprain or a strain as a fracture. Otherwise, use the procedure shown in Figure 28-11.

First Aid for Sprains and Strains

Rest: *Do not use the injured part.*

Ice: *Use ice packs to prevent swelling.*

Compression: *Wrap the injured part in an elastic bandage.*

Elevation: *Elevate the injured part above the level of the heart.*

(FIGURE 28-11) **Remember the steps for treating a sprain or a strain as RICE.**

Internal Injuries

Following any accident, a victim may have injuries inside the body that you can't easily detect. Internal bleeding is especially dangerous. Pain in the chest or abdomen is cause for concern. When an accident victim seems to deteriorate without obvious reason, suspect internal injuries. The victim may turn pale, or the person's breathing and pulse may be unusually rapid. If you suspect internal injuries, treat for shock and get the victim to a doctor right away.

Review

1. *List and describe five types of wounds.*
2. *What steps should be taken for a fracture until the victim can see a doctor?*
3. *What is the most important thing to remember when giving first aid to a victim with a possible neck or spine injury?*
4. ***Critical Thinking*** *Assuming both wounds were minor, would it be more important to have a doctor examine a puncture wound or an incision? Explain.*

ASSESS

Section Review

Have students answer the Section Review questions.

Alternative Assessment

Wounds and Their Treatment

Have students make posters that include drawings of the five major types of wounds and a description indicating how each type of wound should be treated. Display the posters in the class and throughout the school.

Closure

First Aid for Injuries

Have students mention signs that indicate an injury to the neck or spine, then signs that indicate an injury to the head. List them on the chalkboard. Have the students compare the first-aid treatment for each type of injury.

Section 28.3 Choking, Heart Attack, and Other Emergencies

Objectives

- *Describe the first aid for a heart-attack victim.*
- *Explain what to do if you find a person unconscious from an unknown cause.*
- *Know how and when to perform the Heimlich maneuver.*
  LIFE SKILLS: Intervention Strategies

The most serious emergencies are those in which the victims would die or suffer permanent damage without intervention. For example, a classmate sitting next to you in the cafeteria could start choking. It is also possible that an individual could collapse in your presence from a heart attack or a stroke. Knowing what to do and acting quickly could save a life. The information in this section will help prepare you to give aid, should a life-threatening emergency occur.

Choking

A person chokes when something, such as a piece of food, gets stuck in his or her airway and prevents breathing. To save a choking person's life, you must act immediately. You don't have time even for a telephone call. Brain cells die when they are deprived of oxygen for even a few minutes. Unless the obstruction is removed immediately, a choking victim will die or suffer permanent brain damage.

Signs of Choking A choking victim will usually grab his or her neck. The victim may be breathing very shallowly, or not at all, and he or she may be trying to cough but be unable to do so. If you think someone is choking, do the following:

- Ask the person if he or she is choking and needs help. Because people need air to talk, a person who can talk is not choking.
- If the choking person is able to cough at all, encourage him or her to continue coughing as hard as possible.
- If other people are nearby, send someone to call for medical help.
- If the victim is unable or barely able to cough, take immediate action to dislodge the object blocking the airway.

The Heimlich Maneuver You can often dislodge an object from a person's airway by using the **Heimlich maneuver,** which is a series of sharp thrusts to the abdomen. These thrusts compress the lungs, forcing the air out. The air, in turn, sometimes pushes the obstruction out of the airway. The procedure to use when performing the Heimlich maneuver for a conscious person is shown in Figure 28-12.

If a person becomes unconscious, lay the person on his or her back. Using your finger, dislodge any obstruction from the person's throat. Alternate a rescue breath with 8 to 10 abdominal thrusts and a finger sweep until the obstruction is dislodged or help arrives. Don't give up hope. As the victim's body becomes starved for oxygen, the muscles in the throat will start to relax. You may suddenly be successful even after you have started to think it is too late.

Heimlich maneuver: *a series of sharp thrusts to the abdomen, used to dislodge an object from a choking person's airway.*

Section 28.3 Lesson Plan

MOTIVATE

Journal 28F
Choking

This may be done as a warm-up activity. Have each student privately recall a situation in which someone choked momentarily on something that he or she had swallowed. Have the students describe the incident in the Student Journal. Encourage them to include a description of their reactions to the incident. Finally, have them record whether they were prepared, at the time, to help the person dislodge the swallowed item.

TEACH

Reinforcement
Choking

Remind students that choking causes more than 3,000 deaths a year in the United States. Most people choke on food, but some, especially small children, choke on objects inhaled by mistake. It is important to keep toys with small parts, stuffed animals with button eyes, and small, hard pieces of food out of the hands of children younger than three.

Role-Playing
The Heimlich Maneuver

Select a student to play the role of a choking victim and a second student

Background

Stroke

A stroke generally affects one side of the brain. In cases where paralysis of the limbs occurs, it generally affects one side of the body. Since the left side of the brain controls the muscles on the right side of the body, a stroke on the left side of the brain paralyzes the right side of the body, and vice versa. A person who shows paralysis on the right side of the body is also more likely to suffer losses in the ability to speak, read, and understand speech. In most people, these functions are controlled by the left side of the brain.

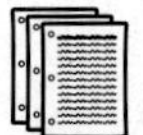

Life Skills Worksheet 28A

Responding to an Emergency

Assign the Responding to an Emergency Life Skills Worksheet, which has students apply first-aid knowledge in a hypothetical health emergency.

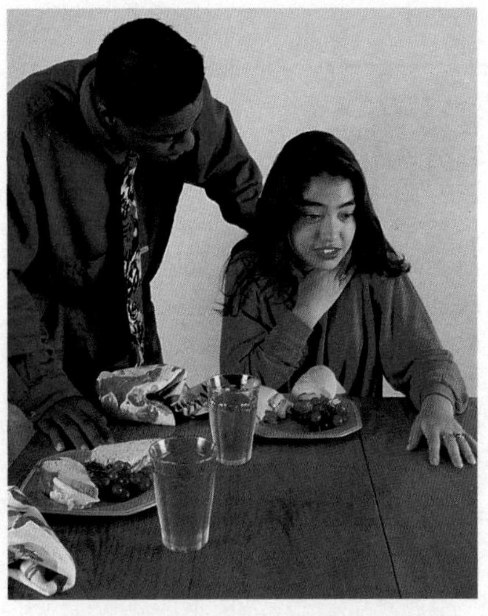

1. Have the choking person stand up, positioning yourself behind him or her.

If a baby is choking, lay the baby face down on your lap with its head slightly lowered. With one hand supporting the baby's head, slap the baby's back forcefully four times. Then turn the baby on its back and give four *chest* thrusts to its breast bone, using only two fingers instead of your fist. Alternate back blows with chest thrusts until the baby's airway is clear. If the baby becomes unconscious, stop after each set of chest thrusts to check the airway and attempt to give a rescue breath.

If *you* are choking, you can perform the Heimlich maneuver on yourself. To do this, lean over the back of a chair, fence, or similar object, and thrust your abdomen into the object, hard, as shown in Figure 28-13.

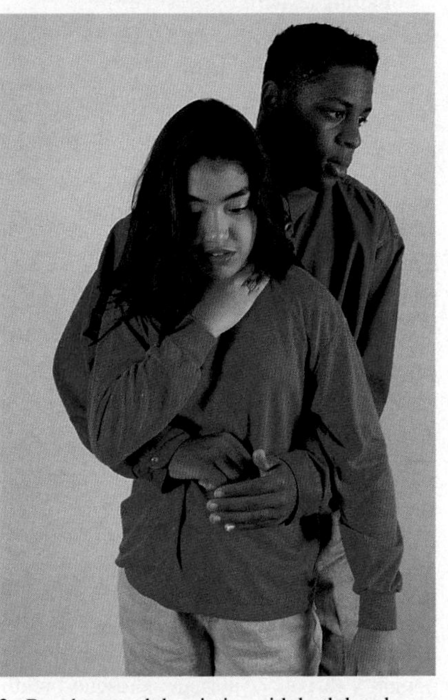

2. Reach around the victim with both hands, placing one fist with its thumb side against the abdomen, a little above the navel and below the rib cage. Grasp the fist in your other hand.

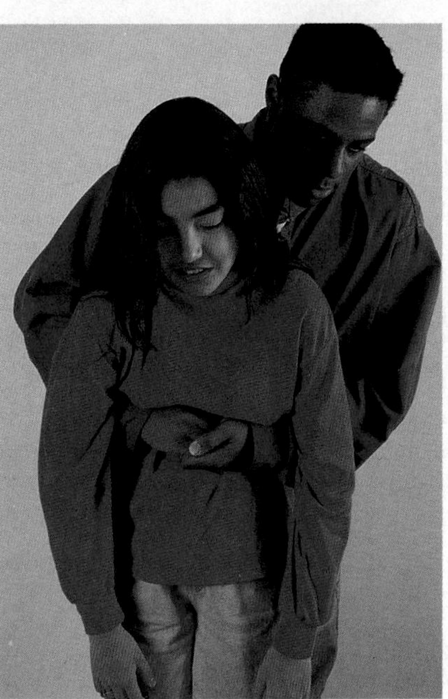

3. Make a sharp, hard thrust with your fist into the abdomen and up toward the rib cage. Continue making hard, vigorous thrusts until you dislodge the obstruction, or until the victim collapses and becomes unconscious.

(FIGURE 28-12) **The Heimlich maneuver. This lifesaving first-aid measure can dislodge an object that is causing someone to choke.**

• • • TEACH continued

to play the role of a passerby who applies the Heimlich maneuver to dislodge the object caught in the victim's throat. Have the choking victim begin by giving the universal sign that he or she is choking—hand held to the throat. The rescuer can refer to Figure 28-12 when applying the Heimlich maneuver. Caution students to demonstrate the position and action but not to apply pressure against the abdomen. Have several teams of students practice the maneuver.

Reinforcement

Rescue Breathing for Heart Attack Victims

A person who suffers a heart attack may stop breathing. Have students review the procedure, described in Figure 28-2, for determining whether a victim is breathing and for administering rescue breathing.

Reinforcement

Remember Your ABCs

Have students recall from Section 28.1 the initial steps in treating a person who is unconscious. Check the ABCs:

- Airway—Place the victim on his or her back and gently lift the chin and tip the head back.
- Breathing—Place your cheek next to the victim's nose and mouth and listen and feel for breathing; watch the chest to see if it rises and falls. Start rescue breathing if necessary.

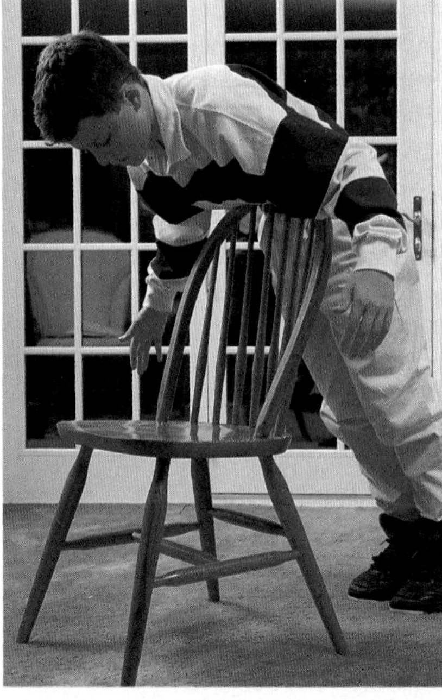

(FIGURE 28-13) **If you begin to choke on an object while you are alone, you can use the Heimlich maneuver on yourself. One technique for doing so is being demonstrated here.**

In a choking emergency, you need to act immediately. Therefore, you may wish to practice the Heimlich maneuver in advance with a friend. However, you should fake the thrusts. You can cause damage by thrusting too hard when it is not needed.

Heart Attack

During a heart attack, part of the heart is not receiving enough blood, and the heart is not pumping well. The signs and symptoms of a heart attack include:

- sudden pain in the chest under the breastbone, possibly radiating into the arms, shoulders, side of the neck, or jaw
- weakness, nausea, or sickness
- rapid, weak, or irregular pulse
- pale or blue skin
- perspiration, anxiety, or fear

To treat a heart attack, follow the steps in Figure 28-14. **Cardiac arrest** may follow a heart attack, meaning that the heart will stop working altogether. In case of cardiac arrest, perform CPR if you are trained.

cardiac arrest:

condition in which the heart stops working.

Steps in Treating a Heart Attack

1. *Sit or lay the victim down, propping up the head.*
2. *Help administer any heart medication the person may have, unless the person is unconscious.*
3. *Immediately send for an ambulance equipped with oxygen, and contact the victim's own doctor if possible.*
4. *Stand by in case rescue breathing becomes necessary.*
5. *In case of cardiac arrest, perform CPR if you have been trained.*
6. *Treat for shock.*

(FIGURE 28-14) **In the event a person suffers a heart attack, you could save his or her life by acting quickly and following these steps.**

SECTION 28.3

Background

Aspirin and Heart Attacks

In a recent study, researchers found that among the subjects of the experiment (all men), those who took one aspirin tablet every other day had fewer heart attacks than those who took a placebo. This is due to aspirin's effect on the formation of blood clots: it reduces the accumulation of platelets, and consequently, the formation of a blood clot when bleeding takes place. Because heart attack results from the blockage of a coronary artery by a blood clot, aspirin's action to reduce clotting is beneficial. But some people should not routinely take aspirin—for them it could be harmful. These include people who have had a stroke resulting from a cerebral hemorrhage, those who have high blood pressure, a history of stroke in the family, a bleeding disorder, ulcers, or impaired liver or kidney functions.

- Circulation—Determine whether the person's heart is beating by trying to find a pulse. Administer CPR if needed and only if you are trained to do so.

Demonstration

Convulsions

To give students an idea of what witnessing a convulsion might be like, set up several situations around the room. In one, a student plays the role of a five-year-old who has a convulsion while in the care of a teenage babysitter; in another, a middle-aged teacher has a convulsion while teaching geometry; in the third, a young woman has a convulsion while standing on a crowded subway platform. In each case, students should ask questions to ascertain the situation and evaluate what actions to take.

Class Discussion

Signs of Stroke

Have a student read aloud the list of symptoms that a stroke victim may experience. Point out that not all stroke victims will experience every symptom and that strokes vary in severity, as do heart attacks. Finally, have students review the procedure for treating a stroke victim, as described in Figure 28-16. **Why should the victim's feet not be raised?** *[Raising the feet would tend to cause blood to flow toward the head, which is the site of the injury; additional bleeding could result.]*

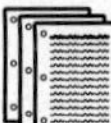

Section Review Worksheet 28.3

Assign Section Review Worksheet 28.3, which requires students to supply information and explain procedures.

Section Quiz 28.3

Have students take Section Quiz 28.3.

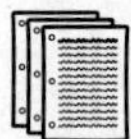

Reteaching Worksheet 28.3

Students who have difficulty with the material may complete Reteaching Worksheet 28.3, which requires them to evaluate the truth of statements about a choking emergency, and complete a Venn diagram comparing treatment of heart attack and stroke victims.

Review Answers

1. Sit or lay the victim down, propping up the head; help administer any heart medication the person may have, unless the person is unconscious; immediately send for an ambulance; contact the victim's doctor if possible; stand by in case rescue breathing becomes necessary; perform CPR if needed, if you have been trained; and treat for shock.

Unconsciousness

If a person becomes unconscious and you don't know why, check ABCs and send for help immediately. Check for medical alert identification that could tell you about any special medical condition. The information might appear on a bracelet, necklace, or anklet such as those shown in Figure 28-15. Some people carry medical alert information on a card, so check the victim's pockets and wallet.

While waiting for help to arrive, treat the individual for shock and stand by in case rescue breathing is needed. If the person vomits, turn his or her head sharply to the side to prevent choking. Use your finger, covered with a cloth if possible, to wipe out the mouth.

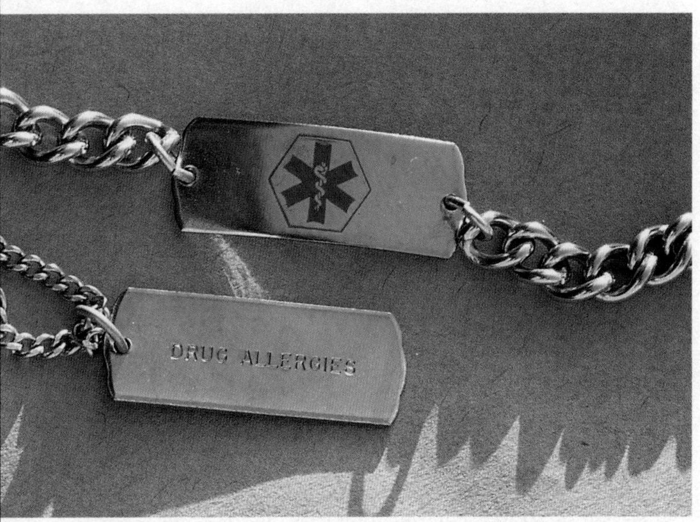

(FIGURE 28-15) **A medical alert identification tag warns of conditions such as diabetes, heart conditions, allergies, or even contact lenses.**

Convulsions

Convulsions may result from epilepsy, poisoning, high fever, or other conditions. During convulsions, every muscle suddenly becomes rigid, then the body starts jerking violently. The victim may also lose control of bowels and bladder. Convulsions can be frightening and upsetting to an observer. It is important to keep yourself calm while attempting to give aid.

Individuals who are convulsing should be prevented from causing themselves injury—for example, from rolling off a

Treatment for Stroke

1. *Send for an ambulance equipped with oxygen, immediately.*
2. *Keep the stroke victim quiet and lying on the side in case of vomiting. If the victim vomits, make sure the head is turned sharply to the side, to reduce the chance of choking.*
3. *Treat for shock by keeping the victim warm, but do not raise the legs.*
4. *Be ready to give rescue breathing if necessary or CPR if you have been trained.*

(FIGURE 28-16) **Some of the symptoms of a stroke are similar to other, less life-threatening conditions. If there is any doubt in your mind, follow these first-aid steps for treating a stroke.**

• • • TEACH continued

Extension

Cafeteria Safety

Have students inspect the cafeteria to see whether instructions for assisting a choking victim are posted. If instructions are posted, have students recommend any needed changes in the number and placement of the signs. If such instructions are not posted, have students find out how to obtain them and have them posted.

sidewalk into traffic. Loosen tight clothing, and remove any objects from the immediate area. Otherwise, there is nothing you can do except wait for the convulsions to stop.

Do not try to put anything into a person's mouth while he or she is convulsing or if he or she is unconscious. If the victim is unconscious, turn his or her head to the side. Observe the victim's breathing, in case you need to provide rescue breathing. The convulsions will go away in a minute or two. If the victim has medicine for convulsions, you may help administer it *after* the convulsions have stopped and *only* if the person is conscious. Victims who are unconscious after convulsions should be laid on their sides. Send for medical help, or take the individual to a doctor.

Stroke

In a **stroke**, also called a cerebral vascular accident, blood supply to part of the brain is obstructed because a blood vessel in the brain has burst or become plugged with a clot. Stroke victims may show some or all of the following signs and symptoms:

- dizziness or loss of consciousness
- difficulty in breathing or talking
- mental confusion or slurred speech
- partial paralysis on one side of the body
- mouth pulled sideways
- pupils of unequal size
- bright red face
- bulging neck veins

Figure 28-16 lists the treatment for stroke.

Something Wrong—Cause Unknown

If a person appears to be ill or in pain but you can't tell what the problem is, treat for shock and send for help. Watch the person in case rescue breathing becomes necessary.

What Would You Do ?

Making Responsible Decisions

Your Best Friend's Mother Collapses

You have just finished studying Section 28.3 of the First Aid and CPR chapter of this book. You are at your best friend's house, and as you close the book, your best friend's mother collapses and gasps that she is having chest pains. Her breathing is rapid and shallow. Her skin is pale and tinged with blue. What would you do?

Remember to use the decision-making steps:

1. **State the Problem.**
2. **List the Options.**
3. **Imagine the Benefits and Consequences.**
4. **Consider Your Values.**
5. **Weigh the Options and Decide.**
6. **Act.**
7. **Evaluate the Results.**

Review

1. *Explain what to do for someone who is having a heart attack.*
2. *What is the first-aid procedure for a victim who is unconscious from an unknown cause?*
3. ***LIFE SKILLS: Intervention Strategies** Describe the steps and purpose of the Heimlich maneuver.*
4. ***Critical Thinking** Is it always possible to determine whether a victim is suffering from shock or a stroke? Explain.*

stroke:

the rupture or blockage of an artery in the brain, leading to oxygen deprivation and damage to brain cells.

What Would You Do ?

Your Best Friend's Mother Collapses

Have students read the What Would You Do? feature. Have a volunteer state the procedure that he or she would follow. Then have the class evaluate the person's procedure, based on what they have read in Section 28.3.

Answer to Question 1 is on p. 632.

2. Send for help, check ABCs, check for medical alert identification, and treat for shock; stand by in case rescue breathing becomes necessary.

3. Answers should agree with Figures 28-12 and 28-13. The purpose of the Heimlich maneuver is to dislodge whatever is obstructing the person's airway so that he or she can breathe again.

4. No. Some of the symptoms of stroke are similar to shock and other injuries, such as a head injury.

ASSESS

Section Review

Have students answer the Section Review questions.

Alternative Assessment

Heimlich Maneuver

Organize students into small groups. Have one student in each group bring a camera (or borrow the school's camera.) Have each group take a series of photos illustrating the steps in the Heimlich maneuver, with students playing the roles of victim and rescuer. When the photos are developed, have each group mount them on cardboard and display them in the classroom.

Closure

Heart Attack and Stroke

As an oral review, ask students to compare the signs of a heart attack with the signs of a stroke. Have them include the steps for treating both emergencies.

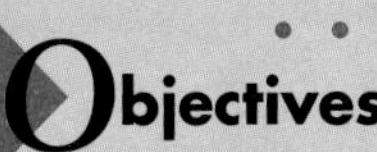

Section 28.4 Common Emergencies

Objectives

- *Contrast two health emergencies caused by heat, and compare their treatments.*
- *Know how to identify and protect your body from cold-related health emergencies.*
  LIFE SKILLS: Practicing Self-Care
- *Describe three types of burns and their treatment.*
- *List the steps to be taken when poison is swallowed.*

This section covers emergencies you could encounter—indoors or outdoors—at school, home, work, or sporting events.

Heat-Related Emergencies

Overexertion in too much heat can lead to emergencies that require first aid.

Heat Exhaustion With heat exhaustion, a person collapses from heat, exertion, and loss of water and salt through perspiration. The victim starts to go into shock, and the body's cooling mechanisms may begin working too hard, actually over-cooling.

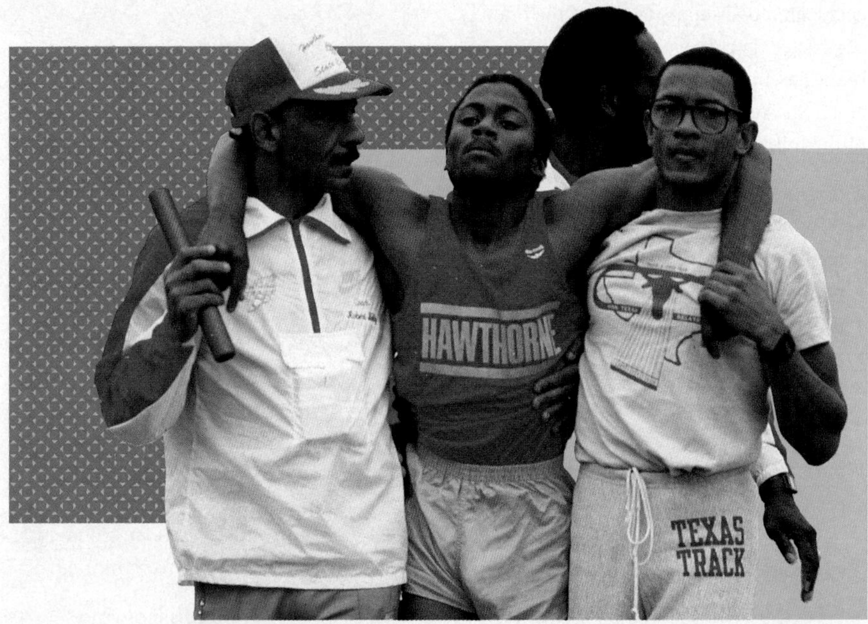

(FIGURE 28-17) **Vigorous exercise or hard work, especially during warm months, can result in heat exhaustion or heatstroke due to overheating and the loss of body fluids and salts. Knowing the difference between these two common conditions could help you save a friend's life.**

Section 28.4 Lesson Plan

MOTIVATE

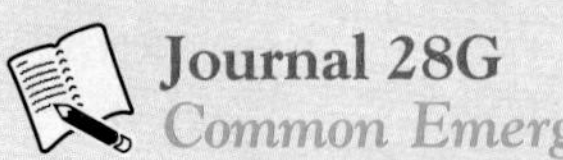

Journal 28G
Common Emergencies

This may be done as a warm-up activity. Encourage students to record in the Student Journal three examples of common emergencies that are likely to occur at home but not outdoors. Then have them record three examples of emergencies that are likely to occur outdoors but not at home. Tell the students to note which, if any, of these emergencies they have experienced and how the emergencies were handled.

TEACH

Class Discussion
Heat Exhaustion and Heatstroke

Stress to the class that heat exhaustion and heatstroke are two very different emergencies. Ask: **How can you tell whether a person is suffering from heat exhaustion or whether he or she is suffering from heatstroke?** *[In heat exhaustion the skin is cool and moist; in heatstroke the skin is hot and dry.]* **What cooling mechanism is working in heat exhaustion but has failed in heatstroke?** *[Perspiring]* Point out that heat exhaustion is related to the loss of water and salts by the body; heatstroke is related to a failure of the body's cooling mechanisms. **Which of these conditions presents a critical emergency?** *[Heatstroke]*

The person's skin will feel clammy (cool and moist). Other signs and symptoms include weakness, dizziness, headache, nausea, rapid and shallow breathing, and dilated pupils.

A victim of heat exhaustion should lie down in the shade and cool off. If the victim is conscious and not nauseated, replace body fluids by giving the victim plenty of drinking water. Suggest that the victim avoid heat and strenuous exercise for a few days, even when feeling better.

Heatstroke (Sunstroke) After working or exercising strenuously in a hot environment, a person can suffer from heatstroke. The skin becomes red and very hot and dry. With heat exhaustion, the body is still trying to cool off by perspiring freely. With heatstroke, the hot, dry skin tells you the body's mechanism for cooling itself is not working anymore. It has been overwhelmed by too much heat and exercise. The internal body temperature becomes very high—106° F or even higher. Heatstroke is life threatening. If the following steps are not taken to cool the body, the victim will die.

- Move the victim out of the heat, indoors if possible.
- Put the victim in cool (not cold) water, or apply wet cloths all over the body to cool it off.
- If conscious, the person should drink water in small quantities.
- Take the victim to a hospital emergency room as quickly as possible.

Heat Cramps A cramp is a sudden, very painful knot in a muscle, often a leg muscle. Heat cramps are caused by exercising in conditions where too much body salt and water are being lost through perspiration. Generally, a cramp will go away if you stretch out the affected muscle. You can also give drinking water to a person with heat cramps to replace body fluids.

Treatment for Frostbite

1. *Cover the affected area, and provide extra blankets or clothing. Take the victim indoors if possible.*
2. *Gently thaw the frozen part by soaking in warm—not hot—water, wrapping in warm blankets, or treating with a warm object. Any water or object that feels hot on your own hand is too hot for thawing frostbite.*
3. *Stop applying heat as soon as the skin is flushed.*
4. *Avoid damaging tissue. Do not rub the affected area, since this may cause gangrene.*
5. *Keep the victim away from hot fires or stoves.*
6. *Do not allow the blisters to break.*

(FIGURE 28-18) **Frostbite may occur during exposure to extreme cold. If you must give first aid for frostbite, follow these steps, but wait until you are sure the frozen parts will remain thawed.**

Cold-Related Emergencies

Overexposure to cold or the loss of too much body heat can also lead to emergencies that require first aid.

Frostbite With frostbite, ice crystals form in the fluids of soft tissues of the body. Typically, whitish or yellowish spots appear on the nose, fingers, toes, ears, or cheeks. Blisters may develop later. To treat frostbite, follow the steps in Figure 28-18.

Frostbitten tissue has been injured and may take time to heal. Have the person gently exercise any affected parts except the feet. It is better not to thaw frostbitten tissue until you can keep the tissue thawed. Frostbitten tissue can be severely damaged if it thaws out and refreezes before it has a chance to heal. In most cases, a frostbite victim should consult a doctor.

Role-Playing
Treating Frostbite

Select one student to play the role of a hiker who has frostbite of the fingers of both hands. Select a second student to play the role of a person living in a nearby cabin who comes across the victim of frostbite on the hiking trail. Have this student demonstrate the proper procedure for treating frostbite. (Provide a pan of warm water, a blanket, and some towels for the student to use.) The student can refer to Figure 28-18 as he or she treats the victim of frostbite. Allow other teams of students to role-play the incident.

Reinforcement
Heatstroke and Hypothermia

It may be useful to compare the conditions of heatstroke and hypothermia and the recommended treatments, since these emergencies are almost mirror images of each other. You might make a comparison chart on the chalkboard, like the one at right.

	Heatstroke	Hypothermia
Body Temp.	Too high	Too low
Temp. Regulation	Sweating stops	Shivering stops
Treatment	Cool the body	Warm the body
Risk to Life	Critical	Critical

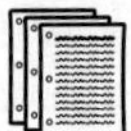

Life Skills Worksheet 28B

First-Aid Supplies

Assign the First-Aid Supplies Life Skills Worksheet, which requires students to decide which first-aid items should be kept on hand for emergency use.

hypothermia: *below-normal body temperature.*

Hypothermia The prefix "hypo" means low, or under. **Hypothermia,** therefore, is a condition in which a person's body temperature is too low. This condition results not just from being exposed to cold but also from losing heat from the body faster than the body can rewarm itself.

As the body loses heat and its internal temperature begins to drop, the body takes steps to protect itself. First, some of the blood flow to the extremities (arms, legs, and head) is cut off. Shivering begins, to rewarm the body, and may become violent. Eventually, the heart rate and breathing rate slow, the victim loses muscle strength and coordination, and other signs and symptoms such as slurred speech, fatigue, confusion, hallucinations, and irrational behavior may appear. Finally, the victim stops shivering. This means that the victim's body has lost the ability to rewarm itself.

Like heatstroke, hypothermia is a life-threatening condition. The treatment for hypothermia is described in Figure 28-19. To find out how to avoid hypothermia, complete the Life Skills activity on page 637.

Treatment for Hypothermia

If the victim is shivering:	***1.*** *A shivering person will recover if you eliminate further loss of heat. Move the victim to a warm place, wrapping him or her in coats, blankets, or sleeping bags to help the body rewarm itself.*
	2. *Give warm drinks to rewarm the body from the inside, if the person can hold the glass alone. Never give alcoholic drinks to a cold person. Alcohol may make people feel warmer, but it actually increases heat loss.*
If the victim has stopped shivering:	***1.*** *A person who has ceased shivering will die unless you rewarm his or her body. Get the person to a hospital if you can do it quickly.*
	2. *Warm the central part of the body first, without warming the extremities. Soak the person in a warm—not hot—bath with arms and legs hanging out, or use warm objects such as water bottles or electric heating pads next to the trunk.*
	3. *Giving warm drinks will help, if the person is conscious and sufficiently coordinated to hold the glass alone. A person whose coordination is too far gone to hold a glass is in danger of choking or breathing liquid into the lungs.*

(FIGURE 28-19) **Follow these steps if you must give first aid for hypothermia.**

• • • TEACH continued

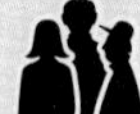

Cooperative Learning
Poisonous Snakes

Obtain several copies of field guides that discuss reptiles. (*A Field Guide to the Reptiles and Amphibians of Eastern/Western North America* is an excellent choice). Then have students meet in small groups, with each group having access to a field guide. Have the groups use the plates and the maps in the field guide to identify the poisonous snakes found in their area of the country. Have students study the pictures of the poisonous snakes in their area so that they can easily identify these snakes on sight.

Demonstration
A Constricting Band

Explain the usefulness of a constricting band in treating a poisonous snake bite. Then cut a piece of cloth about 1 inch wide and about 8 inches long. Have a student assist you in demonstrating where and how to tie a constricting band on your arm. Refer to Figure 28-21 for instructions.

Journal 28H
Insect Stings

Have students record in the Student Journal incidents in which they have suffered insect stings. Have the students describe their reactions in the journal. Encourage students who feel that they may have experienced an allergic reaction to a sting to discuss this fact with their parents or guardians.

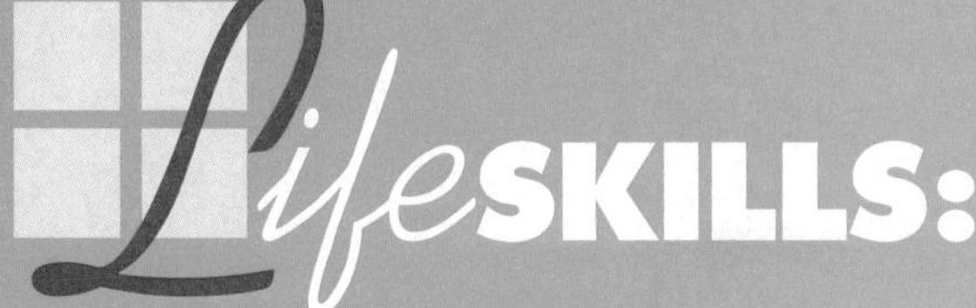

Preventing Hypothermia . . . .

Preventing hypothermia is much easier than treating this life-threatening condition. Remember, it is easier to stay warm than it is to rewarm your body after it has lost heat.

As you get cold, 50 percent of your body's heat loss can be through your head and neck. This is because a large portion of the blood in your body flows though your head and neck, much of it near the surface. Air currents carry away heat as it radiates from your blood.

Water is a better conductor of heat than air is, and if it is cooler than your body temperature, it will conduct heat from your body faster than air. This is why you may feel cold in water that is 70°F , when air at 70°F is comfortable. Even though the water is not very cold, you can develop hypothermia if you stay in it very long. Solids conduct heat even faster than liquids, so you can also lose body heat quickly by lying or sitting on something cold.

Answer the following questions to see if you know how to prevent hypothermia.

1. If you are wearing a warm jacket and start to feel cold, what items of clothing might you add to prevent heat loss?
2. Why do you suppose people wore nightcaps before houses were heated efficiently?
3. Assume you are in water at 70°F, and the air temperature is 70°F. If you start shivering or feeling chilled, what should you do? Why?
4. Why should you put down a blanket before laying an injured person on the ground?

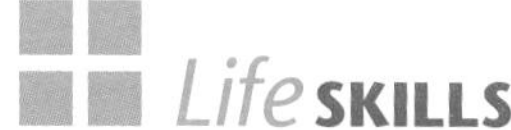

Preventing Hypothermia

Have students read the Life Skills feature. Then tell them to answer the questions. When students have finished, discuss the answers in class.

Demonstration

Safety in the Science Lab

Burns from chemicals and from heat can occur in the science lab. Well-equipped science labs have an eyewash station and may even have a fire shower. If the science lab in your school has either or both of these facilities, have a science teacher demonstrate their uses for the class.

Cooperative Learning

Antidotes for Poisoning

Tell students to check around their homes for substances that have poison warning labels. Have each student copy the names of three poisonous substances and any instructions on what to do if the poison is ingested. Allow students to meet in small groups to exchange information. Each group can prepare a brief list of the poisons that they discussed and the recommended treatment for each. However, point out to students that it is essential to call 911 or contact a poison control center before treating a person for poisoning. The first-aid instructions on labels may not be correct.

Class Discussion

The Dangers of Carbon Monoxide Poisoning

Have students describe conditions under which there is likely to be a danger of carbon monoxide poisoning. *(Run-*

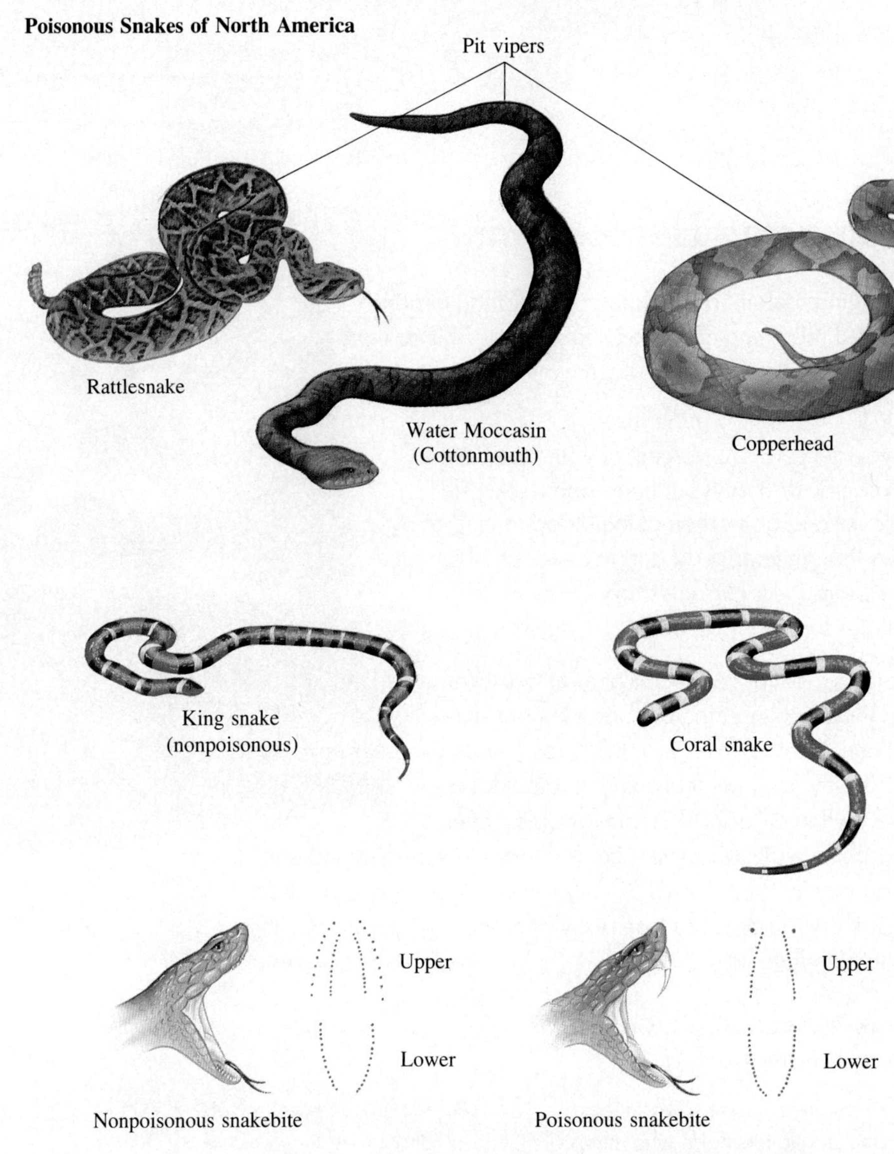

(FIGURE 28-20) **Notice the triangular head of the pit vipers. Any snake with this type of head is poisonous. The coral snake, for which the harmless king snake is often mistaken, is the only poisonous snake in the United States that does not have a triangular head. You can distinguish the coral snake from the king snake by remembering the rhyme: Red on yellow will kill a fellow; red on black does venom lack.**

• • • TEACH continued

ning a car in a closed garage; using an oil space heater in a poorly insulated room; using any charcoal-burning cooking device indoors) Stress that carbon monoxide is odorless and invisible. A person who is being poisoned by carbon monoxide may not realize what is happening.

Role-Playing
Treating Hyperventilation

Have one student play the role of a person who is hyperventilating. Have a second student play the role of a friend who is trying to reassure the victim and treat the hyperventilation. Allow other students to role-play the situation. Have the class critique the treatment given in both cases.

Class Discussion
I Feel Faint

Have students recall incidents in which they felt faint, including factors that contributed to the feeling of faintness, how they felt, and what they did about it. Then have them explain what they would do now if they felt faint.

Demonstration
Treating a Nosebleed

Many people instinctively tilt the head back when treating a nosebleed. Review with students the proper position

Drowning

Drowning may occur in deep water some distance from shore, in a swimming pool a few feet from the side, or even in a bathtub. In a drowning emergency, *do not* attempt to swim to the victim unless you have received the proper training in water-safety and life-saving techniques. Instead, toss a flotation device or rescue line to the victim and then call for help.

Once retrieved, potential drowning victims who have stopped breathing must be given rescue breathing immediately and continually until they begin to breathe. If the victim was in deep water, you should begin rescue breathing as soon as the victim reaches shallow water. If it is necessary, provide CPR if you are trained to do so. Send for medical help immediately.

Procedure for Applying a Constricting Band

1. *Tie the band 2 to 4 inches above any swelling from the bite, but not around a joint. The ideal band would be 1 to $1\frac{1}{2}$ inches wide, but a shoelace would serve if nothing else is available.*
2. *Check snugness. The band should be snug enough to dimple the skin all the way around, but still loose enough for you to slide a finger under it.*
3. *Check for a pulse below the band. If there is none, loosen the band until there is.*

(FIGURE 28-21) **CAUTION: The purpose of a constricting band is to slow circulation just under the skin, where most poison travels, NOT to cut off circulation altogether.**

Snakebite

Out of the hundreds of kinds of snakes in the United States, only four kinds are poisonous. They are pictured in Figure 28-20. One kind of poisonous snake that is rarely seen is the coral snake, which is related to the deadly cobra. The others belong to a family of snakes called pit vipers, which includes rattlesnakes, copperheads, and water moccasins (also called cottonmouths). All pit vipers have a triangular-shaped head and two large fangs in the upper jaw.

A pit viper's bite usually leaves two prominent holes where the fangs went in. The poison is in the fangs, so if you are ever bitten by a pit viper that doesn't leave fang marks, don't worry. Even with a bite that does leave fang marks, a victim may not have been poisoned.

Snakebites are rarely fatal, but they often cause permanent damage that can sometimes make it necessary to amputate a limb. Therefore, a poisonous snakebite should be treated as a serious emergency. Take the following steps to treat a snakebite:

- Wash the wound with soap and water to reduce the chance of infection.
- To slow the spread of poison through the body, keep the person quiet and calm, preferably lying down.
- If the bite is on an arm or leg, keep the affected part below the level of the heart and follow the steps in Figure 28-21 to help slow the spread of poison.

A snakebite victim needs medical treatment within four hours. Whenever possible, the victim should be carried to the doctor, rather than being allowed to walk. Fear and panic can aggravate snakebite symptoms, so you should try to be soothing and reassuring. If you are bitten when you are alone and you must walk for help, you should apply a constricting band and then walk at a slow pace, resting frequently, in order to keep your blood circulating as slowly as possible.

Background
Poisonous Snakes

As the text states, there are four types of poisonous snakes in the United States. However, there are several varieties of each type. For example, there are three varieties of cottonmouths (Eastern, Western, and Florida), all confined to the southeastern section of the country.

With rattlesnakes, the situation is more complex, since a number of different species occur in the United States. The timber rattlesnake is the only one that lives in the populous Northeast. The canebrake rattlesnake, eastern diamondback, and several varieties of pygmy rattlesnakes are found in the Southeast. In the middle of the country are found several types of massasauga rattlesnakes and the prairie rattlesnake. And in the western United States live the western diamondback, mojave rattlesnake, black-tailed rattlesnake, and several other types. Thus, it might be useful to have students become familiar with the rattlesnakes found in their section of the country.

for stopping a nosebleed. To reinforce the proper technique, demonstrate the position that a person being treated for nosebleed should assume.

Reinforcement
Care of the Eyes

Caution students that in attempting to remove a foreign body from their eye or someone else's eye, their hands must be clean, and any item, such as a cloth, used to remove the object must also be clean. Use Figure 28-28 to review with students methods for inspecting both the lower and upper eyelid for the presence of a foreign body.

Extension
Water Safety

Interested students might wish to research water safety or lifesaving techniques for dealing with emergencies in water. They might contact the local office of the American Red Cross or use library references for this information. Suggest that students make a poster that summarizes their findings.

Extension
Rabies in Wild Animals

Have students contact the offices of state parks and forests to request information on the extent of rabies in wild mammals in the state. Such offices should be able to supply information on which animals are likely to be infected, on signs of infection, and to whom suspect animals should be reported. Have students report their findings to the class.

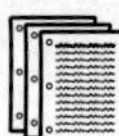

Life Skills Worksheet 28C

Emergency Medical Help

Assign the Emergency Medical Help Life Skills Worksheet, which requires students to gather locations and telephone numbers of sources of advice or care in a health emergency.

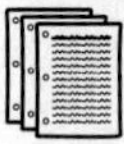

Life Skills Worksheet 28D

Taking the Right Action

Assign the Taking the Right Action Life Skills Worksheet, which requires students to respond to first-aid emergencies in which people are acting on misconceptions or are in need of advice.

Stings

If you have been stung by a bee, hornet, wasp, or scorpion, you know it can cause intense pain, burning, and itching at the sting site. First aid for insect and scorpion stings includes the following steps:

- Examine the sting site carefully. If part of the stinger is still embedded in the wound, *do not* try to pull it out. It may have the poison sac still attached, and by grasping it, you can squeeze more poison into the wound. Instead, scrape it out with a fingernail, broken stick, or the edge of a credit card.
- Use a paste of baking soda, a towel soaked in ammonia, or ice to help reduce the pain and swelling.
- Observe the victim for a while. A small percentage of people are allergic to bee stings and can experience a severe, life-threatening reaction. Victims who are in obvious distress, feeling nauseated, dizzy, faint, or who are having trouble breathing should be treated for shock and be examined by a doctor right away.
- Stand by to perform rescue breathing, if necessary, or CPR if you are trained to give it.

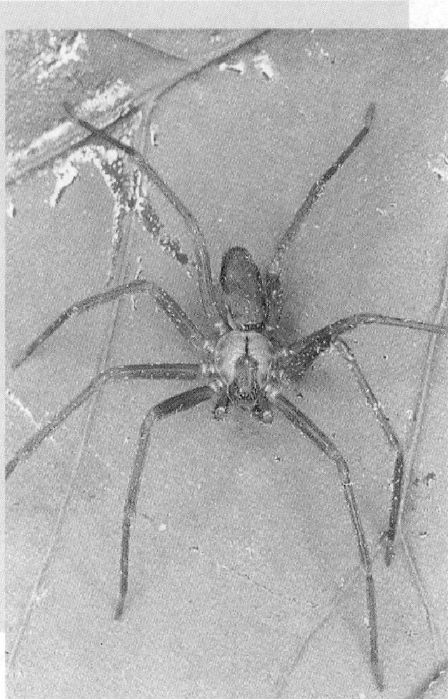

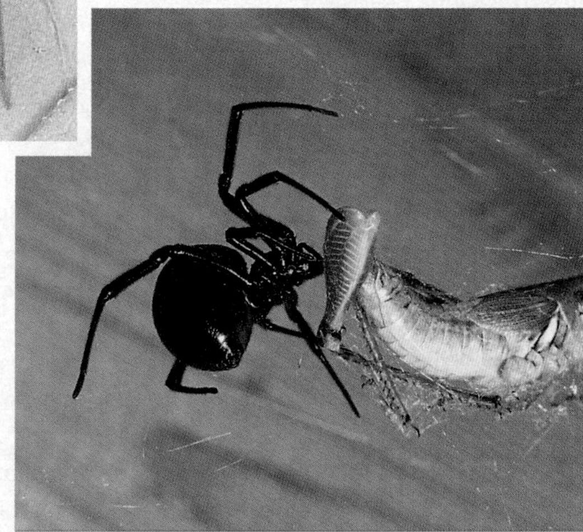

(FIGURE 28-22) **The brown recluse (above) and the black widow (right). Both black widow and brown recluse spider bites require medical treatment. On rare occasions, they can be fatal.**

Spider Bites

Of the thousands of species of spiders in the United States, only two are poisonous—the black widow and the brown recluse. The black widow's bite is painful and will make a victim extremely ill, but it is rarely fatal except to the seriously ill, the very young, or the very old. Only the female black widow is poisonous. The brown recluse spider's bite can form a bad sore in a few hours, but it is not likely to be fatal.

If you must give first aid for a spider bite, follow the steps below.

- Wash the bite with soap and water to reduce the chance of infection.
- Use a paste of baking soda and water, a towel soaked in ammonia, or ice to reduce the pain and swelling.
- Treat for shock and be prepared to give rescue breathing if necessary.
- Seek medical attention immediately.

Human and Animal Bites

The mouths of humans and other mammals are full of bacteria, so their bites carry danger of serious infection. To prevent infection, human and other animal bites should be washed with soap and water, then rinsed thoroughly under running water. Dress a bite as you would any other wound. For severe or infected bites, the victim should see a doctor. Because bites can cause tetanus, bite victims should receive tetanus shots if they are not up to date on immunizations.

The most serious risk from animal bites is rabies. This viral infection of the nervous system is always fatal without preventive treatment. After a bite, observe the animal for unusual behavior or signs of illness. Rabid animals may drool or be unusually calm or excited. If you can do it safely, confine the animal so that it can be examined by a veterinarian or health department official. *Do not* get near the animal in order to capture it, and *do not* handle it. Only a professional should do so. Rabies can always be prevented if treatment is started soon enough. However, the series of treatments is long and painful. Victims can avoid suffering through it if a doctor can be sure that the animal did not have rabies.

Hyperventilation

Hyperventilation is rapid breathing that may be accompanied by chest pains, tingling of the fingertips and around the mouth, dizziness, or fainting. Emotional distress or poor circulation to the brain can precipitate it. Hyperventilation lowers the level of carbon dioxide in the blood. The following treatment is designed to raise the blood level of carbon dioxide to normal.

- Try to calm the victim. Have the person sit and lower his or her head.
- Have the person breathe into a paper bag or cupped hands. Breathing exhaled air helps restore the normal level of carbon dioxide in the blood.
- Seek medical attention if the symptoms persist.

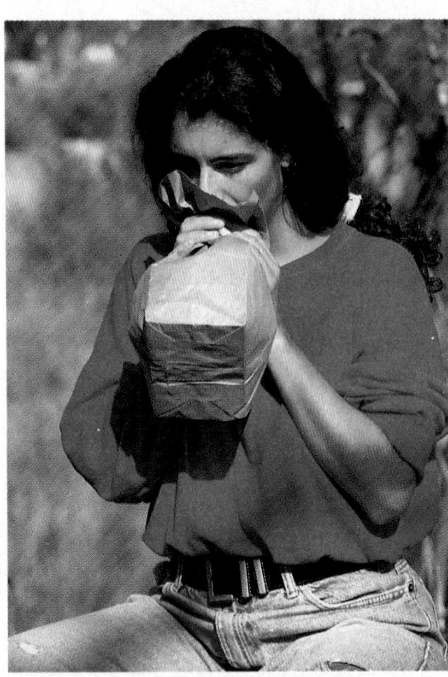

(FIGURE 28-23) **Your breath contains more carbon dioxide than the surrounding air. By breathing into a paper sack for a few minutes, you can raise the level of carbon dioxide in your blood and get rid of the symptoms of hyperventilation.**

Background
Rabies

Rabies is caused by a virus that attacks the brain and central nervous system. It affects mammals, with carnivores such as wolves and dogs being the principal carriers and victims. However, rabies does occur in other mammals and has been transmitted to humans by the bites of insect-eating bats. The rabies virus may also be transmitted via mucous membranes. For example, mammals can contract rabies by breathing the air in caves that have large bat populations.

Rabies is almost always fatal once symptoms develop. Treatment consists of a series of injections that builds up immunity in the victim. An antirabies serum that supplies antibodies against the disease has recently been developed. The most effective treatment involves receiving both the vaccine and the serum.

Making a Choice 28A

Precaution and Preparation

Assign the Precaution and Preparation card. The card asks students to discuss health emergencies that might arise in common situations.

Making a Choice 28B

Putting Yourself on the Line

Assign the Putting Yourself on the Line card. The card asks students to assess the risks of giving first aid in various circumstances and to compare them with the consequences of not acting.

Nosebleeds

A nosebleed is spontaneous bleeding from a nostril that usually results from drying and cracking of the membranes lining the inside of the nose. Most nosebleeds will stop on their own fairly easily. If the bleeding does not stop soon on its own, use the following procedure.

- Have the victim sit upright, lean slightly forward, and gently pinch both nostrils closed for 10 to 15 minutes.
- Apply cold cloths firmly against the bleeding nostril.
- If the bleeding continues, try putting a plug of rolled-up gauze into the bleeding nostril. Do not use cotton for this purpose, because it could be hard to remove later.
- If the bleeding continues and nothing seems to help, take the victim to a doctor. Something else might be wrong.

Electric Shock

Electric shock occurs when an electric current passes through a person's body. The current may cause cardiac arrest (the heart stops beating) and respiratory failure (the person stops breathing). In case of electric shock, follow the steps in Figure 28-24.

Steps to Take in Case of Electric Shock

1. *Do not touch an electric shock victim who is still touching a live wire or other source of electricity.*
2. *Turn off the current if you can do so quickly and safely. Otherwise, use an object made of a substance that does not conduct electricity (such as wood or plastic) to pull any wires away from the victim. Do not use metal! Stand on insulating material such as paper, wood, or rubber. Be sure your hands and the materials you use are dry.*
3. *Check the victim's ABCs—airway, breathing, and circulation (heartbeat).*
4. *If the airway is open and the victim isn't breathing, begin rescue breathing at once. If there is no pulse, begin CPR as well, if you are trained. If the victim doesn't regain consciousness right away, do not give up hope. Victims who have been struck by lightning, or who have suffered other serious electrical shock, may need rescue breathing for an hour or more before they begin breathing on their own again.*
5. *Send for medical help.*
6. *Treat the victim for shock.*

(FIGURE 28-24) **In addition to these lifesaving measures, an electric shock victim may also need treatment for burns.**

Poisoning

Poisons can cause intense pain, permanent injury, impaired health, and even death. The steps you take immediately after a poisoning can save a life and prevent permanent injury.

A victim of poisoning needs medical attention immediately. Until medical help is available, monitor the victim's pulse and breathing. Be ready to give rescue breathing, or if you are trained, CPR.

Poisoning by Ingestion If victims are conscious and able to talk, you can usually ask what they drank or ate. Sometimes eyewitness accounts can be useful. If a person is unconscious or unable to talk, you should suspect poison if you detect the symptoms in Figure 28-25. For the benefit of the medical personnel who will assist, save the container or label of the suspected poison. If the person vomits, save a sample of the material for examination.

If you must give first aid to a person who drank or ate a poison, do not give anything by mouth or try to induce vomiting until you have determined what the poison is and checked with the nearest poison control center for instructions. They may tell you to dilute the poison by having the victim drink a glass of water or milk immediately. Often they will tell you to induce vomiting. Syrup containing *ipecac* is often recommended for this purpose. However, some poisons that can be swallowed contain strong acids or alkalis that damage tissue on contact. Because they cause as much damage coming up as going down, you will be told not to induce vomiting in those cases.

You can reach the poison control center in an emergency by dialing 911, or O for operator, and asking to be connected. Find out the number of the nearest poison control center in advance and keep it posted by your telephone.

Signs and Symptoms of Poisoning

- *Presence of a poisonous substance or its container*
- *Sudden, unexplained illness or pain, especially in the abdomen*
- *Nausea or vomiting*
- *Burns near the lips or mouth*
- *Odor of chemicals or fuel on the breath*
- *Changes in the pupils (dilation or constriction)*

(FIGURE 28-25) **These symptoms may indicate poisoning. Your first step should be to call 911 or contact the nearest poison control center.**

Drug Overdose Drugs are a common cause of poisoning. Even nonprescription drugs can be poisonous if taken in large doses or in bad combinations. Outdated drugs may be poisonous as well. Follow the same steps for a drug overdose as for poisoning by ingestion. In addition, try to keep the person awake and calm.

Poisoning by Inhalation Many substances can be poisonous if they are inhaled, including a number of chemicals, fuels, and gases. Carbon monoxide is a frequent cause of inhalation poisoning. Produced by incompletely burned fuels, carbon monoxide accumulates in poorly ventilated areas where fuels are being burned or where fuel-burning engines are running. Because it is odorless, it can overcome victims before they are even aware of the danger.

If you attempt to rescue a victim of inhalation poisoning, *exercise extreme caution*. Take several deep breaths before entering a closed space where someone has collapsed, and hold your breath while you

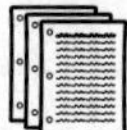

Section Review Worksheet 28.4

Assign Section Review Worksheet 28.4, which requires students to evaluate statements about hypothermia, compare and contrast heat exhaustion and heatstroke, and supply information about treating poisoning.

Section Quiz 28.4

Have students take Section Quiz 28.4.

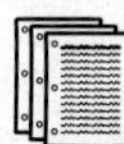

Reteaching Worksheet 28.4

Students who have difficulty with the material may complete Reteaching Worksheet 28.4, which requires them to classify characteristics of burns, to complete a chart showing treatment for three types of burns, and to classify statements as pertaining to heat exhaustion or heatstroke.

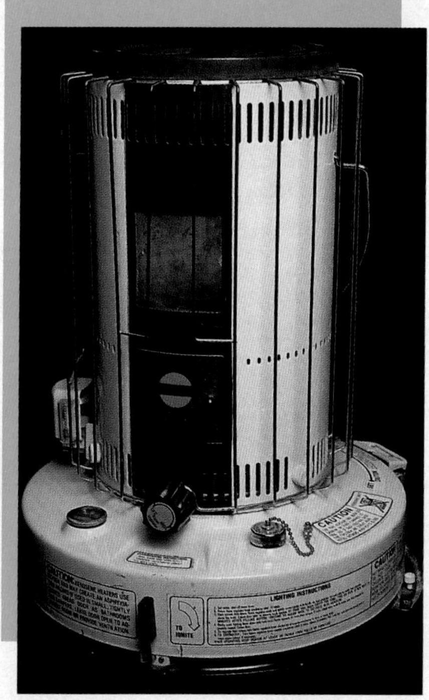

(FIGURE 28-26) **Defective or improperly maintained space heaters and automobile exhaust systems are common sources of poisonous fumes, such as carbon monoxide. Sudden or unexplained drowsiness is a symptom of inhalation poisoning by carbon monoxide.**

immediately move the victim to fresh air. If the person is not breathing, perform rescue breathing. Send for an ambulance equipped with oxygen, and treat for shock.

Contact Poisoning Several types of poisonous substances can burn the skin or be absorbed through it on contact. Treatment for contact poisoning is the same as that for chemical burns: remove clothing and flush the area thoroughly with water for at least five minutes. If the poison is a pesticide, send for an ambulance. Chapter 6 tells you how to treat for contact with poisonous plants such as poison ivy.

Muscle Cramps

A cramp is a sudden knotting of a muscle, usually in the foot, leg, or abdomen. Cramps can be very painful, but they will go away on their own after a few minutes. You can help the cramp go away sooner by massaging or stretching the muscle. If a muscle cramps when you are swimming, tread water while you massage the muscle. Call for help if you need it.

Burns and Scalds

Skin can be burned by fire, sun, hot liquids, heated objects, chemicals, and electricity. Burns are classified by the depth and degree of tissue damage. Figure 28-27 describes the classes of burns and their treatment.

Chemical burns can also be first-, second-, or third-degree, depending on how many layers of skin have been damaged. Take the following steps to treat chemical burns:

- Remove any clothing that covers the affected area or has the chemical on it.
- Hold the burned part under running water for as long as 10 to 15 minutes to wash away all traces of the chemical. If burns are extensive, you may use a hose or shower.
- Once the burn is free of the chemical, you may be able to treat it as you would any other burns. Call a poison control center or doctor to be sure of proper treatment.

If the chemical is in the victim's eye, the eye must be washed out under running water for a full 15 minutes. Hold the person's head under a water fountain or faucet so that the flow of water is away from the nose and toward the ear. Bandage *both* eyes with a soft material to rest the injured eye. If the good eye can see, it will move and the injured eye will move too. Take the victim to a doctor as soon as possible.

1st-Degree Burns

A first-degree burn affects only the epidermis, the top layer of skin. The skin turns red and may hurt but does not blister. Sunburn is the most common first-degree burn. Even without treatment, a first-degree burn will heal in a few days.

▶ Treatment

Cold water and ice can help lower the skin temperature, stop the burning, and relieve the pain. So can pain-relieving preparations you can buy in the drugstore.

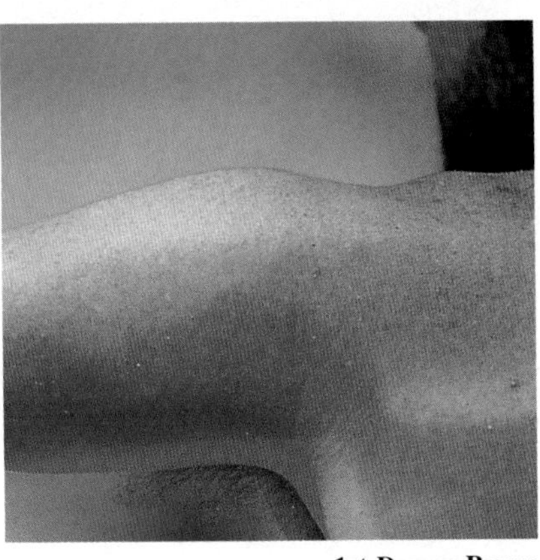

1st-Degree Burns

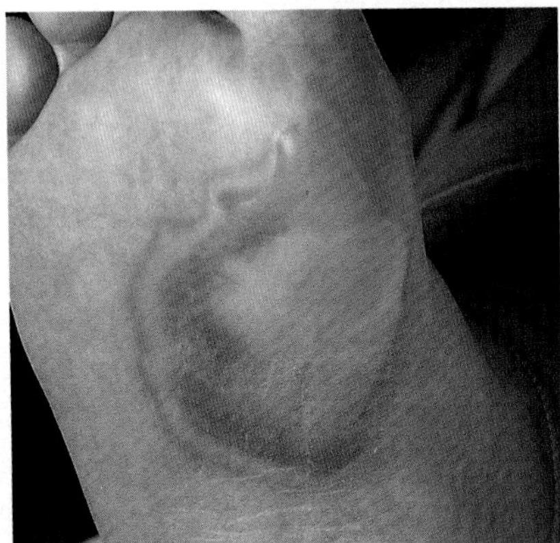

2nd-Degree Burns

2nd-Degree Burns

A second-degree burn forms blisters and affects both layers of skin—the epidermis and dermis. Unless they affect more than 15 percent of the body, second-degree burns are not serious.

▶ Treatment

1. Place the burned area into cool water right away. Cooling it will stop further burning and help relieve the pain.
2. Cover the burn with a clean dressing to prevent infection.
3. Do not pop blisters. The intact skin protects the burned part from infection. Blisters heal on their own in a few days.

3rd-Degree Burns

In a third-degree burn, the dermis and epidermis are destroyed. The tissue underneath is injured and may be partly destroyed as well. Third-degree burns are easily infected. They are typically whitish in color, though they may be charred brown or black. The burns may not hurt at all at first, if the nerve endings have been destroyed.

▶ Treatment

1. Rinse the burned area with cool water only. Very cold water can bring on or intensify shock.
2. Do not apply ointments or creams.
3. Do not remove pieces of clothing stuck to the burns.
4. Cover the burns lightly with sterile dressings or clean cloth.
5. Keep burned limbs elevated, above the heart if possible.
6. Unless victims are unconscious or vomiting, have them drink water to replace fluids lost through the burn.
7. Treat for shock.
8. Monitor breathing.
9. Send for medical help immediately, or take the victim to a hospital or doctor. Third-degree burns will not heal on their own.

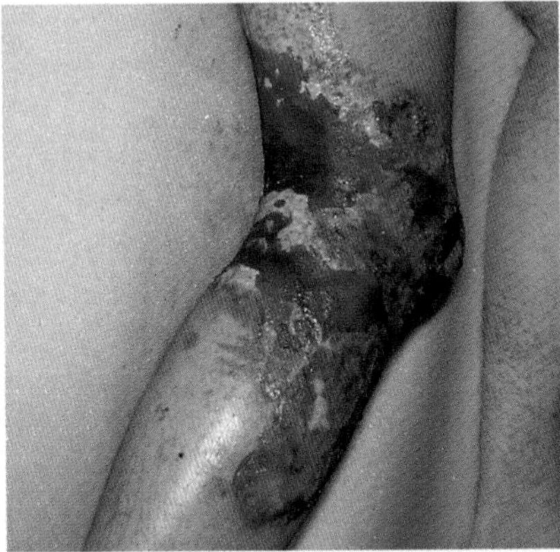

3rd-Degree Burns

(FIGURE 28-27) **First-, second-, and third-degree burns are easily distinguished. Note that the treatment is different for each of these three types of burns.**

Review Answers

1. For heat exhaustion, the victim should lie down in the shade and cool off. If the victim is conscious and not nauseated, the victim should drink plenty of water or an electrolyte replacement solution. For heatstroke, the victim should be moved out of the heat and indoors if possible. The victim should be put in cool water to lower his or her temperature. If conscious, he or she should drink water in small quantities. The victim should be taken to a hospital emergency room as quickly as possible. Heatstroke is more serious than heat exhaustion.

Answer to Question 1 is on p. 645.

2. Answers may include wear clothing appropriate for the weather, such as a warm jacket, hat, and gloves.
3. Answers should agree with Figure 28-27.
4. Answers will vary. Students may answer ask the victim what he or she swallowed, if possible; call the poison control center, give all the information you have, and follow their instructions; monitor the victim's pulse and breathing; administer rescue breathing or CPR if needed.
5. The deep, whitish colored burn is more serious because it is a third-degree burn. Third-degree burns need medical attention, as they will not heal on their own.

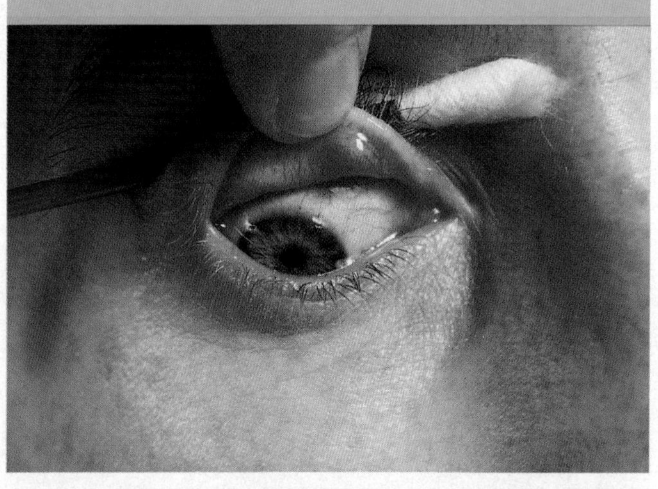

(FIGURE 28-28) **To inspect the upper eyelid, push down gently on the lid with a small stick, such as a matchstick or cotton swab, placed across the lid. Grasping the eyelashes, pull the eyelid upward against the stick and have the person look down while you inspect the lid.**

Foreign Body in the Eye

To remove a foreign body from the eye, first have the victim try blinking several times. Often, blinking and tears will wash the foreign body away. Pulling on the eyelashes of the upper lid may help as well. Gently pulling the upper lid down over the lower lid can permit tears and the lower eyelashes to dislodge the object.

If blinking and tearing don't work, move the person to good light so you can see the eye clearly. To inspect the inside of the lower lid, pull the lid down by pressing on the eyelashes. Use the procedure shown in Figure 28-28 to inspect the inside of the upper lid. If the object is on the inner surface of an eyelid, gently remove it with the corner of a moist, clean cloth or tissue twisted to a point.

If you find an object of any sort embedded in the surface of the eyeball, gently bandage both eyes to restrict their movement. Then take the victim to a doctor.

Fainting

Temporary loss of consciousness is called fainting. Usually, the cause is a shortage of blood flow to the brain. Sometimes a person will be pale and dizzy before fainting. Usually, the victim regains consciousness in a few minutes.

If a person faints near you, keep the person lying down. Elevate his or her feet to increase circulation to the brain. If *you* feel faint, lie down with your head lowered and your feet elevated to increase the blood flow to your brain. If this is not possible, sit down or kneel and bend over so that your head is lower than your heart.

Review

1. *Contrast the treatments for heat exhaustion and heatstroke. Which is more serious?*
2. ***LIFE SKILLS: Practicing Self-Care*** *The temperature is below freezing. You have come in after getting the newspaper and are shivering. You must now walk to school. How can you prevent hypothermia?*
3. *Explain how the treatments for second- and third-degree burns differ.*
4. *What steps would you take if you discovered someone who had swallowed poison?*
5. ***Critical Thinking*** *A burn victim has two burns. One is blistered and painful, and the other is deep and whitish colored but does not hurt. Which is the more serious burn? Explain.*

ASSESS

Section Review

Have students complete the Section Review questions.

Alternative Assessment

Dealing With an Emergency

Allow students to select what they think is the most likely emergency they would encounter among those discussed in this section. Have each student write a brief paragraph discussing how he or she would deal with the emergency.

Closure

Emergencies Differ

Make two columns on the chalkboard. At the top of one column write "Very Serious"; write "Less Serious" at the top of the other. Have students classify the emergencies discussed in this section into these categories.

Highlights

Summary

- Appropriate first aid can mean the difference between life and death or between recovery and permanent injury.
- The steps to take in an emergency are: survey the scene; rescue the victim; send for medical help; treat the life-threatening conditions; identify injuries and provide first aid; remain with the victim, monitoring breathing and pulse until medical help arrives.
- Check the airway, breathing, and circulation (ABCs) of unconscious persons, in that order, before beginning first aid.
- CPR can revive people whose breathing and heartbeat have stopped. It should be attempted only by trained individuals.
- To stop bleeding, apply direct pressure and elevate the wound above the heart.
- All victims of serious injury or illness should be treated for shock. Shock can kill a person even when the injury that triggered it is not life-threatening.
- People with fractures or neck and spinal injuries should not be moved except to be rescued from immediate danger.
- Being calm and reassuring while giving first aid helps prevent panic, which can kill someone even if an injury or illness is not life-threatening.
- Call 911 or the nearest poison control center for advice before giving first aid for poisoning.

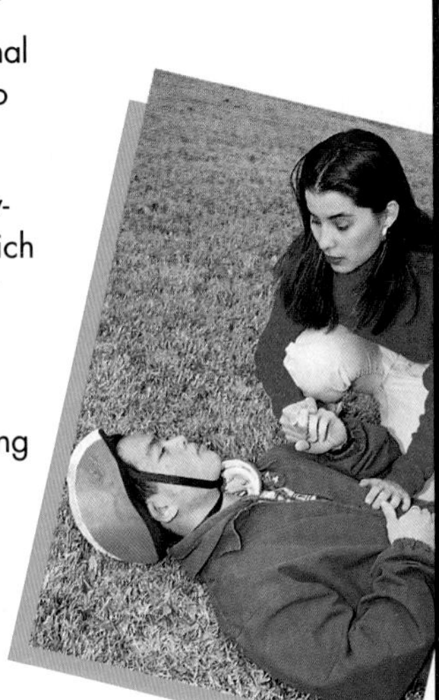

Vocabulary

first aid emergency care given to an ill or injured person before medical attention is available.

cardiopulmonary resuscitation (CPR) a lifesaving procedure designed to revive a person who is not breathing and has no heartbeat.

fracture a broken bone.

dislocation an injury in which the end of a bone comes out of its joint.

sprain a torn or stretched ligament or tendon.

strain a torn or stretched muscle.

Heimlich maneuver a series of sharp thrusts to the abdomen, used to dislodge an object from a choking person's airway.

cardiac arrest condition in which the heart stops working.

stroke the rupture or blockage of an artery in the brain, leading to oxygen deprivation and damage to brain cells.

hypothermia below-normal body temperature.

Chapter 28 Highlights Strategies

Summary

Have students read the summary to reinforce the concepts they learned in Chapter 28.

Vocabulary

Have students write a newspaper account of an accident scene in which they use the vocabulary words from the chapter.

Extension

Have students visit a hospital emergency room, fire station, or other location where paramedics are based. Have them prepare questions covering training, practice, preparation for specific emergencies, equipment, and the experiences workers have had.

Chapter 28 Assessment

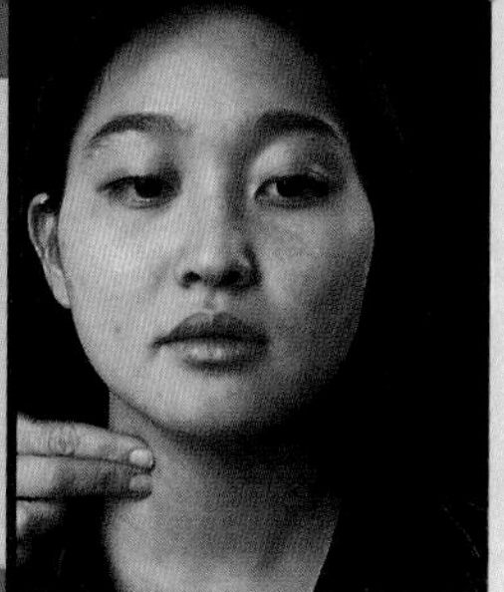

Chapter Review

Concept Review

1. What information should you remember to give when making an emergency telephone call?
2. What are the ABCs of emergency treatment?
3. What is the first-aid treatment for shock and why is this treatment so important?
4. It is important to approach an emergency with the right attitude. How should you behave and why?
5. What are some danger signs to watch for around a wound? What do these signs indicate?
6. What are some symptoms of a head injury? What clues should you look for if you suspect a head injury?
7. What are four symptoms of a heart attack?
8. What is the first-aid treatment for a victim of convulsions?
9. What parts of the body most often suffer from frostbite? What is the most important thing to remember when giving first aid for frostbite?
10. What are the four poisonous snakes in the United States? How soon after being bitten does a snakebite victim need medical treatment?
11. How should the stinger of an insect be removed from its victim? Why? What is the main danger from an insect sting?
12. Why should a person who has swallowed a strong acid be advised not to vomit?
13. Describe the appearance of a first-degree burn.

Expressing Your Views

1. You have started baby-sitting to make some extra money. You are afraid an emergency might arise while the children are in your care. Which first-aid procedures would be important for a baby sitter to know?
2. Do you think the good samaritan laws are fair? Why or why not?
3. Suppose you were bitten by a strange dog while walking near your home. What would you do?
4. You and your friends are planning a camping trip. What do you think should be included in a first-aid kit?

Chapter Review

Concept Review

1. Tell exactly where the victim is; how many people are injured; describe the accident and the injuries; ask what you should do while waiting for medical help.

2. Check airway, breathing, and circulation of blood.

3. Keep the victim calm, lying face up with feet elevated if you do not suspect a head injury. Victims who are unconscious or may vomit should have their heads turned to the side. Keep the victim warm. Untreated shock can lead to death.

4. Behave calmly. Having the victim further upset might cause shock.

5. Pus, pain, redness, fever; infection.

6. Loss of consciousness, nausea, slurred speech, slowed breathing, convulsions, loss of memory, and blood or body fluid leaking from the ears or nose. A clue is whether pupils react to light normally or are dilated.

7. Sudden pain in the chest and possibly radiating to the arms, shoulders, side of the neck, or jaw; weakness, nausea, or sickness; rapid, weak, or irregular pulse; pale skin; perspiration, anxiety, or fear

8. Loosen clothing; remove large objects from the immediate area; if the victim is unconscious, turn his or her head to the side; watch the victim's breathing; if the victim has medicine for convulsions, help administer it; send for medical help or take the victim to the doctor after the convulsion.

9. Fingers, toes, nose, ears, cheeks. It is better not to thaw frostbitten tissue until you can keep the tissue thawed.

10. Coral snake, rattlesnake, copperhead, and water moccasin; within four hours.

11. Scrape the stinger out with a fingernail, broken stick, or the edge of a credit card. If you try to pull the stinger out and the poison sac is still attached, you could squeeze more poison into the wound. Allergic reaction is the main danger.

12. The acid can do as much damage coming up as it did going down.

13. The skin turns red and hurts, but does not blister.

Expressing Your Views

1. Rescue breathing; emergency choking aid; treatment for burns, cuts, and poisoning

Chapter 28 Assessment

Life Skills Check

1. **Intervention Strategies**
   Rescue breathing is a technique that can save lives in a number of different kinds of medical emergencies. If a family member or friend were to stop breathing, what steps would you take to give rescue breathing?
2. **Practicing Self-Care**
   If you suffer from diabetes or epilepsy, what can you do to ensure that others are aware of your condition?
3. **Practicing Self-Care**
   Suppose you want to be an ambulance driver. Knowing that you will have to treat bleeding victims, what steps should you take to protect yourself from a serious disease such as hepatitis or AIDS?

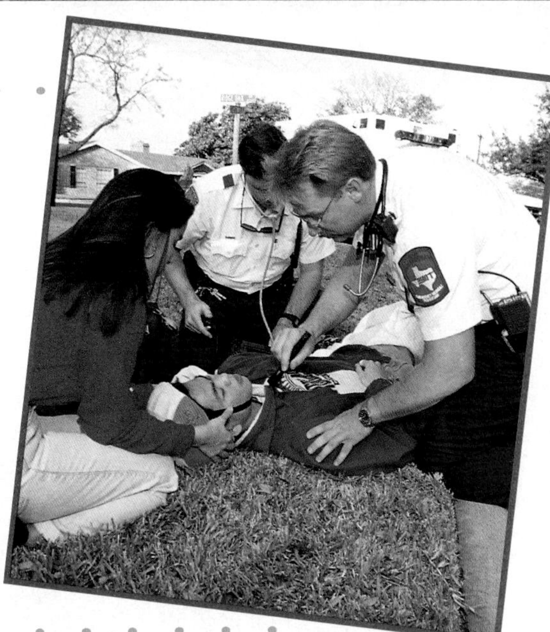

Projects

1. Inventory the first-aid supplies at home, and make suggestions to a parent or guardian about what items are needed. You might also put together a first-aid kit for your car.
2. Working with a group, present a short skit in which a group member experiences one of the emergencies discussed in the chapter. Others in the group should portray people arriving at the scene—police officers, medics, friends, and family members. Without performing the actual techniques, show the audience correct emergency first-aid procedures.
3. Interview an EMT, paramedic, or emergency-room nurse. Ask about the type of training required and the personal qualities they feel are necessary for the job. Also ask the person to relate a particularly rewarding experience he or she has had on the job. Share what you learn with the class.

Plan for Action

First aid and CPR are very important lifesaving skills. Make a list of your activities, and identify the ways you could save lives during an emergency by knowing and using first aid or CPR.

2. Most students should answer yes, as the laws enable a person to administer first aid without worrying about a lawsuit.
3. Wash the bite and call my doctor for further instructions. I would notify the police, and find out whether the dog has had rabies shots.
4. Sterile bandages, antibiotic ointment, elastic bandage, cotton swabs, tweezers, splints, baking soda, ice packs

Life Skills Check

1. Students should respond with the steps given in Figure 28-2.
2. I could wear a medical ID bracelet or necklace identifying my condition.
3. I would put on rubber gloves before treating the wounds. If rubber gloves were not available, I would cover the wound with sterile gauze and then place the victim's hand on top of the material and my hand on top of the victim's hand. Afterward, I would wash my hands.

Projects

Have students plan and carry out the projects for first aid and CPR.

Plan for Action

Have students quiz each other orally in a round-robin fashion. The first student poses an emergency situation, the second describes what first-aid measures should be taken in that situation and then poses a situation for the next student.

Assessment Options

Chapter Test

Have students take the Chapter 28 Test.

Alternative Assessment

Have students do the Alternative Assessment activity for Chapter 28.

Test Generator

The Test Generator (Macintosh® or IBM® format) contains an additional 50 assessment items for this chapter.

Issues in Health

ETHICAL ISSUES IN HEALTH

ISSUE: *Should gun-control laws be passed to reduce the number of violent deaths from gun-shot wounds?*

Have students read the Ethical Issues in Health feature. Ask them to suggest reasons for and against the enactment of gun-control laws. List these in two columns on the chalkboard. Is it difficult to separate arguments and feelings when it comes to gun control? Can students suggest compromises that might be reached in gun-control legislation (for instance, limiting access to certain kinds of guns)?

Ethical Issues in Health

ISSUE: Should gun-control laws be passed to reduce the number of violent deaths from gunshot wounds?

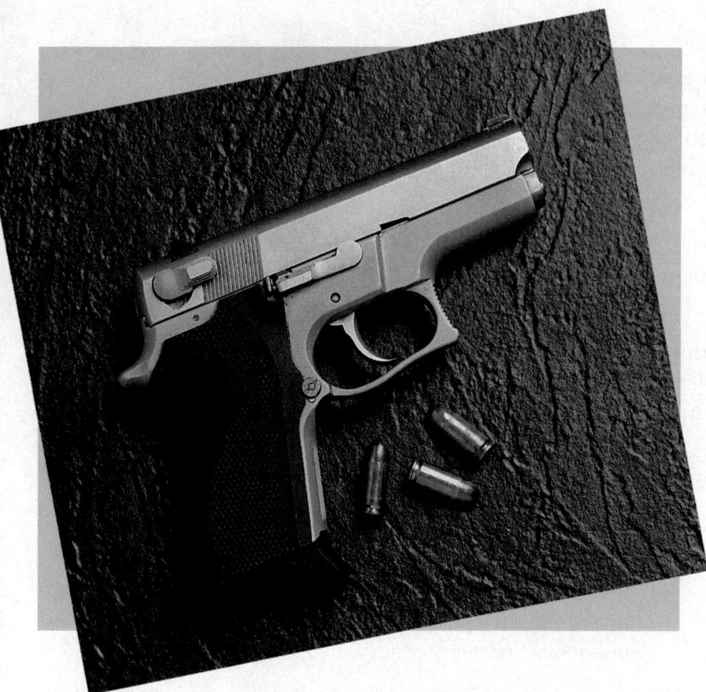

Guns have become a factor that seriously affects teenage health and safety. In a recent survey at an inner-city high school, more than half the students interviewed said they knew someone who had brought a gun to school, and most said they knew someone who had been shot. Sadly, this is not a surprising statistic. Accidents, homicides, and suicides are the leading causes of death among American teenagers. Many of the accidents and a majority of the homicides and suicides of teens involve guns. Statistics from the National Center for Health show that guns were used in more than 70 percent of teenage homicides and in more than 60 percent of the suicides by teenage males. As a result, gunshot wounds are the second leading cause of death among 15- to 19-year-olds in the United States.

To try to stop students and other people from bringing guns to school, schools across the nation are beginning to use metal detectors. In the same way that these devices are used in airports, metal detectors can be installed in a school's doorways so that all students must pass through one of the devices before entering the school. Hand-held metal detectors can also be used to search individuals suspected of carrying a gun or knife. In 1989, nearly half of the students surveyed in one inner-city school agreed that metal detectors should be installed in schools to prevent the entry of guns and other weapons. Many school board members and administrators also believe that as long as guns continue to be a serious problem in schools, metal detectors will be necessary to protect students and school employees.

One reason why guns play such a major role in the deaths of American teenagers may be the large number of guns that are available. Studies show that half of all homes in the United States have firearms (rifles, shotguns, and handguns). It is estimated that 70 million Americans own about 200 million firearms, many of them handguns. Although many people feel that having guns in their homes provides safety, those most likely to be injured by gunshots are the family members of people who have guns. Other high-risk groups include male teens, those who abuse alcohol, and people who frequently get into physical fights to settle arguments.

In an attempt to reduce the impact of guns on the health of all Americans, several laws have been proposed that would control the sale of firearms (handguns, rifles, and shotguns). Some of these laws would require people to obtain a license to own guns. Others would require a waiting period for the purchase of a gun.

Advocates of gun-control laws point out that most people are shot and killed as the result of arguments and fights with family members. They argue that requiring a waiting period before the purchase of a gun would reduce the number of homicides and suicides, because an enraged or depressed person would not have immediate access to a gun. They also argue that licensing would help reduce gunshot injuries, because people with criminal records or histories of mental illness would be denied licenses to own and carry guns.

Those who oppose gun control point out that by itself, a gun cannot kill or injure people—it must be fired by someone. Since most people who own guns use them responsibly, opponents of gun control believe that only those who use guns unlawfully should be punished. Opponents of gun-control laws are also concerned that such laws will not be obeyed by criminals, leaving law-abiding citizens defenseless. The National Rifle Association (NRA) is the most powerful group in the United States that opposes gun-control laws. Citing the United States Constitution, the NRA's philosophy is that all citizens have the right to own and use guns for self-defense, hunting, and recreational purposes.

Situation for Discussion

Mark and George attend the same high school. Last Saturday night, Mark saw George and Wendy dancing and kissing at a friend's party. Mark had been dating Wendy, but they had recently split up. As the party broke up, a loud confrontation between Mark and George began on the front lawn. Several blows were exchanged, but the fight was stopped by other party-goers. As George was leaving, Mark yelled, "I'll see you later, George! You're a dead man!"

a. What is the potential outcome of this situation?

b. Could a gun-control law prevent an injury or homicide in this case? Explain.

c. What other ways are there to protect George, Mark, their families and friends, and other students at their school from injury or death?

d. How could the disagreement be settled without physical harm to either person?

The Nervous System and Its Organs

The nervous system regulates and coordinates body activities in response to changes in the internal and external environment. These changes, called stimuli, initiate impulses in millions of sensory receptors spread throughout the body. The principal sense organs are the eyes, ears, and sensory receptors in the skin, joints, nose, tongue, and muscles.

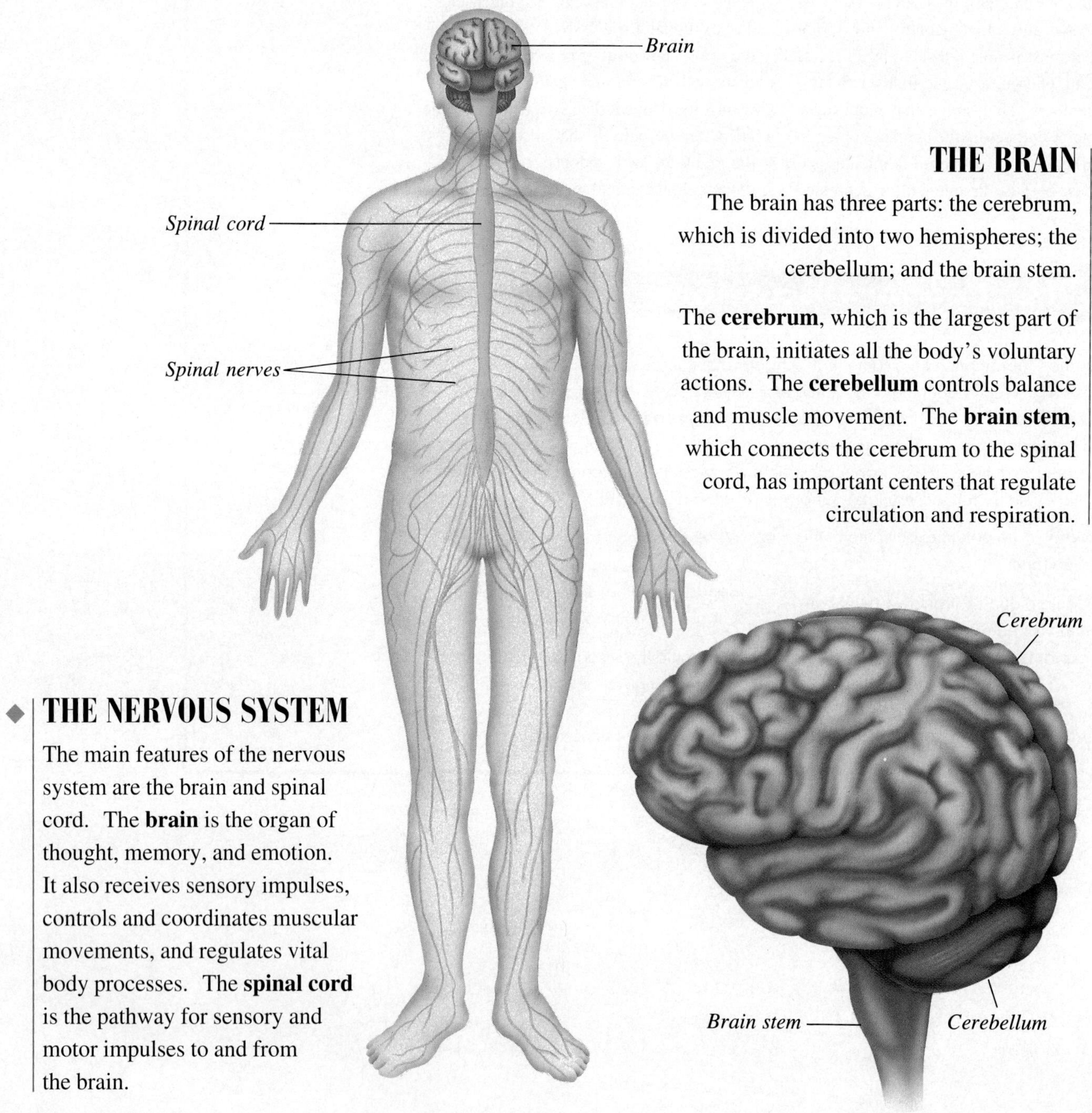

THE BRAIN

The brain has three parts: the cerebrum, which is divided into two hemispheres; the cerebellum; and the brain stem.

The **cerebrum**, which is the largest part of the brain, initiates all the body's voluntary actions. The **cerebellum** controls balance and muscle movement. The **brain stem**, which connects the cerebrum to the spinal cord, has important centers that regulate circulation and respiration.

THE NERVOUS SYSTEM

The main features of the nervous system are the brain and spinal cord. The **brain** is the organ of thought, memory, and emotion. It also receives sensory impulses, controls and coordinates muscular movements, and regulates vital body processes. The **spinal cord** is the pathway for sensory and motor impulses to and from the brain.

A NEURON

A **neuron,** or nerve cell, is the basic unit of the nervous system. A neuron consists of a **cell body**; **dendrites**, which are branched structures that conduct impulses to the cell body; and an **axon**, which is a long fiber that transmits impulses away from the cell body. There are three types of neurons. Sensory neurons send sense signals to the spinal cord and the brain. Motor neurons send signals from the brain and the spinal cord to the body's muscles. Association neurons link sensory neurons to motor neurons.

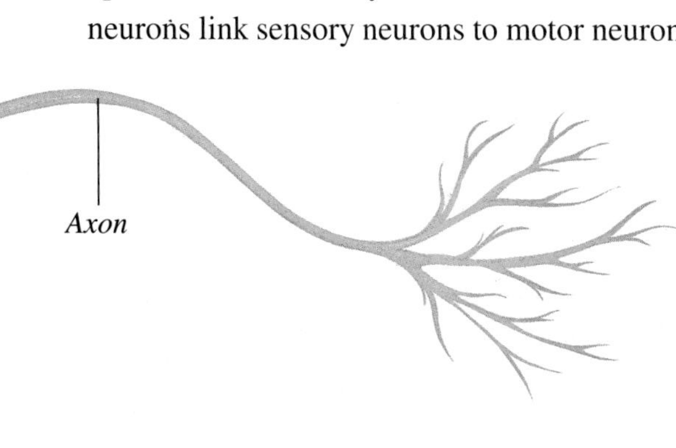

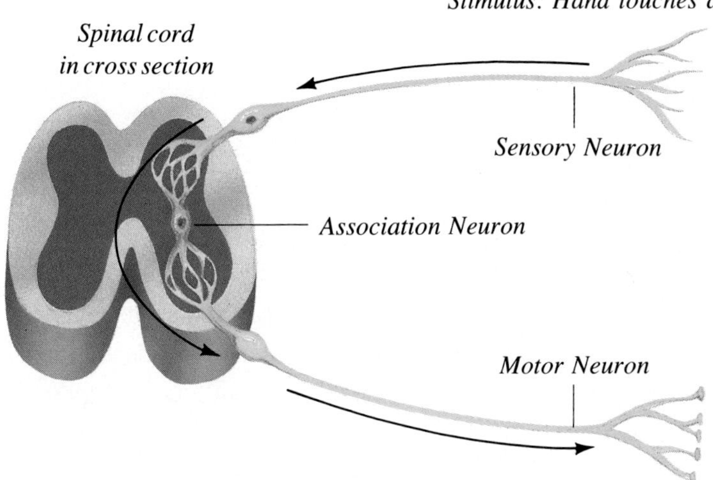

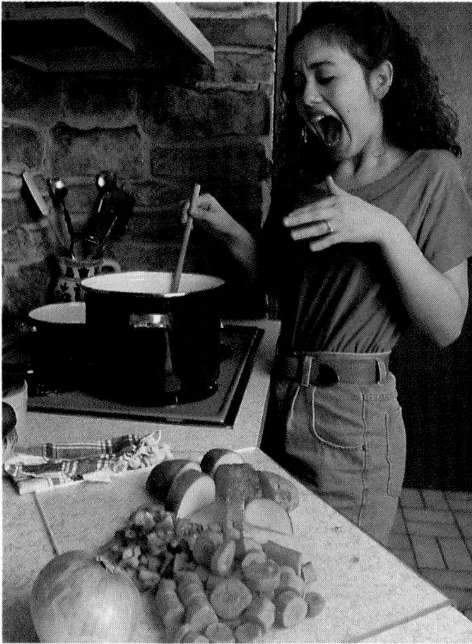

REFLEXES

Some of the body's movements are not controlled by the brain. Let's say you touch a hot stove. A nerve impulse will travel through a **sensory neuron** from your hand to your spinal cord, where it will be transferred to an **association neuron**, and then to a **motor neuron**. The impulse will travel back to your hand through the motor neuron. At this point, you'll know to pull your hand away from the stove. Such an action, known as a reflex, takes only a split second to occur.

SMELL AND TASTE

Sensory receptors in the nose and mouth respond to chemical substances. Olfactory (smell) receptors sense minute amounts of chemicals in the air. Taste receptors sense chemicals in food and beverages, which are classified as sweet, sour, salty, or bitter. Even though taste and smell messages travel separately to different areas of the brain, they often create a combined feeling of pleasure or displeasure when you are eating.

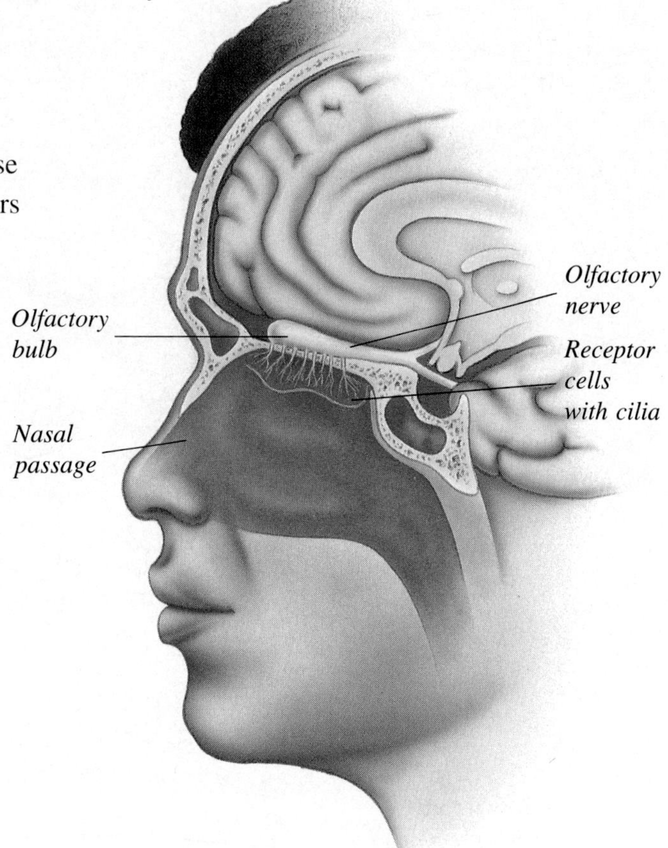

Olfactory receptors are located in thousands of tiny projections from certain cells in the **nasal passages**. These projections—called **cilia**—absorb smells, and the receptors inside transport impulses to the **olfactory bulb**, which relays them to the brain through the **olfactory nerve**.

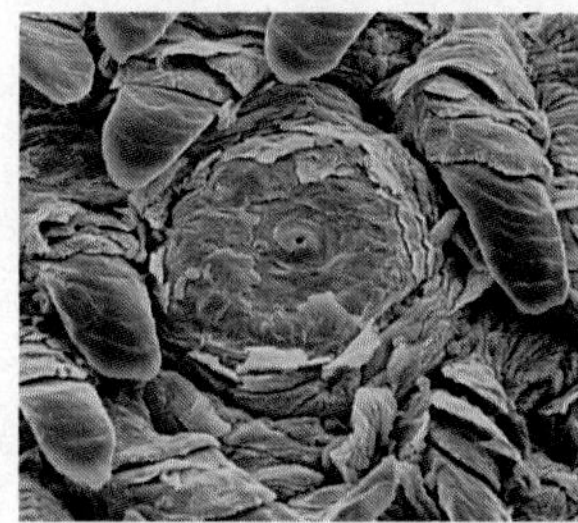

The tongue is covered with small, rough bumps called papillae. Each papilla is covered with taste buds, which contain the sensory receptors for taste. Chewing breaks up food, which is then mixed with saliva and washed across the papillae. Chemicals in the food stimulate the taste receptors in the taste buds.

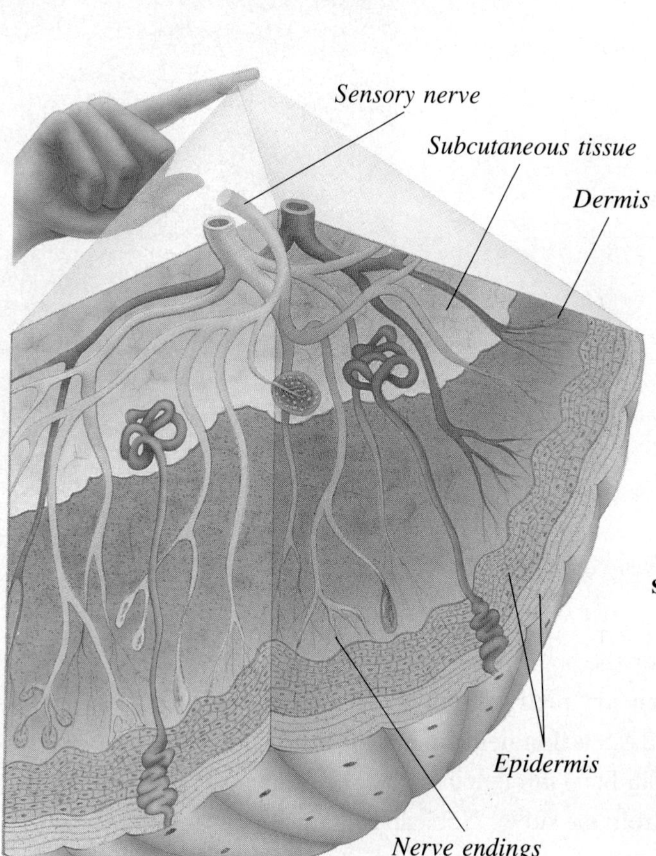

TOUCH

Touch is the sensation produced by pressure on the surface of the body. The skin on very sensitive parts of the body, such as the tongue, lips, and finger pads, has a high concentration of touch receptors.

Touch messages are transmitted by bundles of **sensory nerve** fibers that come through the **subcutaneous layer** underneath the **dermis** (inner layer of the skin). The bundles split into fibers, some of which reach into the **epidermis** (outer layer of the skin). **Nerve endings** in the epidermis are sensitive to pressure and pain. Other sensory nerve fibers end in specialized receptors in the dermis, which sense heat, cold, or pressure.

VISION

Vision is a response to light falling on the eye. The sense of sight interprets the stimulus and triggers a reaction. Light rays from an object enter the eye through the **pupil** and are focused on the **retina**, which converts the rays to nerve impulses that are carried to the brain.

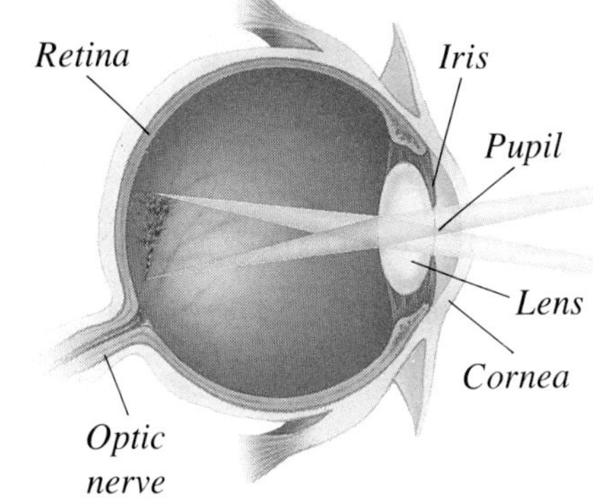

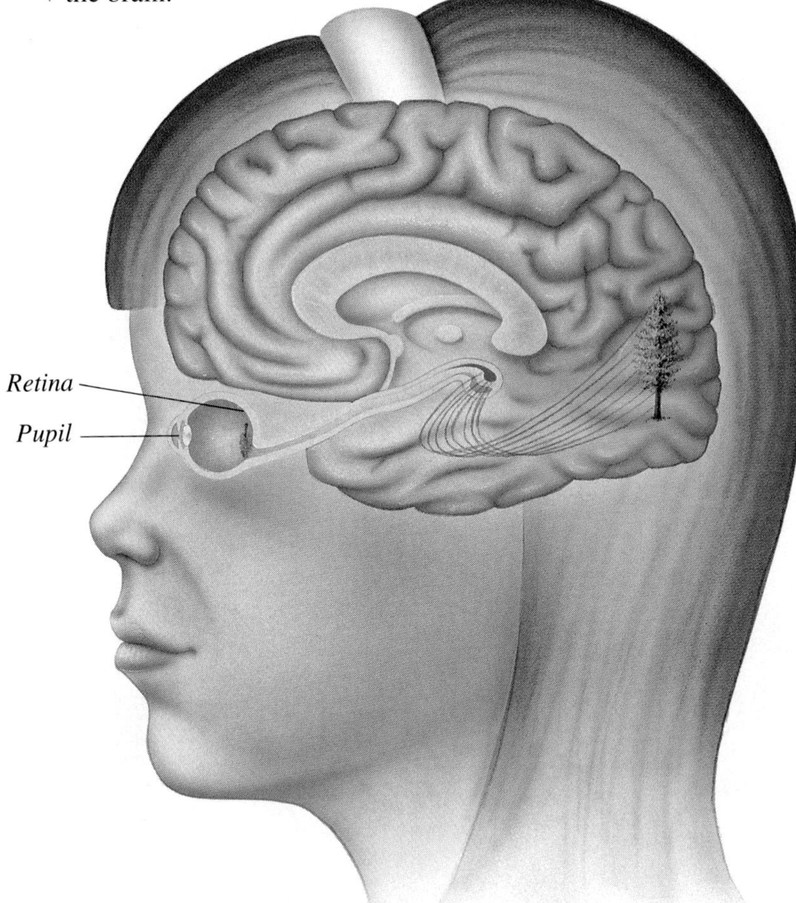

PARTS OF THE EYE

The outer surface of the eye is covered by the **cornea**, a transparent membrane that allows light to enter the eye. Behind the cornea is the **iris**, a thin, colored, circular membrane. In the center of the iris is a hole called the **pupil**. Muscles in the iris dilate (widen) the pupil to let in more light and contract it to let in less light. Behind the pupil is the **lens**, a thick, curved structure that focuses the light rays passing though it on the back of the eye. The **retina** is a thin sheet lining the back of the eye and containing many receptors that respond to light. Nerve fibers from the retina merge to form the **optic nerve**, through which nerve impulses travel to the brain.

HEARING

The ear converts sound waves to nerve impulses. First, the external ear funnels sounds through the **ear canal** to the **eardrum**. Sound waves apply pressure to the eardrum, causing it to vibrate. These eardrum vibrations are then transmitted to the inner ear through three bones known as the **hammer**, **anvil**, and **stirrup**. Once in the inner ear, the vibrations become nerve impulses that travel to the brain.

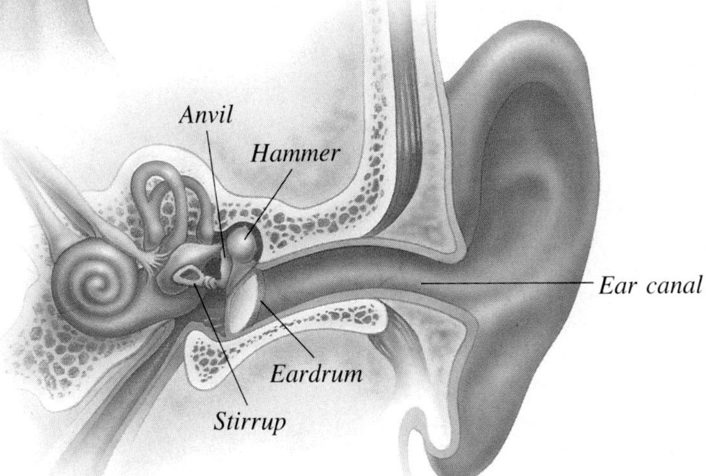

The Skeletal System

The skeletal system supports and protects the soft tissues and vital organs of the body. Without its rigid bones and flexible joints, you would not be able to stand, sit, bend, walk, or run. The heart and lungs are shielded by the ribs, the spinal cord by the vertebrae, and the brain by the skull.

Pairs of muscles attached to bones allow you to move in ways you choose—to toss a ball, jump over a hurdle, or pull a bow over a violin string. One muscle in each pair moves a bone in one direction; the other moves it back.

HUNDREDS OF BONES

Your skeleton contains about 206 bones, depending on which ones you count as separate. The pelvis, for instance, can be counted as a single bone or as 6 bones fused together. There are 24 ribs in 12 pairs, 26 vertebrae in the backbone, and 28 phalanges (finger bones).

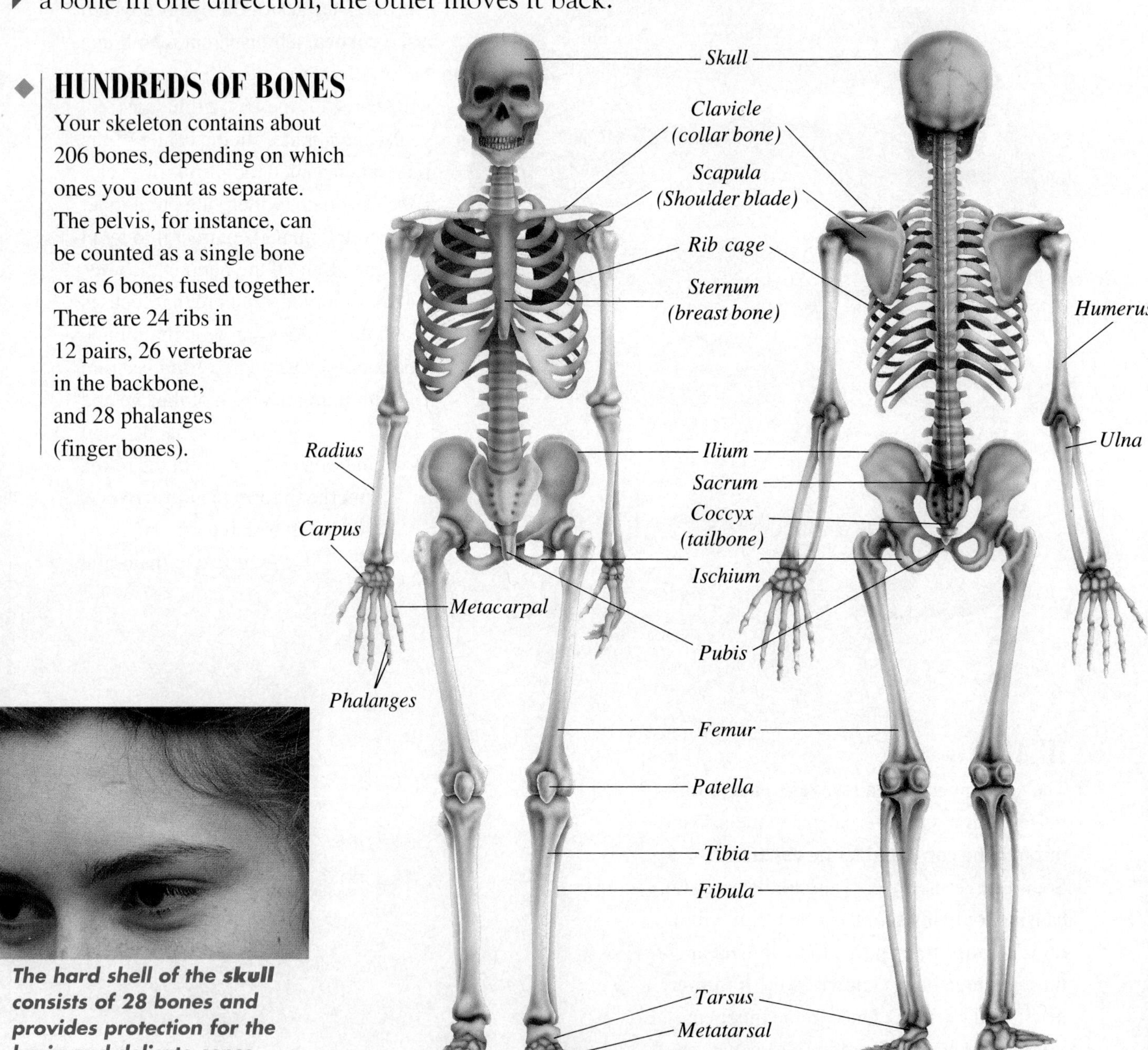

The hard shell of the skull consists of 28 bones and provides protection for the brain and delicate sense organs.

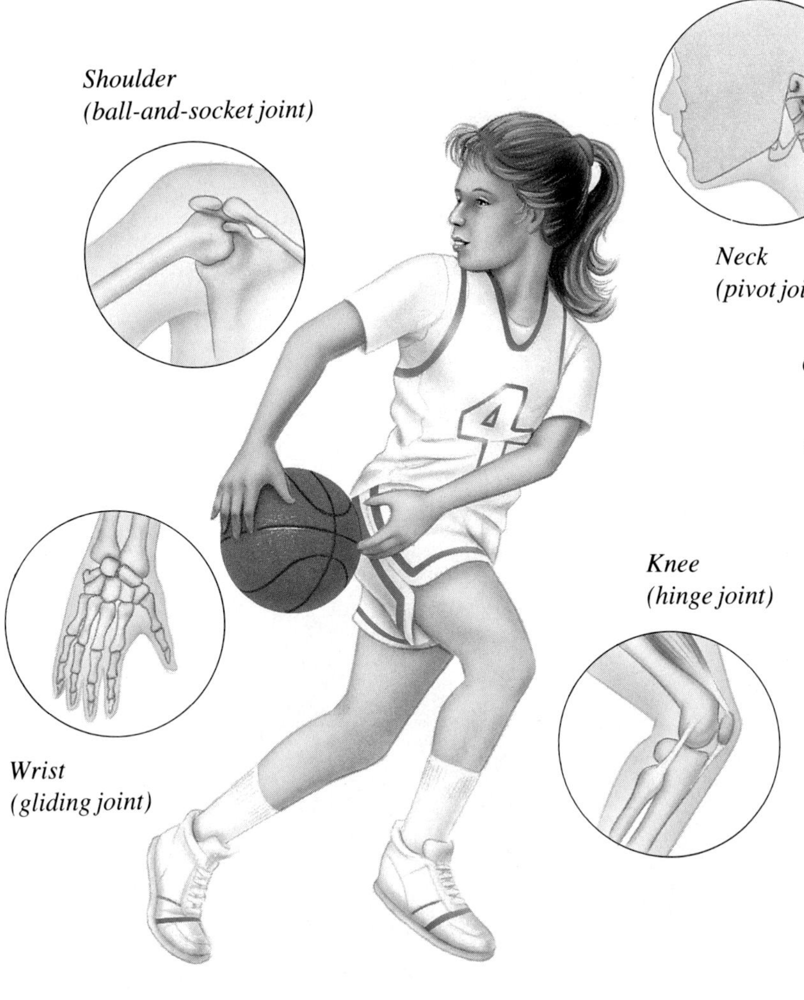

JOINTS

Hinge, pivot, ball-and-socket, and gliding—the names of joints suggest the type of motion each kind allows. Hinge joints, found in the knees and elbows, allow back-and-forth movement—like a hinge in a door. Pivot joints, like those in the neck, let some joints move back and forth and others move up and down. The shoulder and hip joints are ball-and-socket joints, which allow circular movement of the bone. Gliding joints, found in the wrists and ankles, allow for flexibility.

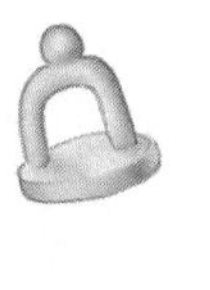

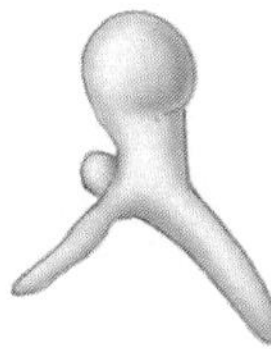

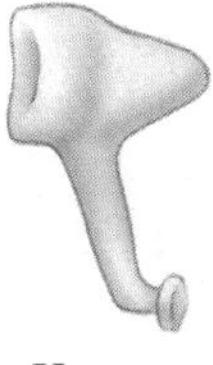

The smallest bones in the body are found in the middle ear. The tiny stirrup, anvil, and hammer bones pass vibrations from the eardrum to the inner ear.

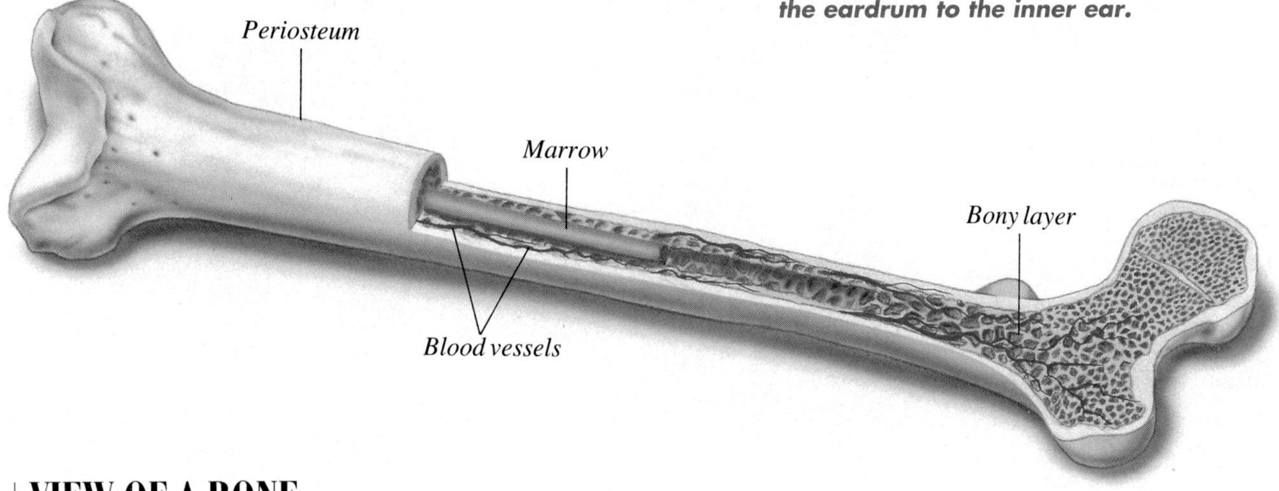

VIEW OF A BONE

They may seem hard and lifeless, but human bones are made of live tissue. The hard outer shell of the bone, called the **periosteum**, contains many nerves as well as **blood vessels** that transport food and oxygen to the bone's many cells. Inside the periosteum is the **bony layer**, which contains more blood vessels, bone cells, and nerves. At the center of some bones is the **marrow**, which makes blood cells.

The Muscular System

The muscular system moves the body. Each muscle consists of muscle fibers that can contract and relax. When a muscle contracts, it pulls the tissue attached to it, resulting in movement of that tissue. The body's large outer muscles also help protect the inner organs. Other muscles help move food, blood, and air.

Your body has more than 600 muscles. Muscles make up about 30 percent of the total mass of an adult female and about 40 percent of the total mass of an adult male.

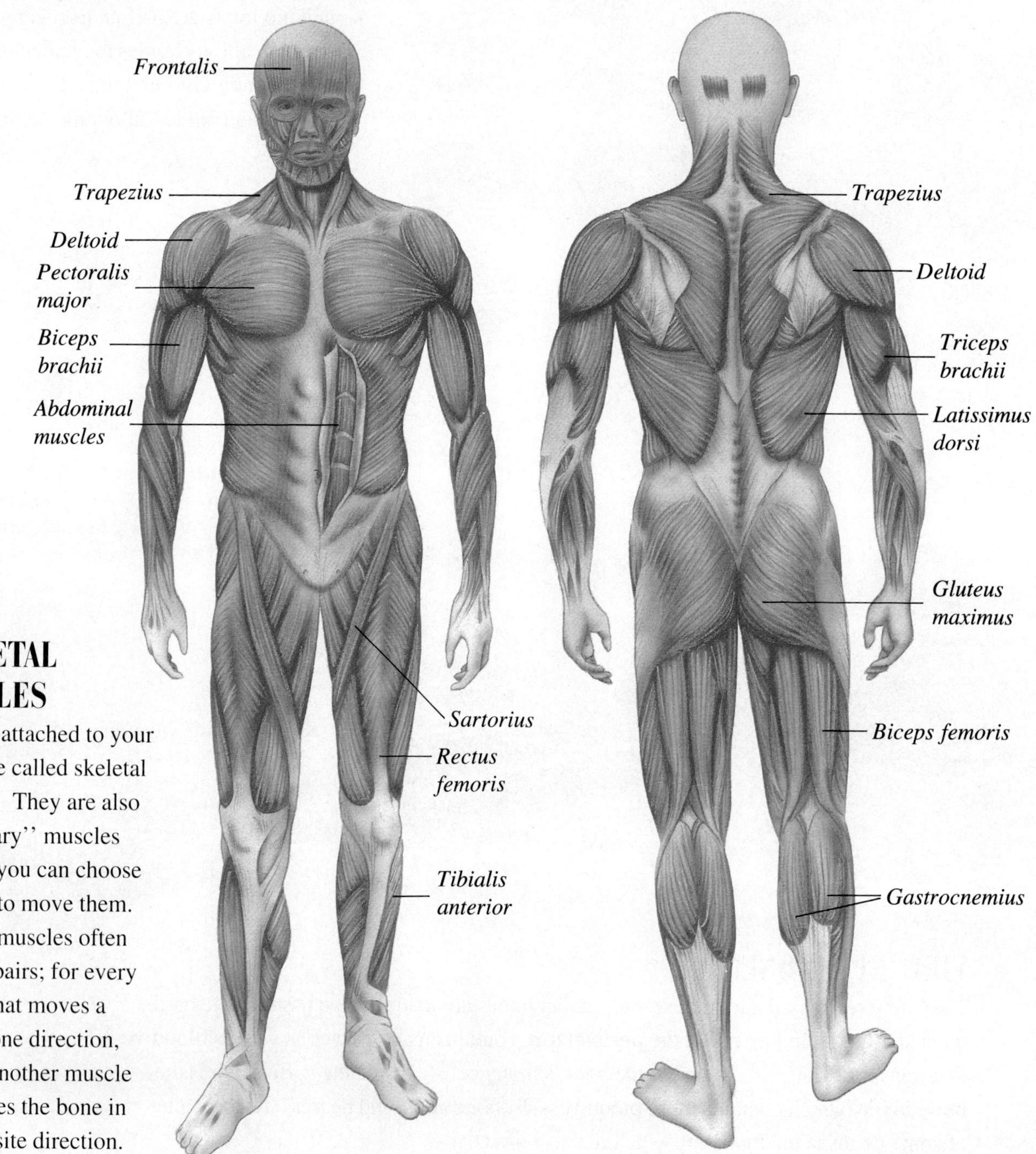

SKELETAL MUSCLES

Muscles attached to your bones are called skeletal muscles. They are also "voluntary" muscles because you can choose whether to move them. Skeletal muscles often work in pairs; for every muscle that moves a bone in one direction, there is another muscle that moves the bone in the opposite direction.

MUSCLE ACTION

Muscles often work in pairs to bend and straighten joints. Whenever you bend and straighten your arm, you are using your biceps and triceps muscles. Contracting your **biceps muscle** bends your arm at the elbow. When your **triceps muscle** contracts, it allows you to straighten your arm.

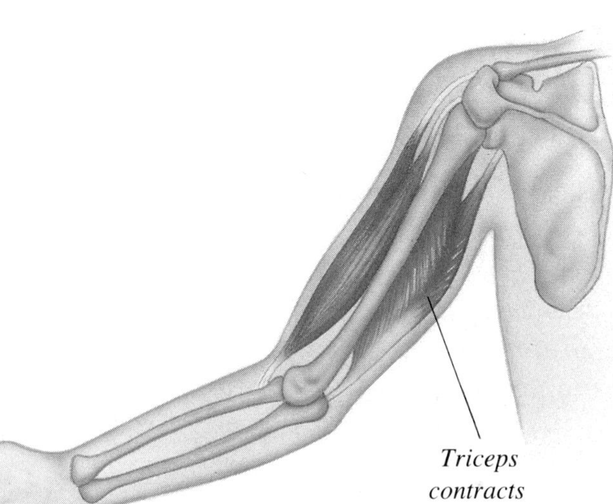

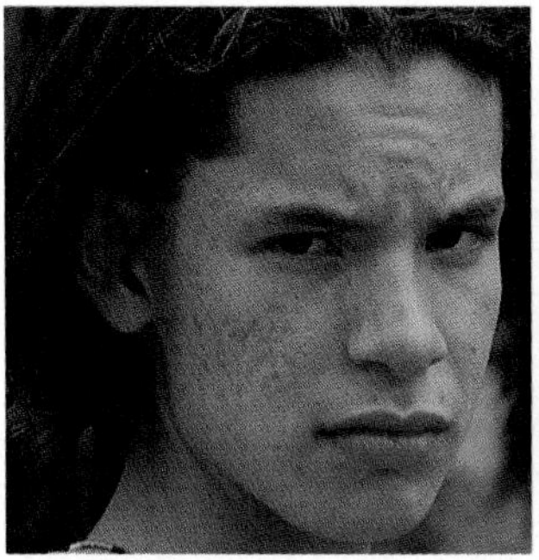

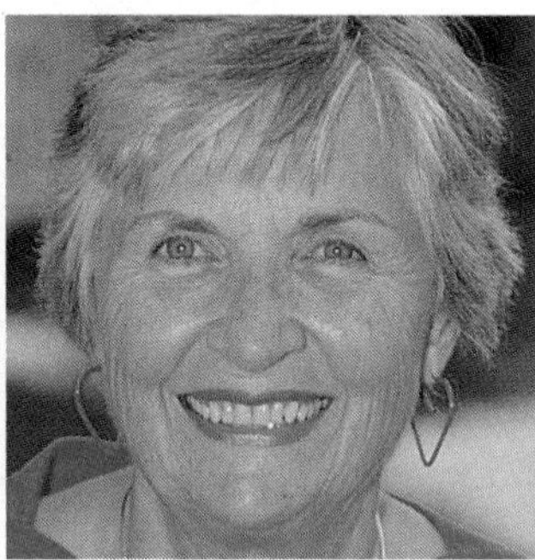

Even the simplest body movements involve the coordination of many muscles. It takes 13 muscles to smile, for example, and 34 muscles to frown.

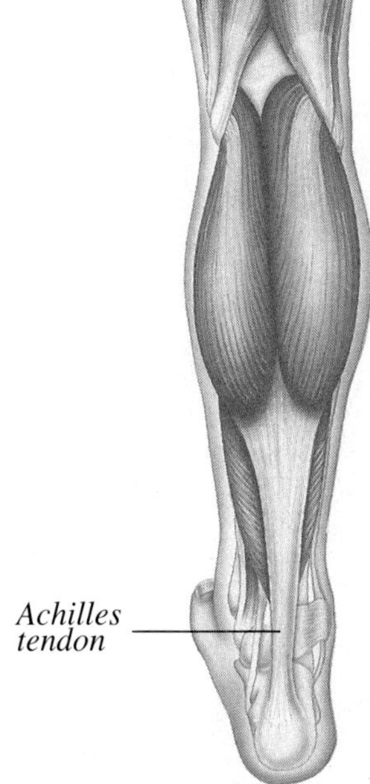

***Tendons and ligaments** are tough elastic bands that connect tissue. The **Achilles tendon** joins the calf muscles to the heel bone. You can feel your Achilles tendon by touching the back of your ankle as you wiggle your foot.*

CARDIAC MUSCLE

The heart is made up of cardiac muscle, an involuntary muscle. You have no conscious control of an involuntary muscle. The contraction and relaxation of cardiac muscle helps pump blood through the body automatically and rhythmically. A normal, resting heart contracts about 70 times a minute. The best way to care for the heart and its cardiac muscle is to get plenty of aerobic exercise and to eat a healthy diet that is low in fat.

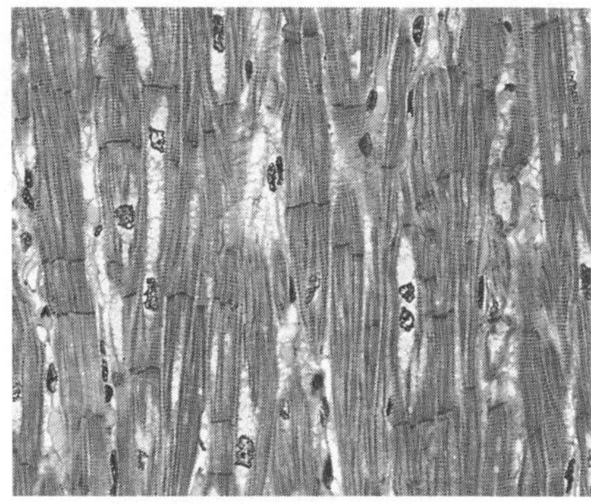

The Endocrine System

The endocrine system consists of nine specialized glands that regulate many body functions. A gland is a body structure that produces and releases chemical substances. Endocrine glands secrete hormones directly into the bloodstream or body tissues. A hormone is a chemically active substance that carries a particular message to a specific part of the body.

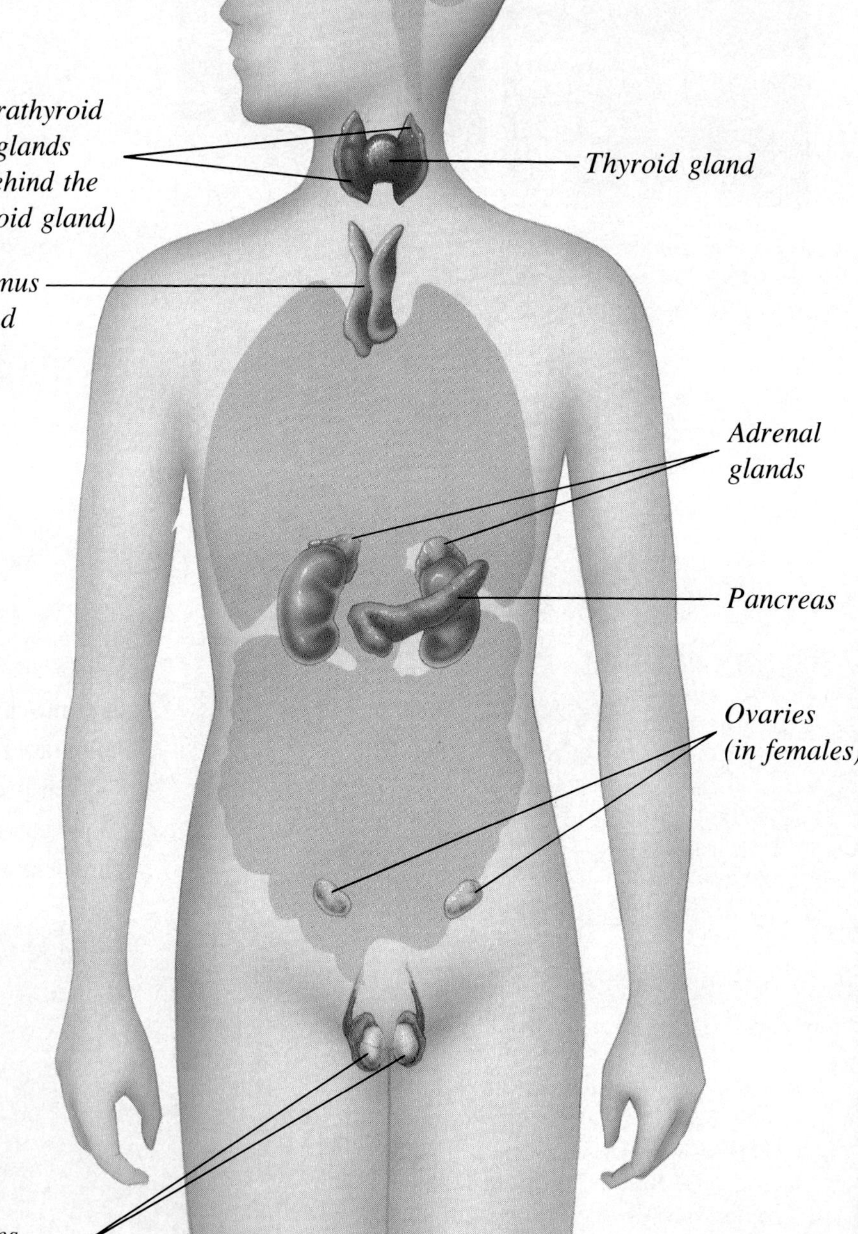

THE THYROID GLAND

The butterfly-shaped **thyroid gland** is located at the base of the front of the neck. It secretes two hormones that play a crucial role in determining the speed at which the body transforms food into energy (metabolic rate) and how quickly the body uses that energy.

Thyroid gland

ADRENAL GLANDS AND "FIGHT OR FLIGHT"

There is an **adrenal gland** located on top of each kidney. The inner layer of each adrenal gland secretes adrenaline and noradrenaline in emergency situations, as directed by the nervous system. These hormones cause a "fight-or-flight" response that prepares the body to take action. The outer layer of each adrenal gland secretes hormones that help regulate the body's metabolism and its salt and water balance.

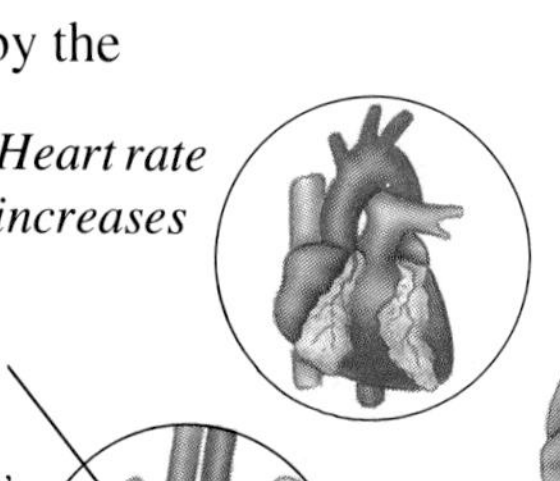

Heart rate increases

Adrenal hormones stimulate other body responses

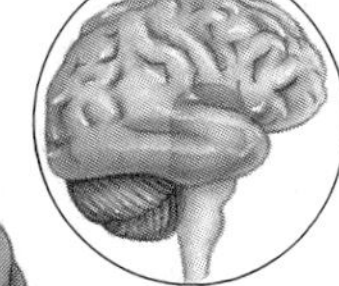

Brain perceives danger; stimulates Adrenal gland

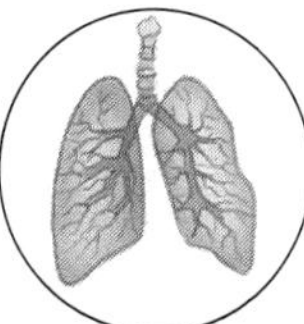

Air passages widen; breathing rate increases

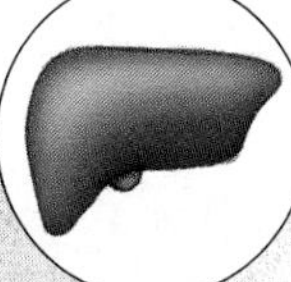

Extra blood sugar released by the liver

Hairs stand on end

THE PITUITARY GLAND

The **pituitary gland** is often called the master gland because it controls many different functions, and even other glands. Hormones released by the pituitary gland regulate growth, direct the reproductive organs, adrenal glands, and the thyroid gland, and—in women—stimulate uterine contractions during childbirth and breast milk release during nursing. The pea-sized pituitary gland, which lies at the base of the brain, consists of two lobes located just below the **hypothalamus**. The hypothalamus is a part of the brain that controls the secretion of pituitary hormones and regulates body temperature, hunger, thirst, and sex drive.

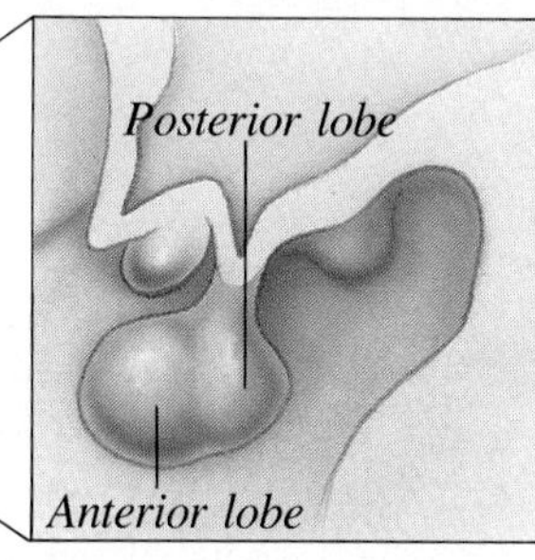

OTHER ESSENTIAL ENDOCRINE GLANDS

Several other endocrine glands aid in maintaining normal body function. The **thymus gland** is important to the development of a child's immune system but has no function in adults. The **pineal gland** is thought to control the body's internal time clock. The **parathyroid glands** control the calcium level in the blood. The reproductive organs—**testes** in males and **ovaries** in females—produce hormones that regulate the development of sex characteristics and initiate the production of reproductive cells.

The Circulatory System

The body's circulatory system includes the cardiovascular system, which consists of the blood, blood vessels, and heart. The lymphatic system, which consists of the lymph fluid, lymph nodes, lymphatic vessels, thymus gland, tonsils, and spleen, is also part of the circulatory system. The circulatory system brings oxygen, nutrients, antibodies, and infection-fighting cells to each cell in the body. It also helps rid the body of wastes.

BLOOD

Blood consists of various specialized cells and a fluid called plasma. The yellowish plasma contains water, nutrients, wastes, and other materials. The cells found in blood include **red blood cells**, which carry oxygen; **white blood cells**, which protect the body against diseases; and **platelets**, which initiate the process of blood clotting.

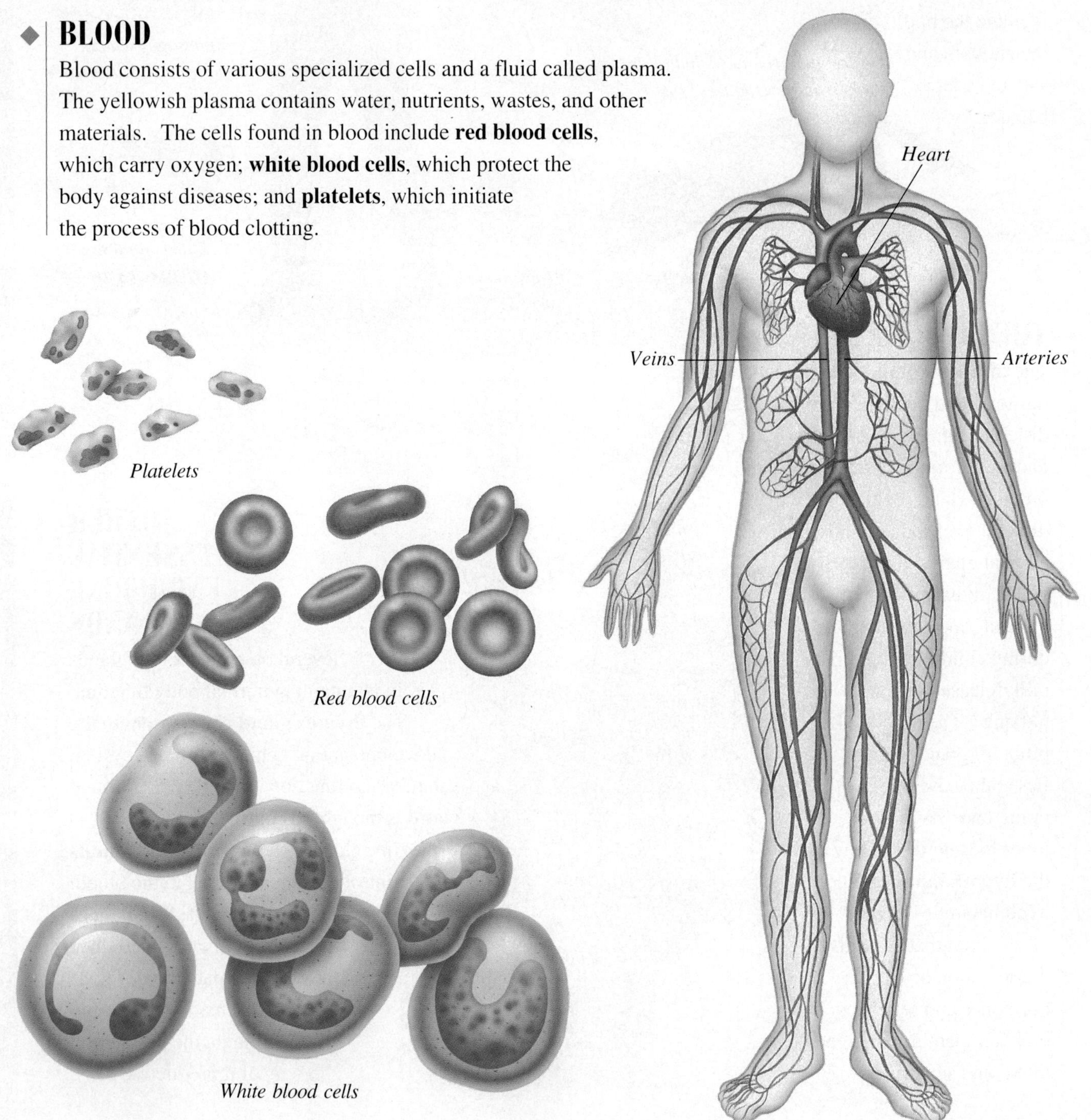

Platelets

Red blood cells

White blood cells

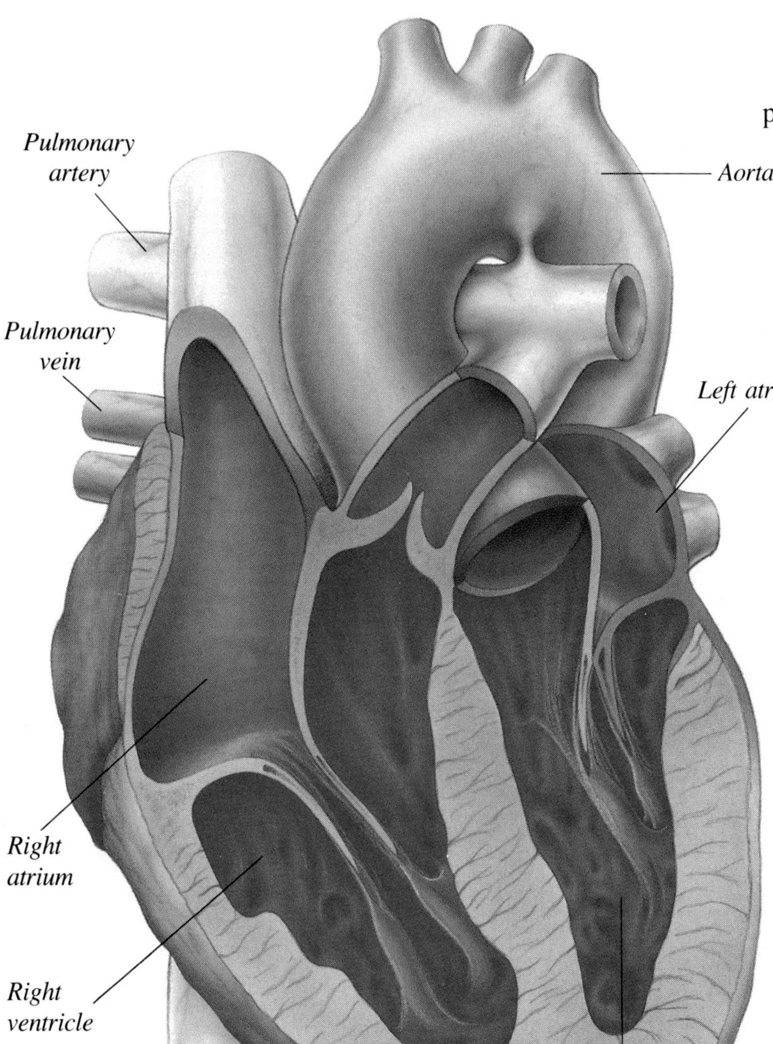

THE HEART

The heart is the circulatory system's pump—the organ that pushes blood through blood vessels to various parts of the body.

Blood travels through the heart in one direction only. It enters the heart through the **right atrium**, and then travels to the **right ventricle**. When the right ventricle contracts, blood is pumped through the **pulmonary arteries** to the lungs, where the blood gives off carbon dioxide and picks up oxygen.

Oxygen-rich blood returns to the heart through the **pulmonary veins**, enters the **left atrium**, and then travels to the **left ventricle**. Then the left ventricle contracts, pumping blood into the **aorta** and out to various parts of the body.

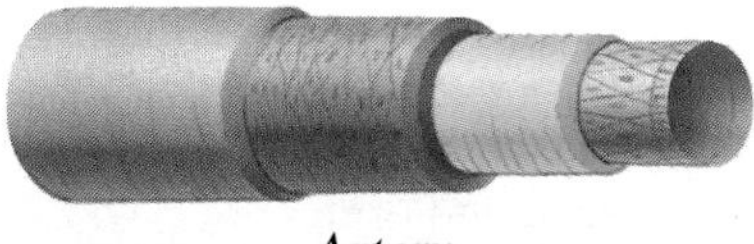

Artery

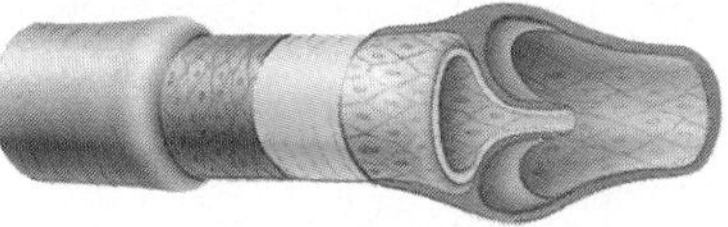

Vein

BLOOD VESSELS

There are three types of blood vessels in the circulatory system. **Arteries** are the thick-walled vessels that carry blood from the heart to all parts of the body. **Veins**, which have thinner walls, carry blood back to the heart from all parts of the body. Veins also contain tiny valves that prevent blood from flowing downward due to the pull of gravity. **Capillaries** link the arteries to the veins. Capillaries are the smallest blood vessels, allowing blood cells to pass through only one at a time. No cell in the body is more than a few cells away from a capillary.

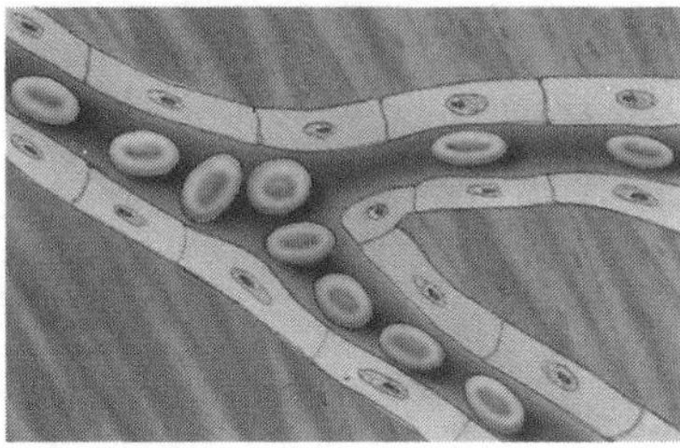

The walls of capillaries are only one cell thick, which allows oxygen and nutrients to leave the bloodstream easily so they can be taken up by the body's cells.

The Respiratory System

Your body's cells need oxygen in order to function. They also produce carbon dioxide, which must be removed from the body. The respiratory system takes in air, separates oxygen from the other gases in the air, and delivers the oxygen to the circulatory system, where it is distributed to the body's cells. At the same time oxygen is entering the bloodstream, carbon dioxide is leaving the bloodstream.

THE RESPIRATORY TRACT

The organs of the respiratory tract provide the body with a way of exchanging gases with the environment. When you breathe through the nose, air enters the body through the **nostrils**. Cells lining the **nasal cavities** secrete mucus, which traps dust and other debris. When you breathe through the mouth, air passes through the **oral cavity**. From the nasal and oral cavities, air enters the **pharynx**, or throat. The air then proceeds to the **larynx**, or voice box, which is found at the base of the tongue. The larynx is attached to an air passageway called the **trachea**. After passing through the trachea, air enters the **lungs**.

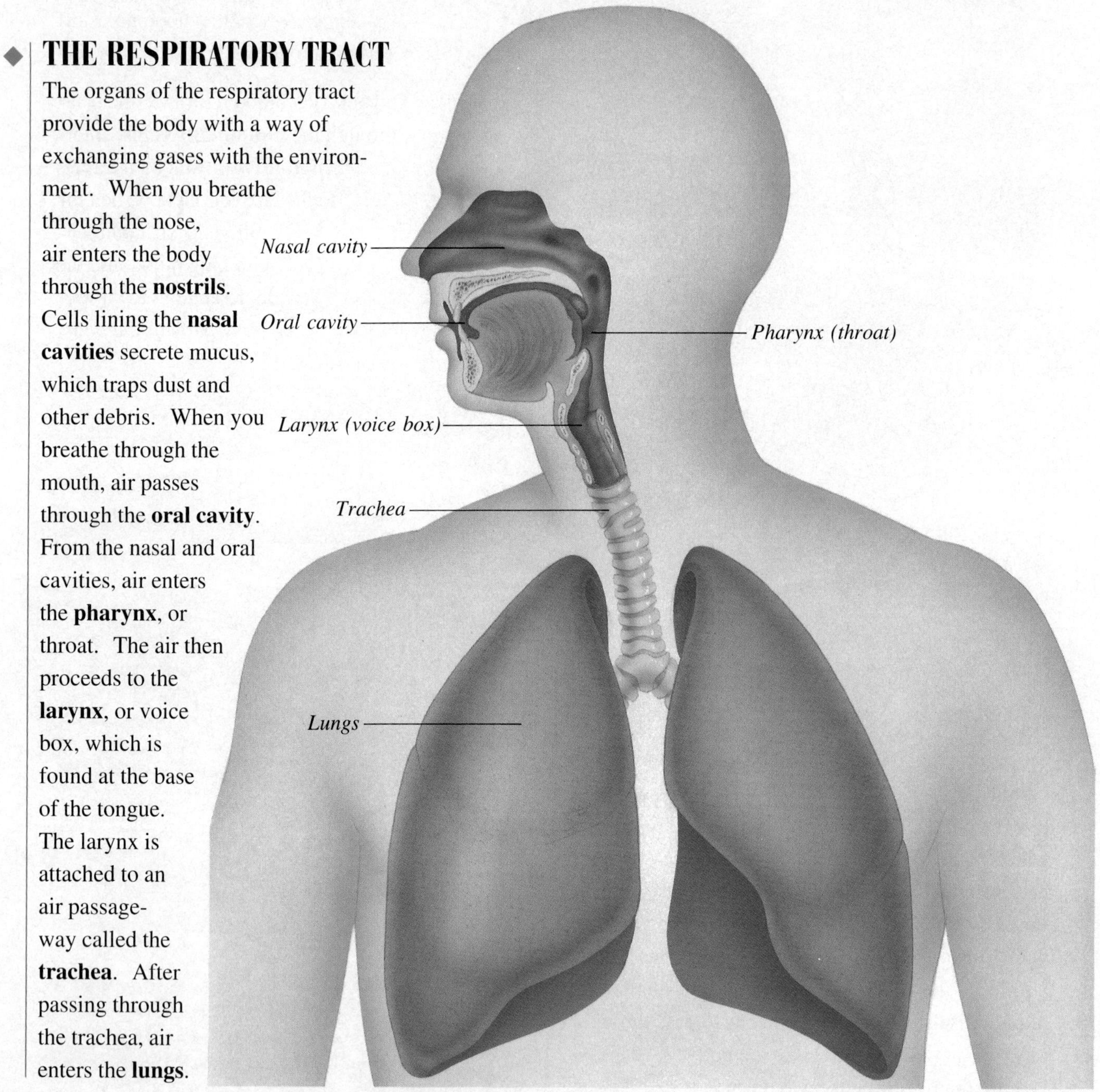

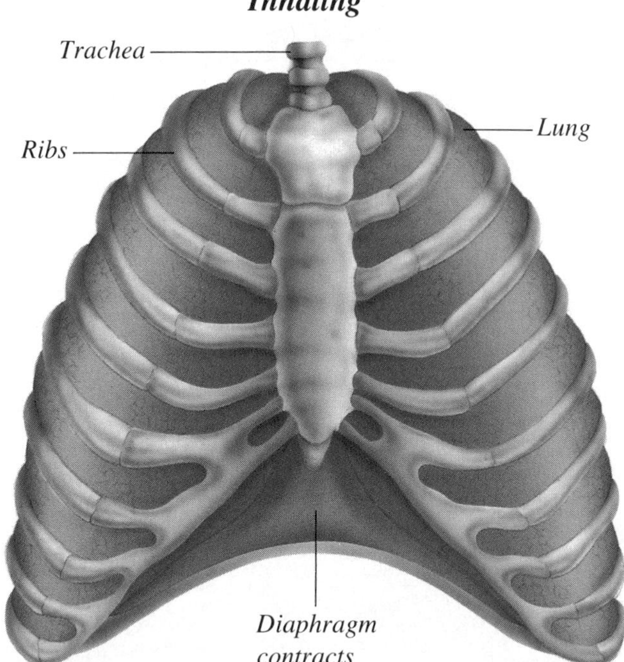

Every time you breathe, your diaphragm and rib muscles contract, expanding your chest and allowing air to enter your lungs. When you exhale, your diaphragm and rib muscles relax, pushing air out of your lungs.

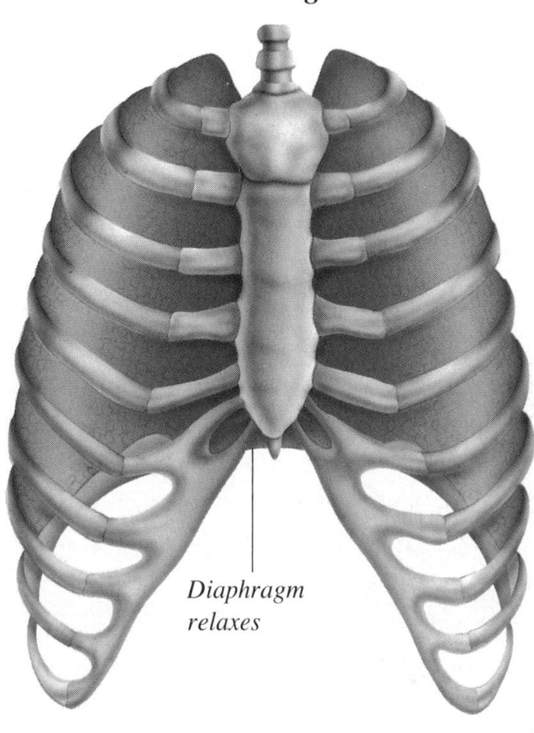

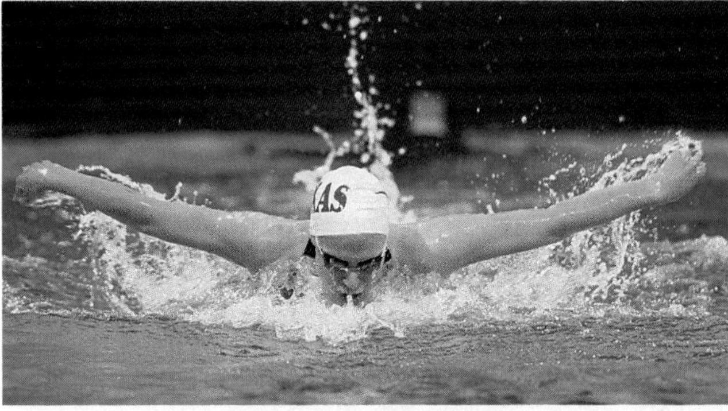

Every breath you take provides your body's cells with essential oxygen.

IN THE LUNGS

Two tubes known as bronchi connect the trachea to the lungs. The bronchi are subdivided many times, forming tiny passages known as **bronchial tubes**. At the end of these passages are clusters of tiny air sacs called **alveoli**, which are surrounded by lung capillaries. The blood in these **capillaries** draws oxygen from the air for delivery to the body's cells. Simultaneously, carbon dioxide in the bloodstream moves from the capillaries into the alveoli, where it can then be exhaled from the lungs.

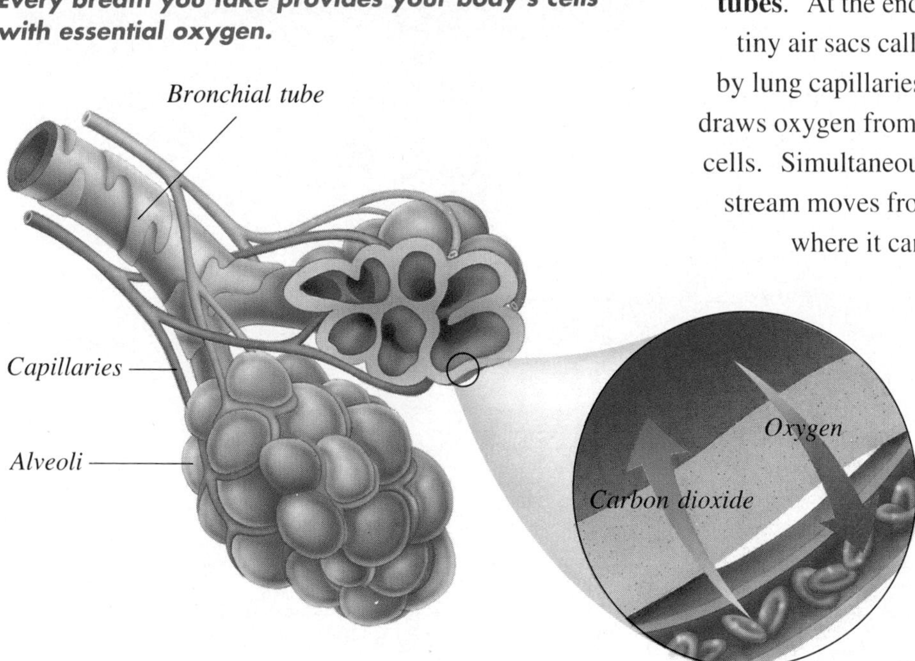

The Digestive System

The digestive system allows the body to take in and process food to nourish its cells. Food passes through the organs of the digestive tract, which begins at the mouth and includes the esophagus, stomach, and intestines. Other organs—the liver, gall bladder, pancreas, and salivary glands—also contribute to the process of digestion.

THE DIGESTIVE TRACT

After food is swallowed, it enters a tube called the **esophagus**. A wavelike motion pushes the food down into the **stomach**. Glands in the stomach lining secrete enzymes that aid in digestion, and a churning action mixes and changes the food into a liquid called chyme. Chyme then passes into the **small intestine**, where digestion is completed by digestive juices secreted by the liver and pancreas. Digested food is absorbed into the bloodstream by capillaries lining the walls of the small intestine. Undigested food moves into the **large intestine** (colon), where water is absorbed from the waste and returned to the bloodstream. The solid waste that remains, called feces, is stored briefly in the **rectum**, then eliminated from the body through an opening called the **anus**.

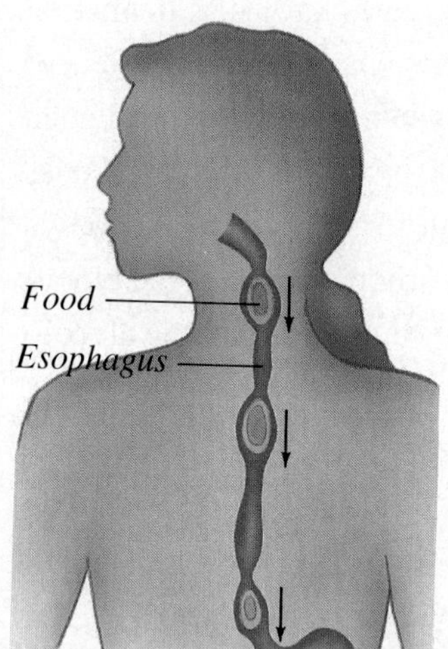

The digestive process begins in the mouth, where three salivary glands secrete saliva, which moistens and softens food.

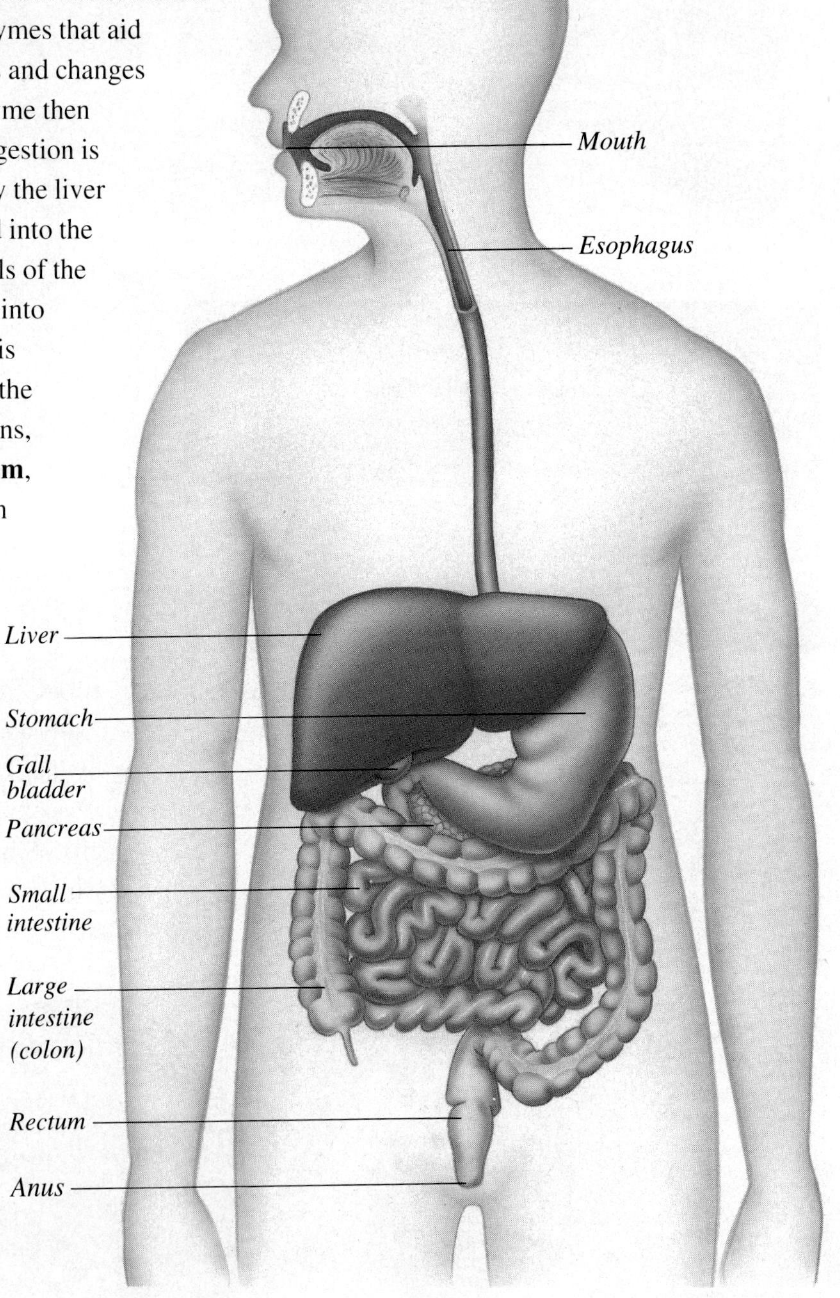

The Excretory System

The excretory system removes from the body the waste products of metabolism as well as excess water and minerals in a process called excretion. The kidneys are the main organs of excretion.

THE KIDNEYS AND THE URINARY TRACT

In addition to its role in digestion, the liver converts the toxic waste products of metabolism into less toxic materials—urea and uric acid. The **kidneys** remove these materials from the bloodstream along with excess salts and water, and turn them into a liquid called urine. Urine leaves each kidney through a tube called the **ureter** and collects in the **bladder**. Eventually, urine leaves the body through the **urethra**.

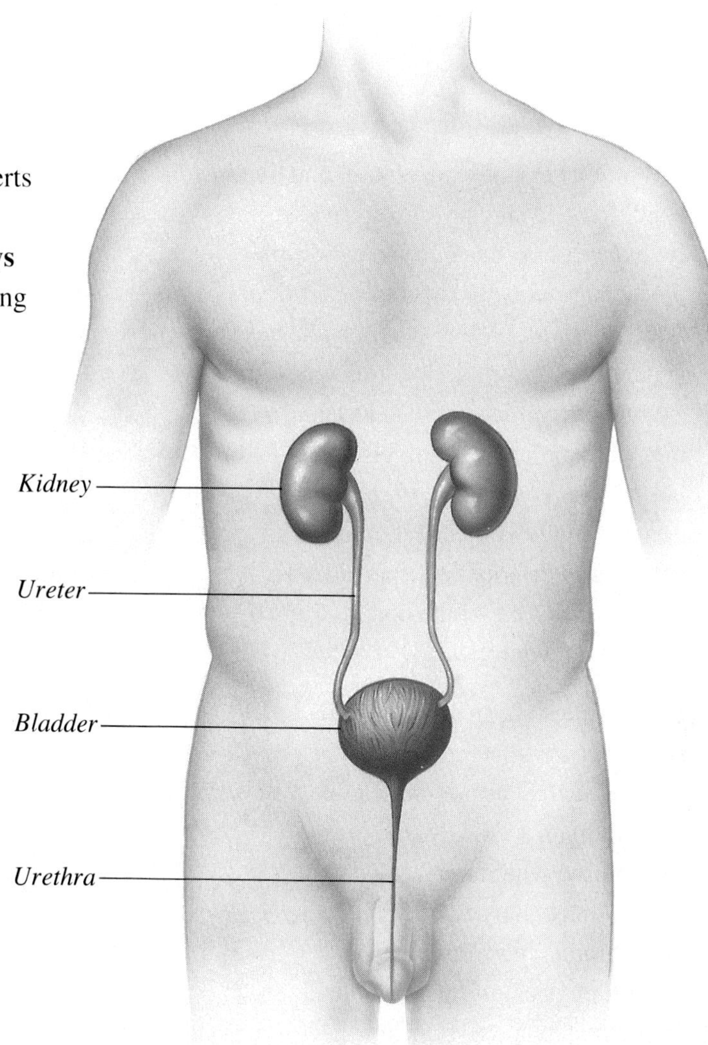

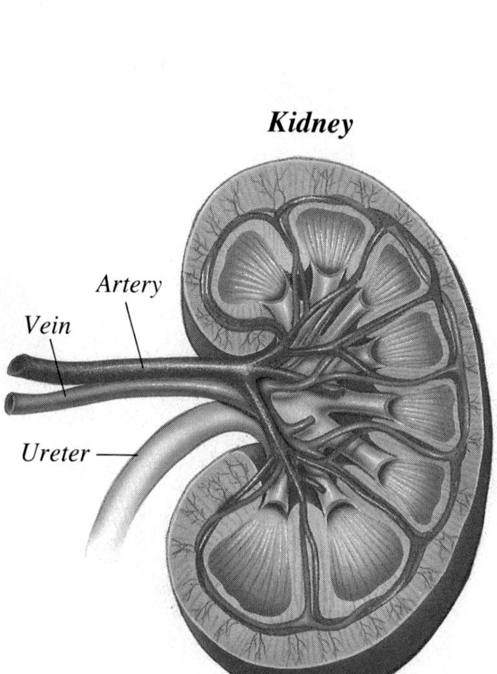

The kidneys maintain the body's internal chemical balance by removing water as well as dissolved wastes and minerals from the bloodstream, and by reabsorbing the amount of water and certain minerals needed by the body.

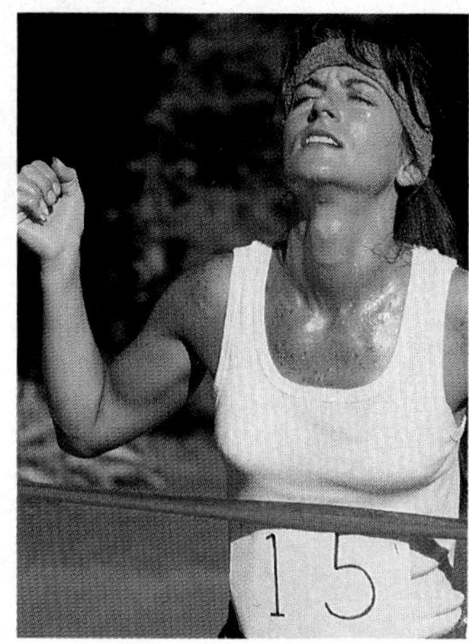

Another waste product, perspiration, is excreted by the skin. Perspiring is also the body's way of keeping itself cool.

Medical and Dental Careers

Many health-care workers provide direct care to help improve a person's health. These highly trained professionals diagnose limitations, illnesses, and injuries; provide necessary treatment; and operate highly specialized medical equipment.

PHYSICIAN

Physicians examine, diagnose, and treat medical conditions. Many physicians treat patients for a variety of illnesses and conditions. Such physicians are called general practitioners, or family doctors. Many other physicians specialize in treating certain types of conditions. For example, psychiatrists diagnose and treat mental disorders, cardiologists treat people with heart ailments, obstetricians treat pregnant women and deliver babies, and orthopedists specialize in treating disorders of the bones, joints, tendons, and muscles.

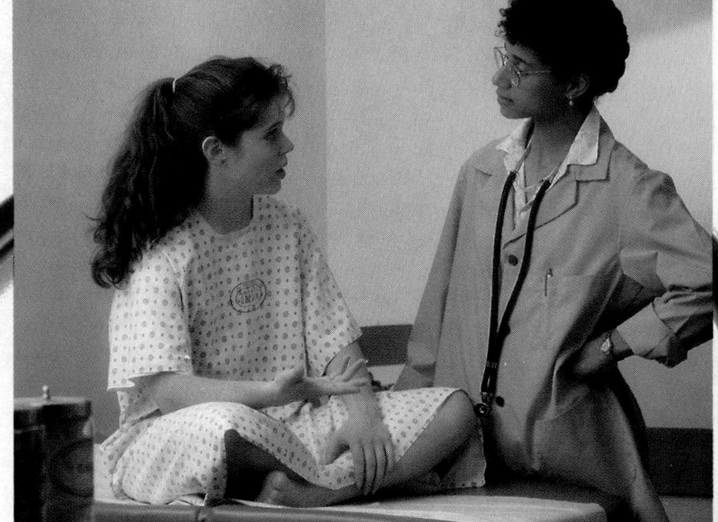

A general practitioner, or family practice physician, performs physical exams and diagnoses and treats a variety of common ailments.

To become a physician, a person must first complete a four-year college degree, usually in science. Four years of medical school follow, during which the medical student may choose a specialty. After graduating from medical school, physicians must complete an internship and a residency at a hospital, during which they receive another three to four years of intense training in both general medicine and their specialty.

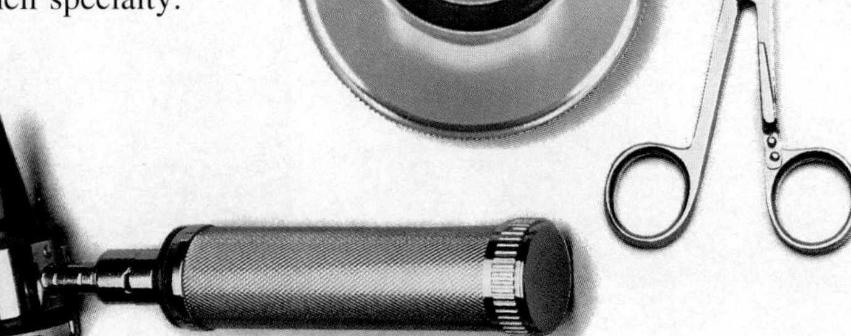

X-RAY TECHNOLOGIST

X-ray technologists operate X-ray equipment. They are often called upon to prepare and administer special formulas that make certain body parts more visible on the X-ray. If, for example, an X-ray is to be taken of the stomach, the technologist gives the patient a drink that highlights the contents of the patient's stomach.

A person who wants to become an X-ray technologist can receive training in college. Most hospitals and technical schools also offer training programs in X-ray technology.

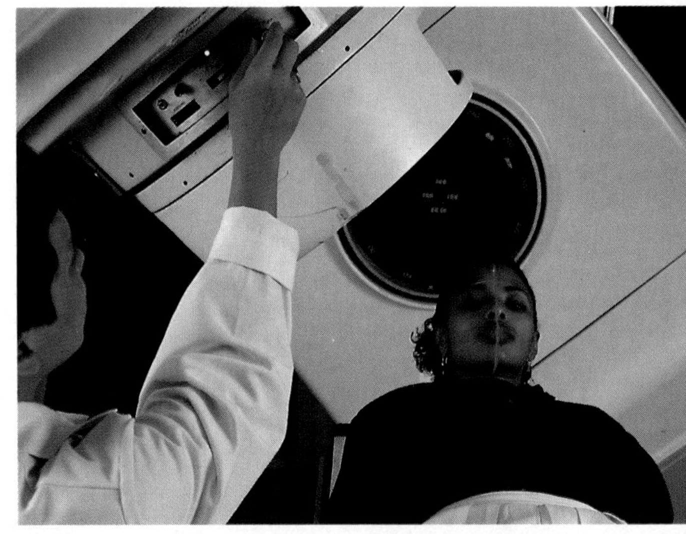

Using high-tech equipment, X-ray technologists work with people of all ages, helping physicians determine the cause of a patient's symptoms.

PHYSICAL THERAPIST

A **physical therapist** helps people with physical disabilities regain the strength to function as independently as possible. People who have amputations, broken bones, nerve or spinal injuries, severe back pain, or diseases such as cerebral palsy or multiple sclerosis can be helped by physical therapy. Therapists use ice packs, hot baths, electrodes, deep massage, exercise, and traction in their treatments.

Physical therapists work in nursing homes, hospitals, and rehabilitation centers. They must have patience, good coordination and physical strength, and good communication skills. Training programs and certification requirements vary from state to state.

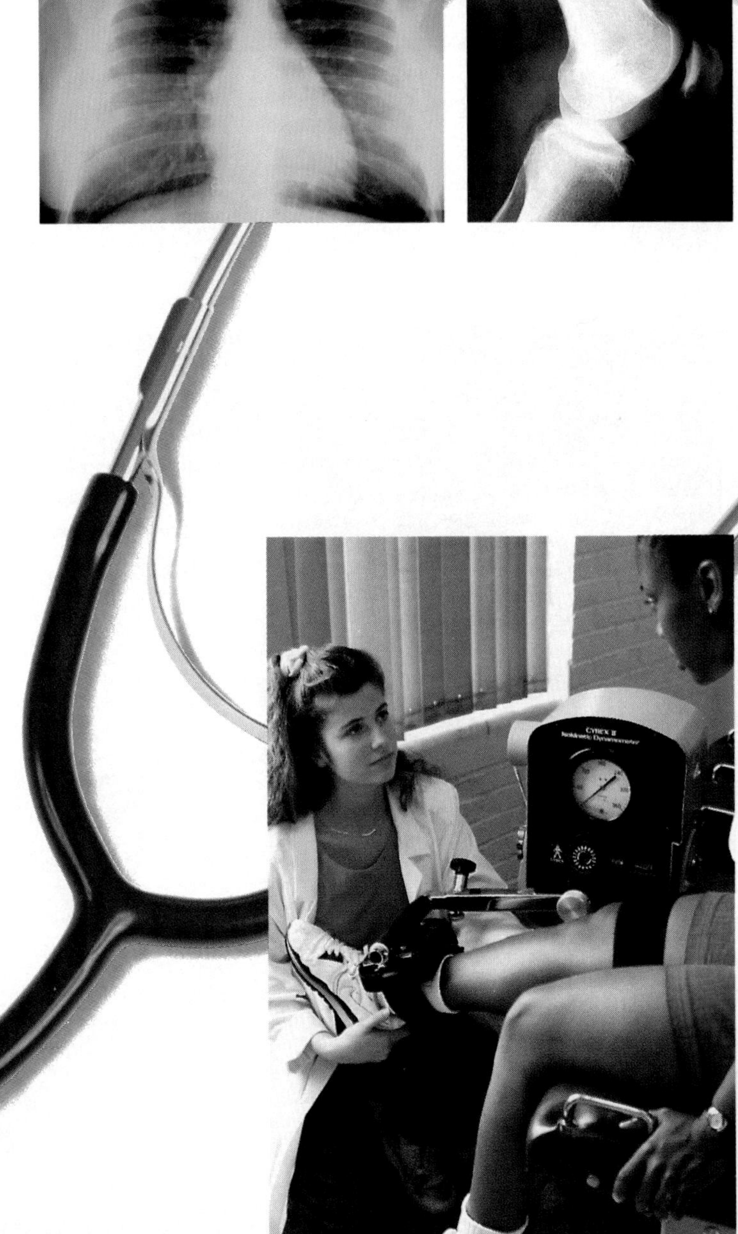

A physical therapist uses massage, exercises, and many other treatments to improve the strength of a person with a physical disability.

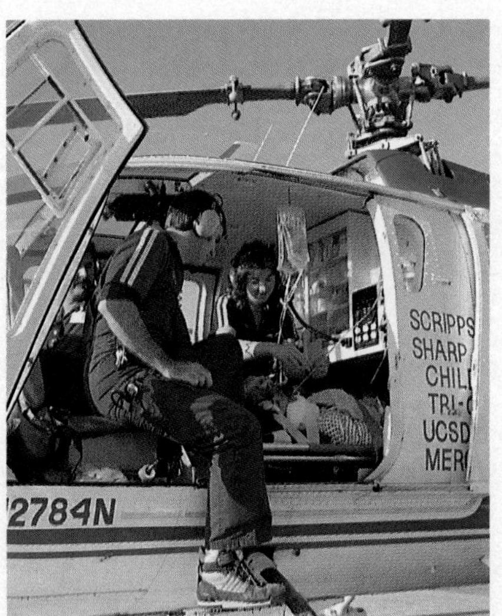

Emergency medical technicians, or EMTs, must react quickly to administer medical care in emergency situations.

EMERGENCY MEDICAL TECHNICIAN

An **emergency medical technician** (EMT) provides quick medical attention in emergency situations, such as automobile accidents. EMTs are trained to assess the seriousness of an injury or illness and to provide care for victims of heart attacks, near drownings, motor vehicle accidents, accidental poisoning, and serious wounds. EMTs treat victims at the scene and often transport them to hospitals for additional medical care.

An emergency medical technician must be at least 18 years old, hold a high school diploma, and have a valid driver's license. After completing an extensive training program, those certified as EMTs find jobs at hospitals, police and fire departments, or with private companies. With advanced training, a person can earn an EMT paramedic rating, which enables him or her to perform more advanced medical procedures.

NURSE

A **nurse** works with doctors to care for those in need of medical attention. Depending on their level of training, nurses perform a variety of duties such as performing physical exams, observing and assessing patient symptoms, administering medication and treatments, and helping patients with proper nutrition, personal hygiene, and general health care.

Registered nurses (RNs) must earn a bachelor's degree in nursing at an accredited college or university. With additional specialized training, an RN may become a nurse practitioner (NP). Licensed practical nurses (LPNs) usually complete a two-year college program or technical school program. In addition to many hours of clinical experience during their schooling, nurses must pass a state board examination before they can be hired.

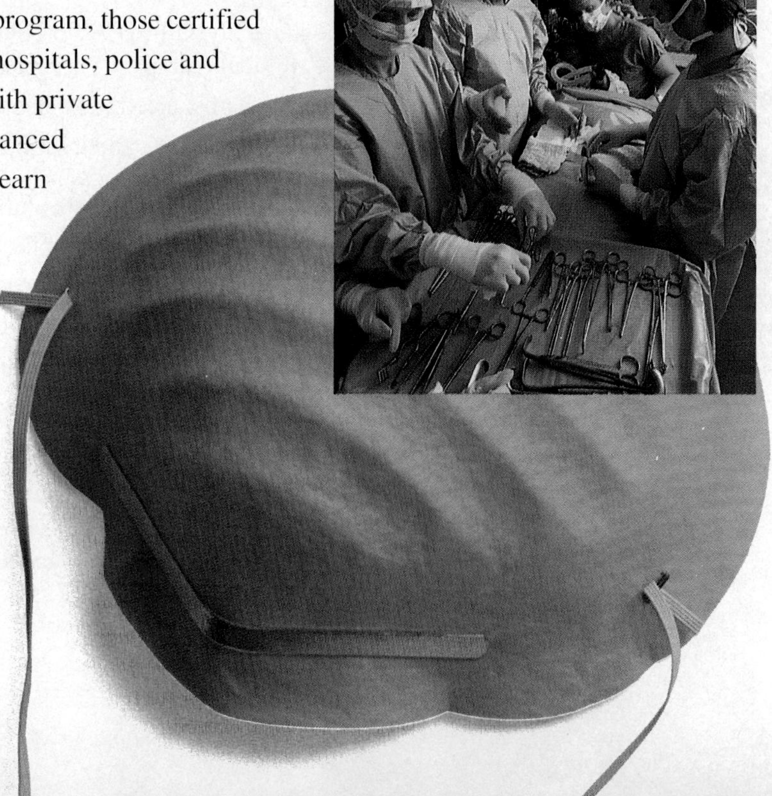

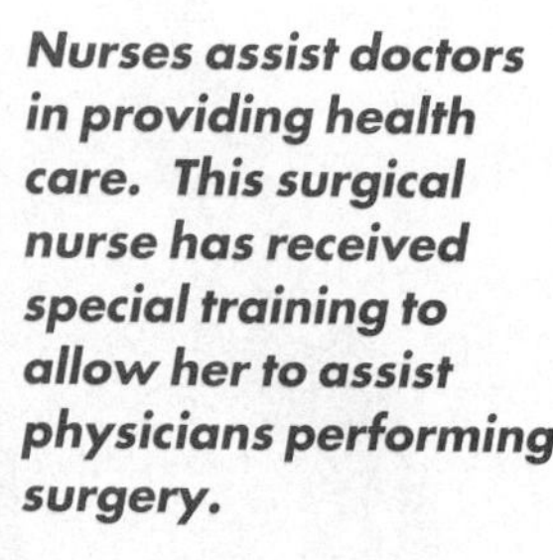

Nurses assist doctors in providing health care. This surgical nurse has received special training to allow her to assist physicians performing surgery.

A dentist treats patients for diseases of the teeth and gums and repairs mechanical damage to the teeth to improve their appearance or function.

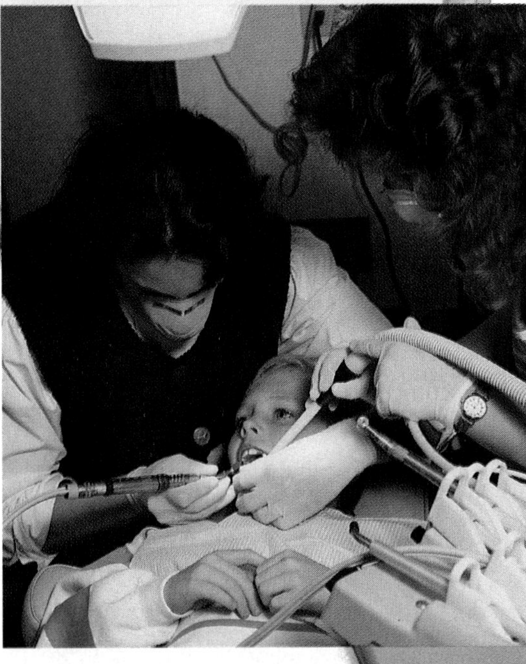

DENTAL LABORATORY TECHNICIAN

A **dental laboratory technician** makes retainers, dentures, braces, bridges, and crowns according to a dentist's exact specifications. He or she must have excellent manual dexterity, because precision and accuracy are crucial to the perfect fit of dental devices.

Most dental laboratory technicians acquire their skills in commercial laboratories. On-the-job training also is provided by hospitals and federal agencies. Schooling without the actual hands-on training takes about two years. Training with no formal schooling can last as long as five years.

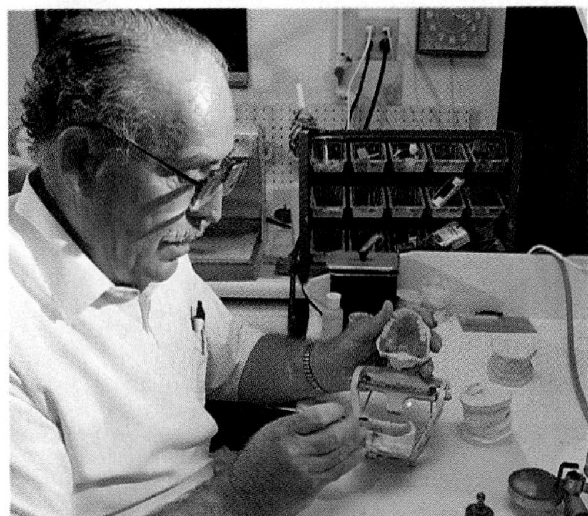

The procedures followed by a dental laboratory technician require manual dexterity and artistic ability.

DENTIST

A **dentist** examines and treats patients for diseases and conditions of the teeth and gums. A general dentist checks teeth for abscesses, fills decayed teeth, determines whether orthodontic devices are needed, and instructs his or her patients on home dental care. He or she also does the preliminary work for fitting a patient with dentures, crowns, or bridges. As with physicians, there are many dental specialties as well.

After successfully completing college and four years of dental school, every aspiring dentist must pass many practical and written examinations as well as a state board exam. Specialists must complete two to three years of additional study and pass exams in their field of specialization.

Careers in Health-Care Administration

Hospitals and other health-care facilities must employ administrators to coordinate the activities of all employees—medical and nonmedical—so that patients receive the best possible care. Health-care administrators range from housekeepers to computer specialists to hospital directors.

MEDICAL RECORDS TECHNICIAN

A **medical records technician** is responsible for what happens to the information recorded by the nurse and doctor on your medical record or chart. They collect the information, classify it, use it to compute statistics, and finally transcribe the data into hospital files.

A medical records technician often holds an associate's degree in this field. However, a person who has earned a bachelor's degree in biology needs only to finish a one-year program for certification. Those who hold bachelor's degrees in medical records administration often supervise medical records technicians.

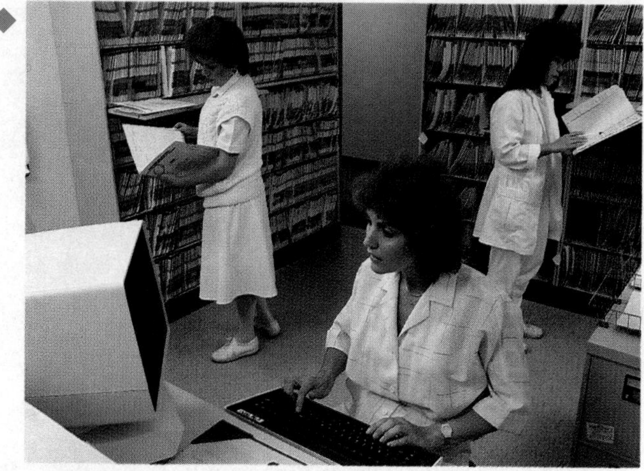

A medical records technician must organize information about many patients and monitor its accuracy and completeness.

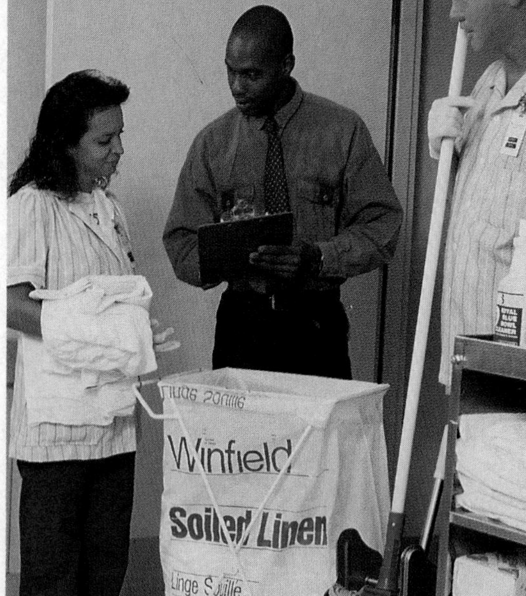

An executive housekeeper in a hospital must see to it that the facility is always clean and sanitary, and in some cases, sterile.

EXECUTIVE HOUSEKEEPER

An **executive housekeeper** trains and manages a hospital's housekeeping staff, which can include custodians, kitchen workers, and laundry attendants. He or she is responsible for assuring that the proper precautions are taken to maintain the sanitary or even sterile environment required in certain areas of a hospital.

A hospital's executive housekeeper must be certified by the National Executive Housekeeper's Association. In addition to several college-level courses, he or she must complete a vocational or technical training program and possibly a management training program.

MEDICAL CLAIMS EXAMINER

A **medical claims examiner** evaluates the charges listed on an insurance claim form to determine whether they are proper and covered by the patient's insurance policy. If the examiner suspects errors have been made, he or she helps work out any problems before making payment to either party. Medical claims examiners work for insurance companies.

Most medical claims examiners hold a college degree. In addition, everyone entering this field should possess a general understanding of medical terms and procedures in order to evaluate each claim properly.

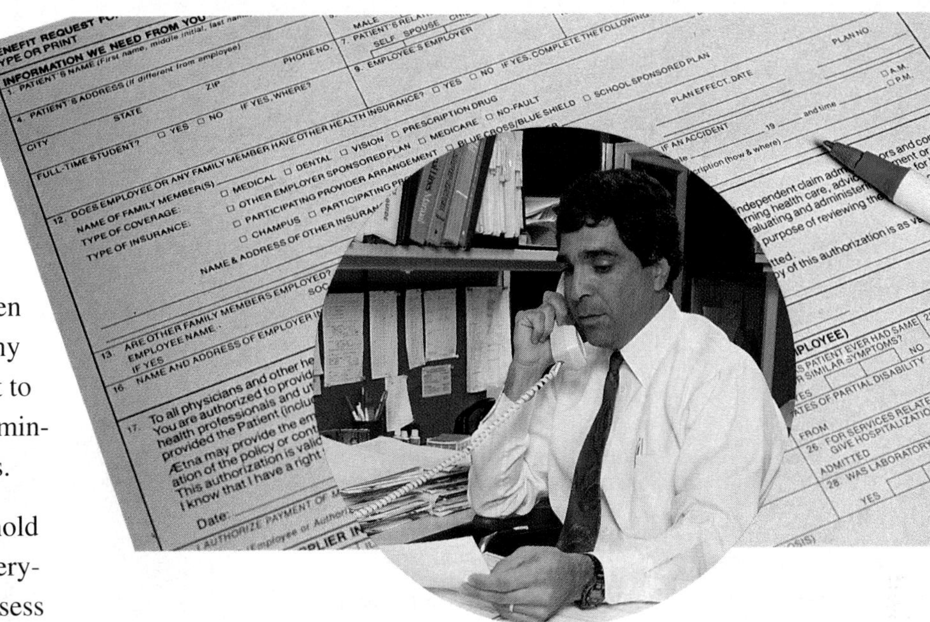

A medical claims examiner spends a great deal of time on the telephone, evaluating the validity of insurance claims and determining whether certain procedures are covered by a policy.

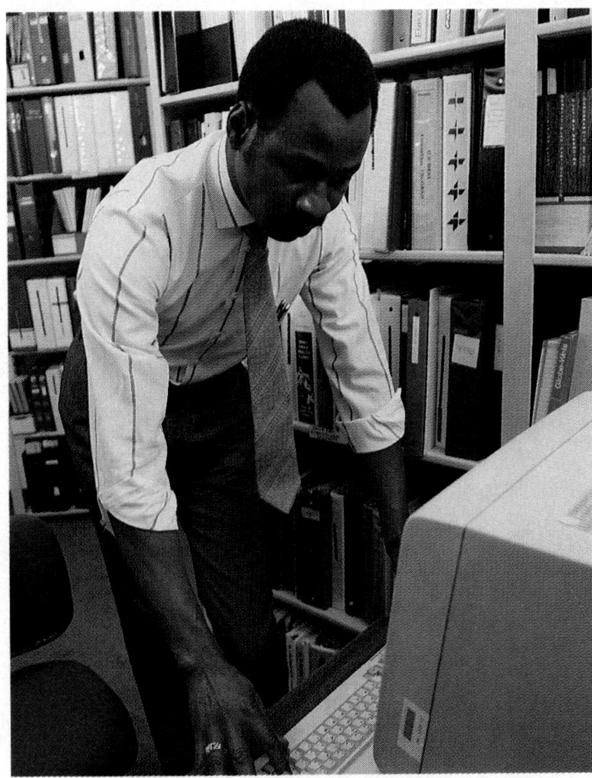

A systems analyst for a health care facility must help meet the changing computer needs of the facility.

SYSTEMS ANALYST

A **systems analyst** evaluates how information should be processed by a computer system. In a health-care institution, he or she is responsible for determining what type of computer system is needed by the facility. The analyst also chooses the printers, terminals, and software that will best meet the facility's current and future needs.

The educational background of a health-care systems analyst can range from a two-year degree with work-related experience to a master's degree in business or computer science. A general knowledge of health-care facilities and the functions they perform is quite useful in this field.

Community Service Careers in Health

Many people assist in the field of health care by providing a multitude of services and products to hospital personnel and patients, and to the general public. Some service careers require extensive training, while others can be started after a few courses beyond high school or with on-the-job training.

PHARMACIST

A **pharmacist** dispenses drugs according to strict specifications provided by physicians and dentists. He or she also discusses possible side effects and drug interactions and advises customers on the proper usage of many nonprescription medications. Most pharmacists work in pharmacies or hospitals.

To become a pharmacist, a person must graduate from a five-year pharmacy program at an accredited college or university. Successful completion of an internship under the direct supervision of a registered pharmacist is also required. Finally, a pharmacy student must pass a state examination to become a registered pharmacist.

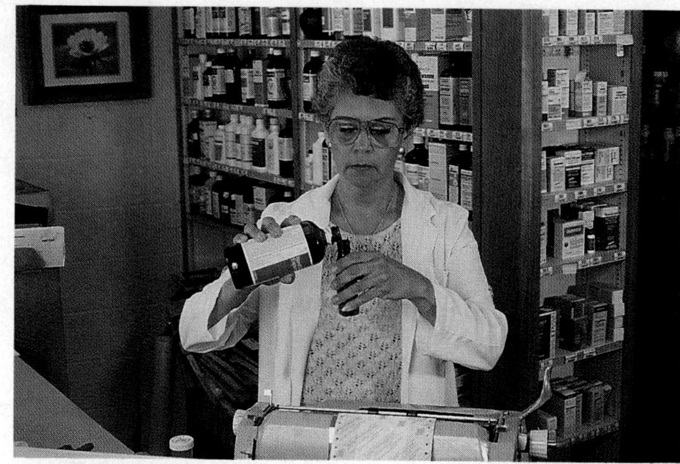

A pharmacist fills prescriptions and advises customers about the use of prescription and nonprescription drugs.

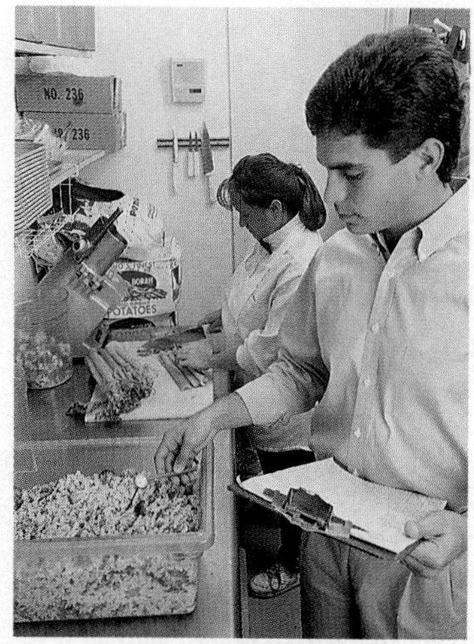

One of the tasks of an environmental health inspector is to check the temperatures of certain foods to ensure that they are safe to eat.

ENVIRONMENTAL HEALTH INSPECTOR

An **environmental health inspector** works for a local, state, or federal government agency monitoring facilities such as restaurants, dairies, and food processing plants. Inspectors routinely test the air, food, and water used in these establishments for harmful bacteria and pollutants to determine whether the facilities are complying with government regulations regarding hygiene.

Environmental health inspectors generally have earned a four-year college degree. Some agencies also require several years of job-related experience.

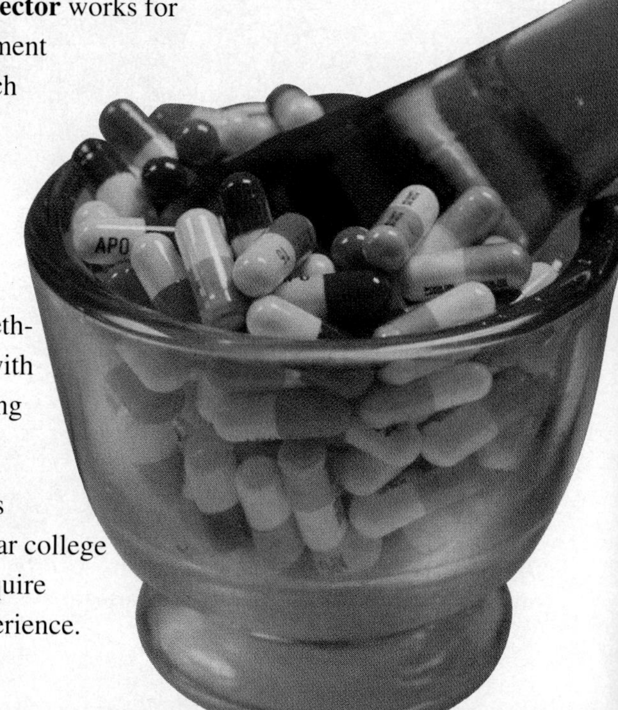

COUNSELOR

A **counselor** works with individuals and families who are having difficulties in their social, economic, and personal lives. He or she helps people overcome the problems associated with drug and alcohol dependency, AIDS, and relationship, marriage, and family issues. A counselor begins by talking to his or her clients about their problems, then assesses the situation and makes recommendations for how the problems might be resolved. The counselor also refers clients to other professionals and organizations if more specialized help is needed.

Most counselors have at least a bachelor's degree in psychology or social work, but a master's degree in one of these fields is usually necessary for employment. In most parts of the country, a state examination is required to obtain a license.

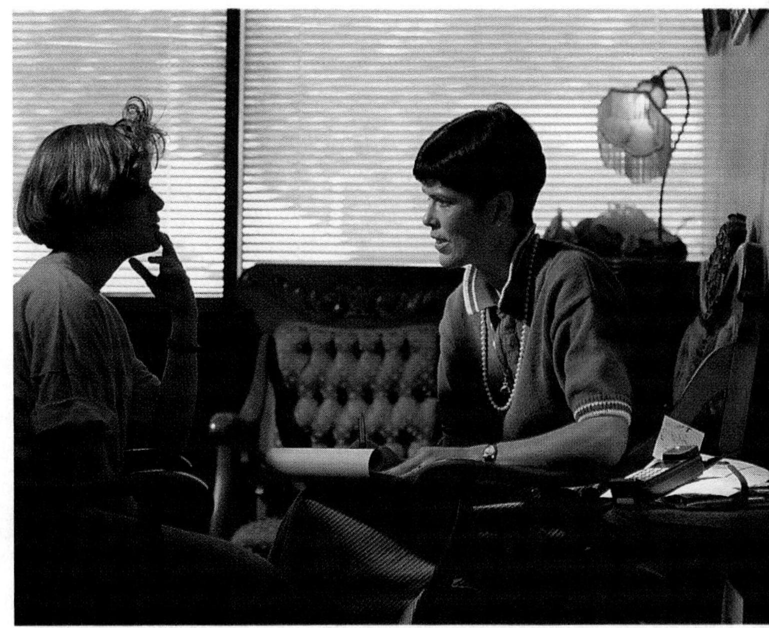

This counselor is telling a young woman how long it will be until her HIV antibody test results are available. She will also answer questions about AIDS and HIV infection.

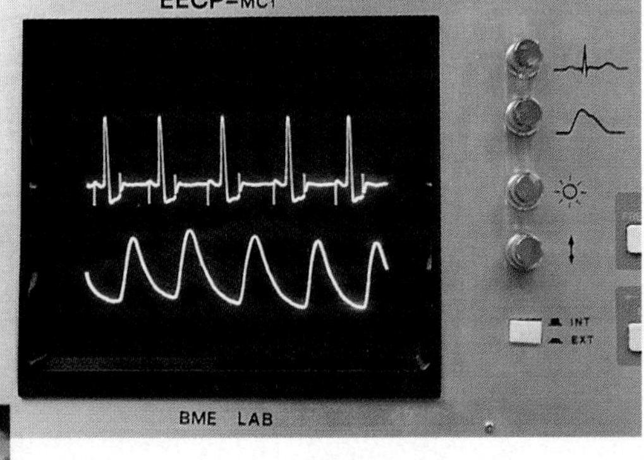

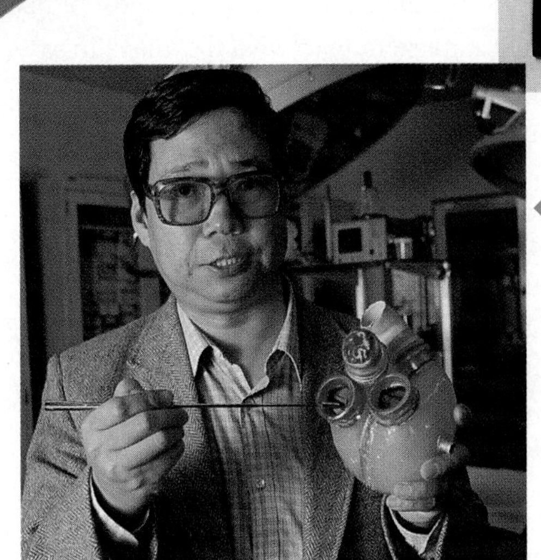

Dr. Kevin Cheng has helped save many lives by designing an artificial heart, which he is demonstrating here.

BIOMEDICAL ENGINEER

A **biomedical engineer** designs new medical equipment and does research to improve existing devices. Biomedical engineers are often assisted by biomedical equipment technicians, who install and service complicated pieces of machinery, such as lasers, electrocardiographs (EKGs), and electroencephalographs (EEGs).

A biomedical engineer usually works for a research facility such as a university, a health-care company, or a large hospital. He or she must have at least a bachelor's degree in engineering with specialization in biomedical training. Research positions require a master's degree or even a doctorate of philosophy in biomedical engineering.

Careers in Health Education

Education is part of any health-care worker's job. However, there are many types of health-care professionals who specialize in educating people about how to improve their overall physical and mental health.

HEALTH TEACHER

A **health teacher** conducts courses on health in public or private schools. He or she helps students understand the material by starting class discussions, delivering lectures on health topics, and giving exams. Often, a health teacher discusses health concerns with individual students who feel uncomfortable talking about their concerns in class.

A health teacher holds at least a bachelor's degree in health education or biology. A strong background in human anatomy and physiology, psychology, sociology, and other health-related topics is also quite useful. Teaching at the college level usually requires a master's degree.

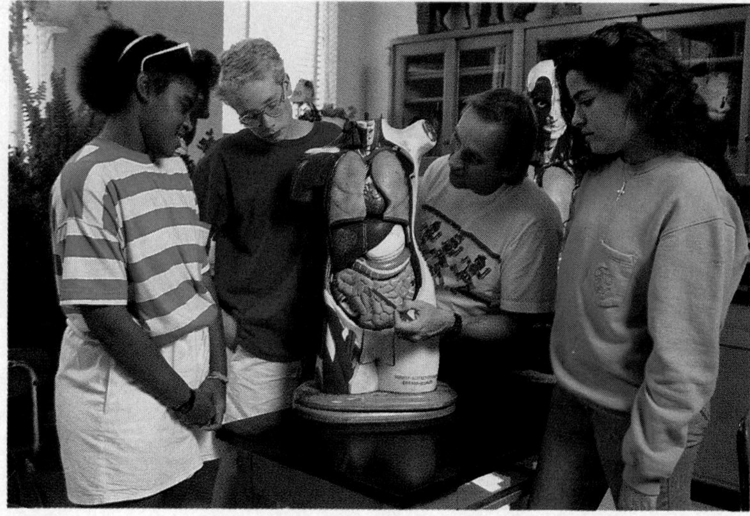

A health teacher gives lectures and answers questions about health-related topics.

SCHOOL PSYCHOLOGIST

A **school psychologist** works closely with students, teachers, and parents to help students overcome social and emotional problems and neurological disorders that might interfere with learning. He or she often administers tests to assess mental health but spends most of his or her time talking to students and listening to what they have to say about their situations. School psychologists also advise a school's administrative body and suggest how policies might be changed to enhance learning.

Nearly all psychologists have at least a master's degree in psychology. Some hold doctorate degrees in psychology, which usually requires eight years of schooling at a college or university. Most psychologists obtain clinical experience during their formal education by assisting and observing other psychologists interacting with patients.

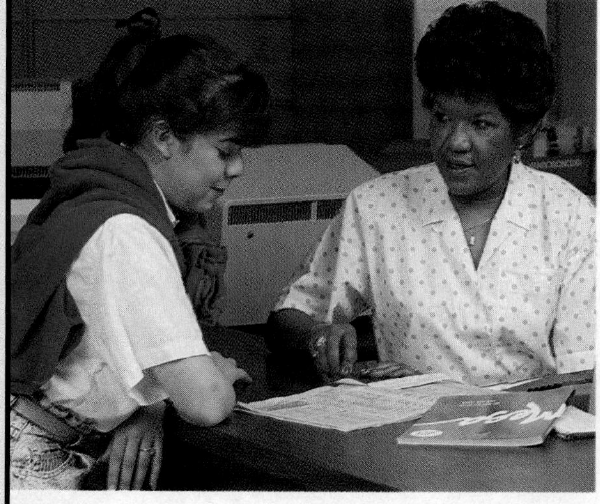

A school psychologist assists students with various problems that might interfere with their ability to learn.

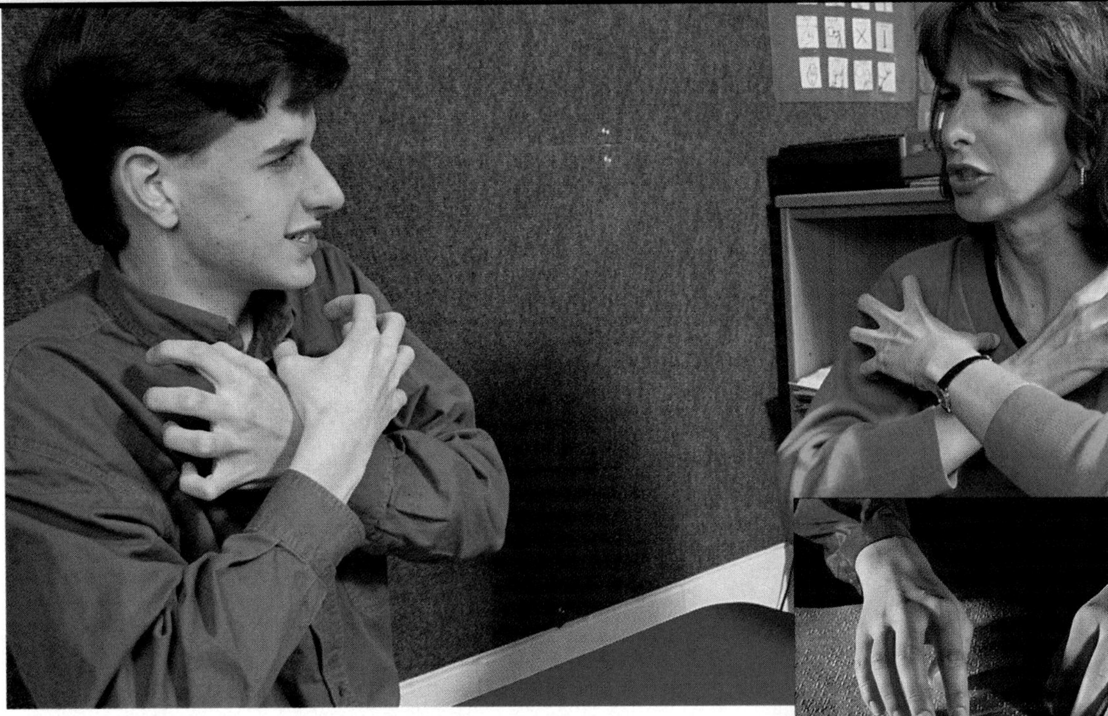

INSTRUCTOR OF THE IMPAIRED

An **instructor of the hearing or visually impaired** uses knowledge of sign language and Braille to help hearing-impaired and visually-impaired people develop better communication skills. Such instructors work in clinics, rehabilitation centers, and schools.

An instructor of the impaired must complete a bachelor's degree in special education. A master's degree with specialization in either the visually or hearing impaired is usually necessary as well. Some clinical work with visually- and hearing-impaired people is required before graduating with either degree.

An instructor of the impaired often works with his or her students on a one-to-one basis. Here the instructor is teaching her student how to say "bear" in sign language.

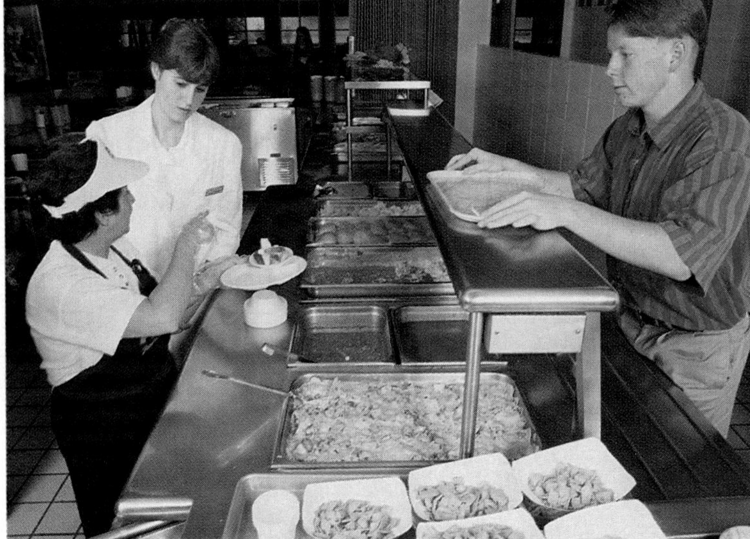

A nutritionist plans meals and manages the food service program of many health care facilities.

NUTRITIONIST

A **nutritionist** manages the food service program in restaurants and cafeterias, hospitals, nursing homes, health-care clinics, private companies, and the military. He or she works closely with the kitchen staff to make sure that nutritious meals are served. Some nutritionists are self-employed and work with individuals to help them improve their eating habits or control certain illnesses through proper nutrition.

A nutritionist must have a bachelor's degree in food science and nutrition. Along with formal education, the American Dietetic Association recommends successful completion of either an internship before employment or an on-the-job training period.

Glossary

A

accident: any unexpected event that causes damage, injury, or death.

acne: a condition in which the pores of the skin become clogged with oil; acne can take the form of blackheads, whiteheads, or pimples.

acquaintance rape: the forcing or coercion of a woman into sexual intercourse by an acquaintance or date.

active listening: the process of hearing the words of the speaker and clarifying anything that is confusing.

addicted: the state of being physically dependent on a drug.

addiction: a condition in which the body relies on a given drug to help it function.

addictive: causing a physical dependence; a person who is addicted to a drug requires that substance in order to function normally.

aerobic exercise: physical activity that increases the heart rate and supplies oxygen to the muscles, and that can be continued for a period of time without resting.

aerobic fitness: the ability to endure at least 10 minutes of strenuous activity.

AIDS: a disease caused by a virus that cripples a person's immune system; AIDS is classified as a sexually transmitted disease, but it can also be spread in other ways, such as through sharing infected equipment for injecting drugs, tattoeing, or ear piercing. AIDS is the last phase of HIV infection.

alcoholism: the state of being psychologically and physically addicted to alcohol.

Alzheimer's disease: an incurable illness characterized by a gradual and permanent loss of memory. Alzheimer's disease most commonly affects the elderly.

anabolic steroid: an artificially made, complex substance that can temporarily increase muscle size.

anaerobic exercise: physical activity that increases muscle size and endurance, and that cannot be continued for a long period of time without resting.

analgesic: a medicine that relieves pain.

anorexia nervosa: an eating disorder in which the person refuses to eat because of a fear of weight gain.

antibiotics: drugs that kill or limit growth of bacteria.

antibodies: substances that stick to the surface of pathogens, slowing their action.

anxiety disorder: a condition in which fear or anxiety prevents one from enjoying life and completing everyday tasks.

appetite: the desire to eat based on the pleasure derived from eating.

assault: a personal attack in which you are threatened or harmed.

autoimmune disease: a disease in which a person's own immune system attacks and damages an organ of his or her own body.

B

B-cells: cells in the immune system that produce antibodies against infection.

bacterium: a microorganism that can cause disease.

basal metabolic rate: energy needed to fuel the body's ongoing processes while the body is at complete rest.

blended family: a family that results when divorced parents remarry; the parents and their respective children from previous marriages live in the home together.

blood alcohol level (BAL): a way to measure the level of alcohol in a person's body.

body composition: the division of the total body weight into fat weight and muscle weight.

body image: the view a person has of his or her body.

brain waves: electrical patterns produced by the brain that fluctuate greatly during the sleep cycle.

bulimia: an eating disorder based on a cycle of bingeing and purging food.

C

calculus: hardened plaque.

calorie: a unit of measurement for energy. 1 nutrition calorie = 1 kilocalorie.

cancer: a disease caused by cells that have lost normal growth controls and that invade and destroy healthy tissues.

carbohydrate loading: consuming large quantities of complex carbohydrates over a seven-day period to provide energy for endurance sports.

carbohydrates: class of nutrients containing starches, simple sugars, glycogen, and dietary fiber.

carbon monoxide: a poisonous gas released by burning tobacco.

cardiac arrest: condition in which the heart stops working.

cardiopulmonary resuscitation (CPR): a life-saving procedure designed to revive a person who is not breathing and has no heartbeat.

cardiovascular disease: progressive damage to the heart and blood vessels.

cervix: the base of the uterus, which bulges down into the vagina; has a small opening through which sperm can enter the uterus.

chewing tobacco: a form of smokeless tobacco that is placed between a person's cheek and gum.

child abuse: mistreatment of a child or adolescent.

chlamydia: the most common STD in the United States; caused by bacteria.

cholesterol: fatlike substance that is part of all animal cells and is needed for the production of some hormones and fat digestion; can block the arteries and cause heart disease.

chromosomes: cell structures that carry hereditary information.

chronic bronchitis: an inflammation of the bronchial tubes in the lungs and the production of excessive mucus.

cirrhosis: a condition in which liver cells are replaced by useless scar tissue. Cirrhosis can be caused by long-term alcohol abuse.

communicable disease: an infectious disease that is passed from one person (or organism) to another.

complete protein: a protein that contains all nine essential amino acids.

complex carbohydrates: a subclass of carbohydrates that includes starches, dietary fiber, and glycogen.

condom: a covering for the penis that helps protect both partners from sexually transmitted diseases and also helps prevent pregnancy.

congenital disease: a disease that is present from birth but is not hereditary.

conservation: the wise use and protection of natural resources.

constipation: a condition in which bowel movements are infrequent or difficult.

contraception: a device or method that prevents the fertilization of a woman's egg.

couple family: a family in which only a husband and a wife live together in the home.

cremation: the complete reduction of the body to ashes by intense heat.

D

decision-making model: a series of steps that help a person make a responsible decision.

deductible: the amount of medical costs an insured person must pay before the insurance company begins paying.

defense mechanisms: techniques people use to protect themselves from being hurt.

defensive driving: driving as though you expect other drivers to drive recklessly.

defensive medicine: use of numerous diagnostic tests to avoid a lawsuit.

degenerative diseases: diseases that result from gradual damage to organs over time.

dehydration: a state in which the body has lost more water than has been taken in.

dental floss: a special string that removes plaque from the teeth.

dependent: having an overpowering psychological or physical craving for a psychoactive drug.

depressant: a drug that slows body functioning.

dermis: the second layer of skin; contains the most important skin structures.

designer drugs: synthetic drugs that are similar in chemistry to certain illegal drugs.

diarrhea: loose bowel movements that occur when food moves too quickly through the digestive system.

dietary fiber: a subclass of complex carbohydrates with a high ratio of plant material that is not absorbed by the body.

disaster: an event that affects the lives and health of people in one or more communities.

dislocation: an injury in which the end of a bone comes out of its joint.

dissociative disorder: a condition in which someone's personality changes to the point that the person believes he or she is someone else.

divorce: the legal end to a marriage.

dose: the exact amount of a drug.

drown proofing: a technique to stay afloat that can be used even by those who cannot swim.

drug: a substance that causes a physical or emotional change in a person.

drug abuse: intentional improper use of a drug.

drug allergy: an unwanted effect that accompanies the desired effect of a drug.

drug misuse: unintentional improper use of a drug.

drug use: taking a medicine properly and in its correct dosage.

dysfunctional family: a family that does not fulfill the basic functions of a healthy family.

E

ecosystem: a system made up of living things and their physical surroundings.

effect: the influence a drug has on the body, the mind, or both.

egg: female reproductive cell, also called an ovum; contains one-half of the instructions needed for the development of a new human being.

elder abuse: physical abuse of an elderly person.

electrocution: death resulting from the flow of electrical current through the body.

embryo: a fertilized egg after it has divided into two cells.

emotional abuse: emotional mistreatment of a child or adolescent.

emotional health: expressing feelings in an appropriate way.

emotional intimacy: sharing thoughts and feelings, caring for and respecting the other person, and gradually learning to trust one another.

emotional maturity: the capacity to act independently, responsibly, and unselfishly. Being emotionally mature requires having compassion, integrity, and self-esteem.

empathy: the ability to understand how another person feels.

emphysema: a disease in which the tiny air sacs of the lungs lose their elasticity.

enamel: the substance covering the crown of the tooth; hardest substance in the body.

endorphin: a substance that is produced inside the brain and has pleasurable effects.

energy-balance equation: eating the same number of calories that you burn each day.

epidemic: an outbreak of disease that affects many people in a particular area.

epidermis: the very thin outer layer of the skin.

essential amino acids: a group of nine amino acids that cannot be manufactured by the body and must be supplied by food.

essential fat: the amount of fat needed for certain metabolic processes to occur.

essential nutrients: six categories of substances from food that nourish the body: carbohydrates, fats, proteins, vitamins, minerals, water.

extended family: a family in which relatives outside the nuclear family live in the same home with the nuclear family.

F

fad diet: weight-loss diet that promises unrealistic results.

fats: a term used to describe a class of compounds in foods called lipids. Fats are energy storage molecules that supply more energy per gram than carbohydrates or proteins.

fertilization: the union of a sperm and an egg.

fetal alcohol syndrome (FAS): a set of birth defects that can occur when a pregnant woman drinks alcohol. These defects include low birth weight, mental retardation, facial deformities, and behavioral problems.

fetus: a developing individual from the ninth week of pregnancy until birth.

first aid: emergency care given to an ill or injured person before medical attention is available.

flashback: unexpected return to an unpleasant LSD experience, often months after the original experience ended.

flexibility: the ability to move muscles and joints through their full range of motion.

food chain: a sequence of organisms that begins with a food producer and continues with one or more organisms, each of which eats the one before it.

food intolerance: a condition in which your body has a negative reaction to food that is not brought about by the immune system.

fracture: a broken bone.

functional disorders: mental and emotional disorders caused by internal struggles.

gene: a short segment of a DNA molecule that serves as a code for a particular bit of hereditary information.

genital herpes: an STD caused by a virus that often causes painful blisters or ulcers; cannot be cured.

genital warts: a viral STD in which warts appear on the genital and anal areas.

global warming: long-term change in temperature (warming) of Earth's climate that is related to air pollution and the greenhouse effect.

gonorrhea: an STD caused by bacteria, which can infect the mucous membranes of the penis, vagina, throat, or rectum.

greenhouse effect: the trapping of heat from the sun by certain gases in the atmosphere called greenhouse gases.

H

hallucination: imaginary sights and sounds, often induced by the use of hallucinogen.

hallucinogen: a drug that distorts a person's senses.

hangover: uncomfortable physical effects brought on by alcohol use. Symptoms of a hangover include headache, nausea, upset stomach, and dizziness.

hazardous wastes: wastes that are dangerous to the health of living things or harmful to the environment.

HDL: "high-density lipoproteins" that remove cholesterol from the blood and transport it back to the liver.

health: state of well-being that comes from a good balance of the five aspects of health.

Heimlich maneuver: a series of sharp thrusts to the abdomen, used to dislodge an object from a choking person's airway.

hepatitis: an inflammation of the liver that can be caused by long-term alcohol abuse. Symptoms of hepatitis include high fever, weakness, and a yellowing of the skin.

hereditary disease: a disease caused by defective genes passed from one or both parents to a child.

heterosexuals: people who are sexually attracted to those of the other sex.

high blood pressure: a condition in which the blood pushes harder than normal against the inside of the blood vessels.

HIV (human immunodeficiency virus): the virus that causes AIDS; also called the "AIDS virus."

HIV-antibody test: a test used to determine whether a person has been infected with HIV.

HIV-positive: the condition of being infected with HIV.

HMOs (health maintenance organizations): organizations that offer subscribers complete medical care in return for a fixed monthly fee.

homeostasis: the tendency of any living thing to maintain a balance in its inner systems.

homicide: a violent crime that results in the death of another person.

homosexuals: people who are sexually attracted to those of the same sex.

hormones: chemical substances, produced by the endocrine glands, which serve as messengers within the body.

hospices: places that offer housing, medical care, and counseling for terminally ill people, and counseling for the family.

hunger: the body's physical response to a need for food.

hypothermia: below-normal body temperature.

I

immune system: the system that protects the body from disease.

immunization: injection of a small amount of a pathogen that will provide protection against an infectious disease.

incomplete protein: a protein that lacks one or more of the essential amino acids.

infectious disease: a disease caused by an agent that can pass from one living thing to another.

inhalants: chemicals that produce strong psychoactive effects when they are inhaled.

insomnia: temporary or continuing loss of sleep.

intoxicated: being affected by alcohol. Effects of intoxication can range from mild lightheadedness to severe and complete loss of judgment and reflexes.

L

LDL: "low-density lipoproteins" are composed mostly of cholesterol and provide a means of transporting cholesterol to cells for cell processes.

lean mass: total body weight minus the weight due to fat.

life expectancy: the number of years a person can reasonably be expected to live.

living will: a document expressing a person's wish to be allowed to die in case of terminal illness or incurable injury rather than be kept alive by artificial means.

M

mainstream smoke: smoke that is inhaled directly into the mouth through a cigarette, pipe, or cigar.

medicine: a substance used to treat an illness or ailment.

mental health: the ability to recognize reality; the feelings you have about yourself and your abilities to deal with problems.

microorganism: a tiny living thing that can be seen only with a microscope.

middle adulthood: the period of adulthood between the ages of 41 and 65.

minerals: inorganic substances that are generally absorbed to form structural components of the body.

mixed message: a message that is sent when the verbal and nonverbal communications do not match.

monogamy: when two people have intercourse with only each other for their entire lives.

mood disorder: a condition in which one mood is experienced almost to the exclusion of other feelings.

mucous membranes: moist, tissues that line the openings of the body; pathogens can enter the body through the mucous membranes, although many are trapped there.

muscular strength and endurance: the muscles' ability to push against a very heavy force over a short period of time (strength) or to apply force over a sustained period (endurance).

N

narcotic: a drug with pain-relieving and psychoactive properties that is made from the opium poppy plant.

neglect: failure of a parent or guardian to provide for a child's basic needs.

nicotine: an addictive chemical found in tobacco.

nocturnal emissions: ejaculations of semen that occur during sleep.

noninfectious disease: a disease that a person cannot catch from another person or any other organism.

nonrenewable resources: natural resources such as coal and oil that cannot be replaced once they are used.

nonverbal communication: nonverbal behavior, such as eye contact, facial expression, and body position, that communicates information.

nuclear family: a family in which a mother, a father, and one or more children live together.

obesity: a condition in which one weighs 20 percent more than the recommended weight.

older adulthood: the period of adulthood past the age of 65.

organic disorders: mental and emotional disorders resulting from a physical cause.

ovaries: female reproductive structures that produce eggs and female sex hormones.

overdose: a serious, sometimes fatal, reaction to a large dose of a drug.

overpopulation: the point at which the population of an area is so large that it can no longer be supported by the available resources.

overweight: weighing 10 percent more than one's recommended weight.

ovulation: the release of an egg from an ovary.

Pap test: a medical procedure in which cells from the cervix are removed and tested for cancer.

Parkinson's disease: an incurable disease characterized by a gradual loss of control of muscle function. Parkinson's disease most commonly affects the elderly.

passive smoker: a nonsmoker who is exposed to the sidestream smoke of a cigarette, cigar, or pipe.

pathogens: agents that cause disease.

pelvic inflammatory disease (PID): an infection of the uterus and Fallopian tubes often caused by STDs; if untreated, may result in infertility.

penis: male reproductive structure that deposits sperm inside the female body.

personality disorder: an emotional condition in which a person's patterns of behavior negatively affect that person's ability to get along with others.

physical abuse: to cause bodily harm to a child or adolescent.

physical dependence: a condition in which the body becomes so used to the presence of a drug that it needs it in order to function.

physical fitness: a state in which your body can meet daily life demands; the ability to perform daily tasks vigorously and to perform physical activities, while avoiding diseases related to a lack of activity.

physical health: your physical characteristics and the way your body functions.

pica: an eating disorder in which the person eats nonfood substances like starch, clay, or soil.

plaque: a film of food particles, saliva, and bacteria on teeth.

positive self-talk: talking in a positive way to yourself about yourself.

premium: payment a person makes to an insurance company in exchange for coverage.

prescription: a doctor's written order for a medicine.

primary care physician: a family medicine physician, pediatrician, or general internal medicine physician.

proteins: class of nutrients consisting of long chains of amino acids, which are the basic components of body tissue and provide energy.

psychoactive drug: a drug that affects a person's mood and behavior.

psychoactive effect: an effect on a person's mood or behavior.

psychoactive substance: a substance that causes a change in a person's mood and behavior.

psychological dependence: a constant desire to take a psychoactive drug.

puberty: the period of physical development during which people become able to produce children.

public health: the health of a community as a whole; the organized efforts of a community to promote the health and well-being of all its members.

Q

quackery: the promotion of medical services or products that are worthless or unproven.

quality of life: the degree to which a person lives life to its fullest capacity with enjoyment and reward.

R

relationship: a connection between people.

REM: (rapid eye movement) the dreaming part of the sleep cycle, in which the eyes move back and forth rapidly under the eyelids.

renewable resources: natural resources such as trees that can be replaced continually.

risk: an action that is potentially dangerous; the chance of injury.

S

safety awareness: knowledge about risks and how to reduce them.

saturated fats: fats that contain single bonds between carbon atoms and the maximum number of hydrogen atoms bonded to carbon.

sedative: a drug that slows down body functioning and causes sleepiness.

sedative-hypnotics: drugs that depress the body system and cause sleepiness.

selective awareness: focusing on the aspects of a situation that help a person feel better (thinking positively).

self-concept: your current mental image of yourself.

self-disclosure: telling another person meaningful information about yourself.

self-esteem: feeling good about yourself and your abilities; pride in and acceptance of yourself; your sense of personal worth.

self-ideal: your mental image of what you'd like to be.

sexual abstinence: delaying or refraining from sexual intimacy.

sexual abuse: sexual behavior between an adult and a child or adolescent.

sexual assault: any sexual contact with a person without his or her consent.

sexual intimacy: breast and genital touching and sexual intercourse.

sexually transmitted disease (STD): a disease that is passed from one person to another during sexual contact.

side effect: an effect that accompanies the expected effect of a drug.

sidestream smoke: smoke that enters the environment from burning tobacco.

single-parent family: a family in which only one parent lives with the children in the home.

social health: interactions with people to build satisfying relationships.

social support: deriving positive feelings from sharing life situations with others.

somatoform disorder: an emotional condition in which there are physical symptoms but no identifiable disease or injury. The physical symptoms are caused by psychological factors.

sperm: male reproductive cell; contains one-half of the instructions needed for the development of a new human being.

spiritual health: maintaining harmonious relationships with other living things and having spiritual direction and purpose.

spouse abuse: physical abuse of one's husband or wife.

sprain: a torn or stretched ligament or tendon.

stimulant: a drug that causes alertness and speeds up the functioning of the body.

storage fat: excess fat stored in the body.

strain: a torn or stretched muscle.

stress: combination of a stressor and a stress response.

stress intervention: any action that prevents a stressor from resulting in negative consequences.

stress response: reaction of the mind and body to a stressor.

stressor: any new or potentially unpleasant situation.

stroke: the rupture or blockage of an artery of the brain, leading to oxygen deprivation and damage to brain cells.

suicidal mindset: the feeling that suicide is the only solution to the problems of living.

suicide: the act of intentionally taking one's own life.

sunscreen: a substance that blocks the harmful ultraviolet rays of the sun.

support group: a group of people who trust each other and can talk openly with each other about their problems.

syphilis: an STD caused by bacteria, which can spread through the bloodstream to any organ of the body.

T

T-cells: cells that regulate the action of the immune system.

tar: solid material in tobacco smoke that condenses into a thick liquid.

testes: male reproductive structures that make sperm and produce the male hormone testosterone.

tolerance: the resistance your body forms to a drug.

U

unsaturated fats: fats that contain one or more double bonds between carbon atoms and have less than the maximum number of hydrogen atoms bonded to carbon.

uterus: the hollow muscular organ that provides a place for the baby to grow before birth; also called the womb.

V

vagina: female reproductive structure that receives the sperm.

values: a person's strong beliefs and ideals.

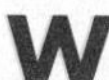

virus: a type of agent that can cause disease.

vitamins: organic substances that assist in the chemical reactions that occur in the body.

W

wellness: optimal health in each of the five aspects of health.

will: a legal document describing what should be done with a person's possessions after the person's death.

withdrawal: the process of discontinuing a drug to which the body has become addicted; the body's reaction when it does not receive a drug it depends upon.

Y

young adulthood: the period of adulthood between the ages of 20 and 40.

Index

E

F

G

Q

R

S

T

U

V

W

PHOTO CREDITS

Abbreviations used: (t) top, (c) center, (b) bottom, (l) left, (r) right.

COVER: Joe Peeples

TABLE OF CONTENTS: Page iv(t), The Stock Market; iv(b), David Young-Wolff/PhotoEdit; v(tc), Tony Stone Images; v(tl), Bruce Ayers/Tony Stone Images; v(c),(b), HRW Photo by Michelle Bridwell; v(b), HRW Photo by Michelle Bridwell; v(b), Roy Morsch/The Stock Market; vi(t), Allen Russell/Profiles West; vi(b), Robert J. Bennett; vii(t), HRW Photo by Rick Williams; vii(c), Tony Freeman/PhotoEdit; vii(b), Thomas Braise/Tony Stone Images; viii(t), Jim Whitmer; viii(b), Rhoda Sidney/PhotoEdit; ix(t), Robert Brenner/PhotoEdit; ix(b), Jon Riley/Tony Stone Images; x(t), David R. Frazier Photolibrary; x(b), Norbet Stlastny/FPG International; 1(t), Julie Bidwell; 1(c), David Young-Wolff/PhotoEdit; 1(b), HRW Photo by Lisa Davis.

UNIT ONE: Page 2(tl), Jerry Howard/Positive Images; 2(tr), David R. Frazier Photolibrary; 2(c), David Lissy/FPG International; 2(bl), Robert Daemmrich/Tony Stone Images; 2(br), Mark Harmel/FPG International; 2-3(background), Spencer Grant/FPG International. **Chapter One:** Page 4, David R. Frazier Photolibrary; 5, HRW Photo by Lawrence Migdale; 7, Steve Vidler/Nawrocki Stock Photo, Inc.; 9, Roy Morsch/The Stock Market; 10, Anthony Edgeworth, Inc./The Stock Market; 18, Steve Vidler/Nawrocki Stock Photo, Inc.; 19, Roy Morsch/The Stock Market; **Chapter Two**: Page 20, HRW Photo by Tony Freeman/PhotoEdit; 21, HRW Photo by John Langford; 23, Norma Morrison; 24, M. Wallace/PhotoEdit; 28, HRW Photo by John Langford; 30, HRW Photo by David R. Frazier; 31, Norma Morrison; 32, HRW Photo by John Langford; 33, HRW Photo by David Frazier; 34, Eric Sander/Gamma Liaison; 35(tr), HRW Photo by John Langford; 35(bl), Mitchell Layton/Duomo.

UNIT TWO: Page 36(t), Ron Rovtar/FPG International; 36(cl), Zao Productions/The Image Bank; 36(cr), Arthur Tilley/Tony Stone Images; 36(bl), Dan McCoy/Rainbow; 36(br), Jerry Howard/Positive Images; 36-37(background), Bruno Joachim Studio. **Chapter Three:** Page 38, Stephen Wade/Allsport; 38, Mitchell Layton/Duomo; 38, Larry Lawfer/Black Star; 39, Myrleen Ferguson/PhotoEdit; 43(tl), Stephen Dunn/Allsport; 43(tr), Bob Martin/Allsport; 45(l), HRW Photo by David R. Frazier; 45(r), HRW Photo by Lisa Davis; 46, HRW Photo by David Frazier; 47, David Young-Wolff/PhotoEdit; 48, Robert Tringali/Sportschrome East/West; 49, HRW Photo by David R. Frazier; 51, Gerry Schnieders/Unicorn Stock Photos; 52, HRW Photo by Lisa Davis; 53, Focus on Sports; 59, John Terence Turner/Allstock; 60, Chris Harvey/Tony Stone Images; 62, Myrleen Ferguson/PhotoEdit; 63, John Terence Turner/Allstock; 64, Bob Martin/Allsport; 65, Chris Harvey/Tony Stone Images. **Chapter Four:** Page 66, David Young-Wolff/PhotoEdit; 67, HRW Photo by John Langford; 68, Robert E. Daemmrich/Tony Stone Images; 71, Sandy Roessler/FPG International; 74(l), 74(r), Frederick C. Skvara, M.D. All rights reserved; 81, Bruce Ayers/Tony Stone Images; 87(t), James Jackson/Tony Stone Images; 87(b), Tony Stone Images; 88, 89(t), HRW Photo by Michelle Bridwell; 89(b), Custom Medical Stock Photo; 90, Karen Leeds/The Stock Market; 91, HRW Photo by John Langford; 92, P. Markow/FPG International; 96(t), 96(bl), Roy Morsch/The Stock Market; 96(br), 101, Richard Embery/FPG International; 102, HRW Photo by John Langford; 103, J. Brenner/FPG International; **Chapter Five:** Page 104, HRW Photo by Michelle Bridwell; 105, David Young-Wolff/PhotoEdit; 107(t), 107(b), Courtesy, University of Texas Adult Fitness Program/HRW Photo by Michelle Bridwell; 108, 110(l), 110(r), 112, HRW Photo by Michelle Bridwell; 113, 114, Tony Freeman/PhotoEdit; 115, HRW Photo by Michelle Bridwell; 117, Courtesy, Anderson High School/HRW Photo by Michelle Bridwell; 119, HRW Photo by Lisa Davis; 121, HRW Photo by Michelle Bridwell; 122, David Young-Wolff/PhotoEdit; 123, HRW Photo by Michelle Bridwell. **Chapter Six:** Page 124, Myrleen Ferguson/PhotoEdit; 125(t), 125(b), HRW Photo by John Langford; 126, George Ancona/International Stock Photo; 128, HRW Photo by Rick Williams; 129, James Stevenson/Science Photo Library/Photo Researchers, Inc.; 129, 130(t), Custom Medical Stock Photo; 130(bl), Francois Gohier/Photo Researchers, Inc.; 130(bc), Tony Freeman/PhotoEdit; 130(br), Gilbert Grant/Photo Researchers, Inc.; 132(l), HRW Photo by Rick Williams; 132(r), Robert Alexander/Photo Researchers, Inc.; 134, J.L. Carson/Custom Medical Stock Photo; 135, Science Photo Library/Photo Researchers, Inc.; 136, Richard Hutchings/InfoEdit; 138, Edward H. Gill/Custom Medical Stock Photo; 141, Tony Freeman/PhotoEdit; 142, Jeffrey Sylvester/FPG International; 144, George Ancona/International Stock Photo; 145, Robert Alexander/Photo Researchers Inc.; 146(r), Michael A. Keller Studios Limited/The Stock Market; 146(l), Clint Clemens/International Stock Photo; 147, Welzenbach/The Stock Market.

UNIT THREE: Page 148(tr), Allen Russell/ProFiles West; 148(cl), Mary Kate Denny/PhotoEdit; 148(cr), Lori Adamski Peek/Tony Stone Images; 148(bl), C. Orrico/SuperStock; 148(br), Mieke Maas/The Image Bank; 148-149(background), Ivan Massar/Positive Images. **Chapter Seven:** Page 150, Bob Daemmrich/Stock Boston; 151, Courtesy of Westlake High School/HRW Photo by Michelle Bridwell; 152, Bob Winsett/ProFiles West; 154(l), 154(r), Courtesy of Westlake High School/HRW Photo by Michelle Bridwell; 158, Courtesy of McCallum High School/HRW Photo by Michelle Bridwell; 161, HRW Photo by Lawrence Migdale; 165, David Young-Wolff/PhotoEdit; 167(l), 167(r), Derek Bayes/Tony Stone Images; 168, Ogust/The Image Works; 169(t), Vince Streano/Allstock; 169(b), HRW Photo by Lisa Davis; 171, Elizabeth Crews/The Image Works; 174, HRW Photo by Michelle Bridwell; 175, HRW Photo by Lawrence Migdale. **Chapter Eight:** Page 176, Richard Hutchings/PhotoEdit; 177, Peter Arnold, Inc.; 178, Yoram Kahana/Peter Arnold, Inc.; 179(l), 179(r), FPG International; 180, Tony Freeman/PhotoEdit; 182, HRW Photo by Lisa Davis; 185, Alan Oddie/PhotoEdit; 186, HRW Photo by John Langford; 187, Alan Oddie/PhotoEdit; 188, Peter Arnold, Inc.; 189, Yoram Kahana/Peter Arnold, Inc. **Chapter Nine:** Page 190, Bob Daemmrich/The Image Works; 191, HRW Photo by John Langford; 192(t), Richard Hutchings/InfoEdit; 192(b), David Young-Wolff/PhotoEdit; 194, Tony Freeman/PhotoEdit; 195(l), HRW Photo by John Langford; 195(r), Walter Chandoha; 196, HRW Photo by John Langford; 198, Michael Newman/PhotoEdit; 201, HRW Photo by John Langford; 203(c), Lawrence Migdale; 203(bl), Robert W. Ginn/Unicorn Stock Photos; 203(br), Neal Graham/Omni Photo; 204, Lawrence Migdale; 205, Robert W. Ginn/Unicorn Stock Photos; 206, Jim Pickerell/Tony Stone Images; 207, HRW Photo by David Frazier; 209, Robert W. Ginn/Unicorn Stock Photos; 211, HRW Photo by David Frazier. **Chapter Ten:** Page 212, Robert W. Ginn/Unicorn Stock Photos; 212, HRW Photo by Michelle Bridwell; 213, Julie Bidwell; 216, Austin Hospice/HRW Photo by Michelle Bridwell; 221, Julie Bidwell; 222, HRW Photo by Michelle Bridwell; 223, Julie Bidwell; 224, HRW Photo by Michelle Bridwell; 225, Julie Bidwell; **Chapter Eleven:** Page 226, Courtesy of McCallum High School/HRW Photo by Michelle Bridwell; 227, HRW Photo by Lisa Davis; 228, Tony Freeman/PhotoEdit; 229, Kobal Collection; 231, Michael Grecco/Stock Boston; 232, HRW Photo by Lisa Davis; 233, Hill/The Image Works; 234, Skjold/PhotoEdit; 236, Robert Brenner/PhotoEdit; 237, Skjold/PhotoEdit; 238, 239, HRW Photo by Lisa Davis; 240, Custom Medical Stock Photo.

UNIT FOUR: Page 242(t), The Telegraph Colour Library/FPG International; 242(tr), Michael Newman/PhotoEdit; 242(cl), Tony Freeman/PhotoEdit; 242(cr), Tony Freeman/PhotoEdit; 242(bl), Robert J. Bennett; 242-243 (background), Zephyr Pictures. **Chapter Twelve:** Page 244, HRW Photo by John Langford; 245, David de Lossy/The Image Bank; 248, HRW Photo by David Frazier; 249, Robert J. Bennett; 254, HRW Photo by John Langford; 256(tl), 256(tr), HRW Photo by John Langford; 257, HRW Photo by John Langford; 258, David de Lossy/The Image Bank; 259, HRW Photo by David Frazier. **Chapter Thirteen:** Page 260, HRW Photo by Lisa Davis; 261, HRW Photo by Michelle Bridwell; 262, HRW Photo by Rick Williams; 266(l), 266(r), Martin Rotker/Photo Researchers, Inc.; 271, Alan Pitcairn/Grant Heilman Photography; 272, HRW Photo by Michelle Bridwell; 273, HRW Photo by John Langford; 276, John Terence Turner/FPG International; 277, George Steinmetz; 278, HRW Photo by Michelle Bridwell; 280, Hank Morgan/Rainbow; 281, HRW Photo by Rick Williams; 282, 283, HRW Photo by Michelle Bridwell. **Chapter Fourteen:** Page 284, HRW Photo by Lisa Davis; 285, Courtesy of McCallum High School/HRW Photo by Michelle Bridwell; 288(l), Harry J. Przekop, Jr. All Rights Reserved/The Stock Shop/MediChrome; 288(r), Biophoto Associates/Photo Researchers, Inc.; 290, Courtesy of Milto's Restaurant/HRW Photo by Michelle Bridwell; 291, Joe Tye/STAT (Stop Teenage Addiction To Tobacco); 292, American Cancer Society; 294, Courtesy of University of Texas Rec Sports Program/HRW Photo by Michelle Bridwell; 296, Courtesy of McCallum High School/HRW Photo by Michelle Bridwell; 297, American Cancer Society. **Chapter Fifteen:** Page 298, 299(t), 299(b), HRW Photo by Michelle Bridwell; 300, P. Cantor/SuperStock; 301, Joe Bator/The Stock Market; 303, 306, HRW Photo by Michelle Bridwell; 307, Bruce Byers/FPG International; 307, Steve Raymer/National Geographic Society; 311, Bob Daemmrich/Stock Boston; 313, Leonard Kamsler/MediChrome/The Stock Shop ; 314, Bob Daemmrich/Stock Boston; 315(t), Courtesy of Austin Community College and Dr. Maria Cisneros-Solis/HRW Photo by Michelle Bridwell; 315(b), Park Street; 316, Jonathan Meyers/FPG International; 320(t), P. Langone/International Stock Photo; 320(b), Mitchell Layton/Duomo; 321, International Stock Photo.

UNIT FIVE: Page 322(tl), Lewis Harrington/FPG International; 322(cr), E. Lettau/FPG International; 322(bl), Thomas Braise/Tony Stone Images; 322(br), Janeart Ltd./The Image Bank; 322-323 (background), Maria Taglienti/The Image Bank. **Chapter Sixteen:** Page 324, Jeffrey Reed/The Stock Shop; 325, HRW Photo by Rick Williams; 328(l), Francis Leroy, Biocosmos/Science Photo Library/Photo Researchers, Inc.; 328(r), L.V. Bergman & Associates, Inc.; 335, David R. Frazier Photolibrary; 339, David Young-Wolff/PhotoEdit; 342(t), 342(cl), 342(cr), 342(br), LENNART Nilsson, A CHILD IS BORN, Dell Publishing Company; 342(bl), CNRI/Phototake, NYC; 344, Penny Gentieu/Black Star; 346(t), Simon Fraser/Princess Mary Hospital, Newcastle/Science Photo Library/Photo Researchers, Inc.; 346(b), James McLoughlin/FPG International; 347, David Young-Wolff/PhotoEdit; 348, Guy Marche/FPG International; 349(t), Francis Leroy, Biocosmos/Science Photo Library/Photo Researchers, Inc.; 349(b), L.V. Bergman & Associates, Inc.; 350, CNRI/Phototake, NYC; 351, Guy Marche/FPG International. **Chapter Seventeen:** Page 352, HRW Photo by John Langford; 353(b), Bob Daemmrich/The Image Works; 353(t), HRW Photo by John Langford; 356, HRW Photo by David R. Frazier; 358, Peter W. Gonzalez; 361, HRW Photo by David R. Frazier; 365, Sidney/The Image Works; 366, Richard Hutchings/InfoEdit; 367, HRW Photo by John Langford; 372, 373, Jim Whitmer; 374, Frank Siteman/Stock Boston; 375, Jim Whitmer; 378, Peter W. Gonzalez; 380, 381, Jim Whitmer; 382, HRW Photo by John Langford; 383, Jim Whitmer. **Chapter Eighteen:** Page 384, Gabe Palmer/The Stock Market; 385, Ken Lax; 386, Tomas del Amo/ProFiles West; 387(t), Robert Brenner/PhotoEdit; 387(b), Frank Staub/ProFiles West; 388, The Stock Market; 390, S. Vidler/SuperStock; 390, Jeffrey Arronson/Network Aspen; 395, Catherine Karnow/Woodfin Camp & Associates.; 398, Tony Stone Images; 399, Catherine Karnow/Woodfin Camp & Associates; 400, Ken Lax; 401, The Stock Market. **Chapter Nineteen:** Page 402, 403, HRW Photo by John Langford; 406, Rosanne Olson/Allstock; 407, The Stockhouse, Inc.; 408, Jose Carrillo/PhotoEdit; 409, Blair Seitz/Seitz and Seitz; 410, Mitch Kezar/Black Star; 411, 414, HRW Photo by John Langford; 415, Rosanne Olson/Allstock; 416, HRW Photo by John Langford; 417, Mitch Kezar/Black Star. **CHAPTER TWENTY:** Page 418, 419, HRW Photo by John Langford; 421(l), Jim Whitmer; 421(r), Robert Brenner/PhotoEdit; 427, Michael Newman/PhotoEdit; 428, Rhoda Sidney/PhotoEdit; 431, 432, 433, HRW Photo by John Langford; 434, Robert Brenner/PhotoEdit; 435, HRW Photo by John Langford; 436(tr), 436(cl) Henry Gris/FPG International; 437, PhotoFest.

UNIT SIX: Page 438(tl), U.N./FPG International; 438(tr), Francesco Reginato/The Image Bank; 438(cl), Robert Brenner/PhotoEdit; 438(bl),Ken Lax; 438(br), Julie Houck/West Light; 438-439 (background), Alan Goldsmith/The Stock Market. **Chapter Twenty-One:** Page 440, Elizabeth Zuckerman/PhotoEdit; 441, HRW Photo by Lisa Davis; 443, Grapes/Michaud/Photo Researchers, Inc.; 444, HRW Photo By Michelle Bridwell; 445, Richard Hutchings/Photo Researchers, Inc.; 446, HRW Photo by Michelle Bridwell; 447, Ellen Dirksen/Visuals Unlimited; 451, Simon Fraser/Science Photo Library/Custom Medical Stock Photo; 452, UPI/Bettmann; 453, Custom Medical Stock Photo; 455, HRW Photo by Lisa Davis; 456, Tony Freeman/PhotoEdit; 457, Courtesy of Dr. Robina Poonawala/HRW Photo by Michelle Bridwell; 458, Custom Medical Stock Photo; 460, Richard Hutchings/Photo Researchers, Inc.; 461, HRW Photo by Michelle Bridwell. **Chapter Twenty-Two:** Page 462, HRW Photo by Michelle Bridwell; 463, Del Valle High School/HRW Photo by Michelle Bridwell; 466(tl), 466(tr), Frederick C. Skvara, M.D.; 466(b), SIU/Peter Arnold, Inc. 467, Alex Bartel/Science Photo Library/Custom Medical Stock Photo; 471(l), Custom Medical Stock Photo; 471(r), L. Moskowitz, M.D./MediChrome/The Stock Shop; 473, Howard Sochurek/MediChrome/The Stock Shop; 474(l), 474(r), Carroll H. Weiss/Camera M.D.; 475, Bob Winsett/ProFiles West; 476, Ginger Chih/Peter Arnold, Inc.; 478, City of Austin, STD Clinic/HRW Photo by Michelle Bridwell; 479, 481, HRW Photo by Rick Williams; 482, SIU/Peter Arnold, Inc.; 483, Bob Winsett/Profiles West. **Chapter Twenty-Three:** Page 484, 485, HRW Photo by John Langford; 491, HRW Photo by Lisa Davis; 492, Courtesy of McCallum High School, Austin, Texas/HRW Photo by Michelle Bridwell; 494, HRW Photo by John Langford; 495, HRW Photo by Lisa Davis; 496, Robert E. Daemmrich/Tony Stone Images; 498, David Pollack/The Stock Market; 499, Gabe Palmer/The Stock Market; 500, HRW Photo by Lisa Davis; 502, Wide World Photos; 503(t), Wil Phinney; 503(b), AP LaserPhoto/Craig Fujii/Wide World Photo; 504, J. Stettenheim/SABA; 506, HRW Photo by John Langford; 507, HRW Photo by Lisa Davis. **Chapter Twenty-Four:** Page 508, Courtesy of American Diabetes Association/HRW Photo by Michelle Bridwell; 509, Jeff Isaac Greenberg/Photo Researchers, Inc.; 511(l), 511(r), Science Source/Photo Researchers, Inc.; 512, Simon Fraser/RVI, Newcastle-Upon-Tyne/Science Photo Library/Photo Researchers, Inc.; 513(l), HRW Photo by Michelle Bridwell; 513(r), Custom Medical Stock Photo; 514, Michael Tamborrino/MediChrome/The Stock Shop; 515, Richard Hutchings/Science Source/Photo Researchers, Inc.; 519, HRW Photo by Michelle Bridwell; 520, Wide World Photos, Inc.; 523(l), M. Abbey/Photo Researchers, Inc.; 523(r), Science Photo Library/Photo Researchers, Inc.; 524, Bill Longcore/Science Source/Photo Researchers, Inc.; 525, Richard Hirneisen/MediChrome/The Stock Shop; 527, HRW Photo by Michelle Bridwell; 528, Courtesy of University of Texas Adult Fitness Program/HRW Photo by Michelle Bridwell; 530, HRW Photo by Lisa Davis; 531, Simon Fraser/RVI, Newcastle-Upon-Tyne/Science Photo Library/Photo Researchers, Inc.; 532, Jeff Isaac Greenberg/Photo Researchers, Inc.; 533, HRW Photo by Lisa Davis; 534, Michael Tamborrino/FPG International.

UNIT SEVEN: Page 536(tl), Sandy Roessler/FPG International; 536(tc), Phil Jason/Tony Stone Images; 536(tr), HRW Photo by Russell Dian; 536(bl), Nigel Dickinson/Tony Stone Images; 536(br), Jon Riley/Tony Stone Images; 536-537 (background), P.R. Productions/SuperStock. **Chapter Twenty-Five:** Page 538, Keith Gunnar/FPG International; 539, 541, HRW Photo by John Langford; 543, J. Van Eps/SuperStock; 544, L. Linkhart/SuperStock; 546, Bill Ross/Allstock; 550, David R. Frazier Photolibrary; 553, Scott Bernef; 554, HRW Photo by John Langford; 555, Jon Riley/Tony Stone Images; 556, HRW Photo by John Langford; 557, Robert Landau/West Light; 559, Ken Karp/Omni Photo; 564, Tor Eigeland/Sipa; 565, Michael Newman/PhotoEdit; 567, HRW Photo by John Langford; 568, Bill Ross/Allstock; 569, Jon Riley/Tony Stone Images. **Chapter Twenty-Six:** Page 570, Ken Lax; 571(t), David Young-Wolff/PhotoEdit; 571(b), Ken Lax; 573, HRW Photo by John Langford; 577, David R. Frazier Photolibrary; 578, Michael Heron/Woodfin Camp & Associates; 581, David R. Frazier Photolibrary; 582, David Young-Wolff/PhotoEdit; 583, Ken Lax; 584, T. Rosenthal/SuperStock.

UNIT EIGHT: Page 586(tl), George Gibbons/FPG International; 586(tr), Denise Deluise/Zephyr Pictures; 586(cl), Patricia J. Bruno/Positive Images; 586(bl), Grafton M. Smith/The Image Bank; 586(br), Norbert Stlastny/FPG International; 586-587 (background), Weinberg-Clark/The Image Bank. **Chapter Twenty-Seven:** Page 588, Spencer Swanger/Tom Stack & Associates; 589, Paul Barton/The Stock Market; 591, 592, HRW Photo by Lisa Davis; 593, Robert J. Bennett; 596, Barbara L. Moore/New England Stock Photo; 599(b), Tony Freeman/PhotoEdit; 599(c), T. Rosenthal/SuperStock; 599(t), 600(l), 600(r), Ken Lax; 601, Clark Linehan Photography/New England Stock Photography; 602, HRW Photo by Lisa Davis; 603, Warren Faidley/Weatherstock; 604, Peter Menzel/Tony Stone Images; 605, Gabe Palmer/The Stock Market; 607, Tony Freeman/PhotoEdit; 608, HRW Photo by Michelle Bridwell; 609, Paul E. Clark/New England Stock Photo; 610, HRW Photo by Rodney Jones; 611, Barbara L. Moore/New England Stock Photos; 612, Paul Barton/The Stock Market; 613, HRW Photo by Lisa Davis. **Chapter Twenty-Eight:** Page 614, Robert Copeland/West Light; 615, Courtesy of Austin EMS/HRW Photo by Michelle Bridwell; 618(tl), 618(tr), 618(cl), 618(cr), Park Street; 619, 628, HRW Photo by Lisa Davis; 630(t), 630(bl), 630(br), Park Street; 631, Ken Lax; 632, Michael Newman/PhotoEdit; 634, Robert E. Daemmrich/Tony Stone Images; 637, HRW Photo by Lisa Davis; 640(t), Ann Moreton/Tom Stack & Associates; 640(b), Buddy Mays/FPG International; 641, HRW Photo by Lisa Davis; 644, Dan McCoy/Rainbow; 645(t), Sinclair Stammers/Science Photo Library/Custom Medical Stock Photo; 645(c), Mike English, M.D./MediChrome/The Stock Shop; 645(b), John Radcliffe/Science Photo Library/Photo Researchers, Inc.; 646, 648, HRW Photo by Lisa Davis; 649, HRW Photo by Michelle Bridwell; 650, Ken Korsh/FPG International.

BODY SYSTEM HANDBOOK: Page 653, HRW Photo by Michelle Bridwell; 654, Bruce Coleman, Inc.; 657, HRW Photo by Russell Dian; 659(l), Tony Freeman/PhotoEdit; 659(r), Tim Haske/ProFiles West; 659(b), Biological Photo Service; 663, Bob Daemmrich/Stock Boston; 665, Michael P. Gadomski/Bruce Coleman, Inc.; 668(c), M.E. Sparks/Profiles West.

HEALTH CAREERS HANDBOOK: Page 668 (background), Tom McCarthy/ProFiles West; 668(t), Rosanne Olson/Allstock; 669(tr), Steve Gottlieb/FPG International; 669(cl), Linda K. Moore/Rainbow; 669(cr), Alfred Pasieka/Bruce Coleman, Inc.; 669(b), Dan McCoy/Rainbow; 670(t), Melanie Carr/Zephyr; 670(bl), Tom Tracy/FPG International; 670(br), Kent Vinyard/ProFiles West; 671(tl), Ken Lax; 671(tr), David R. Frazier Photolibrary; 671(br), Mark Sherman/Bruce Coleman, Inc.; 672(tr), FPG International; 672(bl), 673(t), HRW Photo by Lisa Davis; 673(b), P. Barry Levy/ProFiles West; 673 (inset), HRW Photo by Lisa Davis; 674(t), Bob Daemmrich/Stock Boston; 674(b), Courtesy of Souper Salads, Austin, Texas/HRW Photo by Michelle Bridwell; 675(t), Louis Bencze/Allstock; 675(b), Jack W. Dykinga/Bruce Coleman, Inc.; 675 (inset), Courtesy of Kocurek Elementary/HRW Photo by Michelle Bridwell; 676(t), Grant LeDuc/Stock Boston; 676(b), Melanie Carr/Zephyr Pictures; 677(t), Pat Lanza Field/Bruce Coleman, Inc.; 677(b), Courtesy of Anderson High School/HRW Photo by Michelle Bridwell.

ART CREDITS

All illustrated charts by Precision Graphics.
All anatomical art by Network Graphics.
All tables by Paradigm Design.
Cover and text design by Design Five, New York City.